Practical Manual for

LAPAROSCOPIC AND HYSTEROSCOPIC GYNECOLOGICAL SURGERY

Practical Manual for
LAPAROSCOPIC AND HYSTEROSCOPIC GYNECOLOGICAL SURGERY

THIRD EDITION

Editors

Ibrahim Alkatout PhD MD
Director
Kiel School of Gynaecological Endoscopy
Department of Obstetrics and Gynecology
University Hospitals Schleswig-Holstein
Kiel, Germany

Liselotte Mettler PhD MD
Patroness
Kiel School of Gynaecological Endoscopy
Emeritus Professor
Department of Obstetrics and Gynecology
University Hospitals Schleswig-Holstein
Kiel, Germany

Forewords

Nicolai Maass
Jon I Einarsson

JAYPEE

JAYPEE BROTHERS MEDICAL PUBLISHERS
The Health Sciences Publisher
New Delhi | London | Panama

Jaypee Brothers Medical Publishers (P) Ltd.

Headquarters
Jaypee Brothers Medical Publishers (P) Ltd.
4838/24, Ansari Road, Daryaganj
New Delhi 110 002, India
Phone: +91-11-43574357
Fax: +91-11-43574314
Email: jaypee@jaypeebrothers.com

Overseas Offices
J.P. Medical Ltd.
83 Victoria Street, London
SW1H 0HW (UK)
Phone: +44 20 3170 8910
Fax: +44 (0)20 3008 6180
Email: info@jpmedpub.com

Jaypee-Highlights Medical Publishers Inc.
City of Knowledge, Bld. 235, 2nd Floor, Clayton
Panama City, Panama
Phone: +1 507-301-0496
Fax: +1 507-301-0499
Email: cservice@jphmedical.com

Jaypee Brothers Medical Publishers (P) Ltd.
Bhotahity, Kathmandu, Nepal
Phone: +977-9741283608
Email: kathmandu@jaypeebrothers.com

Website: www.jaypeebrothers.com
Website: www.jaypeedigital.com

Practical Manual for Laparoscopic and Hysteroscopic Gynecological Surgery

First Edition: 2007
Second Edition: 2013
Third Edition: **2019**

ISBN: 978-93-5270-194-0

Printed at: Samrat Offset Pvt. Ltd.

Dedicated to

All patients placing their trust in us

Contributors

Abhishek Mangeshikar MS
Gynecologist
Mangeshikars' MAGIC for Women
Mumbai, Maharashtra, India

Aishwarya Puntambekar
Galaxy Laparoscopy Institute
Pune, Maharashtra, India

Alessandro Loddo MD
Clinica Ginecologica Ostetrica e di Fisiopatologia della Riproduzione Umana
Università degli studi di Cagliari
Caligari, Italy

Alexandros Bader MD FAAOCG FISCG
Consultant (Obstetrician and Gynecologist)
President of European Society of Aesthetic Gynecology (ESAG)
Director
Bader Medical Institute of London
Pelvic Floor Reconstruction, Cosmetic and Aesthetic Gynecology, Endoscopy Surgery
London, UK

Alfonso Rossetti MD
Priv. Doz. Dr. Andreas Hackethal
Frauenklinik an der Elbe, Oberbaumbrücke 1, 20457
Hamburg, Germany

Andrea Tinelli MD PhD
Professor
Department of Obstetrics and Gynecology
Division of Experimental Endoscopic Surgery, Imaging, Technology and Minimally Invasive Therapy
Vito Fazzi Hospital, Lecce, Italy
The International Translational Medicine and Biomodelling Research Group, Department of Applied Mathematics, Moscow Institute of Physics and Technology (State University)
Moscow Region, Russia

Andreas Hackethal
Department of Obstetrics and Gynecology
Universitaetsklinikum Giessen und Marburg GmbH
Giessen, Germany

Antonio Malvasi MD
Professor
Department of Obstetrics and Gynecology
Santa Maria Hospital
GVM Care and Research
Bari, Italy
The International Translational Medicine and Biomodelling Research Group

Artin Ternamian MD
Department of Obstetrics and Gynecology
Faculty of Medicine, University of Toronto
Director, Gynecologic Endoscopy
St Joseph's Health Centre, Toronto, Canada

Bahareh Hamedi MD
Department of Obstetrics and Gynecology
Shiraz University of Medical Sciences
Shiraz, Iran

Bernd Bojahr Pasacica
Head
Department of Gyenocology of the Clinic for Minimal Invasive Surgery (MIC-Klinik)
Deputy of the certified Endometriosis Center of the clinic for MIC-Klinik
Founding Member of Minimally Invasive Teaching Academy of the Clinic for MICC Berlin, Germany
Professor
Department of Gynecology and Obstetrics
University Medicine Greifswald
Greifswald, Germany

Bernd Holthaus MD
Head
Department of Obstetrics and Gynecology
St Elisabeth Hospital
Damme, Germany

Bruno van Herendael
ZNA Stuivenberg
Lange Beeldekensstraat
Antwerpen, Belgium

Carolin Spüntrup MD
Hohe Wacht 77
66119 Saarbrücken

CY Liu MD
Professor of Clinical Obstetrics and Gynecology
Department of Obstetrics and Gynecology
University of Tennessee College of Medicine
Chattanooga, Tennessee, USA

De Wilde RL MD PhD
University Hospital for Gynecology
Carl von Ossietzky University Oldenburg
Germany

Douglas E Ott MD MBA
Adjunct Professor (Biomedical Engineering)
Adjunct Professor (Business and Economics)
Mercer University
Macon, Georgia, USA

Elmar Spüntrup Diplom-Physiker
Hohe Wacht 77
66119 Saarbrücken

Flemming Bjerrum MD PhD
Resident
Department of Surgery
Herlev Hospital
Denmark

Frederike Egberts
Department of Dermatology, Venereology and Allergology
University Hospitals Schleswig-Holstein
Kiel, Germany

Garri Tchartchian MD
Head
Department of Gyenocology of the Clinic for Minimal Invasive Surgery (MIC-Klinik)
Head
Center for Difficult Cases of the Clinic for MIC-Klinik
Berlin, Germany

Goentje Peters MD
Department of Obstetrics and Gynecology
University Hospitals Schleswig-Holstein
Kiel, Germany

Guenter K Noé MD PhD
Priv Doz Dr med
University of Witten/Herdecke
Communal Clinics Rhein Kreis Neuss
Dormagen, Germany, NRW

Hans-Rudolf Tinneberg
Department of Obstetrics and Gynecology
Universitaetsklinikum Giessen und Marburg GmbH
Giessen, Germany

Haytham Elmeligy MBBCH MSc (Alexandria)
Senior Consultant
St Elisabeth Hospital
Damme, Germany

Ibrahim Alkatout PhD MD
Director
Kiel School of Gynaecological Endoscopy
Department of Obstetrics and Gynecology
University Hospitals Schleswig-Holstein
Kiel, Germany

Ingo von Leffern MD
Director of Albertinen Women's Clinics
Head
Department of Gynecology and Obstetrics
Albertinen Hospital Hamburg, Germany

Ivo Meinhold-Heerlein
Professor
Justus-Liebig-Universität Gießen
Universitätsklinikum
Klinikstr 32
Giessen, Germany

J Marek Doniec MD
Private Office for Endoscopic Gastroenterology and Proctology
Kiel, Germany

Jan F Baekelandt MD
Gynecologic Oncology Surgeon
Imelda Hospital
Bonheiden, Belgium

Janesh Gupta MSc MD FRCOG
Professor of Obstetrics and Gynecology
Editor-in-Chief of EJOG
Centre for Women's and Newborn Health
Institute of Metabolism and Systems Research (IMSR)
University of Birmingham
Birmingham Women's and Children's NHS Foundation Trust
Birmingham, England, UK

Johannes Ackermann MD
Department of Obstetrics and Gynecology
University Hospitals Schleswig-Holstein
Kiel, Germany

John E Morrison MD
Louisiana State University Health Sciences Center (LSUHSC)
Department of Surgery
New Orleans, Louisiana, USA

Julia Ionesi-Pasacica MD
Department of Obstetrics and Gynecology
Universitaetsklinikum Giessen und Marburg GmbH
Giessen, Germany

Khulkar Abdusattarova MD
Department of Obstetrics and Gynecology
University Hospitals Schleswig-Holstein
Campus Kiel, Germany

Kubilay Ertan
Department of Obstetrics and Gynecology
Klinikum Leverkusen gGmbH
Leverkusen, Germany

Liselotte Mettler PhD MD
Patroness
Kiel School of Gynaecological Endoscopy
Emeritus Professor
Department of Obstetrics and Gynecology
University Hospitals Schleswig-Holstein
Kiel, Germany

Lotte Clevin MD
Senior Consultant
Department of Gynecology
Bornholm Hospital
Denmark

MacLeod Natalie MD
Department of Obstetrics and Gynecology
Faculty of Medicine, University of Toronto
Director, Gynaecologic Endoscopy
St Joseph's Health Centre, Toronto, Canada

Manfred Schollmeyer MD
Department of Obstetrics and Gynecology
Oschatz, Germany

Marc Banerjee MD
Hohe Wacht 77
66119 Saarbrücken

Maria Fernanda Brancalion MD
Gynecologist
Women Health Reference Centre
Hospital Pérola Byington
São Paulo, Brazil

Mathias SS Löhnert MD PhD
Head of Surgical Department,
Medical Director
Prof Dr med Habil Dr Hc
Department of General and Colorectal Surgery
Clinical Center
Bielefeld, Germany

Mauricio Simões Abrão MD PhD
Professor–Gynecologist
Faculty of Medicine
University of São Paulo
Endometriosis Division
Department of Obstetrics and Gynecology
São Paulo, Brazil

Meenakshi Chate MD
Galaxy Laparoscopy Institute
Pune, Maharashtra, India

Meenu Agarwal MD
National Director
Clinical Board Morpheus IVF
Gen Sec POGS (2017–2018)
Elected Board member-ISGE (2017–2020)
Chairperson
Imaging Science—FOGSI (2018–2020)
Vice- President, POGS (2012–2014)
Elected MCM, IAGE (2009–2011) and (2015–2017)
Life Member, ISGE
Member, SLS
Editor, International Journal of Gynaecological Endoscopy

Michael Stark MD
Professor
Department of Applied Mathematics
Moscow Institute of Physics and
Technology (State University)
Moscow Region, Russia
President
New European Surgical Academy (NESA)
Berlin, Germany

Mohamed Elessawy MD
Department of Obstetrics and Gynecology
University Hospitals Schleswig-Holstein
Kiel, Germany

Munjal Pandya MS (Obstetrics and Gynecology)
Assistant Professor (Obstetrics and Gynecology)
LG Hospital and AMC MET Municipal Medical College
Maninagar, Ahmedabad, India

Nidhi Nagar MD
Consultant Gynecologist and Endoscopy Surgeon
Former Assistant Professor in Obstetrics and Gynecology
LN Medical College
Bhopal, Madhya Pradesh, India

Ospan A Mynbaev MD PhD
Professor
Laboratory of Human Physiology
Moscow Institute of Physics and Technology (State University)
Moscow Region, Russia
The Russian National Research Medical
Moscow, Russia

Parul Kotdawala MD FICOG FICMCH
Endoscopy Surgeon
Department of Obstetrics and Gynecology
VS Hospital and NHL Municipal Medical College
Ellisbridge, Ahmedabad, India

Radmila Sparić MD
Surgeon and Gynecologist
Clinic for Obstetrics and Gynecology
Clinical Center of Serbia
Medical School
University of Belgrade
Belgrade, Serbia

Raviraj Tiruke MD
Galaxy Laparoscopy Institute
Pune, Maharashtra, India

RM Sathe MD
Galaxy Laparoscopy Institute
Pune, Maharashtra, India

Rupinder Kaur Ruprai MBBS MD (Ob/Gyn) FMAS DMIS D Rep Med MA-Gyne MBA
Specialist Gynecologist
GMC Clinics
Medcare Hospital
Dubai, UAE

Saeed Alborzi
Department of Obstetrics and Gynecology
Shiraz University of Medical Sciences
Shiraz, Iran

Sambit Nanda MD
Galaxy Laparoscopy Institute
Pune, Maharashtra, India

Sanjay Patel MD
Gynec-Endoscopic Surgeon
Infertility and IVF Specialist
Director
Mayflower Women's Hospital
Ahmedabad, Gujarat, India

Saša Kadija MD PhD
Surgeon and Gynecologist
Clinic for Obstetrics and Gynecology,
Clinical Center of Serbia
Medical School
University of Belgrade
Belgrade, Serbia

Seema Puntambekar MD
Galaxy Laparoscopy Institute
Pune, Maharashtra, India

Shailesh Puntambekar
Galaxy Laparoscopy Institute
Pune, Maharashtra, India

Shanti I Mohling MD FACOG
Director of Gynecology
Associate Director
Fellowship in Minimally Invasive Gynecology
Department of Obstetrics and Gynecology
University of Tennessee College of Medicine
Chattanooga, Tennessee, USA

Susanne Denny MD
Department of Obstetrics and Gynecology
Krankenhaus St Elisabeth gGmbh
Damme, Germany

Svetlana Spremović Radjenović MD PhD
Surgeon and Gynecologist
Clinic for Obstetrics and Gynecology,
Clinical Center of Serbia
Medical School
University of Belgrade,
Belgrade, Serbia

Tamer Seckin MD FACOG ACGE
Department of Obstetrics and Gynecology
Lenox Hill Hospital
New York, NY, USA

Tejashree Bakre MD
Galaxy Laparoscopy Institute
Pune, Maharashtra, India

Thilo Wedel
Institute of Anatomy
University of Kiel
Kiel, Germany

Thomas Römer
Evangelisches Krankenhaus Köln-Weyertal
Köln, Germany

Wael Sammur MD
Director, Emirates Hospital
Dubai, United Arab Emirates

Foreword

Endoscopic surgery, despite its controversial application in the treatment of malignant tumors, has gained worldwide acceptance not only in gynecological surgery but also in general surgery, orthopedic surgery, urology, ENT and cardiac surgery.

As the Chairman of the Department of Obstetrics and Gynecology, University Hospitals Schleswig-Holstein, Campus Kiel, I wholeheartedly support the publication of the 3rd edition of the *Practical Manual for Laparoscopic and Hysteroscopic Gynecological Surgery* by the Kiel School. The 50 chapters reflect the current knowledge in the field and provide practical advice on the correct implementation of the minimal invasive surgical procedures. The Kiel School of Gynaecological Endoscopy offers training courses in laparoscopic and hysteroscopic surgery and has become an international forum for all the colleagues interested in this field. Our department and the Kiel School have a joint cooperation with the Kurt Semm Center for Laparoscopic and Robotic-assisted Surgery, founded in 2016 as a multispecialty project at the University Hospitals Schleswig-Holstein, Campus Kiel.

Nicolai Maass MD
Professor–Director
Kiel School of Gynaecological Endoscopy
Department of Obstetrics and Gynecology
University Hospitals Schleswig-Holstein
Kiel, Germany

Foreword

Minimally invasive gynecologic surgery has evolved rapidly over the past few decades. Given that, this mode of access is rapidly becoming the standard of care, the relevance of this textbook is greater than ever. We live in an era where the term *minimally invasive* is becoming redundant, and we have to thank the pioneers in the field for getting us there. One of those pioneers is Professor Liselotte Mettler. She has seen the incredible evolution of gynecologic surgery first hand and actively contributed to this evolution. I therefore cannot think of a better author for a textbook in the field. The collaboration between Drs Ibrahim Alkatout and Liselotte Mettler has created an outstanding textbook that offers practical and comprehensive information for the novice and advanced gynecologic surgeons alike. Every chapter is written by authorities in the field and the chapter topics cover the entire gamut of gynecologic surgery. This book is therefore an outstanding resource and will serve the reader well. I would like to congratulate the authors and editors for a well-done job.

Jon I Einarsson MD PhD MPH
Director
Minimally Invasive Gynecologic Surgery
Brigham and Women's Hospital
Associate Professor (Obstetrics and Gynecology)
Harvard Medical School
President
American Association of Gynecologic Laparoscopists (AAGL)

Preface

With pleasure I present this 3rd edition of the *Practical Manual for Laparoscopic and Hysteroscoic Gynecological Surgery* as global masterpiece of the KIEL School of Gynaecological Endoscopy now an integral part of the Kurt Semm Center for Laparoscopic and Robot-assisted Surgery, University Clinics Schleswig-Holstein, Kiel, Germany.

This time with 50 chapters I am rounding up surgical endoscopic challenges primarily in Gynecology, but also in Urology and General Surgery. Based on the ground-braking evolution in this field led by our late colleagues: Raoul Palmer, Kurt Semm and Thoralf Schollmeyer. This book is written by world-known specialists with dedication and passion. Their vigor is best reflected by the Tips and Tricks given for the individual surgical procedures, which are continuously improving the desired outcome. I whole-heartedly thank all authors or their wonderful contributions in text, pictures and videos. The endoscopic surgeons of the world are friends and family, and share their knowledge with the healthy input of new technical developments and recognitions.

The book intends to help all readers to become good surgeons, stay good doctors, and certainly gives a basis for new ideas and developments. All progress may only serve for the necessary treatment of our patients.

I thank our patients trusting in me and carry the responsibility of optimal care.

Liselotte Mettler

Acknowledgments

For the production of this edition, we thank the team of M/s Jaypee Brothers Medical Publishers (P) Ltd, New Delhi, India, under Prerna Bajaj (Development Editor); the Executive Director of the Kiel School, Mr Dawn Rüther; and our Office Manager, Mr Nicole Guckelsberger, for their never-ending patience with the editors, authors, and co-authors.

Contents

SECTION 2 SPECIFIC GYNECOLOGICAL LAPAROSCOPIC PROCEDURES

Video Contents*

**The videos are available on www.emedicine360.com.*

Section 1

Basics and Anatomical Aspects of Endoscopic Surgery

KIEL SCH•OL

1 of Gynaecological Endoscopy

Historical Perspective

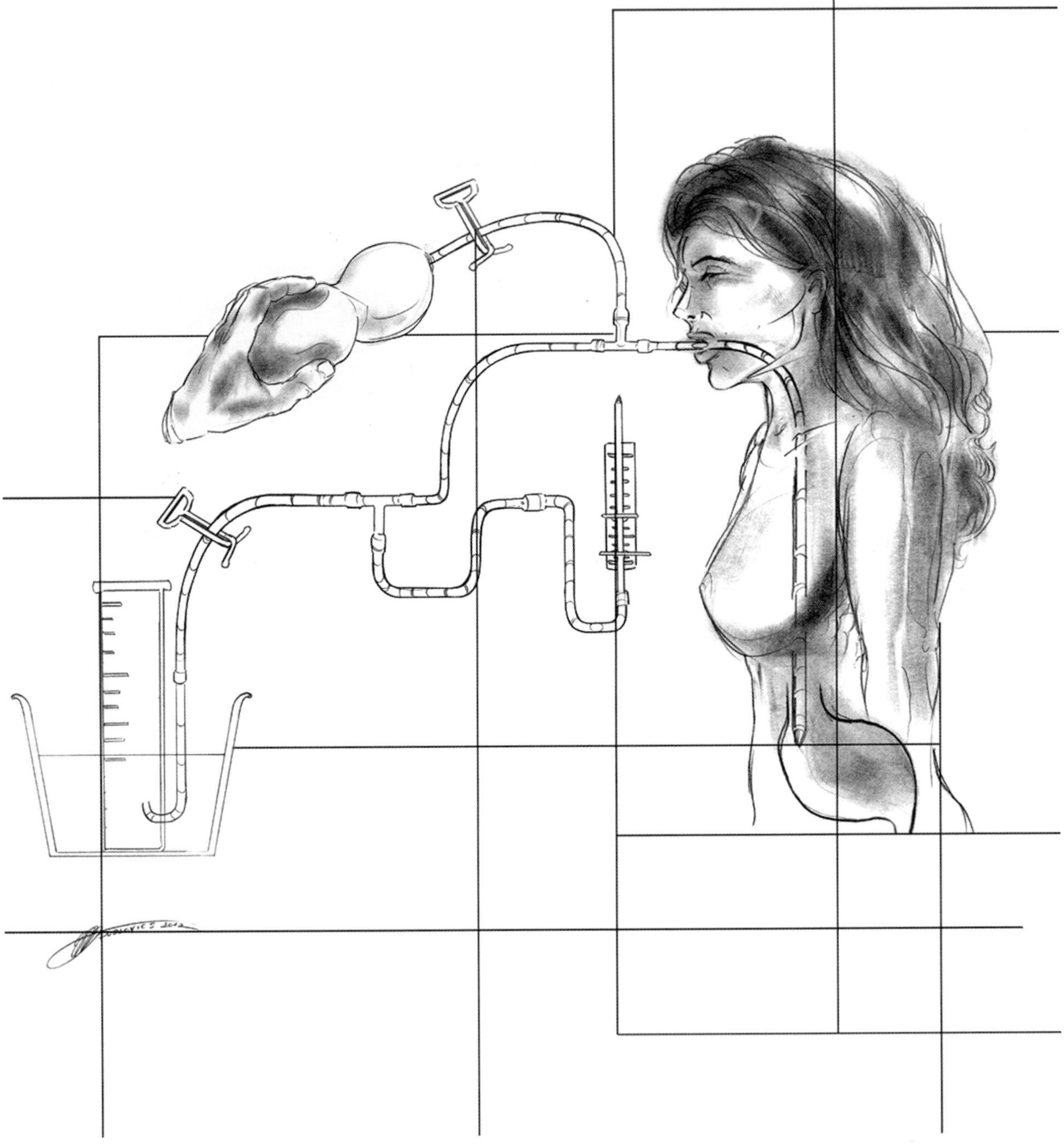

Chapter 1

Historical Perspectives

Liselotte Mettler, Manfred Schollmeyer

Since ancient times, medical men desired to inspect human body cavities and passages to understand their complexity and to treat their diseases. Easily accessible body cavities like mouth, rectum, or even vagina were already inspected in ancient times with the help of speculums.

Accounts of catheters and rectal speculums are handed down from Hippocrates II. The Greek, born on the island of Kos and known for the Hippocratic oath, inserted in vagina tampons with threads using hollowed kalabass. However, the Greeks did not dare to use a speculum to view rectum or inspect vagina.

Erasistos, born in 320 BC in Keos, was first to describe anatomically correct curved catheters. Oreibasis, born in 325 BC in Pergamon, invented an indwelling catheter at Rome in the times of Julius Caesar. He also dilated urethra with a goose quill swathed in swollen parchment.

The origin of endoscopy can be traced back to a reference in Babylonian Talmud. The treatise describes a lead funnel with curved mouth, furnished with wooden outlet (Mechul). Both the parts were inserted into vagina to show, by retraction for the first time to human eyes, cervical os as an internal organ to diagnose uterine bleeding and differentiate it from vaginal bleeding.

A triple-armed vaginal mirror and a rectal speculum were excavated in Pompei. The Syrian gynecologist, Archigenes from Apameia, who practiced in Rome from 95 to 117 BC, wrote a thesis on uterine bleedings. He used a cervical mirror for inspection and commented on various forms of gynecologic palpatory examinations as well as external and internal inspection.

Abu al-Qasim Khalaf ibn al-Abbas Al-Zahrawi, an Arab, is regarded as Middle Ages' most eminent surgeon. Also known as Alsaha-Ravius or Albucasis of Cordoba (936–1009), he used a glass mirror to reflect light to view the inside of vagina. He described his speculum as "two rods, one lying on the top of the other, which is introduced in the cervix (probably meant vagina) to expand it with the help of screws."[1]

The first endoscopic light source can be traced back to Gulio Cesare Aranzi (1530–1589). This Venezuelan used camera obscura (1587) to focus a ray of light to view nasal cavity. He held water-filled spherical glass bottle in front of a hole in a shutter in a darkened room and projected that focused light to view nasal cavity. He recommended an artificial light source on rainy days.

French gynecologist and surgeon, George Arnaud de Rosil (1698–1774), gave new significance to vaginal speculum, which was developed over a century. Arnaud[2] was the first to use endoscopic examination lamp making use of a covered lantern. The light source was a night lamp that was placed in a box painted silver from inside. Similar to camera obscura, light focused through a convex lens could be used to illuminate vagina, which was opened with a speculum.

Philipp Bozzini (1773–1809), who marks the turning point from the old to new medicine, must unquestionably be mentioned for his contributions to development of modern endoscopy. Bozzini studied in Mainz and Jena where he became acquainted with Christoph Wilhelm Hufeland who published the *Journal of Practical Pharmaceutics and Art of Wound Healing*. In 1804 he published first description of his instruments in a small Frankfurt newspaper. The equipment had optical part with illumination device and mechanical part that adapted itself to the

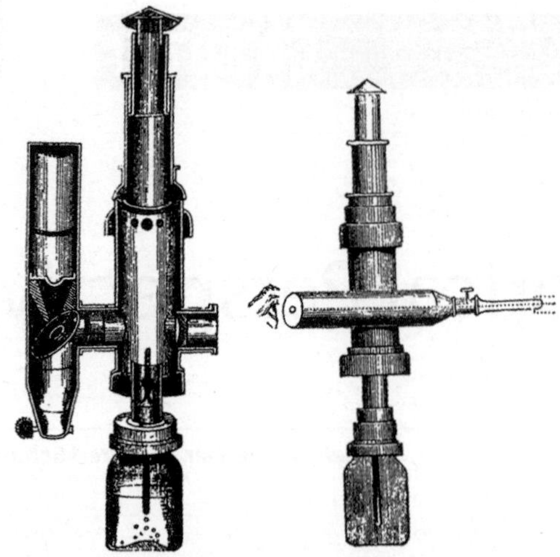

Fig. 1.1: First portable endoscope by Desormeaux.

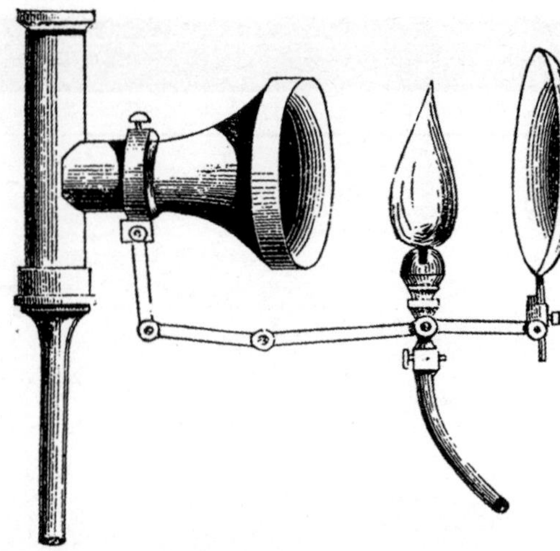

Fig. 1.2: Photoendoscope by Stein.

anatomy of body orifice. In 1806 he published a detailed account of his light guide.[3]

In 1807 the national industrial Comptoir, Weimar, published the monograph, *The Light Guide or the Account of a Simple Device to Illuminate Internal Cavities and Passages of Living Animals.* Bozzini himself made sketches and even engraved them in copper.[4]

Bozzini constructed an instrument for vagina, rectum and oral cavity, including throat. One could see and even operate on a modest scale with it. Even though light source was too weak and visual field too small, all further attempts at cystoscopy in the next 70 years were exclusively based on Bozzini's illumination principle using extracorporeal light source to reflect light. His principle of using artificial light source, reflection of light toward the object to be examined as well as the light conduction and directing the reflection and re-reflection to the observing eye, substantially influenced international discussions on the development of endoscopes.

Antonin Jean Desormeaux (1815–1894) constructed the first portable endoscope[5] (Fig. 1.1) and presented this historic development on November 29, 1843, for which received a part of Argenteuil prize from Academie Imperiale de Medicine. Desormeaux was first to clinically use Bozzini's light guide for which many regard him the "father of endoscopy." His instrument was a system of mirrors and lenses with an open flame as a light source. Skin burns were a most frequent complication. The light guide was essentially used in patients with urological illnesses.

The most important development of endoscopic abdominal surgery is connected with photography and television. Theodor S. Stein (1868) started it in Frankfurt. In 1874 he introduced his "photo endoscope" (Fig. 1.2).[6]

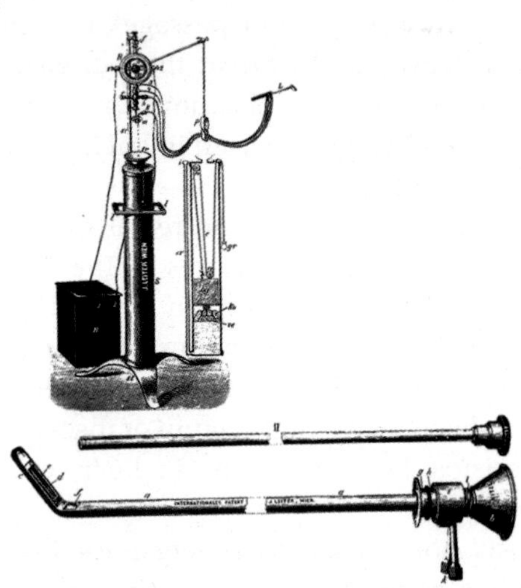

Fig. 1.3: Cystoscope, developed by Nitze and Leiter.

Gynecology was the so to say initiator of the development of operative endoscopy. Apart from Desormeaux,[7] Aubinais,[8] and Pantaleoni[9] must be also mentioned for their attempts to inspect uterine cavity, which is today's hysteroscopy. The technical development of endoscopy to perfection was left to cystoscopy. The plausible cause is that Mignon filament (Edison) at the tip of the cystoscope by Nitze and Leiter[10,11] posed no danger of burns because urine in the urinary bladder ensured appropriate cooling (Fig. 1.3).

In 1881 Johann Mikulicz (1850–1905) and Leiter adopted the principle of rigid optic system developed by Max Nitze and successfully constructed first clinically usable gastroscope.[12] Mikulicz carried out several clinical examinations at Billroth's surgical clinic in Vienna.

Between 1890 and 1900 George Kelling (1866–1945) of Dresden worked on anatomy and physiology of stomach "to determine the size of the stomach."[13-15] He gained experience in oral air insufflation[14,15] and worked on pressure ratio of gastrointestinal tract and abdominal cavity. Simultaneously he worked on improving the techniques of examination of gastrointestinal tract, which resulted in application for a patent.[16]

Kelling's know-how of gastric and esophageal endoscopy and his knowledge of air insufflation were foundation for future attempts to carry out therapeutic and diagnostic examinations in closed body cavities. The brilliant idea of connecting his air insufflation apparatus to Fiedler trocar and Nitze cystoscope led to the birth of laparoscopy.

On September 23, 1901, George Kelling gave the historic lecture on "Tour of the Oesophagus and Stomach by Flexible Instruments" to natural history scientists and doctors' 73rd meeting in Hamburg. He also introduced his new procedure that he called "coelioscopy."[17] Kelling had used his oral air insufflation apparatus for intra-abdominal insufflation (Fig. 1.4) together with a Nitze cystoscope for illumination to see abdomen of a dog, in animal experiment for the time.

I question myself, how the organs will react to the air introduced inside? To find out, I have developed a method to introduce the endoscope in the closed abdominal cavity (Coelioscopy) (Kelling 1901).

After an interval of a century and considering the status of endoscopy today, one can evaluate Kelling's endoscopic work as follows:

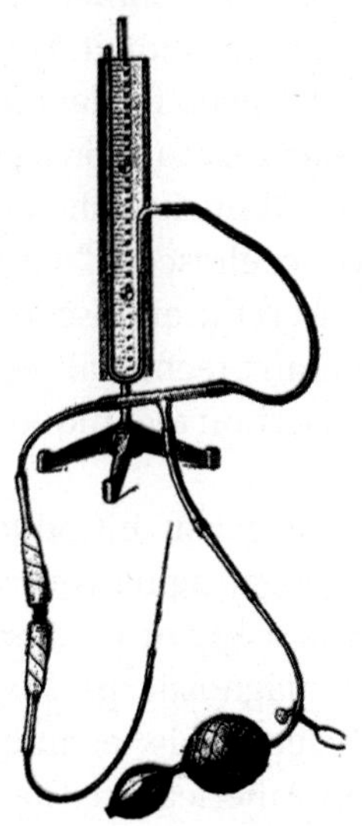

Fig. 1.4: Apparatus for the intra-abdominal insufflation with pump, filter and manometer.

- Contradicting the spirit of times, Kelling had favored endoscopic procedure to exploratory laparotomy.[18]
- With far sight Kelling challenged stagewise treatment of malignancy and for this purpose sent repeated reminders for the primary use of endoscopic procedure.[19]
- Kelling was first to assemble all basic instruments for laparoscopy with insufflation needle (Fiedler trocar), insufflation apparatus (air pump by Politser), optic trocar and telescope (Nitze's cystoscope) and described the method.[20,21]
- Kelling, for the first time in 1901, formulated indications and contraindications of coelioscopy/laparoscopy.
- Kelling demonstrated for first time the possibility of intraabdominal diagnostics by endoscopic inspection and palpation.[21]
- In 1901, Kelling advised, clearly foreseeing the problems in training young doctors, to practice endoscopic procedures on cadavers. A hundred years ago, dummies were not available to the pioneer of endoscopy.
- Kelling, a visionary, had predicted use of endoscopic interventions, particularly laparoscopy as daycare procedures (1901).[22]
- Ahead of his time, Kelling had recognized profitable economical aspects of endoscopic surgery.[23]

In 1911 internist Hans Christian Jacobaeus (1879–1937), from Stockholm, introduced the term "laparothoracoscopy."[24] He was first to view thorax and abdominal cavity by endoscopy and recommended endoscopic technique to view other body cavities. In contrast to Kelling, he inserted the trocar directly without creating pneumoperitoneum. Jacobaeus began like Kelling by breaking down adhesions under thoracoscopic vision.

Bertram M. Bernheim (1880–1958) of Johns Hopkins Hospital introduced endoscopic surgery in the United States in 1911. He called the procedure "organoscopy."[25] His instrument consisted of half-inch proctoscope and a simple light.

Heinz Kalk (1895–1973), a gastroenterologist from Berlin, known as founder of German school for laparoscopy, developed a 135° lens system and double trocar.[26] He used laparoscopy as a diagnostic method in diseases of liver and gallbladder. In the publication of his experiences in 1939, he reported over 2000 liver punctures under local anesthesia with no fatalities. He broke down adhesions by laparoscopy.

Constant improvements in laparoscopic methodology smoothened the way for its wider operative use. The important steps in the process were use of harmless carbon dioxide (CO_2) for pneumoperitoneum by Zollikofer in Switzerland (1924), coagulation of adhesions by Fervers in Germany (1933)[27] and intra-abdominal use of monopolar current by Ruddock in the United States (1934).

Boesch, from Swiss Aarau, reported in his paper on laparoscopy about "wonderful perspective of the feminine, not deformed genitals of woman and about the exposure of hidden organs, e.g., the ovaries with an elevator (palpation probe)."[28] He noted further: "with the laparoscope we have obtained a way to carry out the tubal sterilization for the given indication without laparotomy. With a suitably insulated coagulation clamp, the tubes can be coagulated at multiple places in 3–5 minutes under endoscopic vision." Frank H. Power and Allen C. Barnes developed in 1941 the same technique in the United States; however, they used a peritoneoscope for tubal sterilization.[29]

The insufflation of abdominal cavity by instruments was problematic for a long time. Kelling carried it out with Fiedler trocar, which had a blunt "mandrin" to avoid injuries; Otto Goetze (1886–1957), who coined the term "pneumoperitoneum" in 1918, produced a similar instrument with spring mechanism (Fig. 1.5) for air insufflation for contrast radiograms.[30]

In 1938, the Hungarian Janos Veress (1903–1979) (Figs. 1.6 and 1.7) developed a special canula with spring mechanism aiming to create pneumothorax and consequently to treat tuberculosis, which was prevalent at that time.[31] With little modifications Veress needle is used still today to create pneumoperitoneum for laparoscopy. Its special mechanism prevents injury to internal organs during needle insertion through anterior abdominal wall.

In 1960, gynecologists first began small operative interventions. However, French gynecologist Raoul Palmer had already carried out laparoscopy in Trendelenburg position in 1944. In this position intestines were displaced out of pelvis and consequently could be better assessed during operation. Additionally, he required continuous gas insufflation, which was controlled automatically. Palmer also carried out the first laparoscopic sterilization in Paris.

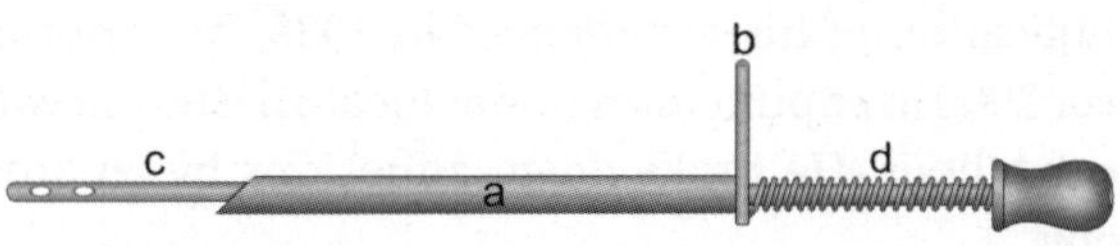

Fig. 1.5: Atraumatic needle by Goetze.

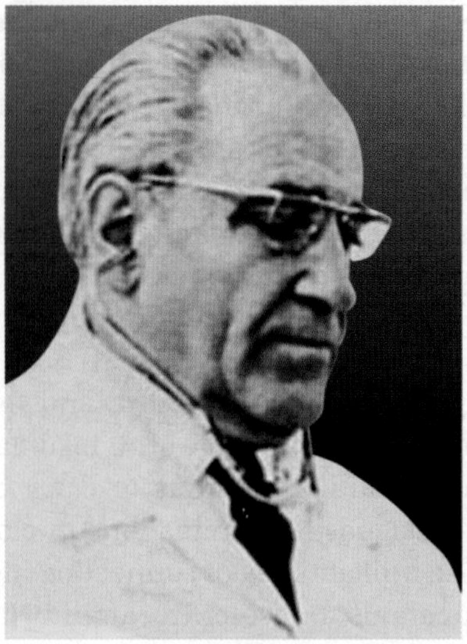

Fig. 1.6: Janos Veress (1903–1979).

From the internal department of Komitats hospital, in Hungary

New instrument for carrying out punctures of chest or abdomen and treatment of pneumothorax.

By Dr Janos Veress Medical Superintendent.

Undoubtedly, an important moment of pleural and peritoneal puncture is the moment when the needle punctures the pleura or the peritoneum, because the vulnerable lungs or intestines are exposed to injuries with the pointed instrument. The sharp tip on the puncture instrument, to penetrate the thoracic or abdominal wall easily, is of great importance, but only till the moment when the needle reaches the cavity; then, in the cavity, the sharp tip is superfluous, even dangerous.

Fig. 1.7: Publication by J. Veress about the Veress needle developed by him.
Source: German Med Sci. 1938; 41:1480.)

Piercing of umbilicus for laparoscope by Raoul Palmer in 1946 was a groundbreaking procedure in gynecology. Like Kelling, he called endoscopic diagnostic procedure "coelioscopy" and developed several methods to insert the endoscope. The abdominal access involved many technical difficulties because of mainly blind insertion technique through anterior abdominal wall.[32]

Decker, an American, introduced laparoscope transvaginally through vaginal fornix.[33] He called this procedure Douglasscopy or culdoscopy (Figs. 1.8A and B). From a diagnostic perspective, Douglasscopy was insufficient. This technique that was initially prevalent in America later lost its importance. In 1998 it was team of Brosens et al[34] that brought about a renaissance of this procedure as transvaginal hydrolaparoscopy for diagnosis of sterility.

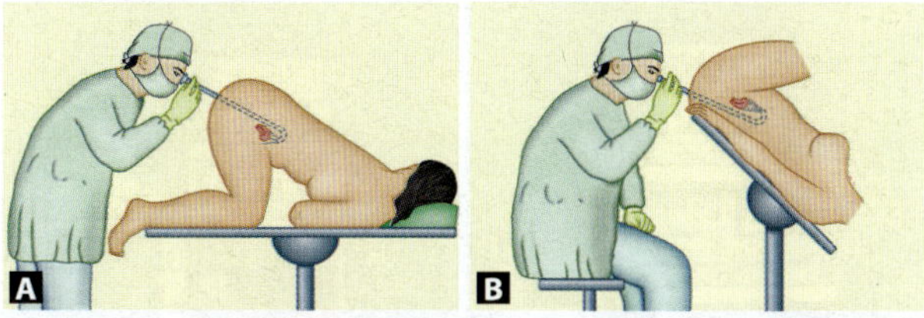

Figs. 1.8A and B: Douglasscopy in the (A) knee-elbow position and in (B) extreme head-low position.

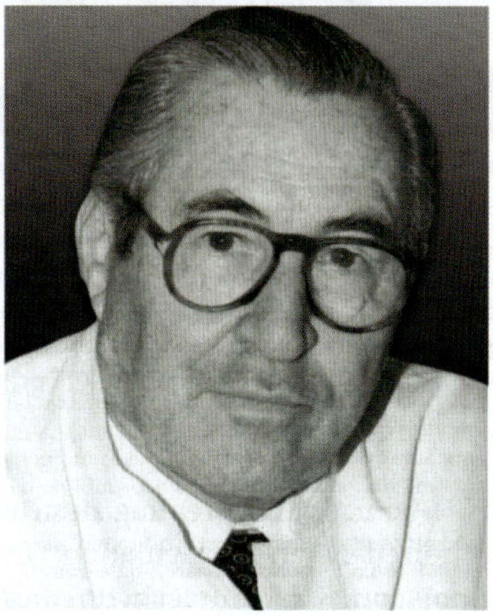

Fig. 1.9: Hans Frangenheim (1920–2001).

Hans Frangenheim (1920–2001) and Kurt Semm (1927–2003) helped in a special way to develop laparoscopy in Germany after the Second World War.

In 1950, Hans Frangenheim (Fig. 1.9) began his training in gynecology at Anselmino and in 1951 came in contact with laparoscopy for first time. He was called to medical clinic in Cologne where a lower abdominal tumor was diagnosed during hepatoscopy and further line of treatment had to be decided. Looking back he wrote:

> I sensed there, that a new aid had presented itself for the field of gynecology and so began to look into literature. A remark made by Kalk in a textbook had impressed me the most, which said, it is certain that gynecology would open a big field of indications for laparoscopy.

After his appointment in October 1955 to the post of assistant medical director of the National Gynecological Hospital at Wuppertal, Frangenheim attended lectures by Palmer in Paris and realized that laparoscopy was clearly superior to culdoscopy, which was still practiced in Germany. Then he concentrated on regulating uncontrolled gas insufflation, developing new instruments and photographic documentation of endoscopic findings. He had difficult time with German endoscopy firms. Finally, with modified anesthesia equipment from Draeger, he succeeded in reducing gas pressure from customary 50 to 15 mmHg. and restricting CO_2 gas flow to maximum of 5 L/min. Frangenheim even defined indications for diagnostic laparoscopy in extrauterine pregnancy, chronic lower abdominal pain, sterility and ovarian tumors.

His monographs, *Laparoscopy and Culdoscopy in Gynecology,*[35] *Laparoscopy in Gynecology, Surgery and Paediatrics,*[36] *Diagnostic and Operative Laparoscopy in Gynecology—Atlas with Colour Illustrations*[37] as well as countless publications and lectures contributed to further spread of the method.

In 1966 he was medical superintendent of gynecological clinic at Konstanz and European Congress for Endoscopy was held under his presidency in Konstanz and from that event laparoscopy received further impetus. In 1982 Frangenheim received First Order of Merit of the Federal Republic of Germany for his outstanding work. On the occasion of his 80th birthday Semm praised Frangenheim for his contribution with these words: "Today the name, Frangenheim is inseparably associated with the gynecologic laparoscopic methods. His achievements for Germany and for the world are epoch making and will go down in the annals of history."[38]

The Kiel University clinic for women under Semm (1927–2003) (Fig. 1.10) is regarded as birthplace of modern endoscopic surgery. Semm, collaborating with Richard Fikentscher (1903–1993), developed a new universal insufflation equipment[39,40] for the diagnosis of tubal patency, i.e., blowing through fallopian tubes by Rubin.[41] Befitting his knowledge of tubal insufflation, Semm developed an apparatus called "CO_2 Pneumo" for insufflating CO_2 gas during

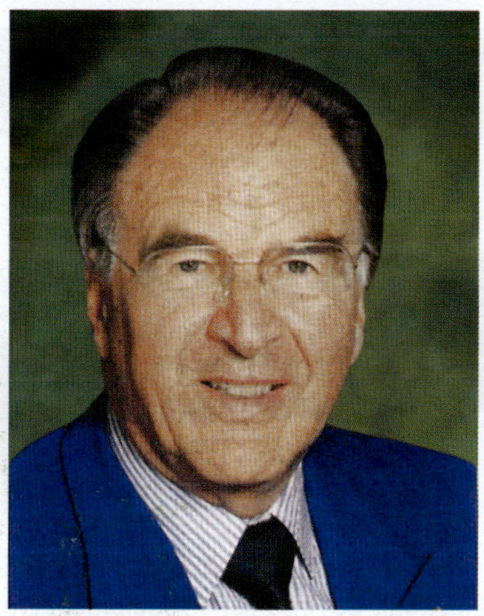

Fig. 1.10: Kurt Semm (1927–2003).

laparoscopy to minimize operative risks of endoscopy.[42] The instrument was in use from 1964 onward at the second university clinic for women in Munich and created pneumoperitoneum automatically.[42] The cold light (extracorporeal light that shone across a bundle of fiber glass) was simultaneously developed. Together, they eliminated intestinal burns and gas embolus, which were main dangers of gynecological laparoscopy. In spite of all progress world over, gynecological diagnostic laparoscopy was universally rejected. So, Semm selected the word "pelviscopy" to project that a new technique was developed. Starting from 1965, within three years, this new method spread quickly within Germany as a diagnostic procedure of female infertility. In 1976, Semm developed an electronic version of CO_2-Pneumo with the quadrotest for operative pelviscopy[43] (Figs. 1.11 and 1.12).

After Semm demonstrated "CO_2-Pneumo" at the Congress of American Fertility Association in Washington in 1969, Cohen published a book on this procedure in 1970. In the United States, acceptance of this new method of pelviscopic procedures in gynecology was phenomenal. Even though the method was used a million times, it was employed in 95% of the cases only for tubal sterilization, unlike in Europe,[44] where Boesch already accomplished this 35 years before.[28] The ignorance about the laws of physics while using the high-frequency (HF) energy in closed body cavities was the cause of many grave accidents causing burns to the internal organs like intestines and ureter. Such incidents once more deeply incriminated this method.

Fascinated by the idea that pelviscopy can be used not only for sterilization but also for other operative purposes,[45] Semm introduced it in his new regimen for hemostasis in New Orleans in 1974 (Figs. 1.12A to I).

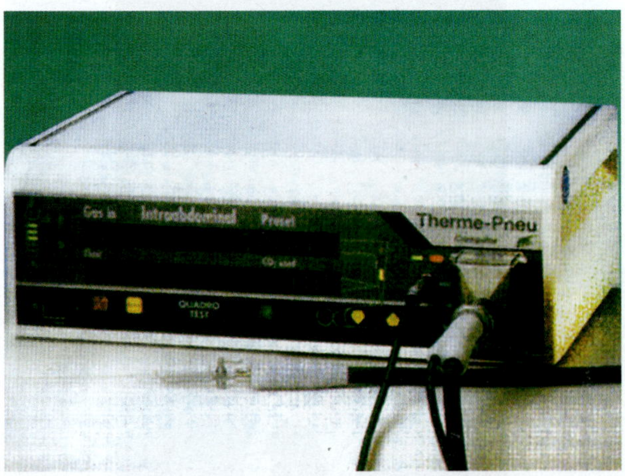

Fig. 1.11: Electronic CO_2 insufflation equipment (Therme-Pneu Electronic, WISAP Gmbh).

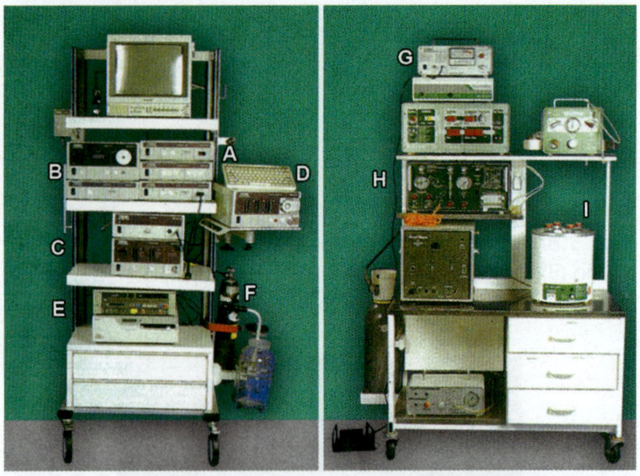

Figs. 1.12A to I: Equipment cart for gynecological endoscopy: (A) Video camera system, monitor, digital video camera; (B) Cold light source; (C) CO_2 insufflation equipment—thermoflator®; (D) Hysteroflator for hysteroscopy; (E) Video recorder and video printer; (F) Suction irrigation equipment; (G) Coagulation equipment for monopolar and bipolar coagulation—endocoagulator; (H) Equipment for CO_2 pertubation; (I) NaCl bottles, warmed up to 37°C.

The use of HF current for creating destructive heat was not required in endocoagulation. The human body did not come in contact with the electrical energy. Optimally controlled hemostasis takes place at 110°C. Between 1970 and 1980, the HF current in the monopolar and bipolar techniques using inadequately covered apparatus led to uncontrollable burns; today, in clinical endoscopic practice also, it is ensured that the electrical energy used under supervision does not lead to burns. The modern coagulation and cutting equipment, which work on mono- and bipolar current, have control mechanisms that minimize risk of unintentional burns. Bipolar and monopolar instruments have a controlled, restricted coagulation zone.[46]

Semm, who produced his own instruments, as he was a skilled instrument maker himself, built an automatic CO_2 insufflator in 1963, introduced thermocoagulation in 1973, and used for first time Roeder loop to stop arterial bleeding. For laparoscopy he developed special suction irrigation equipment and an electronic insufflator. Difficult interventions were possible because of methods of hemostasis (endosuture with intra- and extracorporeal knots) developed by Semm and his range of instruments. However, many physicians, gynecologists as well as surgeons criticized Semm for his vehement use of so-called keyhole surgery. They were of the opinion that due to the modern anesthetic techniques, big operations by laparotomy posed no problems and Semm had exaggerated the problems with subsequent adhesions.

Some treated news of the new spectrum of operations (oophorectomy or the removal of complete uterine appendages, treatment of tubal pregnancy) with disbelief and concluded that Semm has started his operation as laparoscopy and then ended it as conventional operation by laparotomy.

Semm was exposed to most intense hostility of the German gynecologists (and endoscopic surgeons) when he carried out first laparoscopic appendectomy in 1983.[47] The surgeons especially saw no need to abandon established operative method and to replace it with technically more difficult one. Semm's first attempt at publishing his method therefore met with rejection. The fact that a gynecologist wanted to show the surgeons how an operation should be carried out was simply unthinkable at that time. Semm had crossed the limit that was till then considered as sacrosanct. But he knew that endoscopic surgery had enormous potential not only in gynecology but especially in surgery and therefore continued with his endeavors in laparoscopy, unperturbed toward the goal, of reducing the surgical trauma to the patients. Two German surgeons, Friedrich Gotz and Arnold Pier, followed Semms's intent and provided a wider base to laparoscopic appendectomy.[48] In the early 1990s they had already carried out hundreds of appendectomies in this way and perfected the technique, which they could now use even in acute appendicitis.[49]

In 1977 a 10-mm morcellator (Semm) was produced for pelviscopy purposes. However, in today's operative pelviscopy where even fist-sized myomata is removed from uterus with little blood loss, this instrument is not very effective. So in 1988, manually operated serrated edged macro morcellator (Semm) of 15–20 mm diameter was introduced. The instrument could reduce a myoma of about 5 cm size to small pieces within a few minutes. The posterior colpotomy for removal of myoma or even a small abdominal incision was not required any more.[50] Since the introduction of horizontal morcellation, the morcellators are motorized and are available in 10 to 24 mm diameters.

Just like laparotomy, intra-abdominal irrigation equipment are necessary in laparoscopy also to guarantee good view. The acquapurator of 1974 gave way to CO_2 aquapurator in 1990. Today the aquapurator biotherm has removed many problems of hypothermia, even in operations of longer duration. In 1994, insufflation of preheated CO_2 was introduced to preserve isothermia.

In September 1985 a surgeon from Böblingen, Erich Mühe (1938–2005), performed laparoscopic cholecystectomy for the first time in the world using Semm's instruments.[51] In 1986, Mühe reported 97 successful laparoscopic operations.[52] In 1989, Reich et al. described the first laparoscopic-assisted vaginal hysterectomy.[53] In 1991 Mouret carried out the first cholecystectomy by video laparoscopy.

In the 1970s and 1980s most surgeons simply ignored the development of laparoscopic operations because of introduction of new medicines, impressive results of intensive care and innovations in anesthesia that facilitated extensive surgeries. The basic concept, that a big problem (disease) requires a big solution (abdominal incision), was so deeply rooted in surgeon's thinking that there was no place for "keyhole surgery." This is why surgical fraternity refused to accept and modify gynecological instruments for their use.

However, contrary to general development some surgeons accepted the challenge and accelerated introduction of laparoscopic techniques in surgery. A group of German surgeons was particularly active in this process and in December 1976 started Chirurgische Arbeitsgmeinschaft für Endoskopie und Sonographie (CAES) in Hamburg. In the United States, the Society of American Gastrointestinal Endoscopic Surgeons (SAGES) was set up five years later. In the following years both organizations laid foundation for the introduction of endoscopy in clinical practice.

Prompted by Dr. Bernd Manegold, a surgeon from Manheim and one of the founders of the CAES, the first edition of scientific journal *Surgical Endoscopy* was published in 1987 under the direction of many leading endoscopists. Just the following year the first World Congress for Surgical Endoscopy was held in Berlin, which was a great success where 500 experts from all over the world participated. This finally led to acceptance of endoscopy in surgery.

In 1983, British urologist John E. A. Wickham (born in 1927) used the concept of "minimally invasive surgery" for the first time. The concept attracted attention in 1987 after Wickham published his vision of extensive endoscopic treatment in the famous *British Medical Journal.*[54] In spite of the strong criticism it mirrored the general trend of the 1980s as minimally invasive techniques had greatly fascinated doctors and their patients.

This development was further accelerated by crucial technological innovations. The introduction of new light sources (Palmer 1953), Hopkins-optics (1960) and cold light source had already improved illumination in endoscopic operations in 1960.[21] The video technique was also important. The new video camera was much smaller and therefore easier to manage than its predecessor and the videocassettes also were simpler for everyday use than the 8 or 16 mm film. In 1980s more surgeons used video cameras, but even the latest and smallest of the camera together with endoscope proved unwieldy because it altered the balance and made precision work difficult. Electronic minicamera brought the breakthrough: a 4-mm optoelectronic transducer (CCD) converted the view from inside body cavity to electronic impulses and transferred them to a monitor. The combination of optic trocar and video camera opened new possibilities for surgeons because now with both hands free, they could operate ambidextrously and simultaneously follow on the monitor what was happening along with the entire team.

The years that followed were molded by a lively exchange and reciprocal stimulation. Video laparoscopy of cholecystectomy in 1987 in Lyon by Philipe Mouret (born in 1937) and his presentation of the procedure in the SAGES meeting in Louisville triggered a downright boom in France and also encouraged surgeons across the world to tread this path further.

Another milestone was realization of appendectomy by laparoscopy, which Kurt Semm started in patients that showed besides their gynecological problems subacute appendicitis. Although we performed laparoscopic appendectomies since 1981 and numerous German general surgeons had visited Kiel for that purpose, only when Semm presented his laparoscopic appendectomy in Baltimore in 1988, JB Mckernan and W. B. Saye took it up and in June 1988 they reported first laparoscopic cholecystectomy in the United States using Semm's instruments and combining the procedure with laser technology. As a result many successful endoscopists visited both protagonists in Nashville to learn the new technique. At the same time, Sung Tao Ko from Chicago upheld the laparoscopic appendectomy by Semm and brought his instruments to America. A paper on laparoscopic appendectomy that Kurt Semm and I submitted to the *American Journal of General Surgery* was rejected by declaring this as an unethical surgical technique. We also had the same experience in Germany when a lecture of Kurt Semm to the College of General Surgeons on Laparoscopic Appendectomy was rejected as an unacceptable technology. The news about these sensational methods reached even the media in the United States. During a TV talk show it was made public with the help of gallbladder operation. After that the Nashville surgeons received hundreds of calls not only from the patients but also from doctors.

In October 1989, when Douglas O Olsen and Eddie Joe Reddick announced their courses casually at the congress of American College of Surgeons (ACS) for laparoscopic cholecystectomy, they were booked in shortest time and new courses had to be planned. Many American observers felt that laparoscopy has pervaded the entire surgical fraternity in the United States. In the following weeks, a wave of enthusiasm about this new technique passed through the nation and training courses sprung like mushrooms. The industry was confronted with an abundance of orders so that waiting period rose up to six months. In the beginning leading endoscopists tried to canalize the development and to warn about the risks of injudicious use but soon they realized that it was not possible. No one had thought before 1989 that one of the most established operative method in surgery, cholecystectomy, would change so radically within just a few months. Even surgeons who had substantially contributed to this development were surprised by the speed. Literally thousands of surgeons had to restrain themselves. The courses were booked for months and the shortage of instruments was an unheard of phenomenon in the Western medicine. In the following years with the spread of laparoscopy, as the experiences increased, new operative methods quickly developed in many operative specialties.

The production of endoscopic instruments in the industry showed an upswing and the interaction and interest of the various medical specialties—surgery, urology, and gynecology—increased. Today the interest of the industry, doctors and patients worldwide is reflected in a common endeavor—betterment of surgery in many aspects through modern technology. That is reflected in further developments in the use of digital picture control, robotic instruments, computers, and telesurgery. Numerous specialities that have emerged and which deal increasingly with oncological fields also reflect these efforts. That is why in 1965 the German Society for Gynecologic Endoscopy and in 1971 the American Society for Gynecologic Endoscopy were founded. The World Society for Gynecologic Surgery (1986), the European Society for Gynecologic Endoscopy (ESGE, 1990), the Asian Society of Gynecological Endoscopy, the International Society for Gynecologic Endoscopy and the International Society of Gynecological Endoscopy (ISGE, 1991) came into being with yearly or two-yearly meetings.

The development of hysteroscopy and falloposcopy must be mentioned here. After Lindemann

(1971) and Semm (1974) established the CO_2 hysterectomy, the real breakthrough in the operative hysteroscopy came after 1980 basically as fluid hysteroscopy. Today hysteroscopy is a routine procedure and one cannot imagine diagnostic and therapeutic interventions without it.

From today's point of view, the ideal entry for viewing the tubal lumen is by hysteroscopy through a transcervical and transuterine catheter with 0.8–0.3 mm thick telescope or flexible falloposcopes.

When one compares the gynecologic endoscopic surgical work of the 1980s, primarily the sterilization, conservative operations on the adnexa and the enucleation of myoma were described. As against that, from 1989 the publications on adhesiolysis, appendectomy, lymphadenectomy and laparoscopy-assisted vaginal hysterectomy in different variations frequently appeared. In surgery, besides gallbladder resection, fundoplication, and hernia operations, extensive splenectomies, bowel resections, and great advances in surgical oncology and neurosurgery are described. In orthopedics, the operations on knee are improved further. In urology, there are reports on nephrectomies and the first robotic prostatic resection. In gynecology, robotic optic holders and instruments are employed.

The worldwide evolution for improvement of endoscopic surgery has begun; its end is still not in sight.[55] The aim of this surgery is to achieve at least the same, if not better results as with conventional operative techniques. On the wider international level mention should be made of Jordan M. Philipps under whose organization Kurt Semm, Liselotte Mettler, and various other team members of the Kiel School of Gynecological Endoscopy, which we really founded in the year 1990 only, but it existed under Kurt Semm's driving patronage since 1970, were able to teach endoscopy courses all over the United States in 1985 and our endoscopic surgery worldwide between 1985 and 2005. In 2005 numerous centers around the world had started to teach their own courses, which they continue to do. Single-port entries and particularly robotics have moved in with high demands and striking results. Contained in bag morcellation has substituted controlled electronic morcellation. Let us see what the future brings.

Jordan M. Philipps (1923–2008) (Fig. 1.13) founded the American Association of Gynecological Laparoscopy (AAGL), now the International Society of Minimal Invasive Gynecology, in 1971 The AAGL is the leading association promoting minimally invasive gynecologic surgery among surgeons worldwide.

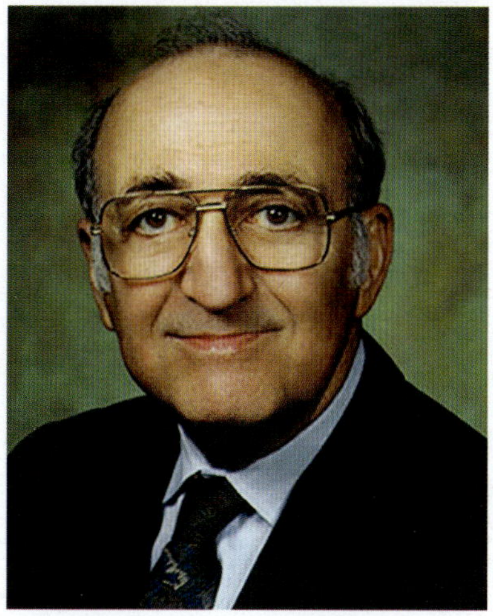

Fig. 1.13: Jordan M. Philipps (1923–2008).

When established in 1971 it was known as the American Association of Gynecologic Laparoscopists. As the field of minimally invasive gynecologic surgery grew, the membership of the AAGL quickly expanded around the globe and came to encompass more than laparoscopy alone.

Although the organization had outgrown its American roots, its name and acronym AAGL had become highly recognized worldwide. To best portray its expanding mission and international constituency, while still preserving its heritage and brand recognition, the organization eventually dropped its full name, "American Association of Gynecologic Laparoscopists" and became known simply as the AAGL, along with the phrase "Advancing Minimally Invasive Gynecology Worldwide."

Today with a membership extending to over 110 countries, the AAGL is an internationally recognized authority in minimally invasive gynecology. With over 7,000 members worldwide, the association counts among its membership the foremost authorities in gynecology and pioneers in technique and procedures and continues besides renowned and as active other previously mentioned international and national societies in our field.[56]

As extremely active colleagues on the American continent in the United States since 30 years, let me also mention the three Iranian pioneers in endoscopic gynecologic surgery who influenced our field like none others by their intuition, love and dedication to their work, the laparoscopic surgery, totally dedicated to their new country, the United States, the Nezhat brothers: Camran, Farr and Ceana Nezhat.[57]

Our late German colleague Thoralf Schollmeyer (1964–2014) was from 2007 onward the director of

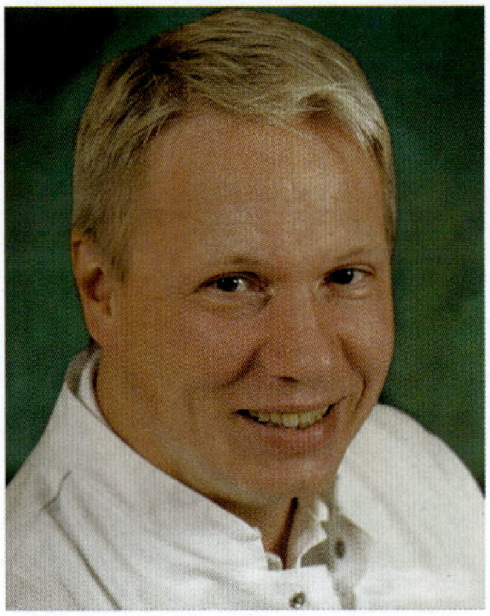

Fig. 1.14: Thoralf Schollmeyer (1964–2014).

the Kiel School of Gynecological Endoscopy and the president of the German Society of Gynecological Endoscopy (AGE) when he died in 2014. He deserves to be especially mentioned in an historical outline as his professional life was fully dedicated to the education in endoscopic gynecological surgery. He was the first editor of our second edition of this book and a truly believing endoscopic surgeon till the end of his early death by the age of 50 years in 2014 (Fig. 1.14). Being a patient himself over eight years he showed us how dedication to the profession and family moves rocks. The development of gynecological endoscopy in clinic, research and science and the support of young researchers characterized his life. He followed his own way, which was marked by extreme passion, audacity and endurance of pain with high ethical and medical values.

In conclusion, it must be stressed that the history of laparoscopy and hysteroscopy and its introduction in the surgical practice is a story of many researchers, who for years battled against prevalent general thinking and partly against rejection of their brainchild of performing "gentle operations." Many of the pioneers were ignored, called dreamers or regarded as crazy. It is only through their persistence, tenacity, strong personalities and intense dedication to life and love that they could stand firm in the face of adversities.[58]

The history of laparoscopy is a unique mixture of various trends in different fields, spurred by the activities of established societies as well as opportunities of their publication and influenced by the world's progress, recession, war, peace and the love of the individuals for life. The influence of industry, which has kept pace and actively supported this development for years, is the driving force besides the heroes of doctors and engineers that bring up new ideas. Without suitable technology, this dissemination would not have been possible. Endoscopic development and its future does depend on new inventions, on the audacity of leading heroes, their input into this field but also on their management of life to continue to survive and on a healthy and successful cooperation with the medical technical industry and the governments of our countries, which grant us the freedom of research and development for the best care of all our patients.

REFERENCES

1. Toellner, R. Illustrierte Geschichte der Medizin. Salzburg: Andreas & Andreas; 1986.
2. Arnaud de Ronsil G. Memoires de chirurgie, avec quelques remarques historiques sur l'etat de la médecine et de la chirurgie en France et en Angleterre. Paris: Londres chez J. Nourse; 1768.
3. Bozzini P. Lichtleiter, eine Erfindung zur Anschauung innerer Theile und Krankheiten nebst der Abbildung. J Practis Arzneyk Wundarzneyk. 1806;24:107-24.
4. Bozzini P. Der Lichtleiter oder die Beschreibung einer einfachen Vorrichtung und ihrer Anwendung zur Erleuchtung innerer Höhlen und Zwischenräume des lebenden animalischen Körpers. Verlag des Landes Industrie Comptoir, Weimar. 1807.
5. Desormeaux, AJ. Sitzungsbericht der Societe de Chir. Paris: Gazette de Hope; 1865.
6. Stein ST. Das Photo-Endoskop. Berliner klin. Woch. schr. 1874:31-3.
7. Desormeaux AJ. De'Lendoscope et ses applications au diagnostic et au traitement des affections de l'urethre et de la vessie. Baillière; 1865.
8. Aubinais EJ. Un Med Provence. 1864;24:591.
9. Pantaleoni DC. On endoscopic examination of the cavity of the womb. Med Pres Circa. 1869;8:26.
10. Nitze M. Über die Behandlungsmethode der Höhlen des menschlichen Körpers. Wien Med Wschr. 1879; 24:851-8.
11. Leiter J. Elektro-endoskopische Instrumente. Wien. 1880.
12. Mikulicz J. Gastroskopie und Oesophagoskopie. Verh dt Ges Chir. Berlin. 1882;11:31-8.
13. Kelling G. Ueber die Ermittlung der Magengroesse. University Leipzig: Leipzig; 1890.
14. Kelling G. Ein einfaches Verfahren zur Bestimmung der Magengrösse mittels Luft (I). Munch Med Wochenschr. 1892;18:1160.
15. Kelling G. Ein einfaches Verfahren zur Bestimmung der Magengrösse mittels Luft (II). Munch Med Wochenschr. 1892;18:1191.
16. Kelling G. Durch Zug und Drehung streckbares gegliedertes Rohr zum Einführen in das Körperinnere. Patentiert im Deutschen Reiche vom 07. 1897.
17. Kelling, G. Über die Besichtigung der Speiseröhre und des Magens mit biegsamen Instrumenten.

in 73. Versammlung der Gesellschaft Deutscher Naturforscher und Ärzte. Hamburg. 1901.
18. Kelling G. Endoskopie für Magen und Speiseröhre: 2. Gegliedertes, winklig streckbares Gastroskop mit rotierbarem Sehprisma. Münchner Med Wochenschrift. 1898;45:1556.
19. Kelling G. Endoskopie für Magen und Speiseröhre: 3. Schluss. Münchner Med Wochenschrift. 1898;45:1591.
20. Litynski GS, Paolucci V. Origin of laparoscopy: coincidence or surgical interdisciplinary thought? World J Surg. 1998;22(8):899-902.
21. Schollmeyer M, Schollmeyer T. Georg Kelling und die sächsischen Wurzeln der Laparoskopie-100 Jahre Laparoskopie. Siebenlehn: Verein Oschatzer Frauenärzte e.V., Druckerei Wagner, Verlag und Werbung GmbH; 2001.
22. Schollmeyer T, Soyinka AS, Schollmeyer M, et al. Georg Kelling (1866-1945): the root of modern day minimal invasive surgery. A forgotten legend? Arch Gynecol Obstet. 2007;276(5):505-9.
23. Kelling G. Zur Cölioskopie und Gastroskopie. Munch Med Wochenschr. 1923;70:1054.
24. Jacobaeus HC. Ueber die Möglichkeit, die Zystoskopie bei Untersuchung seröser Höhlungen anzuwenden. Vorläufige Mitteilung. Munch Med Wochenschr. 1910;57:2090-2.
25. Bernheim BM. IV Organoscopy: cystoscopy of the abdominal cavity. Ann Surg. 1911;53(6):764–7.
26. Kalk H. Erfahrungen mit der Laparoskopie (zugleich mit der Beschreibung eines neuen Instrumentes). Z Klin Med. 1929;111:304-48.
27. Fervers C. Die Laparoskopie mit dem Cystoscop. Ein Beitrag zur Vereinfachung der Technik und zur endoskopischen Strangdurchtrennung in der Bauchhöhle. Med Klin. 1933;29:1042-5.
28. Boesch P. Laparoskopie. Schweiz Z Krankenhaus Anstalt SW. 1936;6:62-3.
29. Power F, Barnes A. Sterilization by means of peritoneoscopic tubal fulguration: a preliminary report. Am J Obstet Gynecol. 1941;41:1038-43.
30. Goetze O. Die Röntgendiagnostik bei gasgefüllter Bauchhöhle; eine neue Methode. Munch Med Wochenschr. 1918;65:1275-80.
31. Veress J. Neues Instrument zur Ausführung von Brustoder Bauchpunktionen und Pneumathoraxbehandlung. Dtsch Med Wochenschr. 1938;64:1480-1.
32. Palmer R. La coelioscopie gynecologique. rapport du Prof. Mocquot. Acad De Chir. 1946(72):363-8.
33. Decker A. Pelvic culdoscopy. In: Meigs JV, Sturgis SH. (Ed.). Progress in Gynecology. New York: Grüne & Stratton; 1946. pp. 95-9.
34. Brosens I, Gordts S, Campo R, et al. Transvaginal access heralds the end of standard diagnostic laparoscopy in infertility. Hum Reprod. 1998;13(7):1762-3.
35. Frangenheim, H. Die Laparoskopie und die Culdoskopie in der Gynäkologie. Stuttgart: Thieme Verlag; 1959.
36. Frangenheim H. Die Laparoskopie in der Gynäkologie, Chirurgie und Pädiatrie: Lehrbuch und Atlas. Stuttgart: Thieme Verlag; 1970.
37. Frangenheim H. Diagnostische und operative Laparoskopie in der Gynäkologie: ein Farbatlas. München: Marseille Verlag; 1980.
38. Litynski GS. Hans Frangenheim - culdoscopy vs. laparoscopy, the first book on gynecological endoscopy, and "cold light." JSLS. 1997;1(4):357-61.
39. Fikentscher R, Semm K. [Contribution on the method of utero-tubal pertubation]. Geburtshilfe Frauenheilkd. 1955;15(4):313-22.
40. Fikentscher R, Semm K. [A portio adapter for persufflation and hysterosalpingography]. Geburtshilfe Frauenheilkd. 1959;19:867-70.
41. Semm K. Zur Technik der Eileiterdurchblasung. Z Geburtsh Gynäk. 1964;162:48-53.
42. Semm K. [Laparoscopy in gynecology]. Geburtshilfe Frauenheilkd. 1967;27(11):1029-42.
43. Semm K. Pelviskopie und Hysteroskopie. Farbatlas und Lehrbuch. Stuttgart, New York: Schattauer Verlag; 1976.
44. Semm K. Methoden der Sterilisation der Frau. Therapiewoche. 1976;26:3931-41.
45. Hulka JF, Fishburne JI, Mercer JP, et al. Laparoscopic sterilization with a spring clip: a report of the first fifty cases. Am J Obstet Gynecol. 1973;116(5): 715-8.
46. Semm K. Die moderne Endoskopie in der Frauenheilkunde. Frauenarzt. 1972;13:300-7.
47. Semm K. Endoscopic appendectomy. Endoscopy. 1983;15(2):59-64.
48. Gotz F, Pier A, Bacher C. Modified laparoscopic appendectomy in surgery. A report on 388 operations. Surg Endosc. 1990;4(1):6-9.
49. Pier A, Gotz F, Bacher C. Laparoscopic appendectomy in 625 cases: from innovation to routine. Surg Laparosc Endosc. 1991;1(1):8-13.
50. Semm K, Mettler L. Technical progress in pelvic surgery via operative laparoscopy. Am J Obstet Gynecol. 1980;138(2):121-7.
51. Litynski G. Erich Mühe and the rejection of laparoscopic cholecystectomy (1985): a surgeon ahead of his time. JSLS. 1998;2(4):341-6.
52. Mühe E. Die erste Cholecystektomie durch das Laparoskop. Langenbecks Archiv. 1986;369: 804.
53. Reich H. Laparoscopic hysterectomy. Surg Laparosc Endosc. 1992;2(1):85-8.
54. Wickham JE. The new surgery. Br Med J (Clin Res Ed). 1987;295(6613):1581-2.
55. Mettler L, Clevin L, Ternamian A, et al. The past, present and future of minimally invasive endoscopy in gynecology: a review and speculative outlook. Minim Invasive Ther Allied Technol. 2013;22(4): 210-26.
56. Linda M, Loffer F. Remembering Jordan M. Phillips, MD. J Minim Invasive Gynecol. 2008;15(6): 656-9.
57. Nezhat CR. My Journey with the AAGL. J Minim Invasive Gynecol. 2010;17(3):271-7.
58. Mettler L, Law EW. Lovers to Spouses. Boston, MA: Branden Books; 2017.

KIEL SCH•OL

2 of Gynaecological Endoscopy

Clinical Anatomy for Gynecological Laparoscopic Surgery

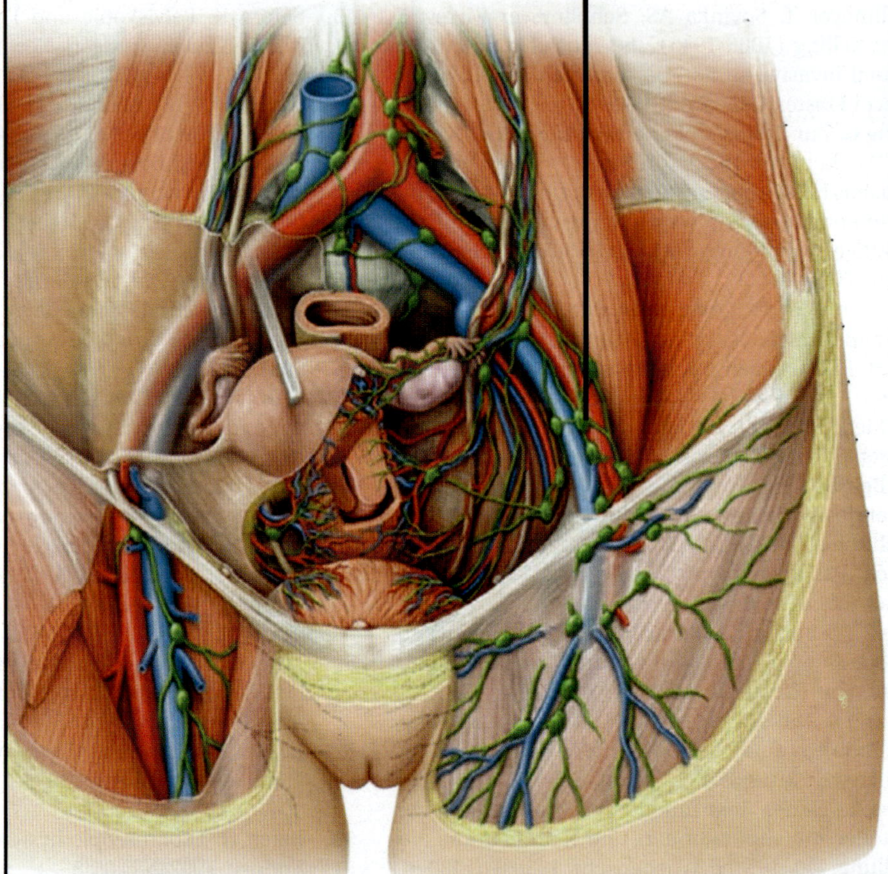

Chapter 2

Clinical Anatomy for Gynecological Laparoscopic Surgery

Johannes Ackermann, Ibrahim Alkatout, Thilo Wedel

INTRODUCTION

Knowledge of human anatomy is a fundamental part in medical education of every physician. In particular, before disturbing the integrity of human body by surgical interventions, an awareness about anatomical structures and landmarks is of utmost importance. This prerequisite holds true especially for laparoscopic procedures in which anatomical structures are approached and addressed differently as compared to open surgery. Thus, the aim of this chapter is to highlight the topographic anatomy of female pelvis, providing a basis for both efficient and safe laparoscopic operations.

ABDOMINAL WALL AND TROCAR PLACEMENT

Abdominal wall is the first natural barrier to be penetrated to gain access to peritoneal cavity or retroperitoneal space. Typical entry sites are predetermined by the topographic architecture of muscles, fasciae and blood vessels. The anterior abdominal wall is composed of three lateral muscles (external and internal oblique muscles, transverse abdominis muscle) and one ventral muscle (rectus abdominis muscle) on both sides separated along the midline by a connective tissue band (linea alba). From inside, abdominal musculature is covered by fascia transversalis, preperitoneal fat and peritoneum itself. Below umbilicus, the peritoneal layer displays five folds: median umbilical fold (obliterated urachus), two medial umbilical folds (obliterated umbilical arteries) and two lateral umbilical folds (inferior epigastric vessels) (Fig. 2.1).[1]

The first trocar entry to create pneumoperitoneum is usually performed at the lower part of umbilicus. After the incision of cutis and subcutis, abdominal wall is lifted up and Veress needle is placed at a 45° angle to penetrate into abdominal cavity. Other systems provide an ability of direct entrance without the use of Veress needle. Nevertheless Veress needle represents state of the art for entering abdominal cavity. While crossing the abdominal wall layers, two successive losses of resistance ("jolts") are perceived, as the needle or trocar pierces muscular fascia and peritoneum. This twofold loss of resistance indicates correct access into peritoneal cavity avoiding a false inflation of pre- or extraperitoneal space.[2]

Placement of additional trocars depends on different procedures to be performed. Normally, trocars are placed in a triangle 10–15 cm lateral and inferior of umbilicus in the region of inguinal fossa. During passage of the abdominal wall, care has to be taken not to injure urinary bladder, especially when not completely emptied or closely attached to the abdominal wall by adhesions and intestine, in particular when peritoneal adhesions are present (Figs. 2.2A and B). Moreover, inferior epigastric vessels are at risk for injury, which can lead to significant bleeding.[2] Inferior epigastric vessels originate medially to the deep inguinal ring and ascend underneath the peritoneum and transversalis fascia to reach and enter rectus abdominis muscle.

FEMALE PELVIC CAVITY AND ORGANS

The female pelvic cavity is divided into three compartments: an anterior compartment with urinary bladder and urethra, a middle compartment with uterus, adnexa and vagina, and a posterior compartment with rectum and anal canal (Fig. 2.3).[1-4] The *anterior compartment* is delimited in front by pubic

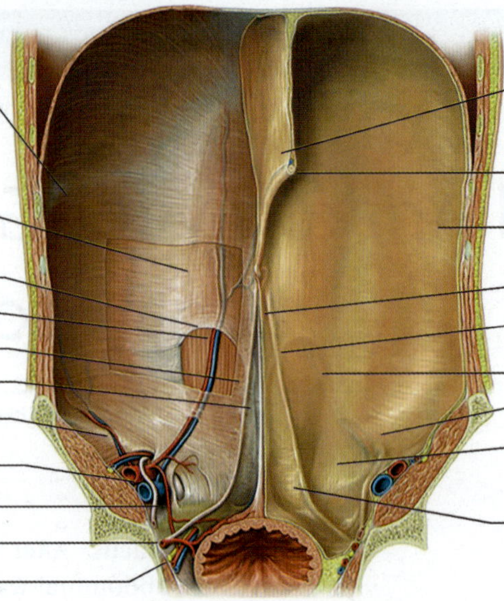

Fig. 2.1: Back side of the anterior abdominal wall. Reproduced from Schünke et al.[13]

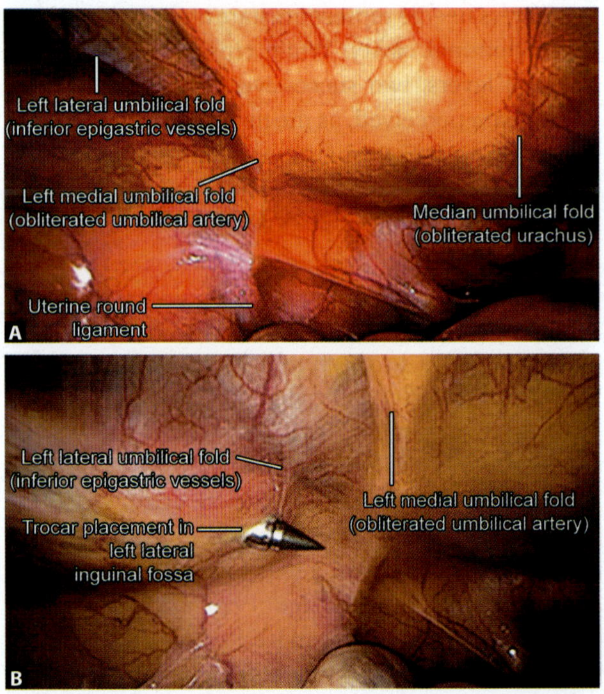

Figs. 2.2A and B: Laparoscopic view onto the left anterior abdominal wall. The three umbilical folds are discernible (A); the entry site of the trocar (B) is lateral to the lateral umbilical fold.

bone and prevesical space and laterally by pelvic sidewall comprising pectineal ligament (Cooper's ligament) and internal obturator muscle. Between the dorsal wall of urinary bladder and urethra and the anterior vaginal wall extends the vesicovaginal/urethrovaginal septum. The *middle compartment* extends between vesicovaginal/urethrovaginal septum and rectovaginal septum and contains uterus, uterine tubes, ovaries and vagina. Ureter crosses the middle compartment at the level of uterine cervix to reach vesical trigonum. Behind rectovaginal septum extends the *posterior compartment* containing anorectum surrounded by perirectal fascias. The dorsal compartment is delimited posteriorly by the concave surface of the sacral bone covered by presacral fascia and blood vessels.[5]

The uterovaginal complex is supported by pelvic floor and additionally fixed to pelvic wall by *uterine ligaments* (Fig. 2.4). Uterine ligaments comprise broad ligament, uterine round ligament, transverse cervical ligament, uterosacral ligament and pubocervical ligament. The *broad ligament* is a wide-stretched connection between the middle pelvic compartment and pelvic sidewall. It displays three peritoneal folds on each side converging from different origins of inner abdominal and pelvic walls toward the uterine cornu. These folds include funicular meso (anterior fold), mesosalpinx (middle fold) and mesovarium (posterior fold). The *uterine round ligament* extends from uterine fundus below and lateral to uterine cornu to deep inguinal ring and is accompanied by a branch from uterine artery and lymphatic vessels draining into superficial inguinal lymph nodes. The *transverse cervical ligament (cardinal ligament of Mackenroth)* connects uterine cervix and vaginal fornix to pelvic sidewall. Besides its mechanical function, it represents a main route of vascular, lymphatic and nervous supply to uterus. The *uterosacral ligament* attaches to uterine cervix and upper vagina and extends along rectal sidewall

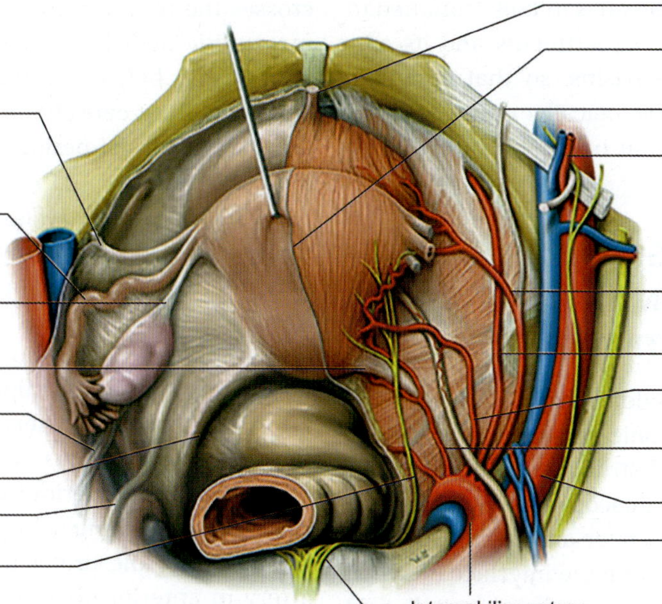

Fig. 2.3: Cranial view into the female pelvic cavity. The peritoneum, uterine adnexa and parametrial tissue are removed on the right side to expose the pelvic arteries, ureter and pelvic autonomic nerves.
Reproduced from Schünke et al.[13]

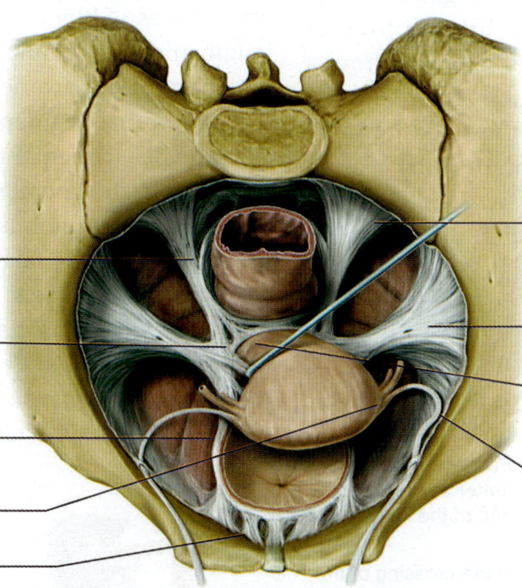

Fig. 2.4: Uterine ligaments. The rectum and urinary bladder are cut transversely, the uterus is shifted to the left side.
Reproduced from Schünke et al.[13]

toward sacrum before inserting at lower sacral vertebrae. The *pubocervical ligament* connects the pubic bone with uterine cervix running along urethra and bladder neck.[6-9]

Mesometrium is an embryologically defined tissue compartment comprising the neurovascular supply and major lymphatic drainage routes of the uterus. The clinical significance of mesometrium has received special attention after the introduction of total mesometrial resection (TMME) for uterine cancer. Mesometrium can be subdivided into vascular mesometrium containing the uterine blood vessels and surrounding lymphofatty tissue with mesometrial lymph nodes and ligamentous mesometrium corresponding to uterosacral ligaments and rectovaginal septum. Surgical approach is based on the concept that tumor spread is initially confined to permissive ontogenetic compartments and its corresponding lymph node basins, so that complete removal of these embryologically defined tissue compartments results in an optimal tumor control with low morbidity.[10,11]

ANATOMIC TOPOGRAPHY, VASCULARIZATION AND INNERVATION OF THE URETER

As ureter crosses the middle pelvic compartment, knowledge of its topographic anatomy and relationship to other organs and structures is essential for safe and considerate laparoscopic surgery. Reasons for high vulnerability of ureter are its considerably long course (25–30 cm) along the interface between retro- and intraperitoneal space, its morphological appearance and size similar to vascular structures, as well as relatively common congenital anomalies (e.g., ureter duplex, ureter fissus, crossed ureter, retrocaval ureter).[2,12]

Abdominal segment (Fig. 2.5) originates from renal pelvis and extends to pelvic brim in front of psoas muscle. The course of ureter may vary from a paravertebral position close to either the vena cava or aorta to a lateral position along the outer border of psoas muscle. Ureter is crossed anteriorly by ovarian blood vessels and posteriorly by genitofemoral nerve. On the left side, ureter additionally undercrosses the root of sigmoid mesocolon and inferior mesenteric pedicle. On both sides, there is a close relationship between ureter and infundibulopelvic ligament. Thus, care should be taken to protect ureter underneath its peritoneal fold when mobilizing uterine adnexa.[12]

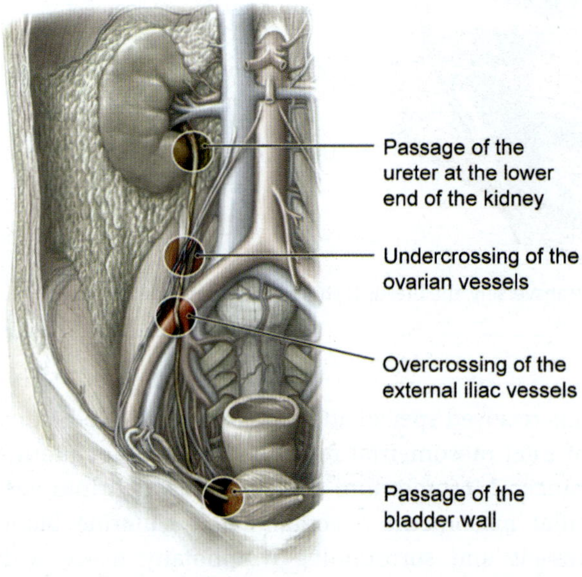

Fig. 2.5: Anatomical relationships of the ureter. Localization of common ureteric injuries.
Reproduced from Schünke et al.[13]

The *pelvic segment* (Figs. 2.3 and 2.5) enters pelvic cavity anterior to common iliac artery on the left side and anterior to external iliac artery on the right side. Ureter further descends underneath peritoneum and is related laterally to the branches of internal iliac artery (obturator, superior vesical and uterine artery) and obturator nerve and medially to uterosacral ligament and its corresponding rectouterine fold as well as to inferior hypogastric plexus (*see* Fig. 2.8). Before reaching urinary bladder via vesicouterine ligament, the ureter has to undercross uterine artery in anterior oblique direction at the angle of vaginal fornix (para- cervix). Because of its close relationship to uterine cervix and artery, great attention has to be paid to this area for the integrity of the ureter.[13]

Vascularization of ureter is supplied by various sources of blood vessels due to its considerable length, including branches from aorta, renal, ovarian and internal iliac arteries. Whereas arteries approach the abdominal segment of ureter from the medial side, the pelvic segment is supplied by arteries originating from the lateral side (Figs. 2.6A and B). Consequently, when mobilizing or dissecting ureter, this principle has to be taken into consideration to preserve the blood vessels. Although interruption of one of many blood supply sources can be compensated by an anastomotic system running within the adventitial layer, excessive denudation of ureter over a long distance should be avoided.[2]

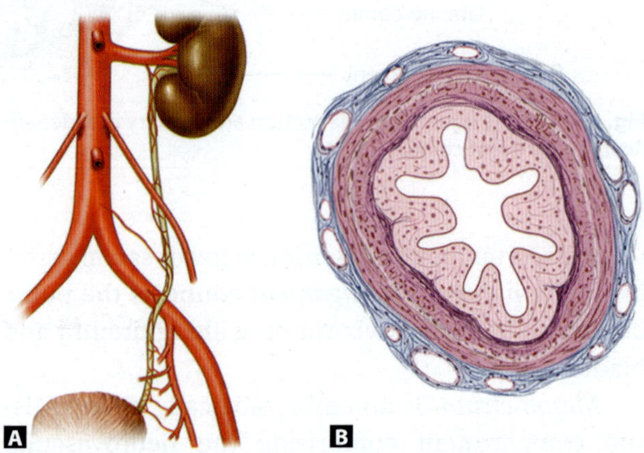

Figs. 2.6A and B: Vascularization of the ureter (A); cross-section of the ureter (B).

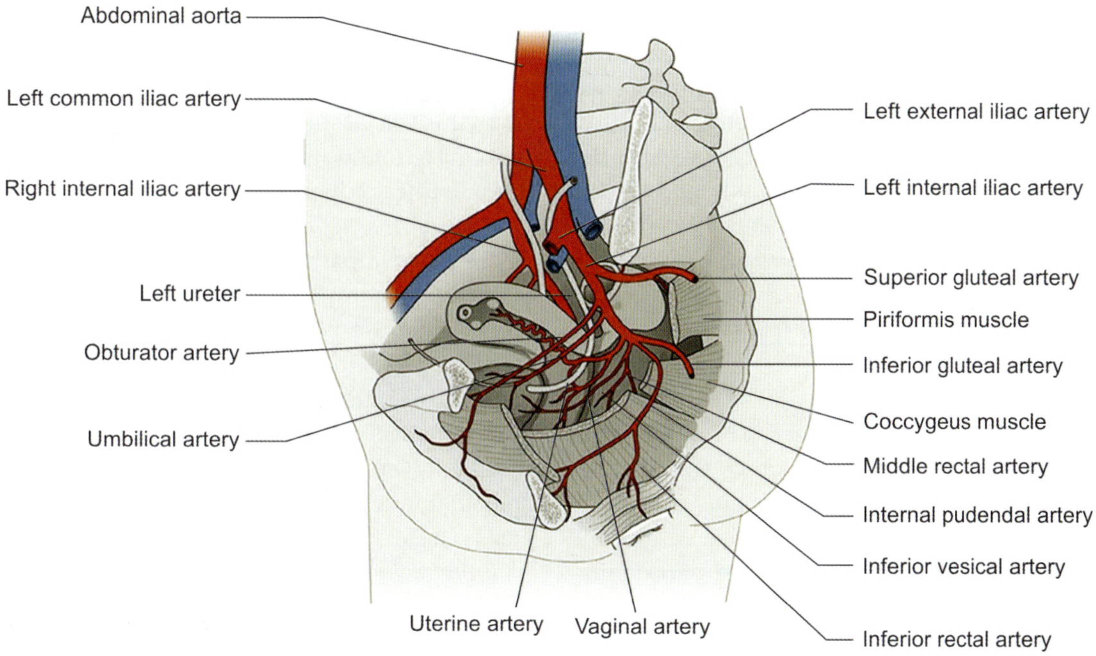

Fig. 2.7: Branches of the internal iliac artery in the female pelvis. Reproduced from Schünke et al.[13]

Nerve fibers responsible for the *autonomic innervation* of ureter derive from renal, superior and inferior hypogastric plexus mediating its peristaltic movements and pain perception. Furthermore, to prevent urinary bladder dysfunctions due to injury of vesical nerve plexus, manipulation of distal ureter at the region of vesicoureteric junction and vesical trigone should be avoided.[12]

VASCULARIZATION OF THE FEMALE PELVIS

Female pelvic organs are mainly supplied by internal iliac arteries (Fig. 2.7). The common iliac arteries originate at aortic bifurcation in front of the left side of fourth lumbar vertebra. They pass along the medial borders of psoas major muscle without giving off major branches and diverge into external and internal iliac arteries. Whereas external iliac arteries follow psoas major muscle until traversing lacuna vasorum through femoral ring to reach the lower limb, internal iliac arteries descend into pelvic cavity in a posterocaudal direction and then divide into anterior and posterior trunk. To expose internal iliac artery, the adjacent and sometimes overlying infundibulopelvic ligament and ovary have to be shifted upward. The common, external and internal iliac veins are located medially or dorsomedially to their arterial counterparts.[3]

The anterior trunk of internal iliac artery comprises the following branches: superior vesical artery, uterine artery, vaginal artery, middle rectal artery, obturator artery, internal pudendal artery and inferior gluteal artery (Fig. 2.7). Frequently, an anastomotic connection between obturator and inferior epigastric artery is provided by a pubic branch running across the pubic bone over pectineal ligament. This anastomotic branch is also termed as corona mortis ("crown of death"), because in earlier times of surgery, an inadvertent injury of this vessel led to serious bleedings during inguinal or femoral hernia repair.[3] The posterior trunk of internal iliac artery comprises iliolumbar artery, lateral sacral arteries and superior gluteal artery (Fig. 2.7).[3]

As a general rule, larger veins such as the common, external and internal iliac veins follow the course of their arterial counterparts. In most cases, veins run medially or dorsomedially to arteries. The same observation holds true for most of the parietal branches (e.g., obturator, pudendal, gluteal veins) of internal iliac artery; whereas visceral branches display different features: urinary bladder, uterus and vagina are drained by venous plexus, which are interconnected with each other and release blood into multiple vesical, vaginal and uterine veins. These veins do not strictly accompany and run parallel to the arteries until they enter internal iliac vein.[3]

It has to be emphasized that during laparoscopic surgery requiring pneumoperitoneum, pelvic veins often collapse due to intraperitoneal pressure exerted onto the thin venous walls. Thus, special care must be taken to clearly identify and respect pelvic veins, because injury may occur inadvertently and lead to troublesome bleeding sometimes only evident after diminishing the intraperitoneal pressure.[2]

AUTONOMIC INNERVATION OF THE FEMALE PELVIS

The challenge of oncologic surgery is to aim at the highest radicalness to ensure curative therapy and lowest loss of function to maintain quality of life after surgery. Therefore, it is essential to take care of the preservation of pelvic sympathetic and parasympathetic nerves. The integrity of this autonomic nervous system is essential for the maintenance of urinary continence and urinary bladder function as well as of sexual and anorectal functions.[14,15]

The preganglionic *sympathetic nerve fibers* emerge from lower lumbar and upper sacral spinal cord segments and pass along aorta on both sides as periaortal trunks. The periaortal nervous network fuses ventrolaterally to aorta to form inferior mesenteric and superior hypogastric plexus. In front of promontorium and slightly left to midline, superior hypogastric plexus divides into left and right hypogastric nerves. Hypogastric nerves often consist of various nerve bundles and are embedded within parietal pelvic fascia extending in front of the sacral concavity. Gentle traction of hypogastric nerve will lift up this fascial sheath in a tent-like fashion thereby enabling to follow its course along the pelvic sidewall down to inferior hypogastric plexus (Fig. 2.8).[16]

Parasympathetic nerves derive from sacral part of the parasympathetic nervous system residing in sacral spinal cord. Together with ventral branches of sacral spinal nerves S2–S4, these pelvic splanchnic nerves leave ventral sacral foramina and pierce parietal pelvic fascia on both sides to join the hypogastric nerves. Pelvic splanchnic nerves coming from dorsocaudally and the hypogastric nerves coming from dorsocranially converge to form inferior hypogastric plexus (Fig. 2.8).

Inferior hypogastric plexus is a mixed autonomic nerve plexus composed of both sympathetic and parasympathetic nerves and is embedded within parietal pelvic fascia covering the pelvic sidewalls. The nervous meshwork extends medially to internal iliac artery and gives off multiple branches to the pelvic organs. Posteriorly, *rectal plexus* diverges at the level of rectal ligaments and enters the rectal wall accompanied by middle rectal artery. Anteriorly, inferior hypogastric plexus releases a lateral and medial trunk. Lateral trunk corresponds to vesical plexus running toward the bladder—lateral and underneath the ureter. The nerve bundles follow branches of vesical artery and further ramify to innervate distal ure-

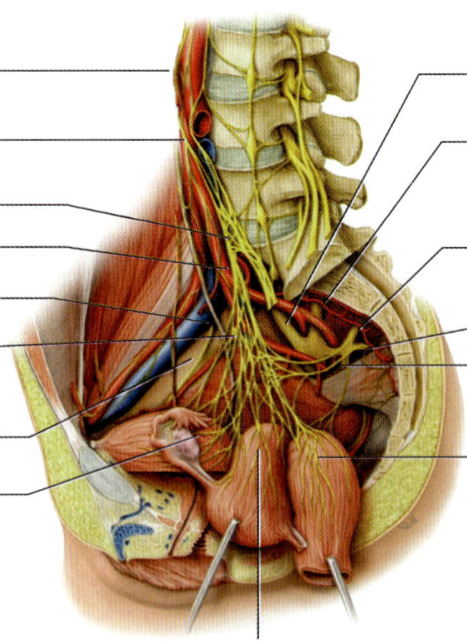

Fig. 2.8: Autonomic nerve supply of female pelvic viscera. Uterus and rectum are shifted to the left side to expose the pelvic autonomic nerve plexus.
Reproduced from Schünke et al.[13]

ter, urinary fundus and neck, and internal urethral sphincter. The medial trunk corresponds to uterovaginal plexus passing to uterine cervix and vagina medial and underneath the ureter. These nerve bundles follow the uterine artery after its intersection with ureter and innervate uterus from both sides (Figs. 2.3 and 2.8)[3]

PELVIC AND PARA-AORTIC LYMPH NODE COMPARTMENTS

Lymphadenectomy is considered to be an integral component of surgical treatment for malignant diseases of female genital organs. Due to topographic complexity of lymphatic drainage and close proximity between lymph nodes and both blood vessels and nerves, pelvic and para-aortic lymph node dissections are challenging and often time-consuming procedures. Therefore, profound anatomical knowledge of different lymph node regions and corresponding anatomical landmarks is required to identify and preserve structures at risk, when removing areolar fibrofatty tissue pads harboring the relevant lymph nodes.[17]

In general, lymphatic drainage follows arterial blood supply of the corresponding organ and is realized by a network of rather thin-walled lymphatic vessels and lymph nodes grouped along the nutrient vascular branches and enveloped by fatty and loosely arranged connective tissues. As blood supply of uterus and uterine adnexa originates from two sources (uterine and ovarian arteries) due to peculiar ontogenetic anatomy of the female genital tract, the main lymphatic drainage is multidirectional involving both pelvic and para-aortic routes.[18]

The *external iliac lymph nodes* (Fig. 2.9) extend from common iliac bifurcation down to femoral ring along psoas muscle. The medial border of the compartment is defined by paravesical and obturator fossa. External iliac lymph nodes can be divided into three subgroups: a lateral group located between external iliac vessels and psoas muscle, an intermediate group between artery and vein, and a medial group between vein and pelvic sidewall. Structures at risk during lymph node dissection are external iliac vessels, in particular the vein when lifted up for harvesting medial lymph nodes, and genitofemoral nerve when harvesting lymph nodes lateral to external iliac vessels. In some instances, minor branches originating from external iliac vessels to supply psoas muscle may be torn and bleed during lymph node removal in this compartment.[3]

The *obturator lymph nodes* (Fig. 2.9) are located within areolar fibrofatty tissue pad extending at the pelvic sidewall along obturator pedicle and internal obturator muscle. The upper border is defined by pelvic brim and the external iliac vessels, the dorsal border by common iliac bifurcation and the medial

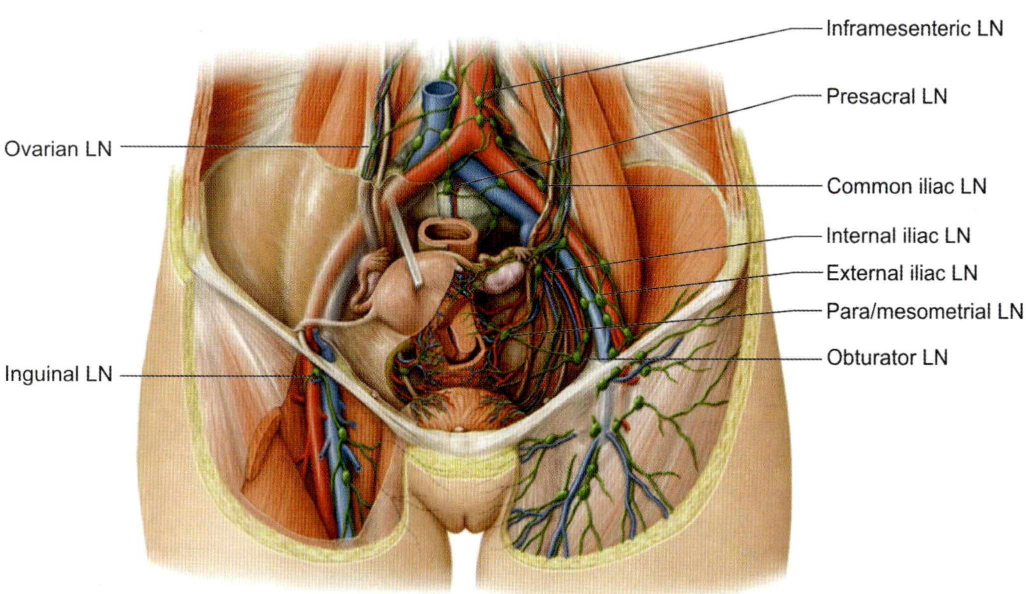

Fig. 2.9: Lymph nodes (LN) and lymphatic drainage of female genital organs. The uterus is shifted to the right side, the peritoneum is removed on the left side and above the aortic bifurcation.
Reproduced from Schünke et al.[13]

border by visceral branches of internal iliac artery. The obturator lymph nodes drain the lymph vessels of bladder, ureter, uterus and upper vagina. A complete lymphadenectomy of obturator fossa also requires subtle clearance of infraobturator nodes located below obturator pedicle at the upper surface of levator ani muscle. Subsequently, care must be taken not to injure the obturator pedicle itself as well as neurovascular pedicles of urinary bladder, in particular vesical venous plexus.

The *internal iliac lymph nodes* (Fig. 2.9) are located between anterior and posterior trunk of internal iliac artery and its corresponding branches. These lymph nodes drain lymphatic fluid from gluteal, perineal and sacral regions as well as from visceral organs like urinary bladder, uterus, vagina and rectum. The compartment originates at common iliac bifurcation and extends dorsally onto piriformis muscle, caudally down to levator ani muscle and ventrally to the origin of visceral arterial branches for urinary bladder and uterus. Most important for lymph node dissection is the direct vicinity of both ureter and delicate branches of inferior hypogastric plexus running medially to internal iliac branches and lymph nodes.[3]

The *common iliac lymph nodes* (Fig. 2.9) are located along the common iliac vessels, extend up to aortic bifurcation and collect lymphatic fluid from external and internal iliac lymphatic vessels. Like external iliac lymph nodes, they can be further subdivided into a lateral group facing iliolumbar fossa, an intermediate group intercalated between the common iliac vessels adjacent to lumbosacral trunk, and a medial group located along pelvic brim underneath the common iliac vein. Structures at risk during lymph node dissection are genitofemoral nerve on the lateral side, lumbosacral trunk and obturator nerve at the dorsocaudal aspect and ureter crossing the common iliac bifurcation.[2]

The *presacral lymph nodes* (Fig. 2.9) are found in front of promontorium and underneath aortic bifurcation draining the bilateral common iliac lymph routes. The presacral compartment extends from aortic bifurcation down to the end of second sacral vertebra. Structures at risk during lymph node dissection are median sacral artery and presacral venous plexus as well as thin-walled common iliac veins, in particular the left one due its exposed course running above promontorium. Moreover, the promontorium region is crossed slightly left by superior hypogastric plexus giving off hypogastric nerves on both sides.[18]

The *parametrial* and *mesometrial lymph nodes* are located next to uterus underneath the broad ligament (parametrium) and intercalated into uterine mesentery (mesometrium) (Fig. 2.9). They are embedded in areolar fibrofatty tissue and follow the branches of uterine artery (vascular mesometrium).[10] Subsequently, ureter is at risk during mesometrial lymph node dissection.

The *para-aortic lymph nodes* are grouped into a readily discernible ventral chain including interaortocaval lymph nodes and less obvious dorsolateral chains. Thus, complete para-aortic lymph node removal requires full exposure of both pericaval and periaortal tissue compartments. However, dissection should be carried out carefully avoiding a too rigorous "cleaning" of large prevertebral vessels to preserve or at least minimize damage of the periaortic autonomic nervous network.[17]

According to the location related to inferior mesenteric artery, para-aortic lymph nodes are subdivided into inframesenteric and supramesenteric lymph nodes. The *inframesenteric lymph nodes* (Fig. 2.9) extend from the origin of inferior mesenteric artery along aorta and inferior vena cava down to aortic and caval bifurcation. The lateral borders of this compartment are defined by ureters running in front of psoas muscles and undercrossing ovarian vessels. The *supramesenteric lymph nodes* are located superior to inferior mesenteric artery and inferior to left renal vein. Like in the inframesenteric compartment, supramesenteric lymph nodes are grouped around and between large vessels. Additionally, lymph nodes from renal hilus drain into this compartment and autonomic nerve fibers derived from aortic nerve plexus diverge to both sides to form renal nerve plexus following the corresponding blood vessels.[17]

REFERENCES

1. Fritsch H, Lienenmann A, Brenner E, et al. Clinical anatomy of the pelvic floor. Adv Anat Embryol Cell Biol. 2004;175:III-X, 1-64.
2. Donnez J. Atlas of Operative Laparoscopy and Hysteroscopy. 3rd edition. Milton Park Abingdon: Informa Healthcare; 2007.
3. Standring S (Ed). Gray's Anatomy: The Anatomical Basis of Clinical Practice. 40th edition. New York: Churchill Livingstone/Elsevier; 2008.
4. Ashton-Miller JA, DeLancey JO. Functional anatomy of the female pelvic floor. Ann NY Acad Sci. 2007;1101:266-96.
5. Schollmeyer T, et al. Practical Manual for Laparoscopic and Hysteroscopic Gynecological Surgery.

2nd edition. New Delhi: Jaypee Brothers Medical Publishers (P) Ltd; 2013.

6. Ramanah R, Berger MB, Parratte BM, et al. Anatomy and histology of apical support: a literature review concerning cardinal and uterosacral ligaments. Int Urogynecol J. 2012;23(11):1483-94.
7. Samaan, A, Vu D, Haylen BT, et al. Cardinal ligament surgical anatomy: cardinal points at hysterectomy. Int Urogynecol J. 2014;25(2):189-95.
8. Touboul C, Fauconnier A, Zareski E, et al. The lateral infraureteral parametrium: myth or reality? Am J Obstet Gynecol. 2008;199(3):242.e1-6.
9. Yabuki Y, Sasaki H, Hatakeyama N, et al. Discrepancies between classic anatomy and modern gynecologic surgery on pelvic connective tissue structure: harmonization of those concepts by collaborative cadaver dissection. Am J Obstet Gynecol. 2005; 193(1):7-15.
10. Hockel M, Horn LC, Manthey N, et al. Resection of the embryologically defined uterovaginal (Mullerian) compartment and pelvic control in patients with cervical cancer: a prospective analysis. Lancet Oncol. 2009;10(7):683-92.
11. Höckel M, Horn LC, Tetsch E, et al. Pattern analysis of regional spread and therapeutic lymph node dissection in cervical cancer based on ontogenetic anatomy. Gynecol Oncol. 2012;125(1):168-74.
12. Frober R. Surgical anatomy of the ureter. BJU Int. 2007;100(4):949-65.
13. Schünke M, Schulte E, Schumacher U. Prometheus Atlas of Anatomy. Vol. 2. Stuttgart: Thieme; 2015.
14. Mauroy B, Demondion X, Bizet B, et al. The female inferior hypogastric (= pelvic) plexus: anatomical and radiological description of the plexus and its afferences—applications to pelvic surgery. Surg Radiol Anat. 2007;29(1):55-66.
15. Raspagliesi F, Ditto A, Fontanelli R, et al. Nerve-sparing radical hysterectomy: a surgical technique for preserving the autonomic hypogastric nerve. Gynecol Oncol. 2004;93(2):307-14.
16. Runkel N, Reiser H. Nerve-oriented mesorectal excision (nome): autonomic nerves as landmarks for laparoscopic rectal resection. Int J Colorectal Dis. 2013;28(10):1367-75.
17. Cibula D, Abu-Rustum NR. Pelvic lymphadenectomy in cervical cancer-surgical anatomy and proposal for a new classification system. Gynecol Oncol. 2010;116(1):33-7.
18. Kimmig R, Wimberger P, Buderath P, et al. Definition of compartment-based radical surgery in uterine cancer: radical hysterectomy in cervical cancer as 'total mesometrial resection (TMMR)' by M Höckel translated to robotic surgery (rTMMR). World J Surg Oncol. 2013;11:211.

KIEL SCHOOL

3 of Gynaecological Endoscopy

Instruments & Equipment
for Laparoscopic Surgery

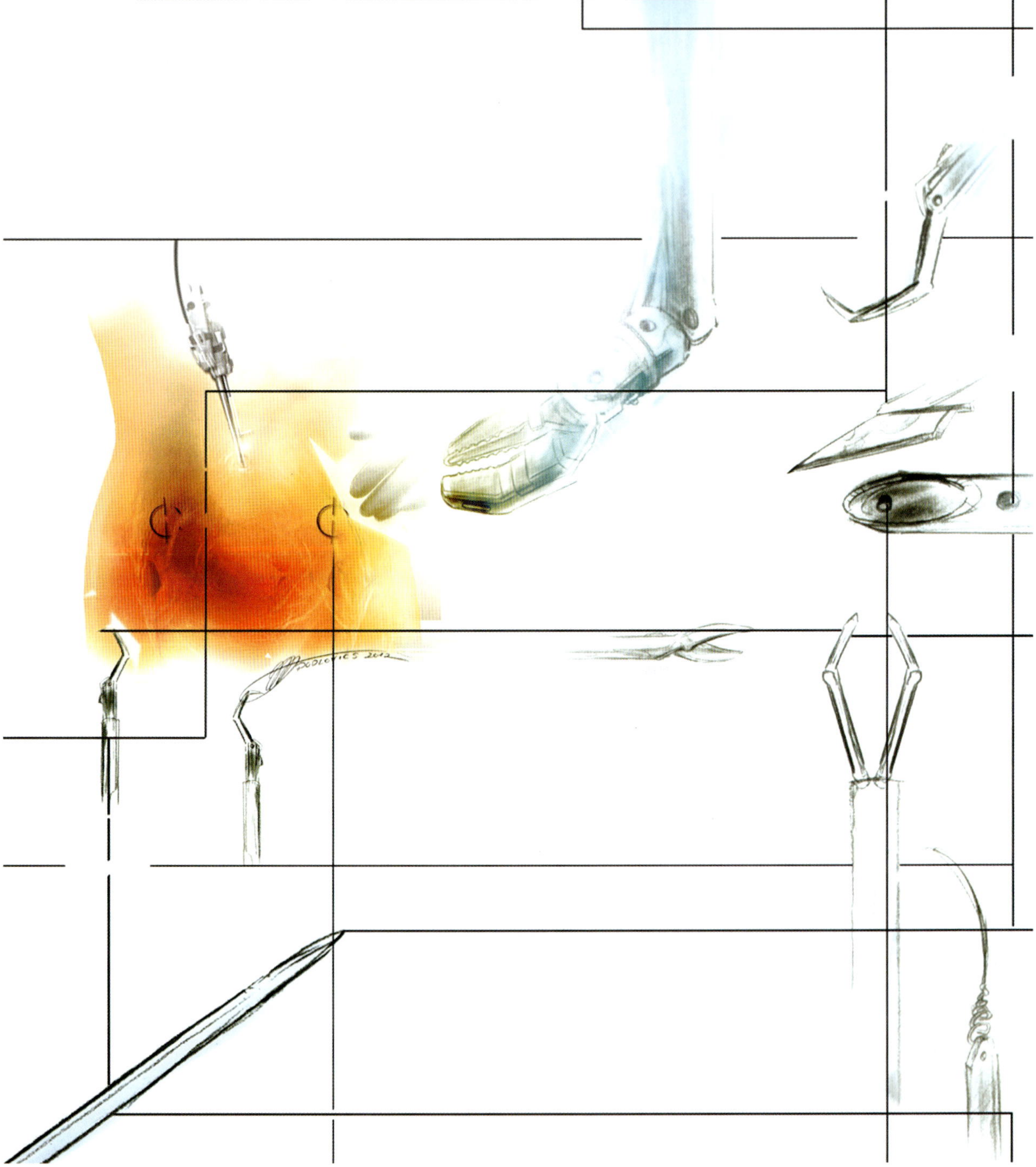

Chapter 3

Instruments and Equipment for Laparoscopic Surgery: Apparatus and Optic Holders

Liselotte Mettler

INTRODUCTION

In the early years of gynecological endoscopy there were only five to ten industrial companies worldwide producing instruments and equipment for laparoscopic surgery. Today, there are over 200 companies offering equipment for laparoscopic surgery. In this chapter, we report on the products of some reliable industrial partners whose products we use or are known to us without any claim to the completeness of the content.

All essential equipment for gynecological and general laparoscopic surgery is assembled on an equipment trolley (Fig. 3.1). For efficient endoscopic work, it is necessary to ensure that the surgeon can check the equipment and settings at a glance. Newer, improved, user-friendly developments are the touch-sensitive panels that are directly operated by the surgeon and the voice-controlled units. Industry is continually developing new technologies to meet surgical requirements.

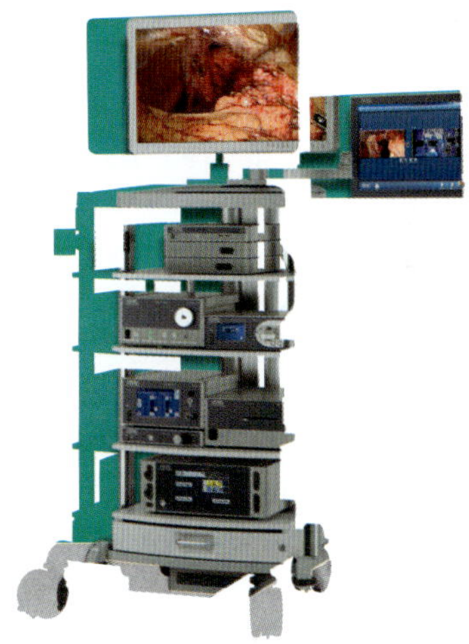

Fig. 3.1: SMARTCART: Equipment cart for gynecologic endoscopic surgery (laparoscopy and hysteroscopy) with electrosurgical unit, CO_2 pneuautomatic with heated gas, light source and HDTV monitor (Karl Storz 3D System) as well as control unit for hysteroscopic surgery (Karl Storz).

The first voice-controlled camera-holding arm, automated endoscopic system for optimal positioning (AESOP),[1] has long been replaced by smaller voice-controlled compact motorized endoscope holders, such as the ViKY® EP Endo Control System (EndoControl, Inc, Dover, USA). More complex robot systems have gained ground mainly in oncologic surgery. The da Vinci system of Intuitive Surgical, Inc. (Sunnyvale, CA, USA) has undergone a remarkable development during the last 10 years enabling a surgeon sitting at a console, a few feet from the patient, to perform delicate and complex operations through a few tiny incisions with increased vision, precision, dexterity and control. The da Vinci Surgical System consists of several key components, including an ergonomically designed console where the surgeon sits while operating, a patient-side cart where the patient lays during surgery, four interactive robotic arms, a high-definition (HD) three-dimensional (3D) vision system and proprietary EndoWrist® instruments. The robot does not substitute the surgeon but robotic-assisted surgery is seen as a possible method of overcoming the technical challenges of conventional laparoscopy. Another telesurgical system is the Telelap ALF-X (Sofar S.p.A., Milan, Italy).

Routine endoscopy trolleys with the units of the late twentieth century have been replaced by "Pan OR endoscopy settings", such as the OR1™ FUSION (Karl Storz GmbH & Co. KG, Tuttlingen, Germany)

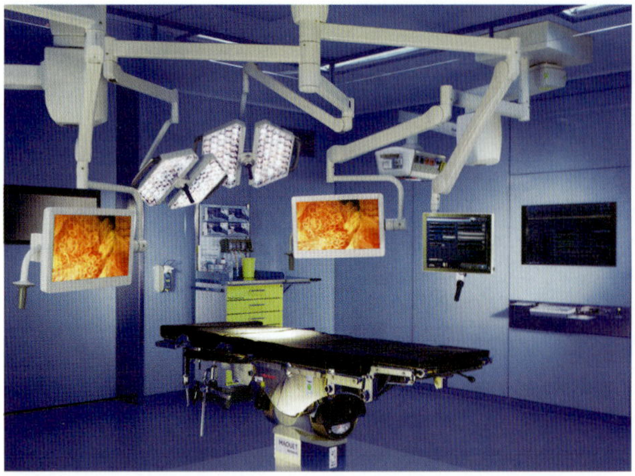

Fig. 3.2: OR1™ NEO (Karl Storz) with panoramic viewing possibilities, integrated commanding functions for all operative procedures and documentation.

(Fig. 3.2). The newly designed KARL STORZ OR1 FUSION® allows all surgical and technical functions to be controlled and monitored from the user interface within the sterile area. The system is able to control KARL STORZ as well as third-party medical devices like surgical tables, endoscopy light sources, insufflators, high-frequency (HF) units, etc., which can be installed either on a trolley or on a boom arm. Moreover, from the same touchscreen it is possible to control advanced features like video communication to external locations, video capture, access to hospital services or video routing.

With video routing the capability to flexibly define is intended where a particular video source (e.g., a surgical microscope) has to be displayed (e.g., on the primary surgical display). KARL STORZ OR1 FUSION® relies on an innovative approach to fulfill this task, as it encodes the video sources in delay and lossless video streams that are distributed on an IP network, instead of directly wiring all sources and destinations. This give the great advantage to be able to route any kind of video (SD, HD, 3D, 4K, ...) of the same infrastructure, thus avoiding cost-intensive upgrade as new technologies hit the market.

The newly designed OR1™ NEO allows all surgical and technical functions to be controlled and monitored from the user interface within the sterile area. The trolley includes all necessary apparatuses to be selected and controlled by the surgeon: endoscopic camera, light sources, insufflators, suction and irrigation pumps, electrical energy systems, AIDA compact NEO documentation systems and OR1™ AV system NEO solutions. AIDA compact NEO uses the highest digital resolution specified for HD of 1920 × 1080 pixels, equal to five times the image information available from today's PAL standard. A new, nearly 3D panoramic view monitor combines the depth of focus with enhanced color brilliance for improved ergonomic viewing. These systems are compatible with third party devices, such as OR lights, energy units (e.g., Erbotom), lasers and modern thermofusion systems.

Other PAN-OR systems are the ENDOALPHA or Visera-Elite of Olympus with the Endo Eye, a fascinating camera system with the camera at the tip of the scope without heat production and the STRIKER unit with the digital documentation system SDC Ultra.

The idea of warming and humidifying the CO_2 gas to avoid damage to the peritoneum has been propagated by Douglas Ott and Philippe Koninckx. The HumiGard™ of Fisher & Paykel Healthcare (Auckland, New Zealand) provides heated, humidified and filtered gas to a patient at a predetermined temperature.

Today every CO_2 pneuautomatic provides up to 37°C heated CO_2 gas, which is controlled by a pressure regulator and within the machine by applying the Quadro-test. In the Quadro-test (*see* chapter "Abdominal Access," Fig. 3.9), the volume of gas flowing through the Veress needle during insufflation, intra-abdominal pressure, total volume and preset filling pressure are measured. Cold light is provided by xenon lamps. The video camera systems are equipped with three-chip camera or HD cameras and can be used for laparoscopy as well as hysteroscopy.

High-resolution video monitors guarantee optimal picture quality. Technological development allows the use of larger monitors in HD quality that facilitate a relaxed working atmosphere for the surgeon.

A realistic, true-to-life 3D picture is possible, because of various technological elements, such as, digital simulation, a second camera system or the use of shutter lens. Digital devices for the video camera control the picture quality and facilitate automatic white balancing. The Karl Storz company already offers the new 3D system that allows real 3D vision by only wearing light sunglasses. The ENDOCAMELEON® laparoscope provides a viewing angle that can be adjusted continuously between 0° and 120° (Fig. 3.3).

Various techniques permit safe cutting as well as coagulation. The earlier thermocoagulator entirely avoided the flux of current through the target tissue and made hemostasis safe by heating it up to

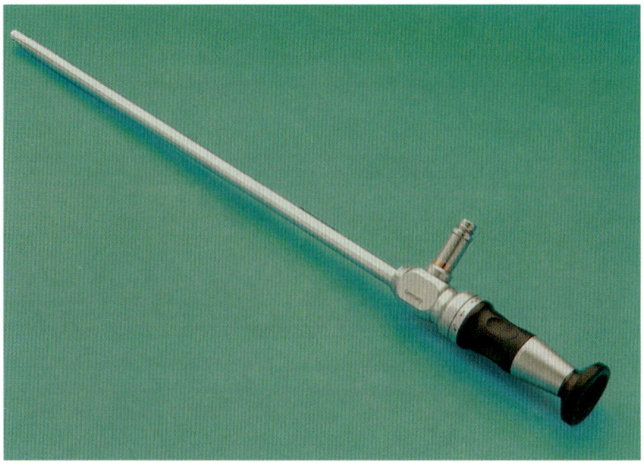

Fig. 3.3: ENDOCAMELEON® laparoscope (Karl Storz).

100–120°C.[2] Today, modern electronic HF systems with monopolar and bipolar currents are widely used. The equipment for other techniques, such as the argon beamer, laser and ultrasonic cutting equipment, is put on an ancillary trolley. Efficient suction irrigation apparatuses remove body fluids as well as abdominal lavage with a warm irrigation solution and are standard equipment for laparoscopy as well as laparotomy.

The universal perturbation apparatus is used for the CO_2 insufflation of the fallopian tubes in gynecology. A cervical adapter can be simultaneously inserted for intraoperative manipulation as well as for hydro and chromopertubation. The hysteroflater facilitates gas or fluid hysteroscopy with control of both inflow and outflow.

Video recorder, photo printers and especially equipped computers are used for documentation. The combination of highly modern charged-coupled device (CCD) cameras and HD cameras with electronic picture capture and document the surgical procedures.

Depending on habit and use, the majority of the equipment is placed either near the head or foot end of the patient vis-a-vis the surgeon. The use of a flexible instrument rack extending from the drapes, which can likewise hold the monitors, is very practical. A voice-controlled camera holder facilitates a fatigue-free positioning of the camera and thus offers a safe working condition.

INSTRUMENTS (BASIC EQUIPMENT)

Until 1960 palpation probes were the only endoscopic instruments available. From 1960 to 1970 the diagnosis and treatment of female infertility and later tubal sterilization were the only procedures performed by gynecological laparoscopy. Therefore, atraumatic forceps and scissors for transection of tubes were the first instruments to be developed for laparoscopy.

From 1970 onward, the demand for thermal coagulation began. Electrical units were not able to catch aberrant electric currency as is possible today. In 2012 all electrosurgical units, once the different and indifferent electrodes have been correctly applied, recapture aberrant electricity.

Cave: *There has to be a complete coverage of the skin by the indifferent electrode.*

Of the multitude of laparoscopic instruments known today, we describe here only a selected few, which are absolutely necessary for gynecological operative laparoscopy and which should be available in duplicate or triplicate on the instrument trolley. Multiple use instruments for cutting, grasping, dissection, pushing, traction, coagulation, irrigation and suction are very helpful.

INSTRUMENTS FOR PERFORATION

- The Veress needle[3] is blindly introduced into the abdomen after lifting the anterior abdomen wall. Trocars of 3, 7, 10, 12, 15, 20 and 24 mm diameter are used for guiding the endoscopes and operative instruments, irrigation, coagulation and during employment of needle holders and morcellators.
- The simple automatic flap valves can leak because of soiling with blood or tissue particles. Therefore they are to be used for single use only. Trumpet valves are stable, but must be always opened and closed. They hinder the introduction of needles and thread.
- Endoscopic lenses must be frequently washed and removed because of soiling during the operation. Therefore, for such trocars we reluctantly use automatic valve, but prefer trumpet valve.
- Primary trocars can be inserted by the Z-puncture technique to prevent dehiscence of aponeurosis and late prolapse of the omentum. The decision, however, depends on the surgeon. We recommend the conical trocars, but are aware that the pyramidal trocars, especially in the so-called safety trocars, are employed as optical trocars. They carry the advantage of a sharp cutting edge (Fig. 3.4).
- Optiview® by Ethicon (Ethicon Endo-Surgery, Cincinnati, USA), Visiport® by Covidien (Mansfield,

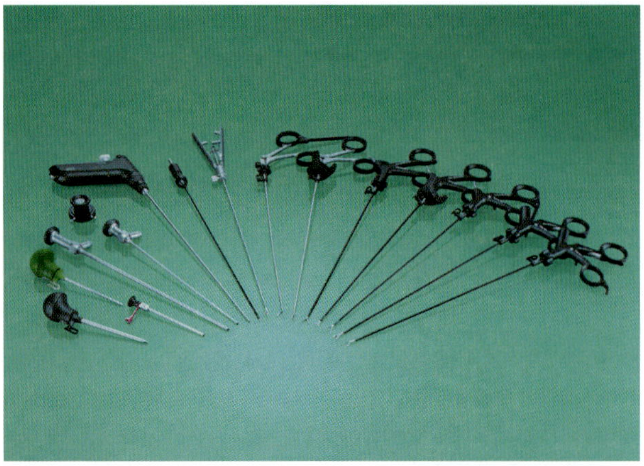

Fig. 3.4: Optics, trocars, needle holder and RoBi® instruments—rotating bipolar grasping forceps and scissors (Karl Storz).

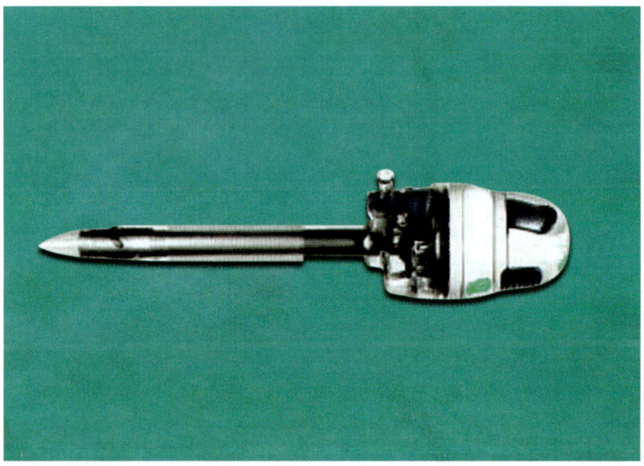

Fig. 3.5: XCEL, a disposable, viewing trocar for *laparoscopic* entry under sight (Ethicon).

MA, USA) and XCEL by Ethicon (Fig. 3.5) offer insertion under vision. At present, only 10–11 mm trocars are available through which the 10 mm laparoscope can be passed under direct vision.

- Optical Veress needles can be inserted under vision. The insertion under vision can be done below left costal margin also; a suitable trocar can be inserted through the umbilicus under vision.
- The linear expansion trocars help controlled widening of a narrow canal by serial dilatation (*see* chapter "Abdominal Access," Fig. 3.19).
- The Endo-Tip is described in the chapter "Abdominal Access" (Figs. 3.1 to 3.4).

DILATATION INSTRUMENTS

It is possible to dilate up to 10, 12, 15 and 20 mm through an introduced rod and a suitable 5 mm threaded trocar (Figs. 3.6A to C).

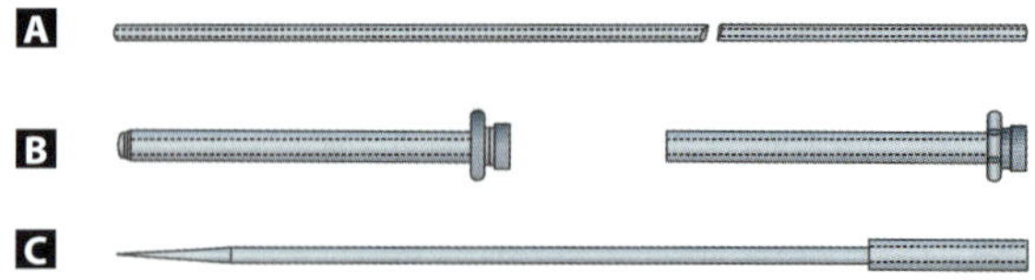

Figs. 3.6A to C: Dilatation instruments. (A) Central introduction rod; (B) Dilators; (C) Mandrin, when the dilator is introduced as trocar.

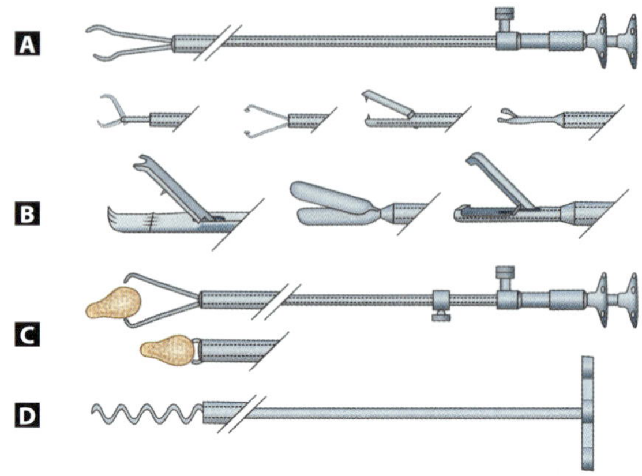

Figs. 3.7A to D: Holding, grasping and drilling instruments: (A) Atraumatic forceps; (B) Various tips of forceps (left to right): two intestinal forceps, lymph node holding forceps, two biopsy forceps, spoon forceps and toothed forceps; (C) Swab holder, before holding and with the swab; (D) Myoma screw.

HOLDING AND GRASPING INSTRUMENTS AND SCREWS

Various types of traumatic and atraumatic forceps are used as endoscopic grasping tools for operations (Figs. 3.7A to D). They are in 5–20 mm in size. In 10 mm size we recommend the big-toothed forceps and lymph node holding forceps to hold the tissues firmly. The 10 mm swab holding forceps are suitable for holding tissues lightly and for pushing. The 5 and 10 mm swab holders are used in tissue dissection. The 5 and 10 mm myoma screw is used for traction on the myoma. The handles shown in Figures 3.7A to D are round-grip handles; however, the handles of the Robi instruments of the Karl Storz company are easier and more ergonomic to use (*see* Fig. 3.4).

CUTTING INSTRUMENTS

Curved scissors (5 mm) and saw-toothed scissors (5 and 11 mm) as well as different microknives with changeable disposable blades are available as doubled-edged models (Figs. 3.8A to C). Mostly, curved scissors are used, but round scissors with electric connection are frequently employed because of their extreme safety. The latter one is often used as a

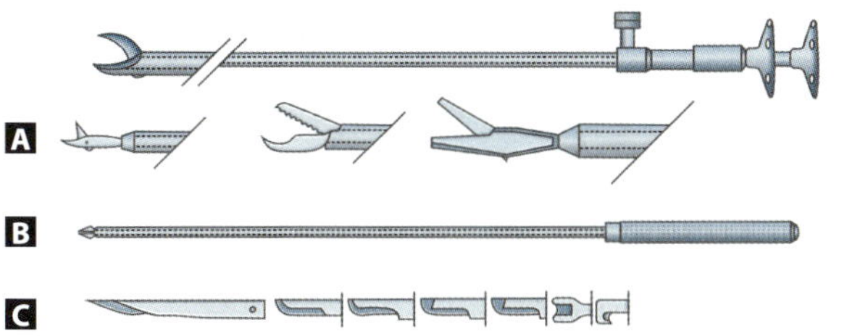

Figs. 3.8A to C: Cutting instruments. (A) Dissection scissors with round handle, as macro- and microscissors (with 2 mm span); (B) scalpel; (C) Changeable cutting blades (single use) of the scalpel.

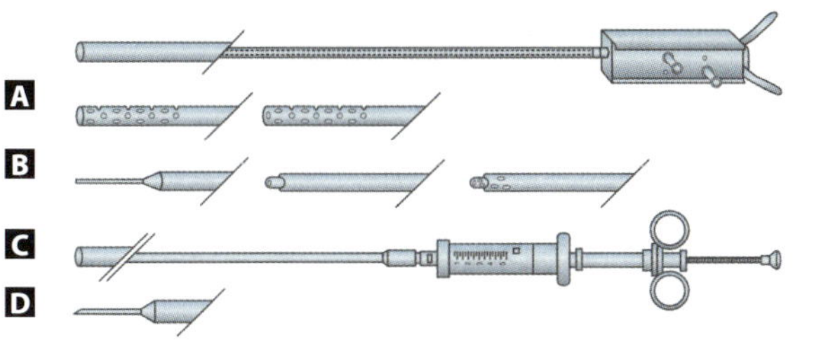

Figs. 3.9A to D: Suction and irrigation instruments. (A) 5 mm suction irrigation cannula with open end; (B) 5 mm suction irrigation cannula with perforated end; (C) Aspiration cannula for cysts; (D) Manual aspiration system for Douglas exudates.

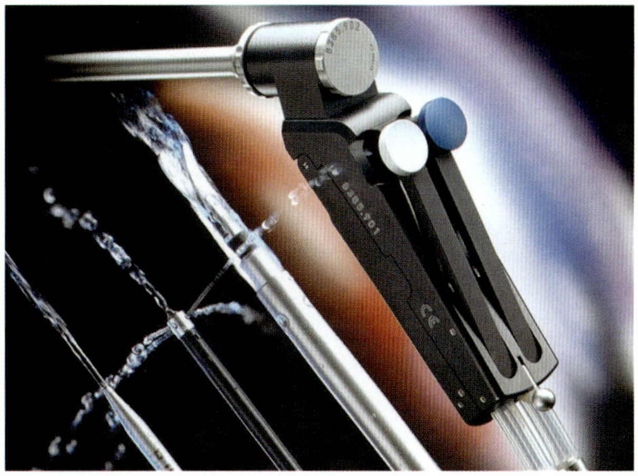

Fig. 3.10: Suction irrigation system (R. Wolf, Knittlingen, Germany).

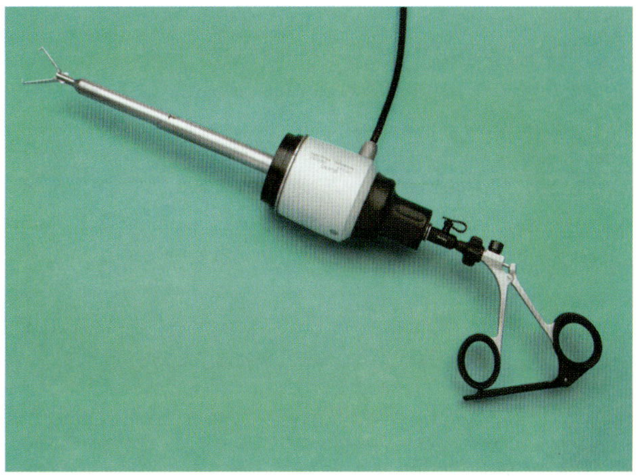

Fig. 3.11: ROTOCUT GI (Karl Storz), morcellation tool with protective shield, available in two sizes (12 and 15 mm).

disposable instrument. Blunt-round scissors are especially suitable for retroperitoneal dissection.

SUCTION AND IRRIGATION INSTRUMENTS

The suction irrigation devices of Karl Storz and Wisap GmbH (Sauerlach, Germany) are well known. The system of Wisap has 5 and 10 mm suction and irrigation tubes (Figs. 3.9A to D). The suction cannula is used either with an open tip or with a perforated tip. Large volumes of fluids in ovarian tumors and ascites are aspirated with these suction irrigation cannula (Fig. 3.10). It is set at an irrigation pressure of up to 300 mm Hg and an aspiration force of up to 1 bar. The normal suction force is maximum 800 mbar; irrigation pressure is 300 mm Hg. With extra-long (50 cm) suction irrigation tubes, it is possible to suck even under the dome of diaphragm from the pelvic region. Many disposable systems are also available.

MORCELLATION INSTRUMENTS

The development of morcellation instruments was slow. In ovarian resection and enucleation of myoma, the tissue was cut with scissors and knives, depending on the size. The specimen can be removed either with big-toothed forceps or a big sponge holding forceps directly through the 11 or 15 mm trocar with conical end. However, the so-called motor drive morcellators in 10, 15 and 20 mm diameters are electrically powered and function well. The tissue is slowly cut electrically, nearly shaved from the surface and pulled into the trocar sleeve. It is particularly suitable for horizontal operations as in vertical use a laceration of bowel or vessels can easily occur. Karl Storz produces the Steiner morcellator®, the Rotocut and a new development, the Sawalhe II Supercut morcellator, all with a tissue protection shield (Figs. 3.11 and 3.12).

Many companies have disposable morcellators. The WISAP electric morcellator was the first on the international market. Alternatively, the surgical specimen from the abdominal cavity is put in an endobag (small plastic bags) with forceps. Morcellation is only advised at present for benign specimens. However, I foresee the transformation of fibroid-like material into powder, which can then be aspirated and examined by the molecular pathologist for malignancy.

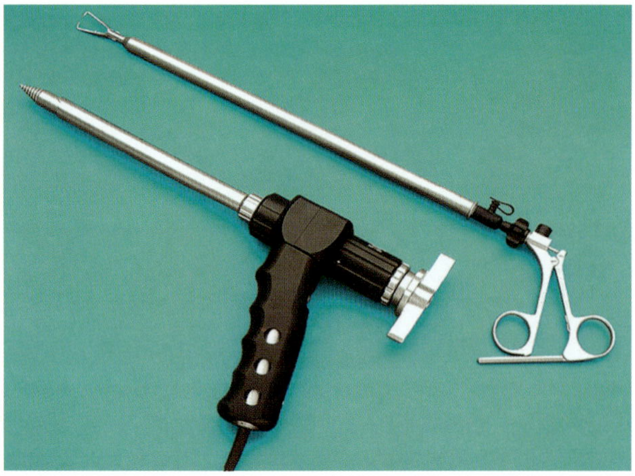

Fig. 3.12: SAWALHE II SUPERCUT Morcellator (Karl Storz).

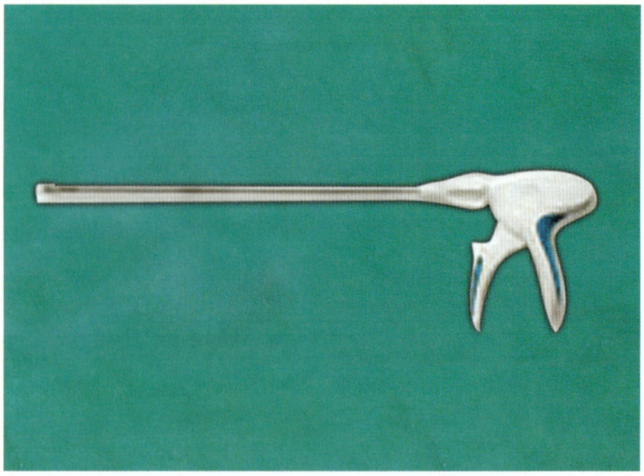

Fig. 3.14: Endo GIA™ Ultra Universal Stapler (Covidien).

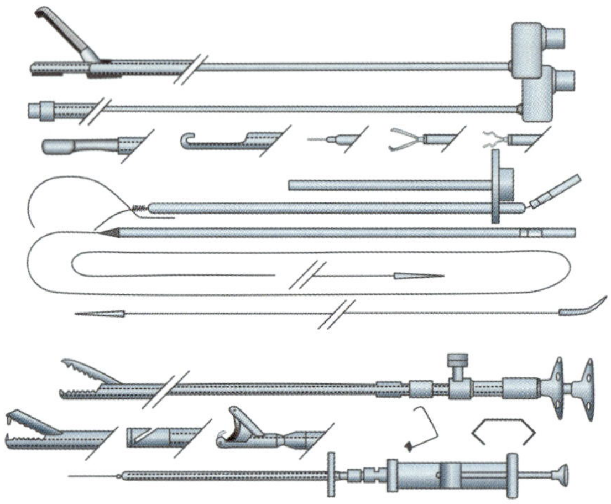

Fig. 3.13: Instruments for hemostasis.

INSTRUMENTS FOR HEMOSTASIS

Instruments for tying the blood vessels, such as the Roeder loop, the endoligature or the endosutures with extra- or intracorporeal knotting are widely known (Fig. 3.13). Needle holders for straight, curved or Ski needles must be available in different variations. Further details are given in a separate chapter on sutures in this manual.

For hemostasis, endocoagulation,[4] heat denaturation at 100–120°C, bipolar coagulation in various forms (*see* section on energy sources in this chapter) and monopolar needle, melting hook, HF scissors or other instruments are suitable. The gentlest methods are endocoagulation at 100°C and bipolar coagulation. For localized ischemia a vasopressin derivative in a dilution of 1:100 is injected subcapsular with an applicator. The hemostasis ischemia set shown in Figure 3.13 may be used or alternatively the Veress needle can be inserted in a separate abdominal incision to inject the vasopressin dilution.

Gynecologists prefer suturing and coagulation devices. However, clips and stapling devices, which are more frequently used by general surgeons, are also used for fixing meshes, for pelvic floor surgery, lymphadenectomy and hysterectomy in our field. Both Ethicon, a Johnson & Johnson company (New Brunswick, NJ, USA) and Covidien have fascinating devices on the market. Let me just mention here Covidien's new Endo Clip Applicator III (5 mm) with easy to be situated clips and a digital clip counter (Fig. 3.14) and the Endo GIA™ Stapler (Figs. 3.15 and 3.16).

INSTRUMENTS FOR CLAMPING LARGE VESSELS: EMERGENCY NEEDLE

Emergency instruments and usual clamps used in routine gynecological operations should not be used for clamping the vessels. Vascular clamps must be readily available (Figs. 3.17A and B). Large-vessel injury must be immediately explored by laparotomy and the bleeding vessel clamped. If a vessel in the anterior abdominal wall is injured (epigastric artery), it is advisable to ligate it at an appropriate place with a large emergency needle.

INSTRUMENTS FOR DRAINAGE

The Robinson drainage is suitable (Fig. 3.18) for abdominal drainage. It works on a gravity basis and as a rule can be left in situ over 24 h. The blind insertion of the secondary trocar is obsolete. Nowadays, the insertion is carried out under vision after making a subumbilical longitudinal skin incision with the knife held parallel to the abdominal wall.

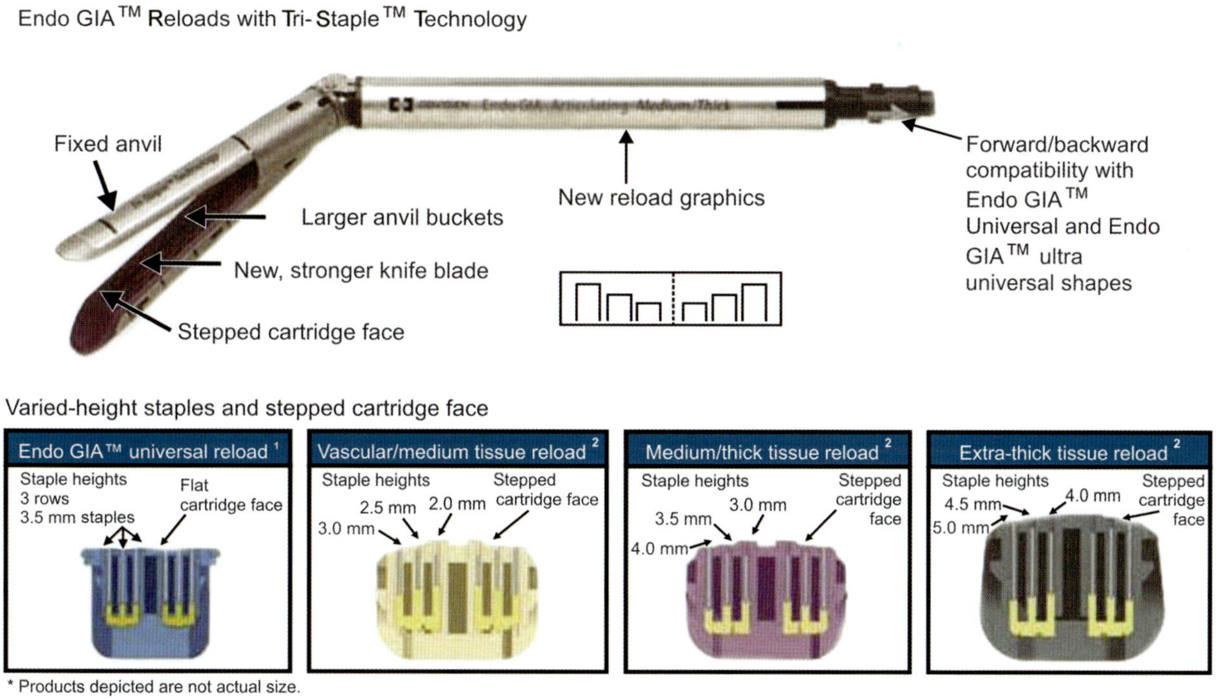

Fig. 3.15: Endo GIA™ reloads with Tri-Staple™ Technology (Covidien).

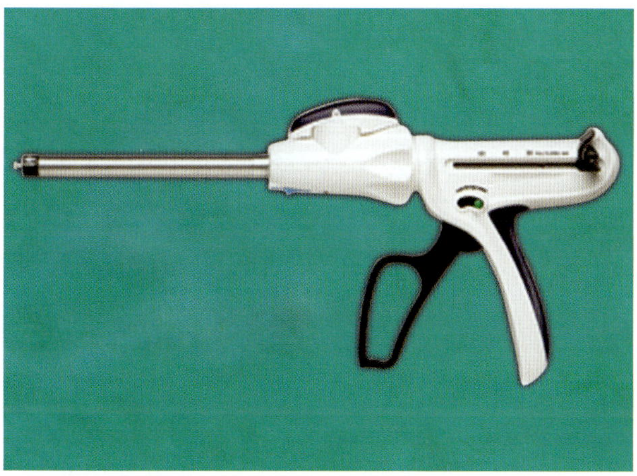

Fig. 3.16: Endo GIA™ Ultra Universal Stapler (Covidien).

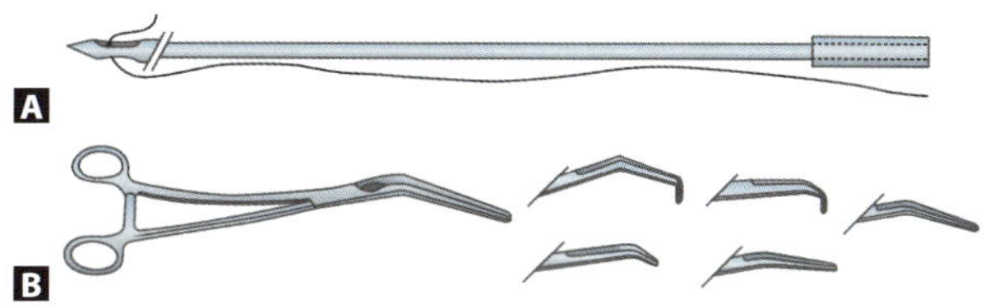

Figs. 3.17A and B: Vascular clamps. (A) Emergency needle; (B) Vascular clamps with different tips.

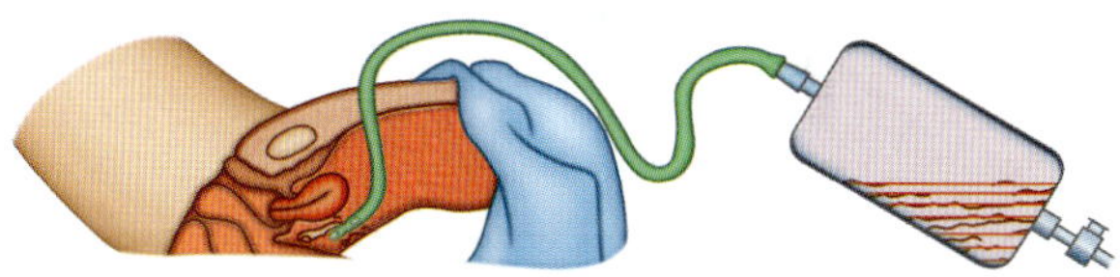

Fig. 3.18: Robinson drainage. The perforated end of the cannula is introduced with a 5 mm trocar and placed in the deepest part of the abdominal cavity. The drainage bottle is fixed to the patient's thigh and collects the drained fluids.

CAVE: *Fatalities have been reported by accidental slitting of the aorta.*

Before insertion of the Veress needle, which is always blind, it is advisable to follow the safety measures described in the chapter on abdominal access in this book.

INSTRUMENTS FOR UTERINE MANIPULATION

Vacuum intracervical probes in the standard three sizes allow only partial movement of the uterus and facilitate tubal chromopertubation.

Various instruments for intrauterine manipulation make it possible to move the uterus in side-to-side, ante and retroflexion as well as rotation movements and sometimes allow the possibility of chromopertubation. Uterine manipulation is required in endometriosis of the pouch of Douglas, for hysterectomies, in bladder dome endometriosis and for enucleation of myoma. The abdominal cavity expander (ACE) serves to elevate the anterior abdominal wall in cases with adhesions. Further versions of this principle are used in the gasless laparoscopy (e.g. as Laparolift®).

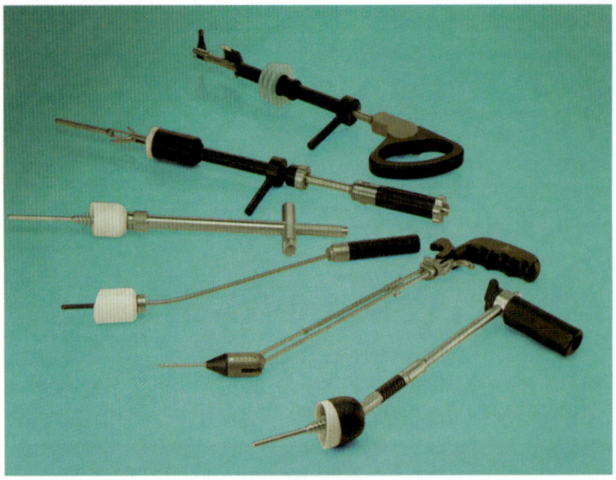

Fig. 3.19: Intrauterine manipulators produced by Karl Storz according to Koninckx, Clermont–Ferrand, Mangeshikar, Hohl, Donnez and Tintara.

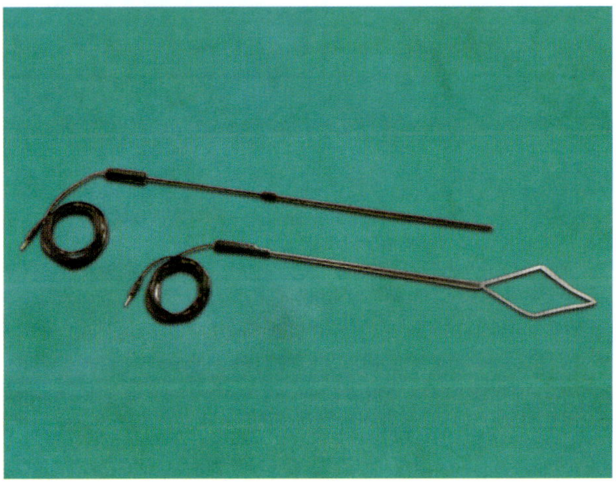

Fig. 3.20: LiNA loop (LiNA Medical).

The Hohl, the Mangeshikar and the Donnez intrauterine manipulators or mobilizers as well as the Konincxk uterine twister are all produced by Karl Storz and have a cup with a well palpable and visible border to visualize the resection level between vagina and cervix for all cases of total laparoscopic hysterectomy (TLH) (Fig. 3.19). This facilitates the intracervical approach of TLH; however, they are not to be used for the extracervical approach and in oncologic cases of hysterectomy. Many companies have disposable manipulators.

Subtotal hysterectomy, such as classic intrafascial supracervical hysterectomy (CISH) or laparoscopic-assisted supracervical hysterectomy (LASH), is facilitated by the use of an electric loop produced by LiNA Medical ApS, Glostrup, Denmark (Fig. 3.20) as the LiNA Loop and by Karl Storz as the Storz Loop (Fig. 3.21).

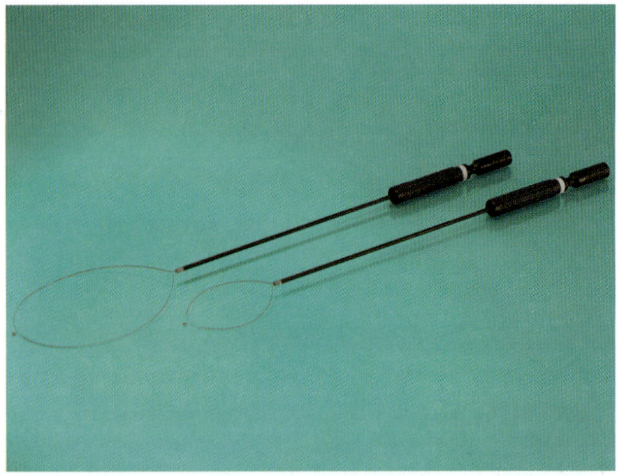

Fig. 3.21: LiNA loop at subtotal hysterectomy.

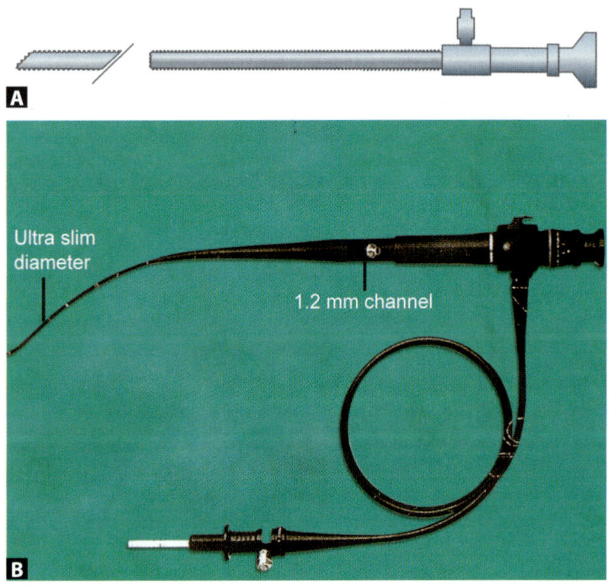

Figs. 3.22A and B: Endoscopes. (A) Rigid standard laparoscope (10 mm) with 30° optic and with 0° optic; (B) Flexible endoscope.

LENSES AND ENDOSCOPES

Scopes are available in rigid and flexible systems (Figs. 3.22A and B). The rigid system is based on Hopkins's experience with a rod lens system, which results in good resolution and depth of focus ratio.[5] Flexible endoscopes are based on the use of optical fiber bundles. The rigid laparoscopes are available in 3–11 mm sizes, e.g., the arthroscope with a 14° angle. Most of the rigid endoscopes are directly connected to the telescope through the camera coupling system. The picture is enlarged so that it looks even bigger on the monitor. In flexible endoscopes, the bundle of fibers is also enlarged. The standard laparoscopes are rigid instruments with a 0° lens. The 30° lens has the

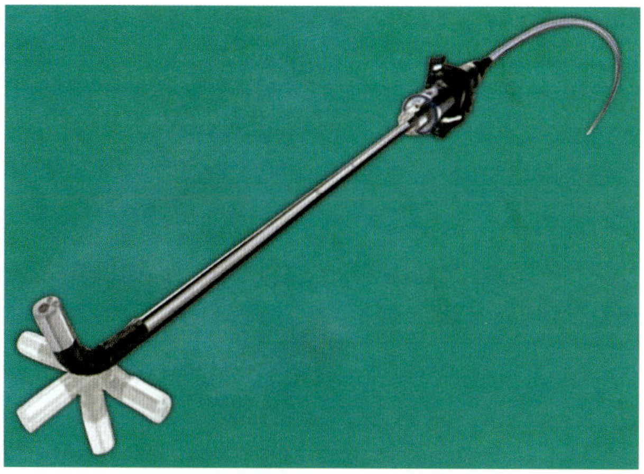

Fig. 3.23: EndoEYE video laparoscope (Olympus).

advantage of a wide panoramic view. With the Endo-Cameleon (Karl Storz) a 120° panoramic view is possible (*see* Fig. 3.3).

Each camera has two components: head and control. A 35 mm coupling system yields a much more enlarged picture than a 28 mm coupler. A direct coupling transmits the picture directly to the camera.

Olympus Surgical (Hamburg, Germany) offers different flexible endoscopes as well as rigid endoscopes with flexible tips with four directions and a 100° bendable performance as chip on the tip (Fig. 3.23). With the chip on the tip of the optic the observation light passes through fewer lenses than on a rigid scope. This allows brighter and sharper images than when the camera is attached to the head of the optic.

ENERGY SYSTEMS FOR OPERATIVE LAPAROSCOPY (ELECTROSURGERY AND THERMOFUSION)

Electrosurgery

Ohm's law, $V = I \times R$ (voltage = current × resistance), is described in terms of current, voltage and resistance. Electrosection, i.e., cutting of tissue between the active electrode and the tissue where an electrical arc is generated, takes place above 200°C. During coagulation and desiccation the tissue is heated slowly. It results in denaturation, evaporation of water and secondary hemostasis. The argon beam coagulator is a monopolar electrosurgical instrument. In principle, noncombustible argon gas (4 L/min) across an electrode cannula acts as a bridge for electrical current to burn the tissue superficially (up to 5 mm depth).[6] As the gas is easier to ionize than air, electrical arcs develop up to 1 cm above the tissue surface. In monopolar electrosurgery, high-density current is used at the active electrode that is conducted to the patient on touching. In bipolar electrosurgery, two small electrodes of same size are used, which lie close to each other and function as active passive electrodes.

Thermal techniques, such as ultrasound coagulation, laser as well as clips and suturing techniques can achieve endoscopic hemostasis. While the use of thermal hemostasis goes back to the glowing iron, according to Paquelin, the development of safe HF current techniques took 40 years. The application of the laser technique, ultrasonic cutting and coagulation techniques and the local thermal effects, such as thermocoagulation, take place in the range of 80–120°C. Suturing and clip techniques are handled in the next chapter.

We differentiate between fulguration and coagulation in HF hemostasis. In fulguration, electromagnetic oscillations across an air bridge produce radiofrequency (RF) between the tip of the electrode and the surface of the organ, i.e., they come in direct contact. The generated heat is limited to tissue surface, i.e., the area visible through the scope. By coagulation we mean the heating of the tissues until intracellular water boils under the influence of HF current.

In addition to the technique used for fulguration and for coagulation, the most important technique in medicine and endoscopic surgery is electrotomy, the cutting of tissue with the so-called electrical knife or the electrical loop. The sustained intermittent or unidirectional HF current, which can be produced with tubes or transistor generator, produces smooth-edged cuts. In bipolar HF current there is tissue destruction between the poles or their contact points. In monopolar current, the current surge arising at the tip of the instrument is used for cutting and generating heat for coagulation.

Semm developed various systems to control the energy output during controlled endocoagulation. The control unit of the Endocoagulator (WISAP company) is switched on or off by a pneumatic foot switch, i.e., without electricity. The desired temperature for coagulation can be preset between 90°C and 120°C just like the acoustically signalled coagulation time. The heated metal mass is reduced to a minimum in the three instruments, point coagulator, crocodile forceps and myoma enucleator, so that the instruments cool off immediately after heating. Deep burns are not caused if the intestines are touched accidently because the thermal energy is too low to emit much heat. The coagulation effects in endocoagulation produce extensive cauterization. They are not selectively controllable.

At present even with HF instruments there is no blind and uncontrolled burning because of the electrical system control. Therefore, we use monopolar current for cutting and bipolar instruments when coagulation is required before cutting big vessels in endoscopic surgery. Most of the systems have an autostop, so that only the required tissue is denatured. It is not set for a very big coagulation zone.

Bi-Clamp for vaginal and open surgery and BiCision (Fig. 3.24) for laparoscopic surgery are the thermofusion devices of Erbe Elektromedizin GmbH (Tübingen, Germany). Their effect is electronically controlled thermofusion and the mechanical separation of tissue.

The electrocoagulation system of Erbe (Fig. 3.25) uses an additional argon beamer, controlled by a foot switch, which facilitates linear coagulation by switching on the argon gas. This gynecological workstation with the HF module VIO 300 D can be connected to any monopolar or bipolar coagulation device. It contains several modules, such as the argon plasma coagulation (APC 2) and the smoke plume evacuator (IES 2). The Erbe electrosurgical unit (ESU) has a color monitor display that provides the user with an on-screen tutorial as well as settings and operational information. The unit has various cutting and coagulation modes with defined effect levels to provide the physician flexibility in interventional applications (i.e., its ability to generate HF current). The system has automatic start and stop features. The equipment is programmable and various accessories (e.g., footswitches, hand instruments, etc.) as well as modes may be assigned to perform specific functions. Upon activation, the energy delivered (in watts) from the ESU to the tissue is displayed on the display screen.

The use of heat in microsurgery can be traced back to Hippocrates who used heat to burn a carcinomatous growth in the neck. Heating the tissue above 45°C causes irreparable cellular damage. Tissue denaturation sets in at 45°C and heating above 100°C leads to typical desiccation with hemostasis. Temperatures above 200°C produce carbonization and disintegration.

Bipolar vessel sealing, also described as thermofusion, combined with pressure between the branches of the instruments, is a new, easy-to-use technique that has been picked up by many companies in the production of disposable instruments with integrated cutting devices, such as LigaSure (Covidien) (Figs. 3.26 and 3.27).

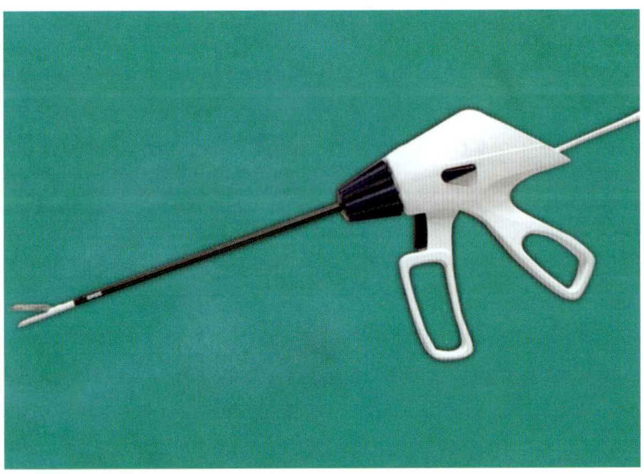

Fig. 3.24: BiCision coagulation and cutting forceps (Erbe).

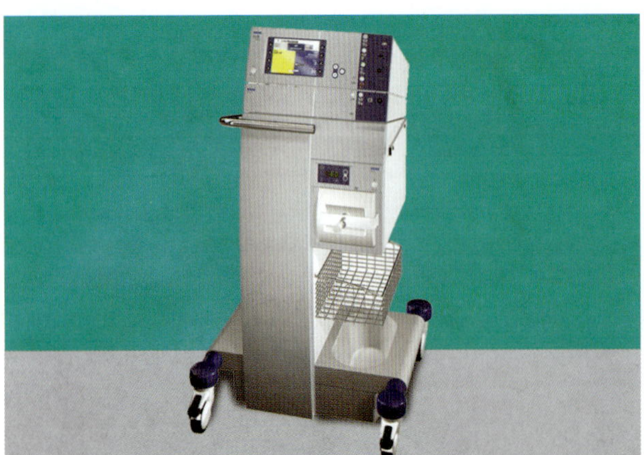

Fig. 3.25: Erbe Gynecological Workstation VIO 300 D.

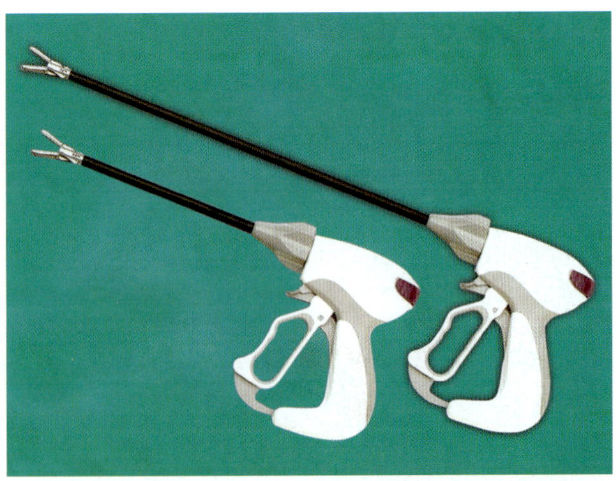

Fig. 3.26: LigaSure (Covidien), bipolar vessel sealing system, 10 mm (Atlas) and 5 mm.

The Nightknife (BOWA-electronic GmbH, Gomaringen, Germany) (Figs. 3.28A and B) is a bipolar vessel sealing device. The instrument incorporates atraumatic tips for secure dissecting and sealing. The integrated cutting system saves changing instruments for tissue separation.

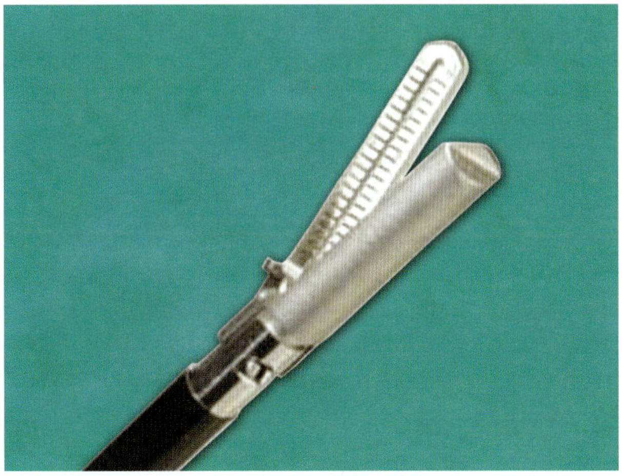

Fig. 3.27: LigaSure (Covidien) jaw providing a combination of pressure and energy to create vessel fusion.

The Gyrus PK (Olympus) technology delivers a proprietary, pulsing ultralow (110 V) and high-current RF energy waveform to create a broad range of tissue effects and allows the tissue and device tip to cool during the "energy off" phase, minimizing sticking and charring (Figs. 3.29A and B).

By means of the smart electrode technology, the ENSEAL sealing instrument (Ethicon Endo-Surgery) permits simultaneous sealing and the possibility of tissue separation, including vessels up to 7 mm (Fig. 3.30). The tip of the instrument has either a 5 mm round tip or a 3 mm slightly curved tip enabling tissue preparation and sealing.

LASER

Laser beam is often described as "light that heals." Laser is acronym for light amplification by stimulated emission of radiation. Fox established the first surgical laser in 1960. Bruhat and his colleagues in 1979 and Tadir and colleagues in 1996 introduced CO_2 laser in laparoscopy. Today, there are enthusiasts

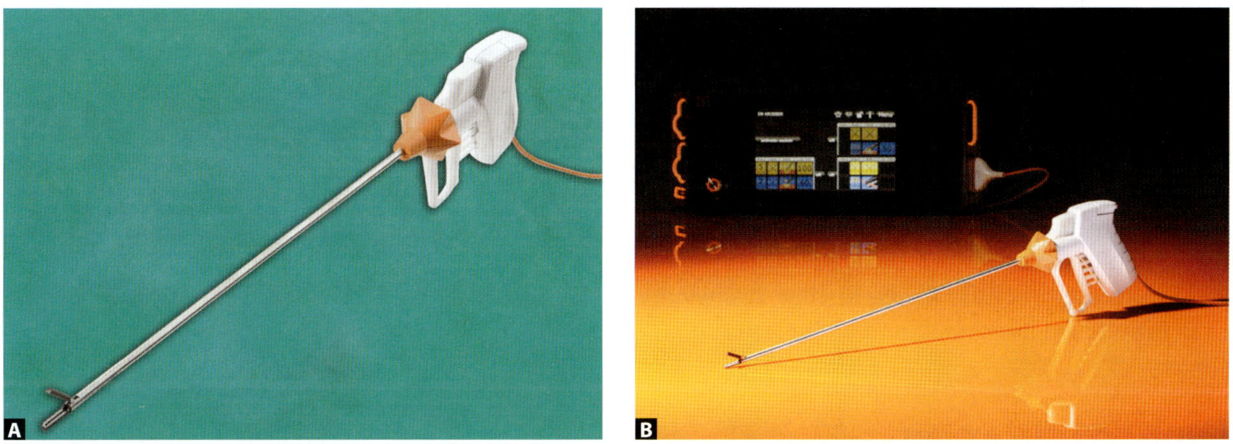

Figs. 3.28A and B: Nightknife (BOWA-electronic).

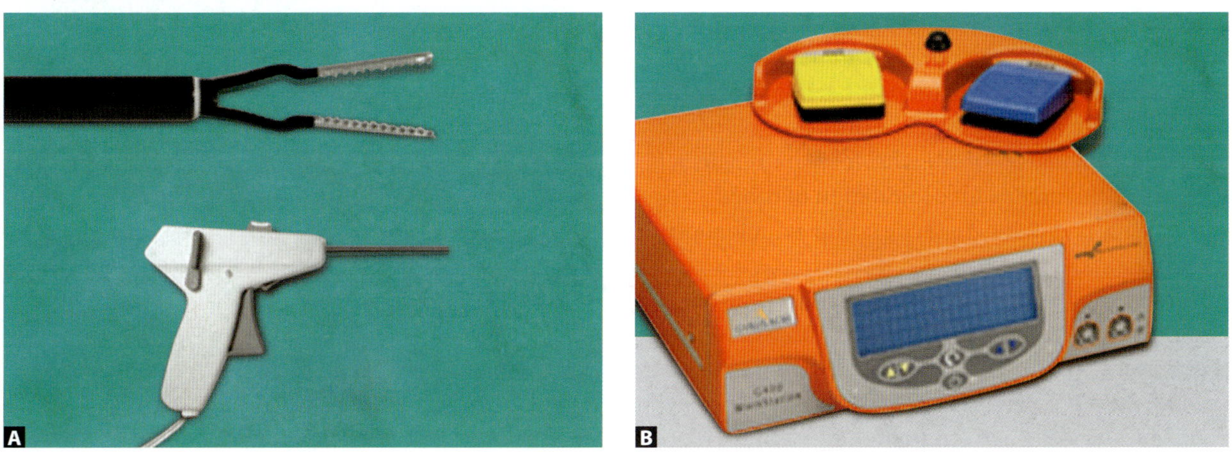

Figs. 3.29A and B: (A) Gyrus PK integrated vessel sealing and cutting system (Olympus); (B) Gyrus PK control unit (Olympus).

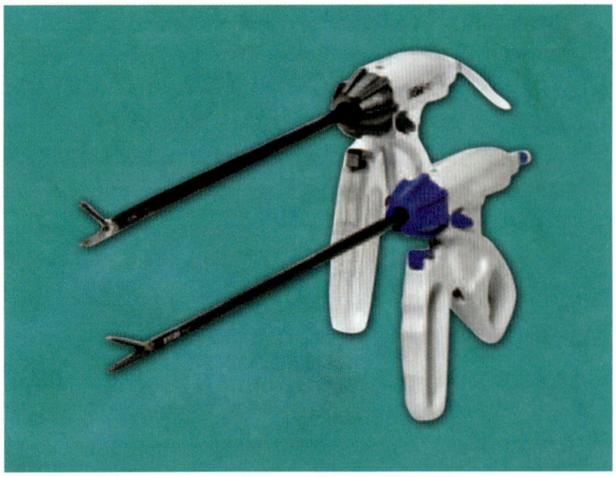

Fig. 3.30: ENSEAL sealing instrument (Ethicon Endo-Surgery).

of laser surgery[7,8] and enthusiasts of electrosurgery. Light energy is amplified to generate increased coherent electromagnetic radiation. Here we mention the three forms of laser used in endoscopic surgery:

- CO_2 laser
- Nd:YAG laser
- KTP lasers.

The neodymium:yttrium-aluminum-garnet (Nd:YAG) laser, the argon laser and potassium-titanium-phosphate (KTP) laser are used for cutting and coagulation. All the tissue effects are produced because of the continuous or pulsing thermodynamic conversion of light in thermal energy. Because of the 15° refraction of the laser beam after arising from the fiber bundle, the effect can be achieved only up to 2 cm from the tip of the fibers. In 1996 Wallwiener et al. introduced laser treatment in the reproductive surgery.[8]

ENDOCOAGULATION

Like the hot plate, endocoagulation takes place as contact coagulation, a heat denaturation by low voltage. A wider coagulation can be more easily employed as compared to point coagulation. The control unit heats three types of probes:

- Point coagulator for specific, focal hemostasis
- Crocodile forceps for coagulation of tubes
- Myoma screw for dissection and enucleation of myomata.

These devices are produced by Wisap but in the practical application are already historic. We used them from 1970 to 2000 in the Kiel School of Gynaecological Endoscopy. Various similar devices using the idea of local heat production are appearing on the market today.

HARMONIC SCALPEL: ULTRASONIC ENERGY

The harmonic scalpel is an ultrasonically activated laparoscopic instrument that uses mechanical energy to cut and coagulate tissues. Today, the harmonic scalpel can be used as 5- to 10 mm cutting blades and scissors. Activation of the titanium blade takes place by a piezoelectric crystal with a frequency of 55,500/s in the hand set. The cutting and coagulation effects are comparable to that of the CO_2 laser.[9] The lateral thermal damage is less than by HF coagulation. Burning and carbonization of tissues are not observed.

The advantages of ultrasound energy in surgical endoscopic instruments produced by Ethicon Endo-Surgery and Olympus are well known today and highly appreciated. As an example, let us focus on the harmonic ace of Ethicon (Fig. 3.31), which with its specific control unit (Fig. 3.32) allows a shorter and a longer effect of sealing. The mechanical energy

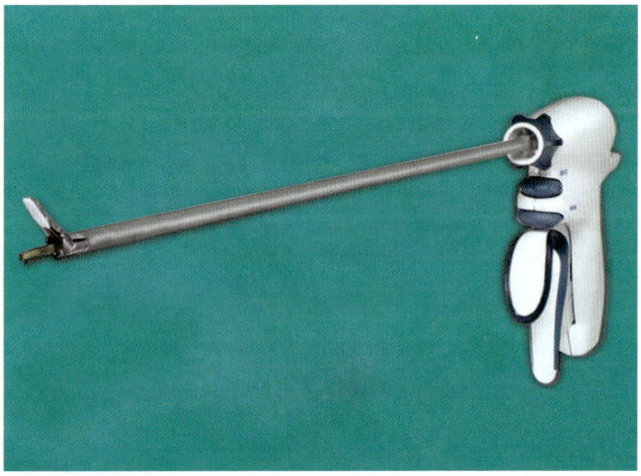

Fig. 3.31: Harmonic Ace forceps (Ethicon).

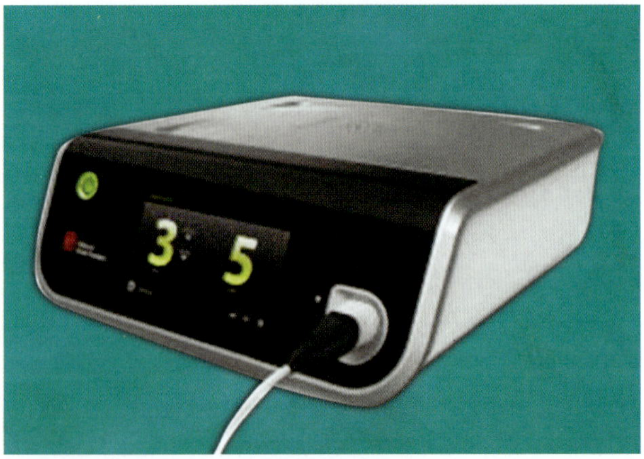

Fig. 3.32: Harmonic Ace control unit (Ethicon).

works with low temperatures, small lateral damage and minimal desiccation of the tissue. The energy is applied parallel to pressure, thus minimizing tissue trauma. The simultaneous cutting and coagulation give a good balance between hemostasis and cutting. A definite coagulation of vessels up to 2 mm is guaranteed. Precise dissection, cutting and coagulation are secured without the patient coming into contact with electricity.

The different harmonic instruments on the market today, such as harmonic shears, forceps and cutting rings, are applied for adhesiolysis as well as any type of adnexectomy, ovariectomy and hysterectomy. It remains up to the surgeon whether he uses them in combination with other sealing instruments or bipolar coagulation.

MICROENDOSCOPY

By rigorously following the concept of minimally invasive access for hysteroscopy and laparoscopy through advances in instrument designing, today optic systems measuring only about 1.8–2 mm including the trocar surrounding them are available. Phase optic and lens optic system with diameter between 1.2 and 2 mm are offered by instrument manufacturers. Common to both of them is that the laparoscope can be passed through the Veress needle or the sleeve. Additional trocar insertion after gas insufflation is therefore superfluous. However, compared to the standard 5 and 10 mm optics, even the most satisfactory of the mini-systems shows deficient lighting efficiency. The instrument trocars are also available in correspondingly small diameters.

The merits of minimal operative trauma and the avoidance of umbilical trocar insertion done by inserting the laparoscope through the Veress cannula, in minilaparoscopies used to have disadvantages, such as the mechanical fragility of the minilaparoscopes and difficult operative sites with a restricted view. Today new optics and stabile instruments have virtually eliminated these disadvantages. Therefore, a set of minilaparoscopic instruments must always be available for use in certain surgical interventions. The small diameter of the mini-instruments contributes toward reducing trauma and pain in children and in smaller surgical procedures.

ROBOTIC ENDOSCOPIC SURGERY

Under the current available robotic systems and instruments, the da Vinci robot has proved to be the most advanced surgical system. Other robotic systems, such as the Telelap ALF-X, are not yet used in patient treatment.

The da Vinci surgical system has been very successfully applied in oncologic surgery and facilitates a faster learning curve for laparoscopists.

A literature survey on robotic-assisted gynecological oncology clearly supports the use of the da Vinci surgical system in laparoscopic oncological surgery. Robotic precision in tumor excision, easier intracorporeal suturing and favorable ergonomics for the surgeon make the da Vinci robot particularly suitable for performing complex laparoscopic, microinvasive surgical operations in gynecological oncology.

Robotic surgery combines the advantages of open surgery and endoscopic surgery. The development of the da Vinci in patient treatment encompasses nearly 10 years and shows continuous improvements in application for urologists, general surgeons, cardiac surgeons and gynecological surgeons.

Figure 3.33 shows the latest da Vinci surgical console and docking station and Figure 3.34 the EndoWrist® instruments. Today, a dual console is available, which allows two surgeons to collaborate during a procedure. The advantages of the system include 3D HD visualization, an integrated surgeon touch pad, which offers comprehensive control of recordings and an extensive array of wristed EndoWrist® instruments with fingertip controls and foot switch performance of various tasks, such as application of energy instruments. A motorized patient cart facilitates quick and controlled docking of the system to the patient.

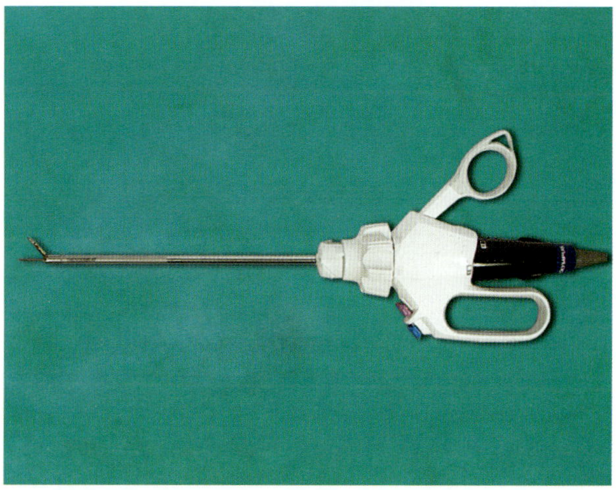

Fig. 3.33: da Vinci Surgical System Si, integrated robotic system with working console, side cart and control unit (Intuitive Surgical).

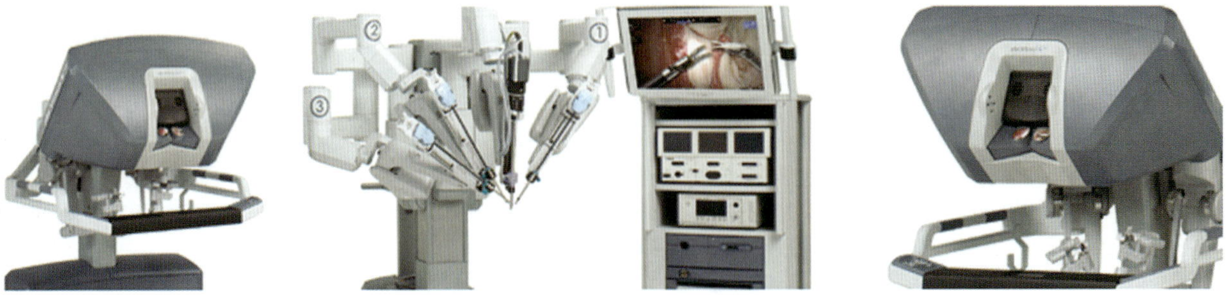

Fig. 3.34: EndoWrist® instruments of da Vinci Surgical System.

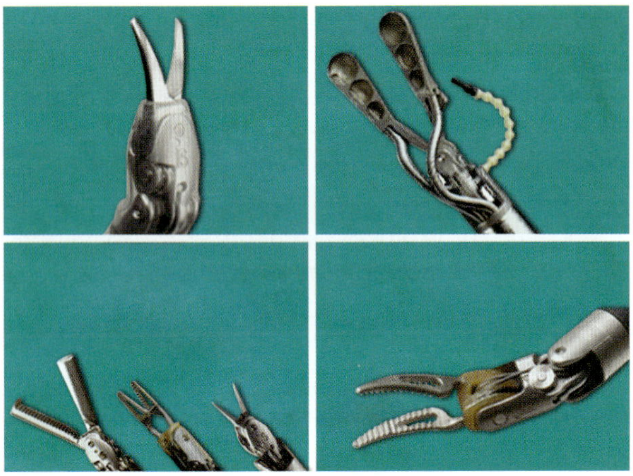

Fig. 3.35: Telelap ALF-X at the operation table (Sofar).

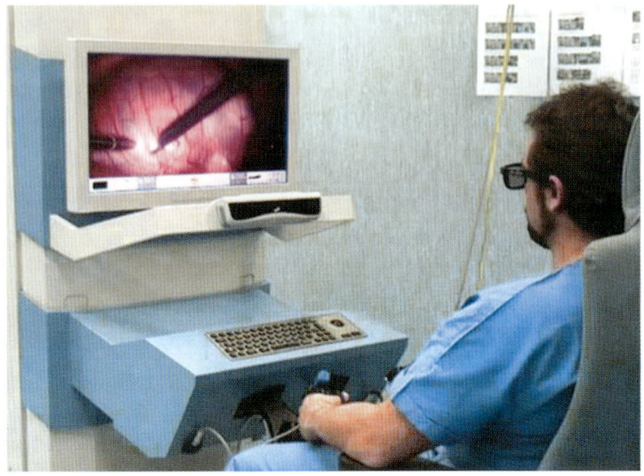

Fig. 3.37: Telelap ALF-X unit for measuring trocar force (Sofar).

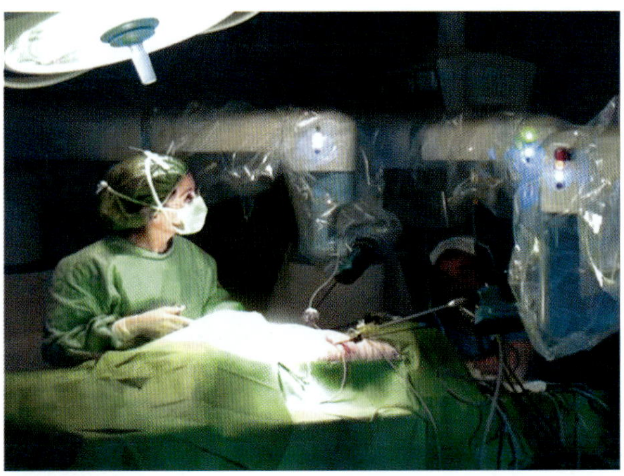

Fig. 3.36: Telelap ALF-X control unit (Sofar).

The Italian robotic system called Telelap ALF-X (Figs. 3.35 to 3.37) incorporates an eye-tracking system, force feedback characteristics and is managed by one surgeon sitting unsterile at a computer console and an assistant interacting with the robotic arms of the second console,[4] which can be easily moved around the table. As a safety function, the system stops when the surgeons ceases to look at the operation site on the computer screen. Activation of any given instrument is performed by gazing at the respective icon on the screen. Each point the surgeon looks at moves to the screen's center. 3D stereo vision simulates the vision of open surgery.

ARTICULATED INSTRUMENTS

Terumo Kymerax System or Terumo "Precision–Drive Articulating Instrument" (Fig. 3.38)

A new motor-driven, handheld system that offers precision-driven articulating instruments, called the Terumo Kymerax System (Terumo, Tokyo, Japan), has recently been introduced in the medical market in Europe.

The System: The three components include a console, a handle and interchangeable instruments. Up to two handles can be connected to the console, which provides power to the motors located within the handle component of the system. The instrument is used under direct surgeon control at the OR table, is

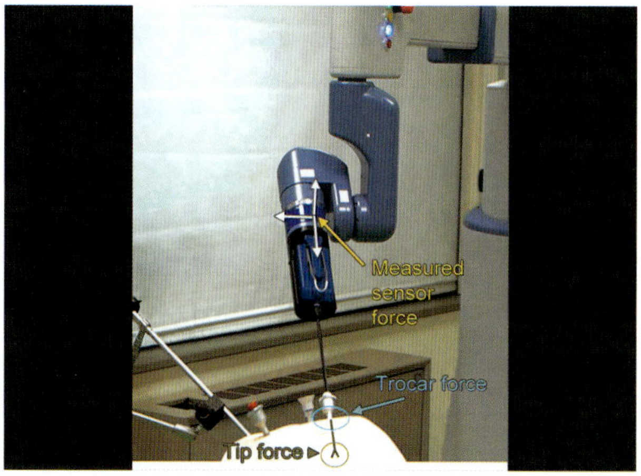

Fig. 3.38: Terumo Kymerax System with control unit and bilateral articulated instruments.

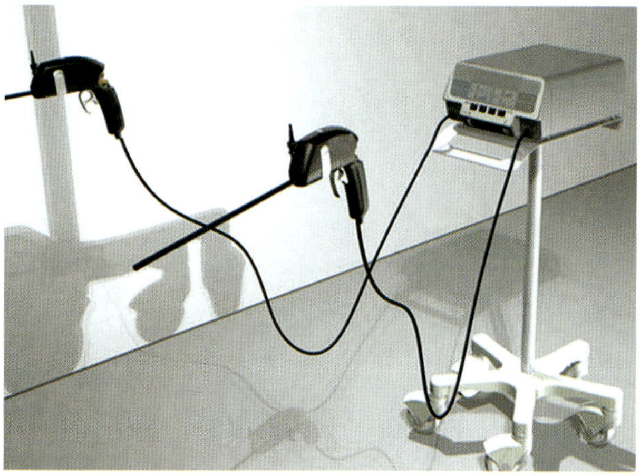

Fig. 3.39: Possibilities of instrument rotation within the Terumo Kymerax S System.

handheld and can be used in conjunction with conventional laparoscopic instruments.

Instruments: The instruments available include a needle driver, monopolar L-hook cautery, monopolar scissors and Maryland grasper and dissector. The instrument's functions are suited for performing general surgical tasks, such as manipulating tissue, ligating, suturing, knot tying, cutting, coagulating and dissecting (Fig. 3.39).

Features and benefits: The tip articulation is computer-assisted and allows the surgeon to control the movements through individual yaw and roll controls on the handle's interface. The speed of the movements can be adjusted to suit each individual surgeon's preference.

The precision-drive articulating instrument provides an additional two degrees of freedom (yaw and roll of the instrument tip, independent of the shaft) to the four degrees of freedom allowed by standard laparoscopic instruments (pitch, yaw, roll and surge). The articulation allows the instruments to efficiently adjust the instrument tip angles to the desired tissue planes for fine dissection and cauterization of tissue while maintaining ergonomic hand positioning. The articulation also facilitates suturing by providing the operator with the ability to adjust the angles for suture placement in the ideal tissue position at the optimal angle. The opening and closing of the jaws or blades are manually controlled through a trigger on the handle. This manual function provides the operator with beneficial haptic feedback:

- Roll: 160° each way (total of 320°)
- Yaw (movement of left and right): 70° each way (total of 140°).

The advantages of the articulated instruments compared to robotics are the following:

- Portability
- By the bedside
- Can be used in conjunction with regular laparoscopic instruments
- Will not cost a fortune
- Precise movement of the tip
- Easy-to-control tip movement by the pushing the button on the handle
- Ergonomic handle (angle of wrist and position of fingers).

r2 DRIVE and r2 CURVE

These instruments are disposable, articulated instruments, which are gaining more and more attention for their use. This Tübingen set of instruments (Tuebingen Scientific Medical GmbH, Tuebingen, Germany) was developed by Gerhard Bues, a creative general endoscopic surgeon.

r2 DRIVE is a handheld instrument that offers all degrees of freedom of a robotic system. Due to the 90° deflectable and infinite rotatable tip, in combination with the infinite rotatable shaft, surgical maneuvers can be confidently and precisely carried out even in difficult angles and tight spaces.

The instrument is primarily controlled with the fingertips, thereby offering utmost precision and comfort for the surgeon. Extensive movements are thus rendered superfluous, which obviates fatigue and discomfort on the part of the surgeon.

The shaft diameter is 5 mm, enabling body access through small incisions.

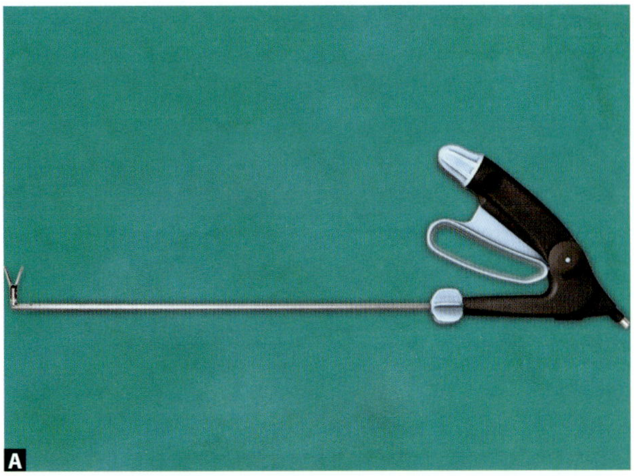

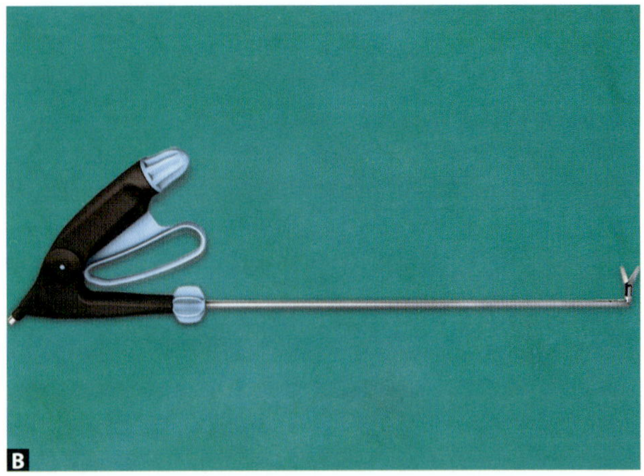

Figs. 3.40A and B: (A) r2 DRIVE handheld instrument, left hand (Tübingen Scientific Medical); (B) r2 DRIVE handheld instrument, right hand (Tübingen Scientific Medical).

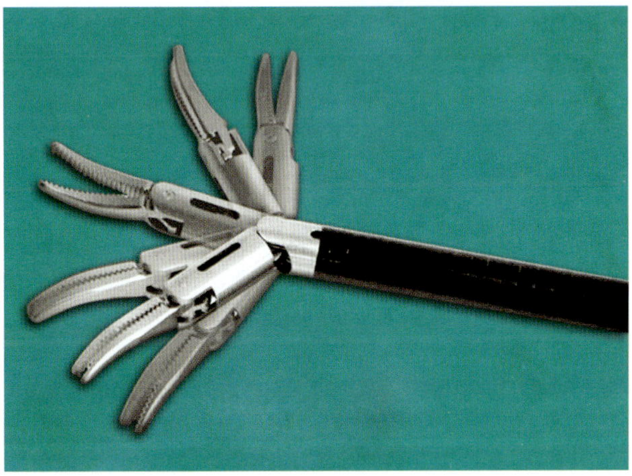

Fig. 3.41: r2 CURVE handheld instruments (Tübingen Scientific Medical).

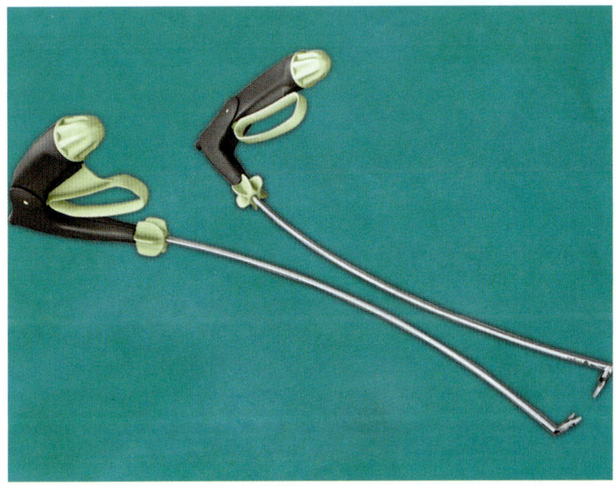

Fig. 3.42: r2 CURVE scissor tip (Tübingen Scientific Medical).

Bipolar HF technology provides secure, reproducible and clearly defined effects in preparation and hemostasis. The instrument is available in various configurations: atraumatic forceps, needle holder, dissector and scissors. The r2 DRIVE is a disposable, one-piece instrument (Figs. 3.40A and B).

The r2 CURVE is a handheld instrument to be used at a single-port entry and offers all degrees of freedom of a robotic system with a special design to support single-port surgery (Fig. 3.41). The unique design of the instruments allows easy and controlled handling and precise and reliable navigation and maneuverability. The combination of the curved shaft with the 360° infinite tip rotation, the tip deflection and the full and infinite shaft rotation gives the freedom needed to perform single port surgery (Fig. 3.42). No sword fighting, no crossover, no mirrored views.

The instrument offers a shaft diameter of 5 mm and bipolar HF technology. The instrument is available in various configurations: atraumatic forceps, needle holder, dissector and scissors. The r2 CURVE is a disposable, one-piece instrument.

SINGLE-PORT ENDOSCOPIC ENTRY (SEL)

See also chapter "Abdominal Access."

Laparoscopy in the 1940s started with the angled laparoscope (optic and one working channel) of Raoul Palmer in France as SEL. Laparoscopy at that time was mainly used for diagnostic purposes and for sterilizations. Kurt Semm in Germany further developed the procedure into operative laparoscopy by using multiple entries and instruments. Semm called the procedure "pelviscopy" to differentiate the technique from the simple liver biopsies that the internists called laparoscopy, as the gynecologist works mainly in the minor pelvis. Thus, the insurance companies

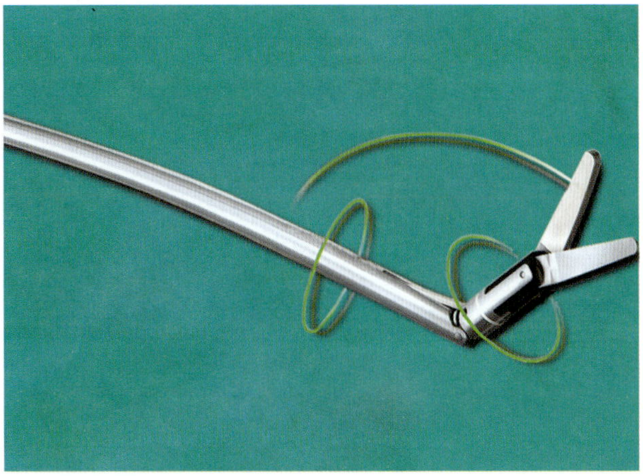

Fig. 3.43: SILS (Covidien).

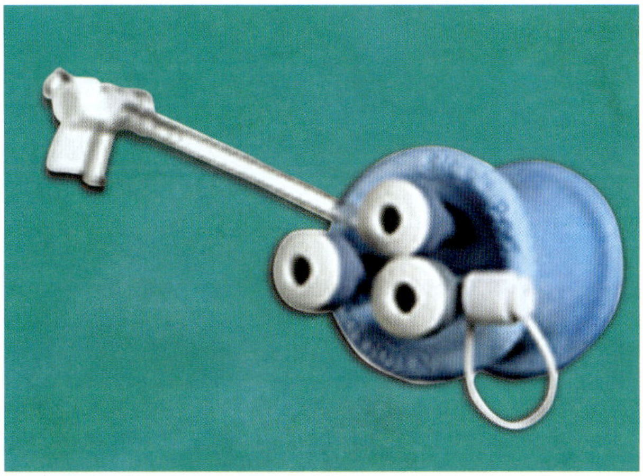

Fig. 3.44: LESS (Olympus).

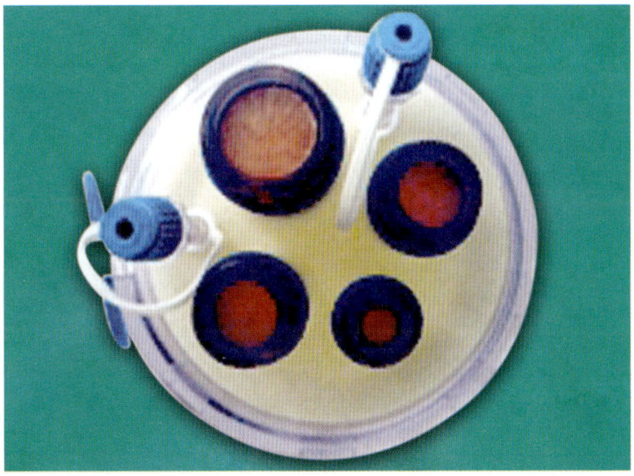

Fig. 3.45: LESS system with EndoEYE and curved instruments (Olympus).

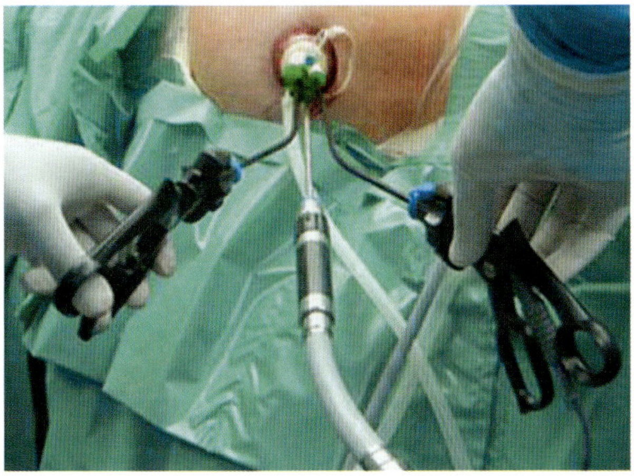

Fig. 3.46: Seven variations of LESS curved instruments (Olympus).

started to pay for these gynecologic laparoscopic procedures in Germany.

With the improved technology of today, SEL takes the idea of the early laparoscopy to new horizons. Of the multitude of SEL ports available, let us mention two disposable and one reusable:

- The SILS port (Covidien) (Fig. 3.43) is a disposable port. Here a silicone port is introduced into the abdominal cavity using a classical curved grasper with a beak of 5–6 cm. The surgeon has the choice of two ports of five mm and one allowing for a large barrel instrument of 10–12 mm or one with four 5 mm ports. The SILS, with the possibility to introduce larger instruments, is suitable for hysterectomies.
- Another disposable port is the LESS QuadPort + (Fig. 3.44) of Olympus, which contains duckbill valves and requires no gel for insertion. Instruments of 5, 10, 12 and 15 mm can be introduced easily for ergonomic surgery. The 5 mm LESS EndoEYE video-laparoscopes provide excellent visualization and help to avoid instrument clashing. Specialized curved HiQ+ LESS instruments allow internal triangulation and mimic traditional laparoscopy (Figs. 3.45 and 3.46).
- As a reusable port we used the XCONE (Fig. 3.47) of Karl Storz. This system is operational in the abdomen with three to five entry channels, one allowing large barrel instruments. Usually the 3 or 5 mm optic is placed into the middle entry and at least one curved instrument on the left or right side. The ENDOCONE® is a special access system developed by the general surgeon Cuschieri in which seven instruments can be introduced simultaneously. Recently the LEROY SPORT® substitutes the XCONE and ENDOCONE (Fig. 3.48).

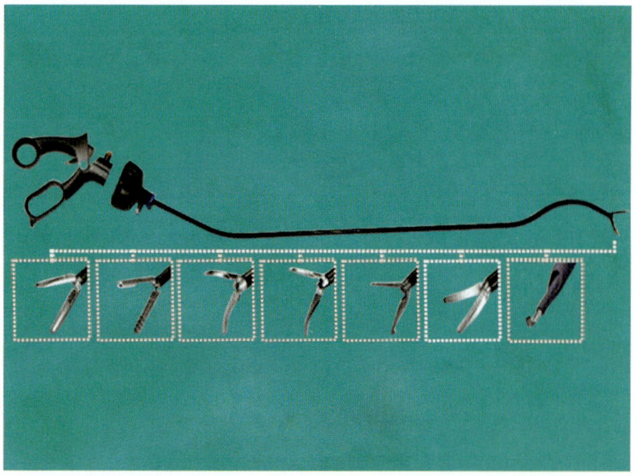

Fig. 3.47: XCONE (Karl Storz).

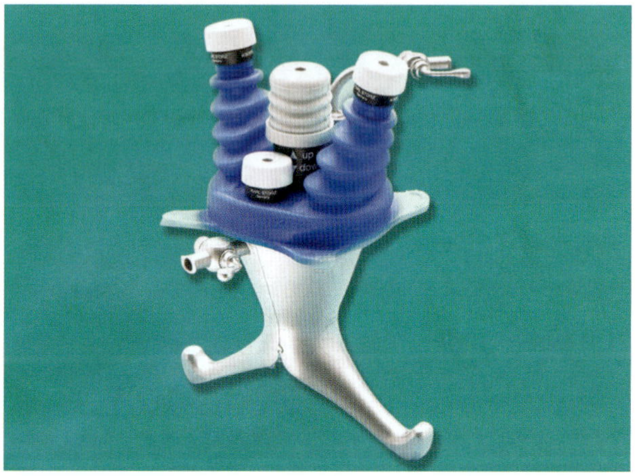

Fig. 3.48: ENDOCONE® (Karl Storz).

Developments are ongoing as can be seen by the ETHOS Surgical Platform™ (Ethos Surgical, Beaverton, USA) (Fig. 3.49), on which the surgeon is postured over the midline of the patient with optimal port triangulation options. New instruments and apparatuses are continuously being appraised. They assist the surgeon but do not replace his knowledge and have always to be critically evaluated and studied before they are applied.

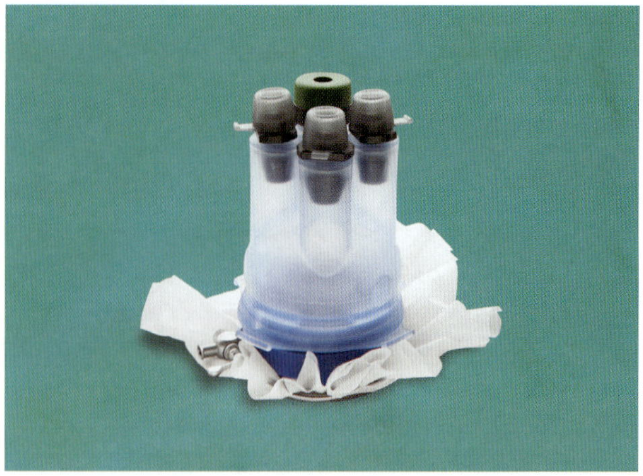

Fig. 3.49: ETHOS Surgical Platform™ (ETHOS Surgical).

REFERENCES

1. Mettler L, Ibrahim M, Jonat W. One year of experience working with the aid of a robotic assistant (the voice-controlled optic holder AESOP) in gynaecological endoscopic surgery. Hum Reprod. 1998;13(10):2748-50.
2. Semm K. Operationslehre für endoskopische Abdominal Chirurgie—operative Pelviskopie. Stuttgart, New York: Schattauer Verlag; 1984.
3. Veress J. Neues Instrument zur Ausführung von Brust-oder Bauchpunktionen und Pneumothoraxbehandlung. Dtsch Med Wochenschr. 1938;41:1480-1.
4. Semm K. Die moderne Endoskopie in der Frauenheilkunde. Frauenarzt. 1972;13:300-7.
5. Hopkins HH. On the diffraction theory of optical images. Proc Roy Soc A. 1953;217:408-15.
6. Brill AI. Energy systems for operative laparoscopy. J Am Assoc Gynecol Laparosc. 1998;5(4):333-45; quiz 347-9.
7. Daniell JF. Tailoring the laser for infertility surgery. Contemp = OB/GYN Special issue. 1987;33-143.
8. Wallwiener D, Maleika A, Rimbach S, et al. The value of laparoscopic and laser-assisted techniques in reconstruction of distal fallopian tube pathology. Zentralbl Gynakol. 1996;118(2):66-72.
9. Schemmel M, Heafner HK, Selvaggi SM, et al. Comparison of the ultrasonic scalpel to CO_2 laser and electrosurgery in terms of tissue injury and adhesion formation in a rabbit model. Fertil Steril. 1997;67(2):382-6.

KIEL SCHOOL

4 of Gynaecological Endoscopy

Practical Approach to Instrumentation

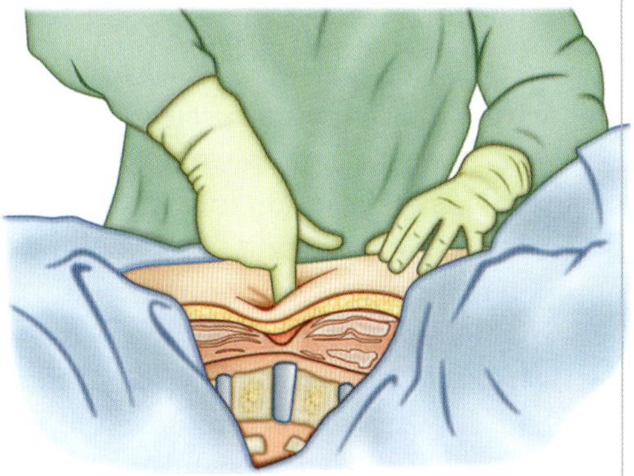

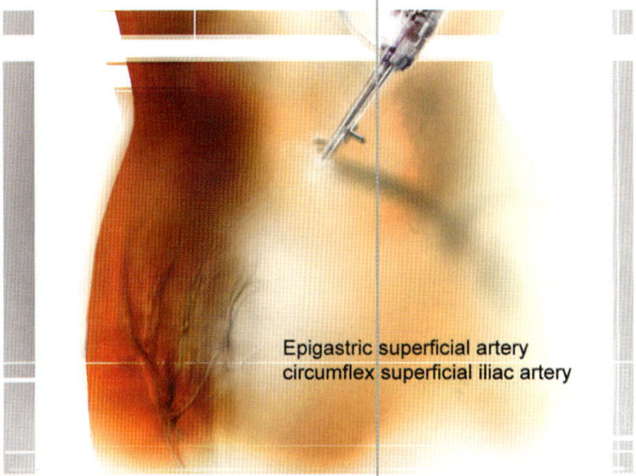

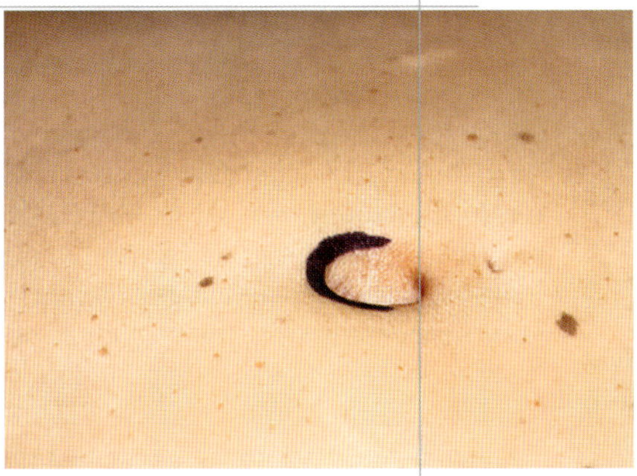

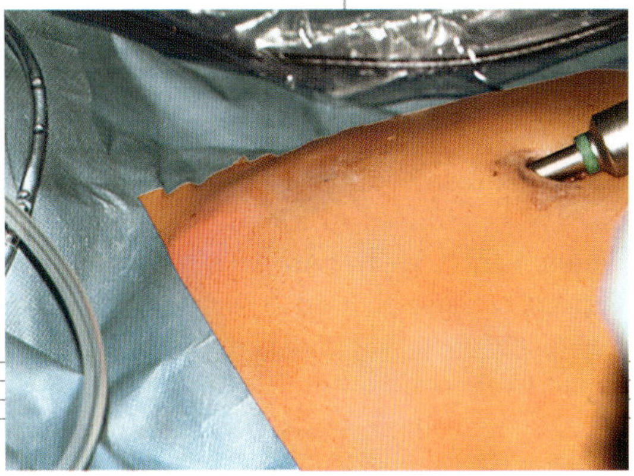

Chapter 4

Practical Approach to Instrumentation

Ibrahim Alkatout, Liselotte Mettler

INTRODUCTION

Minimally invasive surgery has been undergoing a process of consistent and dynamic evolution due to ongoing scientific and industrial improvements. The minimally invasive approach has transformed surgery altogether.[1] The advantages of minimally invasive surgery compared to open surgery as well as vaginal surgery are well-known and widely accepted in our specialty (Table 4.1).[2-4]

Technical advancements, especially those in the last few decades, have led to the development of small instruments and thus reduced the degree of surgical trauma for the patient.[5] The rising quality of image transmission and the establishment of 3D in laparoscopy have made it possible to perform precise and delicate operations with minimal blood loss.[6] Especially the magnification of individual and in part strongly vascularized portions of tissue have made it possible to perform surgery with minimal blood loss while being able to visualize the individual layers of tissue. Complications such as postoperative pain, infection or the formation of adhesions have been reduced to a minimum. Sealing instruments, which, by the aid of ultrasound or bipolar current, can also be used to perform coagulation and transect of tissue are mainly employed as disposable single-use instruments.

Adequate hemostasis is essential for performing safe laparoscopic surgery and obtaining a clear and undistorted view of the operating field, identifying endangered structures like blood vessels, the ureter or the bowel at an early point in time, and protecting these. A number of laparoscopic instruments are suitable for this purpose. These can be used to expose the tissue carefully and visualize individual structures leading to vessels, which are then coagulated and transected selectively and safely.[7] In the event of intraoperative bleeding, the available instruments are also suitable for achieving safe and efficient hemostasis and thus continuing the operation by the laparoscopic approach.[8] Technical advancements have also made it possible to use sealing instruments, which, by the aid of ultrasound or bipolar current, can be employed to perform coagulation and transect tissue as well. These instruments were primarily developed for single use. From the economic point of view, this calls for a complex decision-making process with regard to the acquisition and utilization of instruments. The advantages are primarily the fact that an exchange of instruments is not necessary and coagulation can be performed safely.

The development of instruments for hysteroscopy has also been aimed at reducing complications and instrument size. The reduction of the dreaded condition of hypotonic hyperhydration [transurethral resection of the prostrate (TURP) syndrome] is mainly ensured by the use of bipolar systems and physiological saline instead of electrolyte-free solutions.

LAPAROSCOPY

Laparoscopic interventions are performed through one or more small incisions. The laparoscopic procedure is performed through a closed access (Veress needle, entry under direct viewing) or the open access (Hasson technique). After creating a pneumoperitoneum, one or more ports are placed. The camera system and working instruments are introduced through these ports.

Table 4.1: Advantages of minimally invasive surgery compared to abdominal and vaginal surgery

Vaginal Surgery Compared to Abdominal Operations	
Advantages	Shorter hospital stays (on average 1 day, 95% CI 0.7–1.2) Earlier return to activities of daily living (mean difference, 9.5 days, 95% CI 6.4–12.6) Lower infection rate, lower rate of postoperative fever episodes (OR 0.42, 95% CI 0.21–0.83) Lower rates of complications such as hernia or impaired wound healing Option of using regional anesthesia Best cosmetic outcome after surgery
Disadvantages	No possibility to treat comorbid conditions simultaneously The operation is more demanding because of limited space
Laparoscopic Surgery Compared to Abdominal Operations	
Advantages	Less blood loss (mean difference 45.3 mL, 95% CI 17.9–72.7) Shorter hospital stay (on average 2 days, 95% CI 1.9–2.2) Earlier return to activities of daily living (mean difference 13.6 days, 95% CI 11.8–15.4) Lower infection rate, lower rate of postoperative fever episodes (OR 0.32, 95% CI 0.12–0.85) Lower rates of complications such as hernia or impaired wound healing Less formation of adhesions Better cosmetic outcome Better and enlarged view for the surgeon because of the adjustable distance of the optical instrument Better view for all surgeons and assistants because the operation can be seen on the monitor More delicate surgery due to innovative instruments aligned to the improved view
Disadvantages	Longer operating time (mean difference 10.6 min, 95% CI 7.4–13.8) Longer learning curve; the steps of the operation are more complex Higher rate of complications, such as ureteral lesions, bowel lesions, or vascular lesions (OR 2.61, 95% CI 1.22–5.60) Limited tactile feedback A three-dimensional (3D) image only in exceptional cases Higher costs
Laparoscopic Surgery Compared to Vaginal Surgery	
Advantages	Less blood loss (mean difference 45.3 mL, 95% CI 17.9–72.7) Comorbid organs or structures can be operated on simultaneously Lower infection rate, lower rate of fever episodes (OR 0.32, 95% CI 0.12–0.85) Less formation of adhesions Better and enlarged view for the surgeon because of the adjustable distance of the optical instrument Better view for all surgeons and assistants because the operation can be viewed on the monitor More delicate surgery due to innovative instruments aligned to the better view More independent of the precise preoperative diagnostic investigation
Disadvantages	Longer operating time (mean difference 41.5 min, 95% CI 33.7–49.4) Longer learning curve; the steps of the operation are more complex Limited tactile feedback A 3D view is obtained only in exceptional cases Poorer cosmetic outcome Higher costs

The classical method of entry is described in the following:

Veress Needle Technique

The operating table is placed in horizontal position before introducing the Veress needle. The patient is placed in Trendelenburg position after creating the pneumoperitoneum. In the normal case the Veress needle is introduced in the region of the navel because the layers of the abdominal wall are thinnest at this site. Prior to the skin incision, the course of the aorta and the site of the iliac bifurcation can be palpated in slim persons (Figs. 4.1A to D).[9]

After testing the functionality of the needle it is introduced at a 45° angle to the abdominal wall, in

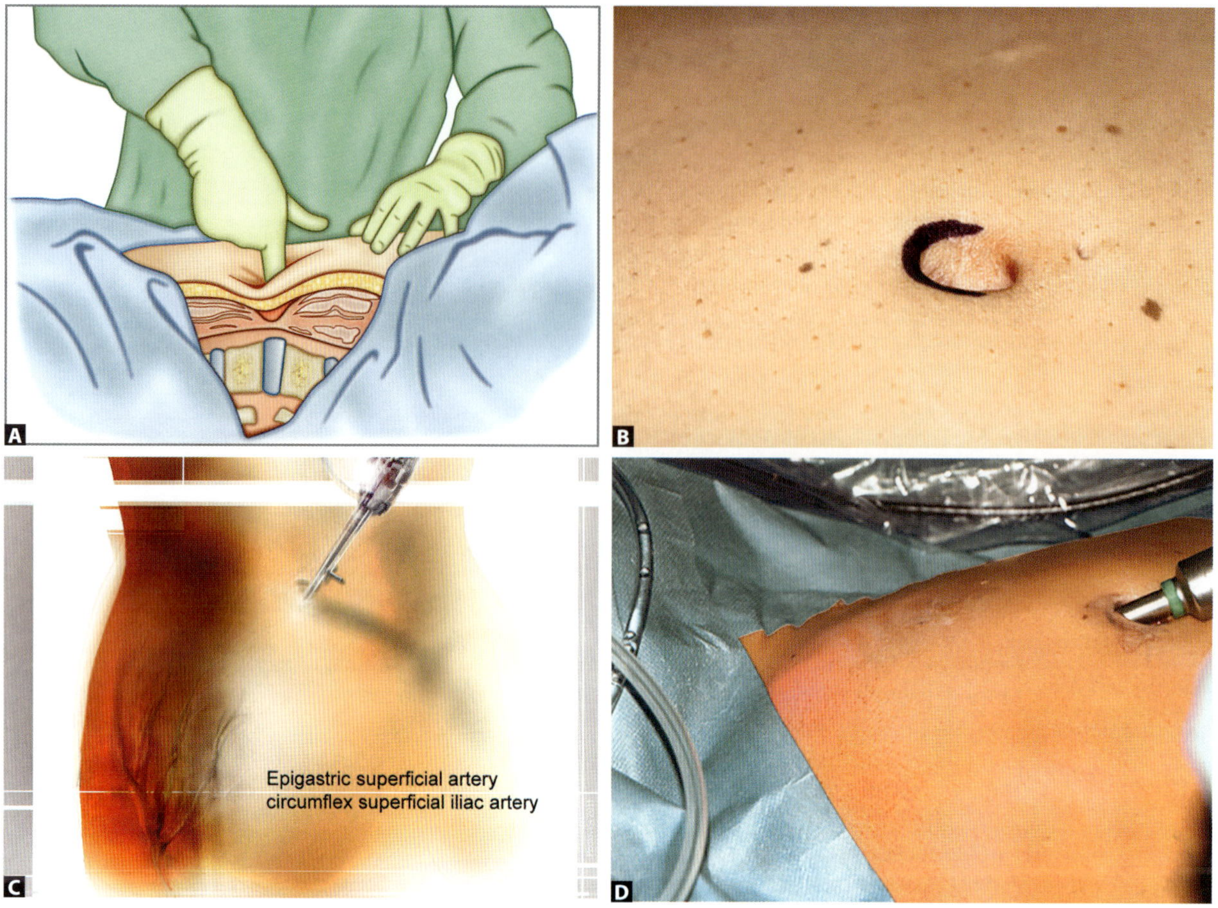

Figs. 4.1A to D: (A) Typical point of palpation in the subumbilical region. The fingertip is pointing to the promontory. Subumbilical incision and local palpation reveal the short distance from the skin to the spine; (B to D). Diaphanoscopy illuminates the region of insertion of the ancillary trocars while demarcating the superficial epigastric artery and the superficial circumflex iliac artery.

the direction of the uterus. The risk of injury to the large vessels or the intestines is thus minimized. Additionally, the abdominal wall is raised slightly (Figs. 4.2A to C). The more obese the abdominal wall, the more steep the angle of entry will be. In patients who have not undergone previous surgery, the surgeon may need to make two attempts before considering an alternative entry technique or introducing the needle at a different entry point.

When introducing the Veress needle, in the normal case one hears two clicks. The first occurs after perforating the muscle fascia and the second after perforating the peritoneum.

Aspiration test: After inserting the needle the surgeon introduces 5 mL of saline solution; this cannot be done when aspiration is attempted. Incorrect insertion of the needle into a blood vessel or the intestines can be observed here by noting the corresponding body fluid.

Hanging drop test and "fluid in flow": Once the needle has been introduced, raising the abdominal wall causes negative intra-abdominal pressure (IAP). A drop of water placed on the opening will be pulled in by the negative pressure. The needle should not be moved after it has been introduced. If the needle has been inserted incorrectly, the small intra-abdominal defect may tear further and turn into a complex and hazardous lesion (torque is caused by the abdominal wall).

Alternative Entry Technique

In the meantime we have several approaches for creating a pneumoperitoneum, even directly through appropriate trocar systems. The first description was provided by Artin Ternemian, who made it possible to enter the abdomen before or after creating a pneumoperitoneum, using a screw mechanism under direct viewing (Fig. 4.3). Alternatively, the pneumoperitoneum can be introduced directly and bluntly into the abdomen under direct viewing, after insufflation through the trocar tip. Thus, the pneumoperitoneum can be set up much faster with fewer

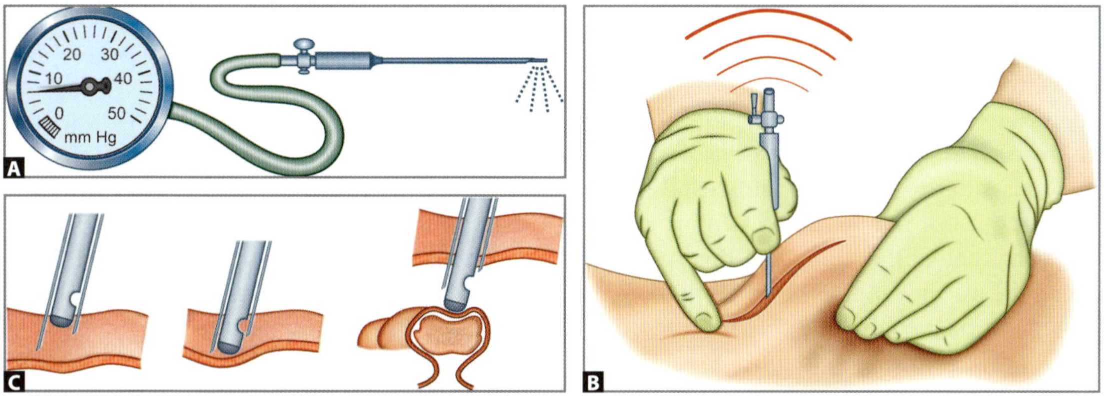

Figs. 4.2A to C: Veress needle and its insertion. The safety mechanism avoids damage or injury to the bowel or vessels.

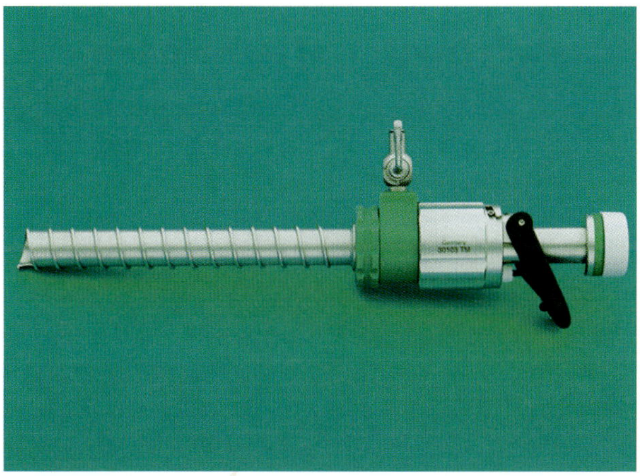

Fig. 4.3: Direct entry mechanism with the EndoTip (Karl Storz Company).

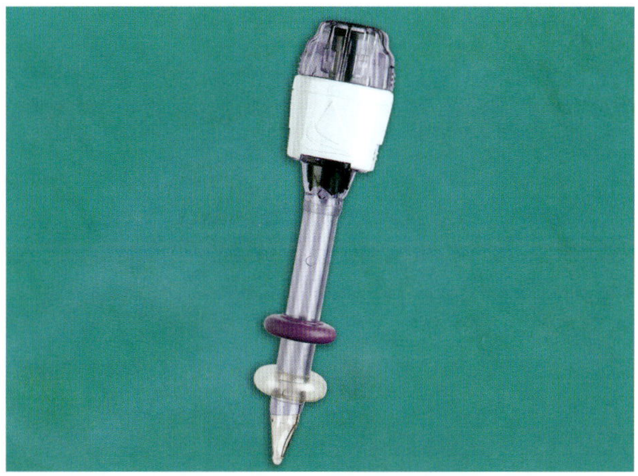

Fig. 4.4: Kii Advanced Fixation (Applied). Offers unsurpassed abdominal wall fixation with minimal depth into the peritoneal cavity. The nonlatex, nonfragmenting balloon provides superior abdominal wall retention compared to other sleeves and ensures minimum penetration of the trocar into the operative field. The retention disk slides down to maintain the sleeve position in the abdomen, securing the trocar in place and virtually eliminating unintentional displacement or forward migration.

instruments, while deleting several (safety) steps (Fig. 4.4).

Insufflation can then be started, initially with 1 liter of CO_2 gas/min, and then increased to 3–5 L/min. The total volume depends on the patient's height and degree of relaxation. Even after the instillation of 300 mL of CO_2 gas distributed uniformly in the intra-abdominal aspect, there is a perceivable *physiological damping of percussion* by the liver. The initial target pressure can be adjusted to 20–25 mm Hg in order to achieve the maximum distance between the abdominal wall and intra-abdominal structures.[10]

A 5-mm optical trocar can be introduced initially, provided this view is sufficient for the planned operation; a 10-mm optical trocar may be introduced instead. The trocar must be introduced by the so-called Z-technique so that it is shifted sideways by a few millimeters subcutaneously in order to achieve functional closure of the fascia and prevent the formation of a hernia after the operation. However, one achieves maximum safety by using the two-step principle. Step 1 consists of the introduction of a 5-mm optical trocar to avoid injury or adhesions. Before dilatation to 10 mm, CO_2 gas is instilled again safely through the intra-abdominal approach. Step 2 consists of introducing a place holder through the 5-mm trocar, followed by the introduction of the 10-mm trocar.[10]

Subcostal Insufflation Technique (Palmer's Point or the Lee–Huang Point)

No entry technique is entirely devoid of the risk of gas embolism, injury to vessels, the urinary tract or the bowel. However, entry through Palmer's point provides maximum safety, especially when the surgeon anticipates umbilical pathologies. In 1974 Raul Palmer described an alternative entry point in the medioclavicular line, about 3 cm below the costal arch. In rare cases, when the patient has undergone previous surgery in the left subcostal region, the Lee-Huang point may be used. This is located in the midline, below the xiphoid. However, when introducing the trocar it should be noted that the falciform ligament may be directly in intra-abdominal location. Besides, gastric suction must be performed before introducing the Veress needle or the trocar (Figs. 4.5A to D).[10]

Introduction of Working Trocars

The patient is placed in the Trendelenburg position before the introduction of working trocars. All working trocars should be introduced under maximum IAP and absolutely clear vision. The inferior epigastric artery is visualized from the inside in the lateral umbilical plica. The region lateral to this point must be screened for superficial arteries (the superficial iliac circumflex artery and the superficial epigastric artery) by performing a diaphanoscopy. From the outside the area is about two finger widths medial to the anterior superior iliac spine. Once the working trocar has perforated the peritoneum, it is swung over to the uterus, thus moving away from the large vessels and the intestines.

The number of working trocars may vary; the same is true of the preferred position. The latter may be symmetrically on the left and right side, or the left and middle, or the left aspect and the left-sided mid-abdomen (Figs. 4.6 to 4.8).[2,10] A number of single-use or reusable trocars are now available for this purpose.

Practical Handling of Instruments

The very specific technical features of the operating field in laparoscopy and the corresponding instruments may even limit the actions of experienced surgeons, especially when the patient experiences significant intraoperative bleeding or the conditions of surgery are rendered difficult by extreme obesity,

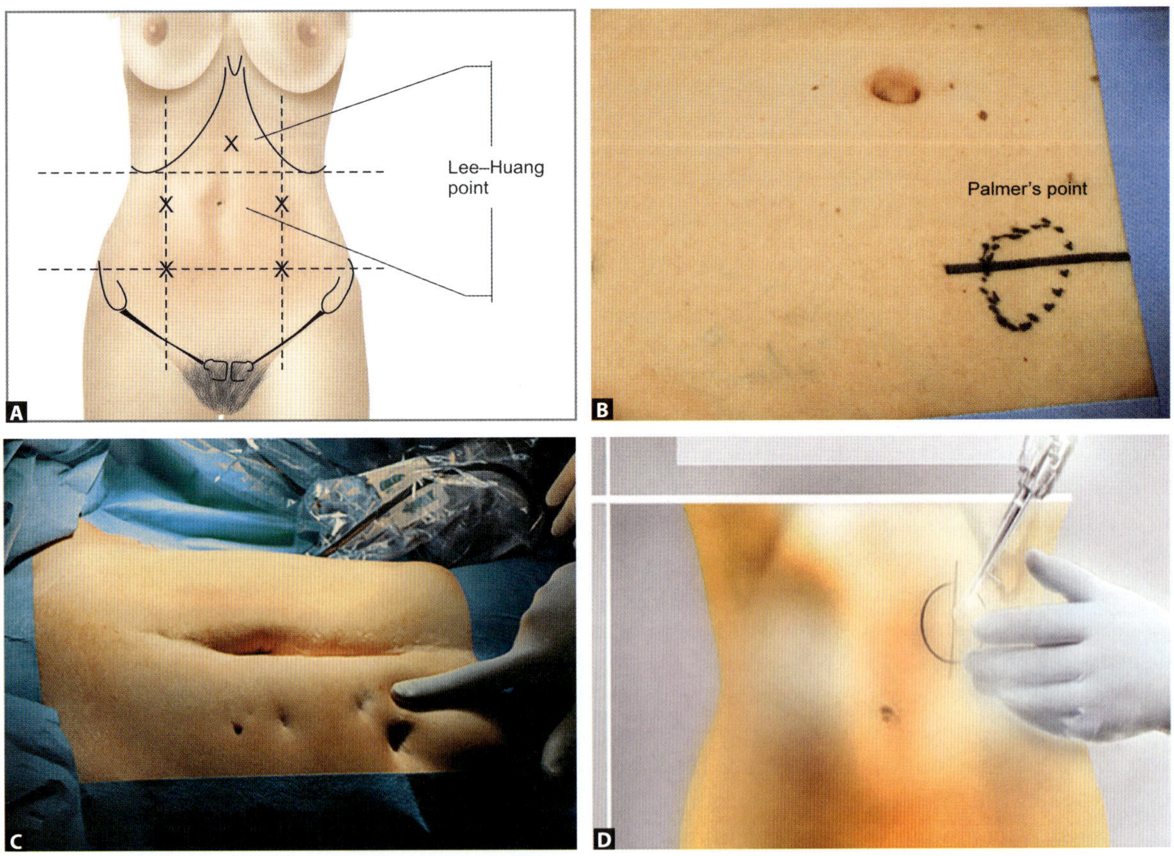

Figs. 4.5A to D: Alternative entry site showing (A), in cases of a large uterus, especially at or above the level of the umbilicus: the Lee–Huang point. This point is recommended for video-assisted laparoscopy or in cases of anticipated adhesions in the region of Palmer's point (C); (B to D) Palmer's point is situated in the midclavicular line, about 3 cm below the costal margin.

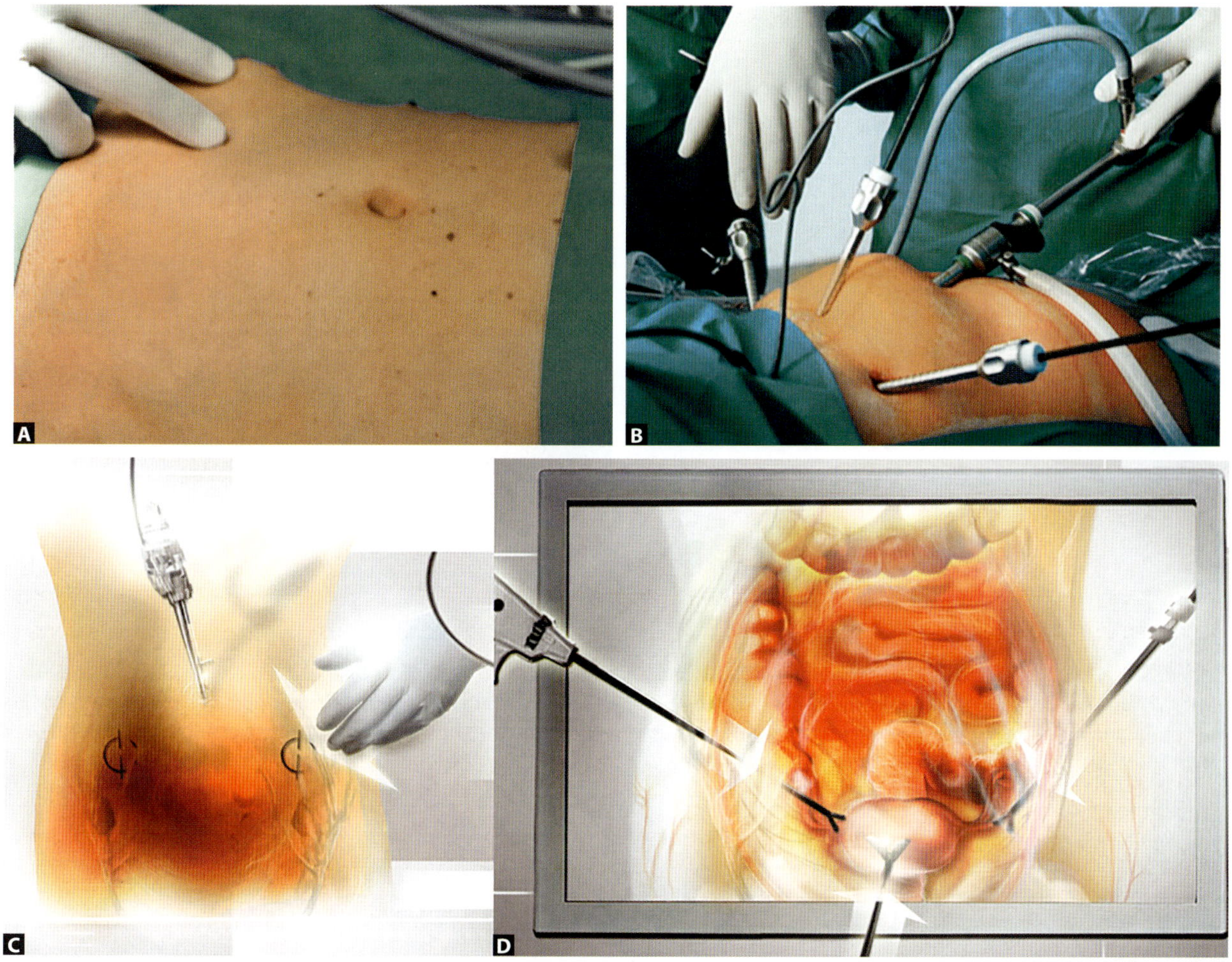

Figs. 4.6A to D: (A and C) Point of insertion from the outside (two-finger widths medial to the anterior-superior spine), at a 90° angle to the surface, with penetration of all layers of the abdominal wall. Trocar insertion site lateral to the lateral umbilical fold; (B and D) Overview after insertion of the laparoscope and three ancillary trocars.

a limited head-down tilt position, comorbid conditions, or adhesions. Compared to open surgery, the surgeon lacks depth perception due to the currently widespread two-dimensional (2D) view. The optical device introduced into the abdomen limits the surgeon's field of vision. As a result, some of the instruments may be withdrawn unobserved from the operating field, or may manipulate or injure tissue without being detected. Concealed bleeding or injury to organs outside the field of vision may not be identified (immediately). Compared to open surgery, laparoscopic instruments are greatly limited in their range of motion. The missing degrees of freedom (four versus seven) and the lever action on the abdominal wall may hinder complete visualization of the operating field as well as that of specific organ structures. Further difficulties include the limited use of instruments and the fact that trocar placement depends on the anatomy of the individual patient.

The view of the operating field may be impaired by impurities in the optical instruments. This may be caused by bleeding, secretion of body fluids, or even vapor or fog on the optical instrument due to coagulation. The port systems have to be opened repeatedly for ventilation, which causes fluctuations of IAP and alterations in the temperature of the CO_2 gas. The illumination system of the optical instrument may limit visibility in cases of extensive blood deposits. The surgeon must get used to semi-paradoxical hand movements, such as left is right, right is left, below is above, above is below, inward is inward, outward is outward, clockwise is clockwise, and anticlockwise is anticlockwise.

HYSTEROSCOPY

In hysteroscopy the entry technique is limited to the setting and dilatation of the cervical canal. This is traditionally achieved by probing and dilating the

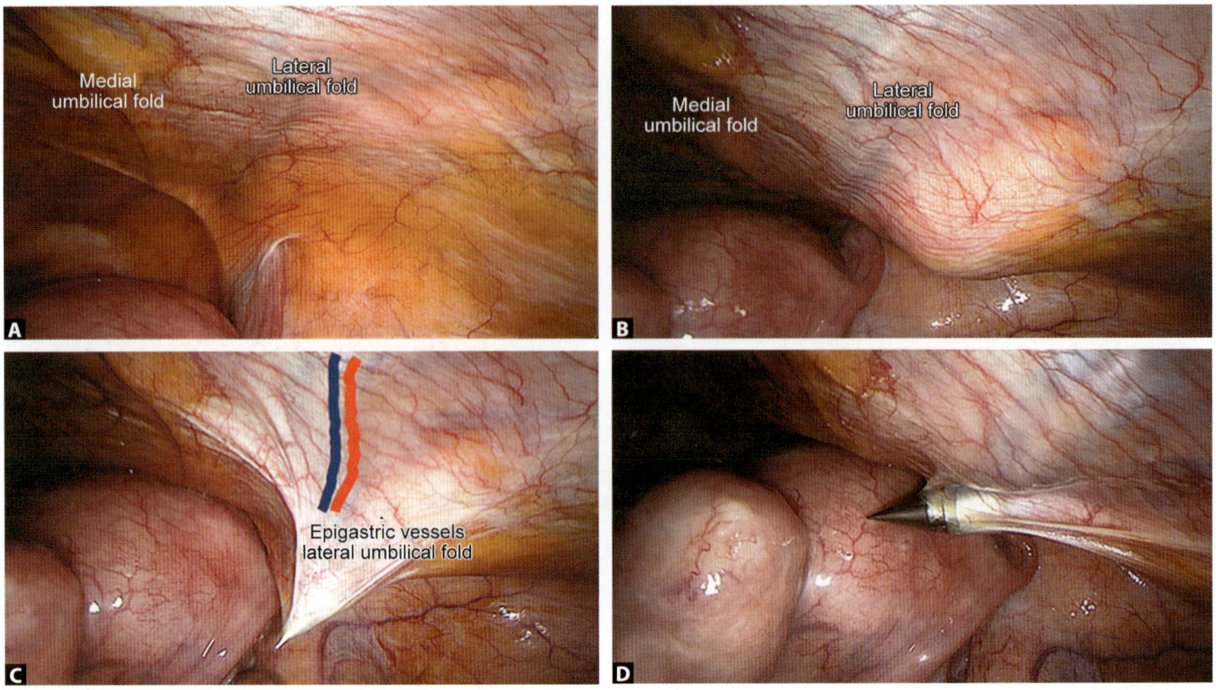

Figs. 4.7A to D: Secondary trocar placement, entry in the right lower abdomen. (A) The three different plicae are visualized; (B) The palpating finger is showing the area lateral to the lateral umbilical fold; (C) Entry of the sharp ancillary trocar in the lateral aspect of the lateral umbilical fold; (D) Once the peritoneum has been penetrated, the trocar points to the fundus of the uterus in order to avoid injury to the major vessels and the bowel.

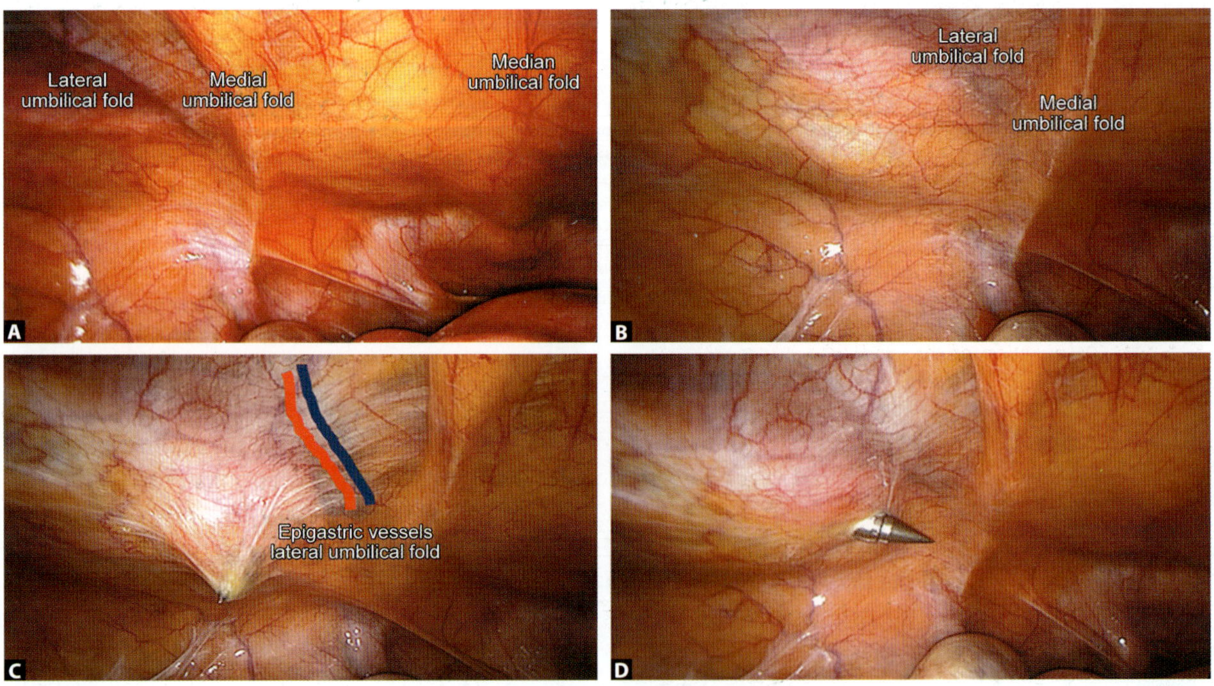

Figs. 4.8A to D: Secondary trocar placement, entry in the left lower abdomen. (A) The three plicae are visualized; (B) The palpating finger is showing the area lateral to the lateral umbilical fold; (C) Entry of the sharp ancillary trocar in the lateral aspect of the lateral umbilical fold; (D) Once the peritoneum has been penetrated, the trocar points to the fundus of the uterus in order to avoid injury to the major vessels and the bowel.

cervical canal to Hegar number 8 for diagnostic hysteroscopy and Hegar number 9 for operative hysteroscopy. Preparation of the cervix with misoprostol (400 µg administered until 12 hours preoperatively) reduces the risk of injury (avulsion injury due to the forceps, perforation, bleeding).

The hysteroscope consists of a single instrument. Techniques of image transmission and light sources were developed for this technique in the same manner as they were for laparoscopy. However, the use of hysteroscopy for the treatment of endometriosis is limited to exceptional cases such as confirmation of the diagnosis or simultaneous operations, including chromopertubation.

IMAGE PROCESSING SYSTEMS

Although minimally invasive surgery is a rather modern surgical procedure, its origins date back to 100 years ago when, in 1901, Kelling first viewed the intra-abdominal organs of a dog with a rigid endoscope. Subsequent advancements were mainly hindered by the absence of adequate light sources. Rapid and simultaneous technological developments, and the immense efforts of the industry were responsible for the success of minimally invasive surgery (Figs. 4.9 to 4.13).[11-13]

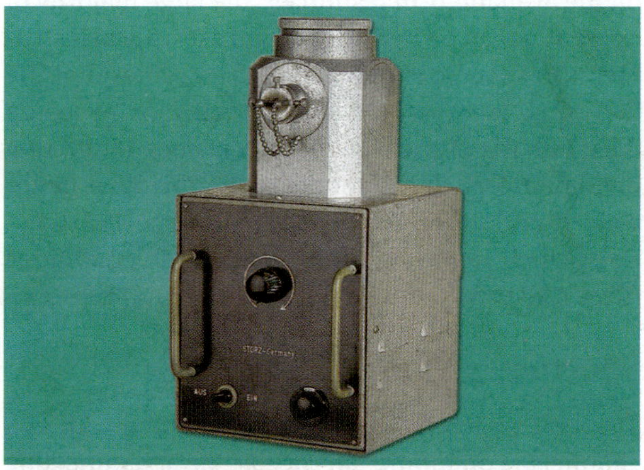

Fig. 4.9: 1960: Invention of the cold light source (Karl Storz Company).

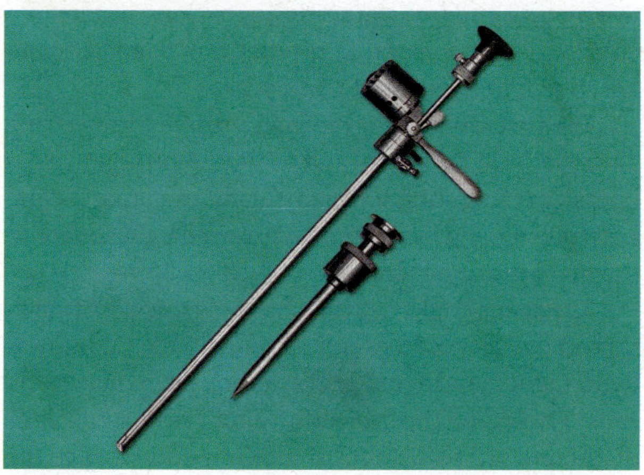

Fig. 4.10: 1962: The beginning of laparoscopy (Karl Storz Company).

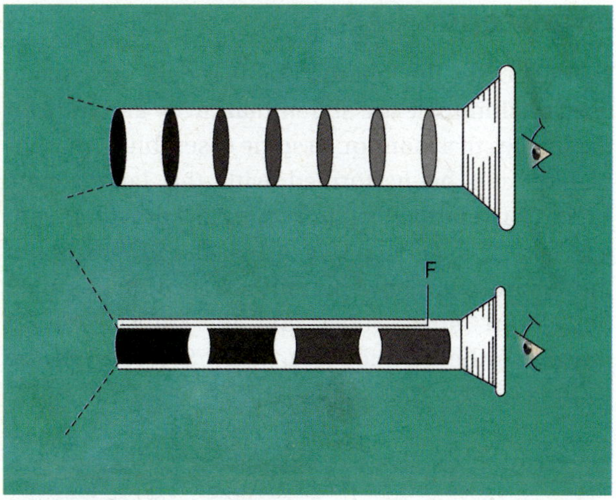

Fig. 4.11: 1965: Introduction of the HOPKINS® rod lens system (Karl Storz Company).

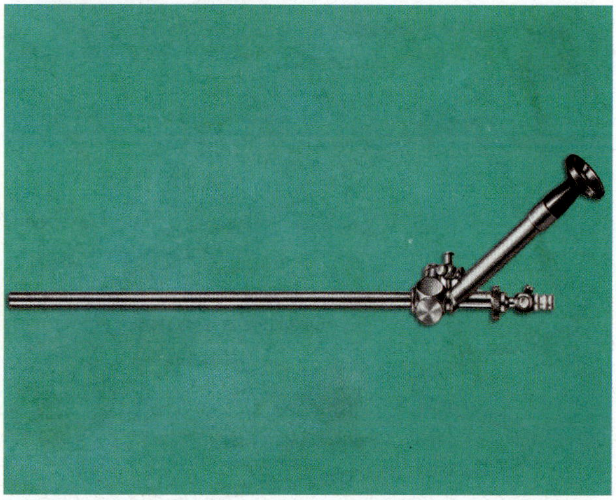

Fig. 4.12: 1973: The beginning of gynecological endoscopy for diagnostic investigation and treatment (Karl Storz Company).

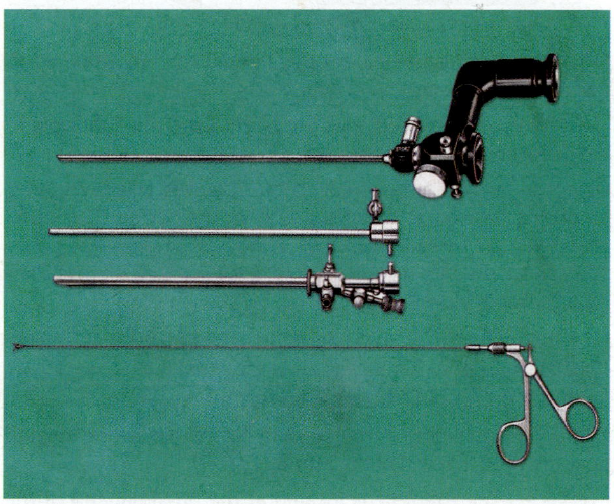

Fig. 4.13: 1980: Introduction of the HAMOU® Micro Contact Hysteroscope with a diameter of just 5 mm (Karl Storz Company).

Endoscope

In most cases the laparoscope is a rigid endoscope used to illuminate the abdominal cavity and transfer the images to a monitor. In some cases, blunt manipulation can be performed with the laparoscope itself. Conventional laparoscopes are provided with a 0° lens or a 30° lens (Fig. 4.14). The innovation of the laparoscope now permits the use of so-called flexible-tip laparoscopes and the transfer of 3D images to the monitor (Fig. 4.15). Selection of the

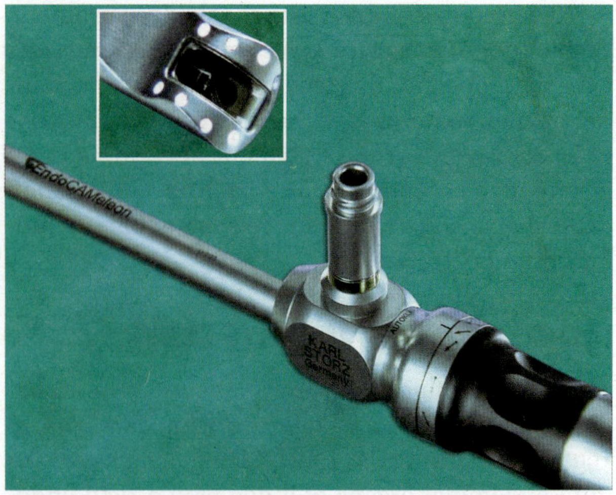

Fig. 4.15: Das EndoCaMeleon (Karl Storz Company) is a special optic device, which, thanks to the swiveled prism, permits the surgeon to set the viewing angle from 0 to 120° during endoscopic investigations.

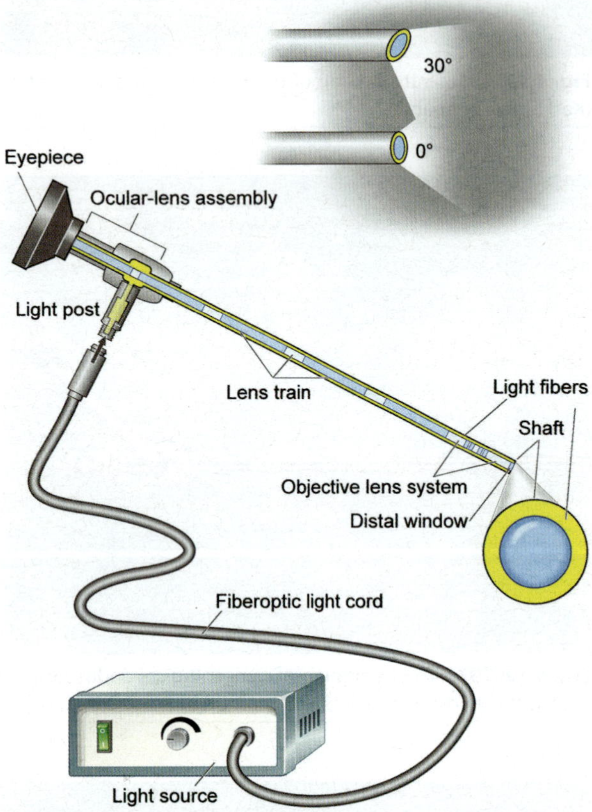

Fig. 4.14: Light post—Fiber-optic light cords are attached to the scope at this site.

Light fibers—Glass fibers that carry light from the light post to the distal end of the scope.

Objective lens system—A collection of lenses, windows, and/or prisms located at the distal end of the scope. The distal objective can be manufactured at angles ranging from 0 to 120°, which enables the operator to see areas that might otherwise be out of view.

Lens train—A series of glass rod lenses and spacers that transfer the image through the shaft.

Shaft—Stainless steel tube that houses the lens train.

Ocular lens assembly—The focusing lens of the scope located near the proximal end of the scope.

Eyepiece—The eyepiece is located at the proximal end of the scope. The image can be viewed through the scope, or the eyepiece can be attached to a camera coupler to view the image on an external monitor.

laparoscope depends on the surgeon's preference and its local availability. Thus, it is also dependent on the availability of resources. The large majority of operations can be performed with a 0° optical instrument. In specific situations, such as removal of the uterus in laparoscopic hysterectomy or exposure deep into the pelvic wall in cases of deep infiltrating endometriosis, the 30° endoscope provides a better view. It permits targeted viewing in a specific direction, which would be less clear under 0° conditions (Figs. 4.16 to 4.19).

Structure of the Rigid Endoscope

The rigid endoscope is a solid metal tube with two channels, containing an ocular or a connecting device to the camera at its proximal end and a camera lens at its distal end, which takes the intraoperative picture and transfers it through a lens system or a chip system. The essential elements of a laparoscope are shown in Figures 4.11 and 4.14.

The first channel of the laparoscope forms a ring along its outer margin and contains bundled glass fibers coursing longitudinally along the laparoscope and transferring light from an external light source to the tip of the endoscope.

The second and central channel consists of several rod lenses made of quartz glass, which conducts light. Light is refracted at the air lenses between the rods. Owing to the powerful light, very small lens diameters are sufficient. In modern endoscopes the central channel is connected to a camera system. Digital chip systems in the camera allow the surgical

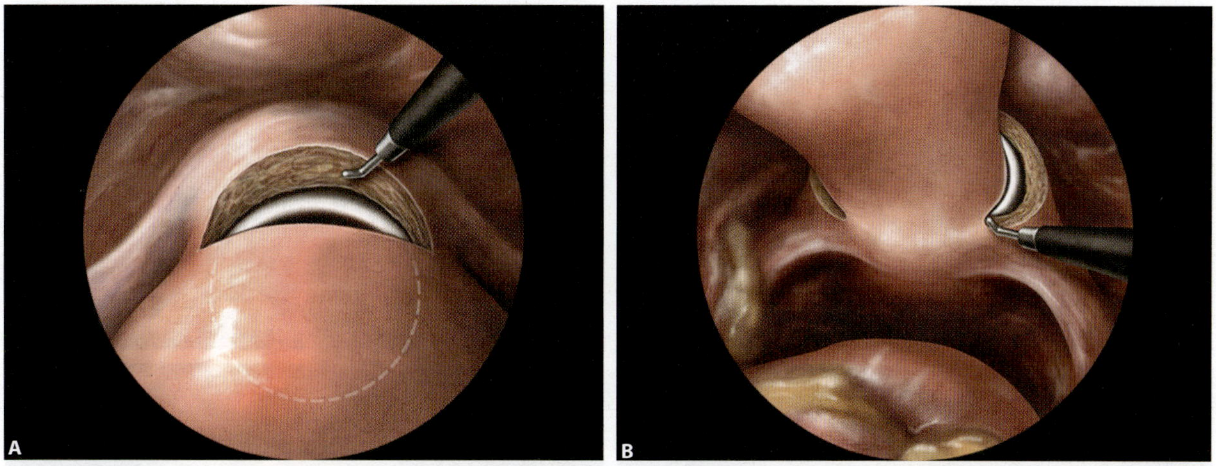

Figs. 4.16A and B: Schematic illustration of uterine dissection. (A) Colpotomy is usually started in the anterior part, on the palpable manipulator cap; (B) Intrafascial hysterectomy can be completed with the sacrouterine ligaments in view.

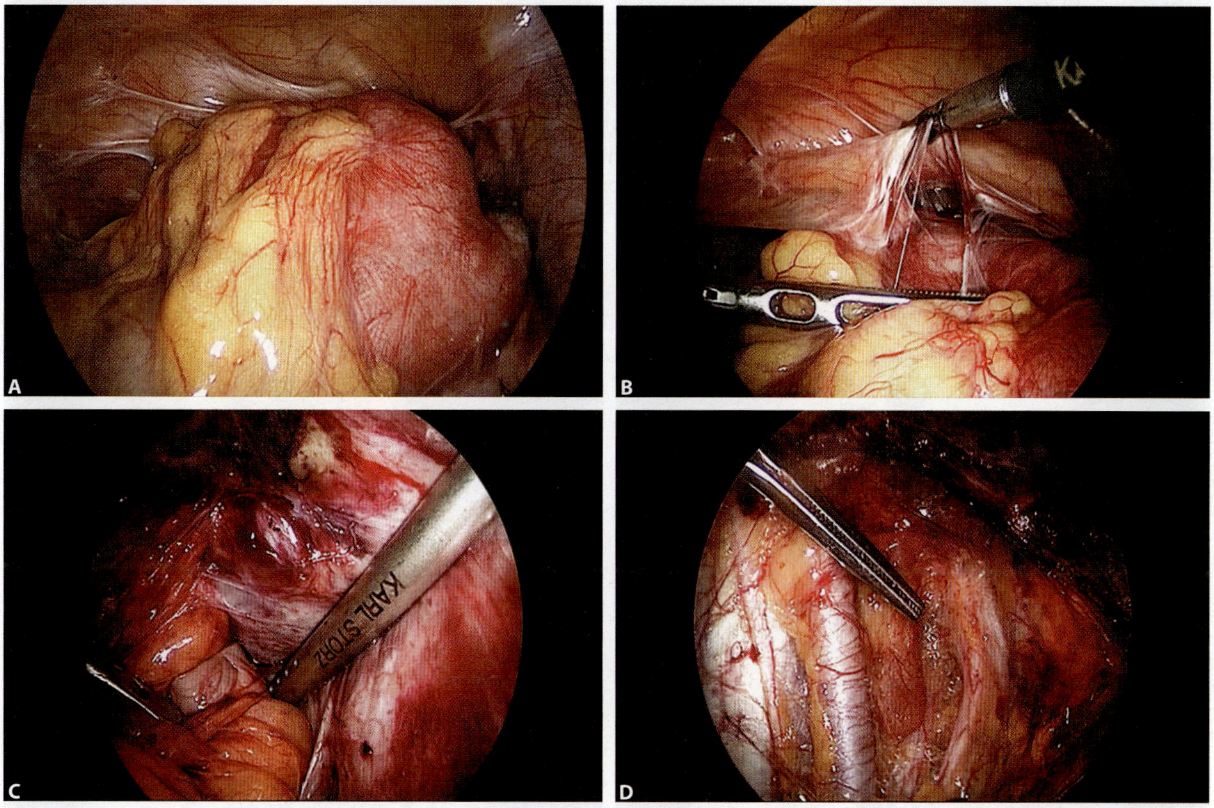

Figs. 4.17A to D: (A) A case of severe adenomyosis of the uterus with subsequent adhesions of the bowel; (B) The bladder peritoneum; (C) Access to the lateral aspect of the uterus is closed; (D) Retroperitoneal access is necessary.

image to be transferred to an external monitor. The diameter of rigid endoscopes ranges between 3 and 12 mm thinner endoscopes provide a weaker image because much less light is able to pass through the central channel.

The lens system is located at the distal end. It may be straight (0°) or angulated (to 120°). The angulation permits the surgeon to view intra-abdominal objects, which would otherwise be outside his or her image frame. The 0° optic system provides a panoramic view while the angulated lens provides viewing angles that permit the surgeon to operate around the targeted surgical structures and work in deeper regions under direct viewing (Figs. 4.20 and 4.21).

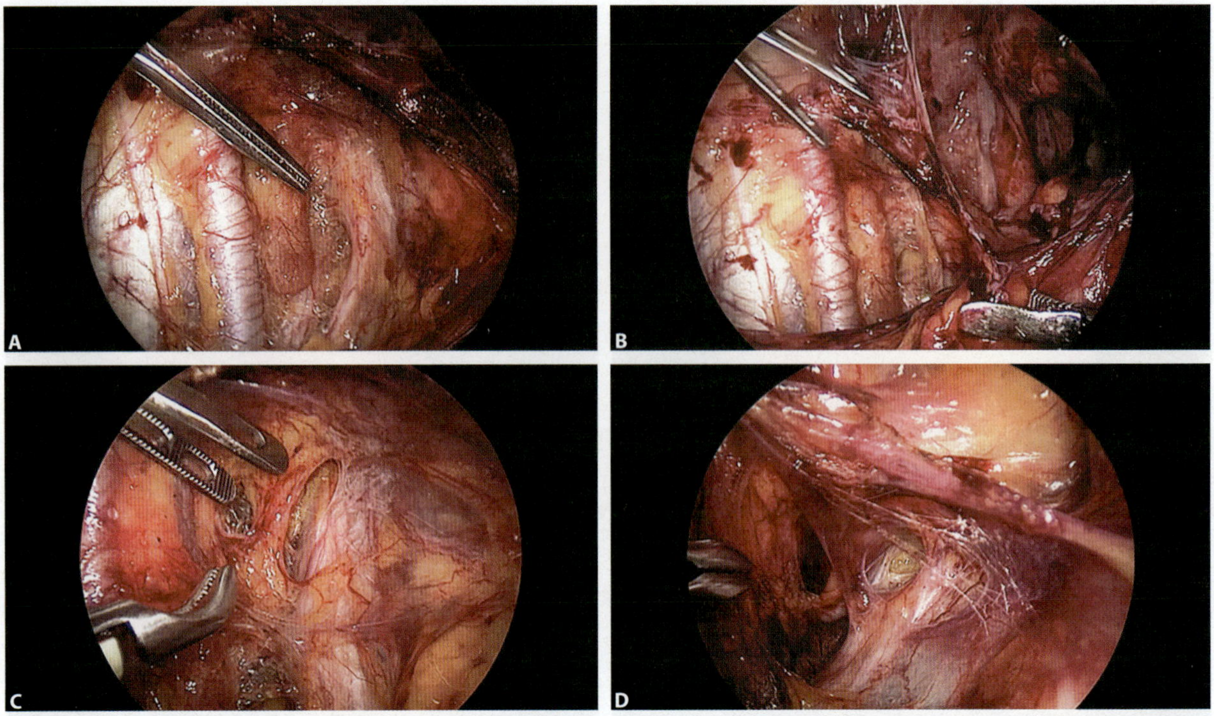

Figs. 4.18A to D: (A) After localization of the external iliac artery, the ureter is usually found adherent to the peritoneum. A major lymph node lies in between; (B) Opening the pararectal and; (C) the paravesical fossa; (D) The crossing point of the uterine artery is demarcated, and the ureter is left in its adventitia to avoid skeletonizing and denudation.

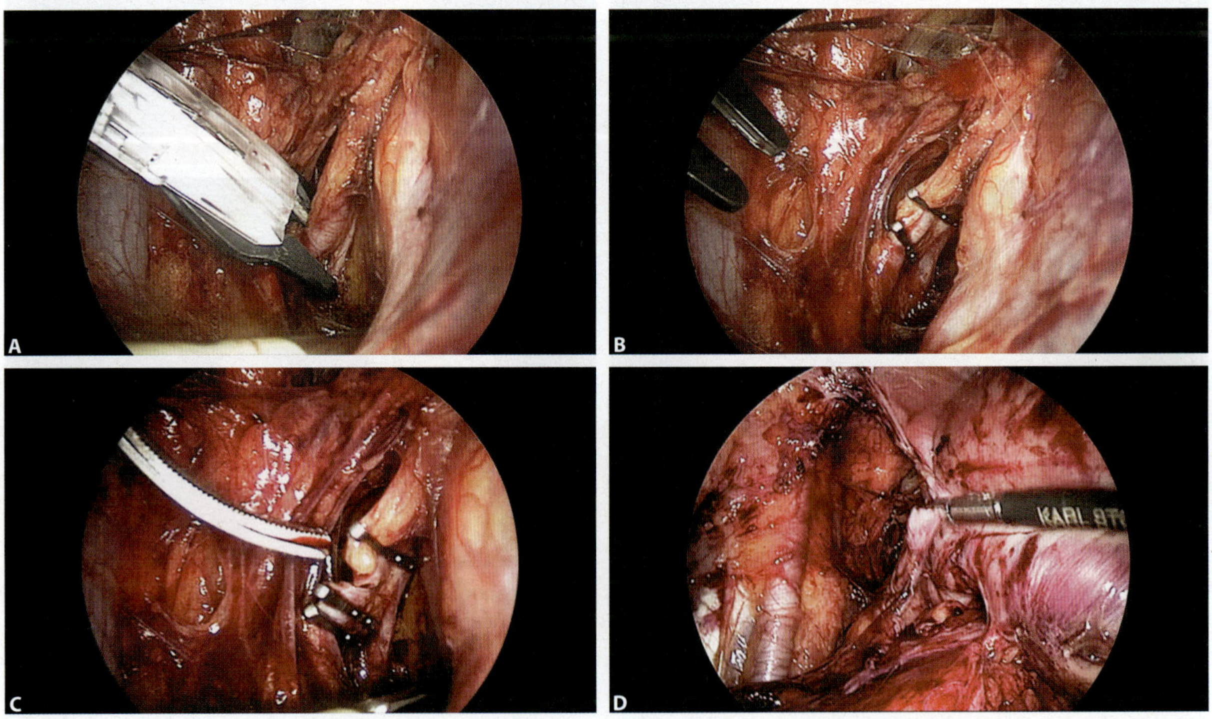

Figs. 4.19A to D: (A and B) Clips can be inserted and the artery can be closed and cut; (C) The uterine vein (deep) is seen just beneath the cut artery; (D) Overview of the exposed situs. To the right you see the uncolored uterus after closure of both arteries.

Light Source and Fiber Optics

Adequate illumination is a prerequisite for a safe operation. In the large majority of endoscopes, the light source is outside the operating field because it needs more space and is subject to excessive warming when in use. Usually xenon lamps are used. These are expensive and do not last long. The technique of

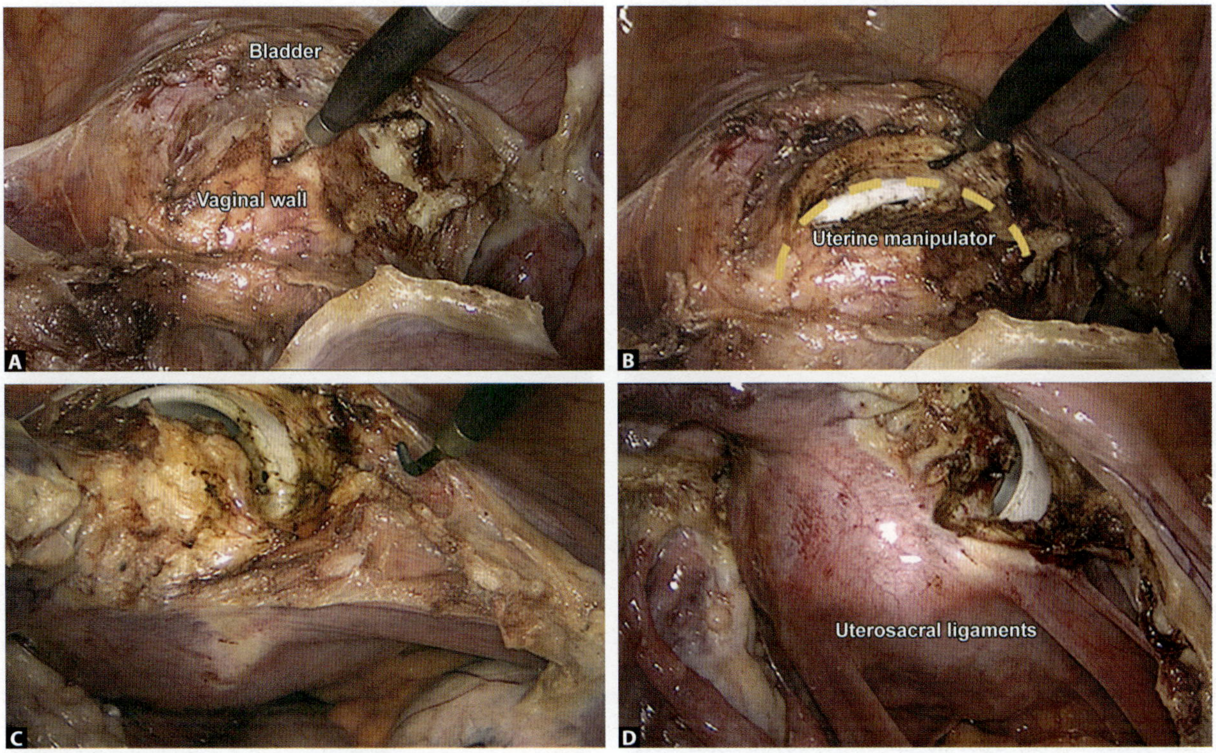

Figs. 4.20A to D: In this case of LTH, the distance between the vagina and the bladder is increased because of exposure of the bladder peritoneum (A); The intrauterine manipulator is firmly placed in the abdomen and dissection of the uterus from the vagina is performed in a stepwise manner (B–D). The conjunction of the sacrouterine ligaments is left in place.

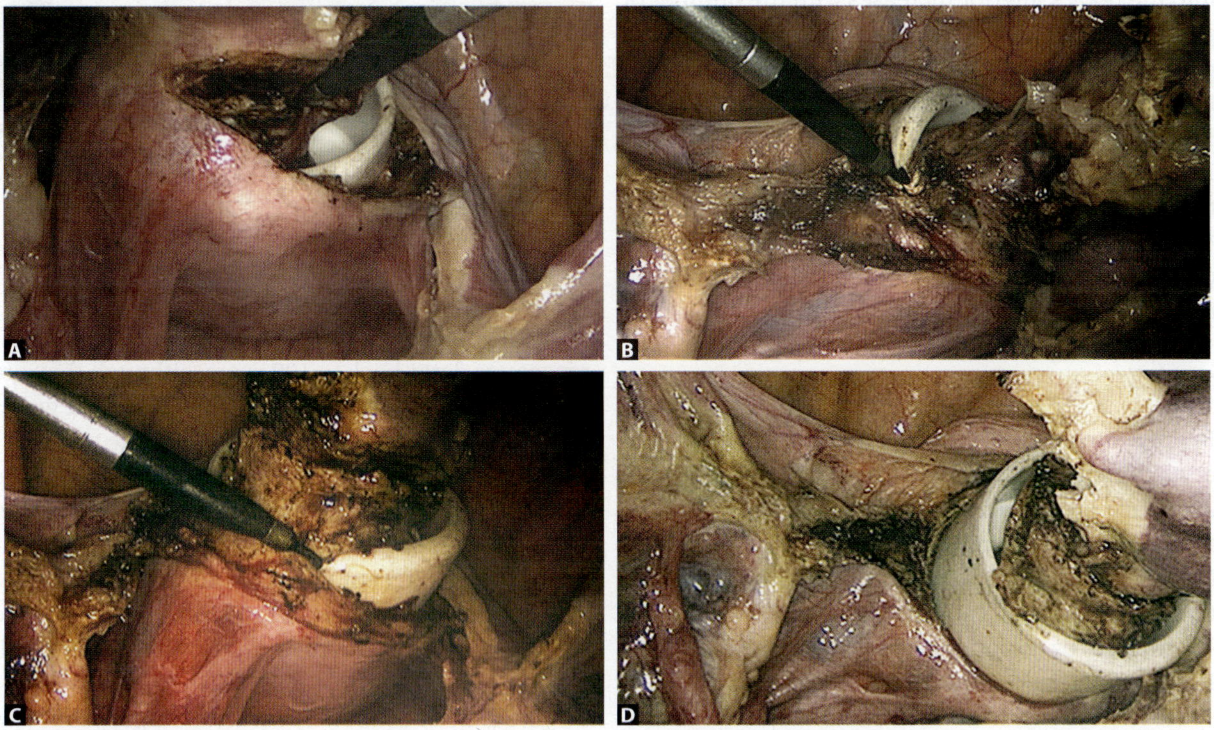

Figs. 4.21A to D: Completion of the dissection of the vagina from the cervix (A to C) and commencement of retraction of the uterine cervix, still grasped by the manipulator forceps, transvaginally. Excessive lens fogging caused by the monopolar current and the sharpness of the monopolar hook makes it necessary to perform precise exposure under full vision. This can be done during simultaneous retraction/manipulation with the use of the 30° optic device. The surgeon's vision may worsen immediately when CO_2 gas leaks through the colpotomy. Visibility may then become extremely poor and the use of monopolar energy hazardous; (D) Final dissection of vagina from cervix to be added at the end.

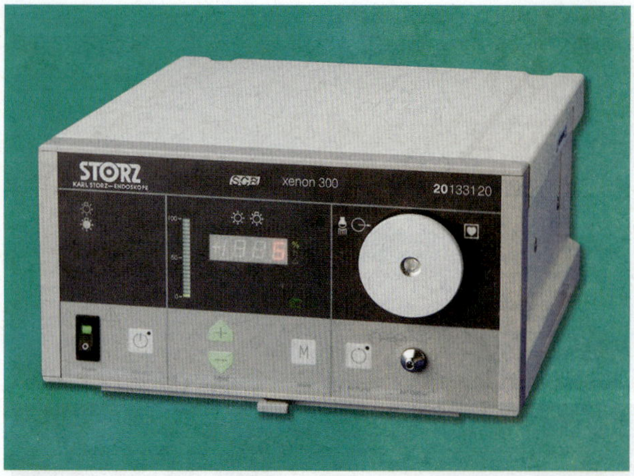

Fig. 4.22: Cold light fountain XENON 300 (Karl Storz Company).

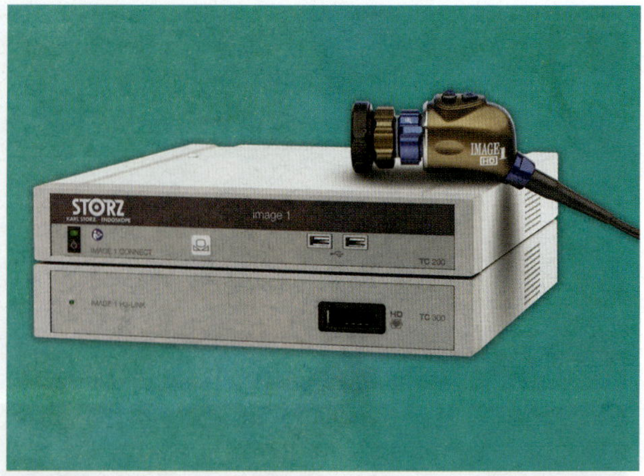

Fig. 4.23: Full high-definition (HD) camera system (Karl Storz Company).

light-emitting diode (LED) lamp system has created entirely new options and is an interesting alternative for experimental applications (Fig. 4.22).

Image Conductors

Fiber glass serves best as an endoscopic light conductor. Gel-filled fiber optics are an alternative; they provide greater luminous efficacy, but cannot be bended and are more expensive. Light transmission into the body's interior increases with the number of glass fibers, their diameter, and the quantity of supplied energy. Image conductors consist of several thousand glass fibers with a thickness of 7–10 μm. Thus, one achieves 3,000 to 42,000 or 75 × 45 to 240 × 180 pixels. Every fiber is able to transmit information about brightness as well as color.

The camera head is provided with an image processor and a mechanical zoom function as well as a focus ring (Fig. 4.23).

Three-Dimensional Imaging

In open surgery as well as in our normal lives, we are accustomed to 3D images. Getting accustomed to the 2D image is one of the greatest challenges faced by surgeons learning minimally invasive surgery. The image is reduced to two dimensions. Depth perception is impossible. The third dimension has to be substituted by experience and imaginative power. However, 3D endoscopy permits the surgeon to view space in a similar fashion as natural vision. This bears the promise of a shorter learning curve, shorter operating times, and fewer complications. Most of all, a 3D endoscope is able to delineate complex structures more clearly, including their location and their relative position in the body.

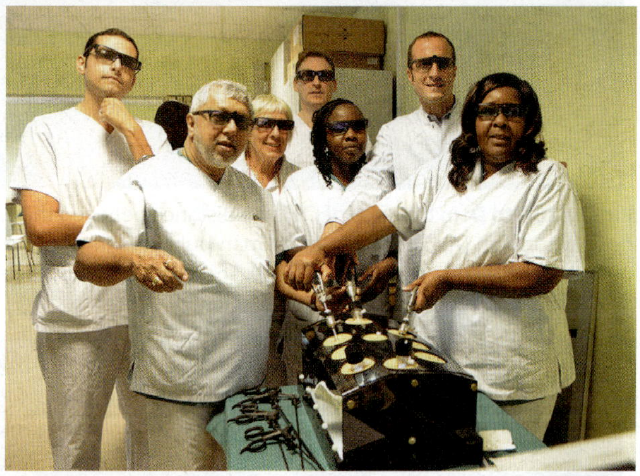

Fig. 4.24: Drilling on the 3D trainer of Karl Storz Company at the Kiel School of Gynaecological Endoscopy.

Special camera systems or so-called stereoscopes utilize two adjacent imaging systems that correspond to the human eye. The development of stereoscopes dates back to 100 years, although they are still not used everywhere. The persistent and greatest technical handicap is the type of image transmission that will permit the human brain to perceive the image three-dimensionally. Wearing 3D glasses is an option, although inconvenient in the operative setup (Fig. 4.24). Recent technical advancements have made it possible to transfer 3D images without the use of 3D glasses. However, such visualization is still in its initial stages and not established everywhere.

The part of minimally invasive surgery that was focused from the very start on 3D work was robotic surgery. Two separate cameras are used within a single optic instrument, and these simulate the human eye. The image is optimized digitally and then transferred to the operation console. The surgeon views

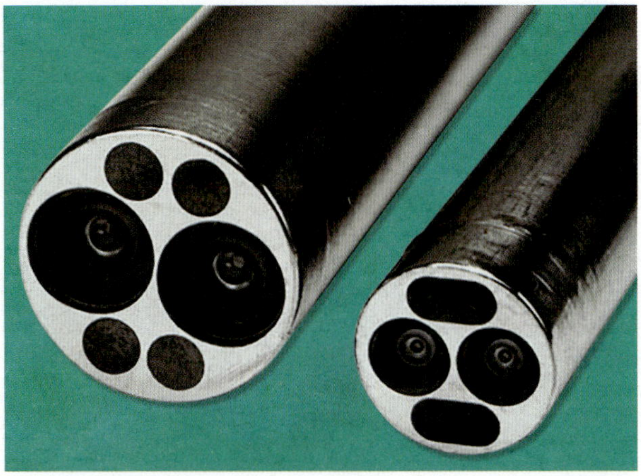

Fig. 4.25: DaVinci Optical system in two sizes. Two adjacent systems within a single optical device provide a three-dimensional image (Intuitive Surgical Company).

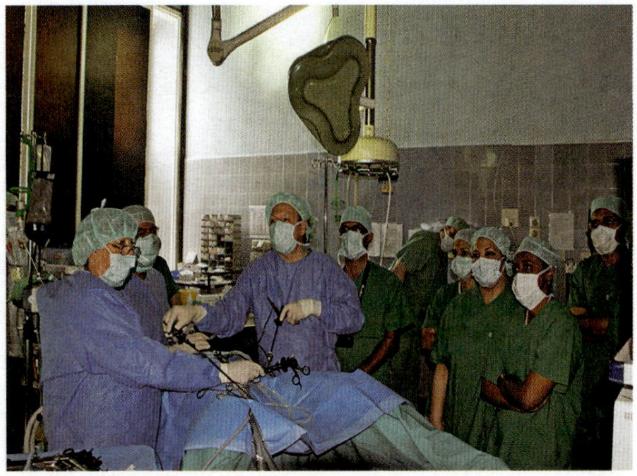

Fig. 4.27: Operation during a training course at the Kiel School of Gynaecological Laparoscopy. The surgeon on the left, the assistant to the patient's right, the operating room nurse to the patient's right, and the anesthetist at the patient's head.

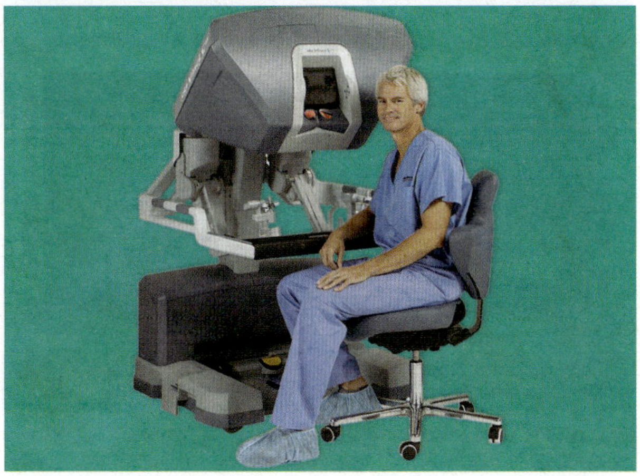

Fig. 4.26: The operation can be viewed with the DaVinci device three-dimensionally by the surgeon when both images are available in processed form at the operation console. The assistant and other observers view the operation in two dimensions (Intuitive Surgical Company).

the 3D image; a monitor is provided for each eye. The forerunner of 3D imaging was the Da Vinci robotic surgical system of Intuitive Company (Figs. 4.25 and 4.26). However, 3D imaging and image transmission are now possible even in conventional laparoscopy.

OPERATING TEAM AND GENERAL INSTRUMENTS

Team

In the usual case the surgeon stands to the patient's left, the camera operator to the surgeon's right, the surgery nurse next to the camera operator, and a second assistant (if needed) between the patient's legs. In certain operations the surgeon stands between the patient's legs and a second assistant next to the surgeon (Fig. 4.27). The anesthetist's position is at the patient's head.

Devices

The devices are positioned such that the surgeon has the most suitable and ergonomic viewing angle to look at the monitor and the other devices on the stack; in most cases this position is between the patient's legs. The monitor is at eye level so the surgeon is able to keep his or her head in a relaxed position. The insufflation devices and the light source are located beneath the monitor, with the suction/irrigation device below. The generator is positioned separately. A stand-in provides any additional instruments that may be needed, if necessary arranged on a separate instrument table.

Insufflation: Pressure regulation is essential for the insufflation of CO_2; this avoids excessively high-pressure peaks or relevant pressure drops. Pre-warming the gas prevents fogging of the optics in the event of a strong gas exchange and is also believed to reduce subphrenic pain postoperatively. The insufflation device shows the IAP (current value), flow per minute, gas reserve, and the total volume of consumed CO_2. The target value can be set manually on the device; it should not exceed 15 mm Hg. IPA may be maximized only at the start of the operation (establishment of the pneumoperitoneum and the introduction of working trocars). However, ventilation is limited under these conditions and sudden bradycardias may occur.

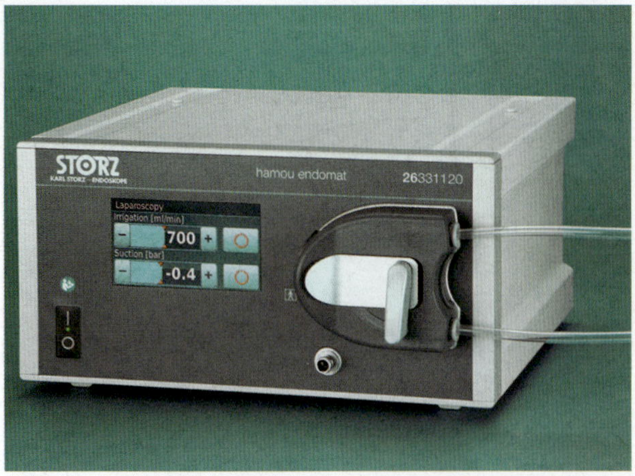

Fig. 4.28: HAMOU® ENDOMAT® (Karl Storz Company).

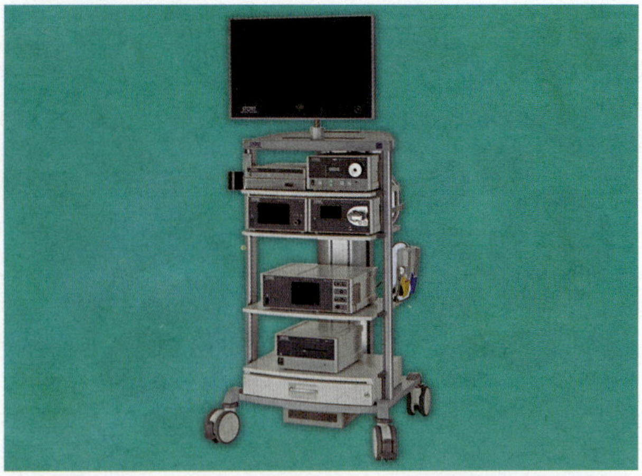

Fig. 4.30: Fully equipped trolley for laparoscopy (Karl Storz Company).

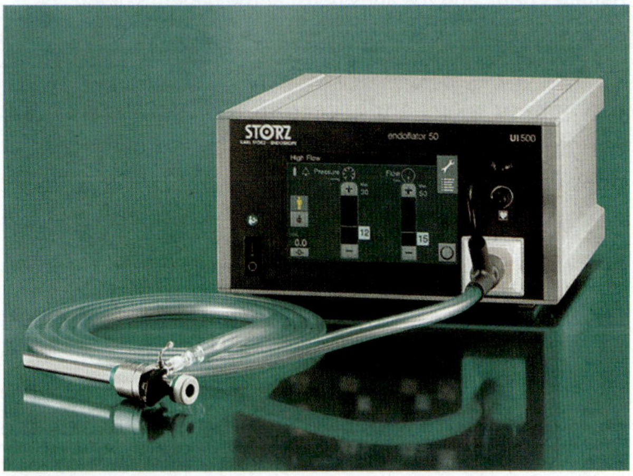

Fig. 4.29: ENDOFLATOR® 50 (Karl Storz Company).

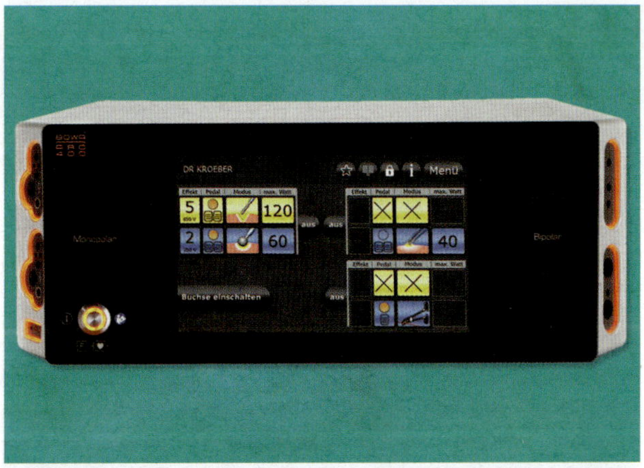

Fig. 4.31: ARC 400, high-frequency generator of Bowa Company.

Suction/irrigation device: Fluid has to be introduced (irrigation) or removed (suction) in many operations (hysteroscopy and laparoscopy). Suction/aspiration devices are provided with a combination of both functions. Warmed irrigation fluid prevents fogging of the optics as well as hypothermia in the patient (Figs. 4.28 to 4.30).

Electric current is provided by a high-frequency (HF) generator (Fig. 4.31) and conducted through a neutral null electrode (Fig. 4.32).

Physics of High-frequency Surgery

In the large majority of endoscopic operations, electric current is used to expose tissue and achieve hemostasis. Knowledge of the underlying physical phenomena is essential in order to use electric current meaningfully as well as estimate and avoid potential risks.

The use of electrosurgery is based on the fact that the human body conducts HF alternating current. The flow of electric current through tissue causes three specific effects:

- *Faraday effect:* The flow of electric current stimulates electrically stimulable cells (muscles and nerves), which causes muscle contractions. The application of alternating current at frequencies above 300 kHz is able to prevent this undesirable effect.
- *Electrolytic effect:* Direct current causes the migration of positive ions to the cathode and negative ions to the anode. In human tissue this effect causes cell damage. However, alternating current at sufficiently high frequencies prevents this effect and causes no more than an occasional ion oscillation.
- *Thermal effect:* The flow of electric current warms human tissue. This is dependent on tissue resistance, current density and exposure time. The thermal effect is the sole desired effect when using electric currents in HF surgery, and is the basis of operative endoscopy.

No relevant cell damage occurs until 40°C. Depending on the duration of exposure, reversible damage of tissue occurs between 40 and 49°C. Irreversible cell damage occurs at temperatures above 49°C. Such damage is caused by the coagulation of cell proteins. Initially the cell matrix remains intact, although individual cells may have perished already. Such damage can be compensated, depending on the regeneration potential of the tissue. Temperatures above 60°C cause desiccation due to the evaporation of intracellular and extracellular water. As long as water particles are present, the tissue temperature remains below the boiling point of 100°C, then rises, and is followed by carbonization effects (blackish discoloration of tissue) (Fig. 4.33).

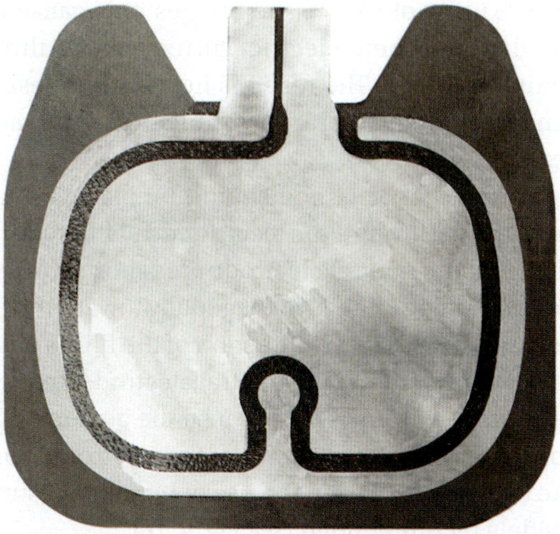

Fig. 4.32: Bowa Easy Universal neutral electrode. Depending on the operating field, the neutral electrode should be placed on the closest upper arm or thigh, but no closer than 20 cm from the operating field and at a sufficient distance from electrocardiographic (ECG) electrodes or implants (such as bone screws, bone plates, or endoprostheses). The neutral electrode should be placed on the supine patient, on the upper side of the body, not in the vicinity of body fluids and also at a distance from the region of sterile washing.

High-frequency surgery employs alternating current of 300,000 to 1,000,000 Hz. The thermal effect is also the therapeutic effect.

Electrocoagulation

A coagulation effect occurs when tissue is heated rather slowly to more than 60°C. Several changes occur during this "boiling" process, such as the denaturation of protein, the evaporation of intracellular and extracellular water, and shrinkage of tissue. Depending on the quality of the current and the type of application, a distinction is made in HF surgery between contact coagulation, forced coagulation, desiccation (coagulation through a pierced needle electrode), spray coagulation (fulguration), argon plasma coagulation (APC), bipolar coagulation and bipolar vessel sealing.

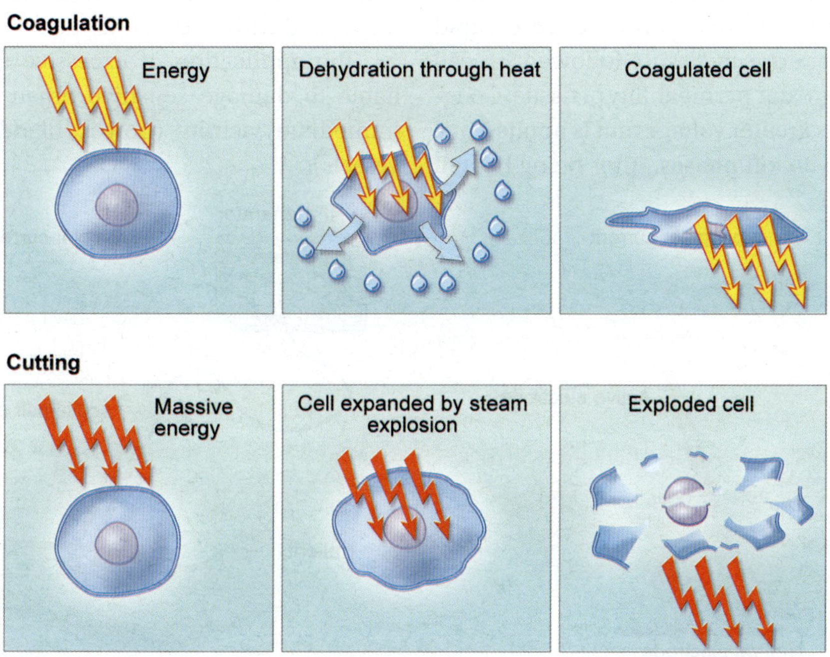

Fig. 4.33: Effects on the individual cell, depending on the electric current used.

Electrotomy

A cutting effect is achieved by rapid heating of tissue to more than 90–100°C. This causes steam in cells, which tears the cell walls and then acts as an insulator. Cutting tension is created between the electrode and tissue, causing (renewed) transmission of sparks from about 200 V onward. A very high current density is present at the base points. The surroundings (air, fluid) are of no importance for the formation of this electric arc. Modulation of the electricity (increased voltage with interruptions) causes additional coagulation of the wound margins. Depending on the intensity, a distinction is made between a smooth incision and a scabbed incision. Further thermal effects of electricity, of secondary importance in HF surgery, include carbonization (from about 200°C onward) and vaporization (at several hundred degrees Celsius) (*see* Fig. 4.31).

Monopolar Technique

When using monopolar electric current, the patient's body is within the electrical circuit (Fig. 4.34). The electric current is made to contact tissue through an active electrode, flows through the body, and departs from the body through a neutral electrode. The ratio of surfaces (active electrode and passive electrode) is shifted in favor of the active electrode, which enhances the thermal effect of the greater current density at this site. The electric current used for resection has a sinewave vibration of relatively low voltage amplitude. This causes a very rapid increase of temperature in tissue, followed by cell vaporization and greater permeability of tissue. Coagulation current has greater voltage and is applied in a rapid exchange of on–off phases. After being heated in the on-phase, the tissue is able to cool in the off-phase. This alternation causes slow tissue heating, which is manifested as coagulation.

Defects in the insulation of instruments or trocars may cause direct coupling of electricity and undetected tissue damage. Likewise, coagulation in the proximity of thin tissue bridges may cause thermal defects when electric current flows through the tissue bridge. The result is heat and undesirable damage at a considerable distance from the actual area of surgery.

The neutral electrode should be placed at a site where the pathway of the electric current between the active and the neutral electrode is as short as possible and runs longitudinally or diagonally toward the body because muscles in the direction of the fibrils possess greater conductivity. The neutral electrode must be in full contact with the skin because the generated heat is proportional to the surface of the electrode. For the sake of safety, however, the use of bipolar HF surgery is widely recommended (*see* Fig. 4.32).

Bipolar Technique

Even in bipolar electricity, warmth is produced in an electric circuit. However, the active and the neutral electrodes are as close to each other as possible and possess the same mass. Thus, only the operating field (tissue between the two branches) and not the entire patient is within the electric circuit. Activation of the electric current causes warming of tissue and coagulation. Therefore, the neutral electrode can be dispensed with (Fig. 4.35).

The application of excessive thermal energy is liable to damage sensitive organ structures in the immediate vicinity (bowel, bladder, ureter, blood vessels).

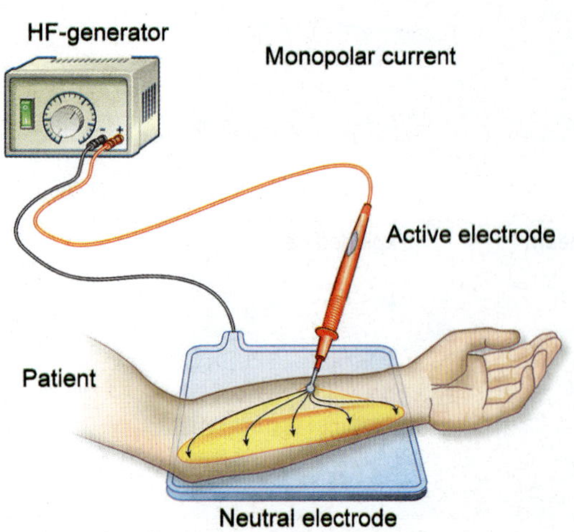

Fig. 4.34: Principle of monopolar current.

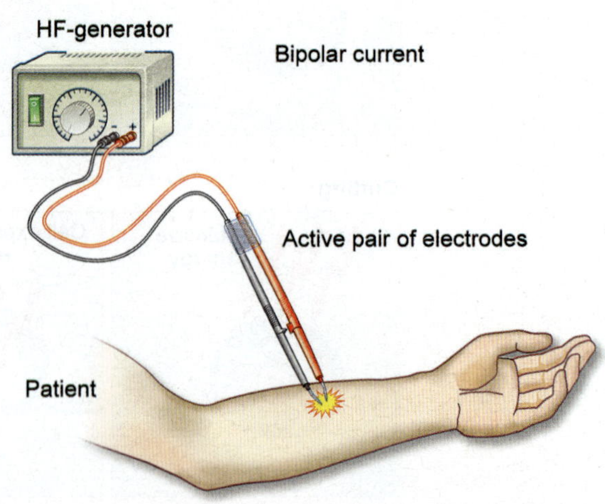

Fig. 4.35: Principle of bipolar current.

Techniques of monopolar and bipolar current are used in laparoscopy as well as hysteroscopy. The application of monopolar current in hysteroscopy permits precise exposure, but at the expense of a higher risk of electrolyte imbalance due to the obligatory use of electrolyte-free solutions.

SPECIAL INSTRUMENTS

Hysteroscopy

The diagnostic hysteroscope is provided with a separate small working channel for exposure and surgery. Microscissors or forceps can be introduced through this working channel. Through a loop, a hook, or a barrel and with bipolar or monopolar current, tissue can be resected and coagulated in a targeted manner (Figs. 4.36 to 4.40). Advancements in hysteroscopy have made it possible to use smaller instruments (office or mini-hysteroscopy) and thus achieve an entirely atraumatic intrauterine access without previous dilatation or anesthesia.

Laparoscopy

Some instruments developed specifically for laparoscopy are introduced in the following, with a few examples of their evolution over the last decades and their future prospects. Overcoming the limits of the 2D image by improving 3D optics has been an essential step in rendering endoscopic operations safer and easier to learn. Two-dimensional projection still is one of the prime arguments against endoscopic surgery compared to the open surgical approach. Having resolved this major problem, one of the prime goals now is to eliminate the handicap of limited degrees of movement by appropriate technical innovations. Open surgery permits seven degrees of freedom for the hands. Endoscopic

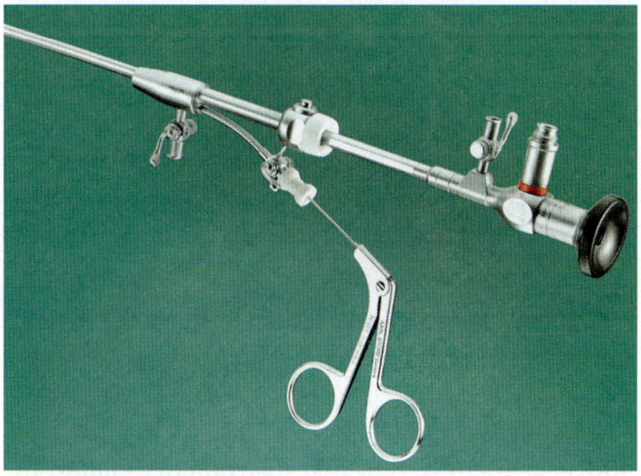

Fig. 4.36: Three Campo Trophyscope® with a 5 Charr. instrument (Karl Storz Company).

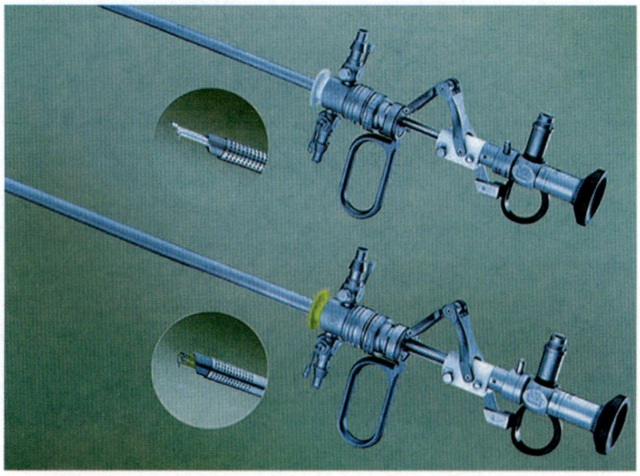

Fig. 4.37: Operative hysteroscope with the corresponding inlay (Karl Storz Company).

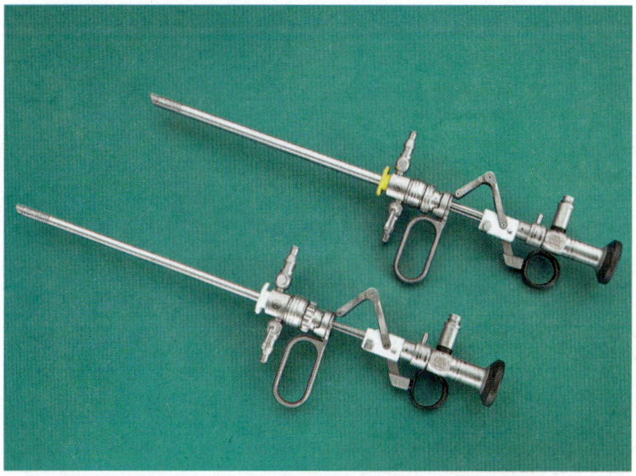

Fig. 4.38: Five Bipolar resectoscopes (22 and 26 Charr.) (Karl Storz Company).

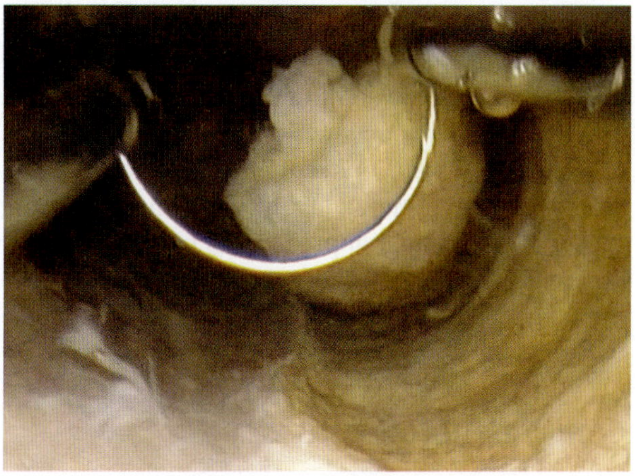

Fig. 4.39: Hysteroscopic chip removal from the uterine wall.

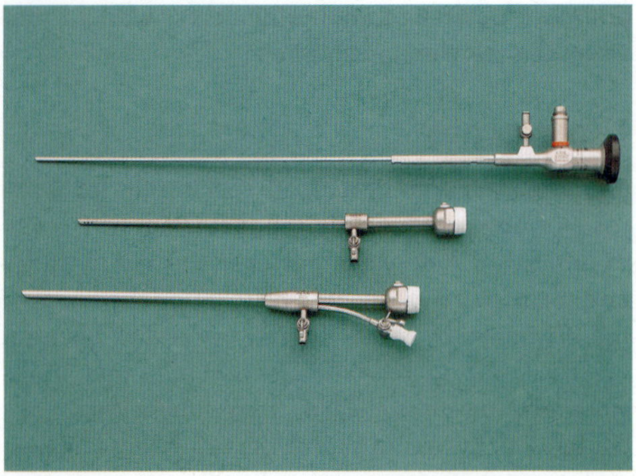

Fig. 4.40: Campo Trophyscope® with a diagnostic and surgical shaft (Karl Storz Company).

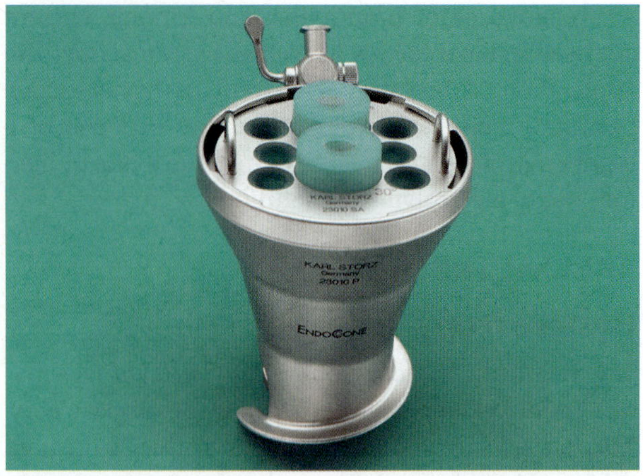

Fig. 4.41: Single-port system of Karl Storz Company (Endocone).

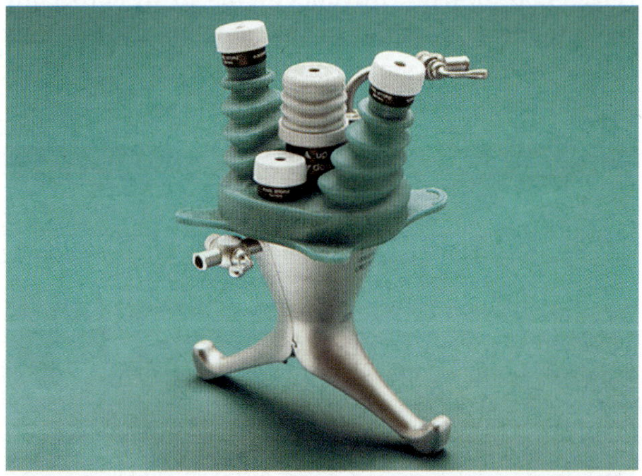

Fig. 4.42: Single-port system of Karl Storz Company (XCone).

instruments, on the other hand, provide only four degrees of freedom. This problem was overcome by robotic-assisted surgery. All conventional attempts (such as those of Terumo Company) have not been able to gain acceptance so far. Therefore, the development of instruments and their innovative options are of decisive importance for the user.

Single-port Laparoscopy

Single-port laparoscopy has not been fully accepted yet. The main advantage of introducing the optics and the working instruments through a single trocar, which is usually placed in a subumbilical location, is that it prevents further scars. These application systems are now provided by the large majority of companies in various forms (Figs. 4.1B, 4.41 to 4.43). The disadvantage of this technique, however, is the much larger incision, which calls for an open entry technique and obligatory fascial closure. Furthermore, the desirable open angle for the instruments cannot be achieved per se. The instruments are introduced in very close proximity to each other so that the angles between the working trocars as well as the angle between the working trocars and the optics is very sharp. This renders handling of instruments more complex and involves a new learning curve. Therefore, the approach has not been widely accepted despite the fact that angulated instruments and bent shafts have largely overcome these barriers.

Conventional Laparoscopy

Karl Storz Company introduced the first collapsible instruments in the 1990s (Fig. 4.44). More precise and user-friendly reusable instruments enable the surgeon to perform delicate and complex operations (Figs. 4.45 to 4.53). As regards the future, the question remains as to whether reducing the size of instruments for “mini-laparoscopy” will gain widespread acceptance (Fig. 4.54).

Complex anatomical structures which are usually difficult to access (Figs. 4.55 and 4.56) can be visualized well when using high-resolution laparoscopes equipped with several-fold magnification. The surgical view (Fig. 4.57) is shared equally by all surgeons. This signifies much better work in the surgical team compared to open or vaginal surgery. Thus, many operations can be performed very precisely with minimal bleeding while ensuring tissue protection, as shown here in an instance of myoma enucleation with reconstruction of the uterine wall (Figs. 4.58 to 4.63). The combination of angulated optical instruments, magnification, and the

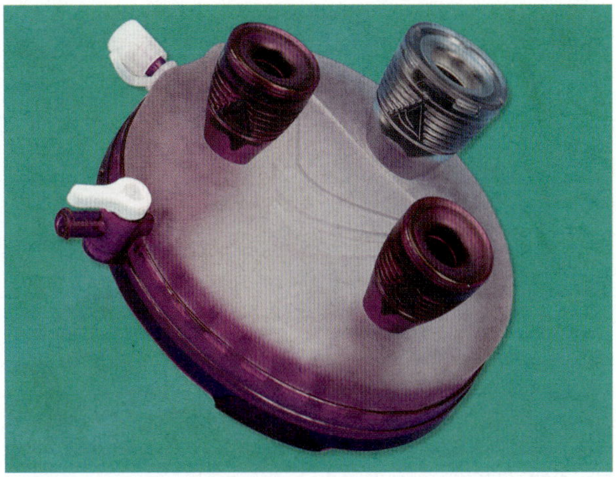

Fig. 4.43: GelPOINT advanced access platform. The GelPOINT advanced access platform permits a single-incision approach by facilitating the triangulation of standard instrumentation through a single incision, while potentially enhancing the cosmetic outcome for the patient. By offering a larger range of motion, the GelPOINT platform provides maximum versatility and access for a wide range of procedures. The GelPOINT platform accommodates a variety of abdominal wall and incision sizes, provides continuous access, and ensures better articulation of 5-mm to 12-mm instruments (Applied Medical).

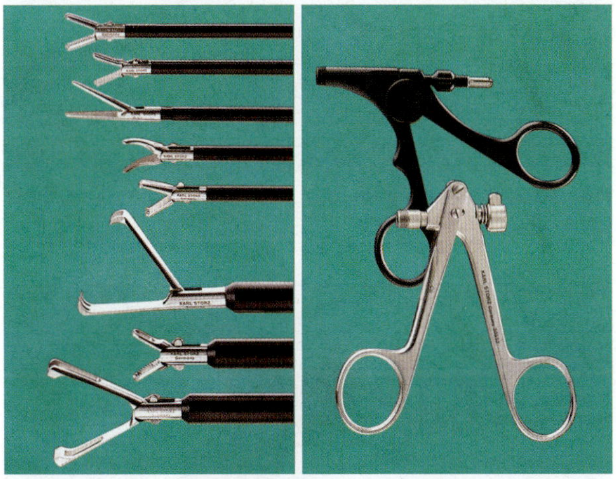

Fig. 4.44: 1992: Karl Storz Company introduced the first collapsible TAKE-APART® manual instruments for laparoscopy (Karl Storz Company).

variable proximity of the optics to the target organ is also helpful. Even in complex situations (such as voluminous organs, adhesions, endometriosis or obesity) this permits safe surgery when using the appropriate working instruments. Once the learning curve has been overcome, the surgical steps that were initially time-consuming can be performed very well with the appropriate instruments, as demonstrated here in a total laparoscopy hysterectomy of a large myomatous uterus (Figs. 4.64 to 4.70).

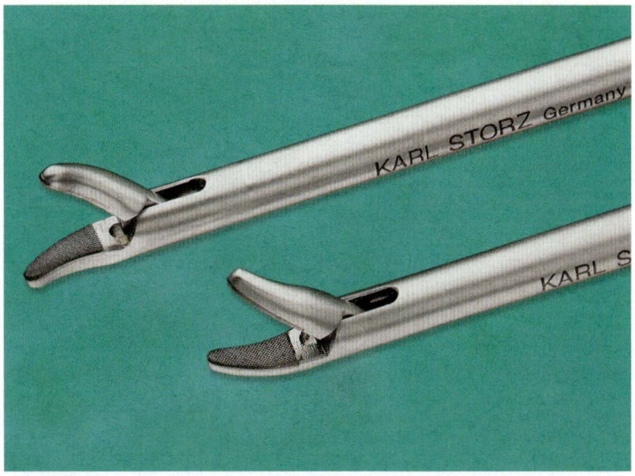

Fig. 4.45: Koh macro needle holder (jaws) (Karl Storz Company).

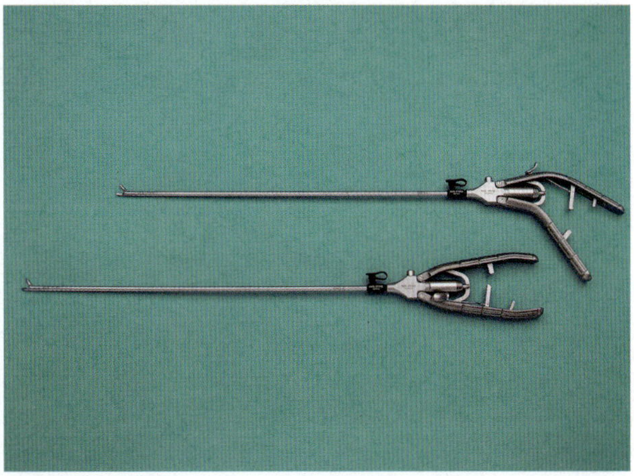

Fig. 4.46: Koh macro needle holder (complete) (Karl Storz Company).

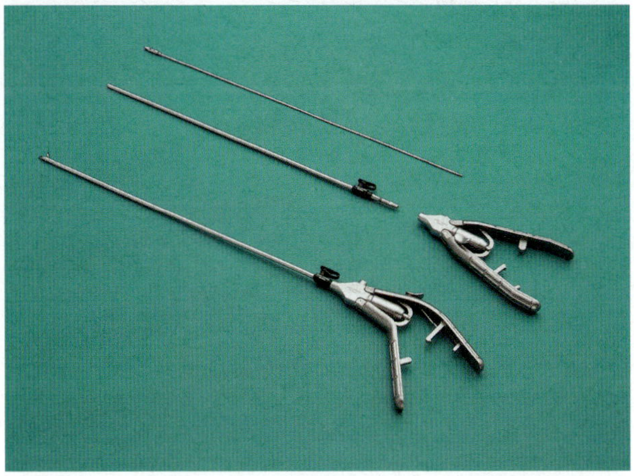

Fig. 4.47: Koh macro needle holder (taken apart) (Karl Storz Company).

Vessel Sealing

Vessels beyond a diameter of about 2 mm cannot be treated by conventional electrocoagulation.

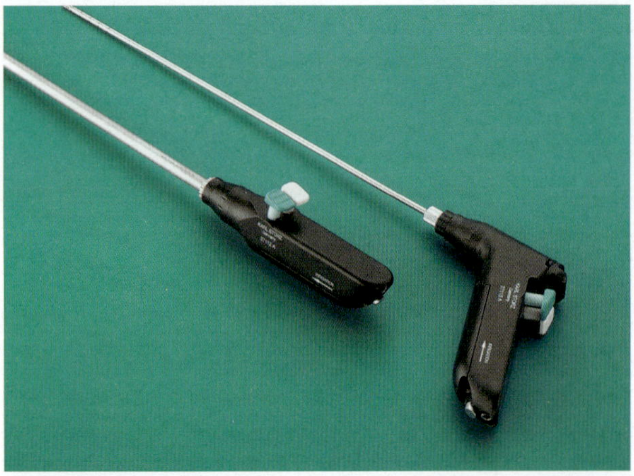

Fig. 4.48: Suction-irrigation tube (Karl Storz Company).

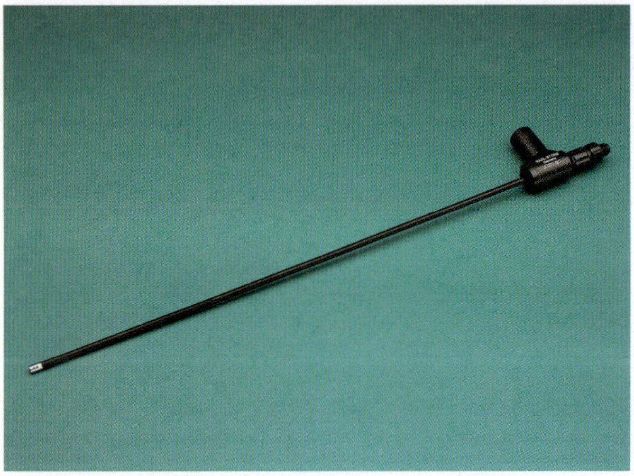

Fig. 4.49: Suction-irrigation tube (Karl Storz Company).

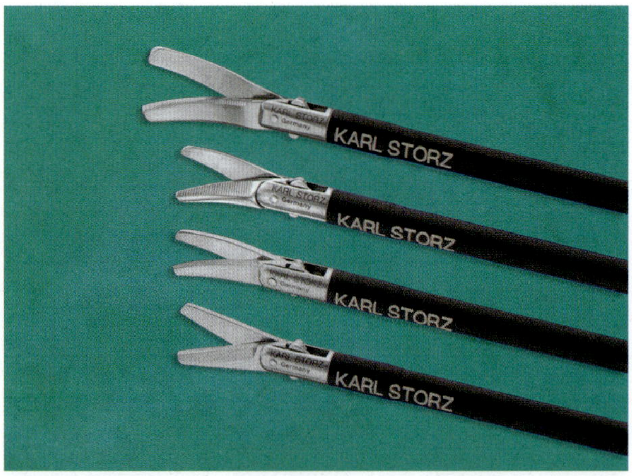

Fig. 4.50: CLICKline scissors (Karl Storz Company).

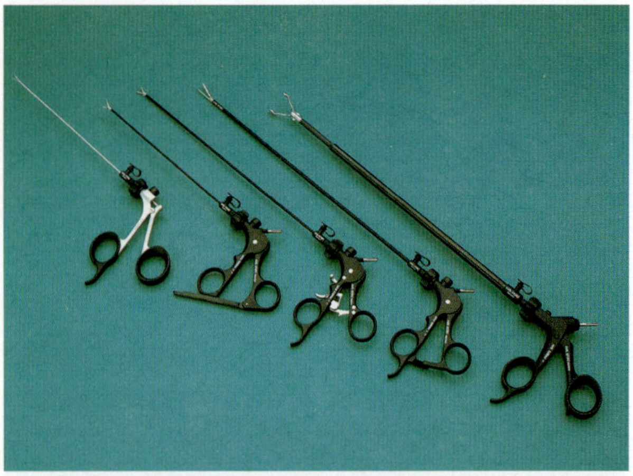

Fig. 4.51: CLICKline set (Karl Storz Company).

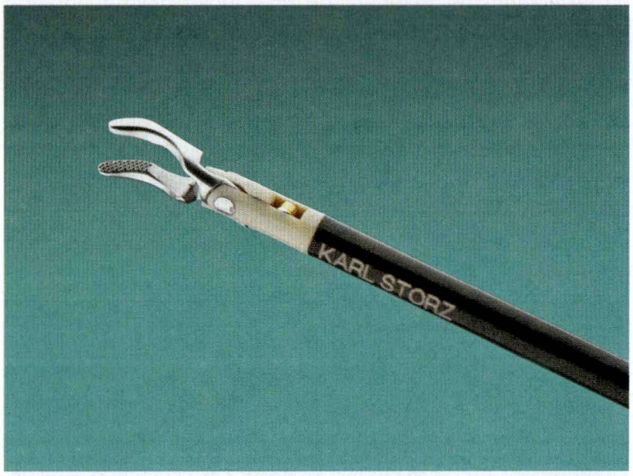

Fig. 4.52: RoBi Kelly bipolar Overholt clamp (Karl Storz Company).

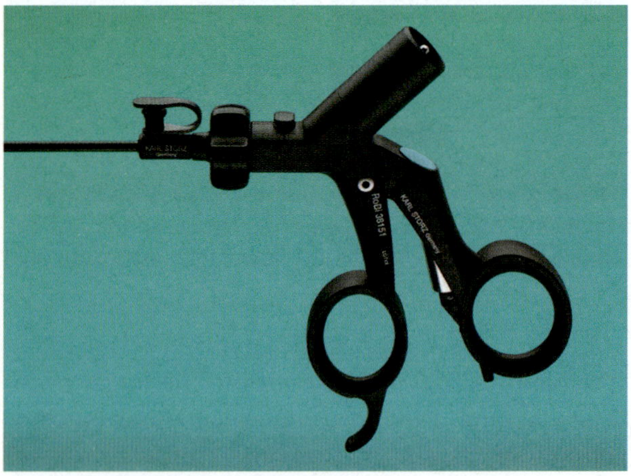

Fig. 4.53: RoBi Kelly handgrip (Karl Storz Company).

Reliable hemostasis and permanent closure can be only be achieved by performing bipolar vessel sealing or ligation. The vascular or tissue bundle is grasped with a special instrument and compressed constantly at a predefined pressure level. Several automatically regulated current cycles with variable electrical parameters, depending on the grasped tissue, "fuse" the mutually opposing tissue walls. Exact preparatory

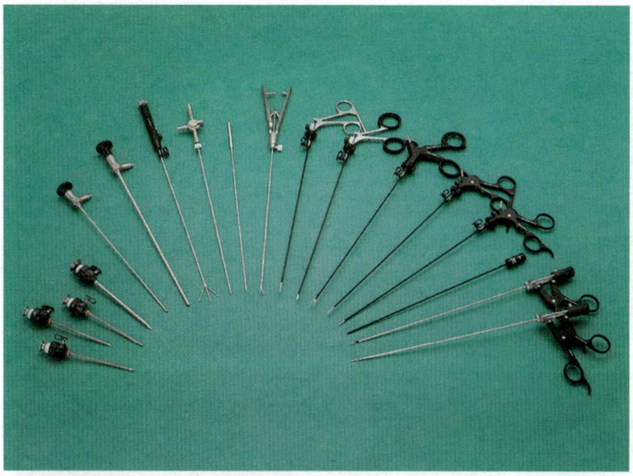

Fig. 4.54: Minilaparoscopy set (Karl Storz)

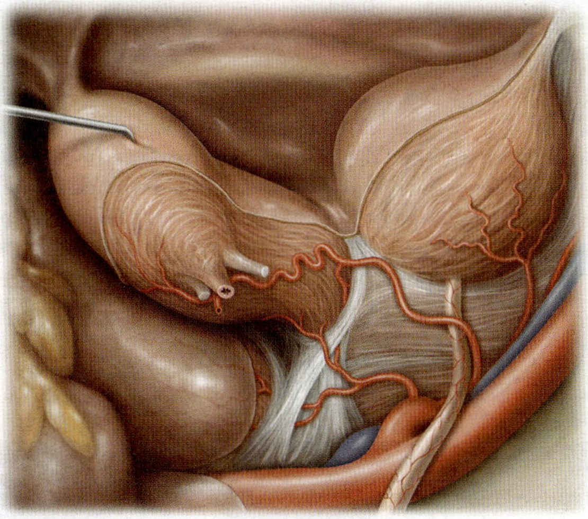

Fig. 4.55: Anatomical illustration showing the relation of the uterine vessel to the ureter in the pelvic wall, compared to its location close to the uterus. The helical course of the ascending branch of the uterine artery can be easily followed. The uterus, bladder, and rectum are embedded in a ligament-based pelvic floor.

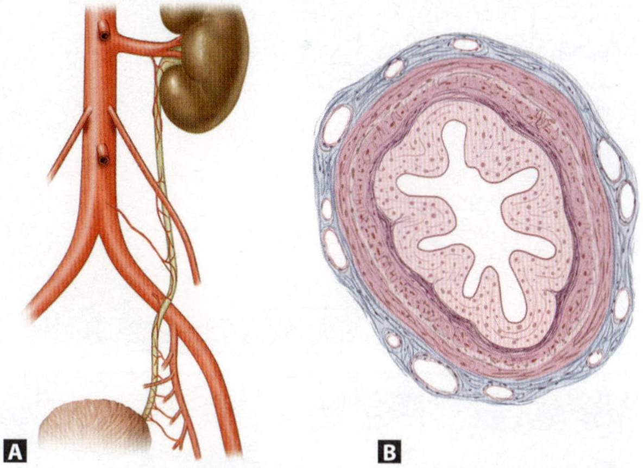

Figs. 4.56A and B: The anatomy of the ureter provides crucial information. (A) Vascularization is effected from the upper part: the renal artery, the ovarian artery, and the aorta. In the lower part the ureter is supplied by lateral vessels: the iliac vessels and the uterine artery. Blunt dissection causes minor bleeding at the respective location; (B) The histological cross-section shows that vascular supply is located in the adventitia. Therefore, electricity or manipulation causing destruction of the adventitia may lead to secondary fistulas and/or leakage.

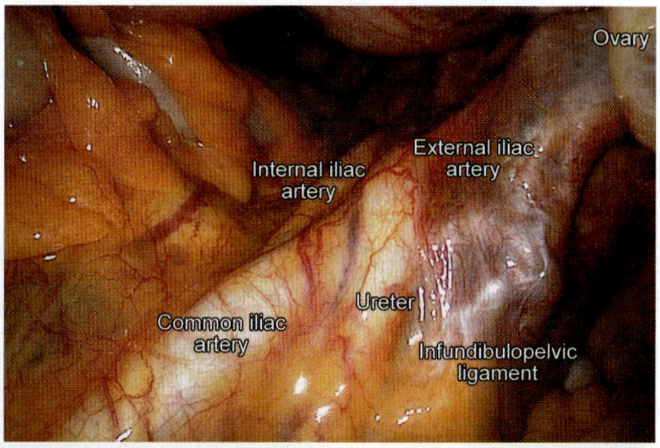

Fig. 4.57: Preliminary inspection of the uterus and the surrounding organs. The lower pelvis as well as the ligaments, vessels and the ureter can be differentiated in relation to the uterus. In slim patients, the crossing of the ureter and the common iliac artery can be seen. The infundibulopelvic ligament is identified and held towards the lateral wall in order to obtain a better view of the field of surgery.

visualization of vessels is usually not necessary. One can grasp entire tissue bundles containing vessels, and seal these. Technically, bipolar sealing can be achieved to a vessel diameter of about 10 mm; it has been clinically validated for a diameter of 7 mm. Due to warming of the instrument tip, it should be performed at a safe distance from sensitive tissue structures. Care should be taken to ensure that no inadvertent coagulation occurs due to contact or when setting the instrument aside. The blade of the ultrasound scalpel becomes much hotter than that of insulated bipolar instruments. In more than 90% of cases, the burst pressure is higher than 400 mm Hg (up to 900 mm Hg) and thus usually much higher than the clinically observed blood pressure values of about 130 mm Hg.

Histologically it was found that, in conventional coagulation, shrinkage of the wall and the formation of a thrombus are involved in hemostasis. In contrast, vessel sealing is associated with the denaturation of collagen and the fusion of opposing layers while the elastic internal membrane, whose fibers are denatured at a temperature beyond 100°C, are largely preserved. Lateral to the sharply margined

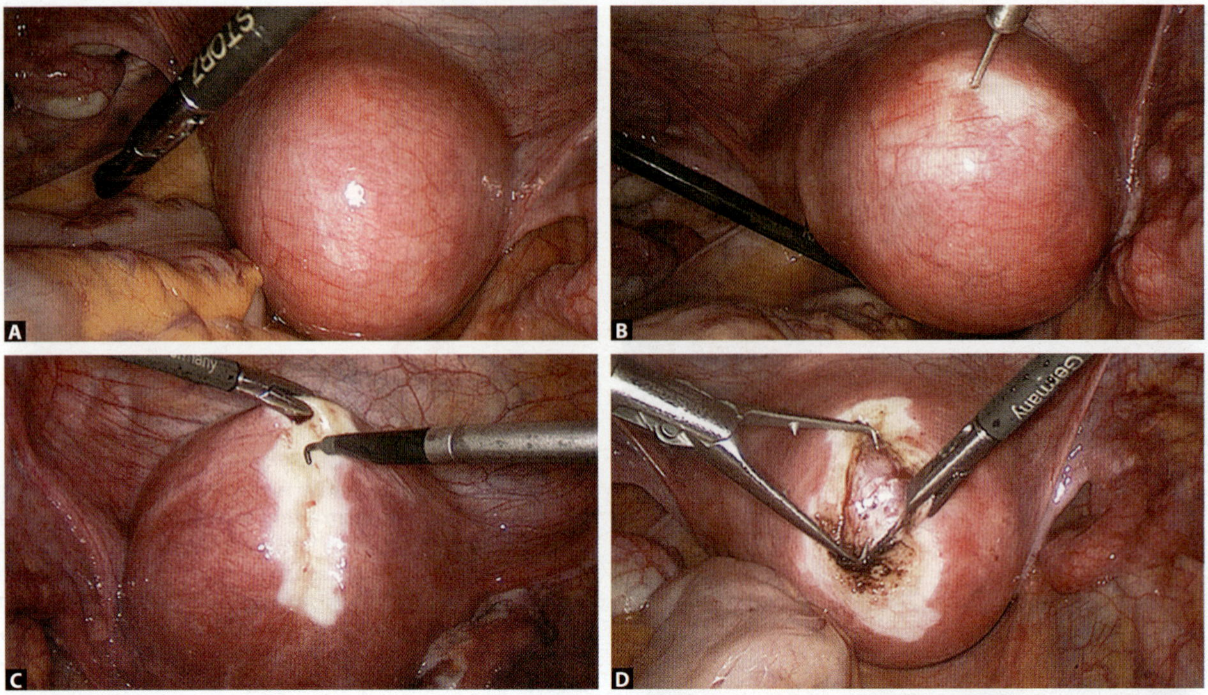

Figs. 4.58A to D: Laparoscopic myoma enucleation. (A) Situs of a fundal/anterior wall fibroid; (B) Prophylactic hemostasis with 1:100 diluted vasopressin solution (glycylpressin) in separate wells between the superficial and healthy tissue of the myometrium, and the capsule–fibroid surface. The purpose of the injection is to separate the pseudocapsule from the fibroid and reduce bleeding; (C) Bipolar superficial coagulation of the longitudinal incision strip and opening the uterine wall above the myoma with a monopolar hook or needle until one reaches the myoma; (D) Grasping the fibroid and starting the enucleation. The pseudocapsule remains within the uterine wall and is pushed off bluntly.

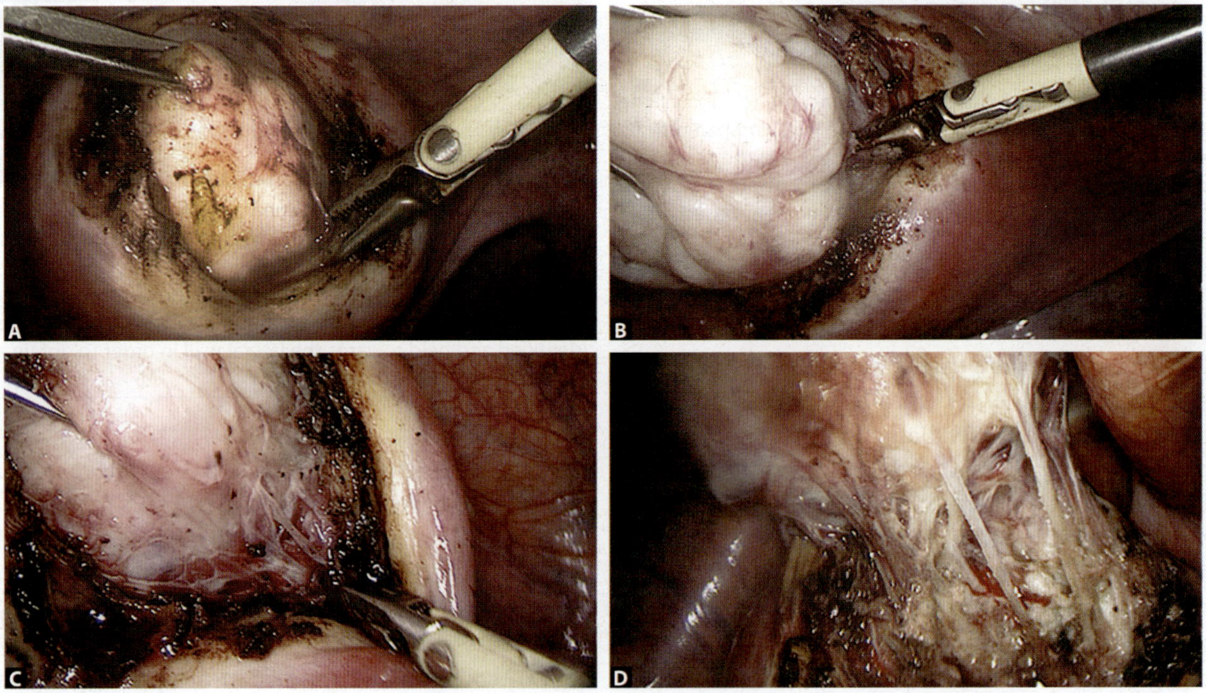

Figs. 4.59A to D: Laparoscopic myoma enucleation. (A) Traction of the fibroid with a tenaculum and blunt demarcation from the capsule; (B) Focal bipolar coagulation of basic vessels; (C) Continuous enucleation of the fibroid under traction and specific coagulation of capsule fibers containing vessels; (D) Magnification of the remaining capsule fibers to be coagulated and cut.

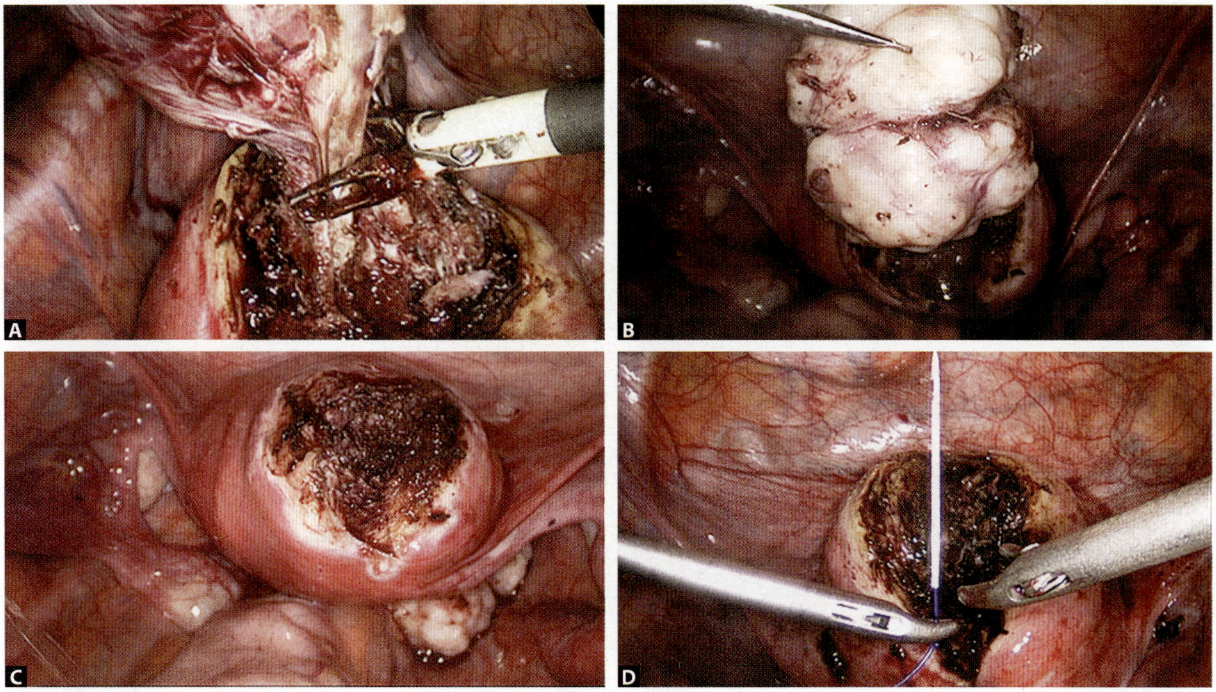

Figs. 4.60A to D: Laparoscopic myoma enucleation. (A) Final coagulation of the capsule vessels; (B) Double belly fibroid after complete enucleation; (C) Minimal coagulation of bleeding vessels under suction and irrigation; (D) Approximation of the wound edges with a straight or round sharp needle and a monofilar late-absorbable suture.

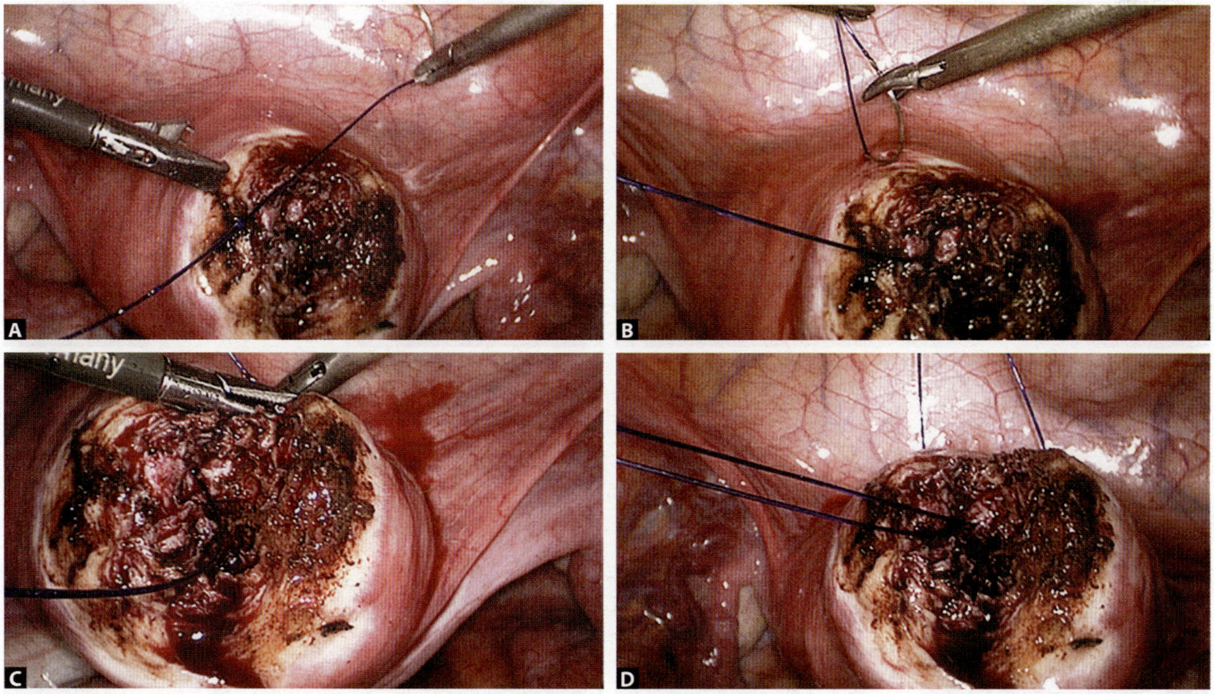

Figs. 4.61A to D: Laparoscopic myoma enucleation. (A) Advantages of a circular needle stitch: a) the wound angle is elevated safely and completely when raised with a Manhes forceps, b) deeper layers of the myometrium can be grasped more easily with a circular needle; (B) Needle exit and simplified re-grasping with the right needle holder; (C) Final stitch to invert the knot; (D) Extirpation of the needle, completing the extracorporeal knot, and preparing to push down the extracorporeal knot.

homogeneous coagulation zone, there is a transition zone of 1–2 mm with thermal damage. On immunohistochemistry its width is about twofold higher. This is followed by a sterile inflammation due to resorption, especially in the surrounding connective tissue, with no sign of any (even temporary) failure of the

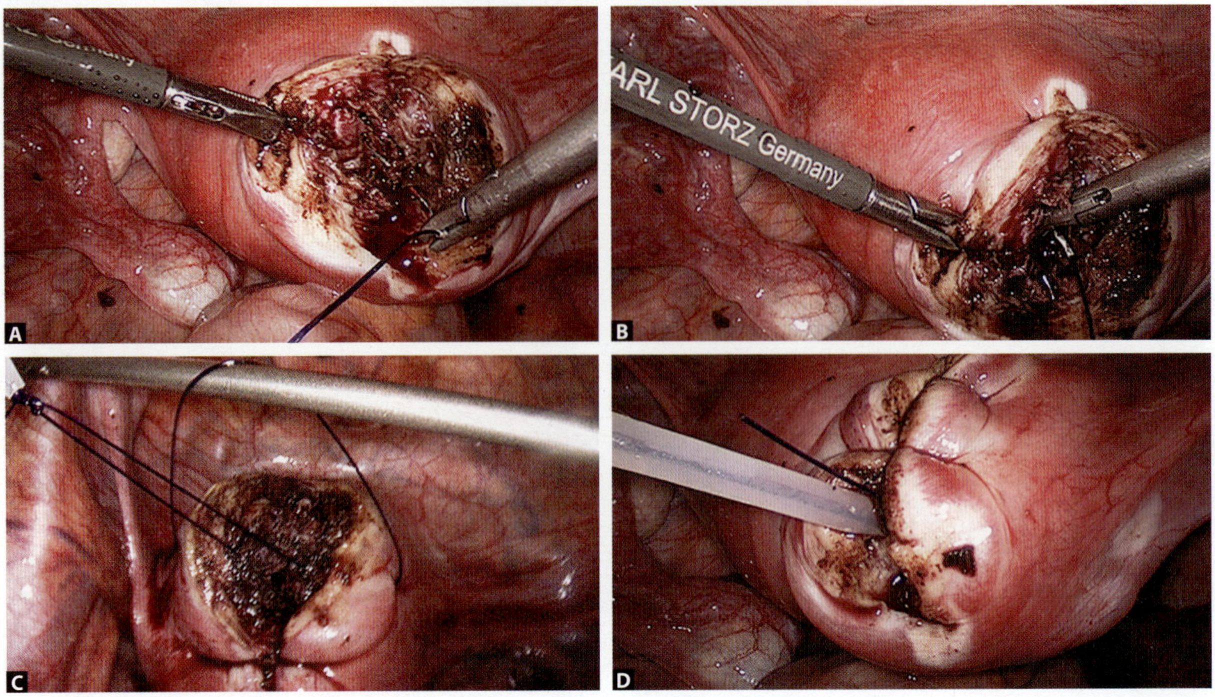

Figs. 4.62A to D: The extracorporeal "von Leffern" knot. (A) Pulling out the suture, removing the needle, half hitch; (B) Holding the knot with the left hand and reaching over with the right hand; (C) Grasping the short end from below and leading it back, exiting before the half hitch; (D) Turning back the knot. Holding the straight suture and tightening the knot.

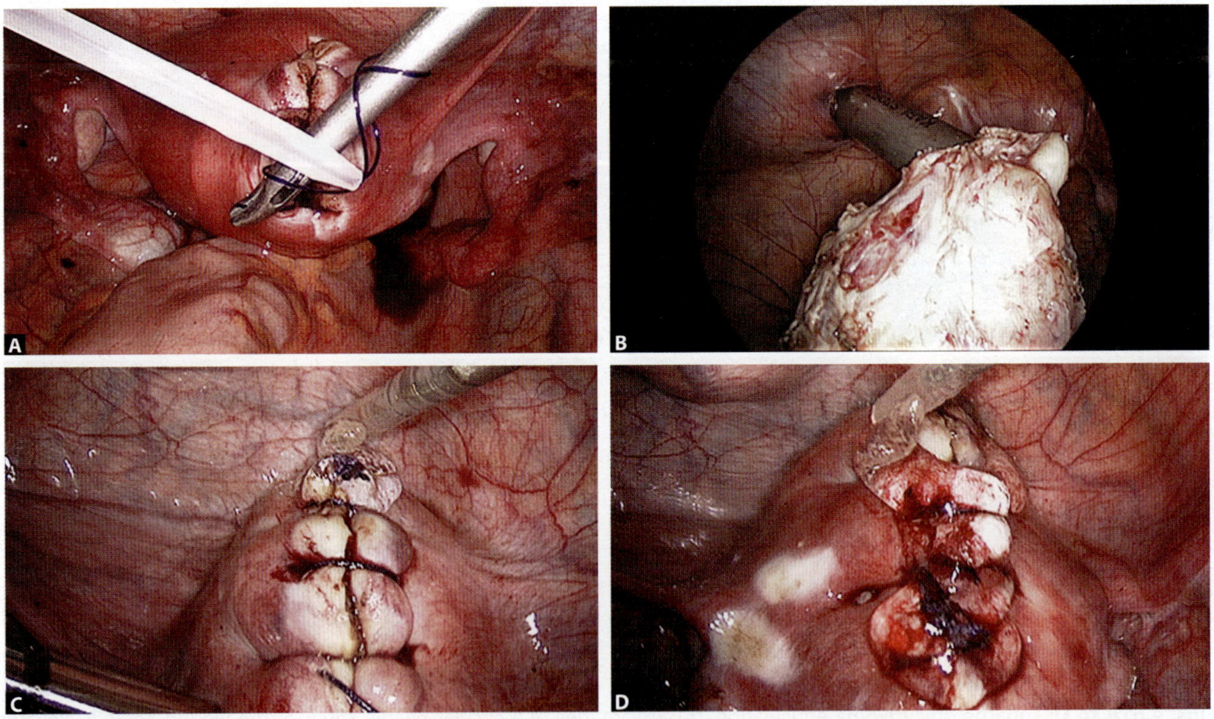

Figs. 4.63A to D: Laparoscopic myoma enucleation. (A) Second single suture starting as deep as possible in the uterine wound; (B) Morcellation of the specimen; (C) Final view of the extracorporal sutures; (D) Application of Hyalubarrier, as anti-adhesive gel.

sealing. The advantages of bipolar vessel sealing compared to other procedures such as ligature or a suture and the use of clips are mainly fast exposure, rapid and safe vessel closure, the absence of foreign material remaining in the operating field, and lower costs. This results in shorter operating times and less blood loss as well as less stress for the patient. Therefore, these instruments are now also used widely in open surgery and vaginal surgery (Figs. 4.71 and 4.72).

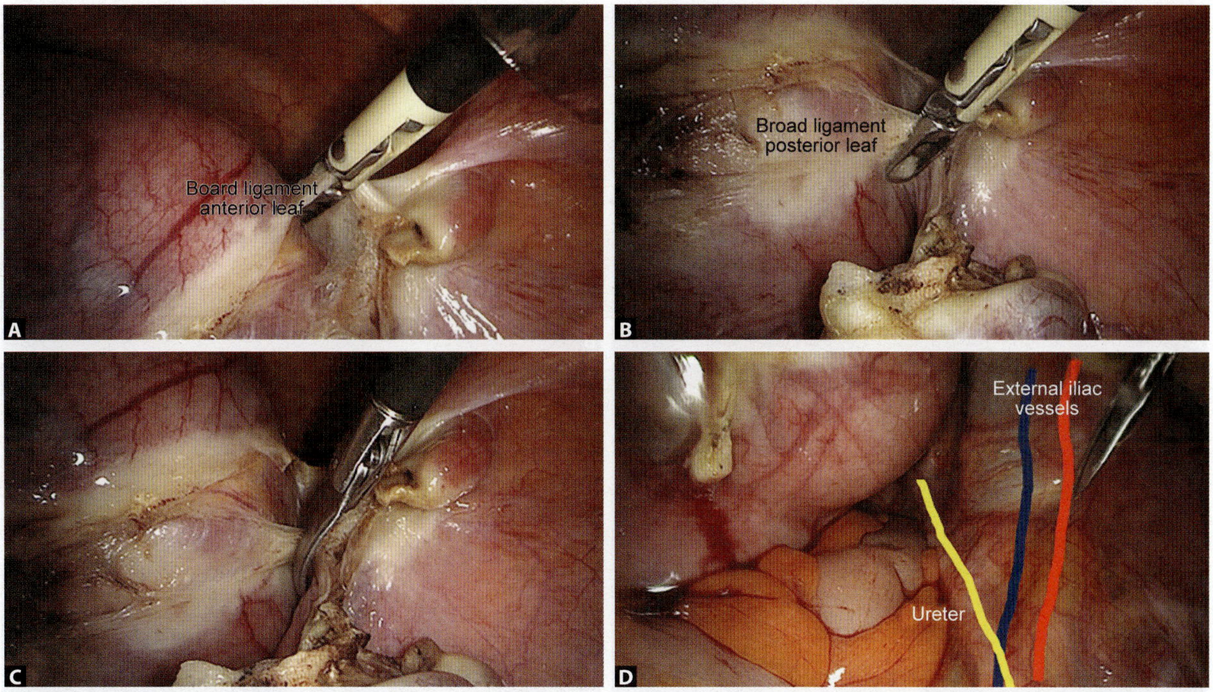

Figs. 4.64A to D: Separation of the anterior and posterior leaf of the broad ligament (A to C) in relation to the ureter and the pelvic vessels (D). (A to C) The broad ligament is coagulated and dissected as close to the uterus as possible without affecting the uterine artery. As the two leaves are separated, the ascending branch of the uterine artery can be visualized easily and omitted. The tip of the scissors is directed strictly away from the uterine wall using the curved blade.

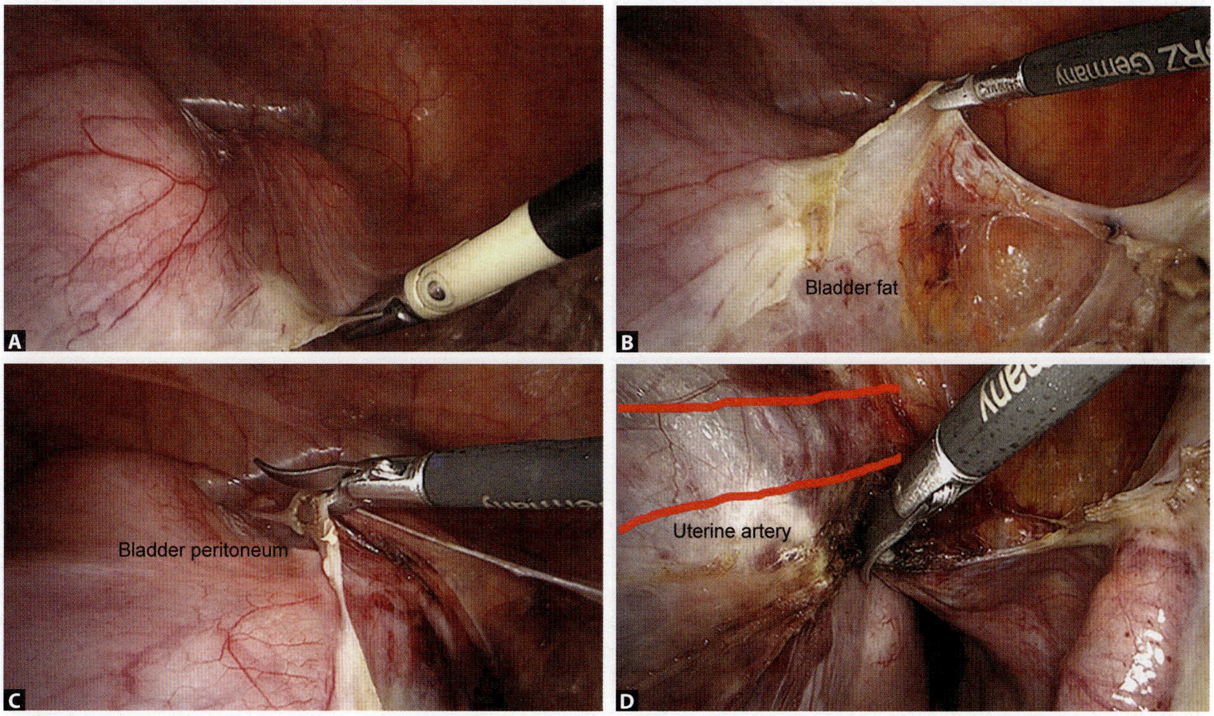

Figs. 4.65A to D: Opening the bladder peritoneum from the right side (A to C). The beginning of the bladder peritoneum can be easily demarcated; the cutting line should be neither above this zone nor too far into the caudal aspect. Gas enters the created space and shows the beginning of the bladder pillar. The uterine vessel bundle (D) is freed by coagulating and dissecting above and below it. The ureter is at a safe distance lateral to this area of exposure.

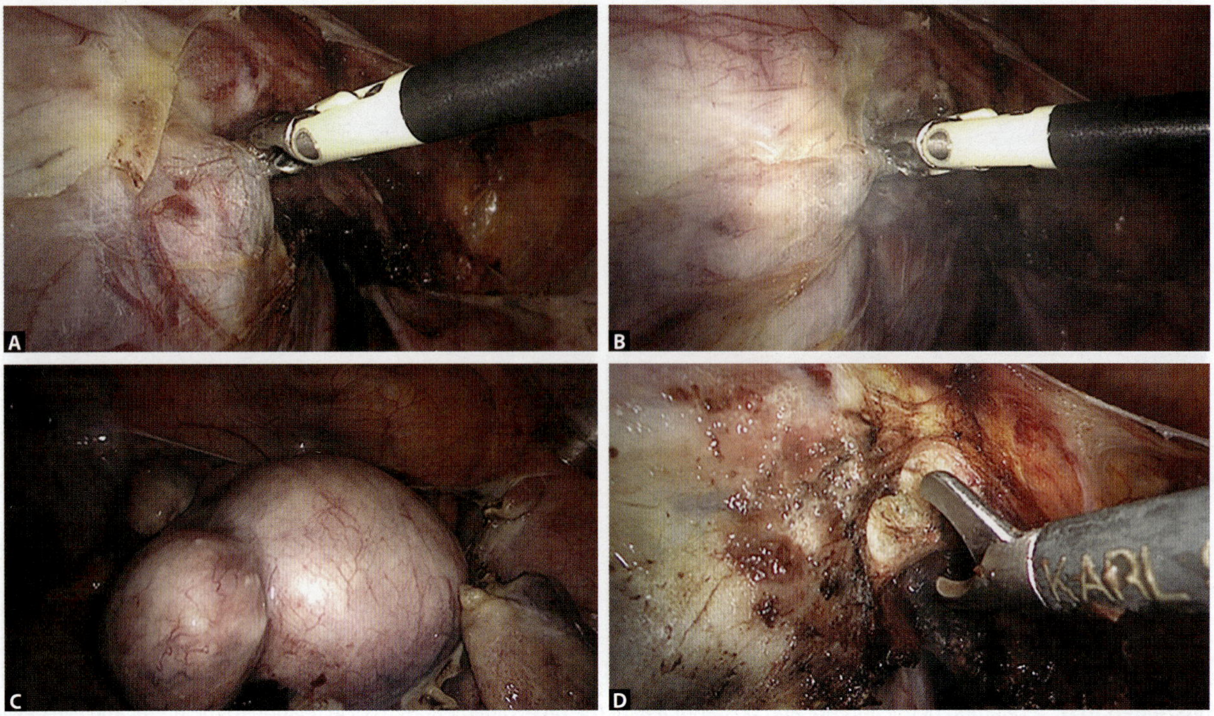

Figs. 4.66A to D: (A and B) Bipolar coagulation and dissection of the uterine vessels. The area of coagulation must include the upper part of the artery to avoid retrograde bleeding after dissecting the vessel; (C) The color of the uterus changes to whitish/gray; (D) A deeper cut can be avoided by using the hook scissors; the uterine artery is dissected in two steps. This allows further coagulation of the tissue lying just behind the artery and avoids cumbersome venous bleeding.

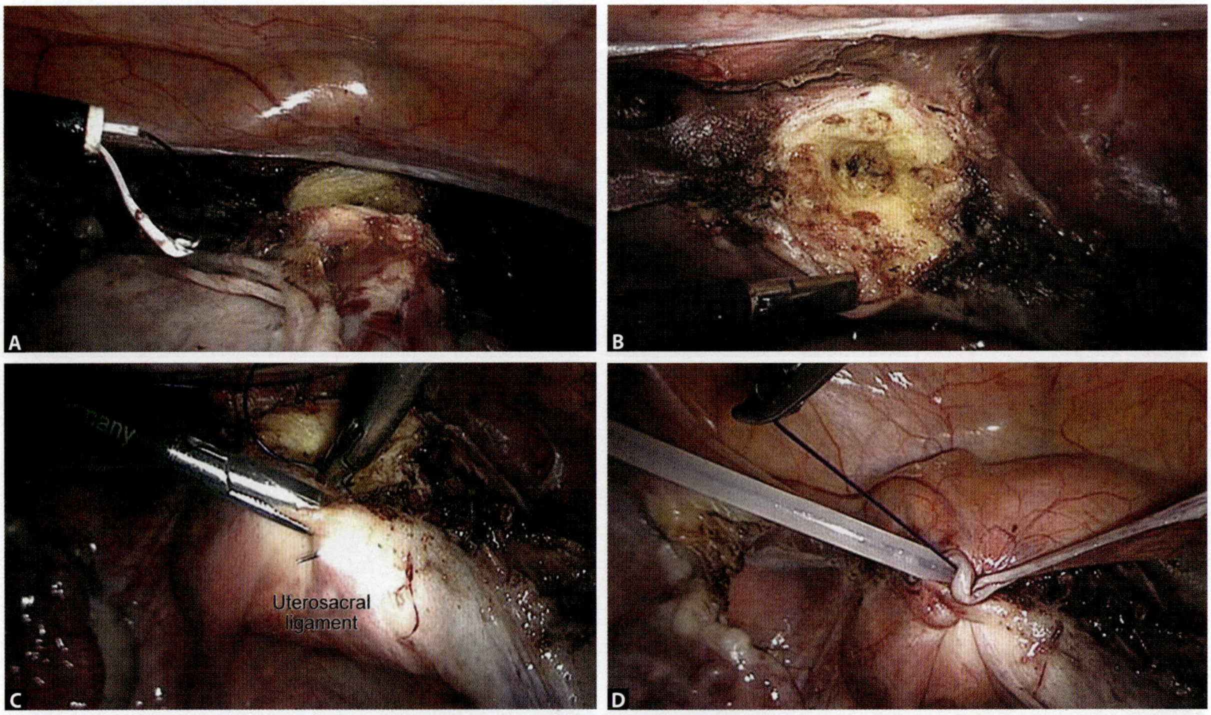

Figs. 4.67A to D: (A) Selectively, the uterine corpus is cut from the cervix; (B) The cervical stump is left with a retrograde cone as the monopolar loop cuts straight and easily under tension; (C) Closing the peritoneum is optional, but when using this technique, a cervicopexy can be performed simultaneously to prevent prolapse (D).

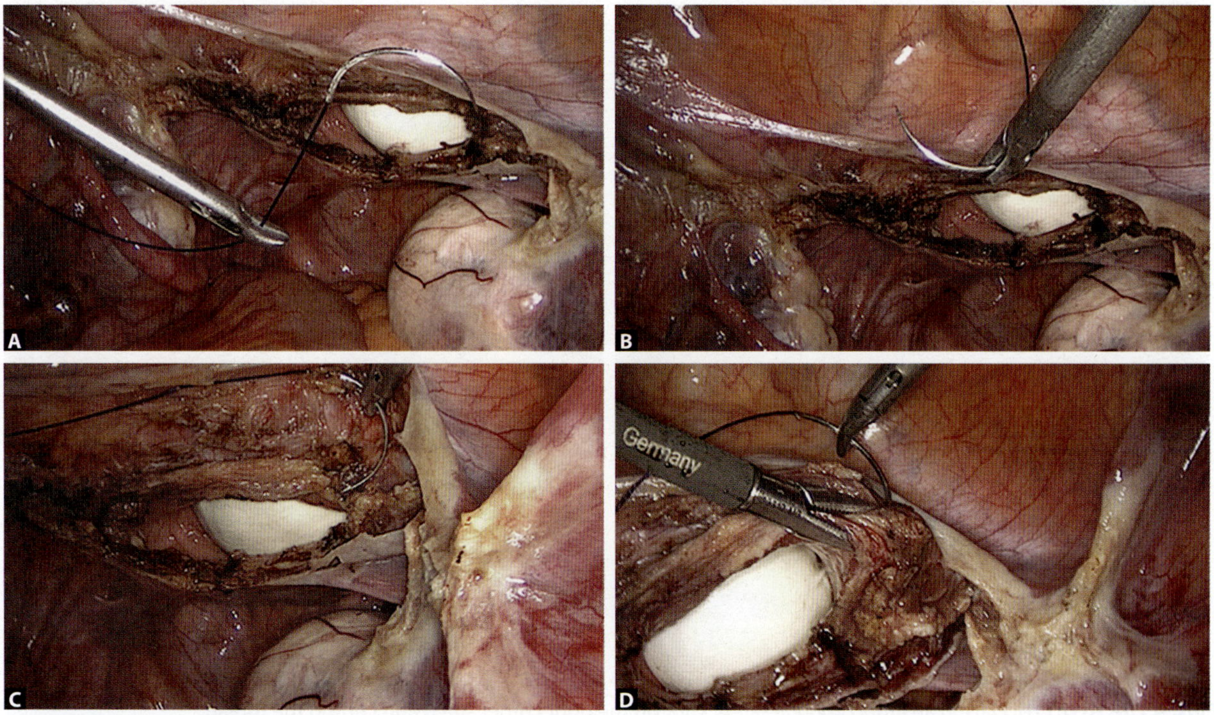

Figs. 4.68A to D: LTH: Right corner suture uniting the anterior and posterior vaginal wall, the posterior peritoneum, and the right sacrouterine ligament. The bladder can be omitted under sight. The forceps must be sharp in order to securely grab the vaginal epithelium. When the suture incorporates the vaginal wall alone and omits the epithelium, there is a high likelihood of postoperative granulomas.

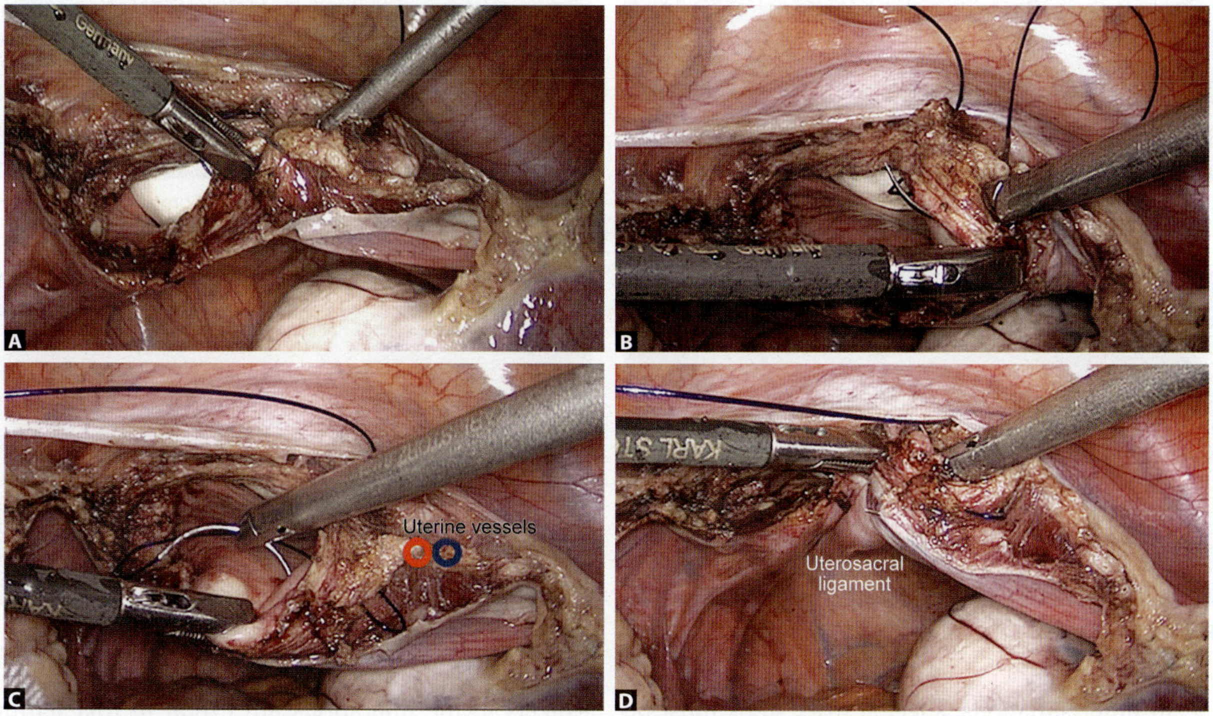

Figs. 4.69A to D: LTH: Continuation of the right corner suture while grabbing the right sacrouterine ligament. The vessel stumps are omitted and lateralized. When using this type of suture, the vessels are compressed mechanically.

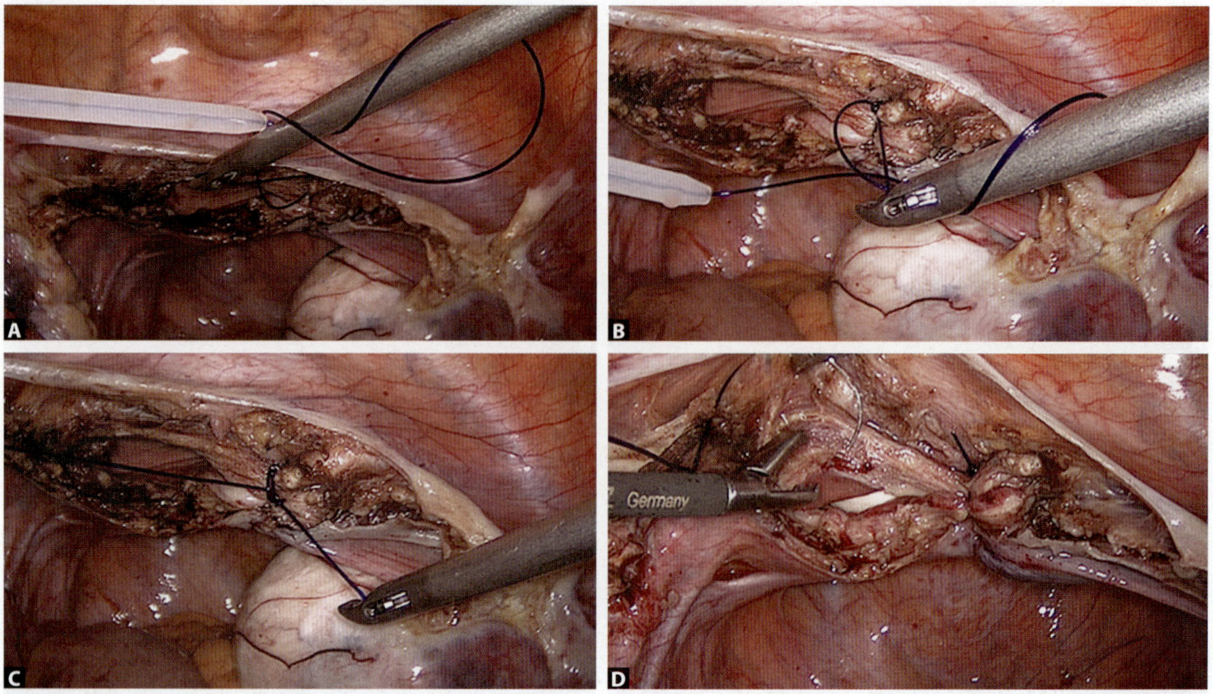

Figs. 4.70A to D: LTH: Placing an intracorporeal safety knot on the right corner stitch and cutting the thread.

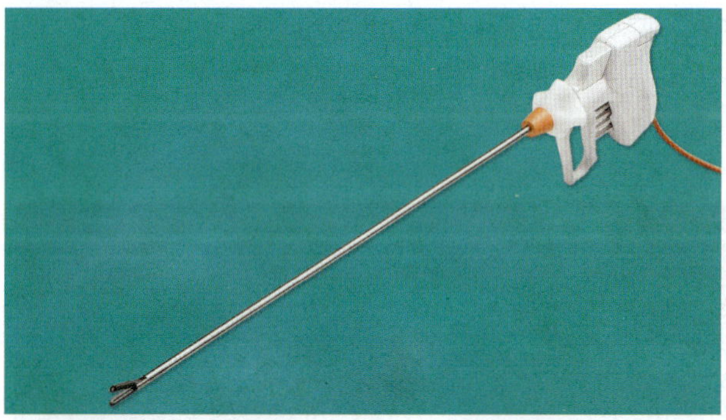

Fig. 4.71: Ergo 310D oblique view (Bowa Company).

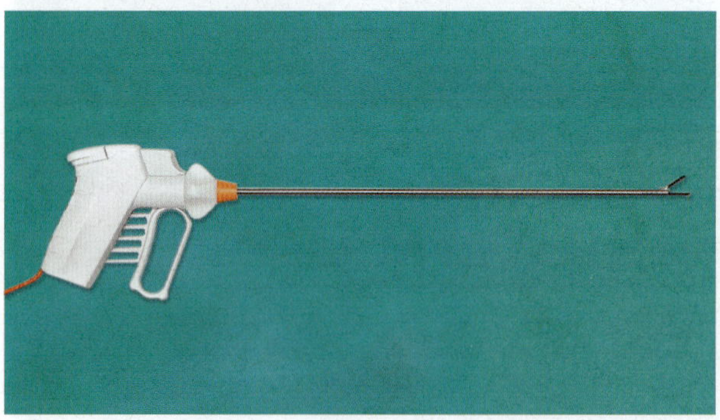

Fig. 4.72: Ergo 310D, lateral view (Bowa Company).

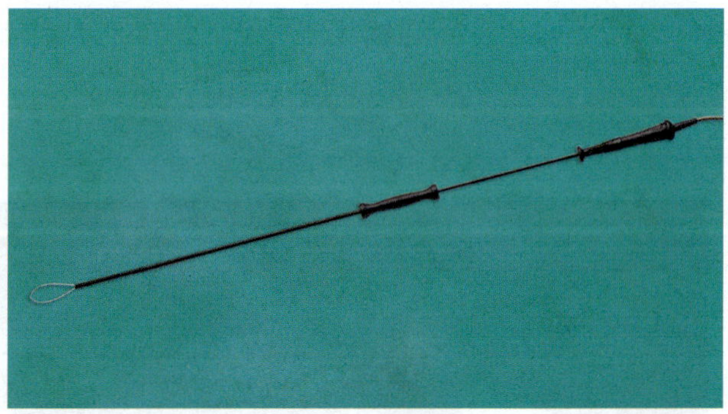

Fig. 4.73: MetraLoop, lateral view (Bowa Company).

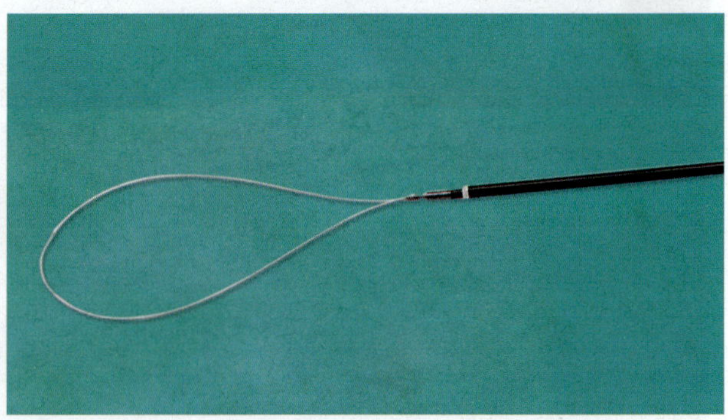

Fig. 4.74: MetraLoop, extended loop (Bowa Company).

In other situations, specific work steps must be taken into account along with the use of physical strength or the natural wear of instruments. Innovative instruments exactly oriented to the limiting aspects of the operations are useful in this setting (Figs. 4.73 to 4.76). Laborious processing of the handle and the instrument tip permits very precise exposure and user-friendly application, thus minimizing

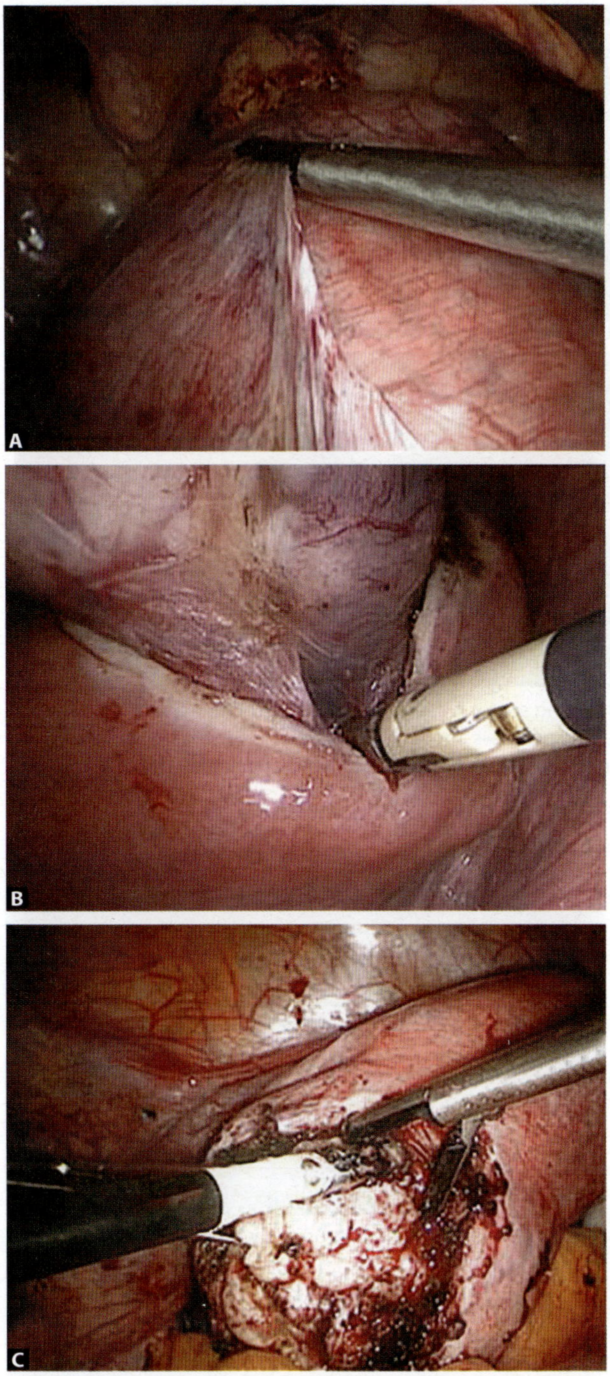

Figs. 4.75A to C: (A) The surface of the intact serosa and myometrium is coagulated and cut with a vessel sealing instrument, ERGO 310D (Bowa Electronic Company, Gomaringen, Germany). There is low thermal spread and high coagulation power compared to monopolar current. The integrated knife is able to simultaneously cut the coagulated tissue parts; (B) Usually the myoma is placed under traction with one hand (left hand in this case) while the other hand manipulates, coagulates and cuts the myoma capsule. This leads to high stress on the manipulating instrument (right hand in this case) because bipolar instruments are not designed for forceful manipulation; (C) Inexpensive single-use sealing instruments permit leverage of voluminous myomas with no risk of instrument breakage.

the risk of heating and damage to adjacent organs, reducing the operating time, and avoiding the exchange of instruments during the operation, which would be needed otherwise. Knives that permit precise cutting through a manual mechanism are integrated in the device.

Depending on the type, strength and frequency of the electric current, it exerts an electrolytic (disintegrating), Faradaic (stimulating nerves and muscles), or thermal effect. Alternating currents with a frequency of at least 200 kHz are used in HF surgery, and the thermal effect is dominant. It mainly depends on the exposure time, current density, and the specific resistance of tissue, which, to put it simply, drops with increasing water content or rising perfusion. The quantity of electric current flowing alongside the target site, which may warm and damage other areas, is also important in the practical setting (such as during irrigation, when using the monopolar technique rather than the bipolar one).

A FEW SUPPLEMENTARY INSTRUMENTS AND THEIR SPECIFIC USES

Johnson & Johnson Company was a forerunner in ultrasound-assisted procedures. The harmonic scalpel is used in several specialties and permits simultaneous hemostasis and cutting with the use of ultrasound technology (Figs. 4.77 and 4.78).

In addition to this instrument, whose tip is now very thin and permits the surgeon to perform very delicate steps in the operation, a flexible sealing tool can be used in very inconvenient anatomical locations as well as in single-port surgery (Fig. 4.79).

Additional substances such as hemostatic agents are needed in laparoscopy because prolonged active compression cannot be achieved with abdominal surgical belts. Besides, electric current should still be used as stringently as possible in very sensitive locations (close to the ureter or the bowel). In these regions the surgeon must frequently resort to additives such as TachoSil provided by Takeda Company (Figs. 4.80 to 4.82). Carriers developed specifically for laparoscopy can be introduced and used easily. They provide additional protection and safety for the patient (Figs. 4.83 to 4.85).

In gynecological surgery performed for benign indications, common reasons for the operation are

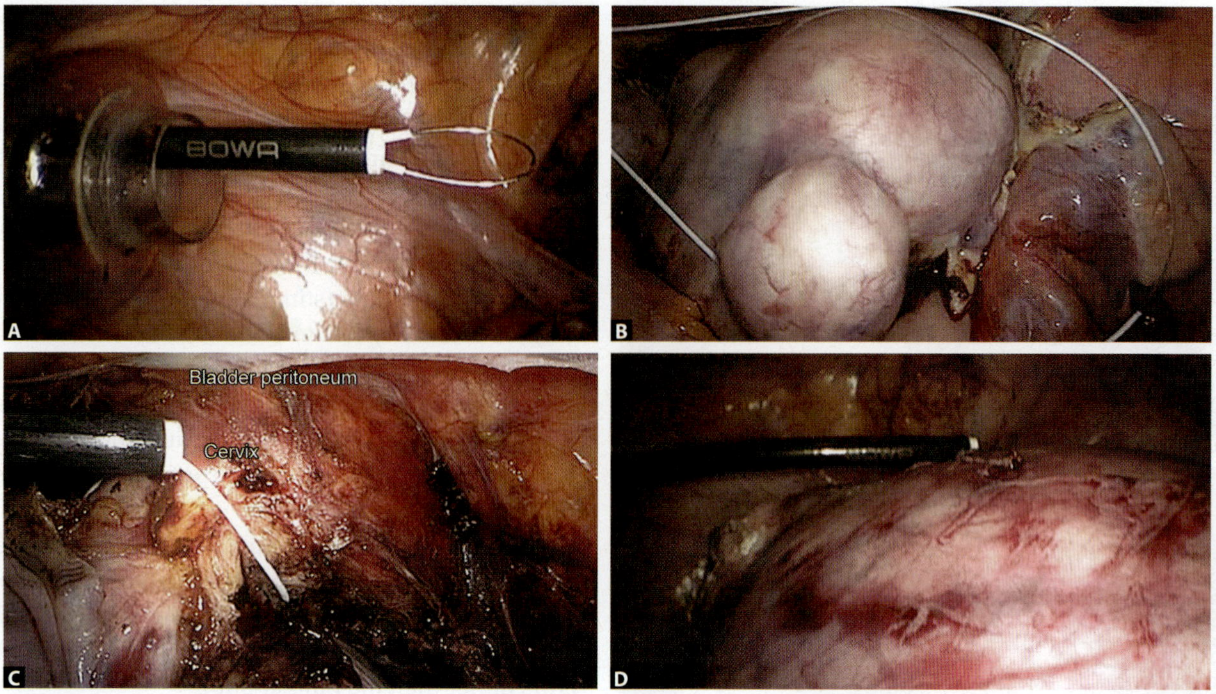

Figs. 4.76A to D: (A) The Bowa Metraloop is inserted and the small cutting sector is seen on the tip; (B) The two application sizes of the loop allow subtotal hysterectomy even of large uteruses; (C) The cutting line is above the cervix and medial to the vessel stumps; (D) The glass fiber-reinforced tube of the outer shaft allows even large uteruses to be pulled upward and avoid contact of the monopolar current with the bowel or the pelvic sidewalls.

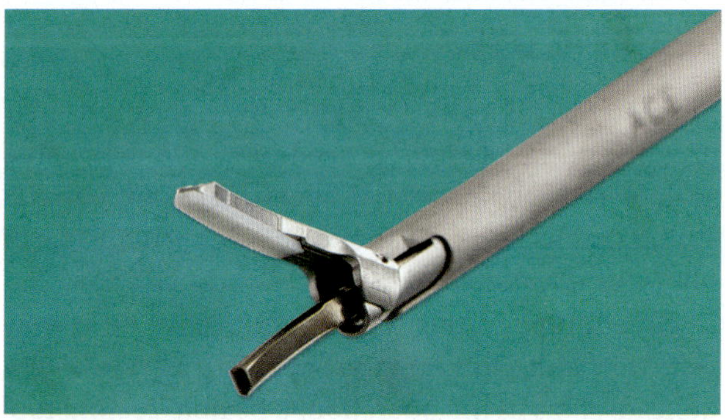

Fig. 4.77: Harmonic ultrasound scalpel (Ethicon/Johnson & Johnson), frontal view. The isolated branch is above, and the heated branch below.

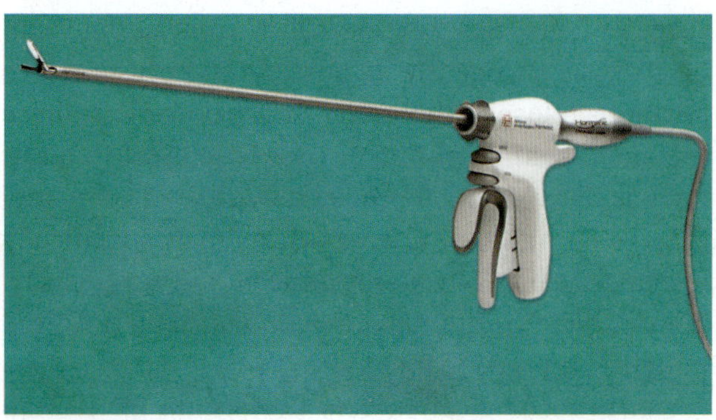

Fig. 4.78: Harmonic ultrasound scalpel (Ethicon/Johnson & Johnson), lateral view.

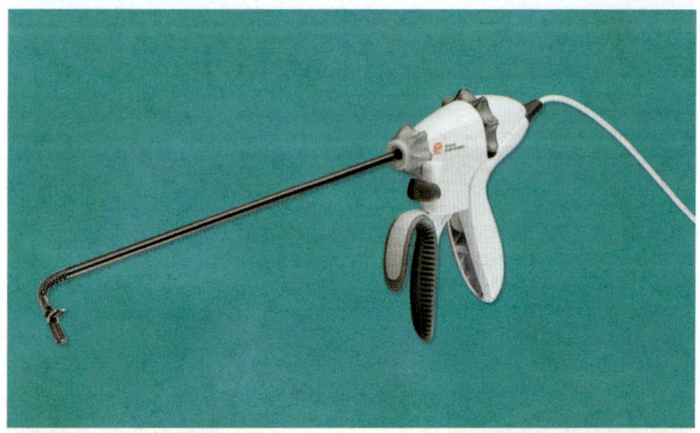

Fig. 4.79: EnSeal sealing instrument with a flexible tip (Ethicon/Johnson & Johnson).

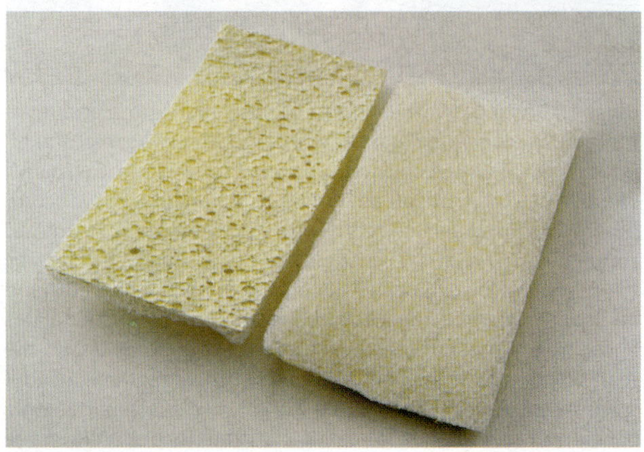

Fig. 4.80: TachoSil (Takeda Company): angles from above and below.

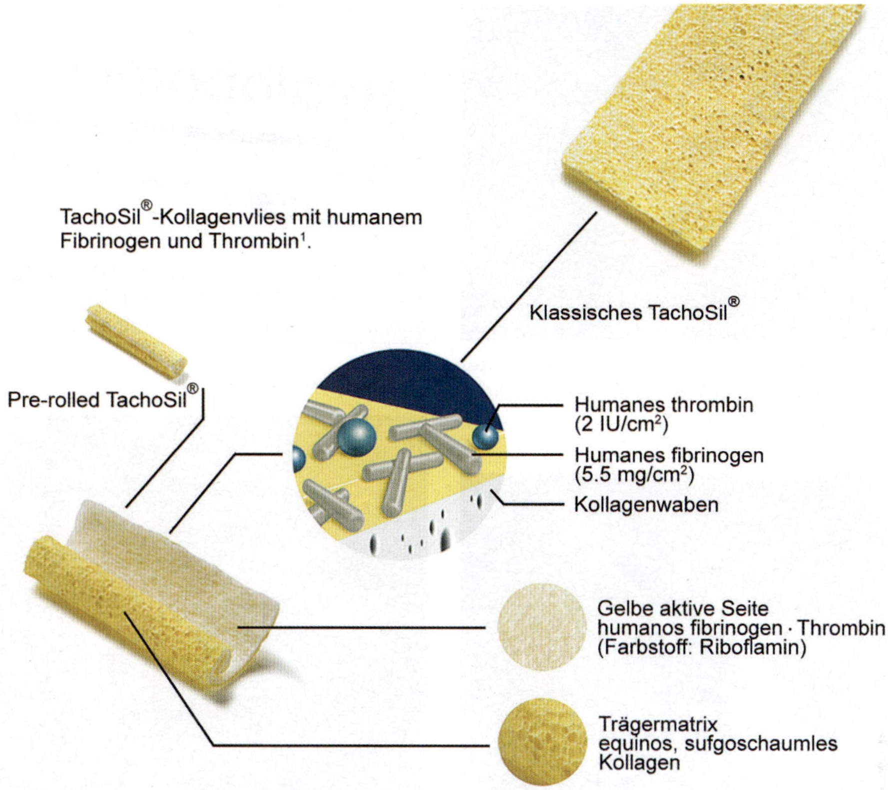

Fig. 4.81: TachoSil: Composition and mechanism of action (Takeda Company).

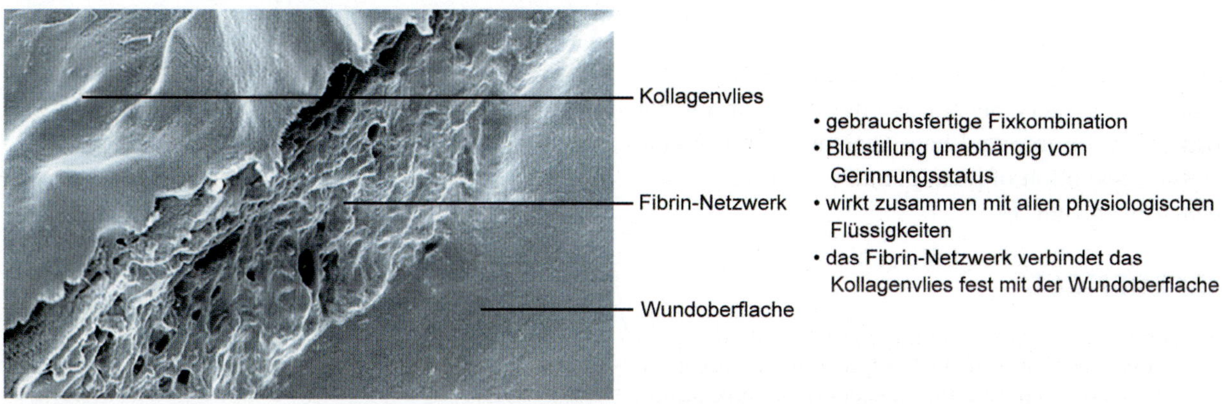

Fig. 4.82: Electron microscopy image of TachoSil's (Takeda Company) principle of action on tissue.

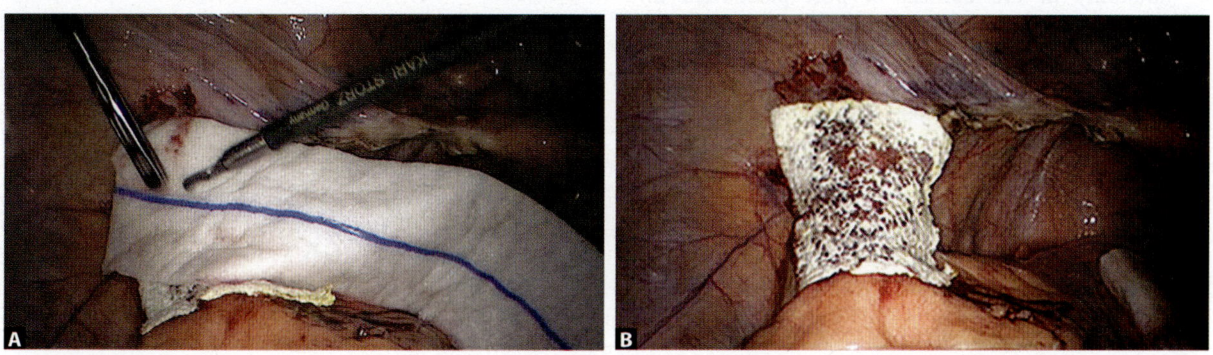

Figs. 4.83A and B: (A) Endoscopic use of TachoSil (Takeda Company) on the pelvic wall; (B) Moistened gauze pad pressing the patch on slightly bleeding tissue until the tissue is fully moistened.

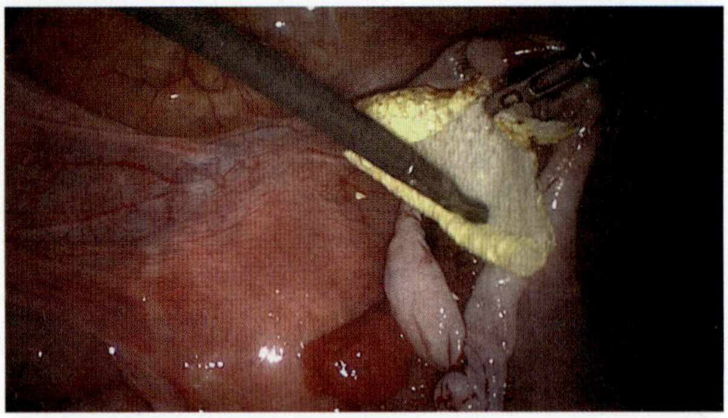

Fig. 4.84: Use of TachoSil (Takeda Company) at the ovary after removal of the endometrium. Hemostasis is achieved without destroying follicles due to electric currents.

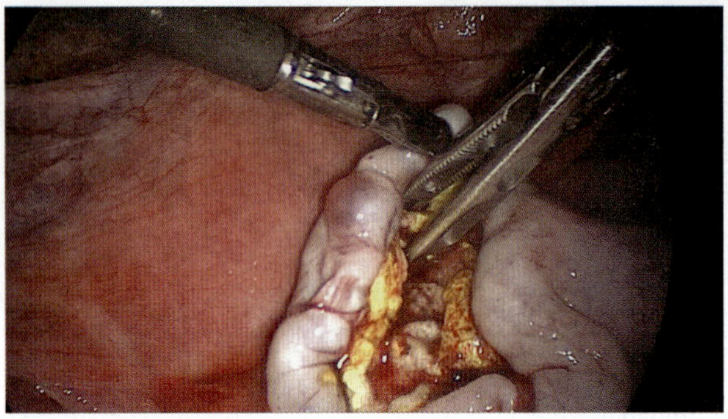

Fig. 4.85: Ovary after removal of the endometrium, with a TachoSil patch in place (Takeda Company).

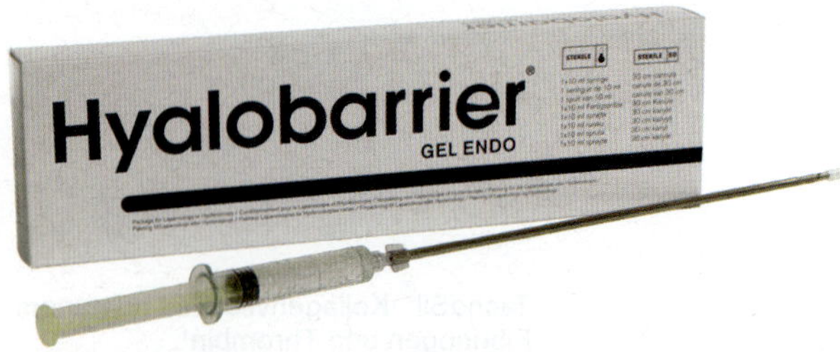

Fig. 4.86: Hyalobarrier (Nordic Pharma Company): A hyaluronic-acid-based gel for open intrauterine and laparoscopic application, for the purpose of preventing adhesion.

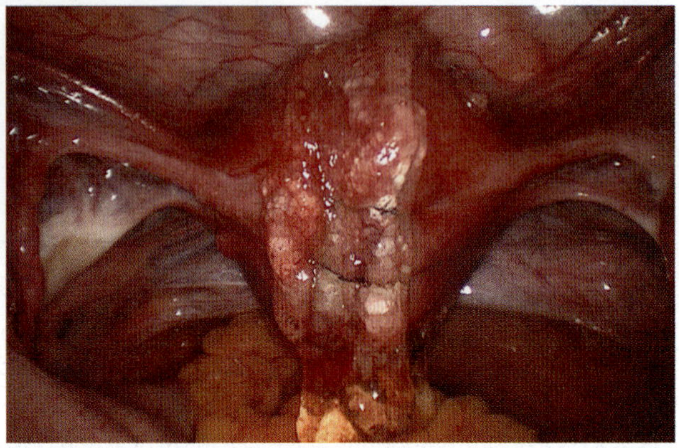

Fig. 4.87: Use of hyalobarrier (Nordic Pharma Company), such as after myoma enucleation.

the presence of adhesions or the undesired sequelae of previous surgery. Several agents in fluid or powder form, or hyaluronic acid-based gels are now available for the prevention of postoperative adhesions (Figs. 4.63, 4.86 and 4.87).

REFERENCES

1. Mettler L, Clevin L, Ternamian A, et al. The past, present and future of minimally invasive endoscopy in gynecology: a review and speculative outlook. Minim Invasive Ther Allied Technol. 2013;22(4):210-26.
2. Alkatout I, Mettler L, Maass N, et al. Abdominal anatomy in the context of port placement and trocars. J Turk Ger Gynecol Assoc. 2015;16(4):241-51.
3. Azziz R, Steinkampf MP, Murphy A. Postoperative recuperation: relation to the extent of endoscopic surgery. Fertil Steril. 1989;51(6):1061-4.
4. Mettler L, Eckmann-Scholz C, Semm I, et al. Factors to consider in gynecological surgery. Womens Health (Lond). 2014;10(3):323-38.
5. Mettler L, Schollmeyer T, Alkatout I. Adhesions during and after surgical procedures, their prevention and impact on women's health. Womens Health (Lond). 2012;8(5):495-8.
6. Alkatout I, Egberts JH, Mettler L, et al. [Interdisciplinary diagnosis and treatment of deep infiltrating endometriosis]. Zentralbl Chir. 2016; 141(6): 630-8.
7. Tinelli A, Mettler L, Malvasi A, et al. Impact of surgical approach on blood loss during intracapsular myomectomy. Minim Invasive Ther Allied Technol. 2014;23(2):87-95.
8. Alkatout I, Schollmeyer T, Hawaldar NA, et al. Principles and safety measures of electrosurgery in laparoscopy. JSLS. 2012;16(1):130-9.
9. Veress J. Neues Instrument zur Ausführung von Brustoder Bauchpunktionen and Pneumothoraxbehandlung. Dtsch Med Wochenschr. 1938;40:1480-1.
10. Semm K. [Hysterectomy via laparotomy or pelviscopy. A new CASH method without colpotomy]. Geburtshilfe Frauenheilkd. 1991;51(12):996-1003.
11. Schollmeyer T, Soyinka AS, Schollmeyer M, et al. Georg Kelling (1866-1945): the root of modern day minimal invasive surgery. A forgotten legend? Arch Gynecol Obstet. 2007;276(5):505-9.
12. Spaner SJ, Warnock GL. A brief history of endoscopy, laparoscopy, and laparoscopic surgery. J Laparoendosc Adv Surg Tech A. 1997;7(6):369-73.
13. Stellato TA. History of laparoscopic surgery. Surg Clin North Am. 1992;72(5):997-1002.

KIEL SCH•OL

5 of Gynaecological Endoscopy

Current Laparoscopic **Training** Models

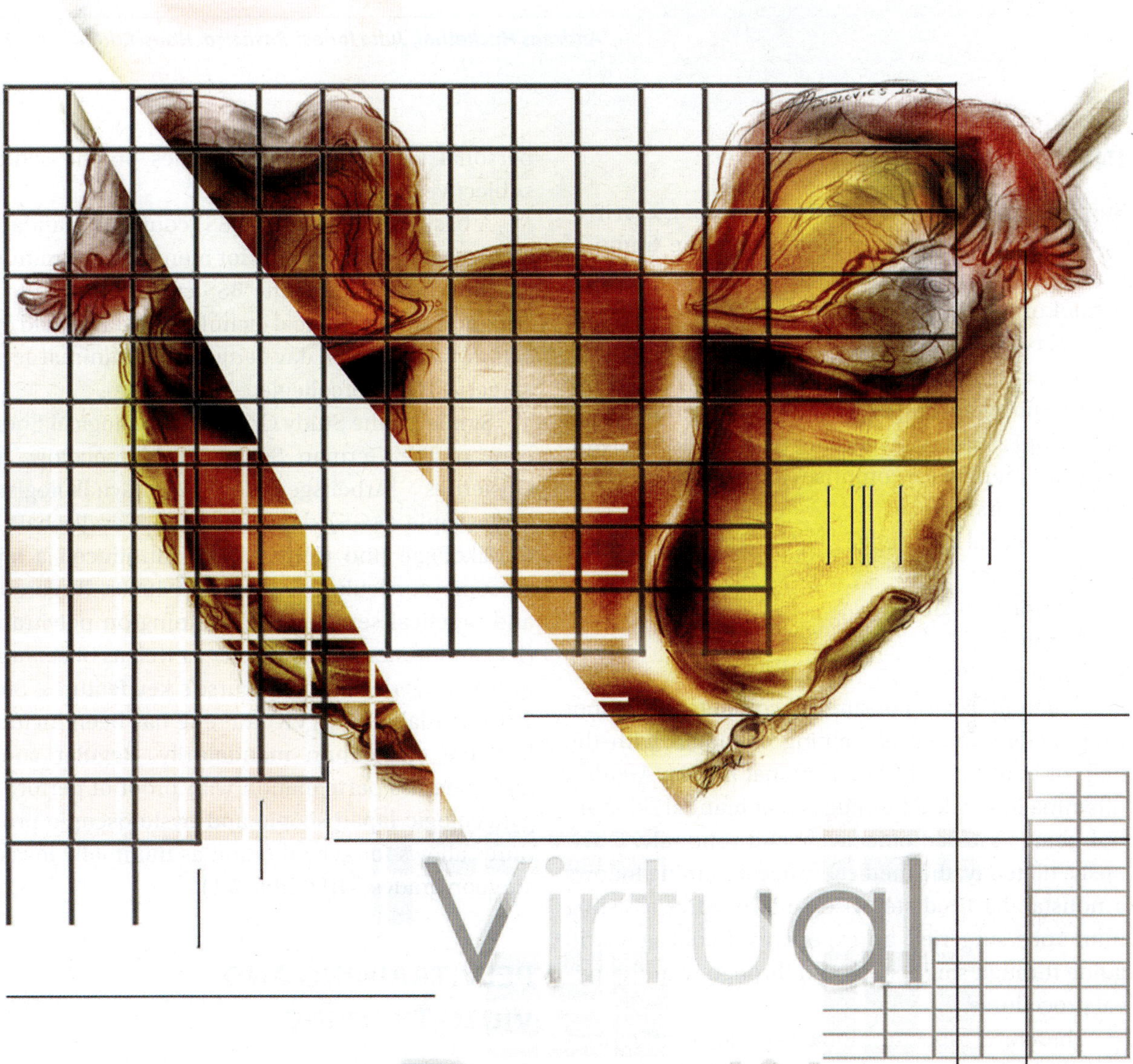

Virtual Reality

Training Models

Chapter 5

Current Laparoscopic Training Models

Andreas Hackethal, Julia Ionesi-Pasacica, Hans-Rudolf Tinneberg

INTRODUCTION

Surgical competence is a must for every surgeon irrespective of the specialization. Within the frame of our international teaching activities at the Giessen School of Endoscopic Surgery in collaboration with the Galaxy Group of Endoscopic Surgery from Pune, India, and many others, we observed many postgraduates who were desperate for effective training in endoscopic surgery. According to Patil and Baldwin, surgical competence comprises a combination of following factors:[1,2]

- Theoretical knowledge
- Experience
- Decision making
- Teamwork
- Manual skills.

Different aspects of surgical competence cannot be provided apractical training or taught with the help of books or other educational media. Another dilemma in surgical training is that manual skills are not being assessed objectively and routinely. Obviously, till today, the medical surgical training follows a nonstandardized stepwise pattern. After assisting numerous surgeries, an experienced colleague will guide through single steps and through whole surgical procedures.

Therefore, the educational process is influenced and limited by various factors. First, the patient, as the most important factor for surgical education, is supposed to receive best medical treatment from experts and not from novices. Second, the health systems worldwide are in financially fierce situations, resulting in tight time schedules, which hardly allow for slower teaching surgeries. More than that, there is a decrease in working hours for junior doctors resulting in less exposure to surgical cases.[3] In general, the personal surgical education relies on the seniors' subjective benevolence.

A basic surgical skills (BSS) course is mandatory since 1996 in Great Britain for membership examinations of the colleges.[4] The BSS course aims to teach "safe and sound surgical techniques" and is held over 3 days, with the final day dedicated to minimal access surgery (The intercollegiate BSS course).

Similarly, the Study Group Gynecological Endoscopy of the German Society for Gynecology and Obstetrics [Arbeitsgemeinschaft Gynäkologische Endoskopie (AGE) der Deutschen Gesellschaft für Gynäkologie und Geburtshilfe] introduced a laparoscopic curriculum in the mid-1990s. Theoretical and practical sessions with training on pelvitrainer (PT) and hysteroscopy trainer as well as observation of live surgeries are the course's key features. Since 2010, virtual reality (VR) training has been included into the curriculum mandatorily. Regular course and congress participation with proof of performed gynecologic laparoscopic and hysteroscopic procedures allows for accreditation as minimally invasive surgeon grades I–III (Table 5.1).

PELVITRAINING AND VIDEO TRAINING

Basic skills of laparoscopic surgery can be taught and trained with laparoscopic equipment used on plastic abdominal cavities, the so called PT. Pelvitrainer training provides the possibility to optimize the motorical aspects and depth perception outside the operating room in an adequate learning environment.[5-9] A visible abdominal wall allows a three-dimensional (3D) intra-abdominal vision for beginners, and the use of video equipment facilitates the

Table 5.1: Study Group Gynecological Endoscopy of the German Society for Gynecology and Obstetrics [Arbeitsgemeinschaft Gynäkologische Endoskopie (AGE) der Deutschen Gesellschaft für Gynäkologie und Geburtshilfe] Minimally invasive surgery accreditation Grade I to Grade III and the surgical performance.

MIC grade	Laparoscopies	Hysteroscopies
I	Diagnostic procedures 20	Diagnostic procedures 20
II	Operative procedures 200	Operative procedures 50
III	Operative procedures 800	Operative procedures 100

Abbreviation: MIC, Minimally Invasive Surgery

Table 5.2: Summary of three different training models, the task and evaluation criteria.

Training model	Training tasks	Evaluation criteria
LASTT[11] and	*Three tasks:* • Camera navigation • Camera navigation and forceps handling • Bimanual forceps handling	*One per task:* Time for task completion or number of transferred objects
MISTLES[10]	*Five tasks:* • Peg transfer • Pattern cutting • Endoloop • Extracorporal knot • Intracorporal knot	*At least 2 per task:* Time for task completion and penalty score according to structured assessment
GBS-Training	*Four tasks:* • Pea transfer • Needle transfer • Pattern cutting • Intracorporeal knot	*At least 18 per task:* Structured assessment of task completion with quantitative and qualitative criteria In total 64 criteria

Abbreviations: LASTT, Laparoscopic Skills Testing and Training; MISTLES, McGill Inanimate System for Training and Evaluation of Laparoscopic Skills; GBS, Giessen Bench Station.

transfer of 3D movements to the two-dimensional TV screen. This setting is often referred to as video training.

Different bench station training environments have been proposed and evaluated to train beginners and assess learning curves [Laparoscopic Skills Testing and Training (LASTT) by Molinas and Campo 2010, McGill Inanimate System for Training and Evaluation of Laparoscopic Skills (MISTELS).[10,11]] Important drawbacks of most training environments are limited and insufficient assessment criteria, such as time for task completion (Table 5.2).

A standardized training environment has been introduced at the Giessen School of Endoscopic Surgery in 2006. The Giessen Bench Station (GBS) training comprises four separate tasks, which address hand–eye coordination, 3D understanding and tissue handling. The performance is being videotaped and quantitatively and qualitatively evaluated by third parties with the help of 60 criteria. The advantage to other training environments is the objective assessment tool with defined criteria and the resulting feedback to the trainees. The drawback might be the time-consuming evaluation of tasks. Till today, various laparoscopic training models have proven feasibility in training basic laparoscopic skills. In today's medical education the concern should be put on the availability of adequate training time for young doctors.

New laparoscopic training models on box trainers with automated assessment of different parameter focus on direct objective feedback to the participant.[12] The ForceSense by Medishield can be combined with a conventional box trainer (Fig. 5.1). It has been shown that tissue handling skills of medical students improved significantly when they are given force feedback of their performance. Hence, learning curves can be objectively measured on an intermediate cost level.[13]

VIRTUAL REALITY TRAINING

The VR training is not new to the surgical community.[12] A combination of physically maneuverable instruments and computer-generated environments allows a trainee to operate in a virtual world.[14] First simulators, such as the minimal invasive surgery trainer-virtual reality (MIST-VR), generated abstract

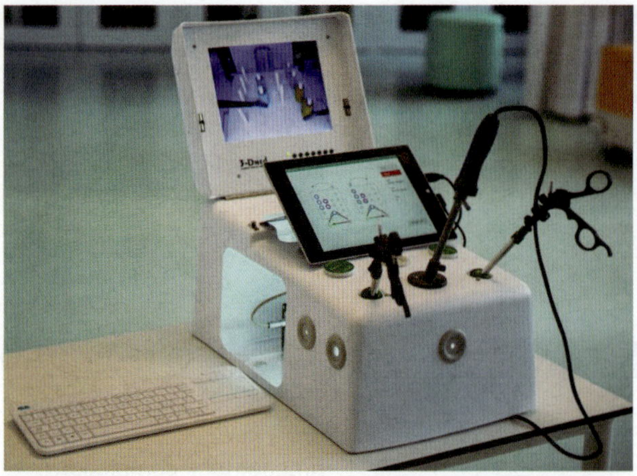

Fig. 5.1: The ForceSense technology can be combined with almost any box trainer

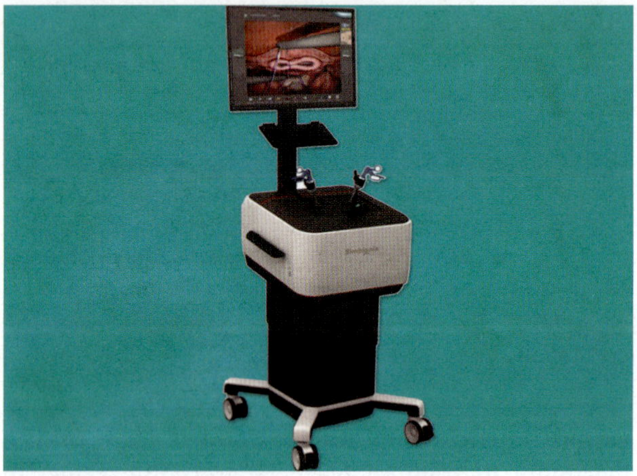

Fig. 5.2: The Simbionix Lap-Mentor (© Simbionix)

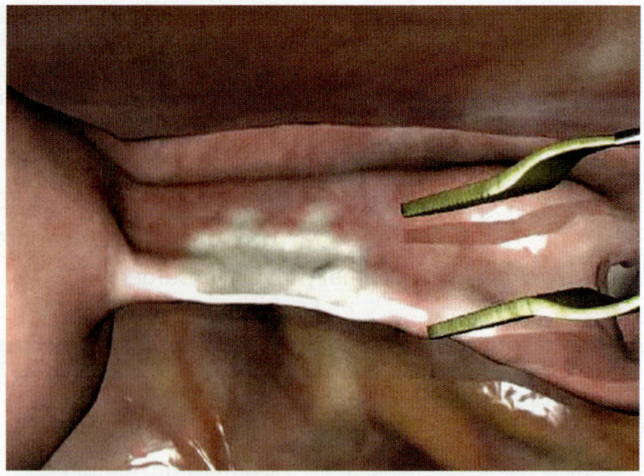

Fig. 5.3: LapSim Simulator with Gyn tubal occlusion task (© Surgical Science)

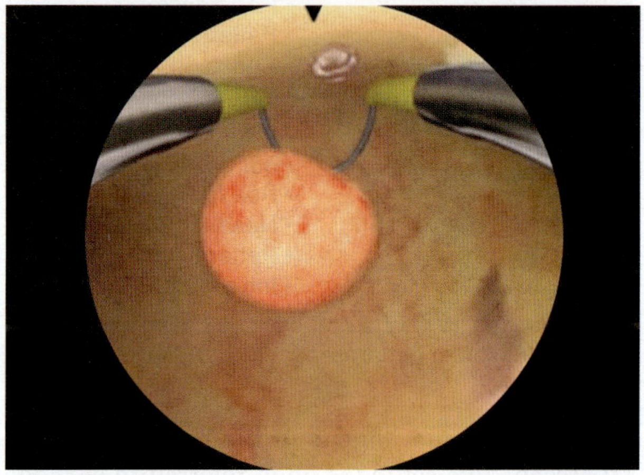

Fig. 5.4: HystSim, Hysteroscopy simulator with myomectomy scenario (© VirtaMed)

environments. Developments of computer hardware and enhanced possibilities of graphic allow almost real surgical scenarios today (Simbionix, Surgical Science, VirtaMed) (Figs. 5.2 to 5.4).

An early study using VR simulators for assessing manual skills was performed in 2001 with the MIST-VR.[15] Torkington et al. showed that the BSS leads to a quantifiable improvement in basic laparoscopic skills, which are measurable with help of the MIST-VR.[16] Hackethal et al. evaluated novices using the MIST-VR and characterized the learning curve and performance stabilization for one MIST-VR scenario.[17] A typical learning curve is shown in Figure 5.4. Meanwhile, numerous studies have shown the impact of VR training on skills and theater performance.[17-20]

Studies comparing conventional laparoscopic training, video training and VR training have been evaluated by a Cochrane Review. Although most of the evaluated trials had the risk for bias, the conclusion states that VR training can supplement the standard laparoscopic training and is, at least, as effective as video trainer training.[21] Various other studies conclude VR training being beneficial because of standardized repetitive training possibility and the objective feedback on training scores. Nevertheless, VR trainers are prone to hardware problems and need extra care and attention. However, the benefits of VR training allowing for independent, structured, multimedia training with objective feedback and benchmarking of results sets the new training standard for this century. This recognition and need for adequate trained surgeons will overcome the high cost of VR trainers.

CONCLUSION

Unlike the education of pilots, surgeon's training has been left to exposure of certain operations and random competence gaining. It is the right of every patient to expect a highly qualified surgeon. Therefore, training models have to be offered that allow for teacher independent skills acquisition. The evaluation of the learning curve and final results have to be objectively assessed. Certain parameters need to be measured and evaluated for surgical competence. Furthermore, above average competence will most likely be achieved by high exposure to difficult surgical cases which at present might be impossible to be simulated in VR.

REFERENCES

1. Patil NE, Stephen WK, Cheng MS, et al. Surgical Competence. 2003;1-5.
2. Baldwin PJ, Paisley AM, Brown SP. Consultant surgeons' opinion of the skills required of basic surgical trainees. Br J Surg. 1999;86(8):1078-82.
3. Sarker SK, Vincent C, Darzi AW. Assessing the teaching of technical skills. Am J Surg. 2005;189(4):416-8.
4. Thomas B. Basic surgical skills courses: an educational success story. Ann R Coll Surg Engl. 1999;81 (4 Suppl):195-6.
5. Torkington J, Smith SG, Rees B, et al. The role of the basic surgical skills course in the acquisition and retention of laparoscopic skill. Surg Endosc. 2001; 15(10):1071-5.
6. Reznick R, Regehr G, MacRae H, et al. Testing technical skill via an innovative "bench station" examination. Am J Surg. 1997;173(3):226-30.
7. Radetzky A, Bartsch W, Grospietsch G, et al. [SUSILAP-G: a surgical simulator for training minimal invasive interventions in gynecology] [Article in German]. Zentralbl Gynakol. 1999;121(2):110-6.
8. Seymour NE, Gallagher AG, Roman SA, et al. Virtual reality training improves operating room performance: results of a randomized, double-blinded study. Ann Surg. 2002;236(4):458-3.
9. McDougall EM, Kolla SB, Santos RT, et al. Preliminary study of virtual reality and model simulation for learning laparoscopic suturing skills. J Urol. 2009; 182(3):1018-25.
10. Fraser SA, Klassen DR, Feldman LS, et al. Evaluating laparoscopic skills: setting the pass/fail score for the MISTELS system. Surg Endosc. 2003;17(6):964-7.
11. Molinas CR, Campo R. Defining a structured training program for acquiring basic and advanced laparoscopic psychomotor skills in a simulator. Gynecol Surg. 2010;7:427-35.
12. Rodrigues SP, Horeman T, Sam P, et al. Influence of visual force feedback on tissue handling in minimally invasive surgery. Br J Surg. 2014;101(13):1766-73.
13. Horeman,T, Rodrigues SP, Jansen FW et al. Force measurement platform for training and assessment of laparoscopic skills. Surg Endosc. 2010;24(12): 3102-8.
14. Taffinder N, Sutton C, Fishwick RJ, et al. Validation of virtual reality to teach and assess psychomotor skills in laparoscopic surgery. In: Westwood RJ, Hoffman H, Stredney D, Weghorst S (Eds). Technology and Informatics 50: Proceedings of Medicine Meets Virtual Reality. San Diego, CA: IOS Press, Amsterdam; 1998. pp. 124-30.
15. MacDonald J, Williams RG, Rogers DA. Self-assessment in simulation-based surgical skills training. Am J Surg. 2003;185(4):319-22.
16. Torkington J, Smith SG, Rees B, et al. The role of the basic surgical skills course in the acquisition and retention of laparoscopic skill. Surg Endosc. 2001;15(10):1071-5.
17. Hackethal A, Immenroth M, Bürger T. Evaluation of target scores and benchmarks for the traversal task scenario of the Minimally Invasive Surgical Trainer-Virtual Reality (MIST-VR) laparoscopy simulator. Surg Endosc. 2006;20(4):645-50.
18. Datta V, Bann S, Beard J, et al. Comparison of bench test evaluations of surgical skill with live operating performance assessments. J Am Coll Surg. 2004;199(4):603-6.
19. Anastakis DJ, Regehr G, Reznick RK, et al. Assessment of technical skills transfer from the bench training model to the human model. Am J Surg. 1999;177(2):167-70.
20. Jordan JA, Gallagher AG, McGuigan J, et al. Virtual reality training leads to faster adaptation to the novel psychomotor restrictions encountered by laparoscopic surgeons. Surg Endosc. 2001;15(10): 1080-4.
21. Gurusamy KS, Aggarwal R, Palanivelu L, et al. Virtual reality training for surgical trainees in laparoscopic surgery. Cochrane Database Syst Rev. 2009;21(1):CD006575.

KIEL SCH•OL

6 of Gynaecological Endoscopy

Learning by Doing:
How to Teach Laparoscopic Surgery

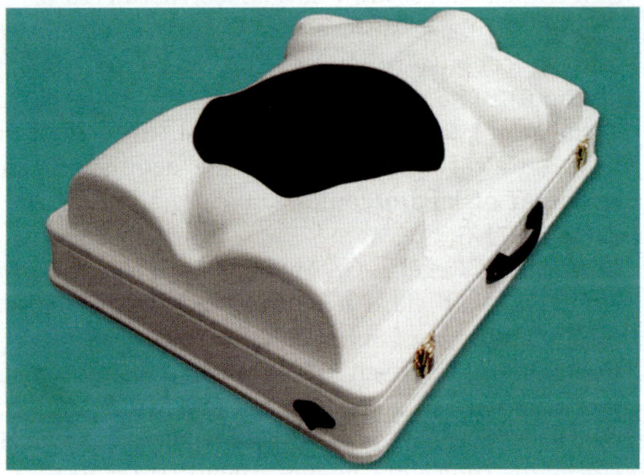

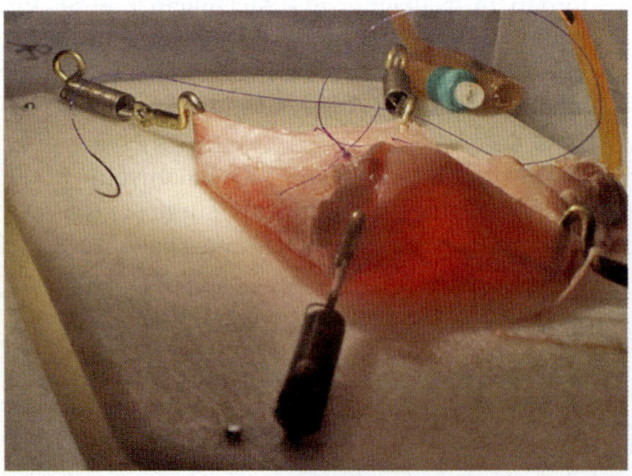

Chapter 6

Learning by Doing: How to Teach Laparoscopic Surgery?

Carolin Spüntrup, Marc Banerjee, Elmar Spüntrup

INTRODUCTION

Surgical education was traditionally transferred using a learning by doing apprenticeship model in real patients. Ethical aspects and other factors made it necessary to innovate this model. The benefits of simulated training for pilots induced the development of simulated skill trainers also for surgeons. Using these trainers several educational strategies, based on findings of behavioral sciences, have been described during the last decades. This chapter summarizes the findings on modern surgical training and coaching methods.

OPTIMIZED LEARNING AND COACHING PROCESS USING BEHAVIORAL SCIENTIFIC FINDINGS

Operative learning is a complex and multifactorial process.[1,2] It has been estimated that the performance of a skillful operation depends in 75% in decision making and only in 25% in manual dexterity.[3] Decision making itself requires theoretical fact knowledge (knowledge of anatomic landmarks, knowledge of operative steps and pathologies, theoretical knowledge on procedure, biochemisty, etc.), a good intraoperative survey and other factors which are summarized under the behavioral scientific term "cognition." Cognition itself is composed of a multitude of factors: perception, attention, information processing, information storage (including organization), and retrieval from long-term memory at the appropriate time.[4-6]

Manual dexterity training (common skills, guidance of instruments, etc.) has been done for a long time. But cognition can also be trained. By repetition mental schemes are induced and psychic stability to manage specific situations increases.[5] In the style of pilot training during the last decades specific training systems have been developed focusing on both cognition and manual dexterity. Surgeons are trained to handle different situations, for example, the step-by-step training of a routine intervention or the management of complications occurring during such an operation. Ideally the trainee reaches step by step a point where many of his or her psychomotor skills and spatial orientation have been automated leading to a constant and optimized performance and finally to a reduction of errors.[3,5,7,8] This status can be reached by repetition. The benefit of repetition of specific interventions to iatrogenic injury is well analyzed (Flowchart 6.1). But repetition also seems to correlate to operative time, operative result, etc. This indicates that repetition is a central factor for the surgeon's education (Flowchart 6.1).

TRIPARTITUDE OF NOVICE, JUNIOR AND EXPERT: DEFINITION OF TRAINING AIMS AT DIFFERENT TRAINING LEVELS

The number of repetitions has been used for the definition of experience of a surgeon.[10] The tripartitude into novices (no experience), juniors (10–100 operations) and experts (more than 100 operations) is a recurrent classification in literature and seems suitable to summarize training aims for an entirety concept respecting both manual dexterity and cognition (Flowchart 6.2).[4,9,10]

Novices are inexperienced in all fields. For novices, training aims are the implementation of automatisms concerning basics: anatomical basics, intraoperative anatomical orientation, handling of

Flowchart 6.1: Interactions in simulated trainings. Repetition is the central factor and influences in all fields.

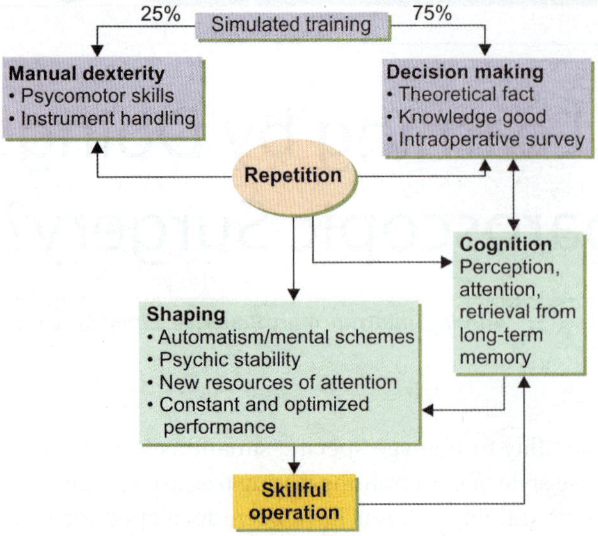

Flowchart 6.2: Tripartitude of novice, junior and expert. Trainees have different trainings aim, depending on their level. Automatisms are growing from level to level. With increasing experience, operations in living patients and need of supervision are reciprocal.

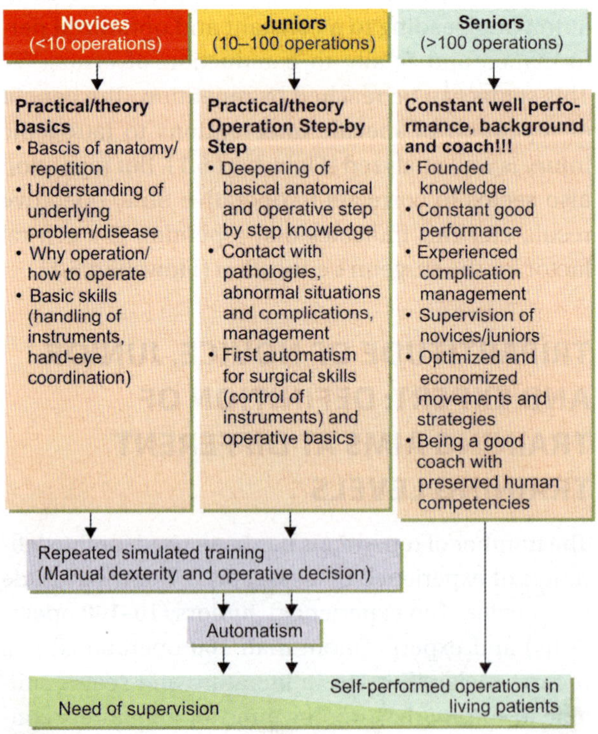

the surgical instruments, basic skills, understanding of the aim of the surgical procedure (that means why is the procedure done, how is it done and what is the final aim).[4,9,10]

Juniors are low experienced with a beginning survey on operative procedures and extended skills. Defined subordinated targets can be accomplished. The training aims of juniors are the implementation of automatisms concerning the single steps of a certain operative procedure, internalizing specific subordinate targets and the progress in control of instruments. With an increasing experience on the way to become an expert, juniors will also learn automatisms concerning pathological situation, complications and other difficult intraoperative situations.[4,9,10]

Experts (more than 100 procedures) are involved in automatisms for operative basics, have a founded knowledge and internalized pathways for many intraoperative situations. Intraoperative movements and activities are optimized, with a clear defined final aim and several subordinate targets, knowing and respecting the consequences of each movement and activity. In case of complications the expert acts more calm and stringent in order to return to the "normal" operative pathway.

This process that is necessary to reach the expert level is called "shaping" in a behavioral sciences sense. It generates new resources of attention for the trainee.[4] and allows the trainee to focus more on learning of the operation steps itself or the management of complications.[4,7] For the definition of aim of trainings the priority aim should be to reach the expert level with optimized and constant performance as well as a reduction of errors by constant shaping.[4,7] The aims of experts are finally to optimize the education of novices and juniors as well as to supervise operation in real patients and help in case of problems (Flowchart 6.2).[4,7,8,10]

Concerning an optimized trainings scheme for shaping process the distributed short interval training has been described as more effective than single long sessions. According to behavioral sciences the implementation of surgical skills is better consolidated, using an interval between two training sessions.[4,11]

HOW TO CONTROL TRAINING SUCCESS?

Control systems to objectify the success of simulated training are necessary but still rare.[3,6]

Performance of technical skills can be measured using an electromagnetically tracking system (ICSAD).[12] This system measures the economy of hand movements and seems to be appropriate to estimate the degree of shaping. The system can be also used for open approaches.

Control systems to check the individual degree of shaping during education are more difficult. Several predictors have been analyzed concerning their value as objective test parameters. Isolated factors are not good predictors, as various factors interact (time-repetition-operative quality-complications, etc).[4,13] A combination of such parameters (e.g., measuring the difference between the ideal puncture of a suture and the actual stich vs. time) seems to be more suitable and can be evaluated, e.g. by a scoring system.

There is need for further objective control systems evaluating both manual dexterity and cognition.

TRAINING SYSTEMS

Referring to our demonstration in "Hysterectomy"[14] in the following section we give an overview over the existing training systems based on the division into organic (human cadavers or animals) and inorganic trainers (others).[15] Combined organic/inorganic trainers complete this division.[11]

Organic Trainers

Organic trainers summarize simulated training in human cadavers or animals.

Human cadavers have been used as a teaching tool for centuries. The simulation of interventions is possible and operative access is comparable to living patients. In general up to three persons learn on one human cadaver. Therefore not all trainees will perform a complete specific operation during the courses, which limits repetition. A vascular perfusion of the cadaver to imitate blood flow is mostly not possible. Nevertheless access, preparation, coagulation, ligation, sutures, incisions and other steps, which are important during intervention, are similar to a real operation. Pathologies in the operative field can be used as a welcome special challenge during the course, but they cannot be planned and sometimes even limit operation. Operations in human cadavers are very useful to recap morphological and topographical aspects of anatomic structures.

Formaldehyde-based fixation techniques are not appropriate due to the rigid consistency of pelvic organs and abdominal wall and, thus, have to be replaced either by alternative fixation methods or the use of fresh frozen cadavers. Fixation procedures providing good conditions to perform open abdominal or laparoscopic procedures include embalming techniques based on ethanol-glycerin or Thiel fixation.[16,17] Although the tissue properties (e.g., color, water content, consistency, mobility) still differ from the in-vivo situation, virtually all surgical procedures including the use of electrocautery and ultrasound devices are feasible applying these alternative fixation methods. Decision making, acquiring operative survey, guidance of assistance as well as single steps (appropriate use of coagulation, preparation, sutures, hand eye-coordination, etc.) are training aims, which can be learned using this setting.

Disadvantages of the use of human cadavers are the risk of transferring certain infections during the procedure and the partly unpleasant odor. The transvaginal access is sometimes limited either by natural factors as the higher age at the time of death (associated with narrow and thin walled vagina) or by a certain disgust of the trainees.

Simulation on Animals

Animals, either living or death, were used for medical learning and education purposes since antiquity. Pigs seems to be most qualified for a couple of organs, as the size and adjacent structures are tolerably comparable to real patients. Operations on living pigs allow a perfusion of the organs, which makes the operation very realistic. Haptic, color and admittance (at least open abdominal or endoscopic) are similar to operations in real patients. All intraoperative steps including admittance, complete steps of intervention and closing the admittance are possible.

Decision making, acquiring operative survey, guidance of assistance as well as single steps (appropriate use of coagulation, preparation, sutures, hand-eye coordination, etc.) are training aims, which can be learned using this system. In living pigs the trainee gets a comparable intraoperative feedback concerning his operative behavior (e.g., via the anesthetist, etc).

Limiting factors are the necessity of a positive ethical votum for each course and the high costs of each pig. In living pigs for ethical reasons pigs must get a general anesthesia. In most courses two to three trainees will operate one pig, so not all participants will operate a complete intervention themselves. Repetition is costly. In general, animals will die after operation. Pathologies cannot be planned. Anatomic and topographic details are only partly comparable

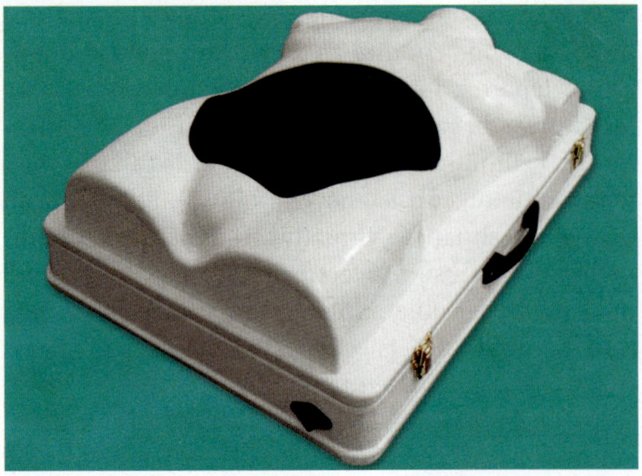

Fig. 6.1: Box trainer (*Courtesy*: Erler–Zimmer).

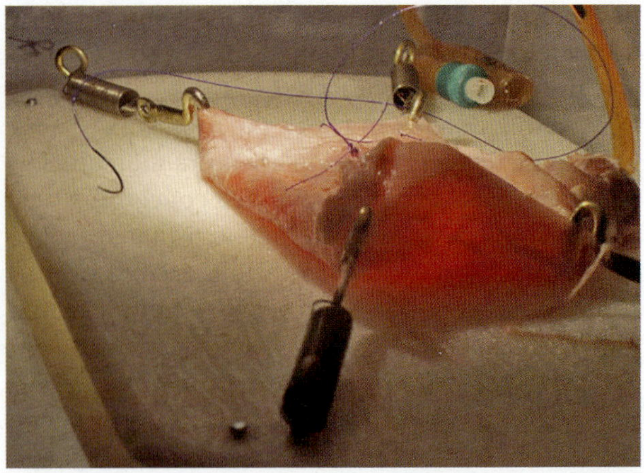

Fig. 6.2: Wet lab: Porcine bladder used for learning knotting and sutures in a simple box trainer (*Courtesy*: Pelvic School, Saarbrücken, Germany).

to human beings. The risk of zoonosis exists, but it is small.

Inorganic Trainers

Inorganic trainers can be divided into classical box trainers, advanced trainers and virtual reality systems (VRT) with the subgroup of robotic assisted VRTs. Most inorganic trainers refer more to the endoscopic approach, but also allow at least an open abdominal access. Some trainers are even equipped with a vagina.

Box Trainers (Fig. 6.1)

Classical box trainers are characterized by a kind of box covered by an exchangeable layer, which simulates the abdominal wall. The box includes possibilities for fixation of artificial layers, structures or even simulated organs. Box trainers are widespread trainings tool and are available in most hospitals. In general they are not associated with a certain operative field. Thus trainee can learn basic steps, such as admittance, hand–eye coordination, instrument handling or knotting and suture techniques. Some box trainers allow the opportunity of a "wet lab," which means the possibility to fix organic parts of animals, such as chicken breast or porcine bladder or guts to perform sutures (Fig. 6.2). Using the box trainer for complex operation in organic material (e.g., gallbladder excision) it offers a kind of simplified entirety simulator.

Advanced Trainers

Advanced (endoscopic) trainers allow the fixation of operative inlays for specific operations. Some endoscopic advanced trainers are additionally equipped with USB connections to overcome the problem of optical system. Genuine endoscopes are no longer necessary to learn on the simulator, but it is possible to adapt the integrated camera, e.g. to the own computer or laptop. Often a mannequin form is chosen with openings on the upper or lower abdomen. Access ports are either determined or can be chosen free on a complete flexible abdominal wall. Operative inlays consist of all important structures and landmarks, which are necessary for specific operations. Inlays are rather expensive, but often two or three organs with pathologies (uterus, ovarian cyst, ectopic tubal pregnancy) are simulated. After operation inlays must be rejected. They can be changed easily and are fixed by a kind of click-in system. They are made completely from inorganic material. This lightens storage.

Decision making, acquiring operative survey, guidance of assistance as well as single steps (preparation, sutures, hand–eye coordination, etc.) are training aims, which can be learned using this system. The use of available training success tool gives the trainee feedback concerning his operative behavior and allows also evaluating the success of learning.

Disadvantage of the systems is that they are not aligned for electrocoagulation or HF surgery. No coagulation of prefunded vessels or electric surgery procedures on tissue (monopolar cutting, sealing, etc.) is possible. Additionally the systems are rather expensive for the daily clinical use and therefor more useful in courses.

Virtual Reality Trainers (Fig. 6.3)

During the last decade for endoscopic procedures a new generation of computer-based simulator has

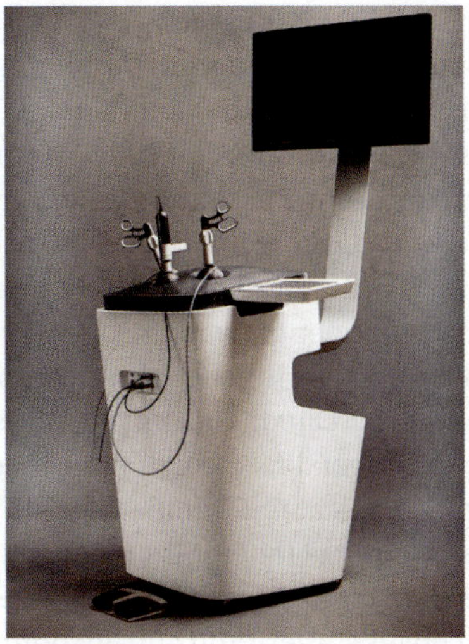

Fig. 6.3: Virtual Reality Systems, LapSim® Laparoscopic Trainer (with permission from Surgical Science).

been introduced. Simplified virtual reality trainers are comparable to a Wi-Fi system, using detectors and microprocessors to convert the movement of surgical instruments into an imaginative movement on the monitor. The underlying imaginative computerized matrix is very realistic and based on real cases.

In first systems sometimes leaps in time or mistakes in converting the surgeon movements occurred, which were meanwhile reduced.

Virtual reality trainers have a large potential, as already every operation and complication can be simulated. Additionally operations can be performed only by the trainee without the need of assistance. Additionally specific hand–eye coordination tools are available.

All procedures that are necessary during an intervention, such as preparation, cutting, sutures, electrocoagulation, monopolar cutting, sealing, etc. are theoretically possible, but must be implemented by the codes.

Decision making, acquiring operative survey and single steps (appropriate use of coagulation, preparation, sutures, hand–eye coordination, etc.) are training aims, which can be learned using this system. The use of additional training success tool gives the trainee feedback concerning his operative behavior and also allows evaluating the success of learning. Using the same training tool, operation can be exactly compared to individual at different trainings levels or interindividual.

A great problem is the lack of haptic feeling. The development of a haptic feeling is a relevant factor for a trainee. Newer systems implemented codes for a kind of haptic feeling, but there is still no solution to copy the original feeling in all situations during the operation.

A further disadvantage is that the coded systems only allow defined steps of the trainee. That means that the system answers with a programmed displacement activity in case of movements of the trainee, which have not been programmed. So an accidental injury of a gut during a hysterectomy is not possible and the gut evades, if the simulated operation has not been coded for the complication "injury of guts."

The fact that in some systems no further assistance is necessary seems to be positive on the first sight. Regarding the trainings aim of intraoperative survey it must be contributed that also the guidance of an intraoperative assistance is a relevant factor and should be trained.

Further disadvantages are the high costs for the systems, which are reasoned in the developing cost for the different tools.

Summarizing virtual reality trainers are at present not seen in the first line of simulated training for novices. They are rather used as control instruments of trainings success in specialized courses. If all "teething troubles" including the lack of haptic will be overcome and a really broad spectrum of intraoperative courses including spontaneous induced complications can be realistically simulated, this system could be the surgical counterpart of simulators for pilots.

Integrated Virtual Reality Trainers in Robotic Assisted Surgical Systems

During the last decade robotic-assisted surgical systems have been introduced for a couple of interventions. The robotic-assisted surgical systems are in general featured with an integrated virtual reality trainer. These "robotic" VRT`s focus on the one hand in general skill training and on the other hand on a training to optimize the use of all function, which are provided by the robotic system.

Moglia et al. published in 2015 a review comparing the different VRTs of robotic systems concerning general skill training and skill transfer to robotic operation.

They found in all analyzed systems a realistic simulation, which made the tool usable and useful for the trainee, but trainings tools are not standardized at all.[18] Robotic VRTs are a useful tool for bimanual wristed manipulation, camera control, master clutching to manage hand position, use of third instrument arm, activating energy sources, appropriate depth perception and awareness of forces applied by instruments for surgeons who intend to use robotic systems.[19]

Concerning the items of general skill training and especially on simulated operations no additional facts than those of VRTs have been reported.

Combined Organic/Inorganic Trainers (Fig. 6.4)

Combined trainers are characterized by a combination of advantages of organic trainers, such as the possibility of electrocoagulation or perfusion with advantages of inorganic trainers, such as reproducible simulation of pathological conditions. By the combination of both components the reälistic simulation of a couple of operative steps is optimized and a more realistic haptic is given.[11] Additional hand–eye coordination tools are available (Figs. 6.5A to D).

In a certain way box trainers with the fixation possibility for organic parts of animals can be considered as a precursor of combined trainers but the characteristic difference is that pathologies cannot be planned and that they are not exactly reproducible. In a real combined trainer organic structures are not used in its entity but only components of organic origin are processed to create reproducible artificial pathological organs. According to bionic sciences characteristics of organic material is analyzed and useful components for each operative step are composed until a fully functional simulation of a certain operation is created. The organic parts are often by-products of vegetable, meat or fish processing.

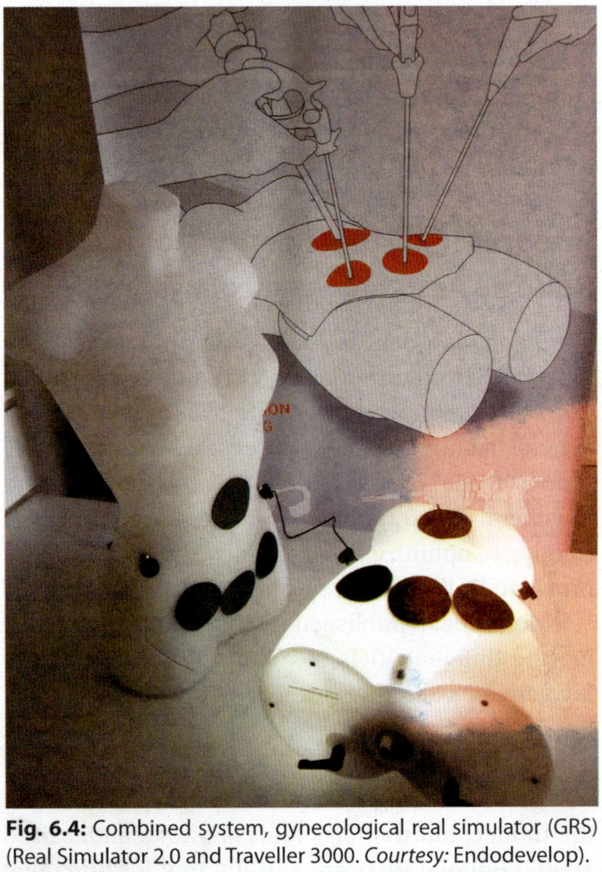

Fig. 6.4: Combined system, gynecological real simulator (GRS) (Real Simulator 2.0 and Traveller 3000. *Courtesy:* Endodevelop).

The gynecological real simulator (GRS) system is a combined trainings tool for frequent gynecological operations (hysterectomy, ovarian surgery, endoscopic descensus surgery and anti-incontinence procedures). The unit consists of three parts:

1. The gynecological real simulator (large or traveler version).
2. Pelvic models available (Figs. 6.5A & 6.6A and D).
3. Operation-specific inlays (Figs. 6.5C, 6.6B to D).

Optionally a USB camera system and light is available.

The real simulator imitates a female torso. It consists of a closable opening on the lower abdomen, a vaginal opening and smaller holes for connection of equipment (e.g. perfusion). Endoscopic equipment is introduced via four defined areas on the classical introduction places. The pelvic models are scaled to the GRS and are fixed by bolted connections. Pelvic models are specific for the simulation of defined operations so different pelvic models are available (hysterectomy model, ovarian cyst model, descensus model, anterior compartment model, Figures 6.6A to E). An additional basic-skills model is available, using classical tools for hand–eye coordination, handling of instruments, knotting and sutures and wet lab training (Figs. 6.5A to D).

Pelvic models consist of all structures that are important landmarks for the specific operations. Depending on the trainings aim learning success tools as well as perfusion or the possibility for the use of electrocoagulative instruments are possible.

The operative area of the pelvic models is recessed for the according inlays and provides fixation mechanisms for the inlays. The inlays are the centerpiece of the simulated operations. They simulate specific operations as realistic as possible, can be changed easily by a click-in system and are thrown away after operation.

The use of additional training success tool gives the trainee feedback concerning his operative behav-

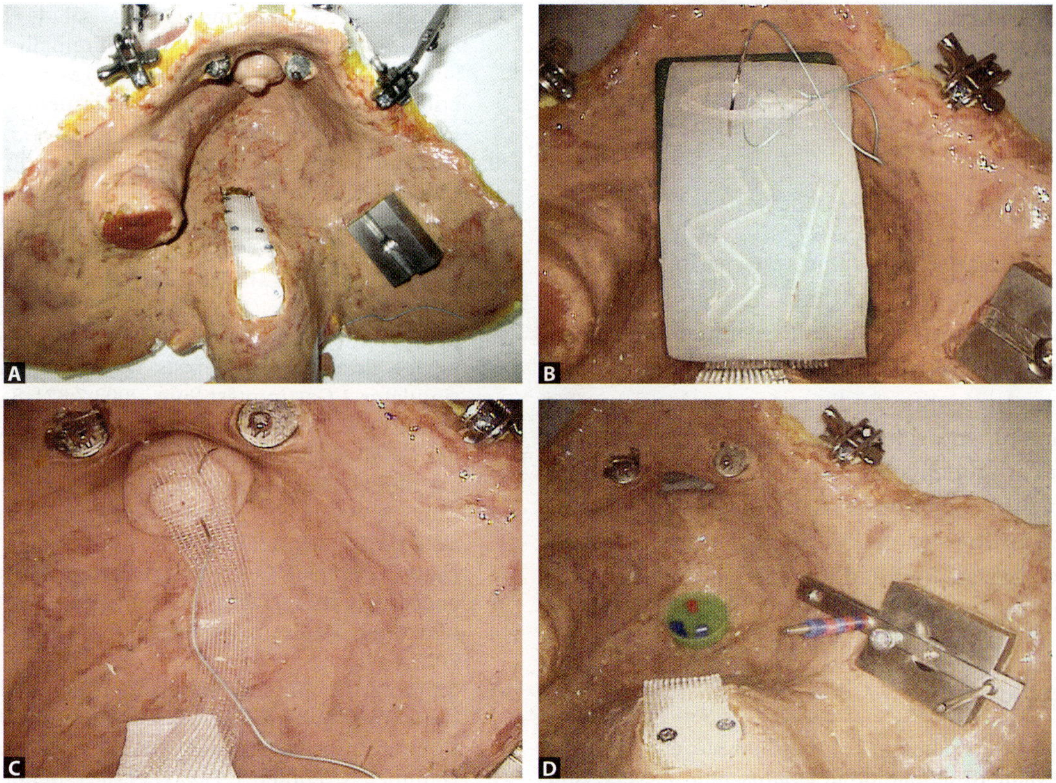

Figs. 6.5A to D: Selection of tools of the multitool Skill training (*Courtesy*: Endodevelop): (A) Basic pelvine model; (B) Suture pad; (C) Simplified sacropexy; (D) Skill training: Pearl tool.

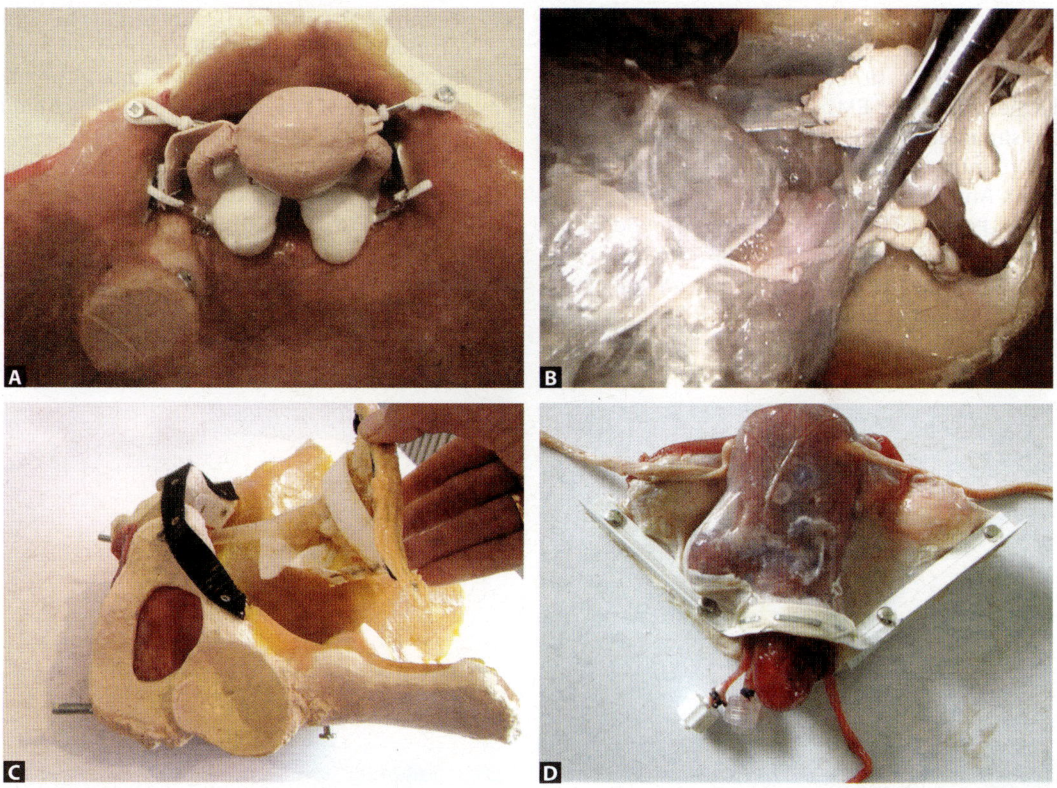

Figs. 6.6A to D: Selection of complete operative tools. (A) Ovarian cysts; (B) Intraoperative real simulator situs: laparoscopic hysterectomy with coagulable uterine artery; (C) Colpo-suspension inlay with endopelvic fascia, bladder, urethra' (D) Artificial hysterectomy inlay with intra-ligamental myoma. Vessels can be prefunded using the lock systems.
(*Courtesy*: Pelvic School, Saarbrücken, Germany)

ior and also allows evaluating the success of learning.

Disadvantages are the necessity of unfreezing inlays before use. Connection of vessels, neutral, etc. is associated with a lead time of about 15 min.

OUTLOOK

Different operative simulator systems focus on different learning objectives and aims. They are not necessarily competitive but often rather synergistic. Modern operative trainings concepts should follow behavioural scientific findings concerning learning and teaching strategies. The consideration of both relevant components for surgical education manual dexterity and cognition is useful for the guided culmination of the expert level with automatisms for operative basics, founded knowledge and internalized pathways.

REFERENCES

1. Fried GM, Feldmann LS, Vassiliou MC et al. Proving the value of simulation in laparoscopic surgery. Ann Surg. 2004;240(3):518-25.
2. Smyth CM. Graduate surgical training in America. Ann Surg. 1945;121(6):793-802.
3. Spencer, F. Teaching and measuring surgical techniques: the technical evaluation of competence. Bull Am Coll Surg. 1978;63:9-12.
4. Gallagher AG, Ritter EM, Champion H et al. Virtual reality simulation for the operating room: proficiency-based training as a paradigm shift in surgical skill training. Ann Surg. 2005;241(2):364-72.
5. Fitts FM, Posner MI. Human Performance. Belmont, CA: Brooks/Cole Publishing Co.; 1967.
6. Esysenck M, Keane M. Cognitive Psychology: A Student Handbook. Erlbaum: Hove; 1995.
7. Gallagher AG, Lederman AB, McGlade K, et al. Discriminative validity of the Minimally Invasive Surgical Trainer in Virtual Reality (MIST-VR) using criteria levels based on expert performance. Surgical Endosc. 2004:18(4):660-5.
8. Hier und heute Reportage 2010 ("nähkurs für ärzte").
9. Gallagher A, Satava R. Virtual reality as a metric for the assessment of laparoscopic psychomotor skills: learning curves and reliability measures. Surg Endosc. 2002;16(12):1746-52.
10. Ritter E, McClusky D, Gallagher A, et al. Objective psychomotor skills assessment of experienced and novice flexible endoscopists with a virtual reality simulator. J Gastrointest Surg. 2003;7:871-8.
11. Spüntrup C, Noé GK, Spüntrup E. Lernprogramme in der Gynäkologie: Learning by doing - aber bitte erst am Modell. Der Frauenarzt. 2012;53(10):952-57.
12. Darzi A, Smith S, Taffinder N. Assessing operative skill. BMJ. 1999;318(188):887.
13. Hanna G, Frank T, Cuschieri A. Objective assessment of endoscopic knot quality. Am J Surg. 1997;174(4): 410-3.
14. Alkatout I, Metller L. Hysterectomy. Berlin: Springer; 2017.
15. Munro MG. Surgical simulation: Where have we come from? Where are we now? Where are we going? J Minim Invasive Gynecol. 2012;19 (3):272-83.
16. Hammer N, Löffler S, Feja C et al. Ethanol-glycerin fixation with thymol conservation: a potential alternative to formaldehyde and phenol embalming. Anat Sci Educ. 2012;5(4):225-33.
17. Hammer N, Löffler S, Bechmann I et al. Comparison of modified Thiel embalming and ethanol-glycerin fixation in an anatomy environment: potentials and limitations of two complementary techniques. Anat Sci Educ. 2015;8(1):74-85.
18. Moglia A, Ferrari V, Morelli L et al. A systematic review of virtual reality simulators for robot-assisted surgery. Eur Urol. 2015;69(6):1065-80.
19. Liu M, Curet M. A review of training research and virtual reality simulators for the da Vinci surgical system. Teach Learn Med. 2015;27(1):12-26.

KIEL SCH•O L

7 of Gynaecological Endoscopy

Training in Minimally Invasive Gynecological Surgery

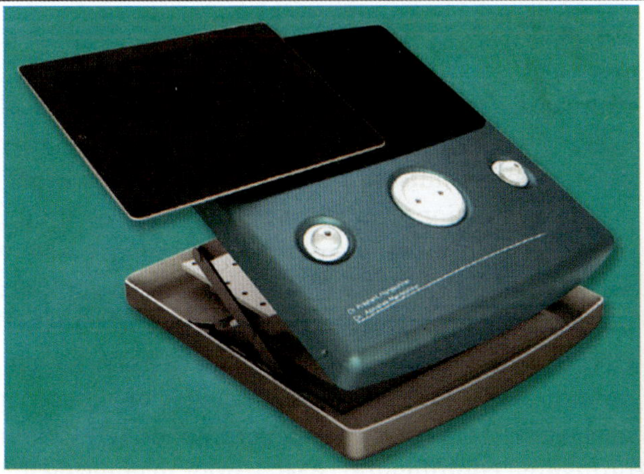

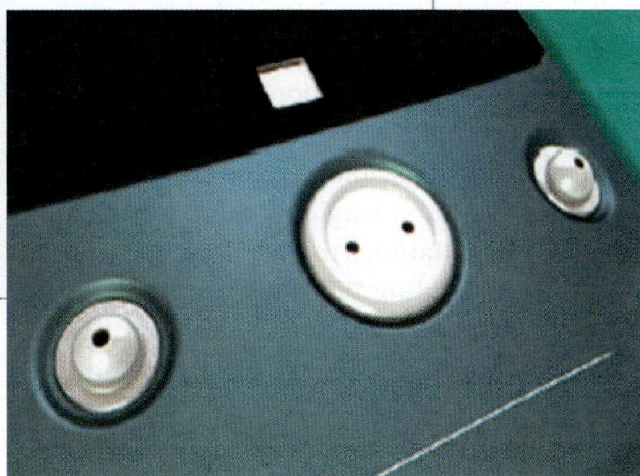

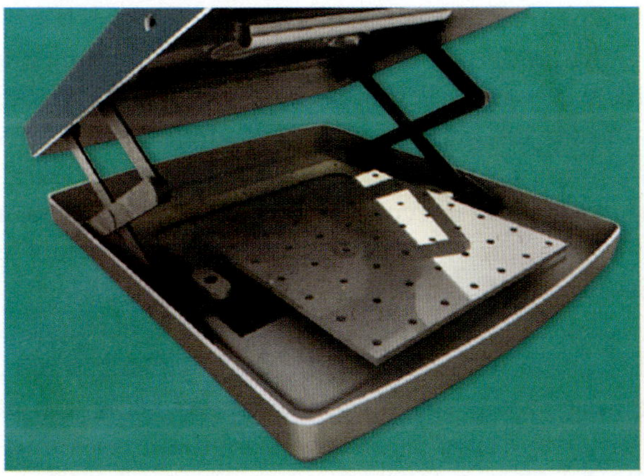

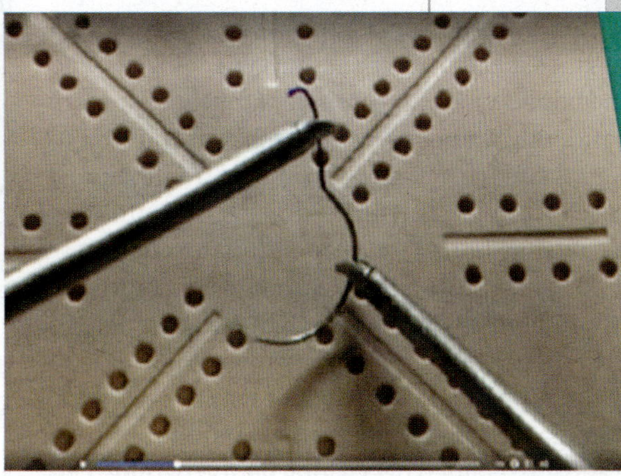

Chapter 7

Training in Minimally Invasive Gynecological Surgery

Abhishek Mangeshikar

INTRODUCTION

A patient's consent for surgery is based upon a trust that the surgeon is sufficiently experienced and technically competent to execute the procedure. Surgical competence includes adequate core medical knowledge, good clinical decision-making skills and judgment, professionalism, keen interpersonal and communication skills, and technical expertise. During the last century, surgical training was completely based on the famous model "see one, do one, teach one," developed by William Halsted, in 1904. Undoubtedly it has produced a generation of good surgeons.[1] However, the language of surgical education has changed over the last 20 years. We are now talking about simulators, objective structured clinical examination (OSCEs), objective structured assessment of technical skills (OSATs), verification of proficiency and fundamentals of laparoscopy, most of which barely existed 20 years ago. The reason being in endoscopic and more specifically in laparoscopic surgery there is a discrepancy between what is taught and what is expected of graduating gynecologists who lack the confidence to perform laparoscopic surgery independently and consider insufficient training to be a significant barrier. Hence, surgical training must be preceded by a structured dry lab skill training with the acquisition of the specific laparoscopic psychomotor skills (LPS). The learning characteristics of LPS are contrary to the surgical competence, in that they do not require constant supervision from a highly skilled surgeon but rely on repetitive practice, and once gained, these abilities shorten the learning curve and are retained over a long period of time. Different studies have proved the benefit of standardized teaching, and the combination of didactic classes with hands-on experience in box trainers, virtual simulators, animals and cadavers improves surgical skills.[2] Drybox training has gained lot of popularity as time constraints and other issues such as medicolegal regulations, increasing patient expectations, efficiency, cost-effectiveness and patients safety make it difficult for trainees to learn these complex procedures on patients in the operating room (OR). Drybox also helps in improving laparoscopic psychomotor skills (LPS), including laparoscopic camera navigation (LCN), hand–eye coordination (HEC) and bi-manual coordination (BMC), prior to entering the OR training program. Nine fundamental manipulations that the surgeon must learn on the drybox are tactile sensation, aspiration/injection, incision, excision, extraction, evacuation, purposeful injury, closure and implantation/transplantation.[3] Even though simulation cannot completely replace clinical learning, the potential benefits of simulation training are widely recognized. Therefore, there is considerable interest in the implementation of surgical simulators in training programs as an adjunct to clinical learning. In recent years virtual reality surgical simulation (VRSS) has become popular; however, lack of tactile sensation and high cost are limitations.

Clinicians, both surgeons as well as gynecologists who perform endoscopic surgery without proper training of the specific psychomotor skills, are at higher risk of increased patient morbidity and mortality.[4]

WHY LAPAROSCOPY NEEDS TRAINING?

- In open surgery, surgeons have direct visual input and stereopsis to ascertain depth. Whereas in laparoscopic surgery a flat screen results in the reduction of depth perception.

- In laparoscopic surgery, the trocar restricts movement by acting as an invariant point and by the fulcrum effect. The range of motion is therefore reduced to four degrees of freedom compared to six needed to perform free motion, negatively affecting the surgeon's dexterity.
- For beginners: poorer hand-eye coordination, variable amplification, mirrored movement, reduced haptic feedback, ergonomics and disorientation are major problems.

LEARNING CURVE FOR LAPAROSCOPIC GYNECOLOGICAL SURGERY

Laparoscopic surgery has a steep learning curve associated with a higher complication rate in the beginning of the surgeon's career. What is the learning curve? The German psychologist Hermann Ebbinghaus first introduced the concept of the learning curve in 1885. In his study of memorization, he realized that the more he repeated the series, the more syllables he could remember, until finally he could recall the whole list. If we want to apply this concept to surgery, we would need to draw a slope, and the definition of learning curve would be beginning of the slope. It is still controversial how many procedures are required by a single surgeon to overcome the technical obstacles and achieve satisfactory performance. As number of procedures is relative and depends on various factors like individual's ability, skills and particularly the type of procedure.

ESSENTIALS OF CURRICULUM-BASED TRAINING

Gynecologic laparoscopic curricula have previously not been developed nor validated using an evidence-based approach. For the most part, gynecologists have adapted laparoscopy curricula from general surgery specialties, which may not be comprehensive with regards to the specific requirements of gynecologic postgraduate training.[5] However, a 7-week laparoscopic curriculum was developed and approved using Delphi consensus methodology, which included four components.[6]

1. Cognitive training consisting of weekly 1-hour didactics lectures covering laparoscopic equipment, electro-surgery, pelvic anatomy, patient selection, medicolegal issues, intraoperative considerations and complications.
2. Low-fidelity simulation to develop productions, production sets and basic technical skills, using 2-hour box trainer sessions (peg transfer, pattern cutting, pre-tied knot, ovarian cystectomy, intracorporeal knotting, extracorporeal knot tying and Roeder knots.
3. Virtual reality simulation is also used to work on the development of productions, production sets and basic technical skills. The included tasks were camera navigation, instrument navigation, coordination, grasping, lifting and grasping, and cutting.
4. High-fidelity operating room simulation to focus on team dynamics, communication, situational awareness, acute stress and decision making under stress.

Role of the Mentor

The mentor plays a key role in creating an effective teaching module and involves two critical aspects: (a) the surgeon-in-training must participate to acquire part of the skills, landscape, and navigational knowledge and utilize the mentor's experience so as to reduce the learning curve and (b) the trainee also should play a significant role in the operation he or she assists in, with part of the responsibility in the evolution and outcome of the procedure. These two aspects are related but not the same. The first is indeed the role of the trainee with his or her mentor, as the two together form an apprenticeship and the trainee can shorten his or her own learning curve by utilizing the mentor's learning curve. Second, the relationship should not be considered as a master/slave relationship, but rather as a partnership in which the assistant provides accurate, precise and adapted vision, anticipating the needs of the operator without leaving the field of attention too quickly or unattended, therefore ensuring the same safety measures as the operating surgeon.

LEARNING MODES

Drybox: Despite the recent surge in popularity of simulator-based training, there is no consensus as to the optimal simulator type or curriculum design. While virtual reality technology holds great promise, trainees may prefer the video-trainer platform because of issues concerning cost effectiveness, tactile feedback and imaging fidelity. New portable and cost-effective laparoscopic trainer has a small, compact and lightweight design to allow storage and portability for home or office. This type of surgical simulator uses real surgical instruments and equipment including video-monitors, cameras and laparoscopes. More laptop-based cost-effective systems have been developed for more widespread dissemination.

The author-designed Mangeshikar MIST allows a portable and collapsible training box without the need for a camera system or a video-monitor. It incorporates the use of a tablet or a phone to simulate the act of laparoscopic movements while looking at a screen. Repetition is key in mastering this and it is of the author's opinion that trainees must first master the skills needed on the dry box before attempting to assist in the OR (Figs. 7.1 to 7.4).

Furthermore the tablets and phones allow video-recording and transmission, which can be electronically transmitted to experts for critical evaluation.

However, the drills developed lack the face validity offered by other systems; the instruments may be real, but the "tissues" used clearly are not.

Virtual reality surgical simulators (VRSS): Current virtual reality (VR) simulators have been inspired by the need for repetition of selected tasks. The toolkit for illustration of procedures includes 3D anatomical representation, instrument interfaces, force feedback and various media such as video-in-the-scene. The system utilizes a six-degree-of-freedom device and a computer with the addition of a haptic feedback device.[7] This device can be modified to accommodate actual laparoscopic instrument handles, which augment the reality of the experience. Another advantage of these trainers is that it can be set up to record and save accurate and objective data for individual performance on specific tasks for later assessment.

Objective measurements such as the time to complete a task, economy of hand motion, dexterity and instrument path length can be easily used as assessment tools to document the progress of laparoscopic skills. Different studies have proved that LapSim[8] and LapMentor[9] virtual reality simulators training of residents resulted in improved performance of basic laparoscopic techniques and transferability of skill from the simulated to the applied environment (Figs. 7.5 and 7.6).[10]

Animal labs: This is the most realistic, nonpatient environment for laparoscopic training. The porcine or canine abdomen is comparable in size to the adult human. Performing a pelvic dissection in this model provides tactile feedback in an environment where technical errors and complications such as bowel perforation or common vascular injury can occur without consequence to a human patient. Even though animal labs are much better tool for learning and refining surgical skills still ethical issues, high maintenance cost and special facility make it difficult to fully integrate into most surgical curricula.

Drybox and VRSS Skill Assessment

To date, very little work has been done for evaluating laparoscopic skills using performance-based standards. Seymour et al.[11] reported good results using a competency standard derived from expert levels for a single virtual reality task. Fraser et al.[5] reported pass/fail scores for the McGill Inanimate System for Training and Evaluation of Laparoscopic Skills (MISTELS) video-trainer tasks for assessment purposes. Korndorffer et al.[12] established a comprehensive set of

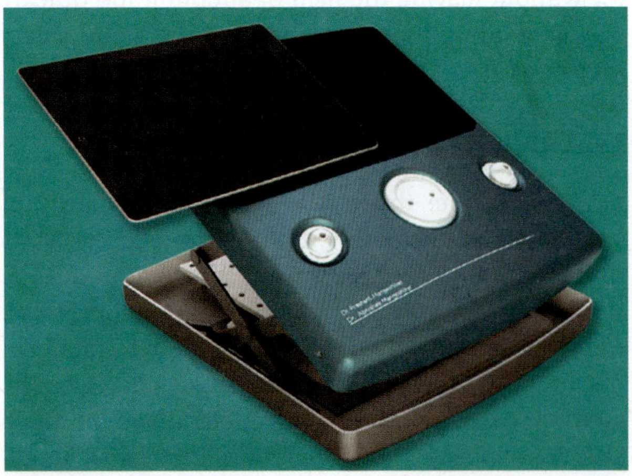

Fig. 7.1: Mangeshikar MIST.

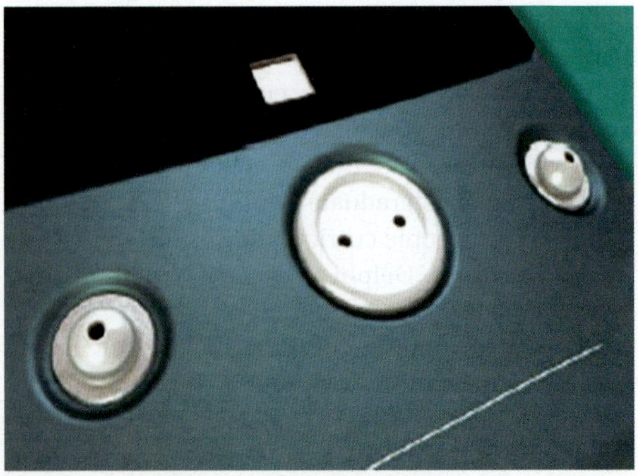

Fig. 7.2: Instrument introducing pathways.

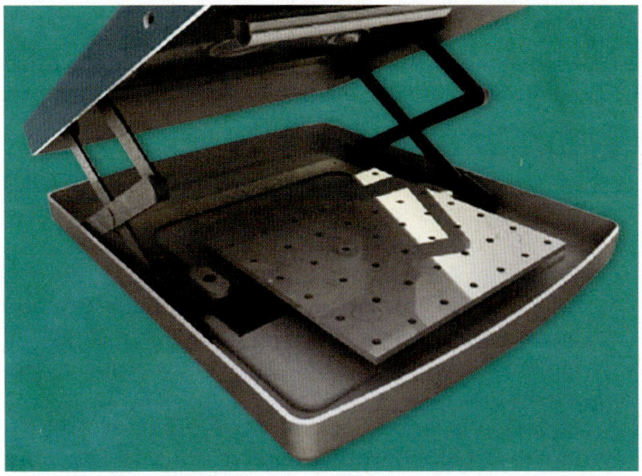

Fig. 7.3: Interior part of training box.

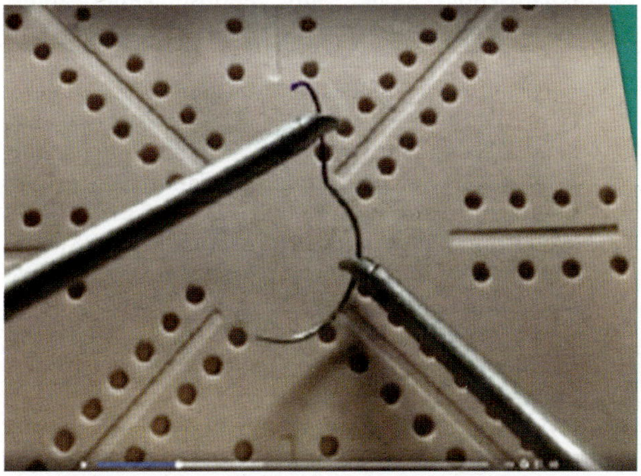

Fig. 7.4: Suture pad and needle grasping prior to sticking.

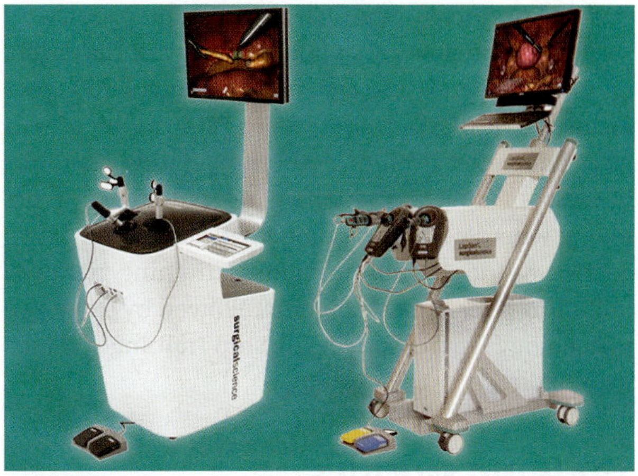

Fig. 7.5: LapSim.

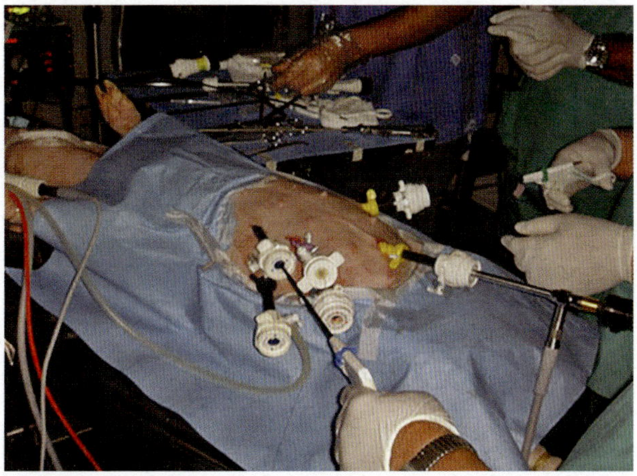

Fig. 7.6: LapMentor.

five tasks (bean drop, running string, checkerboard, block move and suture foam) for assessing Southwestern video-trainer skills.

The question then arises whether trainees who cannot reach competency should be allowed to perform procedures in operating room. High-stakes validation will be required before this question can be answered.

CONCLUSION

Presently, the completion of surgical training is determined by elapsed time in training, general case volume standards and relatively subjective end-of-rotation evaluations by faculty. However, in the era of the 80-hour work weeks, curricula must be not only effective but also efficient; training should maximize the benefit while expending the least amount of time. Current methods of evaluation are highly variable with few standardized training protocols and reliable outcome measures for assessing the competence of residents are not yet well developed. Most curricula use an arbitrary duration or a predetermined number of repetitions as training end points. Since the rate of learning is variable and may be highly dependent on innate visuospatial abilities, arbitrary end points may be neither efficient nor maximally beneficial. Some participants may train longer than necessary, and some participants may not train long enough. An ideal training curriculum would account for variations in ability and tailor the time needed for each individual to acquire a given skill. All individuals must be competent upon completion of training while not spending wasteful hours performing repetitive motions without further benefit.

In the field of surgery, the explosion in technology and the development of minimally invasive techniques have provided both an impetus and an opportunity for developing innovative training programs. Specifically, simulation offers the promise of a safe, nonthreatening training venue with the ability to objectively measure aspects of technical skills performance. It marks a shift in our philosophy of surgical education from one where we threw residents in the pool and expected them to learn how to swim, to one where we are teaching them before they even get to the pool. Thus traditional training pathway including a residency program followed by extensive gynecology laparoscopy fellowship training remains invaluable.

TRAINING MODULE

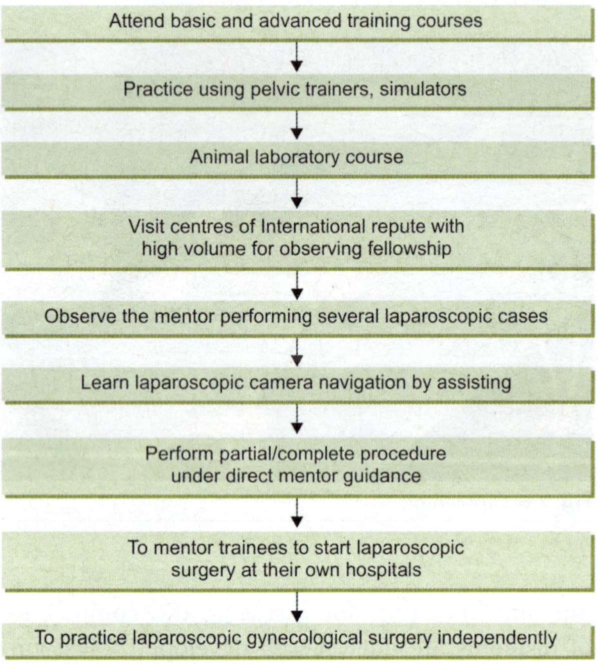

REFERENCES

1. Haluck RS, Krummel TM. Computers and virtual reality for surgical education in the 21st century. Arch Surg. 2000;135(7):786-92.
2. Fernandes CF, Ruano JM, Kati LM, et al. Assessment of laparoscopic skills of Gynecology and Obstetrics residents after a training program. Einstein (Sao Paulo). 2016;14(4):468-72.
3. Gallagher AG, Cowie R, Crothers I, et al. PicSOr: an objective test of perceptual skill that predicts laparoscopic technical skill in three initial studies of laparoscopic performance. Surg Endosc. 2003;17(9): 1468-71.
4. Stefanidis D, Acker C, Heniford BT. Proficiency-based laparoscopic simulator training leads to improved operating room skill that is resistant to decay. Surg Innov. 2008;15(1):69-73.
5. Fraser SA, Klassen DR, Feldman LS, et al. Evaluating laparoscopic skills. Surg Endosc Other Interv Techniques. 2003;17(6):964-7.
6. Cundiff GW. At last, a standardized laparoscopy curriculum for gynecology residents. Am J Obstet Gynecol. 2016;215(2):137-9.
7. Scott DJ, Cendan JC, Pugh CM, et al. The changing face of surgical education: simulation as the new paradigm. J Surg Res. 2008;147(2):189-93.
8. Woodrum DT, Andreatta PB, Yellamanchilli RK, et al. Construct validity of the LapSim laparoscopic surgical simulator. Am J Surg. 2006;191(1):28-32.
9. Andreatta PB, Woodrum DT, Gauger PG, et al. LapMentor metrics possess limited construct validity. Simul Healthc. 2008;3(1):16-25.
10. Hyltander A, Liljegren E, Rhodin PH, et al. The transfer of basic skills learned in a laparoscopic simulator to the operating room. Surg Endosc. 2002;16(9):1324-8.
11. Seymour NE, Gallagher AG, Roman SA, et al. Virtual reality training improves operating room performance: results of a randomized, double-blinded study. Ann Surg. 2002;236(4):458-63; discussion 63-4.
12. Korndorffer JR, Jr., Stefanidis D, Scott DJ. Laparoscopic skills laboratories: current assessment and a call for resident training standards. Am J Surg. 2006; 191(1):17-22.

KIEL SCHOOL

8 of Gynaecological Endoscopy

Current Hysteroscopic Training Models

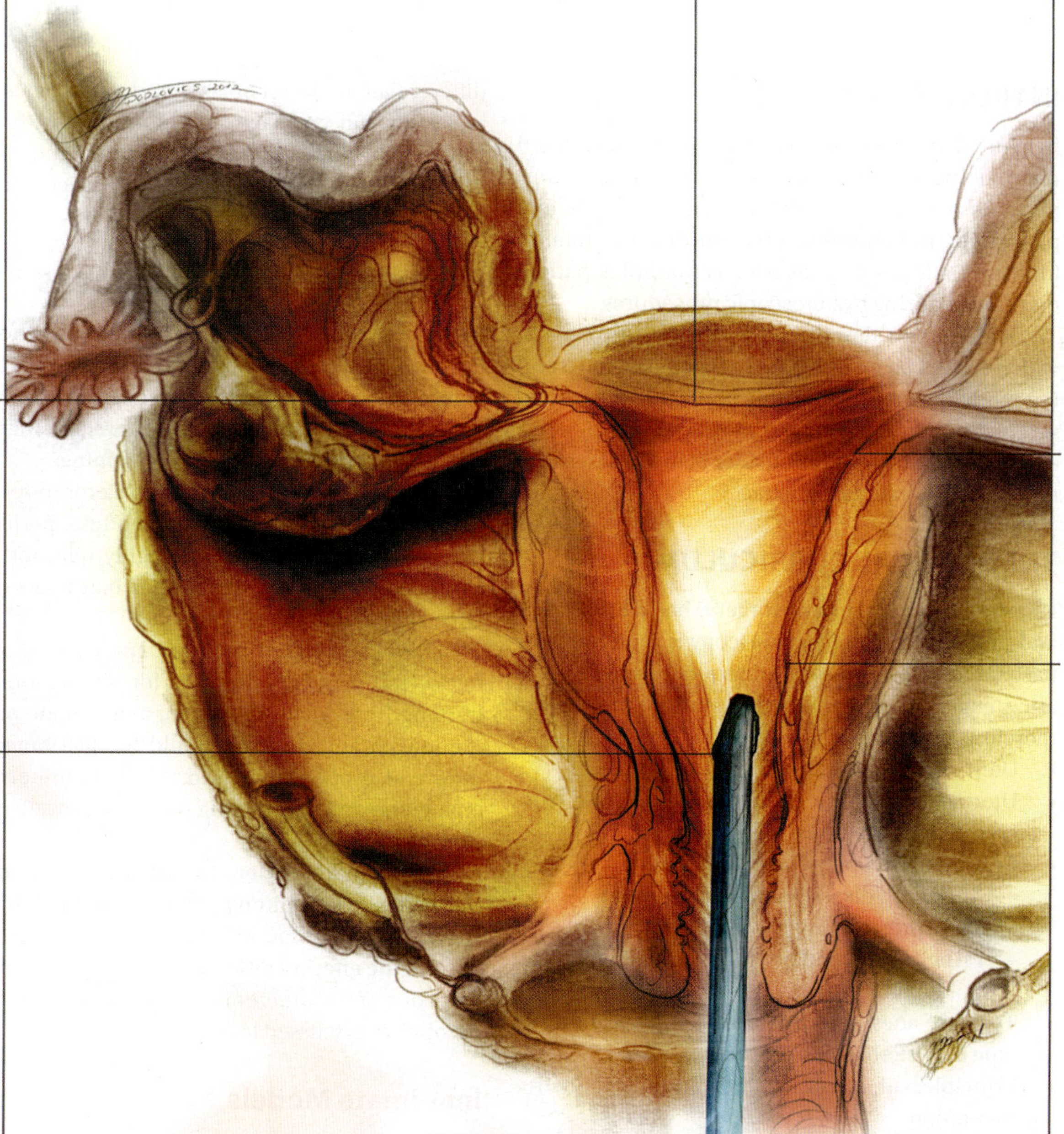

Chapter 8

Current Training Models in Hysteroscopy

Flemming Bjerrum, Lotte Clevin

INTRODUCTION

In general, hysteroscopic procedures are considered reasonably safe; however, in some cases severe complications can arise. For that reason, training before performing hysteroscopic procedures is essential to increase patient safety, as well as minimize patient discomfort during hysteroscopic procedures.

This chapter describes the theoretical content, which should be included in a curriculum, the training models currently available and what to consider when choosing a model, the assessment of hysteroscopic skills and what to consider before trainees are allowed to operate on patients.

THEORETICAL CURRICULUM

Like for all other types of surgery, basic knowledge and understanding of hysteroscopy is a prerequisite for hands-on training and subsequent real-life operating experience. A theoretical curriculum should therefore include the following topics:[1-4]

- Uterine/pelvic anatomy
- Uterine pathology including indications for hysteroscopic procedures
- Knowledge of operating equipment
  - Assembly/disassembly of equipment
  - Basic principles of electrosurgery
  - Principles behind use of distention media and fluid management
- Types of anesthesia required depending on the type of hysteroscopic procedure
- Principles of operating technique and instrumentation
- Management of complications commonly associated with hysteroscopy

Although diagnostic hysteroscopy is a relatively simple procedure, it is important to be able to differentiate between normal and pathological findings. This can be practiced beforehand with use of video recordings, which allows for demonstrating the relevant pathology as well as proper operating technique.

HANDS-ON TRAINING MODELS

In general, simulation-based training has shown to improve surgical skills, although little research has focused specifically on hysteroscopy. It is, however, reasonable to assume that this general finding would also apply to hysteroscopic skills training.

One challenge in teaching hysteroscopy is that there can only be one surgeon at a time performing the procedure. This makes it highly relevant to use simulation-based training to get hands-on experience before operating on patients.[5]

Simulation-based hysteroscopy training should follow the general principles for simulation-based training. This entails the use of a deliberate practice framework and training should be distributed over time and proficiency-based.[6,7] This is important to ensure the optimal training outcome as well as most time efficient training.

A systematic review by Savran et al examined the evidence for training and assessment of hysteroscopic skills and found that there were large variations in the effect of different training tools.[8] The pros and cons of the different training options for hysteroscopy are discussed later.[9]

Inanimate Models

Training of hysteroscopy has been described using synthetic models, vegetables and animal organs to simulate the uterine cavity. Commercially available models generally consist of a uterine model made of

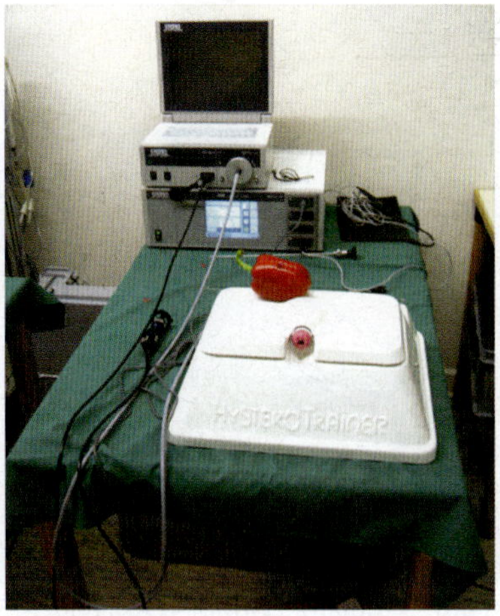

Fig. 8.1: Hysterotrainer.

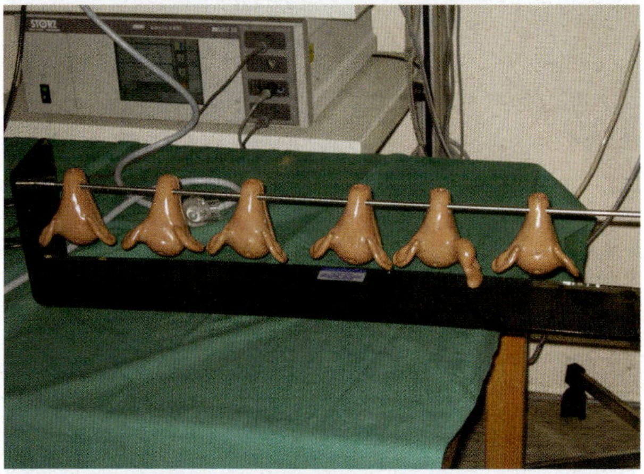

Fig. 8.2: Training model for diagnostic hysteroscopy.

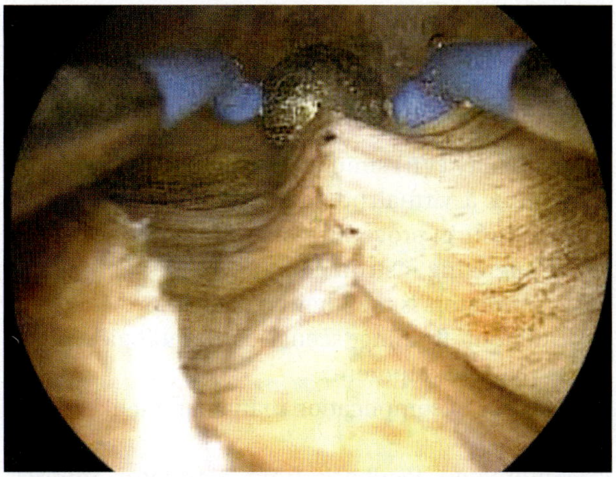

Fig. 8.3: Use of rollerball for endometrial ablation in a pig heart.

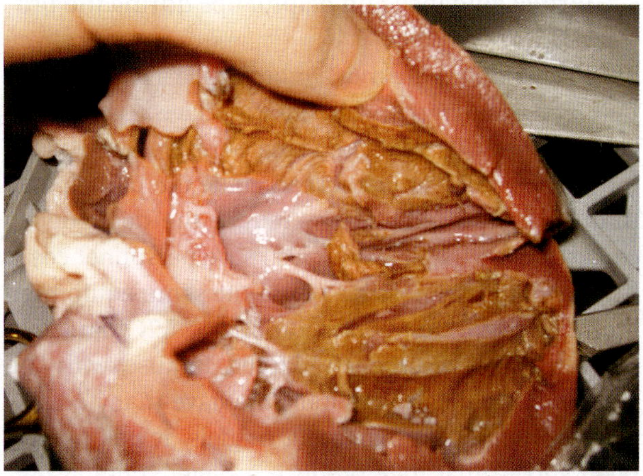

Fig. 8.4: Transsected pig heart after endometrial resection training.

latex, silicone or rubber, which allows for the practice of instrumentation and diagnostic procedures (Figs. 8.1 and 8.2), i.e., the hysteroscopic skills training and testing system.[10] Different models displaying different pathologies can be used to practice diagnostic procedures. Single-use models for operative procedures have also been developed and some of these also allow training the use of distension media.[11,12] Ongoing replacement of these models for practicing operative techniques is, however, associated with higher costs.

Home-made models using a vegetable or fruit, like at butternut pumpkin, to simulate the uterine cavity is less expensive and allows for the use of electrosurgical equipment. However, they are also less useful when practicing the use of distention media because of the reduced flexibility of the material.[13,14]

Using animal organs like cow uteri, sheep bladder or porcine hearts allow for training using electrosurgical equipment[15,16] (Figs. 8.3 and 8.4). However, when using an animal organ to simulate the uterine cavity, you do not get an exact replica of the anatomical structures as you would with commercially available synthetic models. It is therefore difficult to train treatment of specific intrauterine pathologies and these models are more useful in training general operative techniques, i.e., resection. The organ is also not perfused, so bleeding will not be seen as in real operations. Apart from that it is possible to realistically train for resection technique and fluid management. Another advantage is that animal organs for training are relatively cheap.

To avoid complications and delays during operations, it is important for trainees to practice assembly and handling of hysteroscopic equipment. This can be done using all of these models. However, it requires the use of real operating room equipment and instruments. Being able to practice using real instruments could potentially make it easier for trainees to transfer skills acquired in the simulated setting to the operating theater.[17]

Virtual Reality Simulators

Virtual reality (VR) simulators consist of a computer generating a virtual operating field where you are able to perform procedures using an interface simulating operating instruments (Fig. 8.5). The benefits of VR simulators is that they are able to provide:

- Different training scenarios/pathologies using the same equipment;
- Practice of complication management like bleeding;
- Automated feedback from simulator metrics, i.e., estimates of visualization, instrument movements and use of distension media;
- Virtual guidance and helpful tips during the procedure.

VR simulators are much more expensive to acquire than other training models, but they have less ongoing costs as they do not rely on single-use materials. Furthermore, as VR simulators can guide the participants through the procedure, they reduce the dependency on instructors and thus can also save personnel costs. Although it is not possible to use the same equipment that is used in the operating room,[18,19] VR simulators have similar instruments adapted for use with the simulator. Although VR simulators have many advantages compared to inanimate models, it has not yet been shown that they produce a better training outcome.[20] One of the benefits of using a VR simulator is that participants can use the automated feedback from the simulators during training and thereby more easily track their progress. They are also less dependent on an instructor being present.

Currently, the only VR simulator for hysteroscopy available on the market is the HystSim™ (VirtaMed AG, Zurich, Switzerland).[18,19,21-23] With this simulator it is possible to practice a wide selection of procedures, i.e., diagnostic procedures, hysteroscopic biopsies, hysteroscopic sterilization, polyp removal and practice the correct handling of the most commonly used instruments as well as new types such as hysteroscopic morcellators (Figs. 8.6 and 8.7). This simulator also features an anatomic rubber pelvic model with various exchangeable, different shaped uteri and it is able to simulate bleeding, fluid management and complications.

The next level of VR-based training of hysteroscopy is to use full-scenario training, where full procedures and complication management can be practiced alongside operating room staff.

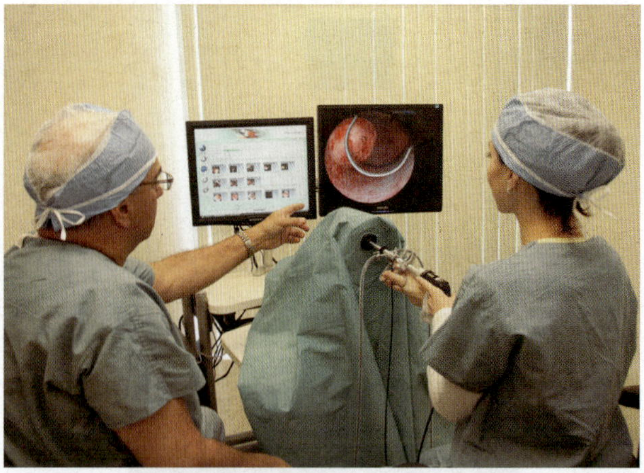

Fig. 8.5: HystSim™ simulator (VirtaMed AG, Zurich, Switzerland) with permission from VirtaMed.

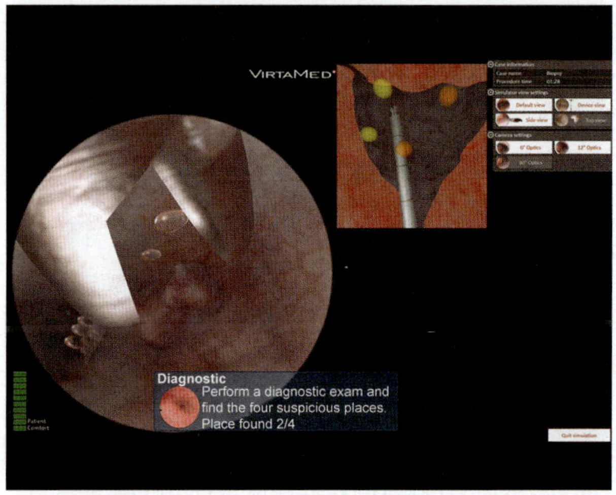

Fig. 8.6: Screenshot of biopsy procedure from the HystSim™ simulator (VirtaMed AG, Zurich, Switzerland) with permission from VirtaMed.

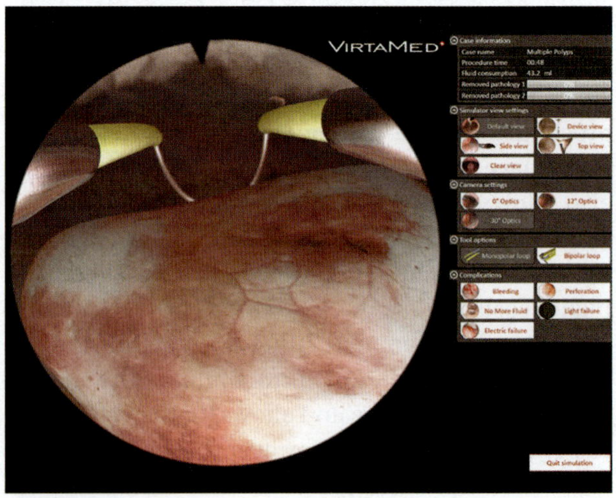

Fig. 8.7: Screenshot of polyp removal procedure from the HystSim™ simulator (VirtaMed AG, Zurich, Switzerland) with permission from VirtaMed.

ASSESSMENT OF HYSTEROSCOPIC SKILLS BEFORE OPERATING ON PATIENTS

Ideally, all surgeons should undergo competence-based assessment of skills before allowing them to perform procedures on patients. This is no different for hysteroscopy.

Assessment of skills can be done using virtual reality simulators metrics, rating scales and checklists.[4,20,24,25]

However, compared to other types of endoscopic surgery, only a limited number of assessment tools have been developed and they are not supported by sufficient validity evidence.[8] This means that currently they cannot be used for certification, but only to provide formative feedback. One example of an assessment tool is The Objective Structured Assessment of Technical Skills consisting of a 20 items checklist to test hysteroscopic proficiency on a hysteroscopy trainer.[26]

Before performing hysteroscopic procedures on patients, the learning curve for hysteroscopy has to be taken into consideration.[27] Trainees will often start by performing diagnostic procedures and when beginning operative procedures appropriate case selection is very important. It is important that trainees begin with simple cases as complications are more frequent in more advanced procedures (Table 8.1).

Initial training should ideally be supervised and trainee performance evaluated using relevant assessment tools to ensure competency before proceeding to perform unsupervised procedures.

Over the last few years there has been major developments in hysteroscopic skills training and this is likely to continue for the years to come. However, compared to other types of endoscopic surgery, much work is still needed in simulation-based hysteroscopic training and assessment.

Table 8.1: Classification of hysteroscopic procedures according to difficulty from the European Society of Gynecological Endoscopy.

Level	Procedures
Level 1	Diagnostic hysteroscopy *Simple procedures excluding the use of electrosurgery:* – Target biopsies – Removal of intrauterine device – Minor intrauterine adhesions
Level 2	Polyp resection Resection of type 0 myoma Endometrial ablation Treatment of uterine septum Tubal cannulation (sterilization)
Level 3	Resection of types 1 and 2 myomas Major Asherman syndrome

REFERENCES

1. Loffer FD, Bradley LD, Brill AI, et al. Hysteroscopic training guidelines. The adhoc committee on hysteroscopic training guidelines of the American Association of Gynecologic Laparoscopists. J Am Assoc Gynecol Laparosc. 2000;7(1):165.
2. Chapron C, Devroey P, Dubuisson JB, et al. ESHRE guidelines for training, accreditation and monitoring in gynaecological endoscopy. European Society for Human Reproduction and Embryology. Committee of Special Interest Group on Reproductive Surgery. Hum Reprod. 1997;12(4):867-8.
3. De Wilde RL, Hucke J, Kolmorgen K, et al. Gynecologic Endoscopy Working Group of the German Society of Obstetrics and Gynecology. Recommendations by the Gynecologic Endoscopy Working Group of the German Society of Obstetrics and Gynecology for the advancement of training and education in minimal-access surgery. Arch Gynecol Obstet. 2011;283(3):509-12.
4. VanBlaricom AL, Goff BA, Chinn M, et al. A new curriculum for hysteroscopy training as demonstrated by an objective structured assessment of technical skills (OSATS). Am J Obstet Gynecol. 2005;193(5):1856-65.
5. Janse JA, Driessen SR, Veersema S, et al. Training of hysteroscopic skills in residency program: the Dutch experience. J Surg Educ. 2015;72(2):345-50.
6. Kolozsvari NO, Feldman LS, Vassiliou MC, et al. Sim one, do one, teach one: considerations in designing training curricula for surgical simulation. J Surg Educ. 2011;68(5):421-7.
7. Gallagher AG, Ritter EM, Champion H, et al. Virtual reality simulation for the operating room: proficiency-based training as a paradigm shift in surgical skills training. Ann Surg. 2005;241(2):364-72.
8. Savran MM, Sørensen SM, Konge L, et al. Training and assessment of hysteroscopic skills: a systematic review. J Surg Educ. 2016;73(5):906-18.
9. Burchard ER, Lockrow EG, Zahn CM, et al. Simulation training improves resident performance in operative hysteroscopic resection techniques. Am J Obstet Gynecol. 2007;197(5):542.e1-4.
10. Janse JA, Tolman CJ, Veersema S, et al. Hysteroscopy training and learning curve of 30° camera navigation on a new box trainer: the HYSTT. Gynecol Surg. 2014;11(2):67-73.
11. Aydeniz B, Meyer A, Posten J, et al. The 'HysteroTrainer'—an in vitro simulator for hysteroscopy and falloposcopy. Experimental and clinical background and technical realisation including the development of organ modules for electrothermal treatment. Contrib Gynecol Obstet. 2000;20:171-81.

12. Wallwiener D, Rimbach S, Bastert G. The HysteroTrainer, a simulator for diagnostic and operative hysteroscopy. J Am Assoc Gynecol Laparosc. 1994;2(1):61-3.
13. Dunkley MP, Brown LH, Robinson JM, et al. Initial training model for endometrial ablation. Gynaecol Endosc. 2001;10(5-6):355-60.
14. Kingston A, Abbott J, Lenart M, et al. Hysteroscopic training: the butternut pumpkin model. J Am Assoc Gynecol Laparosc. 2004;11(2):256-61.
15. Clevin L. A training model for hysteroscopy. Ugeskr Laeger. 2004;166(21):2025-7.
16. Wolfe WM, Levine RL, Sanfilippo JS, et al. A teaching model for endoscopic surgery: hysteroscopy and pelviscopic surgery. Fertil Steril. 1988;50(4):662-4.
17. Courdier S, Garbin O, Hummel M, et al. Equipment failure: causes and consequences in endoscopic gynecologic surgery. J Minim Invasive Gynecol. 2009; 16(1):28-33.
18. Bajka M, Tuchschmid S, Fink D, et al. Establishing construct validity of a virtual-reality training simulator for hysteroscopy via a multimetric scoring system. Surg Endosc. 2010;24(1):79-88.
19. Bajka M, Tuchschmid S, Streich M, et al. Evaluation of a new virtual-reality training simulator for hysteroscopy. Surg Endosc. 2009;23(9):2026-33.
20. Goff BA, VanBlaricom A, Mandel L, et al. Comparison of objective, structured assessment of technical skills with a virtual reality hysteroscopy trainer and standard latex hysteroscopy model. J Reprod Med. 2007;52(5):407-12.
21. Elessawy M, Skrzipczyk M, Eckmann-Scholz C, et al. Integration and validation of hysteroscopy simulation in the surgical training curriculum. J Surg Educ. 2016;74(1):84-90.
22. Neis F, Brucker S, Henes M, et al. Evaluation of the HystSim™-virtual reality trainer: an essential additional tool to train hysteroscopic skills outside the operation theater. Surg Endosc. 2016;30(11): 4954-61.
23. Panel P, Bajka M, Le Tohic A, et al. Hysteroscopic placement of tubal sterilization implants: virtual reality simulator training. Surg Endosc. 2012;26(7):1986-96.
24. Rackow BW, Solnik MJ, Tu FF, et al. Deliberate practice improves obstetrics and gynecology residents' hysteroscopy skills. J Grad Med Educ. 2012;4(3):329-34.
25. Janse JA, Goedegebuure RS, Veersema S, et al. Hysteroscopic sterilization using a virtual reality simulator: assessment of learning curve. J Minim Invasive Gynecol. 2013;20(6):775-82.
26. Alici F, Buerkle B, Tempfer CB. Objective Structured Assessment of Technical Skills (OSATS) evaluation of hysteroscopy training: a prospective study. Eur J Obstet Gynecol Reprod Biol. 2014;178:1-5.
27. Janse JA, Pattij TO, Eijkemans MJ, et al. Learning curve of hysteroscopic placement of tubal sterilization microinserts in 15 gynecologists in the Netherlands. Fertil Steril. 2013;100(3):755-60.

Risk Assessment and Counseling Prior to Laparoscopic Surgery

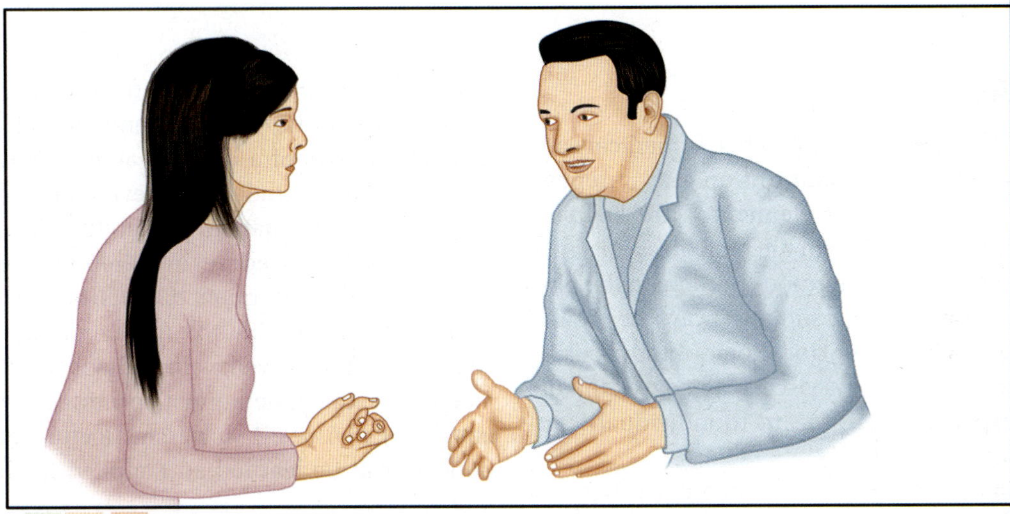

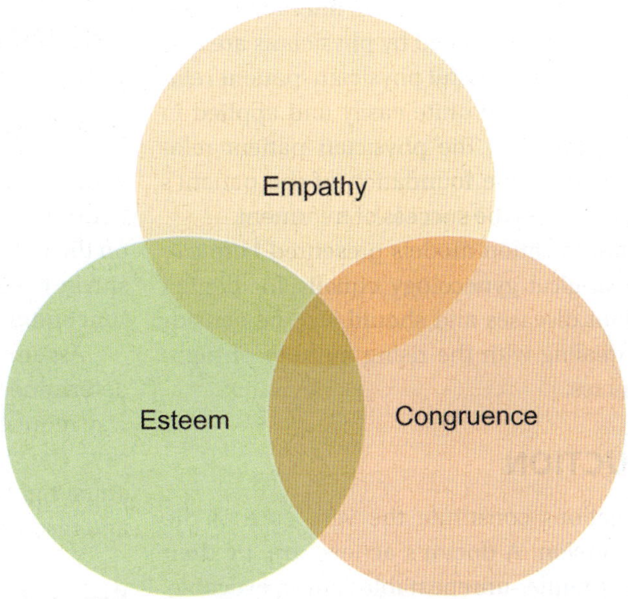

Chapter 9

Risk Assessment and Counseling Prior to Laparoscopic Surgery

Ibrahim Alkatout, Liselotte Mettler

GENERAL

The prime focus of medical practice is medical care. Medical care, by its very nature, is unique, unrepeatable, and irrevocable. The element of irreversibility and permanent contact with the biological existence of a patient impose an enormous burden on the physician. The human being should always be viewed as an integral whole. A doctor should avoid focusing on the illness alone, and is also expected to fulfill the patient's expectations in regard to individual treatment and care.

This chapter addresses the theoretical basis of the doctor–patient relationship and is focused on the patient's autonomy. Fields of interaction and the increasing demands faced by physicians are discussed in detail. A successful physician–patient relationship can be learned quite easily and applied in all medical specialties. The physician–patient relationship constitutes the foundation of the patient's satisfaction as well as the success of treatment.

The communication models presented here can be used in surgical gynecology equally for benign and malignant diseases and should also be considered when dealing with the rising number of high-risk pregnancies.

INTRODUCTION

A doctor's actions constitute the very core of the medical profession. A doctor's actions are, by their very nature, unique, unrepeatable and irrevocable. The element of irreversibility and constant contact with the patient's biological existence impose an enormous burden of responsibility on the doctor's actions.[1] The residual lack of safety and uncertainty, which cannot be eliminated despite most recent discoveries in medical science and technology, still make it almost impossible for the doctor to guarantee the success he or she intends to achieve.[2] The general purpose of a doctor's actions is to cure an ill person. This includes the prevention of disease as well as its cure, the patient's rehabilitation, palliation, the diagnostic procedures required for these measures, and their consequence, which is the treatment.[2] In order to ensure that the treatment addresses the specific disease as well as the patient's right to individual care, the patient must be viewed in his or her entirety at all times. A successful doctor–patient relationship can be learned and applied in all fields of medicine.

THE DOCTOR–PATIENT RELATIONSHIP IS THE BASIS OF ALL FIELDS OF INTERACTION

A positively perceived and productive relationship between the doctor and the patient is primarily based on the following three basic attitudes: empathy (sensitivity), congruence (authenticity), and absolute (unconditional) esteem.[3]

Assuming that the diseased patient is a self-determined individual, his or her autonomy is in no way reduced by the loss of his or her physical integrity. The doctor and the patient are partners with equal rights; each of them has specific competences and responsibilities.

Empathy

Empathy may be defined as understanding the emotional and cognitive processes of another, the ability to recognize a person's conflicts, feelings and attitudes, and be able to experience the emotions of another.[4]

The doctor should, in lieu of the patient, be able to put the latter's feelings into words and determine the patient's needs, which the patient himself or herself may not yet be fully aware of. These processes occur at the emotional and intuitive level in the form of empathy, as well as the cognitive level in the form of comprehension. The therapist's ability to identify himself or herself with the patient for a limited period of time enables the therapist to share the patient's experience. Gestures, facial expression, body posture, the speed of talking, the tone of voice, and other features of nonverbal communication trigger empathy in the interacting partner.[5] Thus, empathy is also an attempt to understand the reasons for another's actions and opinions, based on the latter's view of the world and horizon of experience (Fig. 9.1).[6]

Congruence (Authenticity)

Congruence (authenticity) refers to the therapist's attitude: he or she is entirely sincere toward the patient, without any deception of himself or herself or the patient. The doctor is aware of his feelings at all times and can communicate these to the patient if necessary.[4]

Thus, the doctor–patient relationship incorporates the therapist's authentic communication toward the patient. Authenticity refers to everything the doctor feels and experiences, those parts of his or her feelings and experiences he or she is aware of, and those parts he or she eventually communicates. Thus, the therapist is able to access his own thoughts and feelings toward the client and the therapy situation.[7] The therapy principle of authenticity makes it necessary for the doctor to render his identity (which differs from that of the patient) transparent to the patient, answer questions sincerely, and seek opportunities to face the patient and communicate with him or her.[7,8]

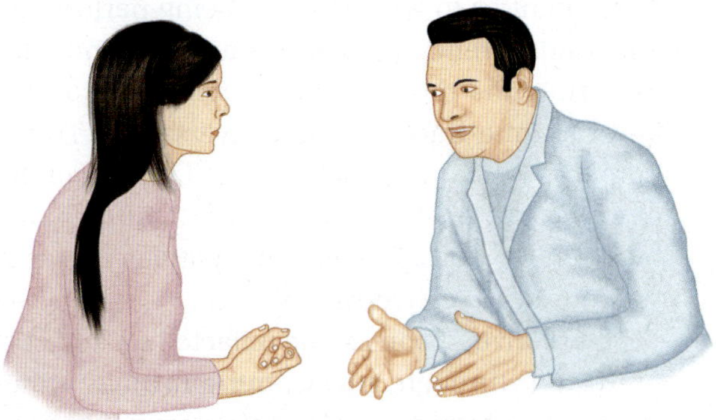

Fig. 9.1: Authentic empathic setting in preoperative counseling contains congruence and esteem.

Unconditional Positive Esteem (Unreserved Acceptance)

A relationship of unconditional positive esteem is marked by trust, appreciation, and respect; these qualities form the foundation of the doctor–patient relationship.[8]

The patient is welcomed and accepted, independent of what he/she says and how he/she behaves at the present time. This unrestricted acceptance is incompatible with an attitude expressing judgment, dislike or disapproval, or even a selectively expressed esteem of another (depending on the contents of the conversation). Unconditional acceptance consolidates the therapeutic relationship, promotes one's experience of self-respect, and mobilizes the patient's own resources. The doctor focuses his entire attention on the patient and confirms the patient's ambitions by acknowledgment, encouragement, and expressions of solidarity and concern. The patient's communication is accepted exactly as expressed by the patient and is not questioned further.[8] This gives the patient the certainty he/she needs in order to fully experience his or her feelings at the moment, although the therapist is still obliged to align his/her experience to his/her values[5] (Fig. 9.2).

CREATING THE DOCTOR–PATIENT RELATIONSHIP

The doctor's professional rule of conduct has existed since the antique ages of medicine: *primum non nocere* (above all, you should do no harm).

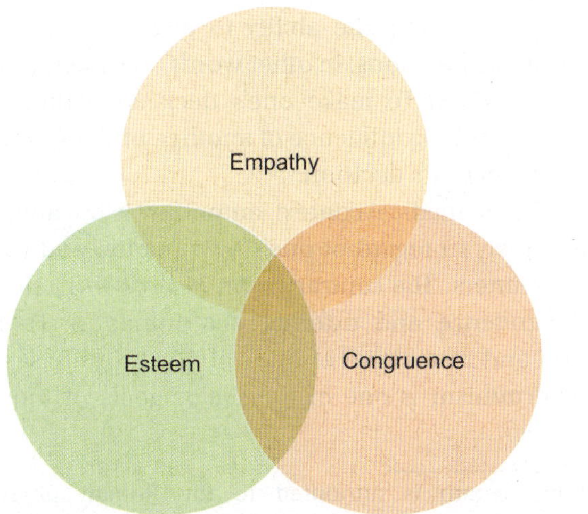

Fig. 9.2: The doctor–patient relationship is the basis of all fields of interaction. It is founded on the three cornerstones of *empathy* (sensitivity), *congruence* (authenticity), and absolute (unconditional) esteem.

*The principle of nonmaleficience or prevention of damage is, in addition to the patient's autonomy, the patient's well-being and justice, one of the four ethical guiding principles of decision-making by a doctor. The art of ethical judgment is derived from a balance of these four basic principles: dispensing with harmful interventions (*primum non nocere*), respecting the patient's self-determined decision (*voluntas aegroti*), ensuring that any medical measures serve the preservation and improvement of the patient's mental and physical health (*benevolence*), and being just in one's actions (*fairness*).[9,10] The four principles incorporate a number of explicit, implicit, and potential standards, which may contradict each other in many ways but result in a coherentistic approach in terms of application.[9,11,12]

Self-Determined Decision (The Patient's Autonomy)

The term *autonomy* is derived from the Greek words *autos* (self) and *nomos* (law, rule), and means self-legislation or self-determination. It was initially used to express the self-determination and self-government of independent city states of the antique period. Kant regarded the autonomy of practical reason as the commitment of human will—driven by the legitimate categorical imperative—to assign greater importance to unconditional obligation than to primordial intentions.

Preconditions for autonomous decisions are the following:

- *Awareness*: Being able to understand the issue in question
- *Competence*: The ability to inspect, judge, and make decisions; in other words, to be competent
- *Freedom*: To make one's decision without the controlling influence of another, and also implement one's decision.

In the medical context, autonomy is the ability to act freely in regard of one's own mental and physical matters. The contrary term *heteronomy* refers to dependence and external determination. Promotion and restoration of one's ability to exercise self-determinism is one of the major goals of medical action.[13] Respect for autonomy, in its minimal form, is expressed as respect for the basic rights of the patient. The relationship between the doctor and the patient must ensure asymmetry between action and suffering on the one hand, and symmetry of self-determinism and freedom of action on the other.[14] The doctor–patient relationship is outlined in three basic models: (1) paternalistic model, (2) contractual or client model, and (3) partnership model. External influences exist due to secularization, economization, and technological developments in medicine, on the one hand, and the changing values of our pluralistic society, on the other. The diverse and variable models of relationship differ especially in regard of the criterion of trust and the actual degree of patient autonomy in the respective interaction. We are concerned with the communication requirements to be fulfilled by the doctor.[15,16]

*The dictum is attributed to the Roman physician Scribonius Largus, court physician of the emperor Tiberius Claudius Nero Caesar Drusus who ruled Rome around 50 AD. A similar phrase is also found in the Corpus Hippocraticum (Epidemics, Book I, Section XI).

TECHNIQUES OF CONDUCTING A DOCTOR'S CONVERSATION WITH THE PATIENT FROM THE VIEWPOINT OF AUTONOMY

The core aspects of a successful conversation conducted by the doctor with the patient include, above all, active listening, determining the structure of the conversation, as well as identifying and resolving difficult patterns of interaction.

- *Active listening*: Techniques of active listening are summarized in Box 9.1.
- *Determining the structure of the conversation*: Transparency is a basic instrument for structuring the conversation and adhering to the time frame. This includes transparency of the elements of the conversation, such as providing information about the steps of the treatment, the necessary medical informatioin, and informing the patient as to why a step is being performed. The transparency of basic conditions includes informing the patient about potential disorders and the time frame of the conversation. Transparency concerning the individual phases of the conversation enables the patient to differentiate between doctor-centered and patient-centered sections of the conversation.
  - The conversation can be reflected on and corrected through metacommunicative statements. Metacommunicative statements concern the content of the conversation, the style

Box 9.1: Techniques of active listening.

Let the patient finish speaking	The first few minutes form the basis of the relationship. Active listening is encouraging and delivers valuable information
Ask open questions	Open questions yield comprehensive information, clarify associations, and provide background data beyond the actual facts of the case
Inquire	Problems of comprehension can be addressed immediately
Balance pros and cons	Helps to determine the patient's priorities or encourages him to think about them. Especially by explaining why a step is being given preferences
Pause	Short pauses (about 3 seconds) have a relieving effect. The patient thinks of data he/she had ignored until now
Encourage the patient to speak further	Echoing or nonverbal communication (nodding, eye contact, body facing the patient) signalizes one's presence
Paraphrase (repeat)	Focus on those parts of the patient's statements that are most significant (verbal accompaniment) and thus open new perspectives
Summarize what has been said	Agreement between the doctor and the patient by expressing longer portions of the conversation in one's own words
Reflect emotions	Address emotions verbally in the form of a suggestion

of conversation, the positions of those conducting the conversation, and problems in the doctor-patient relationship.

- Identifying and resolving complex patterns of interaction. Harmonious communication patterns are oriented to the anticipated reactions of one's counterpart. This calls for a high degree of flexibility and thorough knowledge of role expectations. Interaction may be disrupted by inadequate social competence, fixation on oneself, or distorted perception of social behavior.

INDIVIDUAL REQUIREMENTS OF THE DOCTOR IN A PATIENT-CENTERED DOCTOR–PATIENT RELATIONSHIP

A successful doctor–patient relationship is the foundation of any successful treatment and the breeding ground for sustained satisfaction in the professional existence of a doctor.

The action-guiding obligations of a doctor include the willingness to take responsibility, confidentiality, and authenticity. Action-guiding virtues of a doctor are patience, empathy, compassion, and the willingness to help. Finally, one needs to work out what the various optional decisions mean in terms of obligations towards third parties. In this context one needs to consider the patient's family members and close friends, as well as the entire community of the insured person.[17]

Very urgent decisions and chronic diseases are the easiest to handle from the ethical point of view. In highly acute situations, such as emergencies, the responsibility of decisions is still handed over to the doctor without considering the patient's opinion (accepted paternalism). In this setting the patient is informed of the bare essentials, without disregarding the his or her right of self-determination. Even when the patient's ability to help himself or herself is on the decline and the patient needs help and care to an increasing extent, as in old age frailty and/or cognitive impairment, his or her modified autonomy should be accompanied by a high degree of empathy on the part of the doctor concerning the putative will of the patient. Chronic diseases differ from this approach in that a satisfactory outcome of care and the required degree of compliance can only be achieved cooperatively by the doctor and the patient. The less urgent the decision is, the more responsibility one may assign to the patient; in this setting decisions can be made in accordance with the shared decision-making model (Fig. 9.3).[18] The degree of autonomy depends on the momentary and general condition of the individual patient (such as the patient's mental condition, degree of intellectual differentiation, severity of symptoms, severity of disease), and must be adapted to the current situation. The patient's values (estimation of the disease, will, concept of life) should be viewed along with the values of his environment (the patient's living environment, the treatment team), and the values of society (implicit values, institutionalized values). Even if the patient's living values are clear, there may be ambiguity concerning what is meaningful, appropriate, and beneficial for the patient.

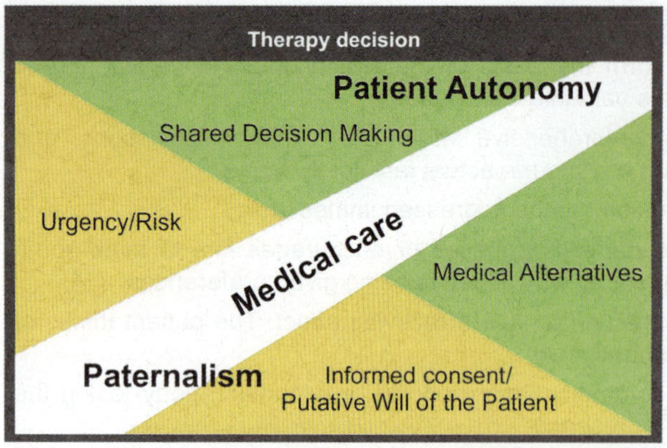

Fig. 9.3: Reciprocal flow diagram of paternalism and informed consent on the one hand, and patient autonomy and shared decision making on the other. Dependent variables are medically equivalent alternatives and the medical urgency or risk for the patient. Medical care should respect the patient's well-being as well as his/her will.

In many medical situations, the relationship between the doctor and the patient remains no more than an idealized behavior pattern. Many situations are rendered complex by the indefinite prognosis of acute diseases, especially when the initiated maximal therapy has not been successful and the doctor contemplates a change in the goals of treatment. However, particularly such extreme situations call for mastery over, and the application of, medico- ethical principles.

Borderline Situations in Dealing with Aged Patients and those with Cognitive Impairment (Dementia)

The rising number of aged patients and those with cognitive impairment (dementia) permits complete patient autonomy in a very small number of cases. However, demographic developments necessitate the establishment of applicable concepts that will do justice to the altered spectrum of morbidity, which includes a rise in chronic diseases and multimorbid conditions. When coordinating the medical reports and other collected data with the individual patient's value system and also when considering the available resources in a specific case, the treatment team needs to employ a high degree of empathy and respect for the patient's autonomy. Again, it may be necessary to re-check and ensure congruency between the medical approach and the patient's concept of living, and make the respective putative decisions anew.[19,20]

Borderline Situations in Dealing with Psychiatric Patients, Young Children, and Mentally Challenged Persons

According to the principle of autonomy, young children, psychiatric patients, and less gifted persons also have the right to be informed comprehensively. On the other hand, a comprehensive explanation may involve potential harm or delay in all three groups. Therefore, in the patient's interest many decisions about him/her are made on his or her behalf. When making serious decisions one must integrate the patient to the greatest possible degree. Consulting and including family members and caregivers is especially relevant in these situations. Showing empathy and sympathy for the patient and the family, answering questions, and explaining the medical treatment are highly valued aspects in this setting.[21]

THE DOCTOR-PATIENT RELATIONSHIP IN ONCOLOGY

Tumor patients are typical candidates for patient-centered doctor–patient communication. Cancer patients need a great deal of information about their disease, its consequences, and the available options. In many cases, the treating doctor and the patient share an intensive and long-term relationship. Therapy decisions are of long duration and have far-reaching consequences on the patient's quality of life and the prognosis of his or her disease. The doctor's task and responsibilities in providing medical assistance for cancer patients involves, to a much greater extent now than ever before, inviting the patient's active participation in decisions regarding treatment.[22]

In 1819 Goethe wrote in *West-Eastern Divan*: "What I thank Allah most for? That he has made a division between suffering and knowing. Any ill person would be desperate if he knew the disease as thoroughly as the doctor does."[†]

Slevin et al were able to show that, in apparently hopeless situations, cancer patients are much more willing to undergo stressful chemotherapy with minimal chances of cure than the medical personnel in charge of their treatment would be willing to subject them to such treatment. Also with regard to the prolongation of overall survival and the improvement of quality of life, the acceptance threshold of severe

[†]von Goethe JW. West-Eastern Divan. Frankfurt am Main; 1999. p. 47.

side effects is highly underestimated (Table 9.1).[23] Although many ill persons will accept a stressful treatment that prolongs their lives by a few months or provides brief symptomatic relief, some patients refuse to undergo a stressful therapy although the prognosis of their disease may be quite favorable.[24] Achievement of the goals of therapy, in this case, is not dependent on the effects or the efficacy of therapeutic measures alone, but is subject to a positive evaluation of the treatment by the patient.[25]

Patient-centered medicine includes the ability to deliver bad news. Communications about impending death and statements about the significance of a disease or death are major challenges for the doctor and the patient. Empathy, congruence, and unrestrained respect for the patient when delivering bad news have culminated, for instance, in the SPIKES protocol described by Baile (Table 9.2).[26]

Questions to establish one's estimation of the patient's perception include, for instance, "What do you know about your medical situation so far?" or "What is your understanding of the reasons we wish to do the investigation?" To better estimate the ability of one's counterpart to receive bad news, it may be useful to ask questions like "How would you like me to give the information about the test results? Would you like me to give you all the information or sketch out the results and spend more time discussing the treatment plan?" To warn the patient before delivering bad news, one could try to steer the conversation, "Unfortunately I've got some bad news to tell you..." or "I'm sorry to tell you that ...". While speaking to the patient, it would be advisable to make repeated and active attempts to optimize the conversation. This includes alignment of one's language to the patient's vocabulary and omitting specialized medical terms. Excessive directness should be avoided, and the required or desired information should be given in small units. The level of communication can be further improved by avoiding phrases like "There's nothing more we can do for you." Empathic statements in these exceptional situations express support. Specifically, the patient is helped when emotions are regis-tered, named, and identified (such as grief, anger, or shock). The patient is also helped when the doctor signalizes that the patient may express himself or herself. Agreeing upon a plan of treatment simultaneously makes the patient feel that his or her wishes are being taken into account; it also avoids misunderstanding, uncertainty, and anxiety (Fig. 9.4).

Table 9.1: The threshold likelihood (in percentage) of cure, prolongation of life, or symptomatic relief: the point from which patients are willing to accept chemotherapy associated with severe side effects and complications. This survey was conducted among cancer patients as well as a group of doctors and nursing staff.

	Patient	Therapist
Chances of cure	1%	10–50%
Prolongation of life	12 months	12–60 months
Alleviation of symptoms	10%	50–70%

Table 9.2: The SPIKES model. A six-step protocol for delivering bad news. This is a tool for obtaining information about the patient's current level of knowledge. He/she can also be informed about medical facts, depending on his/her need for information, support can be expressed, and suitable options can be rendered accessible. Finally, a treatment plan can be drafted in cooperation with the patient.

SPIKES	Steps	Contents
S	1. Setting up the interview	• Arrange for some privacy • Involve significant others • Avoid interruptions • Sit down
P	2. Assessing the patient's perception	• Open questions to assess the patient's current perception (avoid misunderstandings early)
I	3. Obtaining the patient's invitation	• Assess the patient's willingness to receive bad news • Mention that the patient can speak to the doctor at a later point in time
K	4. Giving knowledge and information	• Warning before delivering bad news • Optimizing communication
E	5. Addressing the patient's emotions with empathic responses	• Empathic statements express support
S	6. Strategy and Summary	• Depends on level of well-being • Discuss the next steps

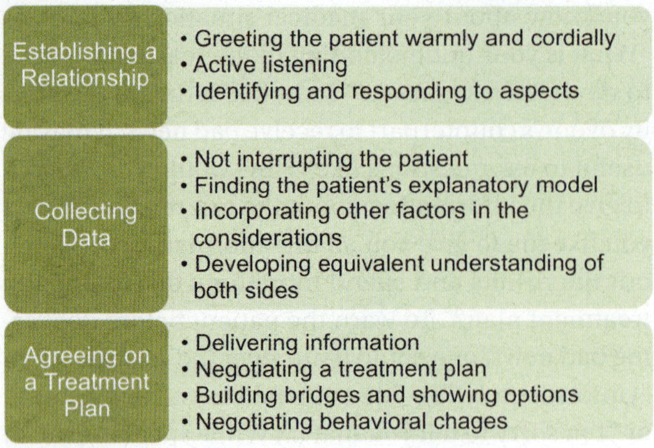

Fig. 9.4: Three functions of a doctor's consultation.

THE DOCTOR-PATIENT RELATIONSHIP IN OBSTETRICS FROM THE INVASIVE POINT OF VIEW

Obstetrics and prenatal medicine constitute an equally important part of our spectrum of activities. In contrast to gynecology, the doctor is called upon to bear responsibilities beyond the patient's scope of action. High-risk pregnancies have risen greatly in the last few years because of improved procedures in reproduction medicine. Maternal diseases may become consolidated or be exacerbated during pregnancy. The increasing complexity of this subject calls for interdisciplinary management and imposes the highest medico-ethical demands on our specialty.

In addition to the medico-ethical questions of the mother, the demands of the unborn child also must be taken into account. A crucial aspect of decision-making when dealing with the unborn child is the moral status an embryo must achieve in order to be granted specific rights—such as the right to live—as a practical subject. The fundamental rights granted to nascent life and the consequent legal protection that goes with these can be described in different ways.[27]

- *The species argument*: All members of the biological species known as *Homo sapiens* and, in fact, only this species, are entitled to human dignity and the comprehensive legal and moral protection that go with it.
- *Potentiality argument*: The potential of entire human development is present in the primary cells. An embryo, which normally develops into a human being, is therefore worthy of protection and possesses the same moral characteristics as the fully developed human being.
- *Identity argument*: The human embryo or fetus has the same rights as the persons they will become in the normal course of life, because the two are basically identical. The identity of the developed individual results from the composite of cells he or she evolves from.
- *Continuity argument*: The process of development that starts with nidation is a continuous process with no sharp divisions and therefore does not permit any specific demarcation of the stages of development. Despite the continuity of human development from the very start, one can identifiy various stages of development whose demarcations, however, are blurred.

Fetomaternal conflicts result from the need to set priorities regarding the well-being of the expectant mother or the future child. Once the moral and ethical status of both parents and their right of self-determination have been established, it will be necessary to register the moral and ethical status of the unborn child. Any decision in favor of one would be accompanied by neglect of the other. Equal treatment of the interests and possessions of the unborn child and the future parents is practically impossible. Once the individuality of the embryo starts to take shape—which would be at the time of insemination or later—the individual possesses complete human dignity and must be protected accordingly. From this time on, the existence of the human being and his or her individuality is determined by the uniqueness of his/her genetic material. Based on the ethical principle of autonomy, one is obliged to justify any hindrance to self-determined life and protect the value of freedom. However, embryos and fetuses are unable to make competent decisions and are therefore incapable of moral, independent, and autonomous action or decisions, which, however, are essential for the self-determined decision-making process. Therefore, competent representatives have to make decisions on their behalf. The representative also has to align the child's value system with general ethical considerations in order to make appropriate decisions in keeping with the presumed life concept of the unborn child. Thus, a person who makes decisions for others is especially obliged to adhere to ethical principles, standards and criteria.

Given these facts, many prenatal diagnostic and obstetric situations pose a dilemma because it is impossible to act in the interests of the embryo or fetus as well as the expectant mother, not do them any harm, preserve their autonomy, and behave in a just manner. The options of action from the medico-ethical point of view would be quite clear if the unborn child's right to live would be ranked secondary to the expectant mother's. These questions are not, by any means, conclusively clarified at the present time.

Since parents are those who have to live with their decisions in favor of one of the courses of action and its respective dramatic consequences, they should be given all of the tools that enable them to make a sustainable decision. These include, in addition to the medical information provided by an interdisciplinary team of doctors (obstetrics, human genetics, prenatal diagnosis, neonatology, pediatrics), information about further decision-making aids and about tools for coping with the conflict-ridden situation.

ENDANGERMENT OF THE DOCTOR–PATIENT RELATIONSHIP

The atmosphere of trust created by both of these parties is currently at risk of being lost forever. Three factors are worthy of mention in this regard. Increasing anonymity is a result of increasingly complex infrastructures. The patient is compelled to surrender his relationship with his treating physician and share his existence as an ill person as well as his doctor (a confidant) with the entire institution. Juridification, by which the doctor–patient relationship is subject to an increasing degree of legal control. The third source of uncertainty is probabilization. Statements about the disease process can only be made with certain degrees of probability.

Industrialization and the enhancement of efficiency in the health care system through measurable performance have, in many instances, reduced nonmeasurable medical services to a minimum. Higher-level optimization processes, technocracy, and bureaucracy are culminating in an unsurmountable pressure of time, which is partly offset by specialized medical services such as those of psychologists, specialized nursing staff, or social workers.

CONCLUSION AND FUTURE PERSPECTIVES FOR MEDICAL PRACTICE

Decision-making in medical treatment is an individual process founded on ethics and can only be rendered possible by a well-functioning doctor–patient relationship. A prerequisite for the latter is communication based on empathy, congruence, and unconditional esteem. With a foundation of this nature, the patient and the doctor will be able to strive for the patient's well-being while preserving the patient's autonomy, avoiding damage or injustice, and treading a common pathway, ideally as partners, which would lead to sustained satisfaction—also from the doctor's point of view—and render the two extremes of paternalism and contractual action unnecessary. In the majority of situations, the basic demands of the two parties must be weighed against each other and may not be achieved simultaneously. In the joint process of decision-making, it will be necessary to strike a compromise between the respective non-negotiable principles.

REFERENCES

1. Wieland W. Strukturwandel der Medizin und ärztliche Ethik—philosophische Überlegungen zu Grundfragen einer praktischen Wissenschaft. Heidelberg: Universitätsverlag; 1986.
2. Gethmann CF. Gesundheit nach Maß? Eine transdisziplinäre Studie zu den Grundlagen eines dauerhaften Gesundheitssystems. Berlin: Akademie Verlag GmbH; 2004.
3. Rogers CR. Therapeut und Klient: Grundlagen der Gesprächspsychotherapie. 20th edn. Frankfurt: Fischer Verlag; 1983.
4. Mittelstraß J. Enzyklopädie: Philosophie und Wissenschaftstheorie. Special Edition edn. Stuttgart: JB Metzler Verlag; 2004.
5. Argyle M. Körpersprache und Kommunikation: Das Handbuch zur nonverbalen Kommunikation. 9th ed. Paderborn: Junfermann Verlag; 2005.
6. Geisler LS. Patient autonomy—a critical concept analysis. Dtsch Med Wochenschr. 2004;129(9):453-6.
7. Rogers CR. Entwicklung der Persönlichkeit. 13 th ed. Stuttgart: Klett-Cotta; 1996.
8. Finke J. Gesprächspychotherapie—Grundlagen und spezifische Anwendungen. 3rd ed. Stuttgart: Georg Thieme Verlag; 2004.
9. Beauchamp TL, Childress JF. Principles of Biomedical Ethics. 6th ed. New York, Oxford: Oxford University Press; 2009.
10. Smith CM. Origin and uses of primum non nocere—above all, do no harm! J Clin Pharmacol. 2005;45(4):371-7.
11. Schöne-Seifert B. Medizinethik. In: Nida-Rümelin J (Ed). Angewandte Ethik. Die Bereichsethiken und ihre theoretische Fundierung. Ein Handbuch. 2nd ed. Stuttgart: Alfred Kröner Verlag; 2005. p. 690-803.
12. Alkatout I, Rummer A. Intrauterines Lebensrecht von Zwillingen mit ungleichen Überlebenschancen—Kommentar I zum Fall. Ethik in der Medizin. 2011; 23(3):233-4.
13. Gabl C, Jox RJ. [Paternalism and autonomy—no contradiction]. Wien Med Wochenschr. 2008;158(23-24):642-9.
14. Marckmann G, Bormuth M. Arzt-Patient-Verhältnis und Informiertes Einverständnis. In: Wiesing U, editor. Ethik in der Medizin. Ein Reader. Stuttgart: Philipp Reclam; 2000. p. 76-85.

15. Krones T, Richter G. [Physicians' responsibility: doctor-patient relationship]. Bundesgesundheitsblatt Gesundheitsforschung Gesundheitsschutz. 2008; 51(8):818-26.
16. von Engelhardt D. Ethik in der Onkologie—Dem kranken Menschen gerecht werden. Im Focus Onkologie. 2006;9:65-8.
17. Marckmann G, Mayer F. Ethische Fallbesprechungen in der Onkologie—Grundlagen einer prinzipien-orientierten Falldiskussion. Der Onkologe. 2009; 15(10):980-8.
18. Krones T, Richter G. Die Arzt-Patient-Beziehung. In: Schulz S, Seigleder K, Fangerau H, Paul NW (Eds). Geschichte, Theorie und Ethik der Medizin. Frankfurt am Main: Suhrkamp Verlag; 2006. pp. 94-117.
19. Wolf E, Lahrmann H. [The seriously affected stroke patient who is not able to communicate—treatment to the best of one's knowledge and ethical principles]. Wien Med Wochenschr. 2014;164(9-10):195-200.
20. Meran JG. Palliative care and quality of life as therapy goal. Wien Med Wochenschr. 2012;162(1-2):1-2.
21. Espinel AG, Shah RK, Beach MC, et al. What parents say about their child's surgeon: parent-reported experiences with pediatric surgical physicians. JAMA Otolaryngol Head Neck Surg. 2014;140(5):397-402.
22. Hahn J, Mandraka F, Fröhlich G. Ethische Aspekte in der Therapie kritisch kranker Tumorpatienten. Intensivmedizin und Notfallmedizin. 2007;44(7): 416-28.
23. Slevin ML, Stubbs L, Plant HJ, et al. Attitudes to chemotherapy: comparing views of patients with cancer with those of doctors, nurses, and general public. BMJ. 1990;300(6737):1458-60.
24. Silvestri G, Pritchard R, Welch HG. Preferences for chemotherapy in patients with advanced non-small cell lung cancer: descriptive study based on scripted interviews. BMJ. 1998;317(7161):771-5.
25. Krones CJ, Willis S, Steinau G, et al. Current patient perceptions of the physician. Chirurg. 2006;77(8): 718-24.
26. Baile WF, Buckman R, Lenzi R, et al. SPIKES—A six-step protocol for delivering bad news: application to the patient with cancer. Oncologist. 2000;5(4): 302-11.
27. Schulz S. Person oder Keim? Der moralische Status des Ungeborenen in der Geschichte der Abtreibungsdiskussion. In: Schulz S, Seigleder K, Fangerau H, Paul NW (Eds). Geschichte, Theorie und Ethik der Medizin. Frankfurt am Main: Suhrkamp Verlag; 2006. p. 303-15.

KIEL SCHOOL

10 of Gynaecological Endoscopy

Peritoneal Access

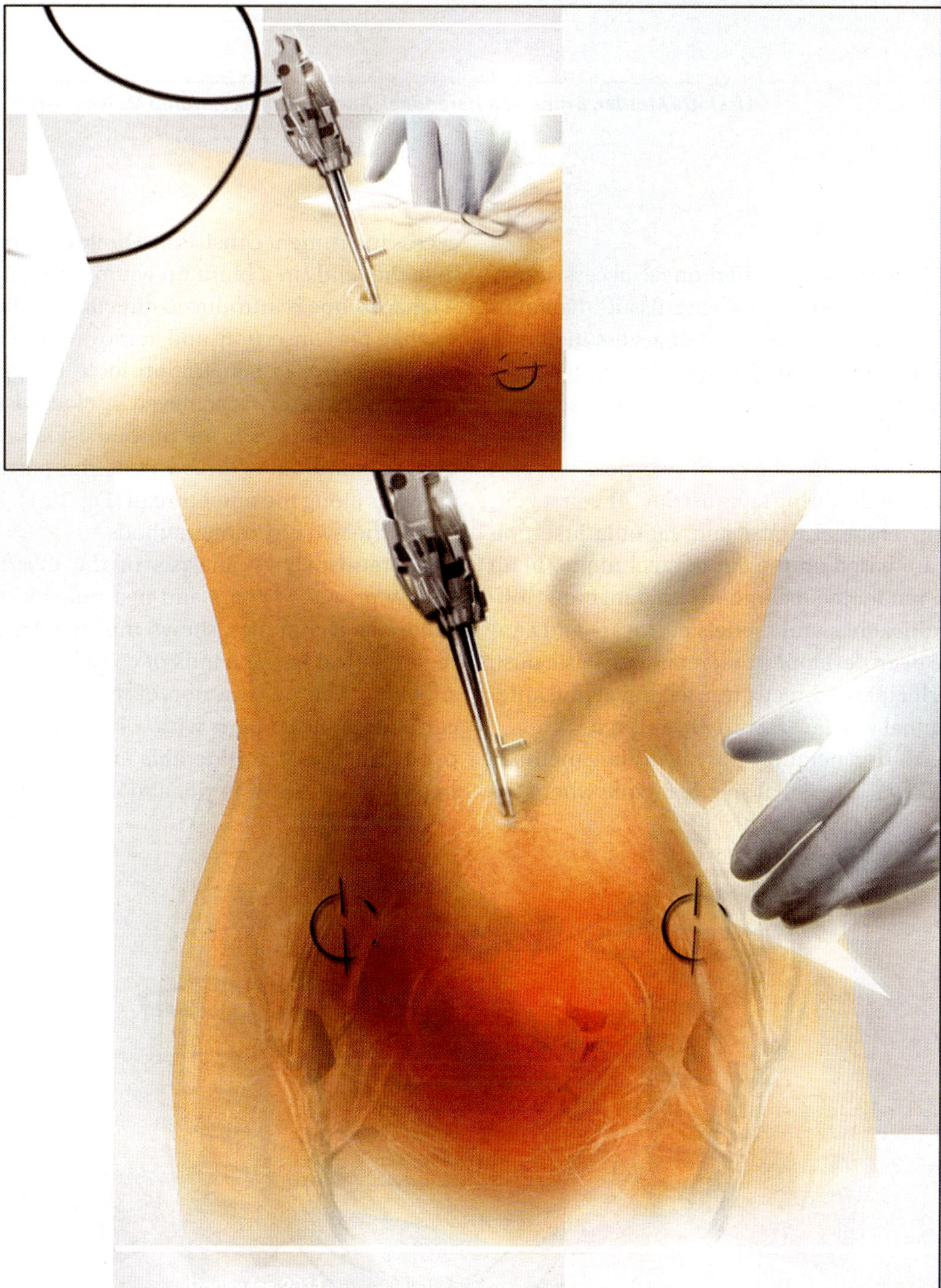

Chapter 10

Peritoneal Access

Liselotte Mettler, Bruno van Herendael, Andrea Tinelli, Antonio Malvasi, Artin Ternamian

INTRODUCTION

The cause of laparoscopic peritoneal access injury can be best analyzed by studying tissue dynamics at insertion site.[1-3] Error analysis of access incidents shows that the interaction between *surgeon, instrument* and *tissue* is important to understand accident causation.

Surgeons have the choice of two possible port insertion methods during laparoscopy. The first generation, conventional trocar and cannula insertion methods, are based on the cutting technique. In an attempt to render the technique less dangerous, different modifications and models of trocars and cannulas have been developed that retain the basic push through principle of directly transecting all the anterior abdominal wall layers with linear force.[4]

The second generation port insertion methods under vision use the radial spin principle where the access instrument consists of a hollow-threaded cannula that ends in a blunt tip without a central trocar. A laparoscope is introduced directly into the cannula so that port insertion and removal is done under vision. No linear penetration force is applied during insertion; entry is achieved by clockwise cannula rotation. Tissue layers are pushed aside radially and the cannula's outer thread pulls the parted tissues upwards along the outer thread (Fig. 10.1). Table 10.1 shows the two insertion methods.[5]

A retrospective analysis of the insertion injuries by primary trocars and instruments using conventional techniques shows the drawbacks of this method even in the hands of competent and skilled surgeons. During insertion of the conventional trocar and cannula, be it with a conical tip or with a pyramidal tip, a considerable amount of axial force must be used. The anterior abdominal wall is pushed

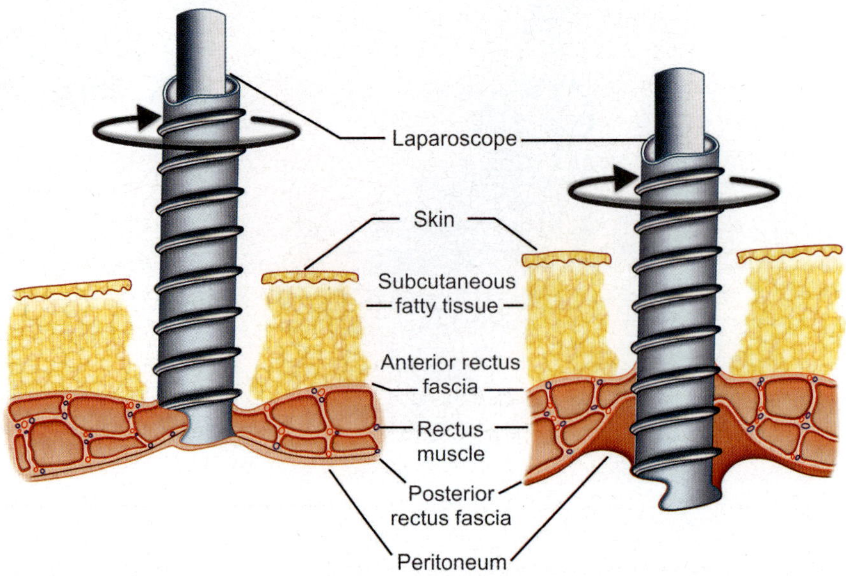

Fig. 10.1: Trocar insertion dynamic with the endoscopic threaded imaging port (EndoTIP) cannula, under vision.

Table 10.1: Classification of peritoneal insertion methods.

First Generation	Second Generation
(Trocar + cannula, cutting principle)	
Closed access • Direct insufflation with Veress needle • Z insertion technique • Radially expanding trocars[12,13] • Higher pressure required	**Optical cannula** (Ternamian 1997) with spin principle • Pre-insufflation with Veress needle • Direct insertion with insufflation later • Extra-peritoneal insufflation
Open access[14] • No prior insufflation by Veress needle • Generous skin incision • Dissection up to rectus fascia • Two Kocher's forceps to lift up the fascia • Incision and insertion of blunt trocar sheath	
Optic trocars • CO_2 insufflation through Veress needle • Optiview and Visiport—so-called safety trocars[15]	
Microlaparoscopy (*optical Veress needle*): • Introduction in left upper quadrant at Palmer point[16,17] • Veress needle (2.1 mm diameter) • Minilaparoscope (1.2 mm diameter)	

against the bowel during straight or Z-insertion. The insertion is blind and uncontrolled if used with CO_2 insufflation or without it. It may work well for experts but cannot be recommended as the optimal technique.

PRINCIPLE OF ENDOSCOPIC THREADED IMAGING PORT (EndoTIP)

In an attempt to understand and avoid inadvertent peritoneal entry injuries, second-generation access systems have been developed. In 1984 Semm attempted insertion under vision with a 5 mm trocar following CO_2 insufflation using the spin principle.[6] EndoTIP is an extension of this technique (Karl Storz GmbH & Co. KG, Tuttlingen).

In 1997, the EndoTIP peritoneal entry method and instrument was developed by Ternamian, at the University of Toronto that realized Semm's vision of controlled visual entry. The EndoTIP entry instrument consists of a 10 or 5 mm stainless steel cannula and a proximal valve section. A single thread runs diagonally on its outer surface, which ends distally in a blunt tip.[7-9] EndoTIP is available in different lengths and diameters for different surgical applications. EndoTIP is a reusable visual access cannula that can be used for closed or open laparoscopy. It can be employed as a primary or ancillary port, for intraperitoneal and retroperitoneal interventions. A reusable sliding ring (telescope stopper) is sheathed on the laparoscope to prevent it from sliding inside the cannula (Fig. 10.2), and fixes the laparoscope about 1 cm short of the cannula's distal end.

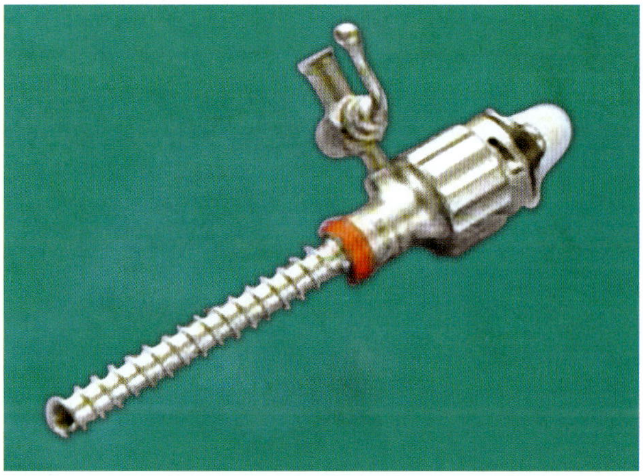

Fig. 10.2: EndoTIP cannula and telescope stopper (Karl Storz & Co. KG, Tuttlingen).

PROCEDURE

With a 15 surgical blade, either a longitudinal or horizontal umbilical incision is made, up to the anterior rectus fascia and the subcutaneous tissue is dissected laterally with retractors. When applying EndoTIP with CO_2 pre-insufflation, the Veress needle insertion is carried out as usual. A 0° laparoscope

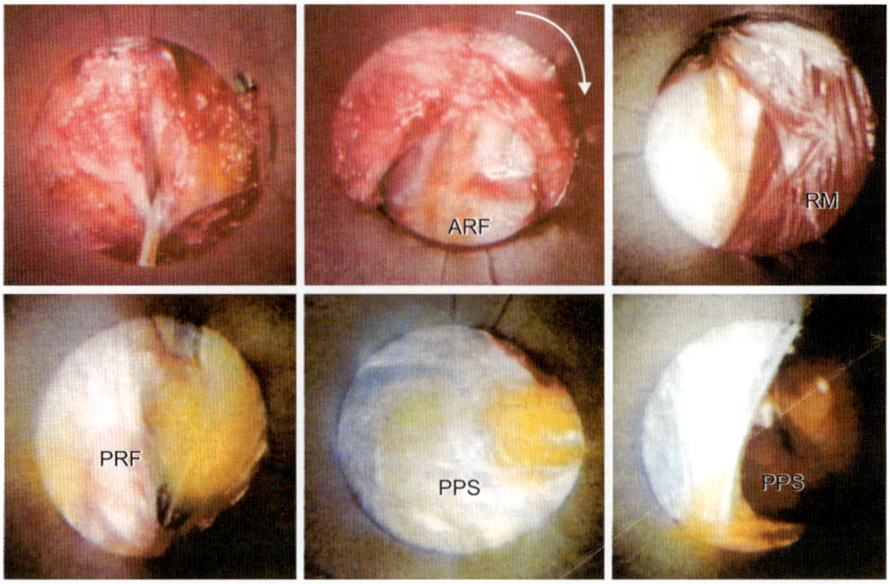

Fig. 10.3: EndoTIP in use. The tissue layers are parted radially when the cannula penetrates the peritoneum.
Abbreviations: ARF, Anterior rectus fascia; RM, Rectus muscle; PRF, Posterior rectus fascia; PPS, preperitoneal space.

is sheathed in the EndoTIP cannula and fixed 1 cm short of the cannula's distal end with the telescope stopper. The white-balanced camera is then focused; the light cable, CO_2 gas and suction irrigation unit are connected. After insufflation the Veress needle is removed and the EndoTIP cannula with blunt tip is placed on to the anterior rectus fascia, at right angle to the supine abdomen. The EndoTIP is rotated clockwise using the dominant hand of the surgeon, keeping the forearm horizontal, while the laparoscope is held with the nondominant hand. The blunt tip traverses the rectus fascia, parts the musculature radially and pulls the tissues layers up along the cannulas outer thread. The rotational movement is carried out till the white posterior fascia and the preperitoneal fatty tissue layers part and the peritoneal membrane becomes slowly visible.

In a normally filled abdominal cavity (with no parietal adhesions), the peritoneum appears gray-blue in color (Fig. 10.3). Vessels, bowel or adhesions are recognized and inadvertent injuries avoided. By further clockwise rotation, the blunt tip enters the peritoneum under direct visual control incrementally, with no cannula overshoot. No axial force is required though the cannula is always held perpendicular to tissues to avoid tissue tunneling. Immediately after entering the abdomen, the standard panoramic viewing is carried out.

Open laparoscopy is carried out in a similar way but the abdomen is not pre-insufflated. Ancillary port insertion is also carried out under vision using EndoTIP as 5 or 10 mm trocar.

EndoTIP REMOVAL

In direct straight insertion with first generation trocars, hernias can develop. Only in the Z-insertion by Semm[6] can herniation be avoided. Moreover, it is important to carry out the removal of all trocars under vision to avoid port herniation. It is not possible to recognize injuries and treat them suitably without carefully observing the port tract during removal of the trocar. Numerous publications quote the incidence of port herniation at 0.3–1.3%.[10,11]

With EndoTIP, the surgeon can observe the tissue dynamics during removal of the cannula. EndoTIP is so designed that during cannula placement, anterior abdominal tissue layers are not transected but parted, consequently, during cannula removal, the anterior abdominal tissue layers recoil back to close the port tract during anticlockwise cannula removal (Fig. 10.4).

At the end of the operation, the tip of the laparoscope is retracted for about 1 cm in the cannula and the telescope stopper fixed again. The camera is focused and the laparoscope is held perpendicular to the patient's abdomen with the non-dominant hand. With the dominant hand the cannula is removed by anticlockwise rotation, while the operator observes the port exit sequence on the monitor. This important

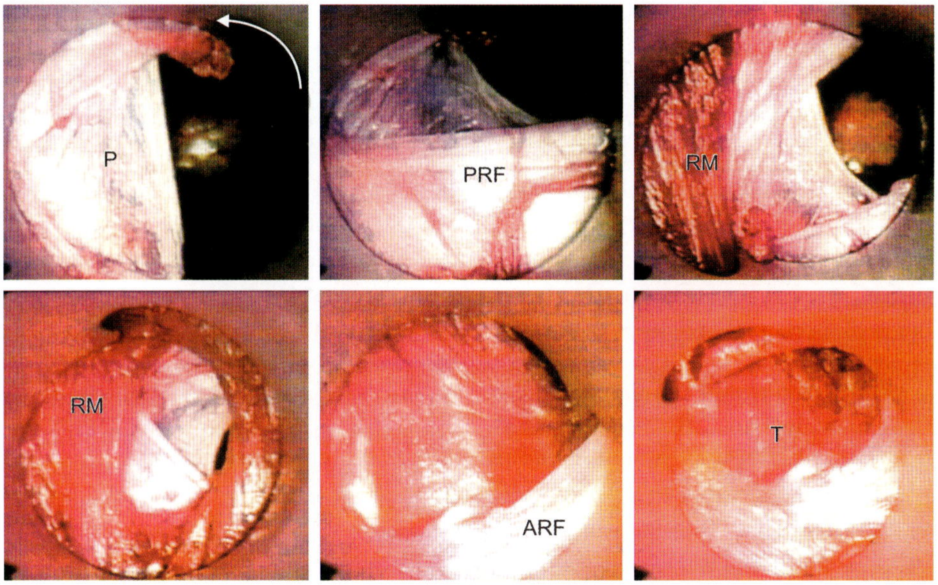

Fig. 10.4: EndoTIP removal. The tissue layers close on retraction of the cannula.
Abbreviations: P, Peritoneum; PRF, Posterior rectus fascia; RM, Rectus muscle; ARF, Anterior rectus fascia; T, Tissue.

step allows the surgeon to determine if reinforcing fascial sutures are required or if abdominal tissues are inadvertently drawn out along the cannula's exit tract. CO_2 is released via an ancillary port to avoid spraying of body fluids onto the telescope's lens.

INDICATIONS

It is very important for every endoscopist to know and use more than one safe peritoneal insertion technique because indications and anatomical requirements vary in every patient. Naturally, every surgeon must select the insertion technique he or she knows to be the safest in their hands. However, the EndoTIP technique suggests that insertion with conventional penetrating trocars and the use of uncontrolled axial force during blind insertion may pose unnecessary additional patient risk. That is why the second generation insertion cannulas offer a less dangerous alternative, where insertion is under visual control using radial penetration force and lifting the tissue layers of the abdominal wall as opposed to pushing it toward the abdomen and offers absolute entry control with no cannula overshoot. Like all new technologies, use of the EndoTIP method must be learnt on easy cases, preferably in the presence of a knowledgeable mentor.

For a competent user the indications are the following:

- History of previous abdominal surgery with many scars and suspected adhesions (adhesiolysis, salpingo and ovariolysis)
- Vague lower abdominal symptoms
- Endometriosis
- Retroperitoneal operations

It is particularly suitable for patients with a past history of more than one laparoscopy, overweight patients with a history of failed laparoscopy or insufflation and patients with conditions, which necessitate insertion under vision (e.g., pregnancy or big tumors).

ADVANTAGES

Unlike the sharp conventional trocar and cannula insertion systems, where the tip of the obturator transects abdominal tissues directly, EndoTIP insertion is under vision and entry overshoot is avoided. Faulty insertion can be immediately recognized and corrected before any injury occurs. This interactive insertion aspect eliminates sharp dissection mishaps and avoids use of axial force at the insertion port site.

As far as the primary trocar is concerned, all endoscopists unanimously agree that insertion under vision is less dangerous and has a considerable safety factor. Systems offering insertion under vision improve our understanding of insertion injuries and reduce recurring mistakes. Second generation insertion systems, such as the EndoTIP, which is inserted under vision, require no sharp trocars and no axial penetration force and allow the recognition of any mistake at the right time. According to a publication by Bogner[2] and in our view also,[11] 90% of all unclassified mistakes in medicine are man-made.

With this background, insertion methods under vision that prevent mistakes or recognize them early are preferred to blind methods. The EndoTIP technique must however be learnt and only after practicing repeatedly, can be employed confidently. In our experience this technique is suitable for most patients.

GYNECOLOGICAL LAPAROSCOPY: IMAGING AND CAPNO PERITONEUM

In 1901, Georg Kelling performed the first "laparoscopy," called "coelioscopy," on a dog using Nitze's cystoscope and air insufflation mechanism in Hamburg, and presented his paper at an Assembly of German Natural Scientists. This technique was developed further by Raoul Palmer, Hans Frangenheim and after 1960 mainly by Kurt Sejm.

Semm initiated diagnostic and operative laparoscopy for gynecologists and operative endoscopic surgery for many other medical specialties and pioneered several innovative endoscopic methods and instruments that we all still use to this day.[6]

Work on "imaging" progressed from camera and light source development to the rod-lens invention, from one chip to three chips, to high-definition (HD) TV and EndoCameleon panoramic cameras (Karl Storz GmbH & Co. KG, Germany) as well as from direct view to 2D or 3D view on the TV monitor. Apparatus and innovative instrument developments, in continuous cooperation with the medical technical industry, brought new features for coagulation, suturing and robotics. Instruments went from two to multiple degrees of liberty, from straight to rotating, multifunctional, articulated and robotic forms.

Precision surgery by means of an enlarged visual image and small or even single-port entries for an instrument set with multiple degrees of liberty has become a reality. Imaging surgery on the video screen is the technique of the future and is already used for most benign and some malignant diseases in the field of gynecology.[18,19]

It is applied for vaginal natural orifice surgery (NOS) and can replace laparotomy in approximately 80% of cases. Only Caesarean sections, hysterectomies for very large uteri and specific cancer surgeries are still performed by laparotomy.

Newer versions of laparoscopic surgery like single-port entry with already quite sophisticated systems, and robotic surgery, using conventional laparoscopic entries, need special attention concerning safety.

The CO_2 pneumoperitoneum = capno CO_2 pneumoperitoneum affects as well the ventilation as the acid–base balance. At an increase of intra-abdominal pressure a cranial dislocation of the diaphragm results. The intra-thoracic gas volume and the functional residual capacity decrease, resulting in a 30% compliance reduction of lungs and thorax. The middle respiration pressure, the plateau level and the peak values may rise and provoke a rise of the pulmonary right left shunt. These alterations are mostly well tolerated from the patient. The p_2CO_2 rises in average due to the transperitoneal resorption by 10 mm Hg in controlled adapted respiration. Only in patients with heavy obstructive lung diseases a critical increase of the carbon dioxide partial pressure may occur: In problems with the pulmonary CO_2 elimination the controlled ventilation can be continued into the perioperative phase.

LAPAROSCOPIC ROBOTIC SURGERY

The growing popularity of laparoscopic surgery focused renewed attention on the need for both improved laparoscopic camera control and instrument range, in terms of motion and dexterity.

The first robotic camera assistant used in endoscopic surgery was the "automated endoscopic system for optimal positioning" (AESOP; Computer Motion, California, USA). This hand-, foot- or voice-controlled arm allows the surgeon to perform complex laparoscopic surgery faster than with an assistant holding the camera.[20]

The next surgical robot was a voice-controlled robot, ZEUS (Computer Motion) that consists of an AESOP to hold the camera and two additional AESOP-like units, which have been modified to hold the surgical instruments.

The modern robot generation named Da Vinci Surgical System is based on the technologies of Computer Motion, which have been developed further by Intuitive Surgical (Sunnyvale, CA). The Da Vinci Surgical System was approved by the Food and Drug Administration (FDA) in May 2005 for clinical use in gynecology and was first used in reproductive gynecology for tubal surgery[21] and later in oncologic surgery.[22,23]

There are four main components to the Da Vinci S Surgical System:

1. *Surgeon's console*: The operator sits viewing a magnified 3D image of the surgical field.
2. *Patient side-cart*: This system consists of three instrument arms and one endoscope arm.

3. *Detachable instruments* (Endowrist instruments and intuitive masters): These detachable instruments allow the robotic arms to maneuver in ways that simulate fine human movements. There are seven degrees of freedom, which offer considerable choice of rotation in full circles. The surgeon is able to control the amount of force applied, which varies from a fraction of a gram to several kilos. Tremor and scale movements are filtered out. The movements of the surgeon's hand can be translated into smaller ones by the robotic device.
4. *3D vision system*: The camera unit or endoscope arm provides enhanced 3D images with the result that the surgeon knows the exact position of all instruments in relation to the anatomical structures. The patients lie in a horizontal position with both arms tucked alongside their body. Four trocars are placed next to the optic trocar. The surgeon sits at the console and the first surgical assistant is seated, in most cases on the patient's left side. This assistant controls the left accessory ports into which the instruments that are used for vessel sealing, retraction, suction, irrigation and suturing are inserted. The middle robotic arm is attached to the optical trocar, with two lateral working arms to the right and one to the left. The robotic arms are connected at the beginning of the procedure and disengaged from the trocars at the end of the operation. The incisions are stitched and the incision lines are reapproximated (Da Vinci S Surgical System). The core technology of the Da Vinci Surgical System has been further refined to now include the Da Vinci S Surgical System and the Da Vinci Si Surgical System.

The Da Vinci Surgical System has captured the imagination of the surgical community worldwide; however, the costs are very high and remain at the same level for each new surgical procedure. On the other hand, smaller innovative robotic systems with instruments with up to seven degrees of freedom are coming on the market. New HDTV systems allow the surgeon to work in what is almost a 3D field.

ABDOMINAL ENTRY SAFETY STEPS

The following safety measures are advised before insertion of the Veress needle for CO_2 insufflation of the abdomen.

- *"Palpation of aorta" test*: If the abdominal aorta can be palpated directly *below* the umbilicus, the bifurcation must be further toward lower pelvis. It cannot be injured by oblique insertion of Veress needle. If the bifurcation is felt *above* the umbilicus, perpendicular insertion with the anterior abdominal wall lifted up is suitable (Fig. 10.5).

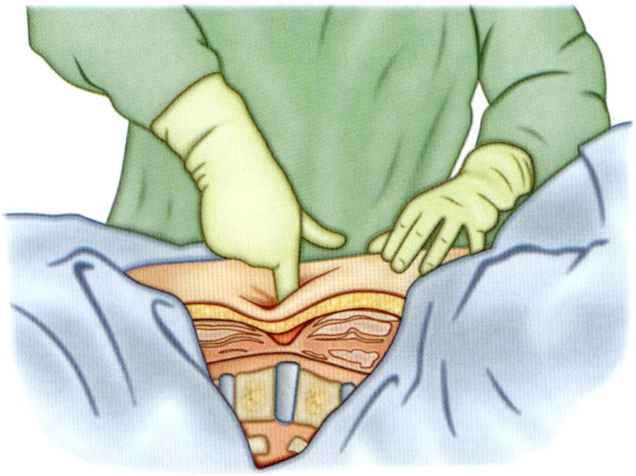

Fig. 10.5: The palpation of aorta test.

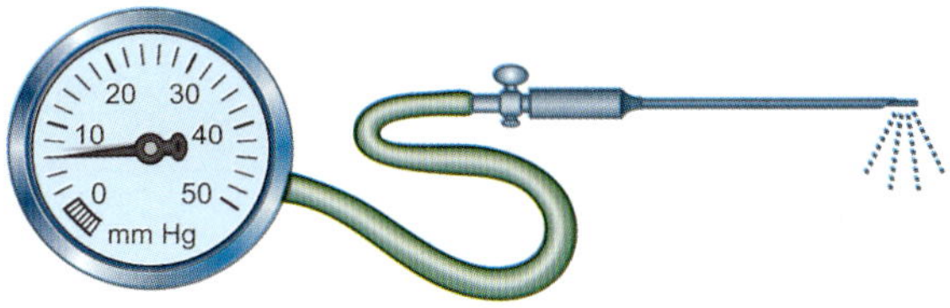

Fig. 10.6: The needle flow test.

- *Needle flow test*: To ensure flawless insertion of the Veress needle, the manometer should be set to a resistance of maximum 4–6 mm Hg with a gas flow rate of 1 L/min. If the resistance is high, there is some obstruction inside the Veress needle (Fig. 10.6).
- *Insertion of the Veress needle*: Veress needle insertion must be always at a right angle (an obliquely inserted needle becomes a scalpel!) Note that the CO_2 must remain in the open position at all times during insertion.
- *"Snap" test*: During insertion of the Veress needle through the skin, subcutaneous fat tissue, fascia, musculature and peritoneum, a snap can be heard because of the CO_2 gushing through the respective layers (Fig. 10.7).
- *Hiss phenomenon*: After successful perforation of the anterior abdominal wall, a soft hissing sound is produced during the insertion of the Veress needle in the elevated abdominal wall as a result of negative pressure in the abdominal cavity.
- *Aspiration test*: Injection of 5–10 mL normal saline solution results in negative aspiration if the Veress needle is correctly placed, but gives

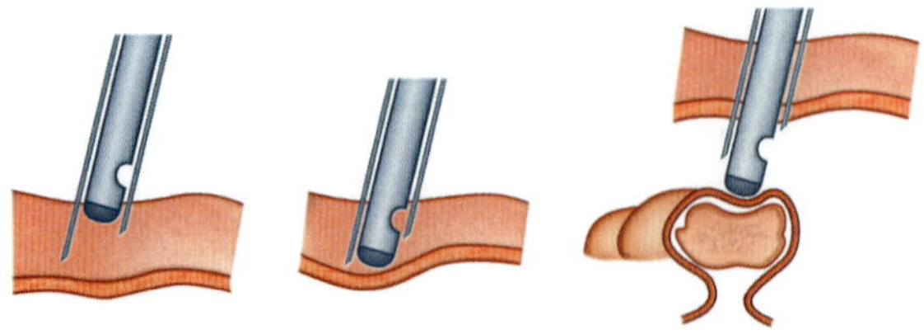

Fig. 10.7: The snap test.

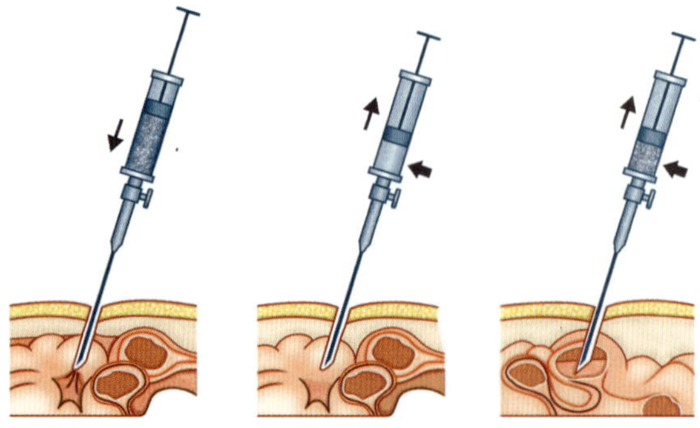

Fig. 10.8: The aspiration test.

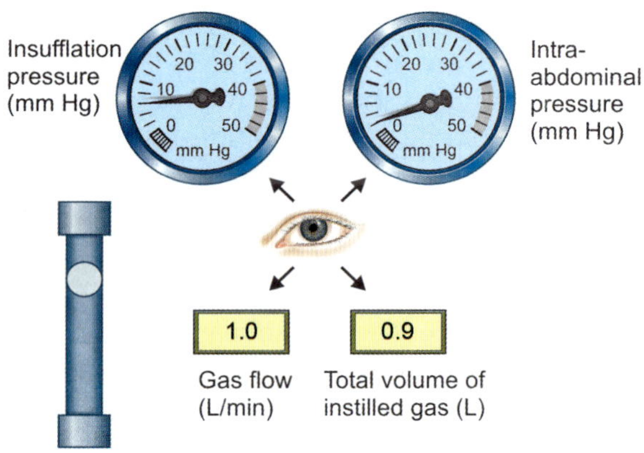

Fig. 10.9: The quadro test.

blood-tinged aspirate or aspirate with intestinal contents if the needle is placed either in a blood vessel or intestine (Fig. 10.8).

- *Quadro test*: The four parameters measured are insufflation pressure, intra-abdominal pressure, gas volume per minute and total volume of instilled gas (Fig. 10.9). When the anterior abdominal wall is lifted up because of the negative pressure created in the abdominal cavity, if the pressure drops to below zero, then only CO_2 should be insufflated up to a pressure of 15–20 mm Hg.
- *Sounding test*: CO_2 is aspirated in a syringe containing 20 mL of normal saline solution and the result examined. When the tip lies free in the abdominal gas, CO_2 bubbles are visible in the normal saline solution during respiration, indicating the position in the free abdominal cavity (Fig. 10.10). When planning Z-insertion, the aspiration must be carried out horizontally toward the right or left and caudally, depending on the planning.
- *Panoramic viewing after Z-insertion*: The panoramic viewing facilitates to uncover any pathological changes in the vicinity of lower pelvis, e.g. in the intestines, liver, gallbladder and spleen (Fig. 10.11).

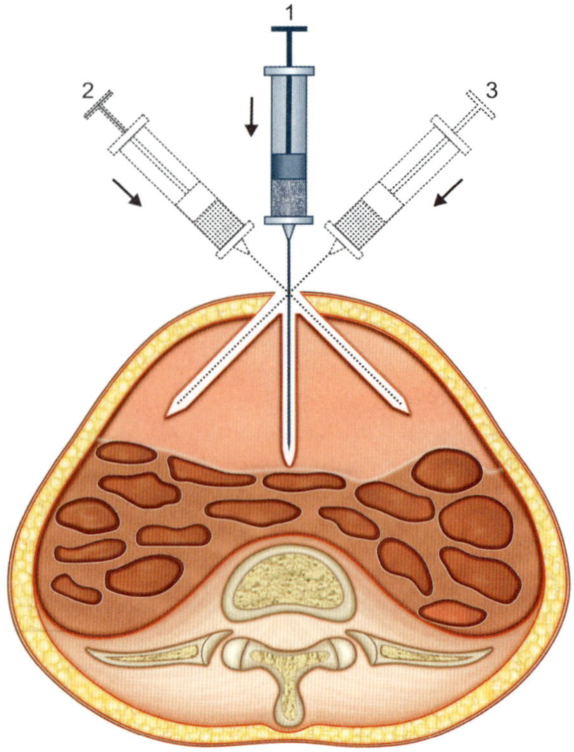

Fig. 10.10: The sounding test.

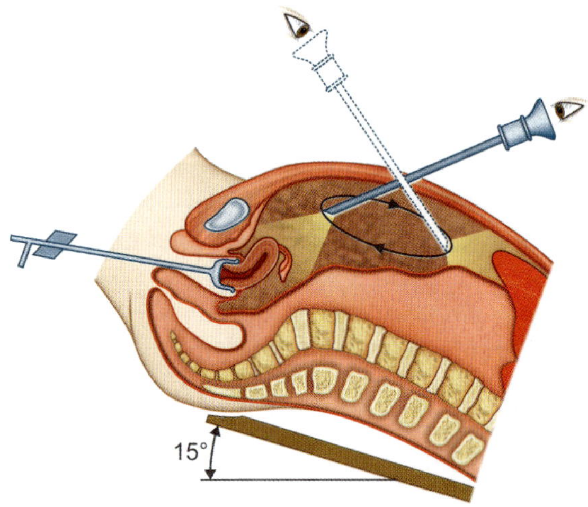

Fig. 10.11: Inspection of the abdominal cavity, after insertion of a laparoscope under CO_2 abdominopelvic distension (panoramic viewing after Z-insertion).

ABDOMINAL ENTRY POSSIBILITIES

Entry possibilities are given for single-port, multiple ports and robotic surgical entries by laparotomy, vaginal access, laparoscopic open and closed approach, blind entry or laparoscopic entry under sight or vision.

The anterior abdominal wall has four muscles that are traversed at all entries:

- Rectus abdominis
- External obliquus abdominis
- Internal obliquus abdominis
- Transversus abdominis.

The transversus abdominis and four structures lead from the medial to the lateral abdominal wall: urachus, inferior epigastric vessels, umbilical lateral ligament and the superficial epigastric vessels. At laparotomy the incision possibilities are transversal with the conventional Pfannenstiel incision in the lower abdomen (Kiel School), a little higher the high fascial opening called the Misgav–Ladach Caesarean section incision described by Joel Cohen and Michael Stark and the longitudinal incision to the umbilicus or around it.

The gynecological surgeon and also the general surgeon have four routes of entry to the Nabdomen to treat intraabdominal disease surgically or by needle puncture with aspiration or instillation. These entry possibilities can remain the same under imaging techniques such as an magnetic resonance imaging (MRI) or computed tomography (CT) scan; however, focussed ultrasound destruction for fibroids controlled by MRI is possible today as well; techniques are changing.[24]

- *Open abdominal*: Laparotomy in its different forms always dissects all abdominal layers to gain enough access to study and heal the respective disease. It always requires the closure of the wound in different layers by sutures.
- *Laparoscopic*: Closed and open—multiple ports, single-port, robotic.

In the closed access technique, the pneumoperitoneum is created by the Veress needle. This is a blind entry and most commonly practiced by surgeons and gynecologists worldwide since the invention of this spring-needle system by the Hungarian internal medicine specialist Janos Veress who used his spring-laded needle to create artificial pneumo-thorax when treating tuberculosis patients (Fig. 10.12).

After pneumoperitoneum, the 5–10 mm conic trocar insertion principles are the following. After making the incision with a scalpel, enter with a 5 mm trocar sleeve and conical mandarin, pushing through the skin, subcutaneous fat tissue and fascia; advance the trocar with a conical tip toward the right with rotational movements through the musculature till the peritoneum is reached; avoid the umbilical aponeurosis and insert the conical elliptical trocar through the peritoneum by rotational movements.

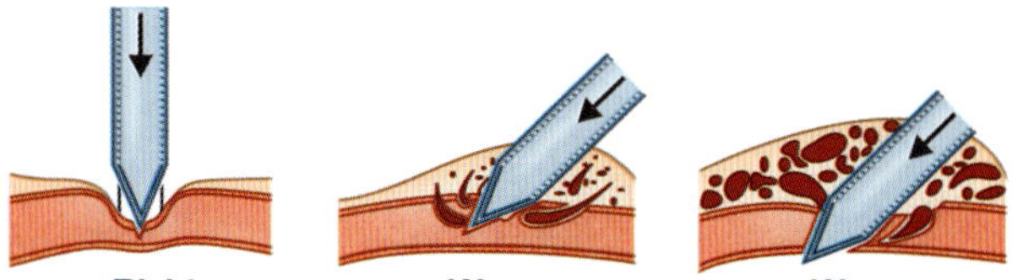

Fig. 10.12: Veress needle entry. After skin incision, Veress needle penetrates into the umbilicus. Through skin and subcutaneous fat tissue, the Veress needle goes up to the fascia and penetrates into the abdomen. In positions 1, 2 and 3, CO_2 is aspirated from the free abdominal cavity.

It is easy to insert the Veress needle and create the pneumoperitoneum mostly through the umbilicus or at Palmer's point (left upper abdomen, about 2 cm under the palpable rib in preoperated patients), but lacerations of vessels and more seldom bowel loops do occur.

Direct access or entry by the open technique, without creating pneumoperitoneum or using insufflators, has been described by Hasson.[14] It is also called the Scandinavian or fielding technique. Some surgeons perform blind trocar insertion without pneumoperitoneum. The vascular lesions and bowel lesions appear to be similar.

- *Conventional vaginal entry*, with colpotomy and single-port systems for transvaginal surgery. Vaginal surgery with colpotomy has a long tradition and is the entry of choice for the gynecologist if the individual patient situation does not require a visual check of the abdominal cavity. Even vaginal hysterectomy is performed by pulling out the organs before transecting them and the vision is poor. Single-port systems for a small 12–15 mm entry through the posterior cul-de-sac are in development.
- *Natural orifice transluminal endoscopic surgery* (NOTES), which includes the transgastric and transvaginal approach and natural orifice surgery: Coming mostly from the field of general surgery, various systems through the entry point stomach and umbilicus are available and facilitate surgical interventions with only one incision: single-port

entries [single-port laparoscopic system (SILS), Covidien], laparoendoscopic single-site surgical technique (LESS, Olympus) and X-Cone or Endo-Cone (Storz, Rochester, New York).

All access possibilities that are done blind through the Veress needle or with the trocar directly (using sharp, edged, conic or blunt trocars) carry a certain danger of risk lacerating structures immediately adherent to the abdominal wall such as adhesions or bowel loops, deeper structures such as bowels or vessels and abdominal organs (stomach, bladder). Entries under sight with the optical Veress needle and with Visiport, Optiview and EndoTIP have been described for closed access and give a certain security; however, basically the open and closed access techniques even under sight give similar numbers of lesions in patients with bowel loops adherent to the anterior abdominal wall.

We think in 2012 entry under sight was required for the primary trocar because this reduces lacerations in all situations in which bowel is not adherent to the abdominal wall.

SINGLE-PORT ENTRY = SINGLE-ENTRY LAPAROSCOPY (SEL)

Technique

- A skin incision of 2.5 cm is made deep in the umbilicus.
- A Veress needle of 18–20 cm is used to create a pneumoperitoneum of 20 mm Hg. CO_2 gas is used at a continuous flow of 4.5 L/min. An intra-abdominal balloon is created in this way allowing a safe opening of the abdominal cavity.
- The fascia of the musculus rectus abdominis is incised and grasped, the peritoneum is opened.
- An open laparoscopy technique is used to grasp the peritoneum under the fascia.
- This peritoneum and the overlying fascia are incised over 4–5 cm.
- The single-entry port is introduced into the abdominal cavity after checking with the fingers that no bowel is adherent to the incision site.
- After access has been achieved, a 30–45° scope is introduced, followed by the necessary instruments needed to perform the surgery.
- Conventional long or specific instruments are used.
- As smoke can be a problem, it is advisable to use sealers as these bipolar instruments of the sixth generation produce less smoke.

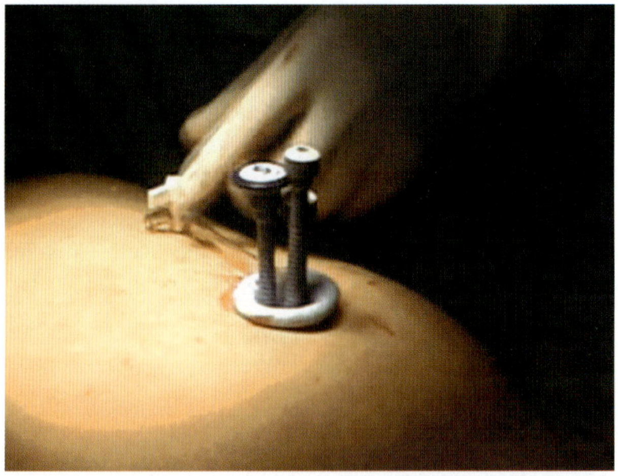

Fig. 10.13: SILS port (Covidien, Norwalk, Connecticut, USA) in place.

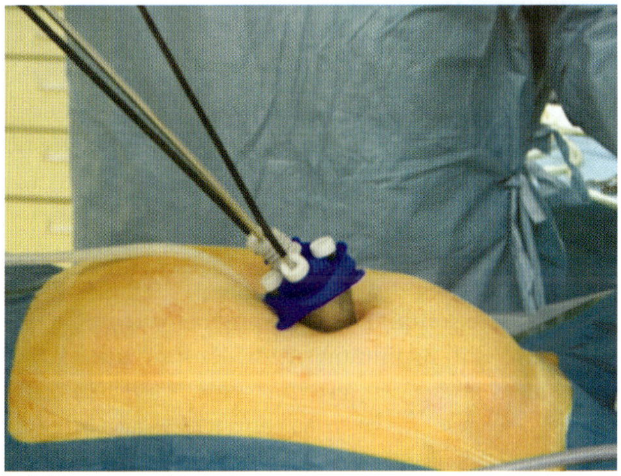

Fig. 10.14: The X-cone (Karl Storz GmbH & Co KG, Tuttlingen, Germany) in place.

A silicone port (Covidien, Norwalk, Connecticut, USA) is introduced into the abdominal cavity. The choice is one or two ports of 5 mm and one of 12 mm or one of four 5 mm ports (Fig. 10.13).

Another port is the X-Cone (Karl Storz GmbH & Co KG, Tuttlingen, Germany) (Figs. 10.14 and 10.15). The advantage of this port of entry is that it is reusable. Here five ports can be used varying from 5 to 10 mm.

SEL Instruments

The instruments have to be adapted for use through SEL ports. These have to be longer than the usual instruments as all have to be used through the umbilicus. The characteristics of the instruments are such that they do not clash with the optic. Therefore, it is easier to have single- or double-bended instruments,

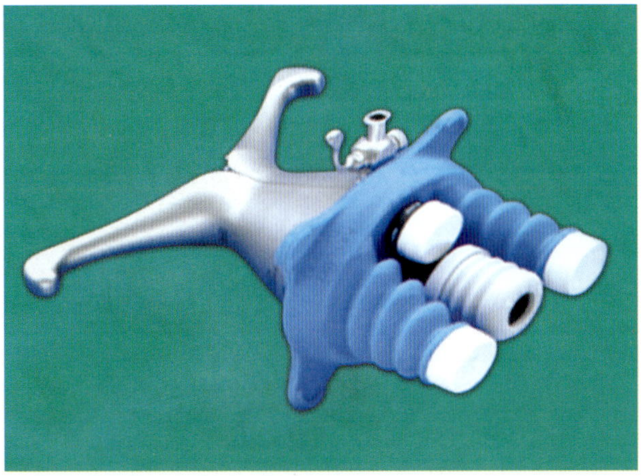

Fig. 10.15: The X-cone (Karl Storz GmbH & Co KG, Tuttlingen, Germany). Note the different seals allowing multiple entries.

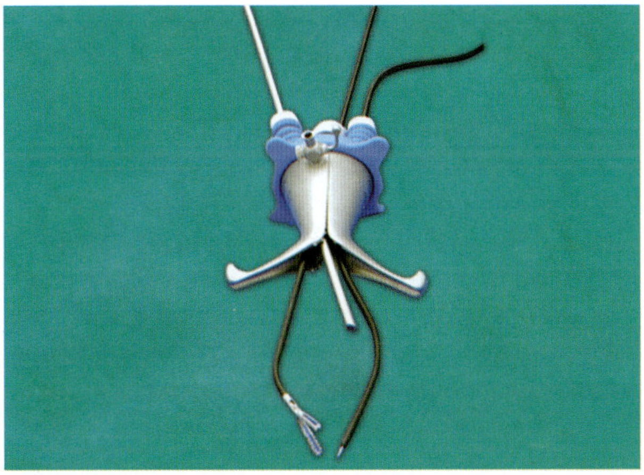

Fig. 10.16: The optic, 5 mm 30°, on the left, in the middle a single-curved instrument and on the right the double-curved instrument.

most of which are reusable (Karl Storz GmbH & Co KG, Tuttlingen, Germany), or single-use instruments that can be bent into the correct position during the operation (Covidien, Norwalk, Connecticut USA).

Scopes have to be adapted. The most frequently used scopes are of 5 mm, 30° final lens of 50 cm. The length of the scope avoids clashes with the instruments (Fig. 10.16).

The long 5 mm scope is seen on the left of the picture. A long single-bend instrument is seen central while a double-bend instrument is seen on the right (Fig. 10.16).

The aim of designing or bending the instruments in this way is to be able to address the objects—the target tissues—in the correct plane to be able perform the necessary manipulations.[25] In Fig. 10.17 single-bend instruments can be seen. Sometimes a single bend is enough to perform the manipulation. The preference depends on the type of instrument and the ability of the surgeon to localize the instrument in space. The localization in space of the instruments is easier with single-use instruments that can be bent to a specific position in space during the intervention. Multiple-use instruments do not have this specific property and hence the surgeon needs more intuition to locate the instrument in the given space.

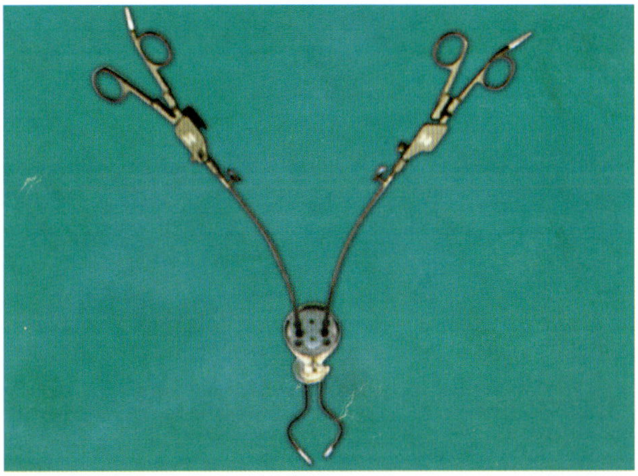

Fig. 10.17: The single-curved instruments in the X-cone port showing the spread from an eventual scope to prevent clashing of the different inserts, while still able to address the target at right angles.

Benefits

- The technique allows for an easy conversion to conventional laparoscopy.
- There is less postoperative pain.
- The recovery time is faster.
- There are less postoperative complications.
- The cosmetic results are even better than after conventional laparoscopy.
- On the macro-economical scale there is a speedier return to classical activities

Disadvantages and Complications

According to the literature search the following complications occur:

- Bleeding complications in 2% of patients.
- Infections of the abdominal wound in 2% of cases.
- Injury to other organs in 1% of cases.
- Herniation at the incisional site occurs in less than 1% of cases.
- Conversions to traditional laparoscopy (5–10%).
- Conversion to open surgery (2%).
- Longer operating time (20–45%).

Table 10.2: Comparison between the types of hysterectomy procedures.[26-28]

Type of hysterectomy	Number of external incisions	Size of external incisions	Number of visible scars	Length of hospital stay	Recovery time
Single entry laparoscopy (SEL) hysterectomy	1 small incision in belly button	20 mm	Potential for invisible scar	Same day to 2 days	2 weeks
Abdominal (open) hysterectomy	1 large incision	150–210 mm	1 large scar	2–6 days	6–8 weeks
Laparoscopic hysterectomy	3–4 small incisions	5–15 mm	3–4 small scars	Same day to 2 days	2 weeks
Laparoscopically assisted vaginal hysterectomy	1–4 small incisions	0–15 mm	1–4 small scars	Same day to 1–4 days	2 weeks
Vaginal hysterectomy	Vaginal incision	Not applicable	Not applicable	Same day to 2 days	2 weeks

- There are additional instrument and training costs, which are difficult to evaluate but substantial.
- The way of access is not yet evidence based.

A comparison of various hysterectomy procedures shows the advantages of single-port entry with a short hospital stay and recovery time (Table 10.2).

PNEUMOPERITONEUM

In early years, air was used for insufflation, but because of the increased risk of air embolism it was quickly replaced by CO_2 or N_2O gas. CO_2 is 200 times more diffusible than O_2. It is rapidly cleared by the lungs and does not support combustion. N_2O is only absorbed in blood up to 68% compared to CO_2 but has the advantage of a mild analgesic effect. Thus, it is preferably used in laparoscopic procedures under local anesthesia. Helium gas, being inert in nature, is also applied in some centers but does not have added benefit over CO_2. Of course, gasless laparoscopy, as advised by some studies, carries no danger of any gas insufflation but requires use of specialized abdominal wall retractors. It does however facilitate the use of conventional surgical instruments.

CLOSED LAPAROSCOPIC ABDOMINAL ENTRY

Surgeons can apply conic trocars, beveled trocars, multi-edged sharp trocars, threaded cannulas such as EndoTIP (entry without force but with feeling, under sight) and visual trocars during first access. After the pneumoperitoneum is established through the Veress needle the optical port is placed.

It is not clear if conical trocars with one point of laceration (the sharp pointed trocar tip) or a multi-edged of laceration (beveled with three sharp edges and a pointed end) is preferred; as the force required to insert a pointed conical trocar is infinitely more that the force required to insert a beveled trocar. Admittedly, beveled trocars need larger incisions.

One of the most important steps for laparoscopic primary port placement is the direction of insertion, as applying entry force in the wrong direction could cause considerable damage (Fig. 10.13).

All the trocars for robotic work need larger incisions because of the 12 cm size of the instruments. Single-port entries all need larger incisions and certain dexterity to access the abdomen safely. Direct trocar application and radially expanding trocars are other systems that can be used for laparoscopic entry. For a safe entry into the abdominal cavity, blind entry can be replaced by sharp trocars under vision. This is also called entry under sight.

After skin incision and penetration through skin and subcutaneous fat tissue with the trocar up to the fascia, insert the scope and reduce the CO_2 flow, cutting through the fascia and musculature to the peritoneum. Under vision, guide the tip of the scope on the peritoneum to a place where there are no bowel loops against it. Perform sharp perforation of the peritoneum under visualization. Turn off CO_2 and inspect the abdominal cavity.

No specific trocars have shown to be superior in preventing vascular and visceral lacerations. EndoTIP is a preferred entry method as no plastic layer is interposed between the end of the laparoscope and the traversed tissues, such as that found with Optiview, Excel or Visiport, as tissue distortion makes situational awareness less reliable and diminishes vision.

RADIALLY EXPANDING TROCARS

Our experience with radially expanding trocars shows that the only advantage in comparison with conventional primary trocar entries is the reduced degree of postoperative pain (Figs. 10.14 and 10.15).

According to a French retrospective study, the incidence of serious trocar accidents was evaluated from 103,852 laparoscopic operations involving almost 390,000 trocars. Seven perioperative deaths occurred (mortality 0.07/1,000), arising almost exclusively from vascular injuries. The incidence of vascular injuries was 0.4/1,000. There were injuries to almost all the abdominal organs and most of the abdominal vascular tree.

COMPLICATIONS AND LACERATION POSSIBILITIES DURING FIRST ACCESS

The following series of drawings compares correct and incorrect needle and trocar positions as well as cutting procedures (Figs. 10.16 to 10.27).

Abdominal Access Complications

Peritoneal entry complications can occur during port placement such as laceration of intraabdominal organs. There can be failure to successfully enter and insufflate the peritoneal cavity, or there can be port competence hernias among others.

During trocar entry, primary bowel lesions of adherent bowel loops to the anterior abdominal wall occur at both laparoscopy and laparotomy. When

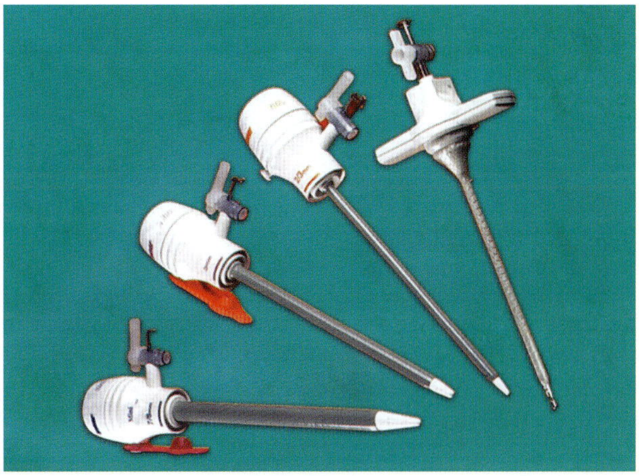

Fig. 10.19: Radially expanding trocars.

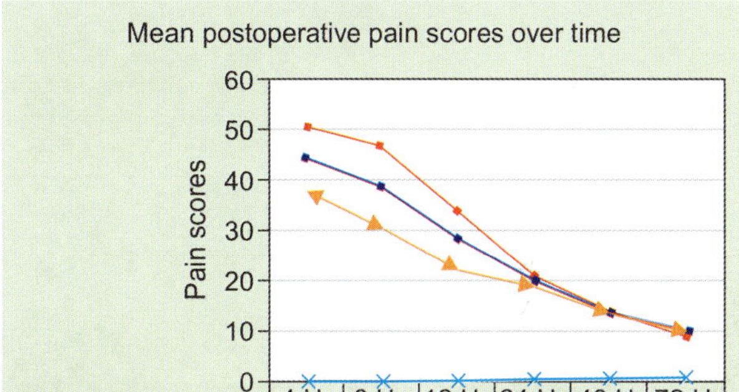

	4 Hr	8 Hr	12 Hr	24 Hr	48 Hr	72 Hr
Overall	44.2	38.6	28.1	19.8	13.5	9.3
Conventional	50.4	46.6	33.9	20.9	13.6	8.9
Step	37.8	30.4	22.2	18.7	13.3	9.8
P-value	0.036	0.004	0.035	0.333	0.701	0.772

Evaluation interval, Hours

Fig. 10.20: Pain score after gynecological laparoscopy conic trocars and radially expanding trocars.

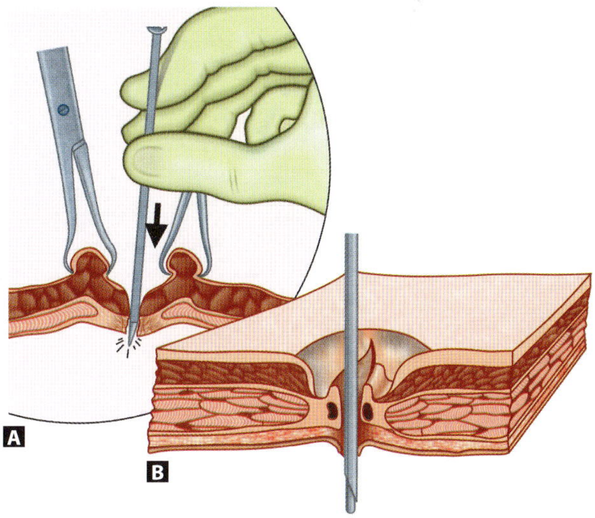

Figs. 10.21A and B: Correct Veress needle introduction through the umbilical fascia by perpendicular direction. (A) Surgeons lift the umbilical area by two Backhaus forceps and introduce the Veress needle; (B) The correct intra-abdominal positioning of Veress needle.

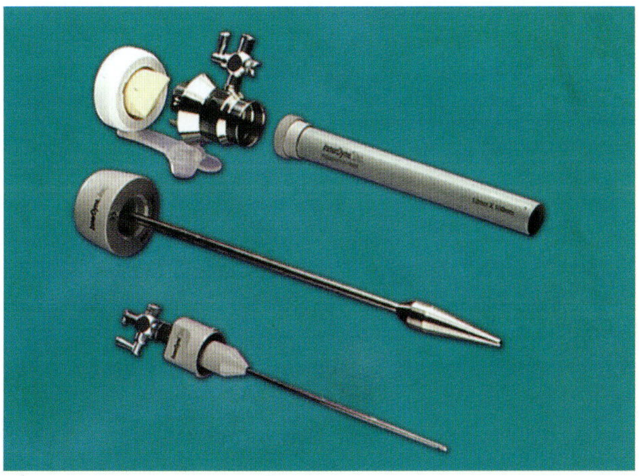

Fig. 10.18: The right direction of trocar insertion at first entry. The first panoramic view after insertion of the laparoscope.

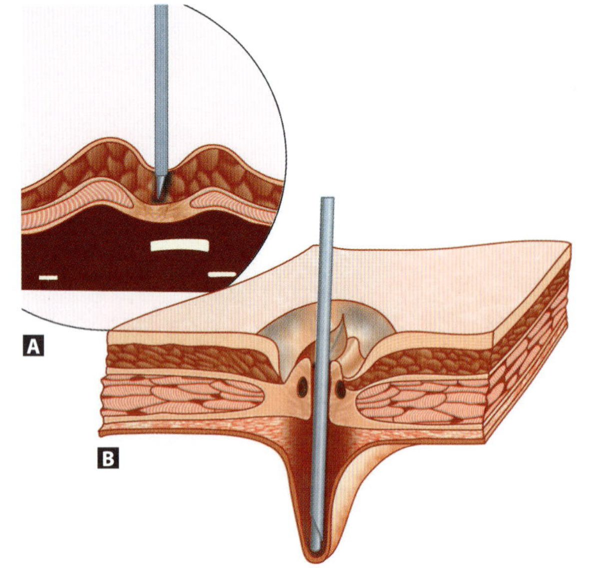

Figs. 10.22A and B: (A) Normal introduction of Veress needle; (B) Wrong introduction of Veress needle in the preperitoneal space with the curtain effect.

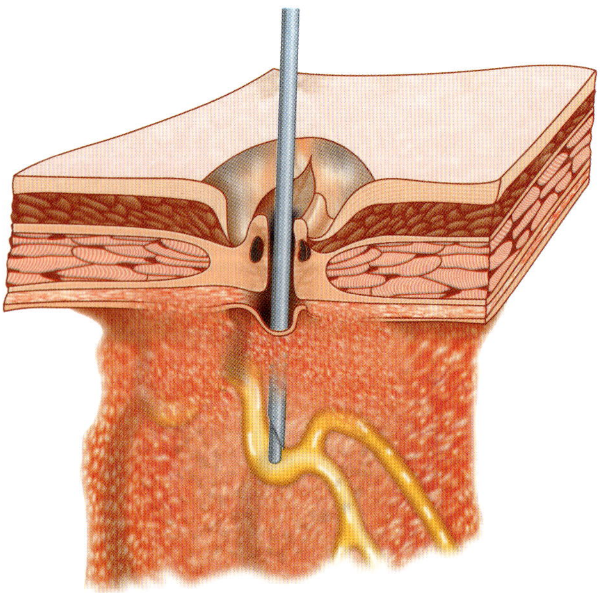

Fig. 10.23: Minor vascular injury. Accidental needle puncture of intraomental blood vessel, adherent to abdominal wall.

placing the Veress needle, a vessel can be lanced inadvertently and intravascular insufflation of CO_2 may occur.

Several mechanisms may lead to gas embolism. Any cut into an abdominal wall or peritoneal vessel can cause CO_2 gas to be forced into the vessel and if the Veress needle is put directly into a vein or a parenchymal organ, this may cause gas embolism.

Lacerations of the epigastric inferior arteries by placing secondary trocars under vision occur repeatedly because colleagues fail to identify the course of the anterior abdominal vessels and they do not use the abdominal translucency technique to determine the presence of vessels. Understandably identification of the vessels course by translucency test in overweight patients may not be easy. The percentage of women requiring more than one attempt at laparoscopic entry is highest in obese and particularly morbidly obese patients. Epigastric arteries and even ureters can be considerably more difficult to identify.

The angle of the optical trocar if under vision or blind should not be more than 45°. It is important to palpate the aorta to find out whether the bifurcation is above or below the umbilicus.

CASE REPORT: PERSISTENT DUCTUS OMPHALOENTERICUS

With the Veress needle at blind entry, I once punctured a persistent, still blood-filled, ductus omphalo entericus that gave a heavy arterial bleeding. The situation was visualized by quickly entering the optical trocar as well as two lower abdominal trocars and the duct grasped and coagulated. The arterial bleeding was immense; the patient had more than 1 L of fresh blood in the abdomen.

Laparoscopic entry lesions are classified as follows:[29]

- *Type 1 Injuries*: Damage by Veress needle or trocar to major blood vessels and normally located bowel (1–4 per 1,000 patients).
- *Type 2 Injuries*: Damage by Veress needle or trocar to bowel adherent to the abdominal wall or vessels in the abdominal wall.

Type 2 lesions may occur whether the mode of access is by laparotomy or laparoscopy. The incidence of primary trocar lesions is 0.4–0.8% and the incidence of secondary trocar lesions is 0.8–0.12%. Bowel lesions occur in 4 per 1,000 cases (obtained from 350,000 laparoscopies in multicentre studies). Even with the most experienced laparoscopic and laparotomic surgeon, bowel lesions are not always avoidable.

Vascular lesions occur in 2 per 1,000 cases. According to the German Laparoscopic Registry (Arbeitsgemeinschaft Gynäkologische Endoskopie, AGE) bowel and vascular lesions are found in 2–4 per 1,000 patients. Open laparoscopy offers no advantage in avoiding these lesions. Immediate action upon recognition of complications guarantees the safety of the patient.

In a retroperitoneal vascular laceration with the Veress needle or the tip of the trocar without an

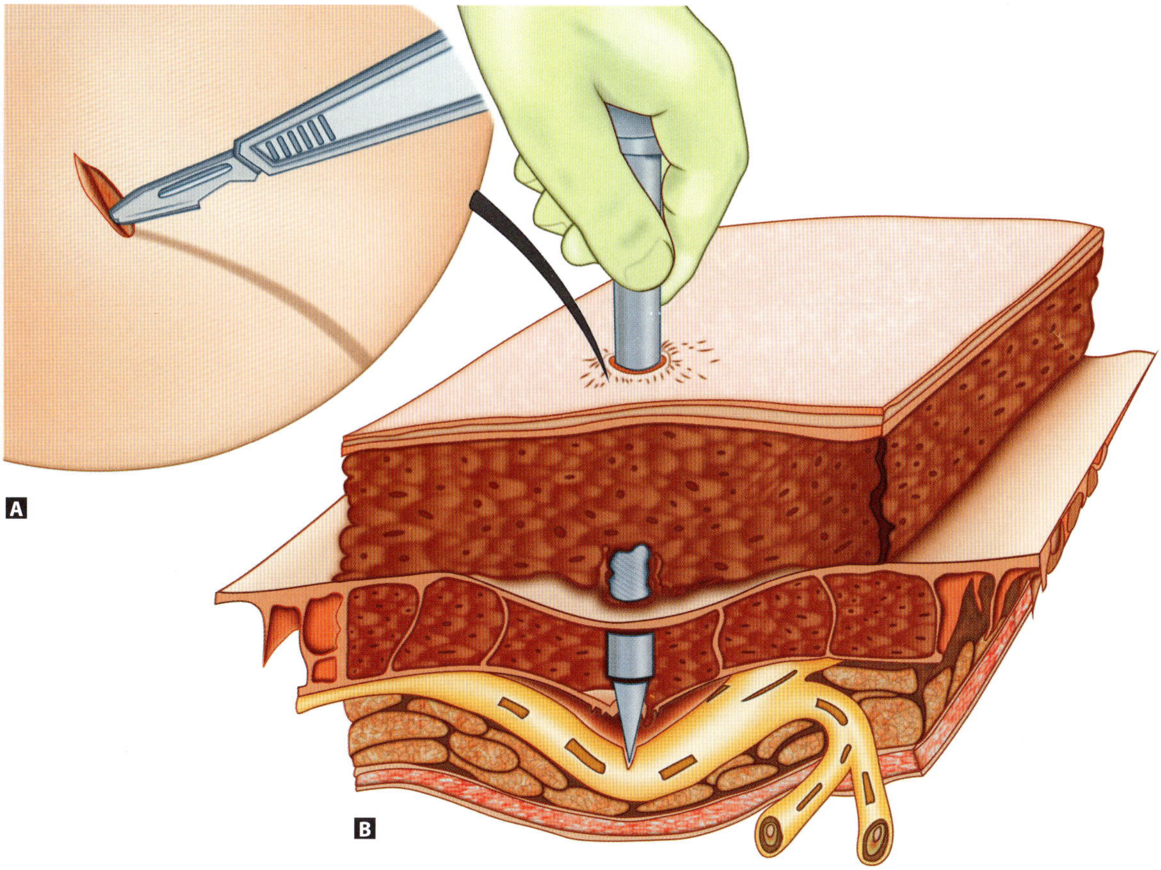

Figs. 10.24A and B: Minor vascular injury during ancillary trocar introduction. (A) Abdominal wall lateral incision to introduce the ancillary trocar; (B) Injury of epigastric artery during the ancillary trocar introduction. This lesion is more frequent in obese women, in whom the Camper's fascia switches the trocar direction.

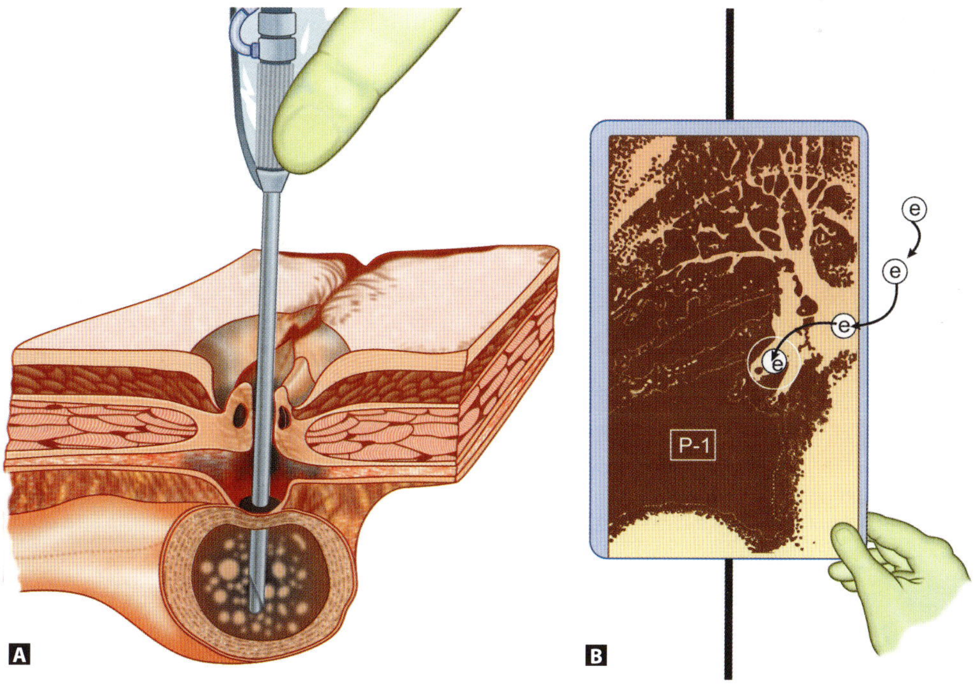

Figs. 10.25A and B: Veress needle entry and possible embolism. (A) Accidental needle introduction into the blood vessel adherent to abdominal wall and wrong CO_2 insufflation; (B) Radiographic image of left lung infarct (e Embolism, P-1 pulmonary infarct).

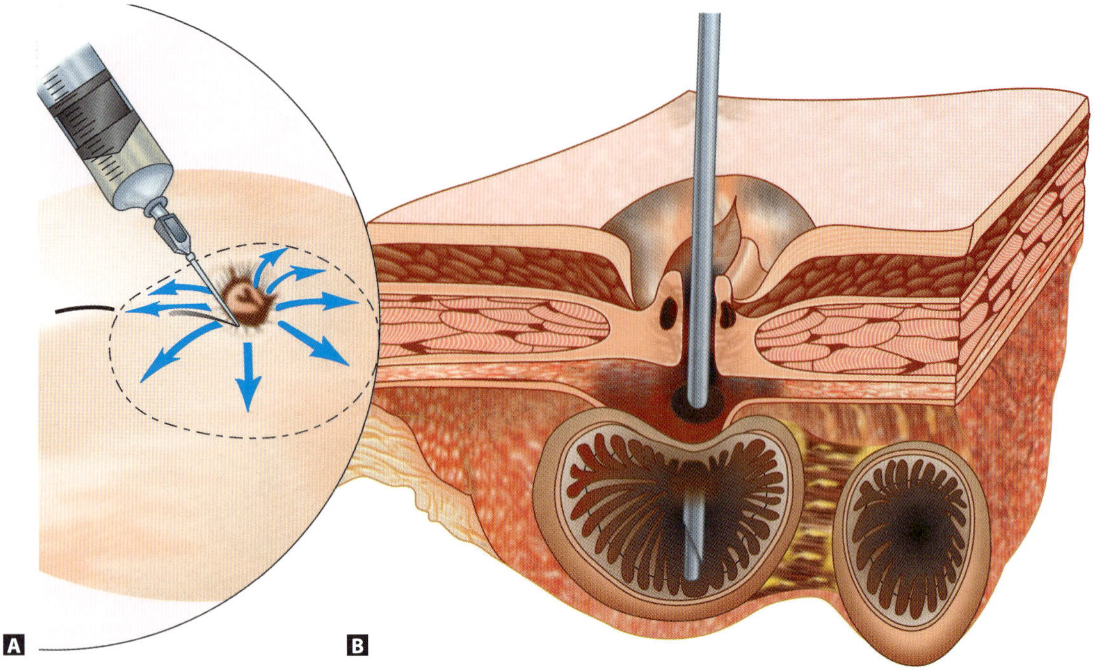

Figs. 10.26A and B: Bowel injury during Veress introduction. (A) Accidental Veress introduction into small bowel, adherent to anterior abdominal wall; (B) Safety maneuver to check correct needle introduction.

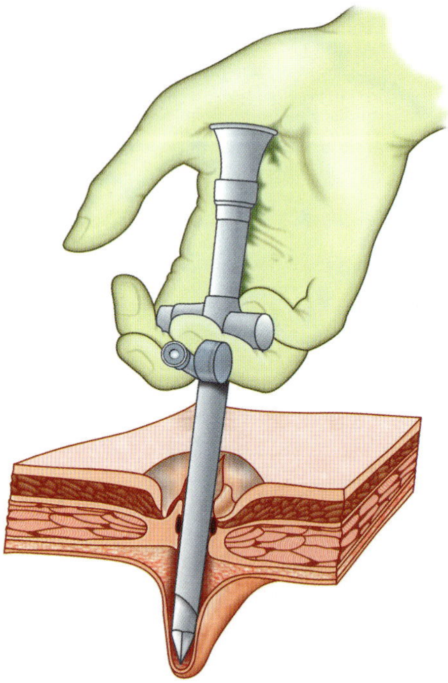

Fig. 10.27: Wrong introduction of a poly-use trocar in the preperitoneal space with the curtain effect.

immediate fast-growing hematoma that requires direct action: Obtain information of anesthesia, call in nurses, call for the help of colleagues and call for a vascular surgeon. A small retroperitoneal hematoma can be carefully observed while performing the planned surgical procedure. A small hematoma does not have to be opened and must not necessarily be revised.

As I learned from my teacher, Kurt Semm,[30] in every laparoscopic operating theater special vascular clamps, such as right-angled Kelly clamps, Adson-Schmidt, DeBakey hemostat or Crawford clamps must be at hand. No attempt should be made to grasp any injured vessel with nonvascular instruments.

IMMEDIATE COMPLICATIONS

These occur during surgical interventions as bowel, vessel, bladder and ureter lesions (Figs. 10.28 to 10.33) as well as anesthesia-related or general complications, such as pulmonary embolism, massive bleedings, as a result of major vessel injuries or intravascular insufflation and heart arrest.

In our gynecological field we have to be aware that even during the clearest laparoscopic hysterectomy and particularly in cancer situation, veins are opened and gas enters into the venous system and may even reach the right side of the heart.[31]

Bowel and some other lesions are not always avoidable, even with the most experienced laparoscopic and laparotomic surgeon. Primary bowel injury occurs by direct cutting, traction at adhesiolysis or as thermal injuries in about 1% of laparoscopies.[32]

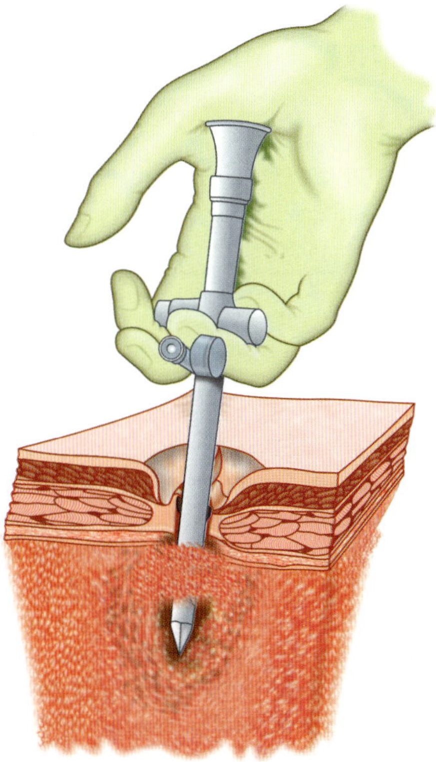

Fig. 10.28: Accidental introduction of a poly-use trocar in the omentum tissue adherent to abdominal wall.

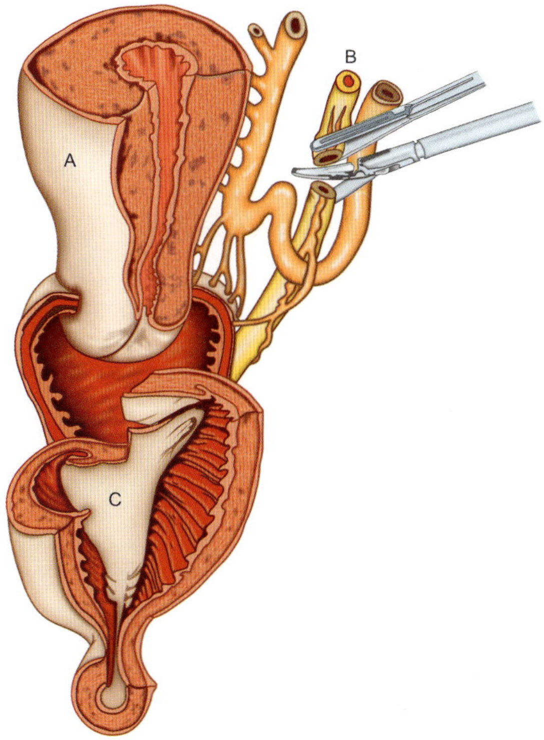

Figs. 10.30A to C: Frontal and sagittal section of uterus. (A) and lower genitourinary system: left ureter (B) and bladder (C). Accidental ureteral section by endoscopic Mayo scissors during laparoscopic total hysterectomy.

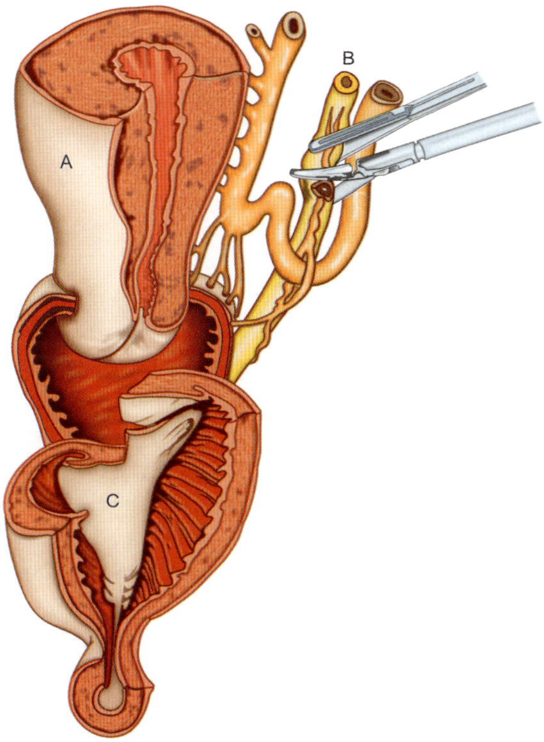

Figs. 10.29A to C: Frontal and sagittal section of uterus. (A) and lower genitourinary system: left ureter (B) and bladder (C). Accidental ureteral partial cutting by endoscopic Mayo scissors during laparoscopic total hysterectomy.

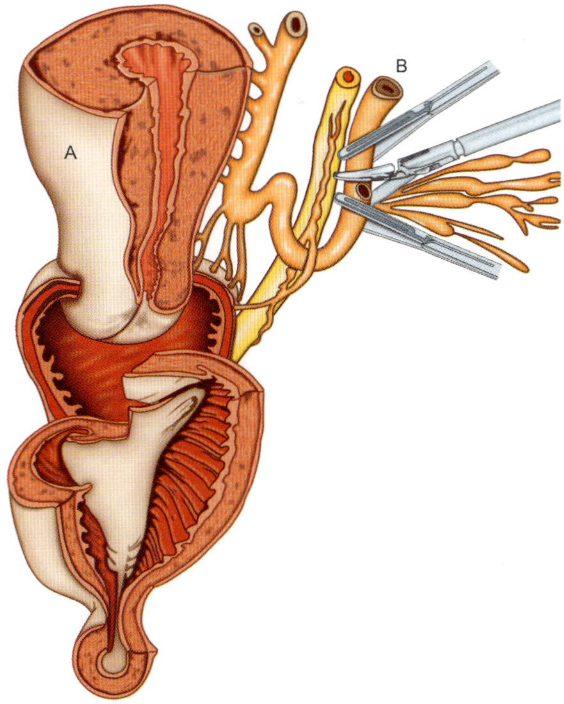

Figs. 10.31A and B: Frontal and sagittal section of uterus. (A) and left uterine artery (B). Accidental partial cutting of descending uterine artery by endoscopic Mayo scissors during laparoscopic total hysterectomy.

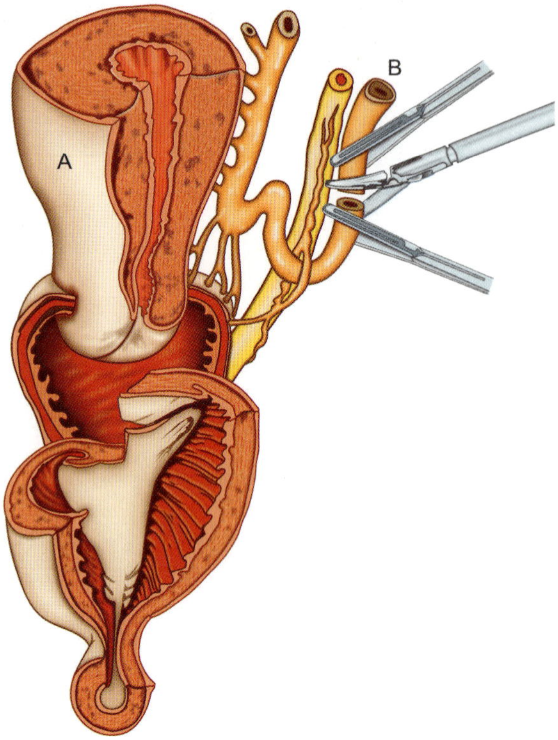

Figs. 10.32A and B: Frontal and sagittal section of uterus. (A) and left uterine artery (B). Accidental total section of descending uterine artery by endoscopic Mayo scissors during laparoscopic total hysterectomy.

CASE REPORT: BOWEL LESION

Here I want to share a report on a bowel perforation recognized at the end of the laparoscopy with entry of the primary optical trocar at Palmer's point and positioning of two lower umbilical trocars under sight.

The case involved a 37-year-old patient with ovarian cancer; stage III, who underwent radical hysterectomy with bilateral adnexectomy, pelvic systematic lymphadenectomy and adjuvant chemotherapy.

At the second-look laparoscopy, the surgeon caused a lesion of the small bowel during placement of a secondary port under suboptimal vision. The question is, Was it avoidable?

After taking a biopsy while performing adhesiolysis and diagnosing all the small cancerous implants, we found that the right secondary trocar had *totally perforated a small bowel loop.*

The surgeons with the assistance of a general surgeon, introduced a Foley catheter through the port, mobilized the bowel loop outside, resected the perforated part and performed an end-to-end anastomosis of the bowel loop (Fig. 10.28).

IMMEDIATE COMPLICATIONS OCCURRING DURING LAPAROSCOPY

Vascular Lesions

Major vessel injuries can occur during the operative part of the surgery and particularly at retroperitoneal dissection. Normally, the distal abdominal aorta and the common, external and internal iliac arteries, lie in the retroperitoneal space. Luckily, lacerations of these vessels occur rarely.[33-35] Most venous injuries, other than to the vena cava, are accompanied by injury of the overlying arteries. The large number of injuries to the aorta and vena cava are surprising as these vessels are above the umbilicus in most women. In most aortic or vena cava lacerations, periumbilical trocars were placed at angles >45° from the plane of the spine.

The first steps in effective management of major vessel injury are early recognition, minimizing the bleeding, performing a laparotomy if the bleeder cannot be laparoscopically compressed or controlled, calling a vascular surgeon and being aware of intravascular insufflation (end-tidal carbon dioxide, decreased oxygen saturation, millwheel murmur, tachyarrhythmia and right-side heart strain with ST-T changes). Direct compression of the bleeder is possible with a midline laparotomy until a vascular surgeon arrives. If an additional surgeon with vascular repair experience is not at hand, tight packing of the pelvis with dry laparotomy pads and temporary abdominal closure as well as transport of the patient to a larger center may be advisable.

Bowel Lesions

Many intraoperative bowel lesions can be sutured. Partial excision and sutures as well as resections of lacerated areas have to be applied, including end-to-end anastomosis. In many cases of endometriotic infiltration of the bowel, a primary resection in planned and the bowel prepared preoperatively. In cases of unprepared bowel, we suggest a careful disinfection of the area and multiple irrigations after the procedure.

Abdominal access and the creation of a pneumoperitoneum carry a significant risk of bowel injuries. Such injuries are more frequent in laparoscopic surgery and are often avoided in open surgery. Although these catastrophic injuries are uncommon, they represent a major reason for mortality from laparoscopic

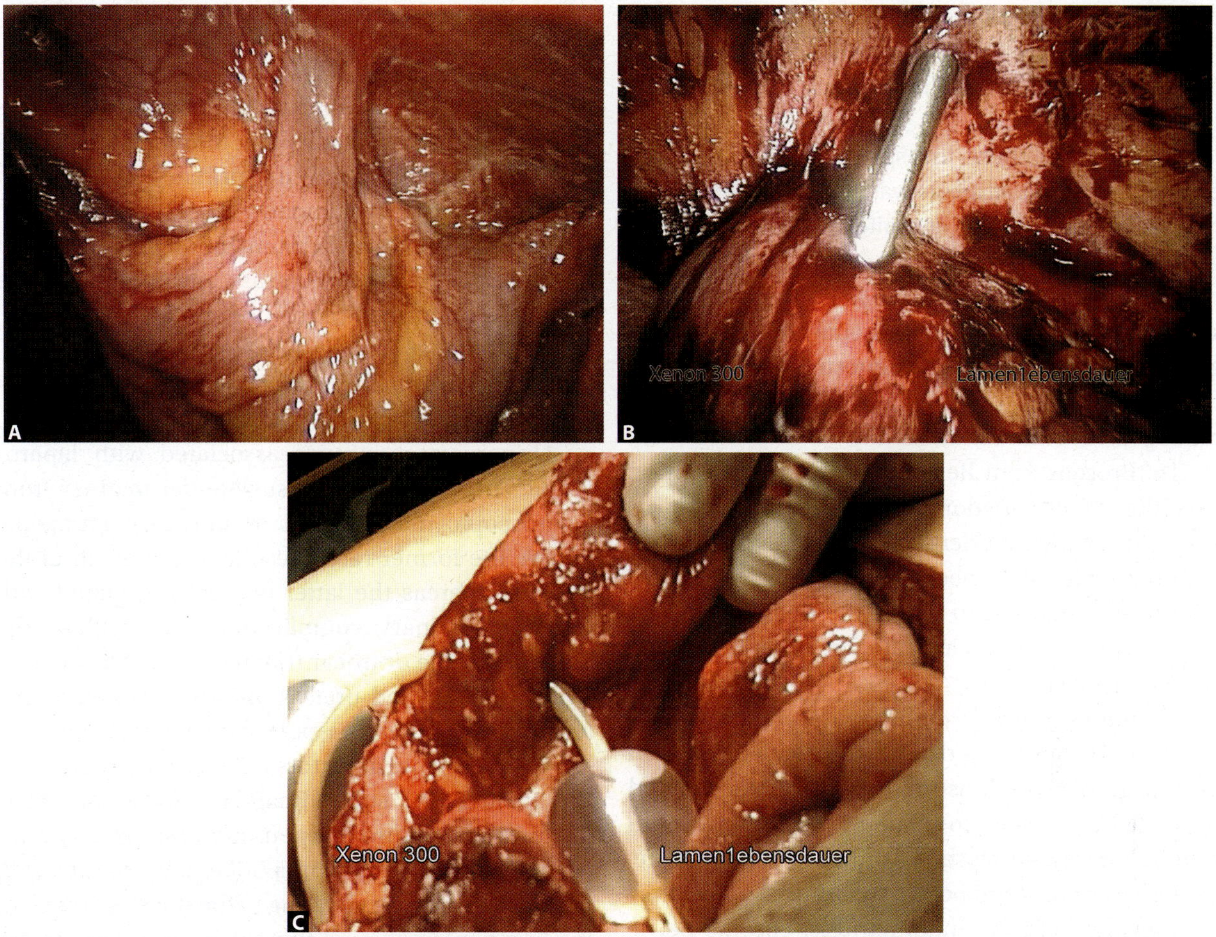

Figs. 10.33A to C: Laparoscopic bowel lesion and repair. (A) A small bowel loop totally adherent to abdominal wall; (B) The secondary trocar totally perforated the adherent small bowel loop; (C) Surgeons entered a Foley catheter through the port and performed the surgical resection of the bowel lesion.

procedures, and a significant source of the morbidity associated with any laparoscopic procedure.

Shea and colleagues examined 78,747 patients in a meta-analysis of 98 laparoscopic cholecystectomy studies. Fourteen percent of 1,400 conversions were from complications such as bleeding and bowel injury.[36]

Despite the rapid evolution of laparoscopic surgery in the past decade, the surgical community has failed to adequately report and study this tragic complication. As a result, most case reports and large series reporting these injuries are derived from older gynecologic literature.

It was generally expected that newer instrumentation and knowledge would reduce the risk of these complications; however, reports from the general surgical literature suggest that this is not the case.

In fact, these injuries occur with greater frequency, however, surgeons have been oblivious to the risk of trocar injury and fail to associate postoperative complication with the possibility of trocar injury, thus failing to recognize bowel perforation until it is too late. Laparoscopic cases are scheduled in outpatient clinics lacking blood, vascular operative instruments and expertise.

Bowel injury is the third cause of death from a laparoscopic procedure after major vascular injury and anesthesia.[37] Unlike major vascular injuries, in which the risk and presentation are immediate and dramatic, many bowel injuries are more insidious and remain unrecognized at the time of the procedure. Consequently, patients present postoperatively, often after discharge, with peritonitis. This delay makes it a significant cause of morbidity and mortality.[38]

A large survey of nearly 37,000 gynecologic laparoscopies in the United States revealed a 0.16% incidence of bowel injury: 39.8% of vascular and intestinal injuries were caused by the Veress needle,

37.9% by insertion of the primary trocar and 22% by the secondary trocar. The remaining gastrointestinal injuries resulted during dissection, electro-coagulation or grasping.[39]

Importantly, these investigators noted that the experience of the surgeon was an important deterring factor in the overall complication rate and in the incidence of intestinal injury.

Surgeons operating on the abdomen and pelvis should be familiar with the management of iatrogenic injuries of the gastrointestinal tract. These injuries should be recognized and appropriately managed, to minimize morbidity.[40]

Dr. Brosens from Belgium and Dr. Alan Gordon from the United Kingdom organized a multinational survey using the experience of members of the International Society of Gynecological Endoscopy (ISGE), who were requested to report the details of bowel trauma over two years and thereby learn from each others' experiences.[41]

A sound knowledge of the laparoscopic anatomy is essential to understand the distorted anatomy often present in disease. Most injuries can be accounted for by failure to keep to tissue planes, blunt dissection, diathermy in close proximity to the intestine, excessive traction and poor visualization.

Previous surgery, endometriosis, chronic pelvic inflammatory disease (PID), malignancy or radiotherapy may distort anatomy and obliterate tissue planes.[42]

All high-risk patients should be warned about the possible risk of gastrointestinal injury. Bowel preparation is advisable before major pelvic surgery.[43]

Injuries may result from mechanical or thermal forces. Damage to the rectum is less common, but carries a higher potential for complications and may occur during pelvic dissection or adhesiolysis.[44]

Injuries with healthy edges can be repaired primarily using tension-free, single-layer, interrupted sero-submucosal 3-0 Vicryl.[45]

For more extensive injuries, resection and primary anastomoses are required. Persistent pyrexia, tachycardia or ileus in the postoperative period should raise the index of suspicion for bowel injuries. Laparotomy followed by resection and defunctioning with an end stoma, may be required.[46]

Proctosigmoidoscopy can be performed at the end of the surgery to evaluate intraluminal integrity or rectosigmoid injury. The pelvis is then filled with isotonic fluid and observed laparoscopically for air leakage.[47,48]

Bladder and Ureter Injuries

Routine intraoperative cystoscopy after many major gynecological operations is recommended as it allows early recognition of inadvertent injury and facilitates immediate repair during the primary surgery with less morbidity for the patient.

The intraoperative demonstration and dissection of the ureter is often necessary and required if the surgery is performed in the ureteric area. Of course, an open bladder can also be detected by direct emission of urine. Sometimes the Foley catheter bag fills with CO_2 and indicates a bladder lesion.

Urinary tract injuries associated with laparoscopic surgery differ in a substantial manner from laparoscopic major vessel or intestinal iatrogenic injury. The former rarely results in the death of the patient, whereas the latter two are associated with mortality. Urinary complications are seldom the result of needle or trocar trauma (i.e., entry related). By far bladder and ureteral injuries happen as the result of the operative aspect of the laparoscopy.[49]

The most cogent factors related to ureteral damage include (1) suboptimal knowledge of pelvic anatomy, (2) failure to open into and dissect retroperitoneally, (3) employment of energy devices with marginal knowledge relating to the physics as well as the tissue interaction of these devices, (4) imprecise application of stapling devices and (5) pelvic adhesions, particularly dense adhesions located in and around the ovarian fossa.[50]

Injury to the ureter sustained is egregiously compounded by late postoperative recognition. Failure to order suitable diagnostic tests (e.g., indigo carmine dye injection, cystoscopy, intravenous pyelogram, retrograde pyelograms) will accrue additional damage.

Bladder injuries may be less serious than ureteral injuries, particularly if lacerations are recognized intraoperatively and are repaired appropriately in a timely manner. As with ureteral injury, the instillation of a dye (e.g., methylene blue) into the bladder will lead to early diagnosis as will intraoperative cystoscopy.

Injury to the trigone may be avoided by performing a cystoscopy before or during bladder laceration closure. Resecting a significant portion of the bladder during a gynecologic surgical procedure reflects a deficit in knowledge of pelvic anatomy.

Similarly, the creation of a vesicovaginal fistula or ureterovaginal fistula is clearly a failure of recognition and is associated with compromise to the blood supply to the bladder or ureter.

A number of recently published reports have quantified the incidence of urologic (bladder and ureter) injuries associated with laparoscopic surgery. These range from 0.3 to 4.0%. The risk of urologic injury was greater with total laparoscopic hysterectomy compared to LAVH: 4.0% versus 0.49%.[46,51-53]

Baggish studied 75 cases of bladder and ureteral injuries over a period of 24 years (1984–2008). Data included single or multi-entry procedures, primary diagnostic or operative procedures, description of pathology encountered, type of bladder or ureteral injury, instrument or device, symptoms and signs, etiologic factor(s) resulting in injury, time of diagnosis, diagnostic tests ordered, performance of ameliorative procedures, results of repair, subsequent surgery, morbidity and follow-up. Of the 75 injuries, the bladder accounted for 33 (44%) and the ureter 42 (56%).

Clearly the majority of entries (trocar)-related injuries were sustained by the urinary bladder. Of the 12 entry injuries, 10 were inflicted by the primary entry trocar and two by means of secondary entry devices. The single ureteral entry injury was caused by a 5-mm secondary trocar ostensibly placed under direct vision. Adhesions between the bladder and uterus were significant in the etiology of bladder lacerations.

Trocar puncture trauma accounted for over one-third of the bladder injuries and thermal devices for another one-third of the bladder injuries. Stapling devices, electrosurgical and ultrasonic devices accounted for 28 = 42% or 67% of ureteral injuries. Depending upon the particular instrument and technique associated with the ureteric injury, the locations of the injury site varied.[54]

Parpala-Spurman et al reported ureteric injuries associated with laparoscopic surgery in three 7-year time periods; between 1986 and 1992, only five injuries were observed, whereas 28 were observed between 1993 and 1999, and 39 were reported between 2000 and 2006. Around 64% of the injuries were in association with gynecologic operations. Only 11% occurred with urologic procedures.[55]

Assimos et al likewise reported a rise of ureteral injuries over a 5-year period in gynecological patients. The rate increased from 13 to 41 per 10,000 admissions.[56]

An analysis of factors contributing to urologic injuries was a high priority goal of the current study. Failure to secure the ureter by exposing the retroperitoneal space and deficient anatomical knowledge of the bladder and ureter, including their relationships, were critical factors associated with complications. The presence of adhesions and particularly a history of Cesarean section placed the patient in a high-risk category for bladder injury.

A history of major intraabdominal surgery and the presence of adhesions were likewise strong indicators for ureteric injuries. The presence of significant endometriosis and accompanying inflammation as well as scar formation were high-risk factors for ureteric complications.[57]

Prevention of accidents and recognition of injury are sentinel pillars for high-quality medical practice standards. Varying opinions have been reported relative to ureteral catheter placement for the prevention of injury during major surgery and particularly relating to laparoscopic surgery.[58]

The latter is cogent because one drawback of laparoscopic surgery relates to a lack of tactile sensation. Late diagnosis of bladder and ureteral injuries may lead to greater difficulties for the patient who underwent surgery as well as the surgeon who performed it.[59]

Although urinary tract injuries are rarely lethal, they can and do lead to significant morbidity, sometimes chronic. The risk of injuries especially to the ureter is increased with the laparoscopic approach and particularly with gynecologic laparoscopic operations. The reason for the higher risk with laparoscopy may be explained on the basis of lack of tactile sensation, decreased mobility, reduced vision, especially depth perception and panoramic view, reluctance of the gynecologist to open into the retroperitoneal space, suboptimal knowledge of pelvic anatomy, and reliance on hemostatic devices, which increase the risk for inadvertent urinary tract injury.

Late Complications

The late complications are secondary bowel lesions associated with peritonitis and massive intraabdominal infection. Often small vascular lesions are not recognized until a hematoma appears and ureter lesions are sometimes only recognized after the development of a urinoma. This may occur many days after the surgery. These lesions occurring in the postoperative period are also called secondary lesions and occur in 0.5%.[32] It is important that patients are informed to immediately report any adverse feelings or situations whether they are still in the hospital or not. Development of port site hernias are also considered to be a related late complications that escapes gynecologist`s domain, as most patients are referred to general surgeons to manage these long-term trocar-related mishaps.

PREVENTION OF COMPLICATIONS AND FUTURE DEVELOPMENTS

To prevent complications you have to know your anatomy and understand the pathophysiology of the disease you are trying to treat. You must know your instruments, work gently and with a plan, be proficient in laparoscopic suturing techniques and not depend on coagulation alone. A defect can occur even with the most modern instruments. Never work alone, but let your assistant both help and criticize you, and certainly train your nurses to help you. Every laparoscopic surgeon needs to know the equipment used coagulation techniques and settings, and must never completely depend on nurses, technicians or colleagues.

Prior to trocar entry we advise palpation of the patient's abdomen to identify bony (anterior superior iliac spine, sacral promontory, iliac crest etc.) and soft tissue landmarks (aortic pulsation, umbilical level etc.) while the patient is in the horizontal supine position.

Always insure proper intraperitoneal Veress placement prior to insufflation. The intraabdominal pressure can be raised to 25 mm Hg before trocar entry but has to be reduced after the trocar is in the right position to 12–15 mm Hg for the continuing surgery.

In high-risk patients, alternate Veress needle placement site can be the Palmer's point, that is the left upper quadrant, and any other area in the abdomen suitable after multiple previous surgeries.

In any type of laparoscopic surgery, the trocar entry points should follow a certain pattern in every team, but the surgeon should be open to schedule different settings for individual cases required by the tumor or the patient's previous surgeries.

If the pathology to remove reaches the umbilical level or beyond, then the optic port has to be placed higher up in the abdomen. When midline adhesions are suspected, the 5 mm trocar could be placed at Palmer's point and if desired, the umbilical trocar placed under sight. This may require extensive adhesiolysis in the umbilical area immediately prior to placement of a trocar in the umbilical area.

After trocar insertion, mostly through the umbilicus, the laparoscope should be rotated through 360°. This circular view affords the possibility of assessing suspected and unsuspected pathology.

Even with all the entry technologies available today, the entry under sight with the EndoTIP cannula of Artin Ternamian (which follows the principle of Kurt Semm), established in early 1980s, represents the method of choice for the primary trocar.

It does take a bit of time and a little larger incision; however, with real good 5 mm optics the entry can be performed by using the threaded 5 mm EndoTIP cannula and a 5 mm optic. For single-port entry and robotic laparoscopic surgery the entries are large in any case. An optical entry of the primary trocar in robotic surgery may be helpful as well.

We compared[60] the safety and efficacy of a modified direct optical entry versus Hasson's method by open laparoscopy in women with previous abdominopelvic surgery in a preliminary prospective case-control study. Statistical differences were found in favor of the direct optical entry in the time span of entry and blood loss. There was no difference in vascular or bowel injuries. The study did suggest direct optical entry to be advantageous in comparison to open laparoscopy in terms of saving time in preoperated patients, thus facilitating a safe visually guided entry for laparoscopy. Hemostasis by modern instrument development became easier as well; however, no technology is without risk.

All abdominal entry possibilities,[61-64] even under direct vision, carry a degree of inherent risk however, as the German thinker Goethe once said "*what one knows one sees*" also applies to visual port entry and exit, where the EndoTIP cannula allows endoscopists to see the anterior abdominal wall anatomy, which they all know so well.

Ultimately, for prevention of complications and improving patient safety, endoscopists can never be careful enough and all need God's protection.

TIPS AND TRICKS

- Be aware of previous surgeries of the patient.
- Use the technique you master, but keep your eyes and ears open, for example, for entry under sight.
- Insert all secondary trocars strictly under vision.
- Primary trocar insertion with patient in a horizontal position.
- Position the trocars according to the pathological situation to be treated.

- Consider left upper quadrant (LUQ) entry in high-risk situations (suspected or known periumbilical adhesions, history or presence of umbilical hernia, after three failed umbilical insufflation attempts). Alternate insertion methods, such as visual entry threaded cannula or open entry is preferred.
- Side to side moving of Veress needle after insertion must be avoided, as this can enlarge an inadvertent bowel or vessel puncture injury.
- Veress intraperitoneal pressure of < 10 mm Hg is a reliable indicator of correct needle placement.
- Abdominal wall lifting during Veress or primary trocar insertion is not routinely recommended, as it does not avoid visceral or vessel injury.
- Veress needle insertion angle should vary according to patient's BMI; 45° in nonobese to 90° in obese patients.
- Volume of CO_2 inserted with Veress needle depend on intraabdominal pressure. Adequate pneumoperitoneum should be determined by a pressure of 20 mm Hg and not by predetermined CO_2 volume.
- In pre-insufflated conventional entry, the abdominal pressure may be increased immediately prior to primary port insertion. High intraperitoneal laparoscopic entry technique does not adversely affect cardiopulmonary function in healthy women.
- Globally, gynecologists prefer Veress pre-insufflated entry as there is no evidence that open entry technique is superior to or inferior to conventional entry.
- Direct sharp blind trocar insertion of primary trocar without prior pre-insufflation is practiced by some but is fraught with potential danger.
- There is no evidence that shielded sharp trocars result in fewer visceral and vascular injuries during laparoscopic access. Some consider them to be outright dangerous.
- Radially expanding trocars are not recommended as being superior to traditional trocars. They do have blunt tips that may provide some protection from injuries, but force required for entry is significantly greater.
- Visual entry cannula system EndoTIP has an advantage over traditional trocars, as it allows clear optical entry, avoids overshoot and requires no sharp or pointed trocars. Entry force is reduced and port size is smaller.

REFERENCES

1. Deziel DJ. Avoiding laparoscopic complications. Int Surg. 1994;79(4):361-4.
2. Bogner MS. Medical devices and human error. In: Mouloua M, Parasuraman R, (Eds). Human Performance in Automated Systems: Current Research and Trends. Hillsdale, NJ: Lawrence Erlbaum; 1994. pp. 64-7.
3. Garry R. Complications of laparoscopic entry. Gynecol Endosc. 1997;6:319-29.
4. Mettler L, Schmidt EH, Frank V, et al. Optical trocar systems: laparoscopic entry and its complications (a study of case in Germany). Gynecol Endosc. 1999; 8:383-9.
5. Ternamian AM, Vilos GA, Vilos AG, et al. Laparoscopic peritoneal entry with the reusable threaded visual cannula. J Minim Invasive Gynecol. 2010;17(4):461-7.
6. Semm K. Operationslehre für endoskopische Abdominal-Chirurgie. Stuttgart, New York: Schattauer; 1984.
7. Ternamian AM. Laparoscopy without trocars. Surg Endosc. 1997;11(8):815-8.
8. Ternamian AM. A second-generation laparoscopic port system: EndoTIP. Gynecol Endosc. 1999;8: 397-401.
9. Ternamian AM. A second generation laparoscopic reusable port system. Gynecol Endosc. 2000;7: 174-80.
10. Crist DW, Shapiro MB, Gadacz TR. Emergency laparoscopy in trauma, acute abdomen and intensive care unit patients. Baillieres Clin Gastroenterol. 1993; 7(4):779-93.
11. Tarnay CM, Glass KB, Munro MG. Incision characteristics associated with six laparoscopic trocar-cannula systems: a randomized, observer-blinded comparison. Obstet Gynecol. 1999;94(1):89-93.
12. Turner DJ. A new, radially expanding access system for laparoscopic procedures versus conventional cannulas. J Am Assoc Gynecol Laparosc. 1996;3(4): 609-15.
13. Mettler L, Maher P. Investigation of the effectiveness of the radially expanding needle system in contrast to the cutting trocar in enhancing patient recovery. Min Invasive Ther Allied Technol. 2000;9(6):397-402.
14. Hasson HM. A modified instrument and method for laparoscopy. Am J Obstet Gynecol. 1971;110(6): 886-7.
15. Mettler L, Ibrahim M, Quang VV, et al. Clinical experience with an optical access trocar in gynecological laparoscopy-pelviscopy. JSLS. 1997; 1(4):315-8.
16. Childers JM, Brzechffa PR, Surwit EA. Laparoscopy using the left upper quadrant as the primary trocar site. Gynecol Oncol. 1993;50(2):221-5.
17. Parker J, Reid G, Wong F. Microlaparoscopic left upper quadrant entry in patients at high risk of periumbilical adhesions. Aust NZJ Obstet Gynaecol. 1999;39(1):88-92.
18. Mettler L. Manual for Laparoscopic and Hysterocopic Gynaecological Surgery. New Delhi: Jaypee Brothers; 2006; p. 184.

19. Mettler L. Manual of New Hysterectomy Techniques. New Delhi: Jaypee Brothers; 2007.
20. Mettler L, Ibrahim M, Jonat W. One year of experience working with the aid of a robotic assistant (the voice-controlled optic holder AESOP) in gynaecological endoscopic surgery. Hum Reprod. 1998;13(10):2748-50.
21. Advincula AP, Wang K. Evolving role and current state of robotics in minimally invasive gynecologic surgery. J Minim Invasive Gynecol. 2009;16(3): 291-301.
22. Mettler L, Schollmeyer T, Boggess J, et al. Robotic assistance in gynecological oncology. Curr Opin Oncol. 2008;20(5):581-9.
23. Bandera CA, Magrina JF. Robotic surgery in gynecologic oncology. Curr Opin Obstet Gynecol. 2009;21(1):25-30.
24. Stewart EA, Gostout B, Rabinovici J, et al. Sustained relief of leiomyoma symptoms by using focused ultrasound surgery. Obstet Gynecol. 2007;110(2 Pt 1): 279-87.
25. Yoon BS, Park H, Seong SJ, et al. Single-port laparoscopic salpingectomy for the surgical treatment of ectopic pregnancy. J Minim Invasive Gynecol. 2010;17(1):26-9.
26. Yim GW, Jung YW, Paek J, et al. Transumbilical single-port access versus conventional total laparoscopic hysterectomy: surgical outcomes. Am J Obstet Gynecol. 2010;203(1):26 e1-6.
27. Lee YY, Kim TJ, Kim CJ, et al. Single-port access laparoscopic-assisted vaginal hysterectomy: a novel method with a wound retractor and a glove. J Minim Invasive Gynecol. 2009;16(4):450-3.
28. Langebrekke A, Qvigstad E. Total laparoscopic hysterectomy with single-port access without vaginal surgery. J Minim Invasive Gynecol. 2009;16(5): 609-11.
29. Garry R. A consensus document concerning laparoscopic entry techniques: Middlesbrough, March 19–20, 1999. Gynecol Endosc. 1999;8(6):403-6.
30. Semm K. Pelviskopie und Hysteroskopie. Farbatlas und Lehrbuch. Stuttgart, New York: Schattauer; 1976e.
31. Kim CS, Kim JY, Kwon JY, et al. Venous air embolism during total laparoscopic hysterectomy: comparison to total abdominal hysterectomy. Anesthesiology, 2009;111(1):50-4.
32. Mettler L. Endoskopische Abdominal-Chirurgie in der Gynäkologie. Stuttgart: Schattauer; 2002.
33. Soderstrom RM. Injuries to major blood vessels during endoscopy. J Am Assoc Gynecol Laparosc. 1997;4(3):395-8.
34. Fuller J, Ashar BS, Carey-Corrado J. Trocar-associated injuries and fatalities: an analysis of 1399 reports to the FDA. J Minim Invasive Gynecol. 2005;12(4): 302-7.
35. Azevedo, JL, Azevedo OC, Miyahira SA, et al. Injuries caused by Veress needle insertion for creation of pneumoperitoneum: a systematic literature review. Surg Endosc. 2009;23(7):1428-32.
36. Shea JA, Healey MJ, Berlin JA, et al. Mortality and complications associated with laparoscopic cholecystectomy. A meta-analysis. Ann Surg. 1996; 224(5):609-20.
37. Tian YF, Lin YS, Lu CL, et al. Major complications of operative gynecologic laparoscopy in southern Taiwan: a follow-up study. J Minim Invasive Gynecol. 2007;14(3):284-92.
38. Kyung MS, Choi JS, Lee JH, et al. Laparoscopic management of complications in gynecologic laparoscopic surgery: a 5-year experience in a single center. J Minim Invasive Gynecol. 2008;15(6):689-94.
39. Chandler JG, Corson SL, Way LW. Three spectra of laparoscopic entry access injuries. J Am Coll Surg. 2001;192(4):478-90; discussion 490-1.
40. Härkki-Siren P, Kurki T. A nationwide analysis of laparoscopic complications. Obstet Gynecol. 1997; 89(1):108-12.
41. Brosens I, Gordon A. Bowel injuries during gynecological laparoscopy: a multinational survey. Gynecology. 2001;10(3):141-5.
42. Schäfer M, Lauper M, Krahenbuhl L. Trocar and Veress needle injuries during laparoscopy. Surg Endosc. 2001;15(3):275-80.
43. Wu MP, Koh L, Chow S. Can bowel injury be prevented during laparoscopic surgery? A case report and literature review. Taiwan J Obstet Gynecol. 2004; 43(4):219-21.
44. Mac Cordick C, Lécuru F, Rizk E, et al. Morbidity in laparoscopic gynecological surgery: results of a prospective single-center study. Surg Endosc. 1999; 13(1):57-61.
45. Leng J, Lang J, Huang R, et al. Complications in laparoscopic gynecologic surgery. Chin Med Sci J. 2000;15(4):222-6.
46. Wang PH, Lee WL, Yuan CC, et al. Major complications of operative and diagnostic laparoscopy for gynecologic disease. J Am Assoc Gynecol Laparosc. 2001; 8(1):68-73.
47. Leonard F, Lecuru F, Rizk E, et al. Perioperative morbidity of gynecological laparoscopy. A prospective monocenter observational study. Acta Obstet Gynecol Scand. 2000;79(2):129-34.
48. Tarik, A, Fehmi C. Complications of gynaecological laparoscopy—a retrospective analysis of 3572 cases from a single institute. J Obstet Gynaecol. 2004;24(7): 813-6.
49. De Cicco C, Schonman R, Craessaerts M, et al. Laparoscopic management of ureteral lesions in gynecology. Fertil Steril. 2009;92(4):1424-7.
50. Baggish MS. Analysis of 31 cases of major vessel injury associated with gynecologic laparoscopy operations. J Gynecol Surg. 2003;19:63-73.
51. Saidi MH, Sadler RK, Vancaillie TG, et al. Diagnosis and management of serious urinary complications after major operative laparoscopy. Obstet Gynecol. 1996;87(2):272-6.
52. Tamussino KF, Lang PF, Breinl E. Ureteral complications with operative gynecologic laparoscopy. Am J Obstet Gynecol. 1998;178(5):967-70.

53. Aslan P, Brooks A, Drummond M, et al. Incidence and management of gynaecological-related ureteric injuries. Aust NZJ Obstet Gynaecol. 1999;39(2): 178-81.
54. Baggish MS. Urinary tract injuries secondary to gynecologic laparoscopic surgery: analysis of seventy-five cases. J Gynecol Surg. 2010;26(2):79-92.
55. Parpala-Spårman T, Paananen I, Santala M, et al. Increasing numbers of ureteric injuries after the introduction of laparoscopic surgery. Scand J Urol Nephrol. 2008;42(5):422-7.
56. Assimos DG, Patterson LC, Taylor CL. Changing incidence and etiology of iatrogenic ureteral injuries. J Urol. 1994;152(6 Pt 2):2240-6.
57. Schonman R, De Cicco C, Corona R, et al. Accident analysis: factors contributing to a ureteric injury during deep endometriosis surgery. BJOG. 2008; 115(13):1611-5; discussion 1615.
58. De Cicco C, Ret Dávalos ML, Van Cleynenbreugel B, et al. Iatrogenic ureteral lesions and repair: a review for gynecologists. J Minim Invasive Gynecol. 2007; 14(4):428-35.
59. Oh BR, Kwon DD, Park KS, et al. Late presentation of ureteral injury after laparoscopic surgery. Obstet Gynecol. 2000;95(3):337-9.
60. Tinelli A, Malvasi A, Guido M, et al. Laparoscopy entry in patients with previous abdominal and pelvic surgery. Surg Innov. 2011;18(3):201-5.
61. Tariq M, Ahmed R, Rehman S, et al. Comparison of direct trocar insertion with other techniques for laparoscopy. J Coll Physicians Surg Pak. 2016;26(11): 917-9.
62. Keheila M, Shen JK, Faaborg D, et al. Percuta-neous externally assembled laparoscopic vs laparoendo-scopic single-site nephrectomy in a porcine model: a prospective, randomized, blinded, study. J Endourol. 2017;31(2):185-90.
63. Johnson TG, Hooks WB 3rd, Adams A, et al. Safety and efficacy of laparoscopic access in a surgical training program. Surg Laparosc Endosc Percutan Tech. 2016;26(1):17-20.
64. Ahmad G, O'Flynn H, Duffy JM, et al. Laparoscopic entry techniques. Cochrane Database Syst Rev. 2012; 2:CD006583.

KIEL SCH•OL

11 of Gynaecological Endoscopy

Risk Management in Gynecological Endoscopy

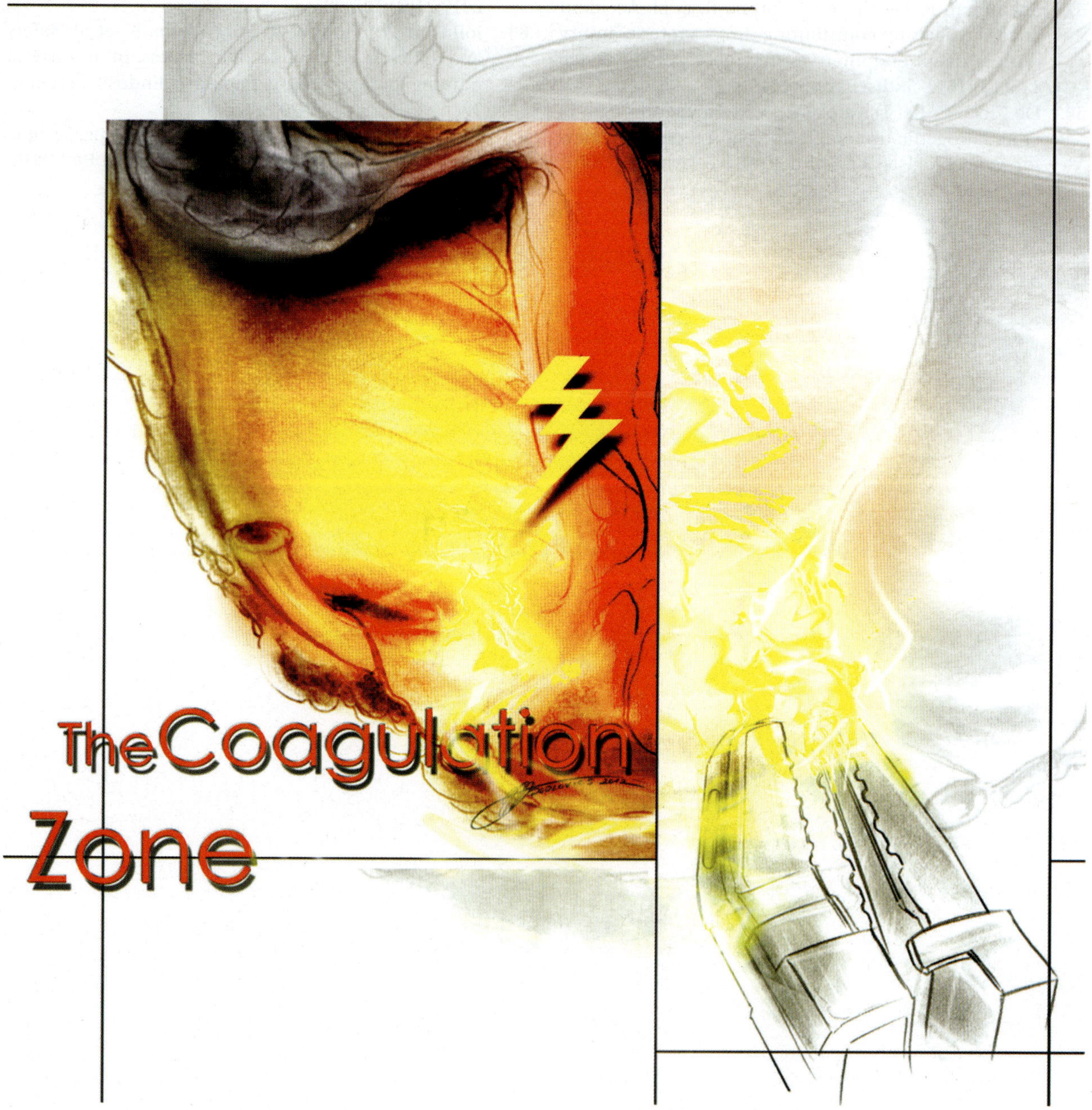

Chapter 11

Risk Management in Gynecological Endoscopy

Artin Ternamian, MacLeod Natalie

INTRODUCTION

Patient safety has been recognized as a public health concern ever since antiquity, when Hammurabi, ruler of Babylon (circa 1740 BC), established carefully conscribed common laws to regulate relationship between patient and practitioner, including fees charged for services rendered and penalties for mishaps.[1]

Surgical interventions now account for a large portion of healthcare expenditure; it is estimated that 187–281 million operations are conducted annually worldwide.[2]

Given such volumes, it is not difficult to fathom potential patient harm caused by unsafe surgical practices. Indeed, research has demonstrated surgical care accounts for just fewer than 50% of all adverse events in hospitalized patients in developed countries and at least one in two of these cases are preventable.[3,4]

Minimally invasive surgery (MIS) is recognized to be less disabling for patients and more enabling for surgeons. It offers superior patient outcomes with reduced perioperative morbidity compared to traditional open surgery.[5]

However, endoscopic surgery is more complex, as it presents operators additional technical challenges, not present during conventional surgery.[6]

Minimally invasive surgery is recognized to be considerably more stressful than conventional open surgery for several reasons, including loss of haptic feedback, altered depth perception, among others.[7]

The ensuing mental fatigue can markedly reduce decision-making capabilities and, therefore, raises error potential.[8] Ultimately, human error is intrinsically linked to vulnerabilities of human memory and attention span.[9]

Given the paucity of research, the relationship between MIS and patient safety has not been clearly delineated to date.[10]

A recent prospective multicenter study found that technological incidents (availability and functioning of equipment and instruments) were major contributors to adverse surgical outcomes, such as blood loss, operative time and complications.[11]

As gynecologic endoscopy evolves and emerging technologies introduce less invasive yet complex remedies to address women's health, the likelihood of inadvertent harm or near misses remains real and not insignificant. Sadly, most health institutions and practitioners remain unaware of the magnitude and costs of such occurrences.

The US New England Healthcare Institute (NEHI) defined waste in healthcare as "Healthcare spending that can be eliminated without reducing quality of care."[12] It is accepted that waste in healthcare exceeds \$1.2 trillion; more than half of all healthcare spending combined, and \$312 billion of which is from clinical waste alone. It is estimated that defensive medicine costs \$210 billion; preventable hospital readmissions costs \$25 billion, medical errors costs \$17 billion, hospital-acquired infections costs \$3 billion and overprescribing antibiotics costs \$1 billion (http://evidencecare.com, May 2017).

In the United States, medical errors, indicating inefficient processes and poor outcomes, are estimated to cost between \$17 and \$29 billion annually.[13]

According to the American Academy of Orthopaedic Surgeons (2008), malpractice suits and defensive medicine practiced in certain North America regions costs the average American family \$1,800 annually or \$140 billion. As practitioners move to lower malpractice jurisdictions to avoid high litigation costs, order unneeded tests and practice defensive medicine, health access is restricted, quality is reduced and health delivery cost is increased.

The Obama administration's proposed Health Reform Bill, required Congress to introduce "no limit on attorneys' fees or no imposition of caps on damages"; this may have been the exact kind of law that would lead to excessive health-related litigation, costs and defensive medicine.[14]

As part of efforts to repeal the Affordable Care Act, recently House Republicans drafted a bill that imposes new limits on lawsuits, involving care covered by Medicaid, Medicare and private health insurance, subsidized by the Affordable Care Act (*R Pear TNYT April 2017*).

Institutions, regulators and practitioners understand that all health systems are capable of erring irrespective. Consequently, efforts to integrate risk management (RM) know-how in contemporary curriculums and teaching initiatives to enhance patient safety in the practice environments are particularly important.

MIS is recognized to be less disabling for patients and more enabling for surgeons; it is considerably more stressful than conventional open surgery for operators, and mental fatigue markedly reduces attention span, decision-making capabilities and raises error potential rendering surgeons vulnerable to lapses and subject to human error.[15-17]

Introduction of competency-based gynecologic endoscopy teaching curriculum that encompasses all aspects of safe endoscopic surgery is essential and deserves special attention.

Current North American Obstetrics and Gynecology residency programs offer cursory formal RM and patient safety teaching content that need to be enhanced, as a comprehensive, contemporary, gynecologic endoscopy teaching curriculum, that emphasizes patient safety and risk aversion is lacking.[18-20]

To improve health quality and outcomes, organizations address and remedy health system failures, rather than take punitive action against individual practitioners,[21] however, when errors occur in healthcare, we still tend to be more interested in *who* did it, rather than *how-why* the mishap occurred.

Over the years, it has been shown that accident causation models developed for high-risk organizations (HRO) apply well for healthcare.[22,23] In effect, we now know that detailed error analysis is essential to identify and understand accident causation.[24]

More importantly, high-risk industries have demonstrated that only data captured concurrently at error point can improve our understanding of accident causation and enhance error analysis, to improve safety.[25]

Endoscopic surgery offers an unprecedented ability to do just that, by capturing operative performance with no limitation, however; surgeons continue to resist recording their endoscopic procedures, for a variety of unsubstantiated reasons and miss out on an incredible teaching, learning and risk aversion opportunity.[26]

Moreover, surgeons scuttle an invaluable real-time archiving and recall opportunity, with no hindsight bias, to learn from near misses and mishaps.[27]

In addition, our age-old operating room mantra of "no harm-no foul" remains the largest obstacle to quality improvement and risk aversion.[28]

Several high risk organizations (HRO) studies, from the aviation, deep mining and nuclear industry, have demonstrated that human error contributes to more than 90% of accidents and equipment now are proven to be more reliable and safer than human performance.[29]

Furthermore, we know that punishment, retraining and motivation are not an effective error management strategy. The decades-old *perfection myth* (if one tries harder, one can eliminate errors) and *punishment myth* (if punished one will commit less errors) have also been shown to be flawed and ineffective.[30,31]

Risk management was initially intended to be a defensive exercise to shield practitioners from litigious exposure; now it offers a broader reach and thrives to improve patient safety and enhance healthcare quality, which is integrally involved with appropriateness and acceptability of treatments offered.[32]

Understandably, RM is only one of a group of organizational remedies whose aim is to enhance quality of care and to reduce inadvertent error. Moreover, RM programs with other quality improvement initiatives help develop a more robust, comprehensive and effective institutional approach to safer health delivery.

In gynecologic endoscopy like other disciplines, performance and mishaps can generally be the result of three types of behavior:

1. The first is when inadvertent error occurs; these are incidents that are truly inevitable and regardless of contingencies, they can occur with any provider or endoscopy team.
2. The second is when risky performance is practiced, where individuals or teams attempt to "take

short cuts or cut corners" for a number of reasons and increase the likelihood of error. Avoidance of this kind of behavior requires system redesign to discourage such uncalled practices and implementation of team or individual audits.

3. The third is when deliberate guideline or policy breaches are practiced, which may require remedial or disciplinary remedies by departmental or regulatory bodies to avoid patient harm.[33]

Given prevailing societal expectations, fiscal constraints and legal vulnerabilities, practitioners, payers and institutions are aware that complex minimally invasive solutions and emerging technologies entail some new and technology-specific potential for unintended harm.

Although our current healthcare underfunding and general economic woes mandate fiscal accountability, health organizations have an established duty of care that dictates that when error prevention is possible, complacency becomes unacceptable and institutions are held negligent if efforts to secure patient safety are not ensured and enforced. (*Thompson v. Nason Hospital Pa. 1991*).

COMMITMENT TO RISK MANAGEMENT

Although every discipline may have its own specific RM policies to enhance patient safety and quality improvement, their approach must be harmonized and tempered by the overarching institutional patient safety strategy, within the context of a larger healthcare delivery framework.

Moreover, it must reflect an absolute commitment to patient safety, quality health delivery and outcomes accountability. A dynamic and comprehensive divisional RM roadmap must be articulated clearly by the unit administrator, updated regularly, posted electronically and presented at different departmental educational events, for all team members to understand and practice.

In addition, other organization-wide dynamic risk awareness efforts (in-house training, mock crisis management, audits, research, complaint management and feedback) are intended to alert all health team practitioners to combat complacency and reinforce the overall institution's unwavering dedication to quality health delivery.

According to the International Organization for Standardization (ISO),[34] "Risk Management Principles and Guidelines on Implementation" (ISO/DIS 31000), the process of RM generally entails these important steps:

- Identify, examine and evaluate risk
- Determine susceptibility
- Recognize risk and evaluate consequences
- Define methods to mitigate those risks
- Prioritize risk aversion measures

The innovative early works on healthcare, quality improvement and RM by Donabedian, established a simple and comprehensive classification of healthcare assessment into three components as targets: structure, process and outcome.[35]

At a time when patient safety and quality of health delivery were not on the forefront, he introduced three fundamental aspects of quality of health delivery; the technical aspects of care, the interpersonal aspects of care and the environment in which healthcare is provided.[36,37]

Deliberate RM strategies, when structured in a similar context, may facilitate understanding and help application of practical measures to minimize inadvertent mishaps, in gynecologic endoscopy.

First, the technical aspect of gynecologic endoscopy care is examined, where care is delivered utilizing an ever evolving cascade of innovative technologies that present a constantly changing risks environment, requiring constant vigilance, audit, retraining and reevaluation.

Second, the interpersonal aspect of gynecologic endoscopy is examined involving human interaction, communication and processes between all stakeholders; patient, ancillary healthcare staff, health administrators and the like.

Lastly, the environmental aspect of gynecologic endoscopy care is examined representing a unique risk environment that includes physical, ergonomic, emotional, administrative and other components.

Establishing a multidisciplinary endoscopy risk management committee (RMC) is an important first step as a deterrent to inadvertent incidents and should include the following members:

- Lead clinician (rotates to include most departmental staff)
- Nursing staff (rotates to include most departmental staff)
- Resident or Fellow in training (if teaching institution)
- Representative from other discipline (pharmacy, anesthesia, central supply)
- Institutional health and safety representative
- Institutional patient advocate

Specific terms of reference and reporting mechanisms can be developed according to departmental and local regulatory requirements, policies and clinical practice guidelines.

Generally, the role of this committee is to facilitate and support health worker's efforts to mitigate risk during everyday practice.

Practically most aspects of RM can be considered in the three quality of healthcare delivery silos described above: the technical aspects of care, the interpersonal facets of care and the environmental components of care where healthcare is provided.

The RMC can assist in several ways including the following important means to identify risk, institute redundancies and develop specialty-specific RM strategies to process mishaps. Establish and update divisional incident and near miss registry to improve recording and reporting compliance. Offer feedback, monitor and convey risk profiles, coordinate departmental risk awareness educational initiatives address high-risk areas identified by specialty organizations and national regulatory bodies and medicolegal associations and supervise compliance with national standards and best practice guidelines.

A. When examining the technical aspects of care, several important and fundamental patient safety aspects become evident. At first one has to acknowledge that gynecologic endoscopy is a technology and skill-driven discipline that relies on complex evolving and emerging technologies and complicated systems, working synchronously, to deliver optimal contemporary care, by a cooperative, skilled surgical team.

Safe endoscopy is contingent on appropriately functioning instruments and systems much more than during open conventional surgery. Given the complexity and number of sophisticated equipment employed, the likelihood of failures may be unavoidable. Moreover, the incidence of technical equipment malfunction during endoscopic surgery remains alarmingly high.[38]

For these and other reasons, it is essential that equipment function perfectly, is maintained in optimal working order and is upgraded whenever a superior innovation becomes available. Additionally, every operating team member should remain credentialed especially when new equipment is acquired.

The process of identifying, examining and evaluating the possibility of mishaps in this complex and evolving environment requires constant vigilance-dedicated faculty and knowledgeable team members, without which a contemporary endoscopy unit is incapable of functioning safely. It is also understood that the actual surgery is only a finite increment in a pathway of care, where operative risk and patient harm can be identified and averted in the pre-, intra- and postoperative stages.

Diligent recording of near misses and deliberate incident reporting is very important to facilitate this process, so that high-risk areas are identified and redundancies instituted in all tenuous segments of gynecologic endoscopy.

Root cause analysis of serious potential or actual incidents will shed more light on specific events that may have serious or permanent negative repercussions on patients and institutions. Certain institutionalized high-risk behaviors may escape detection for long periods of time, unless diligent error analysis and detailed accident causation examination is conducted.

Factors such as lack of or adherence to accepted practice protocols, equipment malfunction, lack of supervision, inadequate technical training, failure to upkeep and communicate, poor incident or near miss reporting, inadequate auditing, all contribute to setting the grounds for recurring unintended mishaps, to the detriment of our patients.

As in all disciplines, gynecologic endoscopy divisions should make sure that new innovative technologies are appropriately evaluated, before adoption and individual practitioners and support personnel are well trained and credentialed in the new method or system prior to integration (robotic endoscopy, single port endoscopy, others).

When establishing outpatient endoscopy facilities, appropriate contemporary monitoring, sterilization and resuscitation equipment that conforms to local health authorities' directives and regulations must be available, before administering health in such environments.

Although in-hospital incidents have worst medicolegal negligence outcomes, the total number of mishaps and inadvertent deaths from out-patient error is much greater (NY State Department of Health's open own investigation + Rivers' death in 2014). In addition, strict pre-procedure surgical checklists and postdischarge follow-up protocols must be established and adhered to in order to avoid complacency and inadvertent lapses. Mislabeling of samples and specimens, lack of communication between health team members and patient, confidentiality slips, delegation and supervision of surgical trainees, among others are all areas of concern and potential mishaps.

Essentially, RM is intuitively practiced anytime endoscopists attend to patient's needs, remain mindful of the potential risks involved and take appropriate measures (action or inaction) to mitigate risk, while attaining the set objective.

B. When examining the interpersonal aspects of care, all stakeholders, including patient, surgical team, administrators, patient advocates and supervisors have to be considered. Crew management methods (CMM), adopted by the aviation industry, has demonstrated the importance and effectiveness of a work environment that empowers individual team members to actively partake in risk aversion without intimidation and hierarchal consideration.[39]

In effect, any one that has to do directly or indirectly with delivery of care before, during and after endoscopic surgery can and does influence outcomes and quality of health delivered. Additionally, the proficient skill and clinical judgment of the entire endoscopy team affects quality of healthcare.

Executive and administrative staff's commitment and understanding of patient safety aspects of care delivery are also important for a risk free endoscopic surgical culture, environment and practice.

Preoperative RM initiatives can impact the likelihood of risk during endoscopy when potential hazards are recognized, addressed or rectified prior to surgery, to improve outcomes and better our understanding of inadvertent mishaps.

Some patient-specific aspects of added surgical risk include the following: patient`s fitness for said endoscopic surgery, extremes of age, comorbidities, such as uncontrolled diabetes, bleeding diathesis, obesity, smoking, use of ancillary or recreational drugs, history of complications during or following previous operations, among other issues.

Moreover, the importance of informed consent (IC) must be stressed as an integral aspect of RM and an essential component in endoscopy that will be addressed later in this chapter.

Intraoperative RM efforts that are also important to consider is the institution of surgical check lists that are tailored to address specific gynecological concerns, such as last menstrual date, fertility wishes, a pregnancy test prior to anesthetic induction and identification of correct operative side in case of adnexal surgery.

Particular care must be exercised to protect vital organs and structures that are in the vicinity of the operative field and are known to be frequently injured because of their proximity or anatomical position (ureter, bladder, bowel, nerve, vessels).

Operative sponge counts, needles, meshes, catheters and broken off parts of endoscopic instruments, all should be recorded and accounted for. A contemporaneous operative note should be dictated soon after the surgery to describe what was done, what was used and how things progressed; detailed description and management of mishaps is also very important.

Gynecologic endoscopy programs, with obstetrics and gynecology residents and endoscopy fellows understand that learning on patients through trial and error is not an accepted surgical skills teaching option any longer.

Although for years the apprenticeship model of surgical skills teaching and training was favored, in this age of simulation and mentored modeling, trainee competence prior to human surgery is safer and a more societally acceptable method of teaching endoscopy.

It has been shown that serious curriculum and training obstacles remain in most obstetrics and gynecology residency programs and integration of endoscopic competencies in the core resident teaching curriculum needs to be addressed and accelerated.[40]

It appears that a shorter work time and lack of learning opportunities (less patients requiring endoscopic surgery because of interventional radiological, pharmaceutical medications or other nonsurgical contemporary remedies) render future endoscopists less technically versed compared to their earlier peers, who trained on patients, worked longer hours and managed a larger patient load.

If unchecked, this may require remedial skills training, longer years of residency, curriculum redesign, credentialing requirements and licensing oversight. In effect, even practicing endoscopists require retraining and re-credentialing, whenever newer technologies are introduced (robotic or single-port endoscopic surgery).

Patients and practitioners understand that endoscopy-related complications cannot be always anticipated or avoided as some are discovered during surgery while others postoperatively.

Generally, in gynecologic endoscopy, certain known areas of surgery are of particular risk such as peritoneal entry injury, electrosurgical thermal accidents, patient positioning related harm, fluid management complications, inadvertent collateral organ mishaps, excessive bleeding, adhesive consequences and others.

The most important issue in all this remains recognition or identification of the mishap, correction of the injury, before the condition escalates to permanent patient harm. Moreover, consultation with other endoscopists, assistance of other discipline, disclosure, contemporaneous accurate documentation of events and careful follow-up are all basic principles of contemporary RM.

Postoperative RM initiatives can also impact the likelihood of risk in gynecologic endoscopy, such as use of antibiotics to prevent infections (wound, urinary, respiratory), adherence to proper sterilization techniques, wound care and use of certain single-use disposable equipment, including other precautions.

Use of prophylactic antiembolic medication and compression stockings when appropriate, early ambulation, adequate nursing follow-up and call-back protocols, readmission or reassessment policies are all important increments to quality care.

Debriefings and other forms of audits are used postoperatively to identify weaknesses in the system and suggest possible solutions instituted, as all failures and near misses are recorded and reported to raise awareness and learn from mishaps.

Postoperative incidents may occur even when the endoscopic surgery itself was uneventful, such as postoperative sepsis, bleeding, vaginal vault dehiscence or adhesions. Serious postoperative complications may develop while the patient is in or out of the hospital, when the most responsible physician may be unavailable. It is therefore very important that surgeons when going off duty, afterhours contact information be known to the patient and hospital, so that they know how and who to get in touch with if need arises. Appropriate transfer of care is equally important and entails communicating pertinent information to the covering endoscopist.

Gynecologists know that although the likelihood of serious endoscopic mishaps is rare but real, and that operative endoscopy carries a potential for serious adverse outcomes, which can result in significant patient harm with medico legal consequences. Acknowledging the possibility of mishaps in all stages of endoscopic patient care will help increase awareness and improve patient safety.

RISK SEVERITY INDEX

Generally, risk is measured by the risk severity index, which includes the severity of harm and the prevalence of such event. However, the probability of risk occurrence is difficult to measure as several risk areas in gynecologic endoscopy is difficult to calculate and reliable estimates are nonexistent; besides, probability does not imply certainty. Additionally, the effect of risk is not easy to estimate as it is usually hard to assess possible injury in the event of error occurrence.

Effective interpersonal institutional risk communication is an important and dynamic interdisciplinary activity that facilitates conveyance of critical risk-related information and feedback in an understandable and sincere way, without offense.

The principal objective of this exercise is to enhance team and member decision-making abilities, as coordinated teamwork and clear communication is known to minimizes error and maximize efficiency.[41]

Failure to communicate effectively among team members may invite team dissonance even in low-risk operations and environments; consequently, risk communication is akin to crisis or natural disaster communication.

Effective communication is particularly critical to ensure safe and seamless transfer of care during provider shift changes, as well as patient transfers to other disciplines, caregivers, or institutions where transfer methods should be recorded and audited periodically.

Considering that a circulating nurse leaves the operating room an average of once every 8 min (33 times per procedure), the importance of team work, communication and meticulous record keeping becomes evident.[42]

Additionally, reducing the number of hand-offs and utilizing technology to establish a robust chain of custody documentation is known to reduce the likelihood of errors.[43]

Individuals and divisions involved in patient complaints, near misses or operative mishaps must be informed of specific outcomes and lessons drawn from these experiences, to avoid recurrent incidents in same or similar areas.

Ultimately, risk communication can have an important preemptive educational objective that the RMC can use as an invaluable teaching opportunity. In essence, endoscopy surgical teams must improve pre-, intra- and postoperating surgery communicating dexterity, to enhance patient safety and minimize mishaps; realizing that use of surgical checklist, briefing and debriefing exercises are all institutional environmental efforts to improve outcomes and mitigate risk.

Important aspects of effective interpersonal risk communication include the following:

[Amended from Covello, VT, Allen, FH. (April 1988). "Seven Cardinal Rules of Risk Communication." Washington, DC: US Environmental Protection Agency. OPA-87-020].[44]

- Engage all stakeholders (patient advocate, administrator, practitioner) as team members.
- Assess and evaluate team initiatives (stress abilities, flaw's opportunities and risks).
- Attend to teams and providers specific concerns.
- Be sincere, truthful, and candid.
- Recruit and collaborate with other disciplines and specialists.
- Address patient advocacy and media queries without delay.
- Communicate plainly with empathy, honesty and consideration.

The path of each patient from initial clinical assessment, investigations, decision making, consenting, preoperative evaluation, anesthetic consultation, endoscopic surgery, recovery, discharge, postoperative care to final clinical resolution and debriefing constitutes a tortuous journey that every patient and caregiver negotiates for safe recuperation and integration.

Health providers appreciate that this circuitous route harbors potential technical, interpersonal and environmental risks, where inadvertent harm can occur and opportunities to avert unintended injury often exists. Empowering endoscopy healthcare team members to act as patient safety advocates along this journey is an important resource to harness and promote.

CONSENTING

Informed consent (IC) is an explicit legal and ethical requirement that is obtained before any kind of heath care is delivered.[45]

Generally, IC has two important and different requirements; a medico legal requirement where provision of factual information is stressed and an ethical requirement where patient autonomy and joint decision-making is practiced.[46]

It is important to appreciate the difference between other kinds of consent (implied, written, substitute, unlawful, and so on) as IC, is really considered an educational process.[47]

While the real purpose of IC is not to persuade patient but to protect patients' choice and autonomy to decide according to her own assessment of competing interests and values. US litigation lawyers in 1957, persuaded courts to expand simple consent to informed consent, so that physician liability for failure to consent appropriately also results in liability for negligence.[48]

Although simple consent negates assault liability, lack of IC exposes practitioners, institutions and insurers to significantly higher financial liability for negligence.

Irrespective, our role as caregivers remain to give good evidence-based advice and it is our patient's right and privilege to accept or reject our advice.

The greatest dilemma in the IC doctrine is the extent and depth of potential risk discussion considering that studies suggest that about 70% of North American patients do not fully read their operative written consents before signing.[49]

According to Association of Adult Literacy, 14% of adults have below basic literacy, 29% of adults have only basic literacy, 44% of adults have intermediate literacy, while 13% of adults are proficient; a total of about 93 million North American adults have insufficient literacy skills to function in society and some of whom are our patients (http://neces.ed.gov/naal/).

So adequacy of consent explanations is judged by what a reasonable patient in that position would have expected to hear before consenting. This approach combines an objective (the reasonable patient) and subjective (this particular patient) approach where they are their own best risk managers.

This is a very important interpersonal communicative exercise in all surgical disciplines, including gynecologic endoscopy, where effective and non-coercive patient consenting requires covering the following five important aspects: explanation of the nature, purpose, benefits, alternatives and risks of the treatment suggested.

The actual signing of the consent form cannot be a substitute but a prompt for covering all five aspects involved in informed consenting.

Team members must realize that any operative procedure performed outside the scope and spirit of the signed document can be construed as assault and may result in criminal or civil action against the endoscopist, as ultimately it is the surgeon who is held accountable in a court of law, if challenged.[50]

A valid IC means that a discussion occurred between provider and patient and that the discussion was recorded on the patient's chart. The patient is informed about several treatment options and alternatives, expected outcomes, risks and limitations. Possible complications are described; additionally, consequences of no treatment are also described.

Consent discussion should be recorded on the patient's chart as a signed consent form itself is not necessarily proof that this discussion took place. She is next given time to consider her options, reading material is provided and electronic websites are offered to help her better understand the available treatment options; remember that signing of the actual form, in the presence of the operating surgeon, is only one minor aspect of this process.[51]

During preadmission interviews, anesthetic consultation and during admission on the day of surgery, the nursing staff must review the signed consent and affirm the patients' understanding of the upcoming surgery. Finally, the signed consent is reviewed as part of the surgical check list prior to anesthetic induction, before starting and upon ending the operation.

Above all, patients must be treated with empathy, respect and dignity during this process and the extent and spirit of their consent must never be exceeded intraoperatively, unless when confronting a life-threatening emergency (oophorectomy during hysterectomy, hysterectomy during endometrial resection, hysterectomy during myomectomy, salpingectomy during ectopic pregnancy).

Occasionally, certain religious or belief-based personal choices, when explicitly articulated, discussed and preoperatively inscribed on the consent form, may limit a surgeon's freedom to do what it takes to save a life. When faced with similar extreme situations, obtaining the opinion of a learned colleague or institutional ethicist prior to or intraoperatively is advisable.

When unexpected pathology is encountered intraoperatively, such as malignancy that requires more extensive or radical surgery, it is prudent not to exceed the consent's limitations and defer definitive surgery to a later date. Unless if the possibility was clearly discussed preoperatively or when a complication of the original operation dictates further intervention.

Ultimately, the onus is on the gynecologist to secure an IC and the institution to ensure that mechanisms are in place to provide a safe work environment to the benefit of patient, hospital staff and surgeon.

ADVERSE EFFECTS TO BE INCLUDED IN RISK MANAGEMENT INITIATIVES

The Royal College of Obstetricians and Gynaecologists (RCOG) published a short list of general gynecologic events that can be included in a clinical RM program. Table 11.1 is adapted to represent a gynecologic endoscopy perspective.[52]

Peritoneal entry injuries, bowel mishaps, vascular accidents, electrosurgical burns, air or gas embolism, distending fluid overload and positioning nerve incidents are all well-documented gynecologic endoscopy serious complications that deserve special attention.[53]

Fortunately, many of these serious gynecologic endoscopy complications are infrequent (e.g., peritoneal entry injuries, large vessel injury, distending fluid accidents, others), however, they can have significant health consequences, and patients and

Table 11.1: Gynecologic endoscopy: adverse effects to be included in risk management initiatives.

Clinical events	Organizational events
Organ injury (ureter, bowel, bladder, nerve, vessel)	Anesthetic complication
Delayed/missed detection	Delay following call for assistance
Deep vein thrombosis	Faulty equipment
Failed procedure (tubal sterilization)	Interpersonal treatment conflict
Unexpected intensive care admission	Potential patient complaint
Omission of planned surgery	Dispensing–administration error
Operative blood loss 500 mL+	Retained surgical product
Unconsented/wrong side surgery	Breach of patient confidentiality
Pulmonary embolism/air/gas	Instrument sterilization mishap
Unplanned readmission or surgery	Surgical specimen mishap
Distending fluid incident	Operative environment ergonomics
Energy mishap	Failure to disclose

Adapted from the Royal College of Obstetricians and Gynaecologists (RCOG) Clinical Governance Advice list.

endoscopists must be aware of these potential risks and alternate accepted less invasive options discussed.[54]

A recent literature review demonstrated that on average, the incidence of a serious vascular injury is one in 2,272 laparoscopic operations and incidence of a serious bowel incident is one in 1,381 endoscopic operations.[55]

The US Food and Drug Administration (FDA) data demonstrated that the majority of deaths associated with trocar injuries are the result of major vascular injury (81%), while only a minority of deaths related to trocar injury are the result of bowel injury (19%). Trocar vascular injuries associated with death involved the aorta in 23% of cases and the vena cave in 15% of cases. Distressingly, more than half the fatal trocar bowel injuries were not recognized intraoperatively.[56]

Fuller et al. reviewed 1,353 serious laparoscopic trocar related injuries and 31 deaths over 5.5 years and concluded that most serious injuries involve the bowel and large vessels.[57]

Consequently, when consenting high-risk endoscopy patients (previous abdominal surgery, morbid obesity, pregnant patient, peritoneal adhesions, others) regarding the probability of peritoneal entry related injury, the possibility of using an alternate entry method (visual-threaded cannula or open), the probability of a different access site (left upper quadrant), or the likelihood of laparotomy must be discussed preoperatively.[58]

Electrosurgical injuries are another rare but serious complication of gynecologic endoscopy, that results either through inadvertent direct contact or as a result of stray current that may not be discovered during surgery.

van der Voort et al. reported a 42% of bowel injuries rate from trocar insertion and a 26% bowel injury rate from electrosurgical injury, with an overall mortality rate of 3.6%.[59]

Often insulation failure and capacitive coupling result in unintended current flow to surrounding tissues. Although technology to prevent this kind of electrosurgical injuries by using active electrode monitoring (AEM) has been available to endoscopists for several years, yet practice patterns have not changed much.

This system prevents injury by shutting off electrical current automatically once a short circuit is discovered. AEM is recommended by the United States Association of Perioperative Registered Nurses and preferred for the prevention of electrosurgical burn risk by the nonprofit ECRI Institute that independently evaluates medical devices.[60,61]

Bioburden and viral contamination is also of particular concern when considering more complex contemporary endoscopic instruments or natural orifice endoscopic surgery, especially when operating on high-risk populations and utilizing reusable surgical instruments.

C. When examining the environmental aspects of care, the importance of a department's or hospital's commitment to patient safety and risk prevention becomes clear. This essential societal obligation and patient advocacy stance must permeate equally all areas of care delivery including gynecologic endoscopy.

Some surgical risks will only require adherence to an already published and available clinical practice guideline or enforcement of a previously established policy that has lapsed to disuse.

Compliance to institutional surgical RM principles must be encouraged if not enforced to combat departmental and team complacency as an important interpersonal and environmental aspect of patient safety. Generally, incidents are infrequent when surgical processes and methods are standardized and reliant on evidence-based guidelines and described best practices.

In this context, auditing becomes extremely important for the RMC to evaluate and identify lapses, offer feedback and advice to all stakeholders, devise remedies to recruit participation and create an environment that encourages and nurtures vigilance.

As errors are unlikely to occur if due process and accepted protocols are followed, all relevant gynecologic endoscopy clinical guidelines, clinical standards, professional association policies and other similar departmental documents should be easily available and accessible, in all clinical areas and on the institution's website.

Here the importance of clear and contemporary documentation has to be emphasized. This applies to all kinds of procedures, where adequate and legible clinical notes, orders, consent, operative notes, discharge summaries are again emphasized as a simple and effective mishap deterrent.

Certain accepted institution wide and standard risk aversion measure are embedded and seamlessly practiced by all health practitioners such as intra- and postoperative policies, protocols, and procedures, electronic forms and charting, digital imaging stations, surgical and other checklists.

Electronic prompts (for preoperative antibiotic, drug reactions, allergies or deep vein thromboprophylaxis), proper contaminated of sharps, biohazard disposal, wearing protective apparels and eye gear, avoiding nonergonomic surgical team environment, instituting safe patient lifting and positioning protocols also create and maintain a safer endoscopy healthcare environment for patients and practitioners.

TRAINING

Appropriate team training is an integral part of contemporary surgery, especially endoscopy; as in all areas of health delivery, a team member must show evidence that they are credentialed and proficient performing a given task and individual members are assessed during such performances and their outcomes evaluated.

Competence is the determination that a team member can perform a given task safely and well, whereas continued competency is a dynamic updating of skills, to accommodate evolving equipment and system changes.

The importance of team training in endoscopy RM cannot be emphasized enough. All staff job descriptions must include reference to responsibility to clinical governance, which is reviewed regularly. Residents and fellows must appreciate the importance and adherence to set protocols and procedures, especially at the beginning of their rotations.

Organizations have a fiduciary societal responsibility to take necessary steps to safeguard patent safety while in their institutions. Teaching departments also appreciate that residents and fellows inevitably require hands on clinical experience, necessary for eventual independent practice.

Residents, fellows and mentors hold a duty of care responsibility toward acting in the best interest and safety of patients. When mishaps occur, the supervising mentor is held responsible and to a standard of care practically expected from any cautious surgeon in similar position.

Residents and fellows are held accountable to a standard of care appropriate to their level of training, experience and specific situation. Whereas the mentor can be held liable for any harm caused by the resident's carelessness, if the supervisor inappropriately assigned a surgery or failed to adequately oversee the student during the operation.

If an incident occurs, it may be complicated to defend the postoperative care provided when the most responsible caregiver is not available or when there is no progress notes recorded. In effect, it is equally important to record when patients do well, in addition to when events deteriorate as they delineate patient's clinical postoperative recuperation.

Several accepted and proven RM steps can reduce organizational exposure such as ensuring appropriate staff skill and knowledge training, enforcing training compliance, applying contemporary evidence-based protocols, matching team skills to task benchmarking, ensuring information is readily available and accessible, securing record keeping standards, conducting regular clinical audits, among others.

DISCLOSURE

When an incident does occur, an open, honest and timely disclosure to the patient and relatives by the surgical team, hospital risk manager and patient advocate, is very important.

Disclosure in plain language of an adverse incident, suspected reasons, possible consequences and suggested remedies along with a sincere apology, without necessarily implying fault may be all that is required initially.

Recording and reporting inadvertent errors and complications to a national or regional database have become compulsory in many jurisdictions. Practitioners and institutions are encouraged to comply without expecting punitive action and offered feedback to implement suggested system changes and recommendations consequent to their reporting.

Generally, only when an incident recurs repeatedly with a given team, when there are laps in reporting, when a police investigation is initiated, and when the local professional association views an incident unacceptable practice standard is disciplinary action warranted.

Although all incidents are expected to be reported, not all events will require an exhaustive investigation. The local RMC must first review and assess the event and make further recommendations to the department head. If a pattern of adverse events or incidents are discovered, then a more detailed audit is required.[62]

Though public outrage has resulted in more transparency in healthcare delivery, lack of disclosure continues to be a significant issue with patient advocates.[63]

It has been shown that disclosure by practitioners and institutions does not increase the likelihood of litigation,[64] although fear of litigation continues to discourage error publication by physicians and institutions alike.[65]

According to the FDA, it is estimated that only 8% of medical errors are reported in the United States and it is known that hospital underreport their adverse events,[66] and for every declared hospital error 20 are unreported.[67]

In gynecologic endoscopy, like all other surgical disciplines, nonphysician team members are more diligent in reporting mishaps and near misses; as a result, they constitute an invaluable asset in the operative team that ensures RM compliance to learn from one's own incidents. Moreover, failure of a robust feedback response to incident reporting is one of the most important factors that undermine prevention initiatives and possibility of future adverse event avoidance.

Some departments have created simple online incident and near miss reporting lists, available to all team members, to use as a template to identify, archive and address redundancies in a given discipline. Establishing an incident registry remains a useful tool to highlight events, raise awareness and motivate teams to take appropriate preventative actions to manage operative risks.

The principal premise of any RM investigation is that the objective is risk identification, accident solving and system change and not individual blaming.

Incident root cause is the failure of a process that, if rectified, can prevent recurring patient error. The upgraded policies and methods must be evaluated and tried to make certain that it has the desired risk aversion effects.[68]

When an event is discovered, several measures have to be taken during the investigation. Senior stakeholders have to be recruited to examine the incident; they have to remain impartial, confidential, compassionate but also consistent. They have to examine system as well as team failures, analyzing digressions from accepted protocols and processes, while remaining nonconfrontational and nonretributional. They must engage those who are most familiar with the incident and summon relevant expertise to identify all roots and causes, analyze evidence base to support incident and actions and give structured feedback of findings to teach ways to avert recurrences.

INFORMATION TECHNOLOGY RISK MANAGEMENT

Electronic patient information in all its forms is increasingly pervasive and ubiquitous in modern medicine, and gynecologic endoscopy practice is not alone. Institutions, surgeons and ancillary healthcare personnel have to be vigilant in information cyber security as more of our practices go electronic and most of patient-related archived private information is subject to vandalism, piracy and misuse.

Information technology risk (ITR) within healthcare organizations is a relatively new entity and deserves special mention in all RM initiatives, as practitioners and hospitals may not be well versed and as diligent in protecting electronic confidential patient identity and information.

Digital archiving of captured operational footage is an important aspect specific to endoscopic surgery, which deserves special notation here, as practitioners are cautioned to secure a separate institutional consent form, prior to digital or still capture, affording operators legal right to obtain and use captured digital footage for research or education, while securing patient identity and information.

Ultimately, some suggest these images to be a part of the patient's chart and may be considered institutional property; however, it appears that most captured information resides with the operator at this time. A representative such consent form is included, courtesy of the Canadian Medical Protective Association (Fig. 11.1).[69]

A number of methodologies have been developed to deal with ITR and involvement of the IT department professionals along with institutional RMC, as they are be best informed to in-service staff before confidentiality breaches, cyberattacks or other ransomware mishaps arise.

RISK ASSESSMENT

A fundamental difficulty in risk assessment is determining the rate of occurrence, since reliable statistical information is not readily available on all kinds of past incidents. Nevertheless, risk assessment should synthesize such information for management of organizations, so that primary risks are easily understood and RM decisions are prioritized.

In 2008, the RCOG in the UK described standards of gynecological care as follows:

PHOTO AND VIDEO CONSENT FORM

To be completed following discussion with the patient

Patient's Name:
Patient's Address:

This authorization grants permission to use your image (still or moving) and/or your spoken words in perpetuity for educational purposes. By signing this document, you agree:

- To allow recording of your image and voice (e.g. photographs, audio or video).
- To distribute your image or recording in any medium, be it print or electronic form, which may include the Internet or other educational social media.
- To grant permission to other entities to reproduce images or recording for educational purposes.
- That there is no reimbursement for the right to take, or to use your photograph, video or recording.

Nature of image and/or spoken words to be recorded:
Purpose of recording, image and/or spoken words, including the intended audience:
Your anonymity will always be secured.
Restrictions and limitations (Specify if applicable):

I have read and fully understand intent and purpose of this document and am signing it without reservation.

Name (please print):
Signature: **Date:** **Witness:**

Fig. 11.1: Sample consent form for digital archiving of captured surgical footage; adapted from the Canadian Medical Protective Association suggested consent form.

There is evidence that RM systems can identify factors that could expose patients, staff, visitors and hospital property to harm. To minimize risk, it is important that a proactive approach is in place within a RM framework that integrates all aspects of clinical governance, including clinical audit, training, complaints handling, research and service development.

Other means of discovering areas of concern stems from review of recent litigations, patient complaints, national professional society publications, medical or nursing protective association recommendations, government health directives, among others.

Certainly times have changed to the benefit of patients, providers and organizations, and will evolve further as our understanding of quality health evolves. Contemporary patient safety-centered principles and perceptions of safe endoscopic practice have replaced old conventional "wisdoms" that seemed to apply well for open surgery.

The following instances describe how far health delivery has evolved. Previously we provided optimum care; now patients receive safe care. Previously doctors were rebuked for errors; now systems are blamed for safety lapses. Previously physicians stressed responsibility as a keystone; now team performance is celebrated. Previously surgeons offered personalized care; now teams provide best practices. Previously we treated diseases; now clients obtain better quality of health. Previously surgeons dictated a care plan; now patients negotiate solutions. Previously operators remedied mishaps; now summoned experts report events. Previously master surgeons honed skills intraoperatively; now skills are perfected in virtual reality surgical skills labs. Previously we operated for countless hours; now we balance work and family. Previously healers handled pathology; now robotic arms remotely manipulate tissues.

RM is an exercise of methodically choosing practical and cost-effective remedies to diminish the likelihood and effects of inadvertent incidents that threatens patient safety. Admittedly, all healthcare risk cannot be totally avoided or mitigated and patients, administrators, as well as health providers acknowledge that some degree of residual risk inevitably remains.

Irrespective of medical advances, our obligation remains to be vigilant and make every possible effort to avert unintended patient harm, confront failures, correct errors and pledge to continually learn from our mishaps. As President JF Kennedy said, errors do not become mistakes until we refuse to correct and learn from them.

This short practical overview of RM in gynecologic endoscopy examines some basic principles and describes solutions to patient safety while delivering contemporary minimally invasive care; our objective remains to raise awareness, invite discussion and encourage research to render our discipline less hazardous to the benefit of all.

USEFUL TERMS

The following definitions and terms are commonly associated with patient safety, RM and medicolegal situations that are important in healthcare.

Risk in healthcare is defined as the likelihood of harm by a hazard, multiplied by the severity of potential harm.[70]

The Occupational Health and Safety Advisory Services defines risk as the product of the probability of a hazard resulting in an adverse event, times the severity of the potential injury.[71]

It can be viewed as the effect of uncertainty on objectives, whether positive or negative. It is a combination of the likelihood of harm and the severity of injury or ill health that is caused by an event.

Risk management is a dynamic process by which health systems proactively identify, assess and treat risk so as to avoid occurrence or recurrence of foreseeable adverse events.[72,73]

In practice, it can be a powerful energetic tool that introduces safety increments and embeds redundancies, so as to mitigate and control likelihood of harm and enhance patient safety during health delivery; conversely, inadequate RM capabilities can have serious and far reaching patient, institution and practitioner consequences.

Numerous RM standards have been developed for HRO; however, definitions and goals vary according to the discipline and context where a given RM method is deployed.[34]

Risk awareness is the ability of a healthcare system to alert patients, providers and institutions of potential danger and combat complacency. It entails identifying vulnerabilities and learning from near misses.

An **adverse event** is an inadvertent act of commission or omission causing injury and usually involves outcomes and patient experiences. Whereas **error** is an inadvertent failure of planed action and often involves processes and health providers. Consequently, an adverse event in healthcare is not synonymous to an error.

Due diligence or the duty to act reasonably, prudently, and in good faith in the best interests of patients is used in reference to a defence by a health provider who would otherwise be liable for inadvertent outcomes.

Duty of care is sometimes also referred to as *reasonable care* and is tied to the concept of due diligence. Health providers must show similar standard of care that would be expected by a reasonable caregiver with similar ability and experience in a particular circumstance.

Indemnity is a guarantee from one party to another that, should a medico legal liability arise; the first party will cover costs of any losses or damages incurred. For example, insurance is an indemnification from a medico legal protective organization, to cover losses in circumstances set out by the policy.

Liability refers to a situation where a provider causes an incident that hurts a patient or costs her financially, and the practitioner is held responsible or liable. This means they can be asked to compensate for damages or losses.

Negligence is fault liability, which means there is an allegation that health delivery (by an individual provider, as a team or organization), erred or failed to provide something that it should have done and an injury or loss ensued as a result.

Standard of care refers to the degree or level of service, attention, care, and protection that a practitioner is obligated toward patients' health and safety, according to the law, usually the law of negligence. The required standard varies according to circumstances of each situation, and determining appropriate standard of care is often not a simple matter.

Vicarious liability is when an organization is held liable for actions of health providers if they practice under the auspices and direction of an institution and acting within the scope of their responsibilities when mishaps occur. In other words, an organization itself does not have to have done anything wrong for it to be found responsible for actions of its healthcare team.

Vulnerable person: This term is used to describe individual patients who have difficulty in protecting themselves and are at a greater risk of unintended harm. Vulnerability may be temporary or permanent and may affect children, youth, seniors, people with disability and those who are victims of crime or harm.

TIPS AND TRICKS

International Organization for Standardization Risk Management Steps

- Identify, examine and evaluate risk
- Determine susceptibility
- Establish risk and evaluate consequences
- Define methods to lessen those risks
- Prioritize risk prevention measures

Seven Cardinal Rules of Effective Risk Communication

- Engage all stakeholders
- Assess and evaluate team's initiatives
- Attend to team's and provider's specific concerns
- Be sincere, truthful and candid
- Recruit and collaborate with other specialists
- Address patient advocacy and media queries
- Address patient advocacy and media queries
- Communicate plainly with empathy, honesty and consideration.

When Error is Discovered and Needs Investigation

- Stay impartial and confidential
- Involve senior stakeholders
- Summon relevant expertise
- Be compassionate but consistent
- Examine system and team failure
- Remain non-confrontational non-retributional
- Recognize digression from accepted protocols
- Identify evidence base to support incident and actions
- Analyze all roots and causes
- Engage those most familiar with the incident
- Give feedback and teach findings for deterrence

Composition of an Endoscopy Risk Management Committee

- Lead clinician
- Nursing staff
- Resident or fellow in training
- Representative from other discipline
- Institutional health and safety representative
- Institutional patient advocate.

Risk Management to Minimize Organizational Error Exposure

- Ensure appropriate staff training skill and knowledge
- Enforce training compliance
- Apply mandatory contemporary protocols
- Match skills to task benchmarking
- Information available and accessible
- Secure record-keeping standards without delay
- Regular clinical audits
- Governance structure

Risk Management in Gynecologic Endoscopy

- Remain familiar with local clinical governance
- Organize Gynecologic Endoscopy RMC
- Develop RM strategy and policy
- Report errors to learn from mishaps
- Register risks and remedies
- Perform risk evaluation and auditing
- RMC to facilitate implementation efforts
- Institute safety protocols when introducing new technology
- Conduct honest disclosure when error occurs
- Senior endoscopist to spearhead learning from near misses and accidents.

REFERENCES

1. Violato C. Editorial: doctor-patient relationships, laws, clinical guidelines, best practices, evidence-based medicine, medical errors and patient safety. Can Med Educ J. 2013;4(1):e1-e6.
2. Weiser TG, Regenbogen SE, Thompson KD, et al. An estimation of the global volume of surgery: a modelling strategy based on available data. Lancet. 2008;372(9633):139-44.
3. WHO guidelines for safe surgery: safe surgery saves lives. WHO. 2014. Available from: http://www.who.int/patientsafety/safesurgery/tools_resources/9789241598552/en/. [Accessed April 30, 2017].
4. Brennan TA, Leape LL, Laird NM, et al. Incidence of adverse events and negligence in hospitalized patients.. Results of the Harvard Medical Practice Study I. N Engl J Med. 1991;324(6):370-6.
5. Gandaglia G, Ghani KR, Sood A, et al. Effect of minimally invasive surgery on the risk for surgical site infections. Results from the National Surgical Quality Improvement Program (NSQIP) Database. JAMA Surg. 2014;149(10):1039-44.
6. Siska VB, Ann L, Gunter de W, et al. Surgical skill: trick or trait? J Surg Educ. 2015;72(6):1247-53.
7. Reason J. Safety in the operating theatre - Part 2: human error and organisational failure. Qual Saf Health Care. 1995;14(1):56-60.
8. Card AJ, Ward J, Clarkson PJ. Successful risk assessment may not always lead to successful risk control: a systematic literature review of risk control after root cause analysis. J Healthc Risk Manag. 2012; 31(3):6-12.
9. Card AJ, Ward JR, Clarkson PJ. Rebalancing risk management—Part 2: The Active Risk Control (ARC) Toolkit. J Healthc Risk Manag. 2015;34(3):4-17.
10. Rodrigues SP, Wever AM, Dankelman J, et al. Risk factors in patient safety: minimally invasive surgery versus conventional surgery. Surg Endosc. 2012; 26(2):350-6.
11. Driessen SRC, Sandberg EM, Rodrigues SP, et al. Identification of risk factors in minimally invasive surgery: a prospective multicenter study. Surg Endosc. 2017;31(6):2467-73.
12. Waste and Inefficiency in the U.S. Health Care System, Clinical Care: A Comprehensive Analysis in Support of System-wide Improvements. New England Healthcare Institute, February 2008.

13. Bentley TG, Effros RM, Palar K, et al. Waste in the U.S. Health care system: a conceptual framework. Milbank Q. 2008;86(4):629-59.
14. Section 2531 Med Liability Alternatives Health Reform Bill HR 3962. p. 1432.
15. Berguer R, Smith WD, Chung YH. Performing laparoscopic surgery is significantly more stressful for the surgeon than open surgery. Surg Endosc. 2001;15(10):1204-7.
16. Zhang J, Patel VL, Johnson TR, et al. A cognitive taxonomy of medical errors. J Biomed Inform. 2004; 37(3):193-204.
17. Weingart SN, McL Wilson R, Gibberd RW, et al. Epidemiology of medical error. West J Med. 2000; 172(6):390-3.
18. Nissen K, Angus SV, Miller W, et al. Teaching risk management: Addressing ACGME core competencies. J Grad Med Educ. 2010;2(4):589-94.
19. Singh SS, Marcoux V, Cheung V, et al. Core competencies for gynecologic endoscopy in residency training: a national consensus project. J Minim Invasive Gynecol. 2009;16(1):1-7.
20. Moreno-Hunt C, Gilbert WM. Current status of obstetrics and gynecology resident medical-legal education: a survey of program directors. Obstet Gynecol. 2005;106(6):1382-4.
21. National Patient Safety Agency (NPSA). Seven steps to patient safety: A guide for NHS staff. 2003.
22. Reason JT. Human error. Cambridge: Cambridge University Press; 1990.
23. Roberts KH, Yu K, Van Stralen D. Patient safety as an organizational systems issue: lessons from a variety of industries. In: Youngberg BJ, Hatlie MJ (Eds). The Patient Safety Handbook. Sudbury MA: Jones & Bartlett; 2004. pp. 169-86.
24. Meister D. Human Factors in Surgery Design, Development and Testing. Mahwah, NJ: Lawrence Erlbaum Associates, Inc., Publishings; 1992.
25. Krizek TJ. Surgical error: reflections on adverse events. Bull Am Coll Surg. 2000;85(7):18-22.
26. Clarke JR. Designing safety into the minimally invasive surgical revolution: a commentary based on the Jacques Perissat Lecture of the International Congress of the European Association for Endoscopic Surgery. Surg Endosc. 2009;23(1):216-20.
27. Calland JF, Guerlain S, Adams RB, et al. A systems approach to surgical safety. Surg Endosc. 2002;16(6): 1005-14.
28. Bender ML, Hirschhorn L. An irreplaceable safety culture. Crit Care Clin. 2005;21(1):31-41. viii.
29. Siddiqui J, Tuffnell D. Minimizing risk in gynaecological surgery. Rev Gynecol Pract. 2005;5:152-8.
30. Reason JT. Human Error. Cambridge, United Kingdom: Cambridge University Press; 1999.
31. Leape LL. Striving for perfection. Clin Chem. 2002; 48(11):1871-2.
32. Reason JT Understanding adverse events: the human factors. In: Vincent C (Ed). Clinical Risk Management. London: BMJ Publishing Group; 2001. pp. 9-30.
33. Marx D. Patient Safety and the "Just Culture": A Primer for Health Care Executives. [Internet]. New York, NY: Columbia University; 2001. Available from: http://psnet.ahrq.gov/resource.aspx?resourceID=1582 [Accessed January 7, 2015].
34. ISO/DIS 31000. Risk Management—Principles and Guidelines on Implementation. International Organization for Standardization; 2009.
35. Donabedian A. Evaluating the quality of medical care. Milbank Q. 2005;83(4):691-729.
36. Donabedian A. The Definition of Quality and Approaches to Its Assessment. Ann Arbor, MI: Health Administration Press; 1980.
37. Moss F. Risk management and quality of care. Qual Health Care. 1995;4(2):102-7.
38. Verdaasdonk EG, Stassen LP, van der Elst M, et al. Problems with technical equipment during laparoscopic surgery. An observational study. Surg Endosc. 2007;21(2):275-9.
39. Powell SM, Hill RK. My copilot is a nurse—using crew resource management in the OR. AORN J. 2006;83(1):179-80, 183-90, 193-8 passim; quiz 203-6.
40. Raymond E, Ternamian A, Leyland N, et al. Endoscopy teaching in Canada: a survey of obstetrics and gynecology program directors and graduating residents. J Minim Invasive Gynecol. 2006;13(1): 10-6.
41. Roberts KH, Yu K, Stralen D. Patient safety as an organizational systems issue: lessons from a variety of industries. In: Youngberg B, Hatlie M (Eds). Patient Safety Handbook. Sudbury, MA: Jones & Barlett; 2004. pp. 169-86.
42. Christian CK, Gustafson ML, Roth EM, et al. A prospective study of patient safety in the operating room. Surgery 2006;139(2):159-73.
43. Nakhleh RE, Fitzgibbons PL (Eds). Quality Management in Anatomic Pathology: Promoting Patient Safety through Systems Improvement and Error Reduction. Northfield, IL: College of American Pathologists; 2005.
44. Covello VT, Allen FH. Seven Cardinal Rules of Risk Communication. US Environmental Protection Agency. Washington, DC: OPA-87-020; 1988.
45. Abed H, Rogers R, Helitzer D, et al. Informed consent in gynecologic surgery. Am J Obstet Gynecol. 2007; 197(6):674-5.
46. Dickens BM, Cook RJ. Patients' refusal of recommended treatment. Int J Gynaecol Obstet. 2015;131(1): 105-8.
47. Chambliss DF, Schutt RK. Making Sense of the Social World: Methods of Investigation, 3rd edn. Thousand Oaks, CA: Pine Forge Press; 2010.
48. Olga Salgo. Administratrix, etc., Respondent, v. Leland Stanford Jr. University Board of Trustees et al., Appellants [Civ. No. 17045. First Dist., Div. One. Oct. 22, 1957].
49. Lobo RA, Gershenson DM, Lentz GM, et al. Comprehensive Gynecology, 7th edn. Amsterdam: Elsevier; 2015. Chapter 24, p. 568.
50. Elliott C. Clinical governance in gynaecological surgery. Best Pract Res Clin Obstet Gynaecol. 2006; 20(1):189-204.

51. Nicholas N, El Sayed M. The changing face of consent: past and present. Obstet Gynaecol. 2006;8(1):39-44.
52. Clinical risk management for obstetricians and gynaecologists. RCOG Clinical Governance Advice No. 2; January 2001. www.rcog.org.uk
53. Groenman FA, Peters LW, Rademaker BM, et al. Embolism of air and gas in hysteroscopic procedures: pathophysiology and implication for daily practice. J Minim Invasive Gynecol. 2008;15(2):241-7.
54. Vilos GA, Ternamian A, Dempster J, et al. Laparoscopic entry: a review of techniques, technologies and com-plications. J Obstet Gynecol Can. 2007;29(5): 433-47.
55. Larobina M, Nottle P. Complete evidence regarding major vascular injuries during laparoscopic access. Surg Laparosc Endosc Percutan Tech. 2005;15(3): 119-23.
56. Bhoyrul S, Vierra MA, Nezhat CR, et al. Trocar injuries in laparoscopic surgery. J Am Coll Surg. 2001;192(6):677-83.
57. Fuller J, Ashar BS, Carey-Corrado J. Trocar-associated injuries and fatalities: an analysis of 1399 reports to the FDA. J Minim Invasive Gynecol. 2005;12(4): 302-7.
58. Ternamian AM, Vilos GA, Vilos AG, et al. Laparoscopic peritoneal entry with the reusable threaded visual cannula. J Minim Invasive Gynecol. 2010;17(4): 461-7.
59. van der Voort M, Heijnsdijk EA, Gouma DJ. Bowel injury as a complication of laparoscopy. Br J Surg. 2004;91(10):1253-8.
60. Managed Care Weekly Digest (2002) AORN panel cites Encision's AEM technology as recommended device. Available at: http://www.newsrx.com/newsletters/Managed-Care-Weekly-Digest/2002-05-27/2002052733315MH. html. May 2002; Accessed January 2016.
61. ECRI. Safety technologies for laparoscopic monopolar electrosurgery; devices for managing burn risks. Health Devices. 2005;34(8):259-72.
62. Vincent C. Taylor-Adams S. The investigation and analysis of clinical incidents. In: Vincent C (Ed). Clinical Risk Management. London: BMJ Publishing Group; 2001.p. 439-60.
63. Gibson. Wall of Silence. Washington DC: Regnery Publishing Co; 2003.
64. Leape LL, Berwick DM. Five years after to err is human. What have we learned? JAMA. 2005;293(19): 2384-90.
65. Munro MG. Laparoscopic access: complications, technologies, and techniques. Curr Opin Obstet Gynecol. 2002;14(4):365-74.
66. Schmidek JM, Weeks WB. Relationship between tort claims and patient incident reports in the Veterans Health Administration. Qual Saf Health Care. 2005; 14(2):117-22.
67. Physicians Insurers Association of America. Claim Trend Analysis 2009 Edition. Rockville, MD: Physicians Insurers Association of America; 2009.
68. Learning from experience. Presentation from www.clinicalrisk.com
69. www.cmpa-acpm.ca.
70. Department of Health. An organization with a memory: report of an expert group on learning from adverse events in the NHS chaired by the Chief Medical Officer. London: The Stationary Office; 2000.
71. Occupational Health and Safety Advisory Services (OHSAS) 18001; 2007.
72. Walshe K. The development of clinical risk management. In: Vincent C (Ed). Clinical Risk Management. London: BMJ Publishing Group; 2001, pp. 45-60.
73. Edozien LC. Risk management in gynaecology. Obstet Gynaecol Repro Med. 2009;20:1-13.

KIEL SCHOOL

12 of Gynaecological Endoscopy

Female Pelvis
Innervation and Vascularization
in Laparoscopy

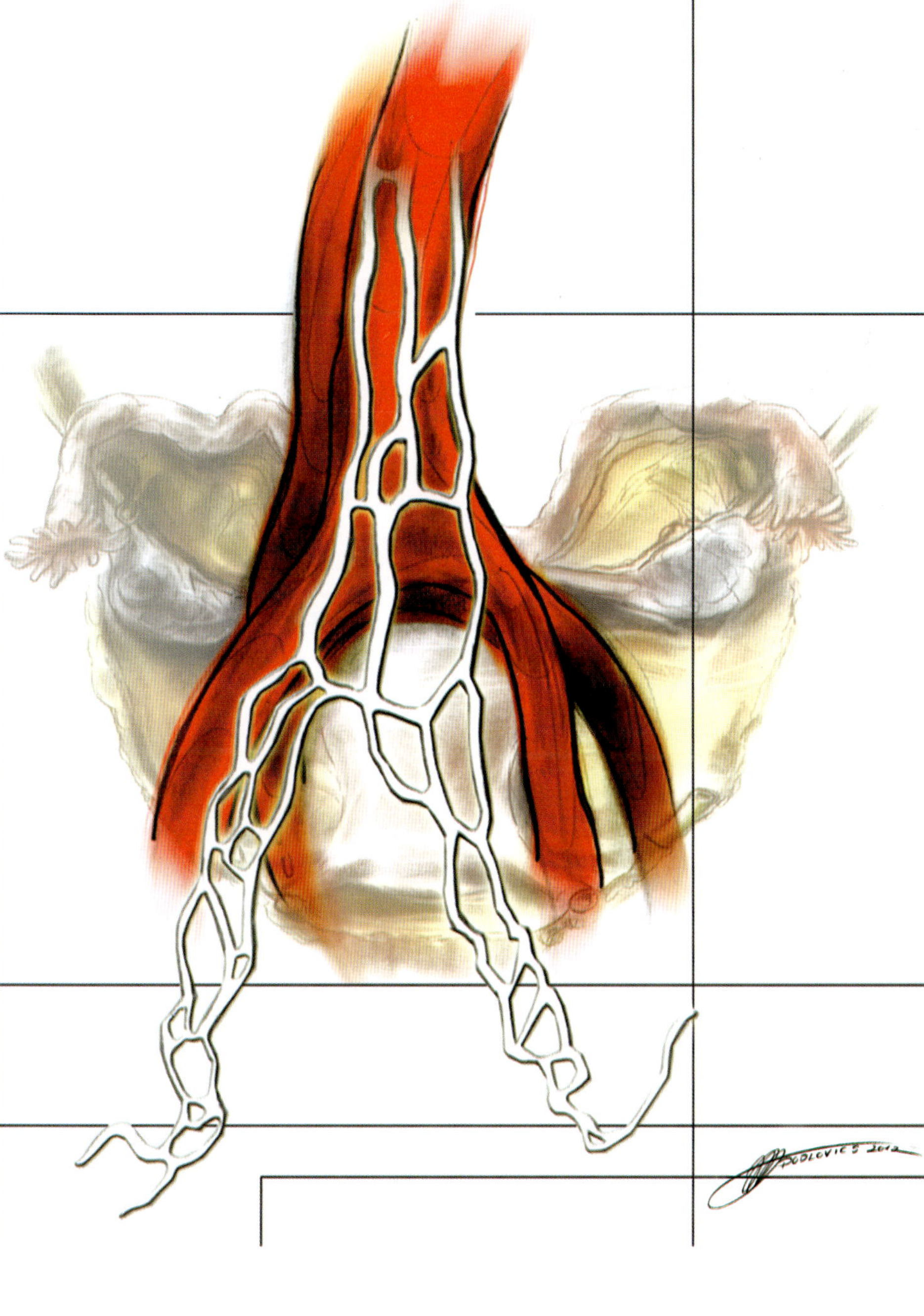

Chapter 12

Female Pelvis Innervation and Vascularization in Laparoscopy

Andrea Tinelli, Radmila Sparić, Saša Kadija, Svetlana Spremović Radjenović, Ospan A Mynbaev, Michael Stark, Antonio Malvasi

INTRODUCTION

The familiarity of the female pelvis anatomy is essential to perform an endoscopic procedure safely, including the opening of the retroperitoneal space. Namely, knowledge on surgical endoscopic anatomy of pelvis and abdomen includes the memorization of spaces, of viscera, of support systems, of vascular-lymphatic trees and nerves. Besides being familiar on the anatomy of the abdominal–pelvic viscera, it is the knowledge of the arrangement of the connective tissue that fills the virtual spaces between pelvic organs, lymph nodes and vessels, called "perivisceral spaces" (Figs. 12.1A and B), which allows the identification of connective structures containing vessels and nerves. This allows to identify areas and anatomical structures usually unknown to laparotomic surgery.[1]

Female pelvic nerves run along in the retroperitoneum and their paths are partly described in anatomical texts on pelvic innervations. It has now been accepted that, in the small pelvic spaces, during some kinds of gynecological surgery performed laparoscopically, especially in cases, such as cancers, endometriosis and pelvic organ prolapse (POP) surgery it is possible to come in contact with some of these (Figs. 12.2A and B), even damaging them.[2]

Nowadays, the laparoscopic technique is getting wide acceptance in gynecological surgery. Thus, many laparoscopic procedures include the opening of the retroperitoneal space, previously possible only by means of laparotomy; therefore, the possibility to interact with retroperitoneal pelvic structures (Fig. 12.3) becomes, day by day, part of the everyday work for gynecological endoscopists.

LAPAROSCOPY IN EXTRA-PERITONEAL SPACES

Numerous laparoscopic interventions are performed without opening the retroperitoneal space, as it is not required for the purpose of the surgery procedure. In some cases, however, the type of

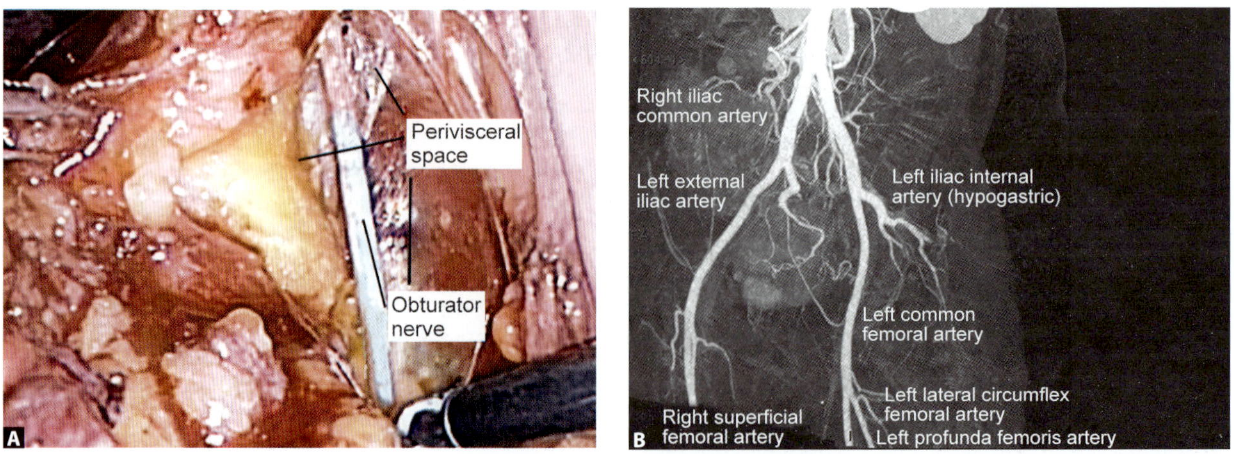

Figs. 12.1A and B: Obturator fossa with the "perivisceral space" surrounding obturator nerve, involving lymph nodes and nerves.

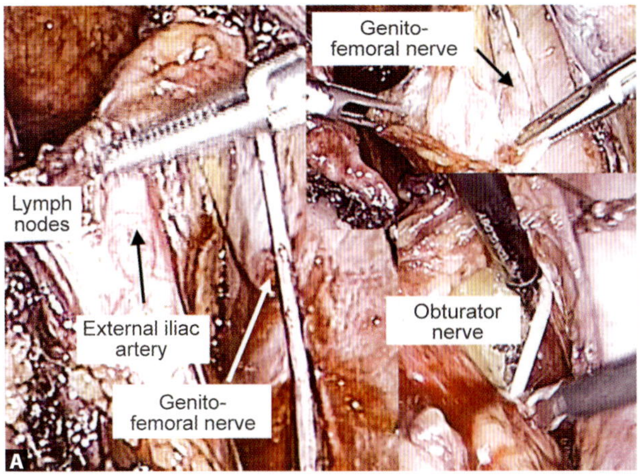

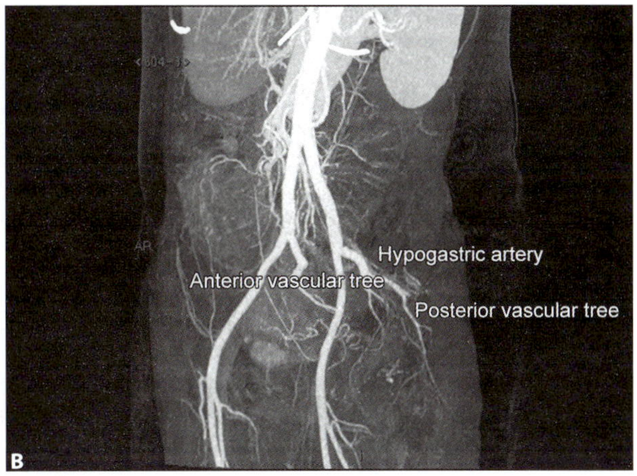

Figs. 12.2A and B: In small pelvic retroperitoneal spaces, it is possible to come in contact with some nerves, as obturator or genito-femoral nerves, during some gynecological laparoscopies.

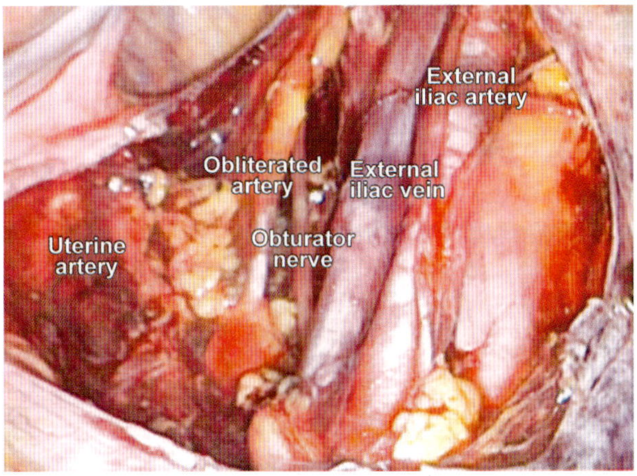

Fig. 12.3: Right retroperitoneal pelvic fossa, which shows, from left to right, uterine artery, obliterated artery, obturator nerve, external iliac vein and artery.

condition affecting the patient, demands a complete surgical management even in spaces not usually investigated by endoscopists.

Several types of interventions that include the opening of the pelvic retroperitoneal spaces, currently performed in women in reproductive age, including the pelvic lymphadenectomy (Figs. 12.4A and B), associated to procedures of surgical oncology, pelvic organ prolapse surgery and the treatment of deep pelvic endometriosis.[2]

In order to perform a laparoscopy that goes across these spaces safely, it is important to be familiar with the location of organs, of muscular-ligamentous and vascular-nervous pelvic supporting organs, to be identified at the beginning of every surgery. These interventions require considerable familiarity with the retroperitoneum and special proficiency on the surgical anatomy.

Pelvic floor disorders affect significant proportion of woman, and with growing life expectancy, more and more women will be affected.[3] These conditions mainly require surgical treatment. Most of the corrective surgical procedures for these conditions were performed transvaginally or transabdominally. With the wide implementation of laparoscopy in gynecology some of these procedures are now performed laparoscopically. The basic principle underlying in POP surgery is to restore the altered morphology of the pelvic floor, correct vaginal anatomy and support and return normal bowel, bladder and sexual function, thus elevating patient's symptoms. These procedures are performed by fixation of the organs to pelvic structures/fixation points, such as uterosacral, sacro tuberous and sacrospinous ligaments either with sutures or by synthetic mesh or graft.[3] Transvaginal approach, by avoiding laparotomy/laparoscopy, is still a major mode of treatment, particularly in women with major comorbidities.

Nevertheless, most of the procedures performed for these conditions could be performed by laparoscopic approach.[3] Laparoscopic approach was introduced into urogynecological surgery since 1991, with the advantages of enhanced visualization of the pelvic structures, lower morbidity and faster post-operative recovery.[4] Further advance of laparoscopic approach includes less vaginal fibrosis, direct visualization of the ureter and minimizing the chance of mesh contamination with vaginal flora, thus reducing mesh infection rates.[4]

The most frequently used procedure is laparoscopic sacrocolpopexy (LSC).[3] The procedure requires opening of prevertebral peritoneum, thus

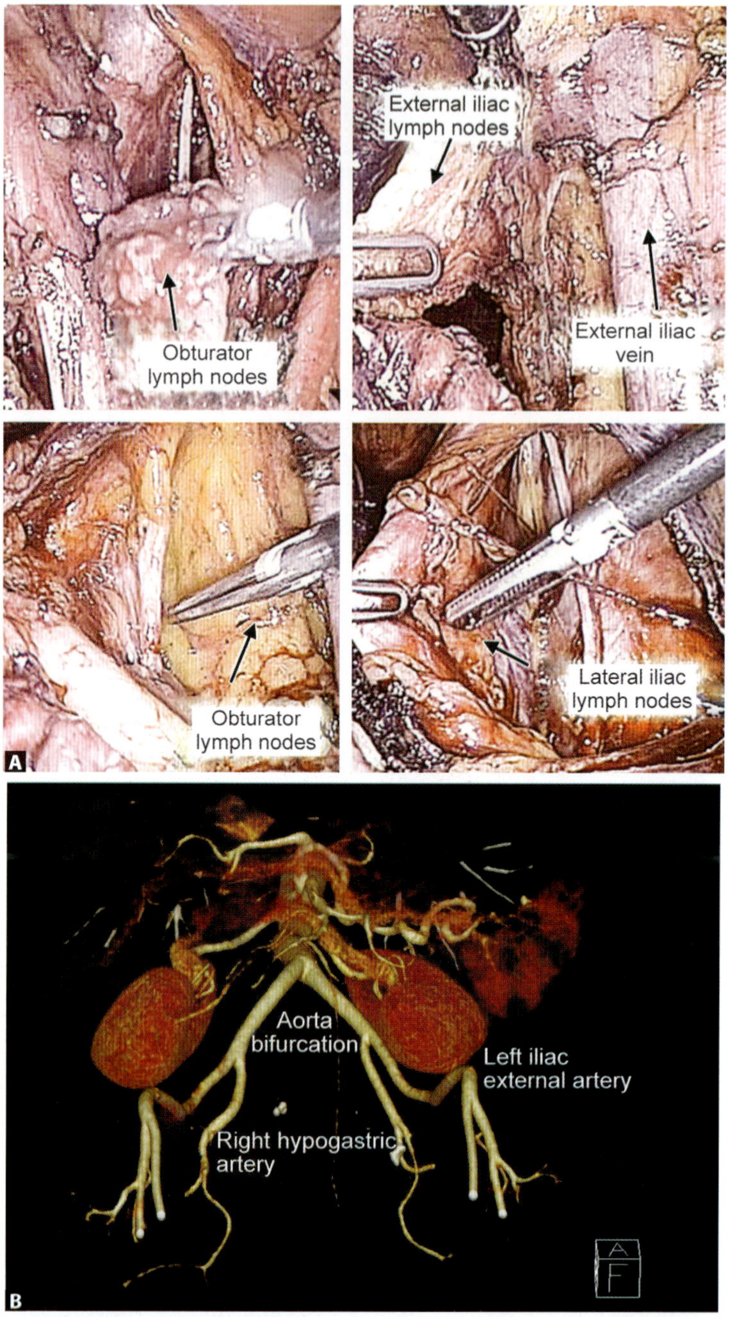

Figs. 12.4A and B: The pelvic lymphadenectomy into the retroperitoneal space starts along the external iliac vein and the lymphatic overlying the external iliac artery was also removed. Dissection then proceeded inferiorly to the obturator fossa, to isolate and preserve the obturator nerve, the obturator artery and vein, and to remove the obturator lymph nodes. Dissection further proceeded proximally to the bifurcation of the common iliac artery where the lymph nodes in the angle between the external iliac and hypogastric arteries were removed, with no closure of peritoneum over vessels after pelvic lymphadenectomy.

requiring wide knowledge of anatomy of presacral and pararectal spaces, as well as rectovaginal and vesicovaginal space and anatomy of muscles levator ani. Laparoscopic approach used for sacrocolpopexy prevents denervation of the rectum, which could further cause defecation difficulties. Unlike laparotomic procedure, LSC provides benefit in terms of sexual functioning by not causing dyspareunia.[4,5] The same procedure can be performed by robotic surgery and also robot-assisted sacrocolpopexy (RSC).

Another POP procedure performed by laparoscopy is laparoscopic sacral hysteropexy, fixating uterus to the promontory.[4,5] Laparoscopic lateral suspension is procedure performed either with or without preservation of the uterus.[4,5]

Data on pregnancies following such procedures are mainly lacking, and in most cases patients had cesarean delivery.[4]

VASCULARIZATION AND LYMPHATIC SYSTEM IN LAPAROSCOPY

During advanced laparoscopy the retroperitoneal vascularization and lymphatic system of pelvis are easily detectable.

In young nulliparous women, it is possible to perform a conservative treatment in the early stages of cervical cancer (IA1, IA2, until IB1 stage). It consists of a laparoscopic lymphadenectomy combined with a wide conization or trachelectomy.[6] Laparoscopy made a big step forward in these complex surgical cases, as this procedure is less invasive than laparotomy, and offers to expert endoscopist surgeons substantial benefits, due to the significant magnification of the intraoperative anatomic view.

This enables the laparoscopist to remove the pelvic lymph nodes accurately, with the minimum damage to the surrounding structures. The pelvic lymphadenectomy consists in removing the lymph nodes around the common iliac vessels (Figs. 12.5A and B), and later in the excision of any others located around the external iliac vessels; the procedure ends with the extraction of the lymph nodes from the obturator fossa (Figs. 12.6A and B).[7]

In some centers, where advanced laparoscopy is practiced, if the pathological condition should require it, also the lymph nodes of the lomboaortic chain can be excised (Fig. 12.7). The magnification of the laparoscopic view permits the endoscopist not only to extract the lymph nodes, but also to coagulate, with bipolar current, bleeding areas within the lymphatic tree or bleeding of the small retroperitoneal vessels.

With the excision of the lymph nodes, the sensitivity of the genitofemoral nerve (Fig. 12.2), running

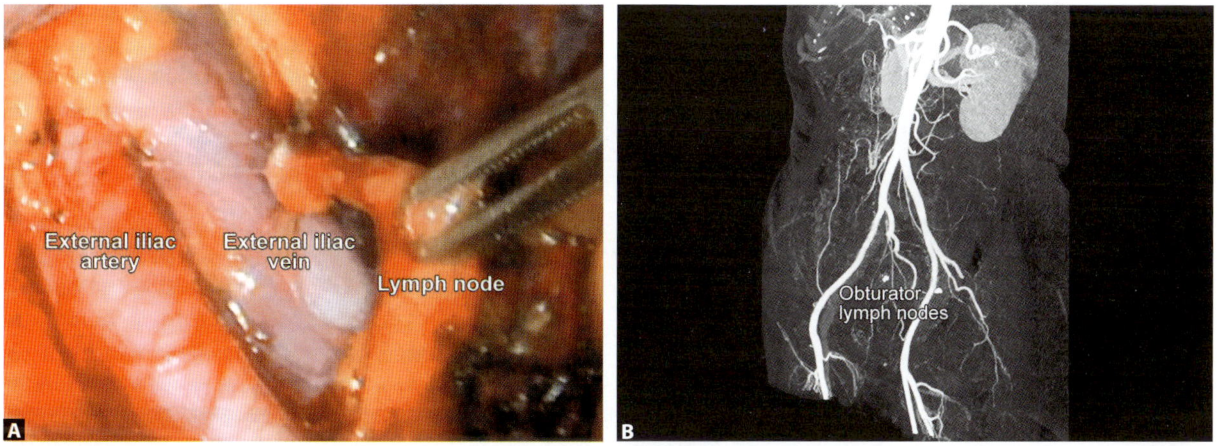

Figs. 12.5A and B: A bulky pelvic lymph node removal along the external iliac vein during a radical laparoscopy for cervical cancer treatment.

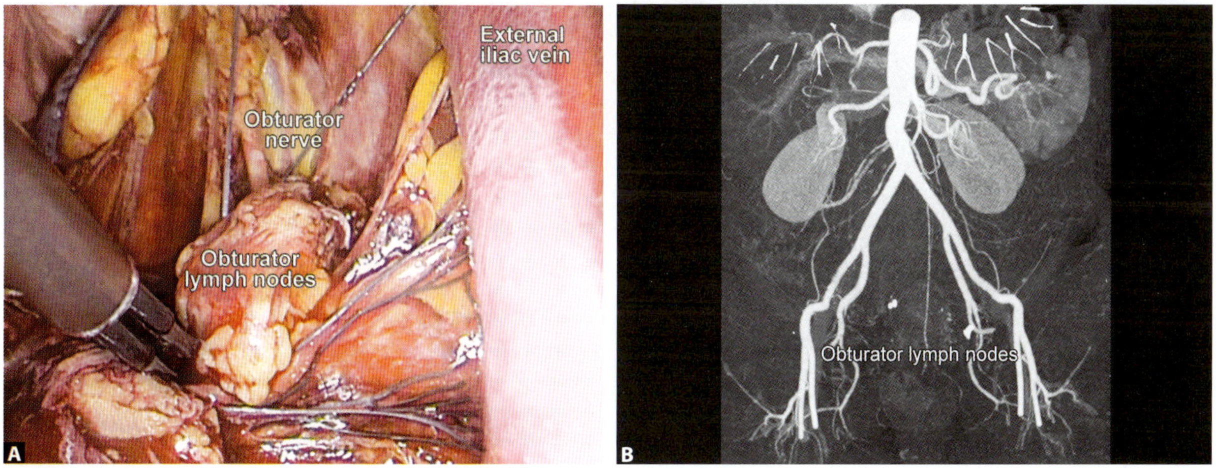

Figs. 12.6A and B: The pelvic lymphadenectomy ends with the extraction of the lymph nodes from the obturator fossa, as shown in the picture with the extraction of the whole package of lymph nodes.

along the iliac vessels, may be preserved integrally. During the laparoscopic procedure, this appears as the most important and crucial nervous structure to be preserved, since the subsequent surgical steps involve major nerves which must not be absolutely injured.[8]

After removing the lymph nodes around the external iliac vessels (Figs. 12.8A and B), the medialization of such vessels is to be, in order to facilitate access to the obturator fossae and to the interiliac lymph nodes, subsequently excised. Access to interiliac and obturator lymph nodes run medially to the external iliac vessels (*see* Fig. 12.4).

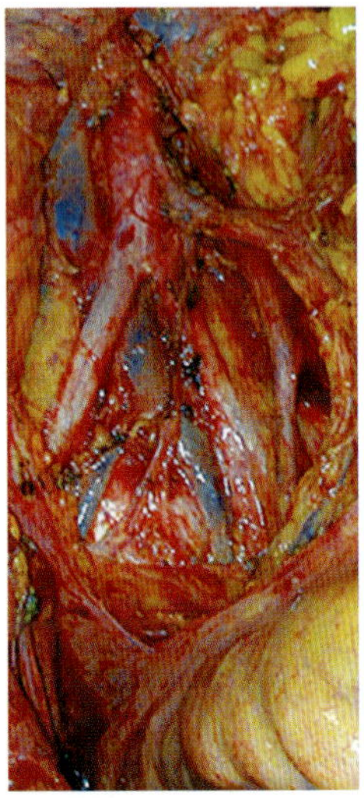

Fig. 12.7: Lymphadenectomy of the lomboaortic chain: in the image is well represented the inferior mesenteric plexus over the aorta bifurcation.

The obturator lymph nodes (Fig. 12.9) surround the obturator nerve (*see* Fig. 12.6), which is rather broad and resistant compared to the surrounding nervous structure. Nevertheless, a superficial and inaccurate preparation might cause injury during the emptying of the lymph nodes from the fossa.

A broad excision of pelvic lymph nodes (Fig. 12.10) will clearly enable the view of some vascular structures, such as the anterior branch of the hypogastric artery (Fig. 12.11), which is further divided into the uterine artery, the upper vesical artery and the obliterated artery (known also as "ligamentum lateralis").[9]

Running parallel and somehow beneath, the uterine artery, there is the profound uterine vein, which converges to the branches of the hypogastric vein. An excessively deep excision of lymph nodes located below this uterine vein might damage the upper portion of the inferior hypogastric plexus (Fig. 12.12) (also called "plexus pelvicus"), which rarely influences the functionality—along the inferior urinary tract—but could lead to hyposensitivity of the cervix and of the dorsal vaginal sheath.

In this type of lymphadenectomies, further damage to the caudal portion of the inferior hypogastric plexus (Fig. 12.13) that might cause rectal and vesical hyposensitivity (or atonia) occurs almost always after laparoscopy.[10]

Pelvic lymphadenectomy in early cervical cancers may be followed by a broad conization[11] or, as mentioned above, by a trachelectomy;[12] hence, the possible influence of the pelvic denervation of the

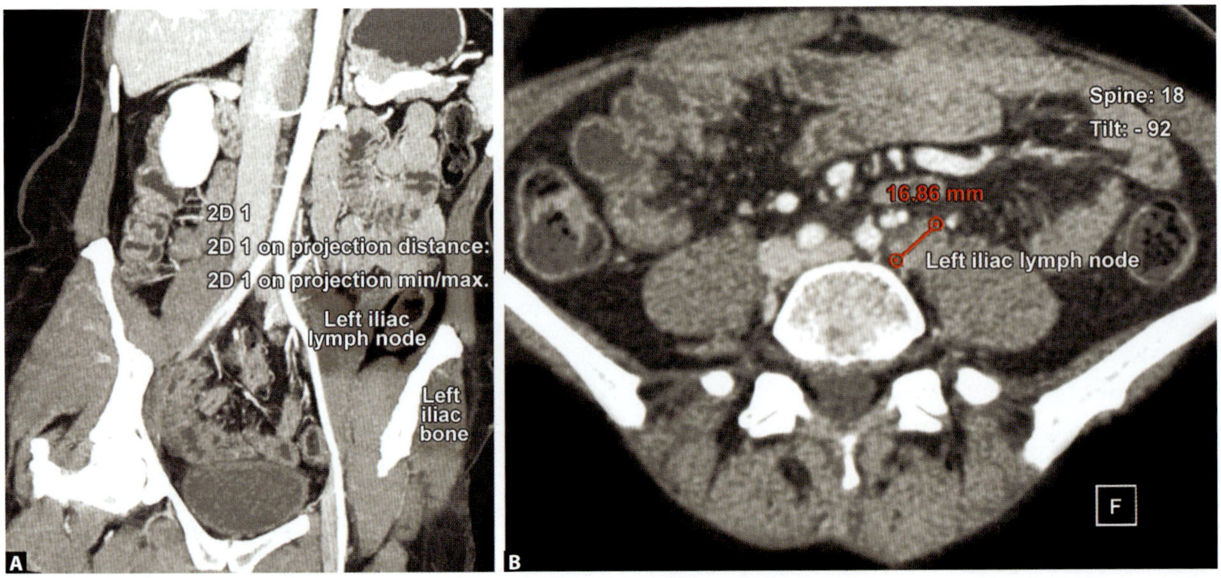

Figs. 12.8A and B: Two angio-tomographic computerized images in sagittal and coronal projections, showing a lymph node on the external iliac vessels of 16 mm diameter.

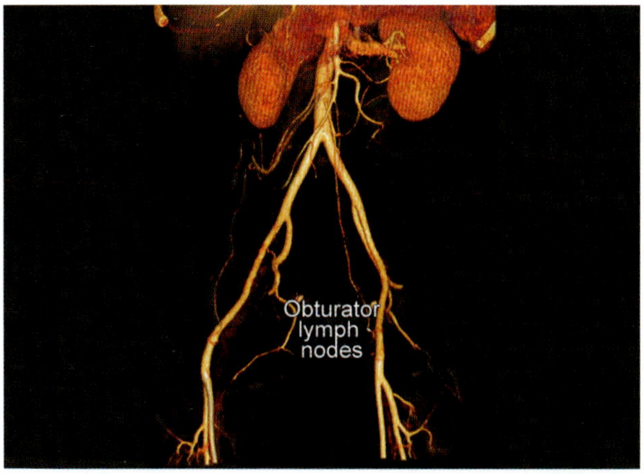

Fig. 12.9: An angio-tomographic computerized image in sagittal projection showing two obturator bilateral lymph nodes.

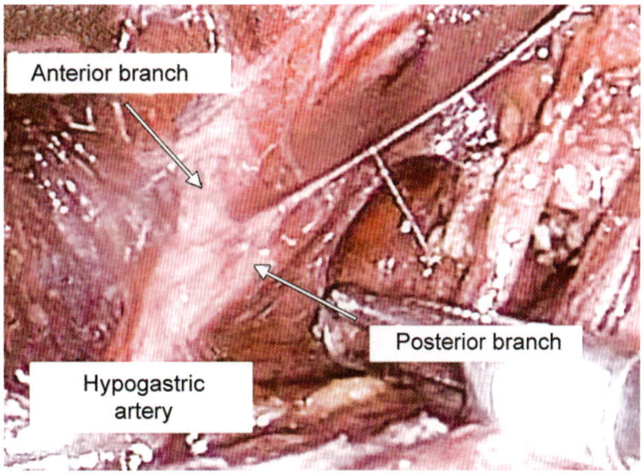

Fig. 12.11: The division of hypogastric artery in anterior and posterior branches; the anterior is further divided into the uterine artery, the upper vesical artery and the obliterated artery.

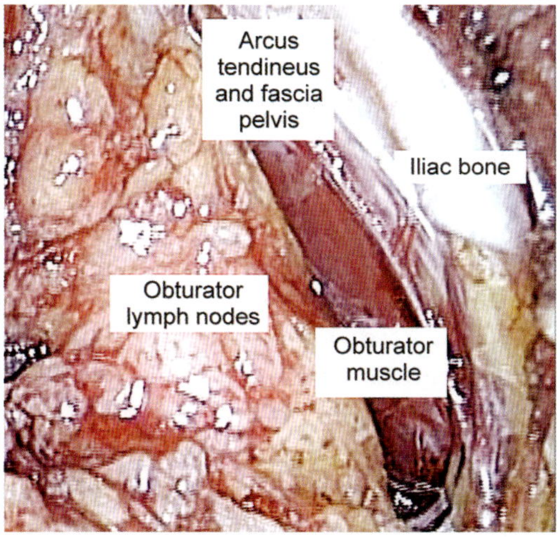

Fig. 12.10: A laparoscopic image of a right-sided lymphadenectomy showing the obturator lymph nodes detached from arcus tendineus and pelvic fascia, adherent to pelvic iliac bone and surrounding to obturator muscle.

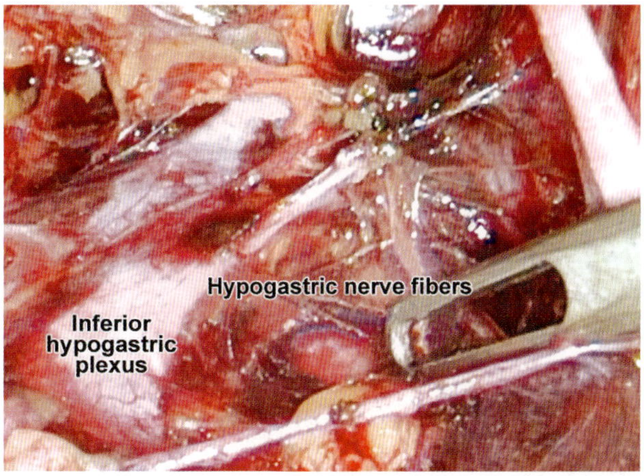

Fig. 12.12: The inferior hypogastric plexus under the hypogastric vein and obturator nerve (on the right), with the hypogastric nerve fibers directed to the lateral pelvic wall.

cervix and of the vaginal sheath in some physiological processes—as in delivery outcome—is difficult to establish.

There is still few information on delivery outcome and the percentage of cesarean sections in women who underwent pelvic laparoscopy with lymphadenectomy and a subsequent conization or trachelectomy.[13] We maintain that this topic should be studied further and follow-up of further clinical and surgical trials should be carried out to better understand the functionality of pelvic innervations in patients treated laparoscopically for retroperitoneal conditions.[14]

Some experimental models on animals have been described to date, whereby the bilateral neurectomy of the cervix may lead to alteration of the angiogenesis and to the sensitivity of some neuronal factors.[15] These, in turn, may influence the regulation of the dynamic microvascularization of the cervical ripening, and might play a major role in ripening proper, as well as in the fetal birth process.

FEMALE PELVIC NERVOUS SYSTEM

Another laparoscopic procedure that might cause damage to pelvic innervations is operative laparoscopy in deep pelvic endometriosis.[16] This is a condition that often gives general symptoms, such as chronic pelvic pain, dyspareunia, dysmenorrhea, menstrual flow alterations and sterility.[17,18]

The treatment of the deep infiltrating endometriosis is essentially surgical—either laparotomic or laparoscopic—although these procedures can be performed only in few surgically experienced centers.

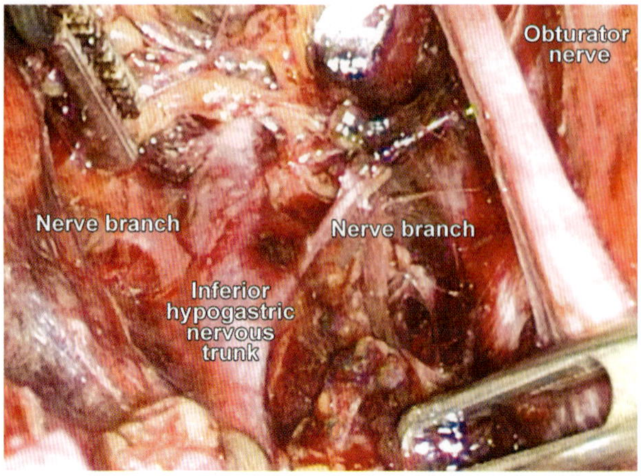

Fig. 12.13: The lateral branches of inferior hypogastric plexus, directed to the medial and lateral pelvic walls.

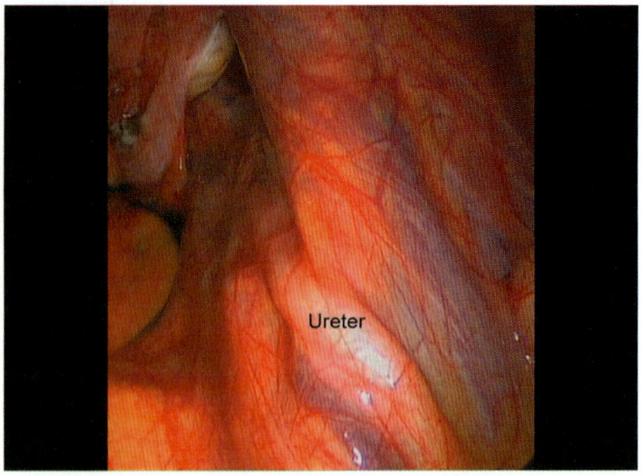

Fig. 12.15: The right ureter exposition under peritoneum crossing right common iliac vessels, prior to preparing the retroperitoneal exposition for deep endometriosis laparoscopic treatment.

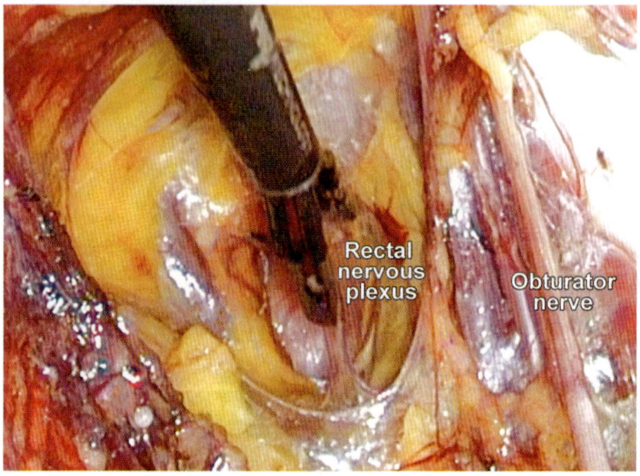

Fig. 12.14: The rectal nervous plexus, enhances by laparoscopic forceps, during posterior parametrium preparation for deep endometriosis treatment.

The latter endoscopic approach offers a number of advantages to the surgeon, if compared to the laparotomic approach, due to the enhanced vision of the surgical field—with a large magnification of the endoscopic anatomy that enables detection the thin and delicate nervous structures to be preserved during the preparation of the surgical areas to be excised.

A complete knowledge of the pelvic anatomy[19] and the experience of the endoscopist, who uses laparoscopic instrumentation, are all advantages needed to eradicate pathological features infiltrating the pelvic and retroperitoneal spaces.[20]

Should the posterior sacrum-uterine wall be affected, it will often be necessary to resort to excision during operative laparoscopy in deep pelvic endometriosis. The preparation of the posterior parametrium with its nerve fibers (Fig. 12.14), which embraces the wall of the sacrouterine ligaments, often comes after a preventive exposure of the ureters of the retroperitoneum (Fig. 12.15).[21]

After opening the retroperitoneal space, the ureter is often accurately isolated and separated, with an excision running superiorly to the large ligament and medially from the medial wall of the pelvic peritoneum of Douglas.

The ureter should always be separated from the surrounding structures it goes across, together with the uterine artery, by means of a careful dissection of the tissues. Another access in pararectal spaces is possible by stretching medially to the posterior parametrium.[22]

This part of the parametria is usually quite delicate. If there is no endometriosis, the posterior parametrium, enveloping the wall of sacrum-uterine ligaments, may be easily divided into two portions, namely the medial and the lateral portions, the former representing the ligament fibers and the latter the hypogastric nerve fibers.[23]

Moreover, if endometrial nodules and scars affect these structures, the resection could become exceptionally difficult (Fig. 12.16), with the resection of the hypogastric nerve. Should this incidence occur bilaterally, there will usually be urine loss, as well as cervical hypoesthesia, since the hypogastric nerve originating in the upper hypogastric plexus contains also this region's sensitive fibers.

Resecting such fibers might explain why there is less postoperative pain or the minor pain due to the nonexcision of the endometriotic nodules. Nevertheless, the total loss of vesical sensitivity seldom occurs, especially due to the fact that some of the sensitive fibers run along the sympathetic splanchnic nerves, which, with the resection of the posterior parameters are not involved.[24]

It is worth mentioning that the resection of the posterior parametria and the simultaneous accidental resection of the hypogastric nerve determine the loss of vaginal lubrication during intercourse, as a consequence of the resection of sympathetic fibers.[25]

In extensive laparoscopic procedures, when the entire rectum is involved, in case of deep infiltrating endometriosis, also the portion of intestine affected will be resected. More nervous fibers might be damaged during surgery, since this procedure requires a complete mobilization of the rectum from the pelvic floor and, dorsally, from the promontory and the sacrum.[10]

The endoscopic procedure usually begins with the opening of the pararectal peritoneum and, subsequently, with the wide dissection of the pararectal space (Fig. 12.17). The massive dissection of the tissues affected might facilitate damage to sympathetic fibers stemming from the sympathetic trunk at the level of the coccyx, to be anatomized with the lower hypogastric plexus, between the hypogastric nervous fibers cranially and the splanchnic nerves caudally.[26]

Should this incident occur, the vesical and rectal sensitivity might be affected, mainly as a loss of the sensation of vesical filling, if the dissection requires further preparation of the tissues of the hypogastric sacral fascia and the extension, laterally, up to the pelvic wall, the possible damage caused to the nervous fibers of S3 and S4 will determine vesical failure. This will be expressed with a hypotonic bladder and the impossible spontaneous micturition.[27]

The sacral roots originating in S3 and S4 provide fibers that shape also the pudendal nerve, which innervates the anal and the urethral sphincter. Damage to such fibers might seriously affect the functionality of the sphincter.[28]

The damage to the hypogastric plexus (*see* Figs. 12.12 and 12.13) might lead, respectively, to the extension of the damage to the plexus, namely the hypoesthe-sia of the vaginal sheath, the loss of the sensation of vesical and rectal filling, to the vesical atonia.[28]

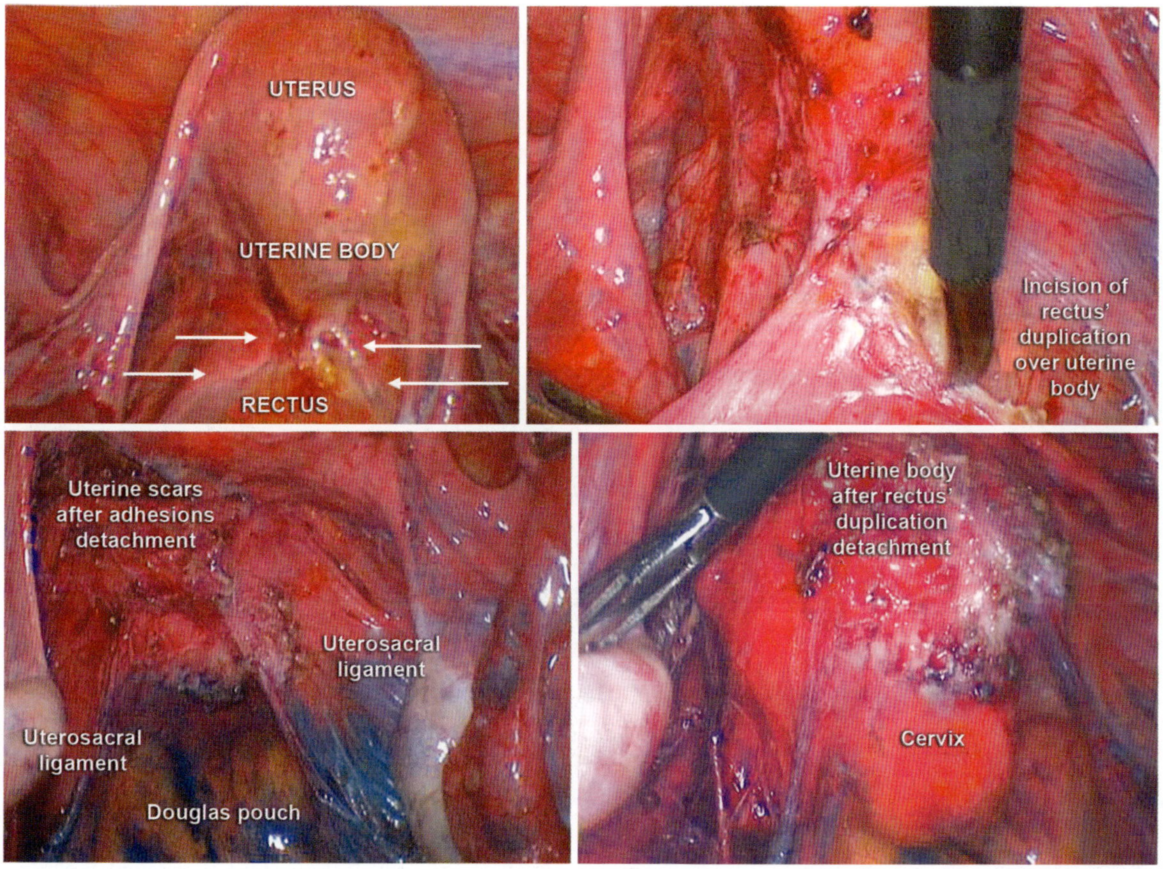

Fig. 12.16: A deep endometriosis laparoscopic treatment: from the upper left box in clockwise fashion it is clearly detectable a tilting of the rectum on the body of the uterus, which is cut and separated into its duplication and out of the uterosacral ligaments to expose the uterine cervix with the upper bloody area.

The damage of 2–3 cm that runs superior to the plexus determines the hypoesthesia of the cervix and of the dorsal vaginal sheath. Another 1–2 cm of further damage might lead to the loss of the rectal and vesical filling sensation. Moreover, the damage of further 3 cm caudally to the Douglas pouch could lead to rectal and vesical atonia.[29]

CONCLUSION

Latest technological advances have revolutionized the realm of patient care and led to remarkable changes in the nature of anatomical knowledge required by a clinician. It has therefore become necessary to review teaching strategies to ensure that these newly desired learning outcomes are addressed. With the advent of modern surgical techniques and operative armamentarium, as laparoscopy or robotics, the nature of living anatomy required for a medical student has changed immensely. There has also been an increasing tendency to replace the hours of dissection with prosected specimens, anatomical models and simulated procedures as a result of the dearth of conventional learning resources including cadaveric material, and the reduction in time allot-ted to anatomy teaching. It has been suggested that this reduced attention to anatomy has resulted in a situation, in many medical schools, where undergraduate education in anatomy is below the minimum necessary for safe medical practice.[30]

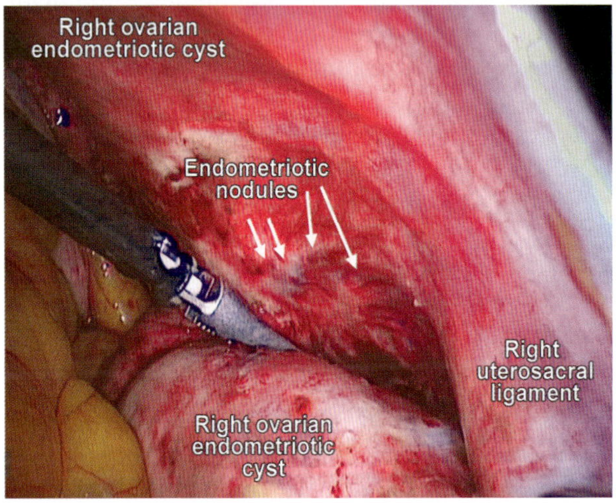

Fig. 12.17: A laparoscopic image of deep endometriosis prior to laparoscopic treatment: under the body of the uterus is clearly detectable a wide endometriotic nodularity directed to pararectal space.

The changing trends in modern gynecological surgery indicate a sharp decrease in percentage of abdominal and vaginal hysterectomies and increasing numbers of laparoscopic and robotic procedures.[31]

For entry into these spaces and maneuvers to circumvent anatomic pitfalls unique to each region, laparoscopic and robotic surgical techniques need to be always performed during these minimally invasive approaches. So a great emphasis needs to be placed on vascular abdominal–pelvic tree (Fig. 12.18) and especially on the course of hypogastric artery and its two branches (Fig. 12.19).

As mentioned above, it is difficult to foresee to what extent damage to the pelvic nerves correlated to a gynecological laparoscopy involving the retro-

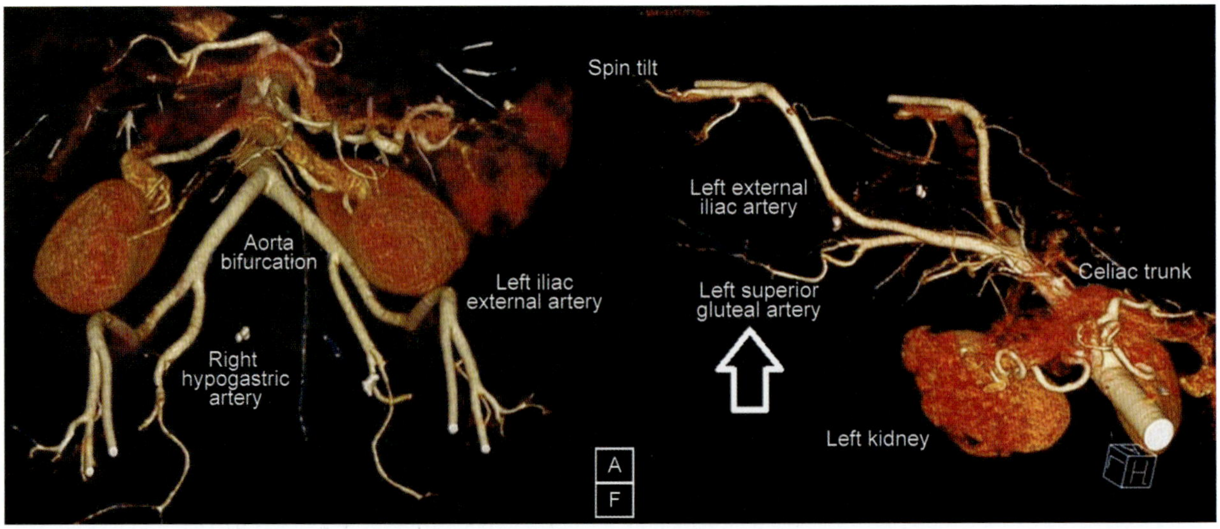

Fig. 12.18: Two angio-tomographic computerized images showing the abdominal–pelvic vascular tree, with great emphasis to aorta bifurcation and to left superior gluteal artery (indicated by a white arrow).

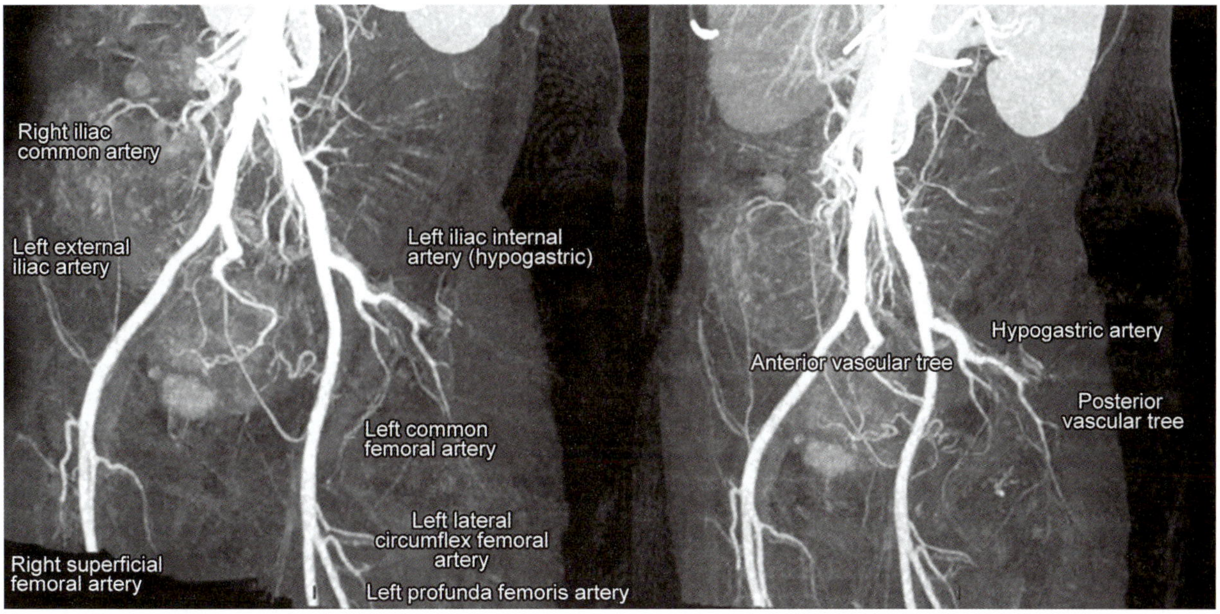

Fig. 12.19: Two angio-tomographic computerized images showing the pelvic vascular tree, with the two iliac internal and external arteries; on the right, they are showed the anterior and the posterior tree of left hypogastric artery.

peritoneal pelvic space,[32,33] may influence the pelvic sensitivity and innervations,[33] which entails the normal processes of sexual intercourse, micturition and defecation.[34,35]

In addition, at the beginning of each advanced laparoscopy, it is mandatory to review the course of the ureter through the retroperitoneum as well as common sites and types of ureteral injury, since it is still one of the most common injuries in gynecologic surgery.[36,37] Injuries typically occur at the pelvic brim and the area where the uterine artery crosses over the ureter.[38]

Finally, another problem has not been tackled to date, namely the association between patients treated laparoscopically for retroperitoneal conditions and delivery mode. In recent years, the number of operative laparoscopies involving retroperitoneal spaces has increased considerably, but the link between nerve sparing and delivery has not yet been established.[31,36,39]

The percentage of cesarean sections after these surgery procedures has never been calculated; neither after some radical pelvic surgeries, nor on pregnancies occurred after these procedures.[40-42]

Some laparoscopic procedures are becoming more frequent in everyday endoscopic surgery[43,44] and in near future we might expect further studies to come out, offering data on the analysis of lymph vascular complications, nerve damages and delivery outcome after advanced retroperitoneal laparoscopy.

REFERENCES

1. Fritsch H, Lienemann A, Brenner E, et al. Clinical anatomy of the pelvic floor. Adv Anat Embryol Cell Biol. 2004;175(III-IX):1-64.
2. Yabuki Y, Sasaki H, Hatakeyama N, et al. Discrepancies between classic anatomy and modern gynecologic surgery on pelvic connective tissue structure: harmonization of those concepts by collaborative cadaver dissection. Am J Obstet Gynecol. 2005;193(1):7-15.
3. Park YH, Yang SC, Park ST, et al. Laparoscopic reconstructive surgery is superior to vaginal reconstruction in the pelvic organ prolapse. Int J Med Sci. 2014;11(11):1082-8.
4. Galczynski K, Nowakowski L, Romanek-Piva K, et al. Laparoscopic mesh procedures for the treatment of pelvic organ prolapse-review of the literature. Ginekol Pol. 2014;85(12):950-4.
5. Weng SS, Liu CY. Laparoscopic pelvic floor repair using polypropylene mesh. Taiwan J Obstet Gynecol. 2008;47(3):312-7.
6. Maas CP, Kenter GG, Trimbos JB, et al. Anatomical basis for nerve-sparing radical hysterectomy: immunohistochemical study of the pelvic autonomic nerves. Acta Obstet Gynecol Scand. 2005;84(9):868-74.
7. Kim HS, Kim K, Ryoo SB, et al. Conventional versus nerve-sparing radical surgery for cervical cancer: a meta-analysis. J Gynecol Oncol. 2015;26(2):100-10.
8. Fröhlich B, Hötzinger H, Fritsch H. Tomographical anatomy of the pelvis, pelvic floor, and related structures. Clin Anat. 1997;10(4):223-30.
9. Shekarriz B, Upadhyay J, Jewett MA. Nerve-sparing retroperitoneal lymphadenectomy using hydro-jet dissection: initial experience. J Endourol. 2004;18(3):273-6.

10. Kihara K. Nerve-sparing retroperitoneal lymph node dissection: control mechanism, technique for nerve-sparing and reconstruction. Int J Urol. 2000; 7(Suppl):S52-5.
11. Maneo A, Sideri M, Scambia G, et al. Simple conization and lymphadenectomy for the conservative treatment of stage IB1 cervical cancer. An Italian experience. Gynecol Oncol 2011;123(3):557-60.
12. Speiser D, Mangler M, Köhler C, et al. Fertility outcome after radical vaginal trachelectomy: a prospective study of 212 patients. Int J Gynecol Cancer 2011;21(9):1635-9.
13. Xu L, Sun FQ, Wang ZH. Radical trachelectomy versus radical hysterectomy for the treatment of early cervical cancer: a systematic review. Acta Obstet Gynecol Scand. 2011;90(11):1200-9.
14. Fritsch H, Zwierzina M, Riss P. Accuracy of concepts in female pelvic floor anatomy: facts and myths! World J Urol. 2012;30(4):429-35.
15. Fritsch H. Topography and subdivision of the pelvic connective tissue in human fetuses and in the adult. Surg Radiol Anat. 1994;16(3):259-65.
16. Ceccaroni M, Clarizia R, Alboni C, et al. Laparoscopic nerve-sparing transperitoneal approach for endometriosis infiltrating the pelvic wall and somatic nerves: anatomical considerations and surgical technique. Surg Radiol Anat. 2010;32(6):601-4.
17. De Nardi P, Osman N, Ferrari S, et al. Laparoscopic treatment of deep pelvic endometriosis with rectal involvement. Dis Colon Rectum. 2009;52(3): 419-24.
18. Kavallaris A, Banz C, Chalvatzas N, et al. Laparoscopic nerve-sparing surgery of deep infiltrating endometriosis: description of the technique and patients' outcome. Arch Gynecol Obstet. 2011;284(1): 131-5.
19. Thomas M, Au-Yong IT. Anatomy of the female pelvis. BMJ. 2011;343:d7823.
20. Fritsch H, Hötzinger H. Tomographical anatomy of the pelvis, visceral pelvic connective tissue, and its compartments. Clin Anat. 1995;8(1):17-24.
21. Kyo S, Kato T, Nakayama K. Current concepts and practical techniques of nerve-sparing laparoscopic radical hysterectomy. Eur J Obstet Gynecol Reprod Biol. 2016;207:80-8.
22. Kavallaris A, Zygouris D, Dafopoulos A, et al. Nerve sparing radical hysterectomy in early stage cervical cancer. Latest developments and review of the literature. Eur J Gynaecol Oncol. 2015;36: 5-9.
23. Schmeiser G, Putz R. The anatomy and function of the pelvic floor. Radiologe. 2000;40(5):429-36.
24. Volpi E, Ferrero A, Sismondi P. Laparoscopic identification of pelvic nerves in patients with deep infiltrating endometriosis. Surg Endosc. 2004;18(7): 1109-12.
25. Long Y, Yao DS, Pan XW, et al. Clinical efficacy and safety of nerve-sparing radical hysterectomy for cervical cancer: a systematic review and meta-analysis. PLoS One. 2014;9(4):e94116.
26. Chen L, Zhang WN, Zhang SM, et al. Effect of laparoscopic nerve-sparing radical hysterectomy on bladder function, intestinal function recovery and quality of sexual life in patients with cervical carcinoma. Asian Pac J Cancer Prev. 2014;15(24): 10971-5.
27. Strohbehn K. Normal pelvic floor anatomy. Obstet Gynecol Clin North Am. 1998;25(4):683-705.
28. Rendón GJ, Echeverri L, Echeverri F, et al. Outpatient laparoscopic nerve-sparing radical hysterectomy: a feasibility study and analysis of perioperative outcomes. Gynecol Oncol. 2016;143(2):352-6.
29. Liu Z, Li X, Tao Y, et al. Clinical efficacy and safety of laparoscopic nerve-sparing radical hysterectomy for locally advanced cervical cancer. Int J Surg. 2016; 25:54-8.
30. Kumar PA, Norrish M, Heming T. Laparoscopic surgery recording as an adjunct to conventional modalities of teaching gross anatomy. Sultan Qaboos Univ Med. J 2011;11(4):497-502.
31. Svets M, Falcone T. Update on gynecologic surgery. The 13th annual Pelvic Anatomy and Gynecologic Surgery Symposium. Womens Health (Lond Engl). 2011;7(2):159-61.
32. Xue Z, Zhu X, Teng Y. Comparison of nerve-sparing radical hysterectomy and radical hysterectomy: a systematic review and meta-analysis. Cell Physiol Biochem. 2016;38(5):1841-50.
33. Puntambekar SP, Lawande A, Puntambekar S, et al. Nerve-sparing radical hysterectomy made easy by laparoscopy. J Minim Invasive Gynecol. 2014;21(5): 732.
34. Park NY, Chong GO, Hong DG, et al. Oncologic results and surgical morbidity of laparoscopic nerve-sparing radical hysterectomy in the treatment of FIGO stage IB cervical cancer: long-term follow-up. Int J Gynecol Cancer. 2011;21(2):355-62.
35. Chen C, Li W, Li F, et al. Classical and nerve-sparing radical hysterectomy: an evaluation of the nerve trauma in cardinal ligament. Gynecol Oncol. 2012;125(1):245-51.
36. Frankman EA, Wang L, Bunker CH, et al. Lower urinary tract injury in women in the United States, 1979-2006. Am J Obstet Gynecol. 2010;202(5):495. e1-5.
37. Hove LD, Bock J, Christoffersen JK, et al. Analysis of 136 ureteral injuries in gynecological and obstetrical surgery from completed insurance claims. Acta Obstet Gynecol Scand. 2010;89(1):82-6.
38. Han CM, Tan HH, Kay N, et al. Outcome of laparoscopic repair of ureteral injury: follow-up of twelve cases. J Minim Invasive Gynecol. 2012;19(1):68-75.
39. de Andrade Vieira M, Cintra GF, dos Reis R, et al. Laparoscopic vaginal-assisted nerve-sparing radical trachelectomy. J Minim Invasive Gynecol. 2016;23(3): 297.
40. Kim JH, Park JY, Kim DY, et al. Fertility-sparing laparoscopic radical trachelectomy for young women with early stage cervical cancer. BJOG. 2010;117(3): 340-7.

41. Abu-Rustum NR, Sonoda Y, Black D, et al. Fertility-sparing radical abdominal trachelectomy for cervical carcinoma: technique and review of the literature. Gynecol Oncol. 2006;103(3):807-13.
42. Abu-Rustum NR, Sonoda Y. Fertility-sparing surgery in early-stage cervical cancer: indications and applications. J Natl Compr Canc Netw. 2010;8(12): 1435-8.
43. Sakuragi N, Todo Y, Kudo M, et al. A systematic nerve-sparing radical hysterectomy technique in invasive cervical cancer for preserving postsurgical bladder function. Int J Gynecol Cancer. 2005;15(2): 389-97.
44. van Gent MD, Romijn LM, van Santen KE, et al. Nerve-sparing radical hysterectomy versus conventional radical hysterectomy in early-stage cervical cancer. A systematic review and meta-analysis of survival and quality of life. Maturitas. 2016;94:30-8.

KIEL SCH•OL

13 of Gynaecological Endoscopy

Suturing and Ligature Techniques at Laparoscopy

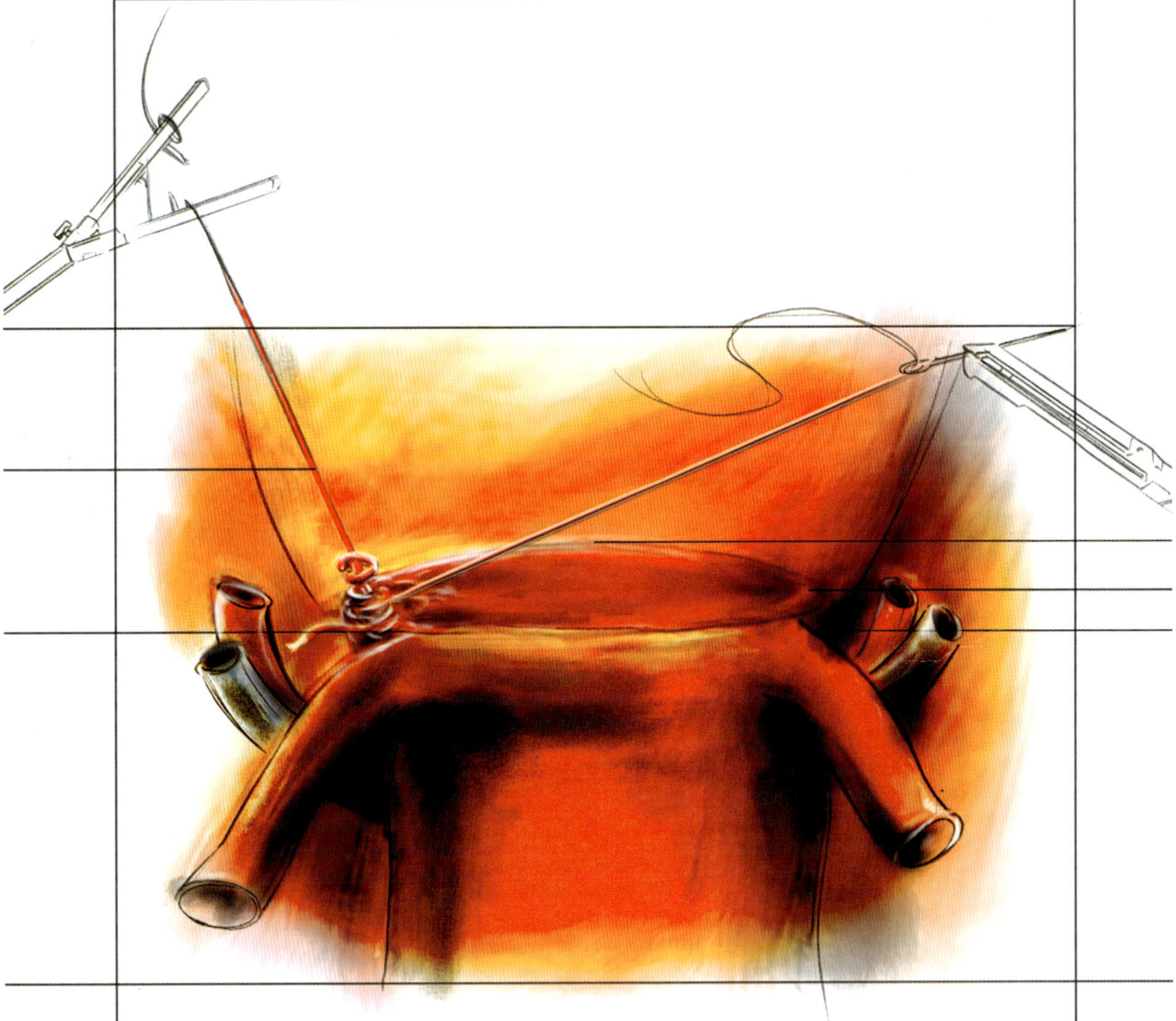

Chapter 13

Suturing and Ligature Techniques at Laparoscopy

Liselotte Mettler, Goentje Peters, Tamer Seckin, Ibrahim Alkatout

INTRODUCTION

Ligatures and suturing techniques represent a safe; and, in many cases, the only method of hemostasis even in endoscopic surgery. In many cases suturing techniques are better suited than thermal methods. Various suture materials, applicators and needle holders with straight, sharp, curved, blunt and curved needles, such as the ski-needle, have been developed for that purpose.

A skill score of 10 for various surgical modalities conventional laparotomy requires a score of 2, microsurgery a score of 4, laparoscopy a score of 6 and laparoscopic suturing a score of 8, while robotic laparoscopic suturing returns to the skill level of general laparoscopic surgery with a score of 6.

Therefore, never get frustrated but understand that laparoscopic suturing requires training.[1-6]

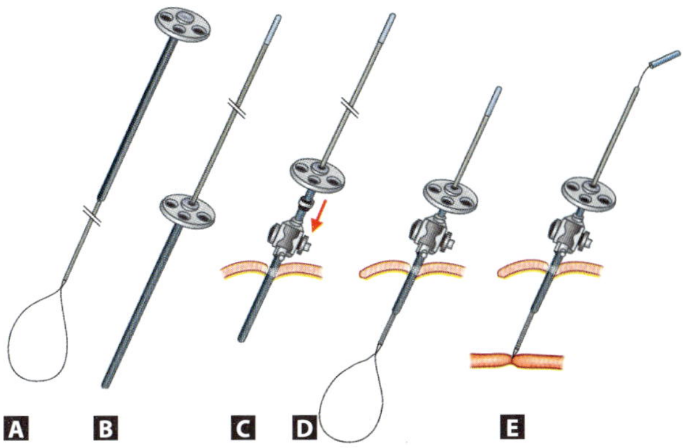

Figs. 13.1A to E: Roeder loop with applicator and illustration of the technique. (A) Loop applicator with partially introduced Roeder loop; (B) Fully introduced Roeder loop; (C) Roeder loop in the abdominal cavity (still completely in the applicator sleeve); (D) Roeder loop in the abdominal cavity (partially introduced); (E) Tightly pulled Roeder knot.

HEMOSTASIS BY LOOP LIGATURES

The sliding loop developed by H Roeder (1866–1918) around the end of the last century for pediatric tonsillectomy in ear, nose, and throat (ENT) is an important addition to endoscopic intra-abdominal surgery. It is marketed in sterile packing as ETHI-Binder® by Ethicon or Endo-Loop® by Autosuture.

In 1976, Semm introduced it with an applicator for the 5 mm ancillary trocar. Figures 13.1A to E show the Roeder loop in a 3 mm applicator. It is introduced into the abdomen to ligate omental or adnexal bleedings. Afterward, the ligature is cut and the projecting tissue resected. It is essential to grasp the target tissue freely and pull it through the loop. The Roeder loops are available as catgut and polydioxanone (PDS) loops and are also made by other companies, e.g. by Serag-Wiesner as Serag-Binder® (safety knots in monofilament material). In valveless trocars, it can also be inserted without an applicator.

The partly electrically powered loops produced by Karl Storz, Brenner Medical and LiNA Medical are ideal loops to cut the cervix from the uterus in cases of laparoscopic subtotal hysterectomies (LSH).

HEMOSTASIS BY ENDOLIGATURE OR ENDOSUTURE AND EXTRACORPOREAL KNOTTING

In many cases it is convenient to ligate vascular bundles, adhesion bundles and similar structures with sling ligatures. Timewise it is worthwhile to tie the vascular omental and intestinal adhesions before cutting because searching for bleeders later can be time-consuming and associated with much blood loss. Primarily, an 80 cm long Ethi-Endoligature® with a plastic knot pusher by Ethicon is used as a ligature.

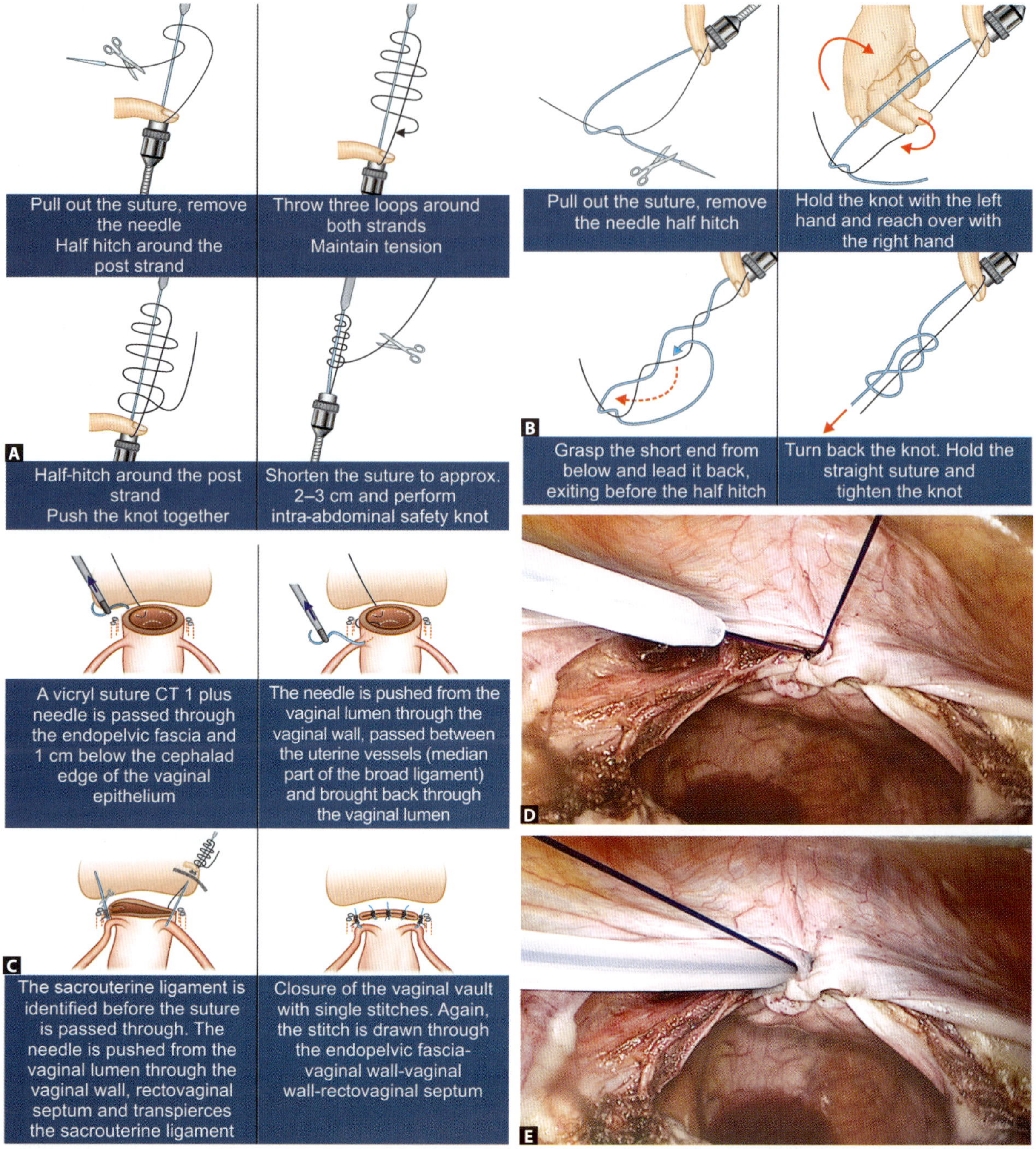

Figs. 13.2A to E: Extracorporeal knotting. (A) Roeder knot; (B) von Leffern knot; (C) Vaginal closure for descent prevention (Te Linde adapted by van Herendael); (D) After having formed the knot extracorporeally, it is pushed down with the plastic knot pusher; (E) To tighten the knot, the other end of the thread is held with some tension while the knot pusher is pressed onto the knot firmly.

As an endosuture, it has a 3 cm long and 0.8 mm thick needle. The endosuture with extracorporeal knotting has a 2.5 and 3.5 cm long sharp needle as well as a 2.5 cm round needle. It is supplied with a suture applicator and a 3 mm trocar in case of using a valved trocar or use a 5-mm trocar without a valve. After taking a purse-string suture, the needle is cut; extracorporeal knots are fashioned and pushed down in the usual way with the plastic pusher (Figs.13.1 and 13.2).

To push the knot, the applicator is pulled up. When it is pushed again into the 5 mm trocar, the plastic tube pushes the knot into the abdominal cavity. The loop is tightened under vision and the wound edges are adapted (e.g., the wound edges of the ovary). Cutting scissors are inserted in place of the 5 mm needle holder to cut the thread. The thread must be long enough to be able to fashion extracorporeal knots outside.

HEMOSTASIS BY ENDOSUTURE WITH INTRACORPOREAL KNOTTING

For intracorporeal knotting, a straight or curved needle with different suture calibers is used. For microsurgical interventions, such as end-to-end anastomosis of the tube, 4-0 to 6-0 sutures are used otherwise 1-0 is adequate. Figures 13.3 A to F show the six steps for making the intracorporeal cross knots with or without a needle. Figure 13.4 demonstrates how the long end of a thread, originally knotted extracorporeally, is wrapped around the needle holder twice while the needle holder is aiming for the short end of the thread to perform an additional, intracorporeal safety knot.

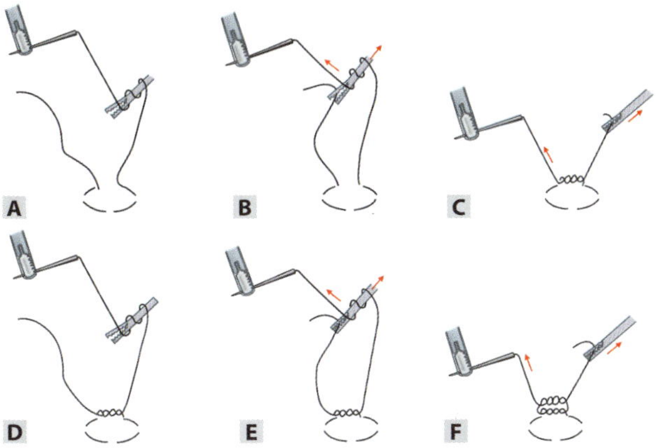

Figs. 13.3A to F: Illustration of intracorporeal knots as double surgical knots in six steps. (A) Wrapping the long end of the thread twice around the needle holder; (B) Holding the short end to form the first surgical knot; (C) Tightening the first surgical knot; (D) Wrapping the long end of the thread for the second time; (E) Holding again the short end to form the second surgical knot; (F) Tightening the second surgical knot.

Among many other intracorporeal suturings, the baseball suture is especially suitable to compress wounds (e.g., after enucleation of huge ovarian cysts). Figures 13.5A to R show the stepwise closure of an ovarian wound caused by an enucleation of a dermoid cyst. Due to this technique of suturing the size of the wound is minimized and along with it the risk of immediate and later bleeding. In addition, the occurrence of adhesions is reduced since the wound is closed toward the surrounding tissue.

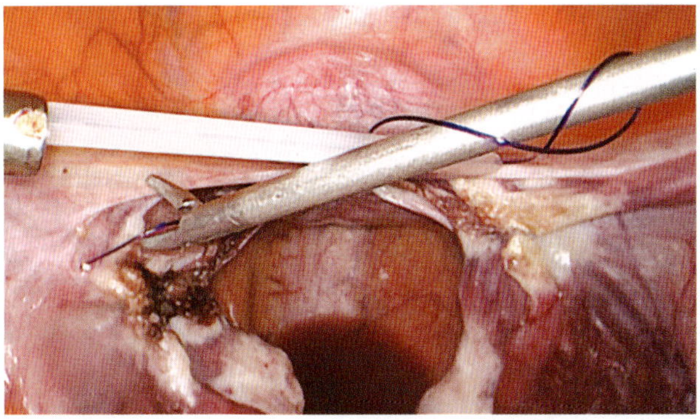

Fig. 13.4: The long end of a thread, originally knotted extracorporeally, is wrapped around the needle holder twice while the needle holder is aiming for the short end of the thread to perform an additional intracorporeal safety knot.

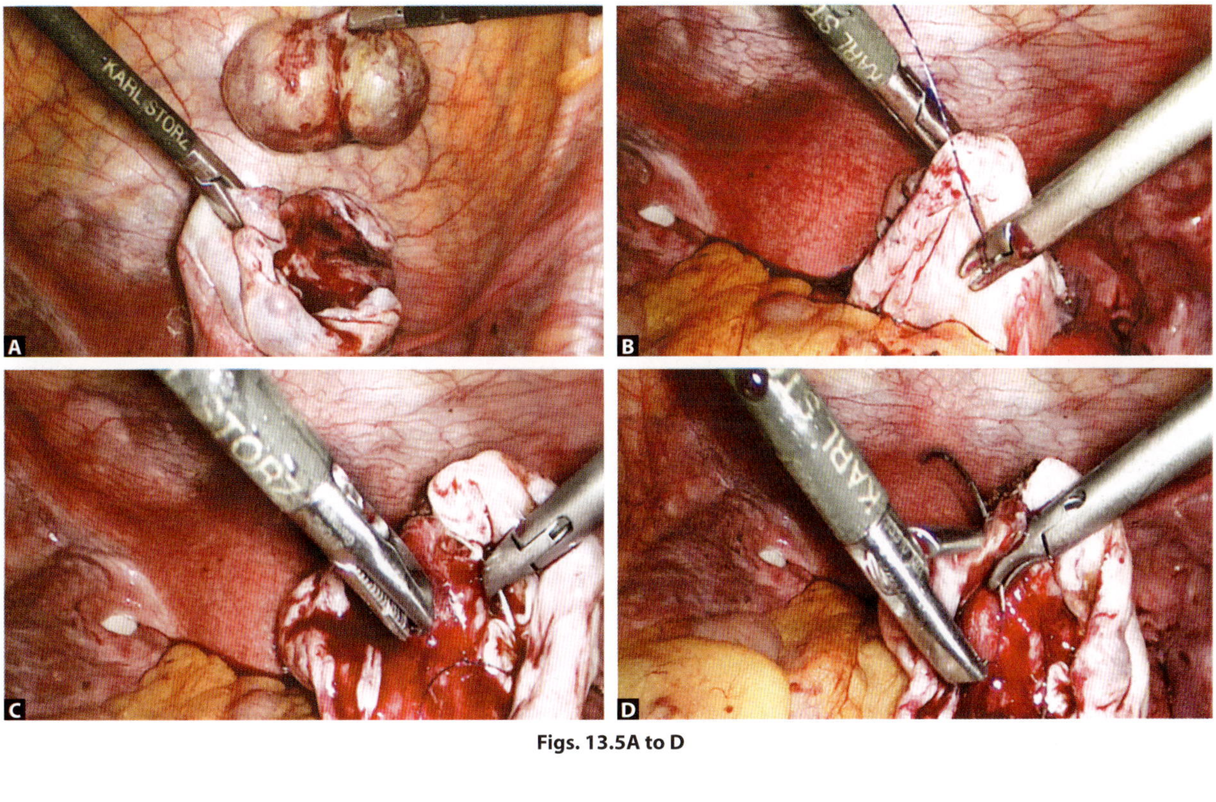

Figs. 13.5A to D

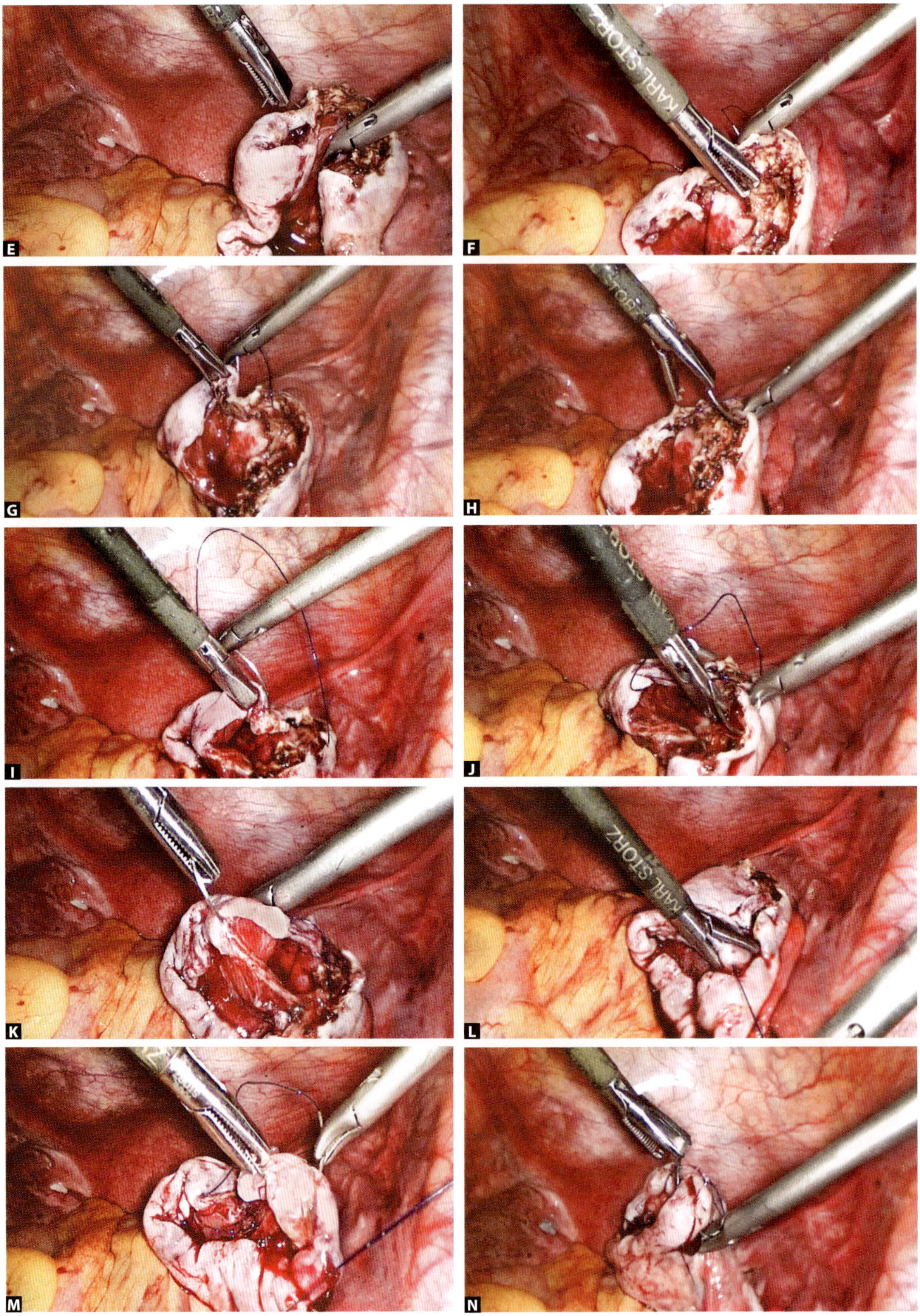

Figs. 13.5E to N

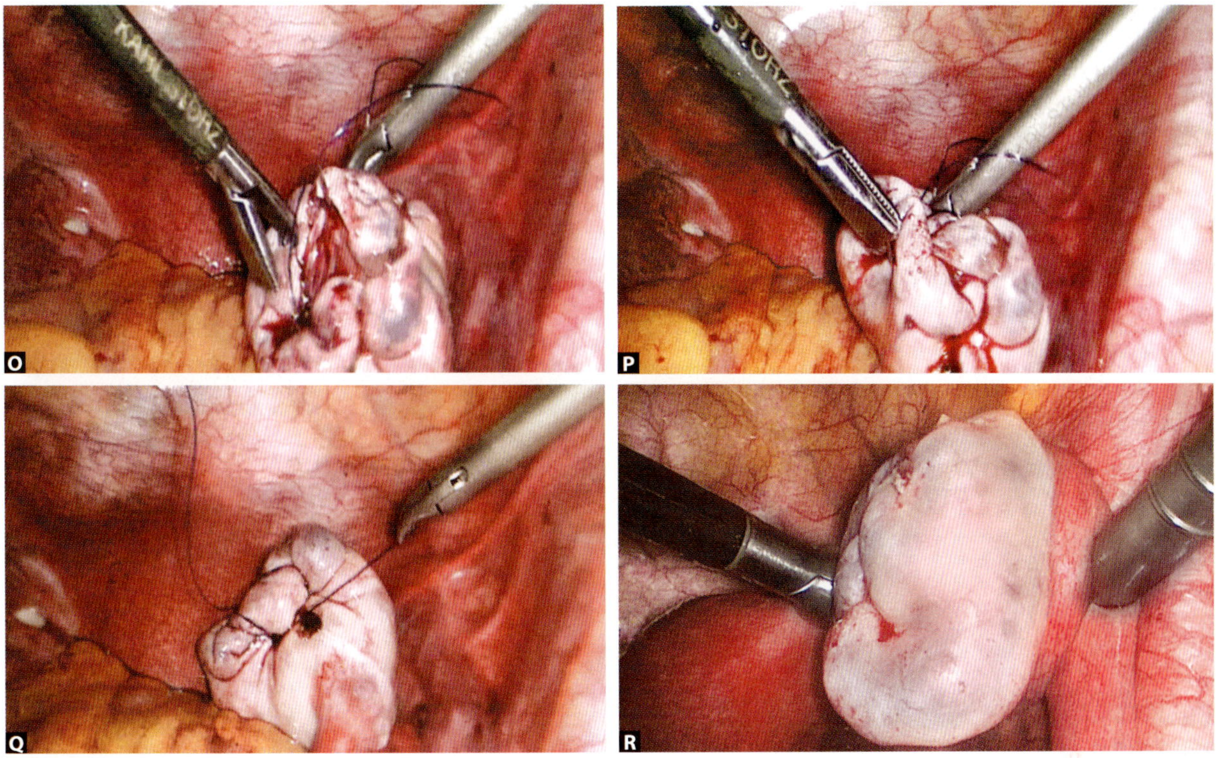

Figs. 13.5A to R: Baseball suture: (A) Enucleation of a dermoid cyst of the right ovary, leaving behind as wound a relatively large, thin layer of ovarian tissue; (B) First stitch of the running suture, starting backhand from outward to inward of the ovarian surface; (C to P) Cording up the tissue by continuing with a stitch in the depth of the wound, followed by stepwise stitches from out to inward of the wound surface, alternating the opponent margins, ending with a stitch outward close to the start of the suture where the other end of the thread can be seen; (Q) Forming an intracorporeal knot with the two ends of the thread; (R) As a result of this kind of suturing the original round shape of the ovary is restored, but more importantly, the surface of the ovarian wound is completely sunk in so that it is less likely to form adhesions with the surrounding tissue (peritoneum, bowels, uterus). Furthermore, the compression that is caused by cording up the wound prevents it from bleeding and forming coagula.

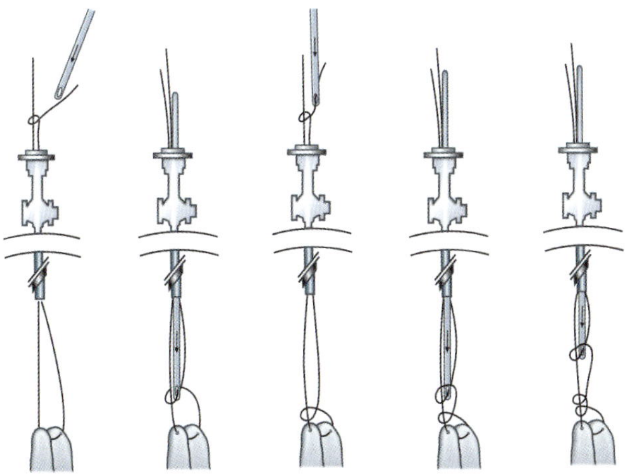

Fig. 13.6: Clark knot pusher for making three extracorporeal half hitches that are pushed in.

HEMOSTASIS BY SUTURE AND TYING KNOT WITH HALF HITCH

The Clark knot pusher is used for this (Fig. 13.6). With both the extracorporeal threads a half-hitch is fashioned and the knot is then pushed down.

NEEDLES AND SUTURES

The correct selection of the appropriate suture is essential. Each surgical procedure requires specific needle configurations and needle-suture combinations.

The following set of suture exercises describes in easy steps the correct and incorrect handling of the needle. The pictures are taken from the suturing course of the "International Society of Gynecological Endoscopy" designed by Tamir Seckin and applied by Ornella Sissi, Alfonso Rosetti and Bruno Van Haerendahl (Figs. 13.7 to 13.17).

Needle Characteristics

- *Handling characteristics*: The ideal needle should be of bicurve design. Different sites require different needle sizes.
- *The tip*: A tapered needle with a small cutting tip is ideal.
- *Diameter and profile of the needle*: The grip should be a well-matched, refined grip. Thicker

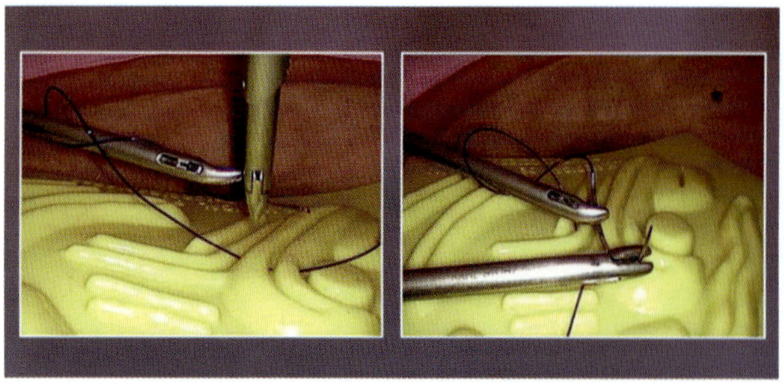

Fig. 13.7: Technique for intracorporeal knot tying.

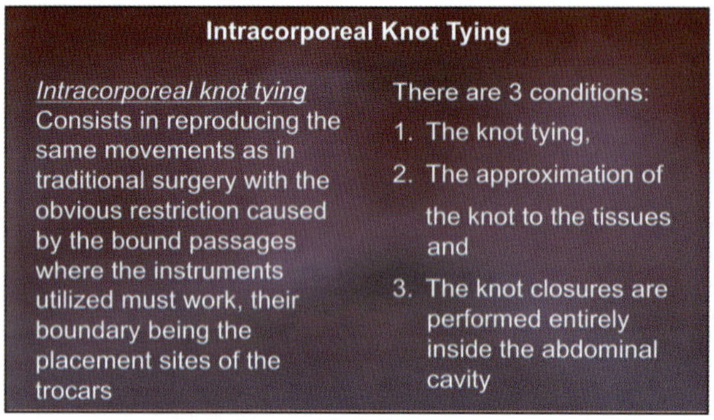

Fig. 13.8: Intracorporeal knot tying.

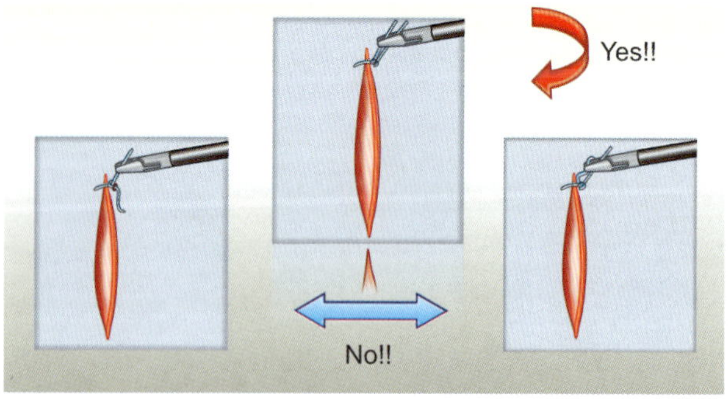

Fig. 13.9: Mistakes to avoid.

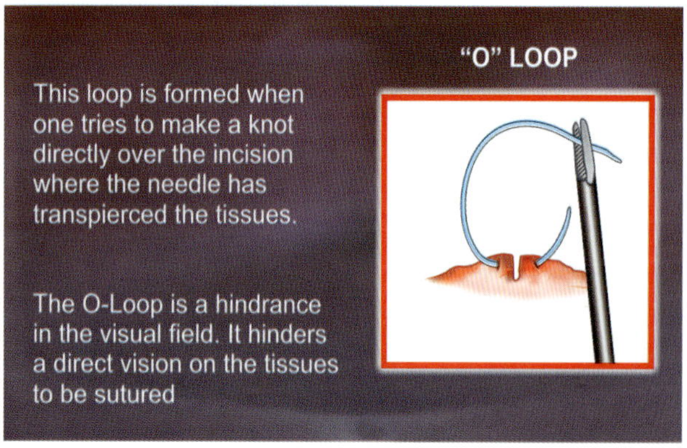

Fig. 13.10: Mistakes to avoid—"O" loop.

tissue layers require sturdier needles; more delicate tissues require smaller thinner needles.

The straight needle was earlier handled by the Semm needle holder. The straight round-bodied needle has limited use with friable tissue and can easily tear tissue at its point of entry.

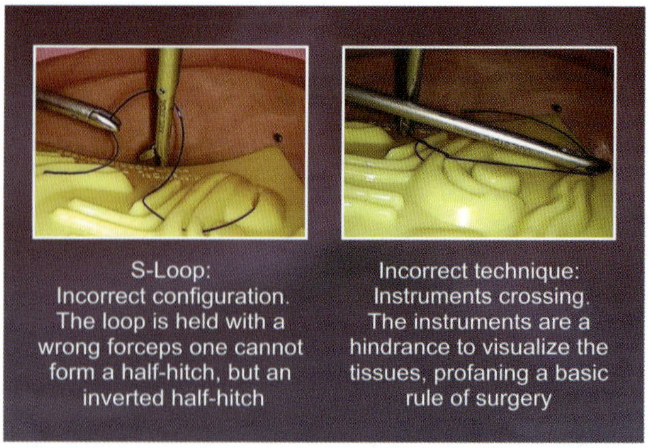

Fig. 13.11: Mistakes to avoid—incorrect configuration and technique.

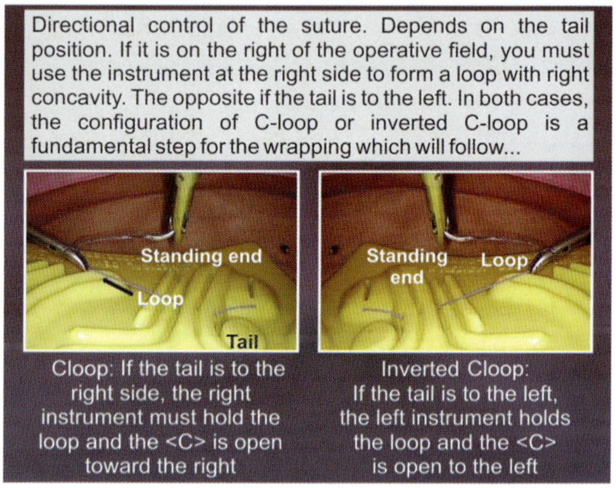

Fig. 13.12: Knot tying technique.

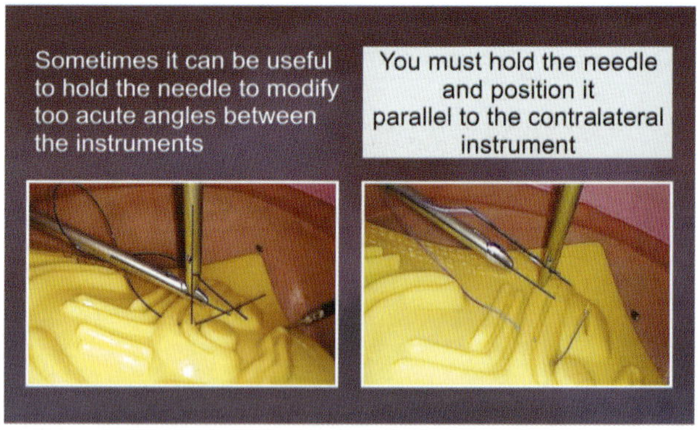

Fig. 13.13: Wrapping technique.

The ski-shaped needle (Fig. 13.18) is rounded near the slightly curved tip and triangular along the straight shaft. The needle is gripped along the triangular shaft and avoids the problem of swivel.

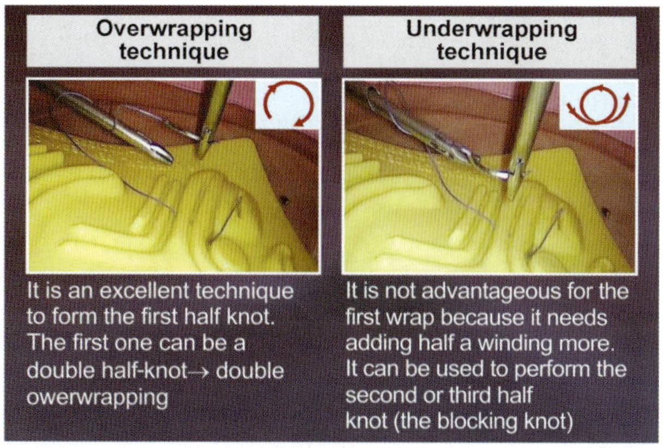

Fig. 13.14: Wrapping technique—overwrapping and underwrapping.

Improved "Ski" needles with flattened cross-section (Dundee) along the shaft can be easily erected by simply grasping them. The flat cross-section has the advantage of improved locking, which increases the fixation of the jaws.

The standard curved needle (Fig. 13.19) is a good alternative to the ski-needle; however, the needle can swivel during suturing.

Suture Characteristics

- Should have a favorable tissue response.
- Good handling/memory characteristics: 2-0 and 3-0 are easiest to handle and tie a secure knot.

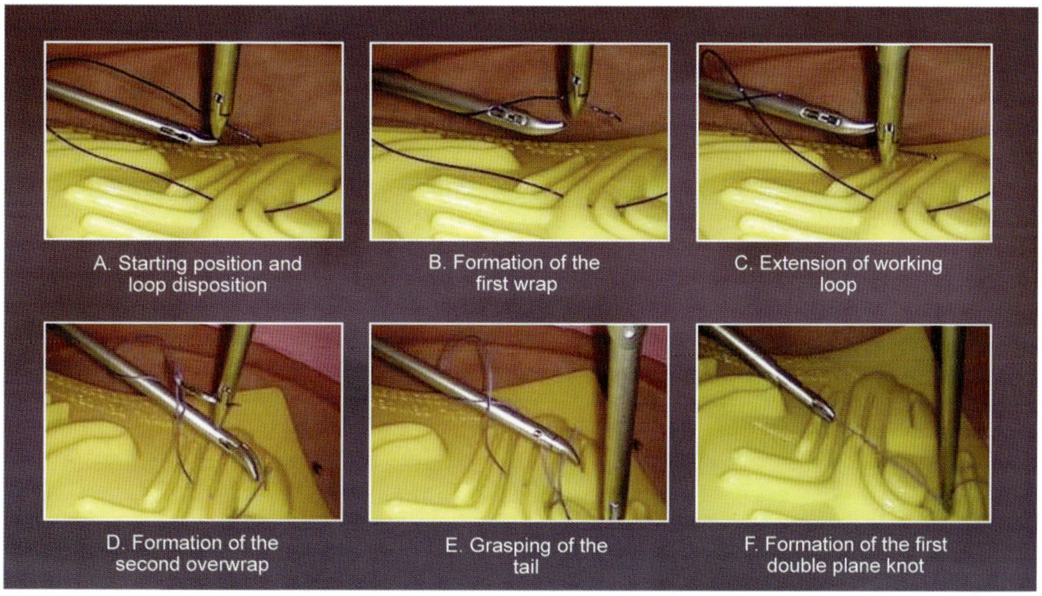

Fig. 13.15: Surgeon's knot: (A) Starting position and loop disposition; (B) Formation of the first wrap; (C) Extension of working loop; (D) Formation of the second overwrap; (E) Grasping of the tail; (F) Formation the first double plane knot.

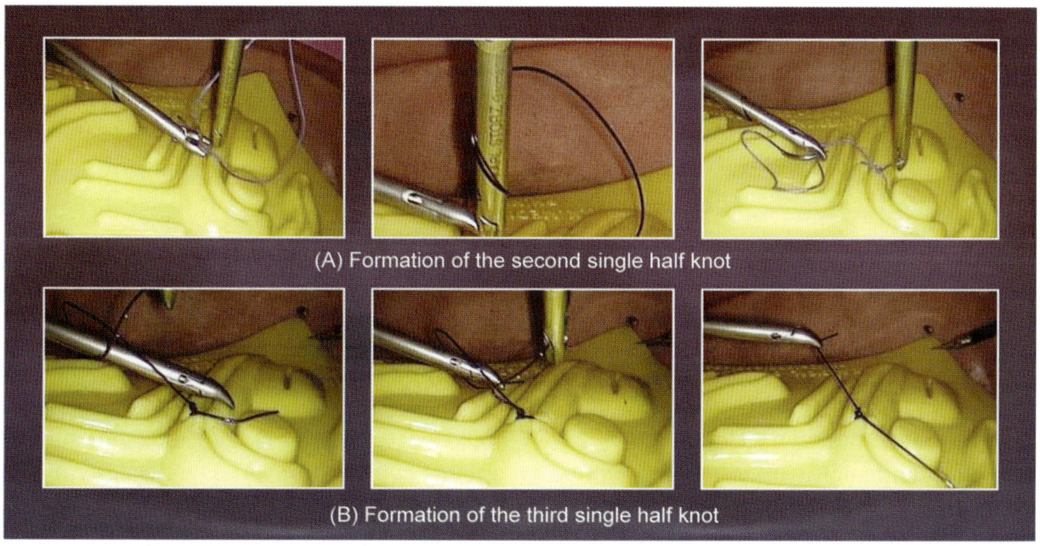

Fig. 13.16: Surgeon's knot: (A) Formation of the second single half knot; (B) Formation of the third single half knot.

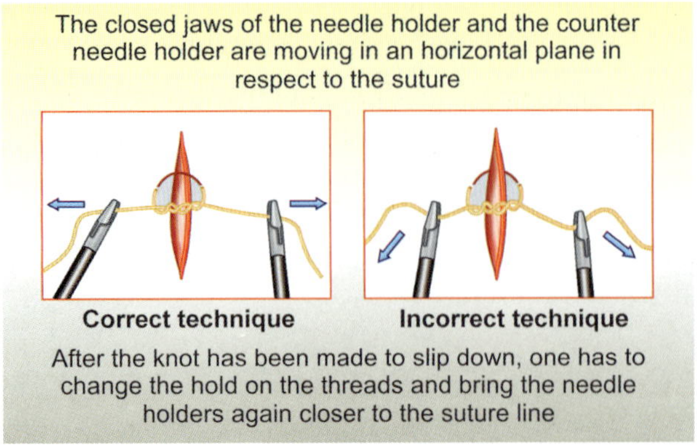

Fig. 13.17: Tightening technique.

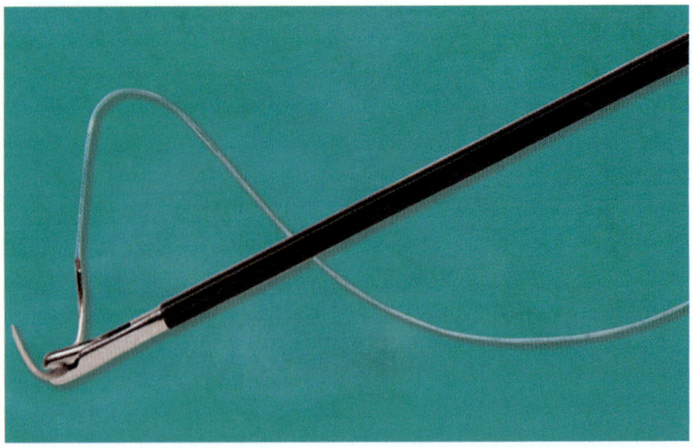

Fig. 13.19: Curved needle.

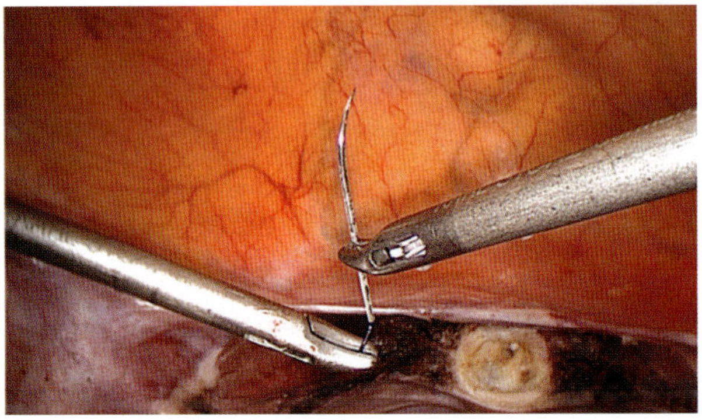

Fig. 13.18: Ski-shaped needle.

The Roeder knot has best results with chromic catgut, is not ideally used for PDS or polypropylene, but serves well for Vicryl.

- Polyfilament sutures should be used for intracorporeal interrupted or running sutures and specifically for intracorporeal knotting.
- Extracorporeal slip knots tied with silk and polyamide have been found to be less secure than equivalent knots tied with Dacron, lactomer and polydioxanone.
- Prelooped intracorporeal knots are available which render intracorporeal knotting an easy and rapid task to achieve.

Needle Holder

The primary role of the needle holder/driver is handling the needle, although suturing and tissue grasping are also part of its function.

- The preferred shape of the tip is a slightly spooning curvature.
- For grasping tissue and looping suture, the tip must be able to reach in almost any direction. This is best accomplished with an aggressively curved or angle tip (e.g., a flamingo beak-shaped tip).
- The jaws should be finely engineered to grasp fine sutures without slipping and have rounded edges to avoid accidental cutting of the suture as traction is applied.
- The dominant needle holder should have a lock that the surgeon can activate or inactivate at will.
- It should be strong and preferably have one moving jaw to reduce suture snagging.
- The lock on the nondominant needle holder should preferably be inactivated.
- Optimal laparoscopic bowel suturing, in terms of the accuracy of suture placement and the integrity of the suture line closure, can be obtained with a 40 degrees handle-to-shaft angle.

First-generation (Semm) Needle Holders: 5 mm and 3 mm

The standard Semm needle holder has handles at a right angle to the shaft and working jaws with a serrated surface. It provides secure manipulation of a straight round-bodied needle. These holders allow curved needles to swivel and, because of the orientation of the handle, the extent of the wrist motion during suturing is exaggerated.

Second-generation Needle Holders (Ethicon, Cook, Storz and Wolf)

Newer needle holders have different grasping mechanisms with improved jaw design and serrations (diamond-shaped). The handles are in line with the shaft or can be opened from any rotational angle (similar to Castro-viejo needle holders). These allow

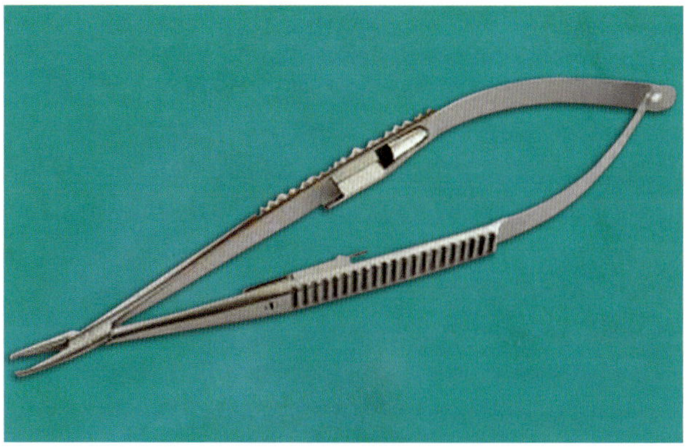

Fig. 13.20: Castroviejo needle holder.

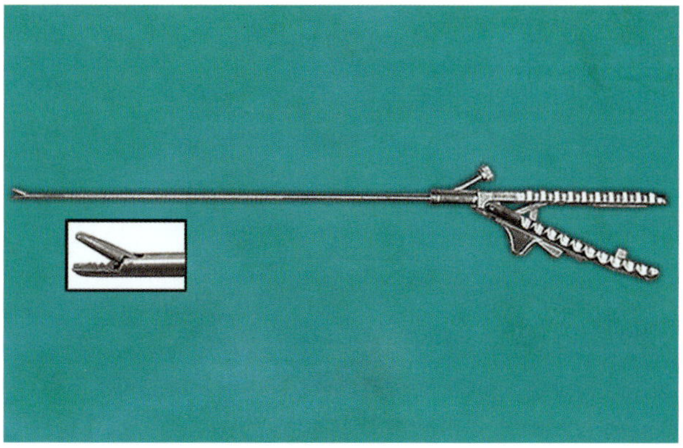

Fig. 13.21: Ethicon needle holder.

a more secure grasping of standard flattened needle shafts and have paved the way for the use of standard curved needles. Introduction of the curved needle requires the diameter of the larger 11 mm port. To improve the delicate handling of both the grip and the locking mechanism, classical and novel design features have been introduced. Figures 13.20 and 13.21 show an original Castro-viejo needle holder and a laparoscopic needle holder with a straight handle by Ethicon.

The most advanced mechanism created by Wolf involves telescopic locking, which functions like a ball point pen: one presses locks and the next releases the grip. Unfortunately, the mechanism cannot be disassembled, which hinders complete and easy cleaning.

The Cook curved needle holder (Fig. 13.22) has an altogether different jaw design, which automatically sets the curved needle in the upright position. It has the advantage of grasping the needle securely but suffers from being a bit awkward to regrasp the needle. However, only one needle position is possible with a particular type of Cook needle holder and there is difficulty with the internal handling of the suture material.

The needle holder by MBG (Gembloux, Belgium) probably has the firmest gripping of the holders available. Its principle is quite simple; it consists of a tube and a pushrod and two tungsten metal rings, which are simply pressed against each other. There are two major disadvantages to its design; it is difficult to tie a knot, because the tip is too long and the opening depth of the jaws is reduced due to the central rod.

Z Szabo and G Berci have designed two instruments: the parrot and the flamingo forceps, which permit excellent execution of internal suturing and knotting. Although the handling is not optimal, the congruently shaped jaws of the instruments facilitate grasping and positioning of needle and thread. The handle is designed like a Castro-viejo needle holder and can be opened from any rotational position. The axial shape enables rotation of the instrument 360 degrees, which allows the precise maneuvering necessary for laparoscopic suturing.

The best Storz needle holders have been designed by Charles Koh and are called the Koh needle holders. The tips point to the left and to the right for the right and the left needle holders, respectively, and the handpieces are slightly angled. A simple but very effective "hold-release" mechanism simplifies its function.

TIPS AND TRICKS

Loading the Needle

- First grasp the thread about an inch from the needle with the assisting grasper.
- Dangle it in a fashion so that the tip of the needle touches the tissue surface.
- The needle is rotated and pivoted until it lines up in the direction required.
- It is then grasped with the needle driver.
- Gripping at the junction of middle and proximal third of the shaft of the needle is best for good suturing.
- Optimal conditions for good suturing include a needle holding angle >90 degrees and an angle of needle insertion into tissue of 80–100 degrees. Figures 13.23 and 13.24 show a ski-shaped needle, held approximately in the middle at a 90 degrees angle so that the tissue, held steadily by a more profiled clamp, can be pierced at a 90 degrees angle also

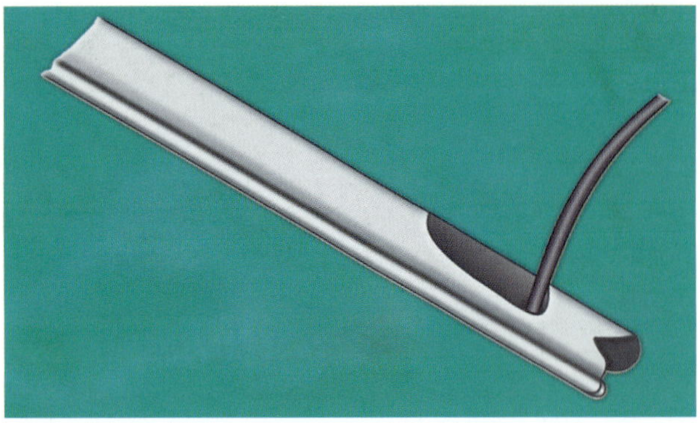

Fig. 13.22: Cook needle holder.

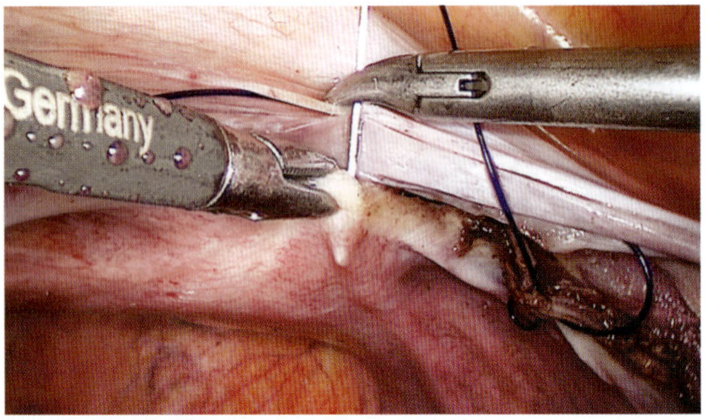

Fig. 13.23: Ski-shaped needle, held approximately in the middle at a 90° angle, while the tissue, held steadily by a more profiled clamp, can be pierced at 90° angle.

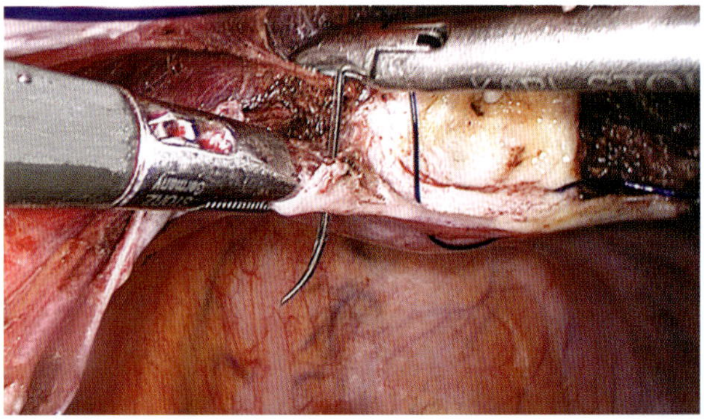

Fig. 13.24: One stitch in a running suture of the peritoneum to cover the cervical stump after having cut off the corpus uteri (LSH), also a ski-shaped needle, 90° angle of needle holder, needle and tissue.

- Tip to tip method: the tip of the scope is taken to the tip of the needle so that the exact direction is known.

Adjusting the Needle

Invariably, beginners attempt to reposition the needle by handling it back and forth between the grasper and needle driver, hoping to adjust it in the process. This technique might seem logical but it requires considerable skill and can become very frustrating.

- A better method is to hook the needle tip into the tissue just lightly enough to fix it, loosening the needle without actually letting it go, then pushing, pulling or rotating the needle driver to pivot the needle into the desired position. This requires skill and concentration.
- Another method is to grasp the needle lightly and brush it backward against the tissue. This movement will sweep the point of the needle exactly opposite of the direction it is pushed.
- Alternatively, the needle can be adjusted by holding the suture near the swaged end of the needle and maneuvering it till the needle is aligned perpendicular to the jaws.
- For erecting the needle, a preferred method is to place the needle on the serosal surface of the viscera, preferably the stomach. By pressing the upper jaw of the open needle holder over the needle, the needle will automatically erect into the correct position for suturing.
- After the ideal position has been reached, the grip on the needle is tightened to lock it into position.

CONCLUSION

Laparoscopic suturing courses from basics to experts for vertical and horizontal suturing, including hands-on training, are offered today all around the world. Laboratory-based practice of basic and advanced laparoscopic suturing can be obtained on dry modules, animal modules and in cadaveric surgery. The advice of our teacher Kurt Semm, that laparoscopic suturing is essential, has been accepted by the endoscopic surgical community. Particularly robotic surgery also includes various suturing training modules. The European Academy of Gynaecological Surgery, American Association of Gynecologic Laparoscopists (AAGL) and the International Society for Gynecologic Endoscopy (ISGE) run continuous programs in laparoscopic suturing. Modern automatic suturing devices have not yet replaced conventional laparoscopic suturing.[7-9]

REFERENCES

1. Berguer R. Forkey DL, Smith WD. The effect of laparoscopic instrument working angle on surgeons' upper extremity workload. Surg Endosc. 2001;15(9): 1027-9.

2. Bhatia P, John SJ, Deed JPS. Step by Step Art of Suturing. New Delhi; Jaypee Brothers Medical Publishers (P) Ltd; 2005.
3. Emam TA, Hanna G, Cuschierei A. Ergonomic principles of task alignment, visual display and direction of execution of laparoscopic bowel suturing. Surg Endosc. 2002;16(2):267-71.
4. Emam TA, Hanna GB, Kimber C, et al. Effect of intracorporeal-extracorporeal instrument length ratio on endoscopic task performance and surgeon movements. Arch Surg. 2000;135(1):62-5; discussion 66.
5. Frede T, Stock C, Renner C, et al. Geometry of laparoscopic suturing and knotting techniques. J Endourol. 1999;13(3):191-8.
6. Joice P, Hanna GB, Cuschieri A. Ergonomic evaluation of laparoscopic bowel suturing. Am J Surg. 1998; 176(4):373-8.
7. Di Saverio S, Birindelli A, Mandrioli M, et al. Intracorporeal anastomoses in emergency laparoscopic colorectal surgery from a series of 59 cases: where and how to do it—a technical note and video. Colorectal Dis. 2017;19(4):O103-7.
8. Naval S, Naval R, Naval S, et al. Tips for safe laparoscopic multiple myomectomy. J Minim Invasive Gynecol. 2017;24(2):193.
9. Jain, N. Book review of State of the Art Atlas and Textbook of Laparoscopic Suturing in Gynecology. J Obstet Gynecol India. 2016;66(2):137-8.

14 of Gynaecological Endoscopy

General Surgery Conditions Techniques for Gyne-Endoscopic Surgeons

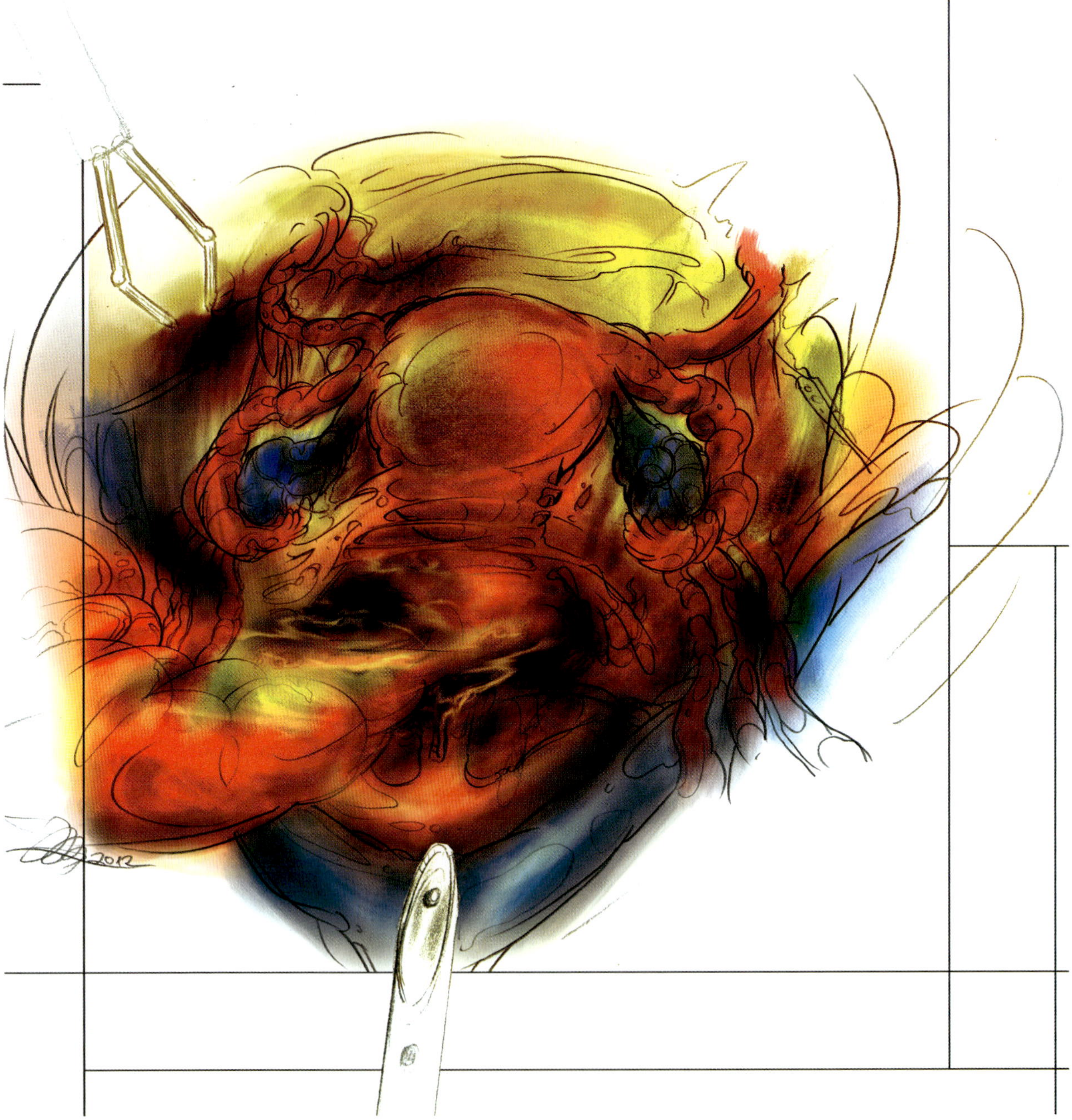

Chapter 14

General Surgery Conditions and Techniques for Gyne-endoscopic Surgeons

John E Morrison

ABDOMINAL AND PELVIC WALL: HERNIAS

The abdominal wall from the umbilicus superiorly to the symphysis pubis inferiorly and laterally to the iliac crests is an area that can be the site of abnormalities that are encountered either upon entering the abdominal cavity or be identified during the performance of laparoscopic procedures. The different techniques used to enter the abdomen are not within the scope of this chapter, but some of these abnormalities when encountered in the abdominal wall may make safe access a challenge.

The most commonly performed surgical procedure by general surgeons is hernia repair. Approximately 800,000 inguinal hernia repairs and over 200,000 incisional hernia repairs are performed yearly in the United States. Primary hernias occur most commonly in the anterior abdominal wall either at the umbilicus or in the inguinal canal. They also may be present lateral to the rectus sheath at the linea semicircularis, the Spigelian hernia. However, this is an uncommon type of defect.

The diagnosis of small incisional or inguinal hernias may be difficult preoperatively particularly if the patient is obese or the defect is small and their presence may not be certain until insufflation is achieved.

Large hernias on the other hand are usually diagnosed preoperatively through a thorough physical exam, or by preoperative imaging, however in the morbidly obese patients this can be a difficult task. When an incisional hernia is suspected, computed tomography (CT) scan of the abdomen and pelvis without contrast is the most sensitive imaging exam for hernia defects and is routinely performed to assess the size and number of defects in order to better plan operative repair and safe access into the abdomen.

The treatment of hernias differs depending on the symptoms, location, size and etiology so their diagnosis, location and size are crucial to planning appropriate care.

Umbilical Hernias

Primary umbilical hernias are usually diagnosed preoperatively and may be symptomatic particularly when small. If abdominal entry is planned through the umbilicus, an open (Hasson) technique is preferred because the fascial defect is already present and can be easily closed when exiting the abdominal cavity. Direct entry through the umbilicus when a hernia defect is present can be a very dangerous task, as omentum or bowel can easily be included in the hernia defect and as such can be injured with the Veress needle or visual port entry device. It is not uncommon for adhesions to form at the hernia site even without prior surgery so caution is advised (Fig. 14.1).

Defects 2 cm or less in diameter are closed primarily with permanent suture and do not require mesh reinforcement. The suture chosen is usually a permanent material, polypropylene or polyester, size 0 and the fascial edges approximated using simple or mattress suture techniques.

If the patient has had an umbilical hernia repaired previously and it is recurrent, then the defect is usually closed utilizing a reinforcing synthetic mesh

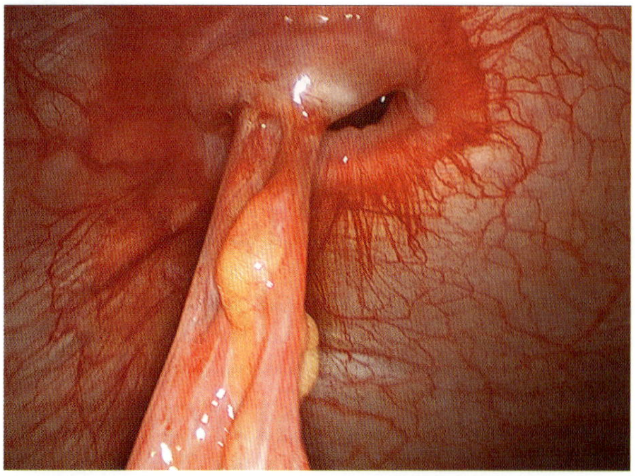

Fig. 14.1: Primary adhesions at the umbilicus.

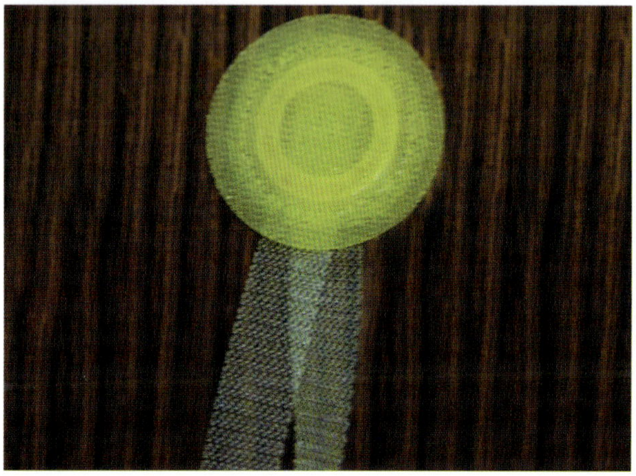

Fig. 14.2: C-QUR V-patch hernia repair system.

material. There are several devices available, which are designed specifically for these repairs. One such design is C-QUR V-patch manufactured by Atrium corp. (Fig. 14.2), which is a circular polypropylene mesh coated with omega-3 fatty acid and is placed in the defect then sutured lateral to the fascial edges making certain that the mesh extends at least 3 cm from the fascial edge in all directions. The defect is then closed primarily over the reinforcing mesh.

Any mesh placed intra-abdominally should have a barrier substance on the surface of the mesh coming in contact with the underlying bowel in order to reduce adhesions to these structures. Several products exist that have absorbable material incorporated onto the mesh to provide this barrier. If the reinforcing mesh is placed extraperitoneally then barrier material is not necessary.

Tips

- Primary umbilical hernias 2 cm or less, close primarily with permanent suture.
- Recurrent umbilical hernias or larger than 2 cm: repair with mesh reinforcement.
- Mesh should extend at least 3–5 cm from the fascial edge.
- Entry into abdomen through umbilical hernia: open technique is safest.

Incisional Hernias

Patients who have had any prior abdominal surgery are potential candidates for incisional hernias. There are approximately 250,000 incisional hernia repairs performed in the US yearly.[1] If the patient is found to have an incisional hernia, then the surgeon can usually anticipate more than one defect being present in the incision. The majority of incisional hernia defects are asymptomatic when they are small < 1 cm. Defects between 2 cm and 6 cm usually are symptomatic and are repaired using a reinforcing synthetic material when they are encountered. There is no difference in treatment of incisional hernias with regards to their location in the abdominal wall whether above or below the umbilicus.

Large defects in the fascia are most often identified on physical exam but the most sensitive method again for diagnosis and measurement of the defect is a CT scan of the abdomen and pelvis.

Primary repair of incisional hernias without reinforcement of mesh has an unacceptably high recurrence rate.[2]

The choices for reinforcement material are either synthetic or biologic. There are certain conditions where the biologic grafts have distinct advantages over synthetic materials but discussion of this topic is out of the scope of this chapter.

Most 2–8 cm incisional hernia defects currently are repaired using the laparoscopic approach. The repair most commonly utilized is referred to as a "bridge" repair where the defect is covered by mesh and the fascial edges are not reapproximated. The fascial defect may be primarily approximated and then covered with mesh but this technique is used less commonly. In both instances a reinforcing material is used.

When an incisional hernia defect is encountered during an "open" procedure, the fascia is closed primarily with suture, either permanent or long-lasting absorbable suture, with synthetic mesh reinforcement. The synthetic mesh can be placed either (1) under the abdominal wall on the peritoneal surface in which instance the material should have an adhesive barrier, or (2) between the posterior rectus fascia

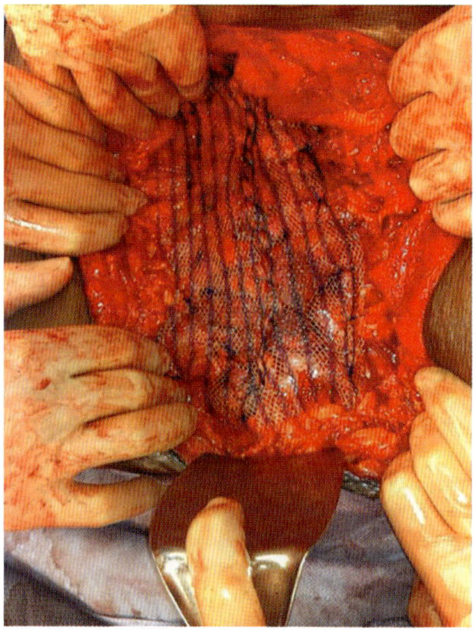

Fig. 14.3: Onlay light weight polypropylene mesh repair.

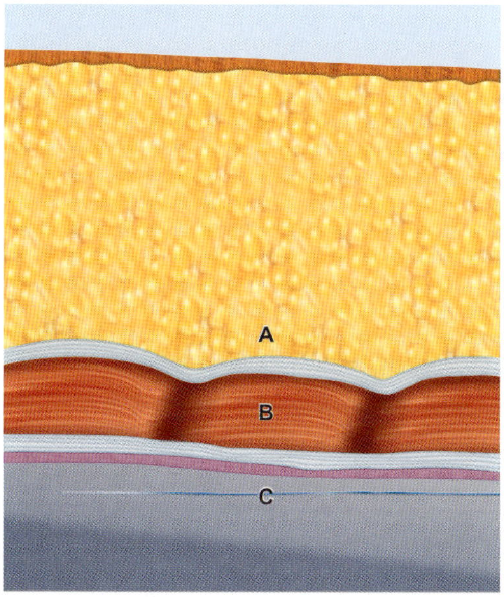

Fig. 14.4: Hernia repair mesh placement sites: (A) Onlay placement; (B) Submuscular placement; (C) Intra-abdominal placement.

and anterior rectus muscle and fascia (retro rectus) or (3) as an onlay where the mesh is simply anchored to the abdominal wall covering the reapproximated midline incision and extending laterally at least 5 to 8 cm from the midline. The onlay method is the easiest and safest approach (Fig. 14.3).

Figure 14.4 demonstrates commonly used sites for mesh placement: (A) is where an onlay graft is placed, (B) is where an inlay graft is placed. It usually lies between the fascia and muscle layers of the abdominal wall, (C) is an underlay. Site C is where placement of laparoscopic mesh is usually performed.

Synthetic Materials Used for Repair

Characteristics of the materials

The materials used in these repairs must have certain properties:

First, the material must have the strength to tolerate pressures that are generated in the abdominal and pelvic cavity.

There are several studies currently ongoing that are addressing the most accurate way of determining the actual pressures generated in the abdominal and pelvic cavities and thus what strength characteristics the synthetic material must have in order to maintain an adequate repair. Over the past several years the density and structure of the synthetic mesh material used has undergone significant change. The main change is one of thinner, lighter weight materials with large pore structure for flexibility and easy incorporation into the abdominal wall tissues.

Figure 14.5 demonstrates the two most commonly used polypropylene mesh types. The mesh on the left is a lightweight mesh and the material on the right of the figure is a medium-weight material. The differences are a combination of pore size and weight of the material used. The trend now is to utilize lighter weight materials; however, in large incisional hernia repairs tearing of this lightweight mesh is being seen with more frequency and there may be a return to using medium or heavier weight materials.

The second characteristic is that the material must adhere securely to the abdominal wall. The material is anchored either with suture or tacking devices or a combination of the two. The anchoring devices assist in preventing slippage of the material while it is being incorporated onto the abdominal

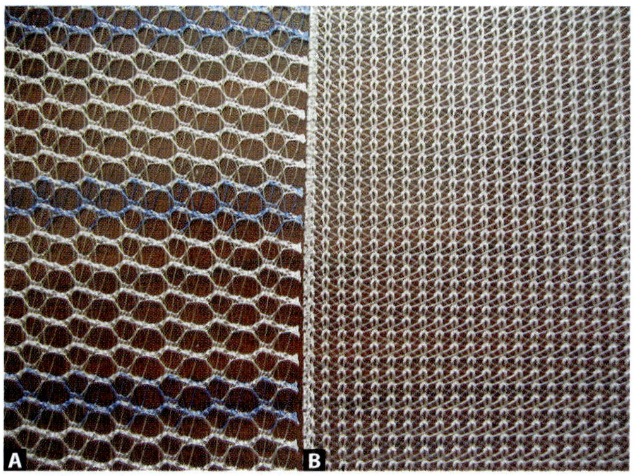

Figs. 14.5A and B: Polypropylene mesh. (A) Light weight; (B) Medium weight.

wall. Depending on the physical properties of the material used, the mesh elicits a reaction that results in scar formation around the material that also assists in incorporation of the material into the abdominal wall and adding to the strength of the repair.

The third characteristic and one of the most important characteristics is that the material must possess a property that reduces adherence to the bowel and any underlying structures. The mesh must have secured onto it a barrier device that helps reduce adherence to the underlying bowel if it is placed intraperitoneally. Synthetic mesh placed into the abdominal cavity without any barrier carries a risk of erosion into the bowel or any other structure it comes in contact with and thus fistula formation. If this does occur, then the synthetic mesh must be removed and the fistula closed. Replacement of the mesh by synthetic materials in this situation is not recommended and a biologic material is usually needed.

The fourth characteristic is that the material should elicit a minimal inflammatory or immunologic response. Research is ongoing in this area and materials are constantly being tested and refined to reduce this reaction.

Materials for Repair

The most frequently utilized synthetic material in hernia repairs is polypropylene mesh. Figure 14.6 is an example of a coated polypropylene mesh used for hernia repair when the mesh is placed intra-abdominally.

Polypropylene has been used for decades and because surgeons have a long experience and great familiarity with it, it is the preferred mesh material. Because of the hydrophilic nature of the material it does result in the formation of a fibrous capsule, which can become firm over time and a source for pain but with reduction of polypropylene mesh weight, this phenomenon is becoming less of a problem.

Polytetrafluorethylene (PTFE) is another material utilized in hernia repair in the abdomen. It has properties of minimal adherence to surrounding tissues and flexibility, but because of its propensity for nonadherence, other materials must be incorporated into the mesh in order to make it adhere to the anterior abdominal wall. Otherwise the material is not incorporated and the repair not secured. Figure 14.7 is an example of a PTFE mesh used for hernia repair.

The PTFE mesh is a microporous material, so seroma formation above the mesh and below the overlying skin and subcutaneous tissue after bridge repair is not uncommon. These seromas usually are asymptomatic and over time resolve; however, if they become infected or symptomatic they can be drained percutaneously or if mature, excised after adequate incorporation of the underlying mesh has occurred. Seroma formation is not uncommon after any bridge type repair regardless of the material used (Fig. 14.8).

When PTFE material is used for repair if an overlying seroma or the material itself becomes infected, it must be removed. The pore size is such that bacteria are able to enter the mesh but neutrophils cannot so the resulting infection cannot be cleared without mesh removal.

All grafts contract over time, but PTFE grafts do contract the most when compared to other synthetic materials, so this characteristic must be taken into consideration when placing the material and ensuring adequate overlapping of the defect.[3]

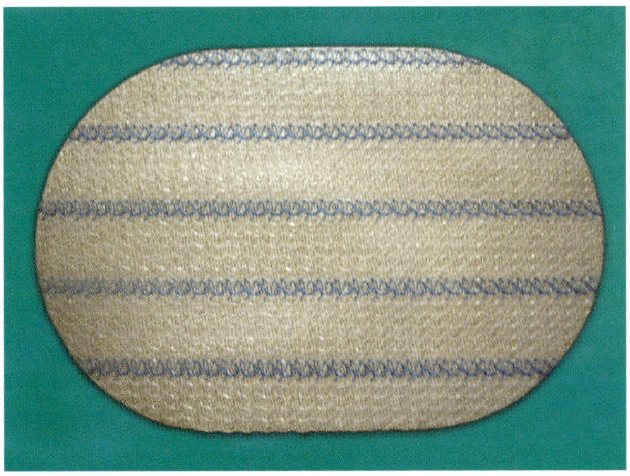

Fig. 14.6: Adhesion barrier-coated polypropylene mesh.

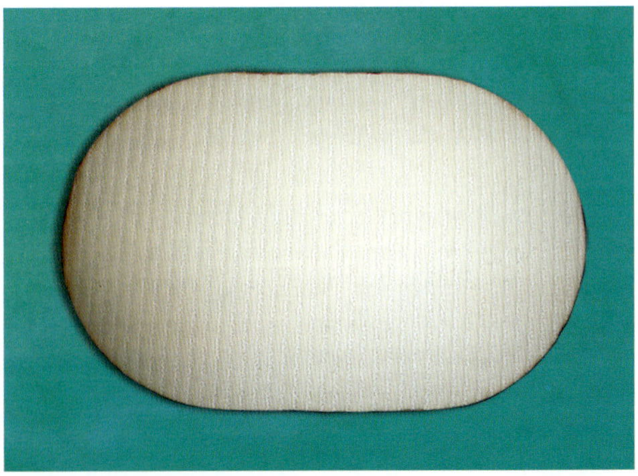

Fig. 14.7: PTFE hernia patch.

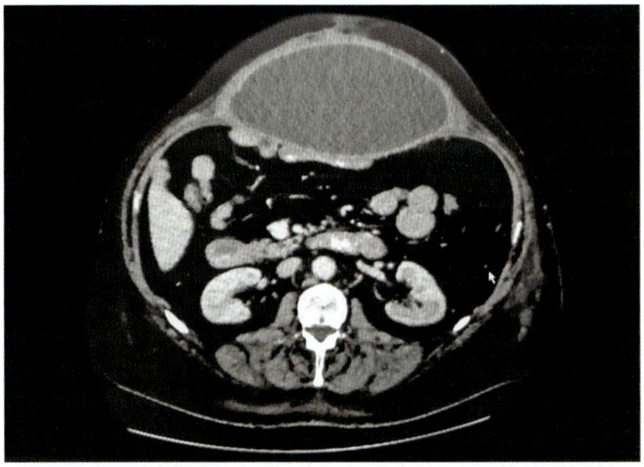

Fig. 14.8: Postoperative seroma anterior to mesh and deep to fascia.

Polyester mesh is also utilized for hernia repair but less frequently. The material is a woven braided polyester fiber that incorporates into the surrounding tissues well. This material has been used for decades in the manufacture of vascular grafts, so its use has a long history in surgery and thus experience with this material is large. It is a hydrophilic material so it does not elicit the intense fibrotic reaction that polypropylene does, but as with any braided material if it does become contaminated with bacteria or infected, it is difficult to clear of bacteria so it may require excision if this does occur.

'WHEN' and 'HOW' for Incisional Hernia Repairs

Defects 2 cm or less may be repaired primarily with permanent suture material as in umbilical hernia repair.

Hernia defects >8 cm may require mobilization of anterior abdominal wall fascial layers with reinforcement by synthetic or biologic material in order to reapproximate the midline fascial edges and restore a dynamic abdominal wall.

To accomplish this there are a number of options that include relaxing incisions in the external oblique muscle bilaterally or in the posterior rectus fascia and transverse abdominal muscle layers in order to mobilize the fascia to get the midline fascial edges together. Discussion of this type of repair is out of the scope of this chapter and these large defects should be referred for definitive repair either before gynecologic procedures are performed or preferably repaired at the time of gynecologic surgery by a general surgeon or plastic surgeon familiar with these types of repairs.

The treatment of choice for repair of incisional hernia defects from 2 to 6 cm currently is via laparoscopy and is usually performed at the end of other surgical procedures. The mesh should overlap the defect by at least 3 cm preferably up to 5 cm or more on all edges and be anchored to the abdominal wall. If during the primary operative procedure the bowel is entered, gross contamination with infected material is encountered or the vagina or bladder are entered and an incisional hernia repair is considered, then the use of synthetic mesh is discouraged and biologic graft used in its place. Biologic grafts may be used in a bridge repair or as a reinforcing material to primary closure but there are no good studies to gauge its long-term success and these materials are very expensive.

Procedure for Repair of Incisional Hernia

All contents in the hernia defect must be reduced into the abdominal cavity and the surrounding fascial edges cleared of overlying tissue, bowel and fat in order to ensure adequate incorporation of mesh into the abdominal wall fascia. Figure 14.9 demonstrates a defect prepared for repair.

The material chosen for repair must have an adequate size in order to overlap all aspects of the defect by 5 cm or more and have a barrier for reduction of adhesions.

If the defect is large and a large piece of mesh is needed for coverage, sutures are placed at the four quadrants of the mesh; the sutures are retrieved through the abdominal wall to align the mesh adequately over the defect for final anchoring of the mesh. These sutures can be used to primarily anchor

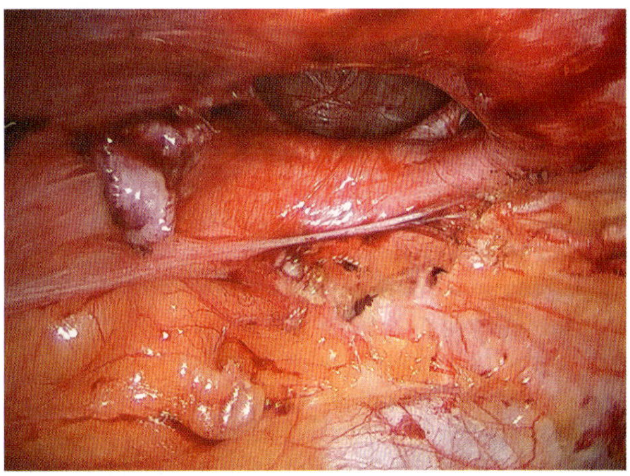

Fig. 14.9: Incisional hernia defect cleared for repair.

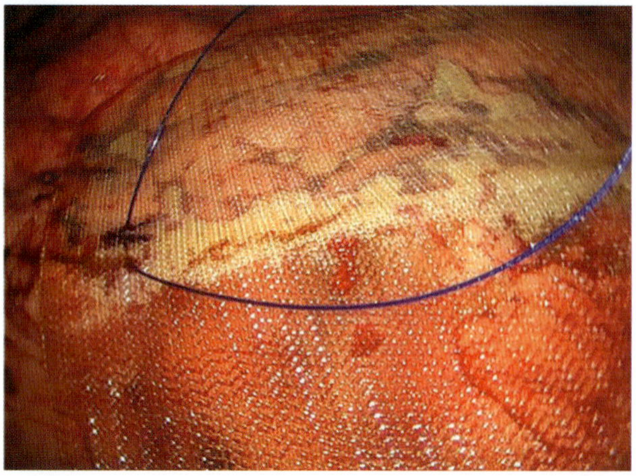

Fig. 14.10: Mesh patch intra-abdominal in preparation for repair.

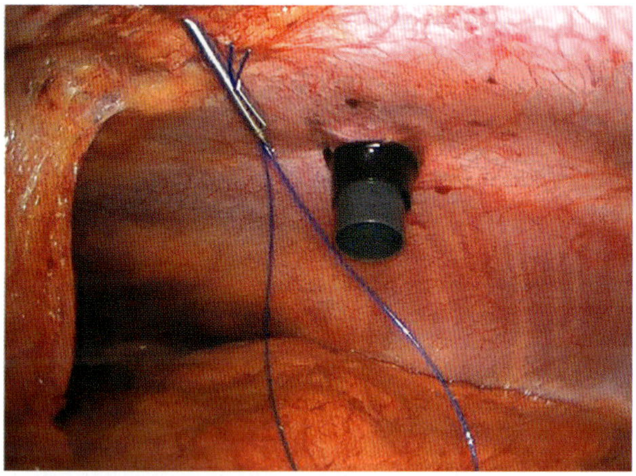

Fig. 14.11: Suture passing device grasping anchoring suture for mesh placement.

the mesh to the abdominal wall. Figures 14.10 and 14.11 demonstrate the mesh with anchoring sutures and retrieval of the sutures through the abdominal wall.

The mesh is then anchored to the abdominal wall with either suture, or tacking devices or a combination of the two. Particular attention is addressed to the edges of the mesh in order to ensure that adequate anchoring of the mesh has taken place and the possibility of bowel herniation between the mesh and abdominal wall tacks does not take place. Figure 14.12 demonstrates anchoring of the mesh with a permanent tacking device.

Abdominal binders are usually placed on the patient immediately postoperatively to give support to the abdominal wall and reduce pain. It is recommended that the patients wear such devices for 6 weeks or more after surgery.

Results with laparoscopic bridge repair of incisional hernias have been very good with comparable

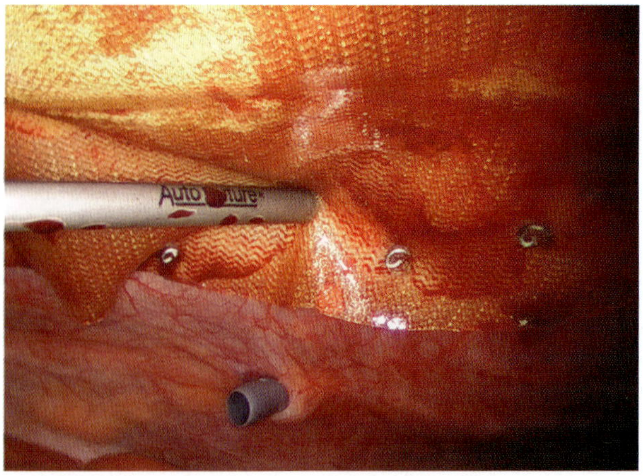

Fig. 14.12: Placement of permanent tacks to secure mesh to abdominal wall.

low recurrence rates when compared to open repair, but with higher major intraoperative complication rates when compared to open repair. Patients do return to normal activities sooner, have less pain and hospital stay is shorter.[4]

Special Considerations after Hernia Repair

If a patient has had prior hernia repair utilizing mesh, then special consideration must be given for safe entry into the abdomen. Despite the application and incorporation of adhesive barriers into the mesh, or even if the mesh is completely covered by peritoneum, the presence of adherent bowel or omentum to the mesh and particularly to the edge of the mesh should be expected.

Entry into the abdominal cavity can be accomplished in these instances either by remote entry, i.e. Palmer's point in the left upper quadrant or other sites outside of the prior surgical field. Entry can also be accomplished through the mesh itself. If a laparoscopic procedure is planned, then open (Hasson) technique is recommended either directly through the mesh utilizing careful blunt dissection of adherent bowel and omentum away from the mesh as the abdominal cavity is entered or at a remote site lateral to the prior incision. Extreme care must be taken around the edges of the mesh as this is the area most involved with adhesion formation. Figure 14.13 demonstrates adhesions at the edge of a previously placed mesh.

Once the procedure is completed, upon closure of the incision if it was made through the mesh, the closure should be accomplished with permanent suture.

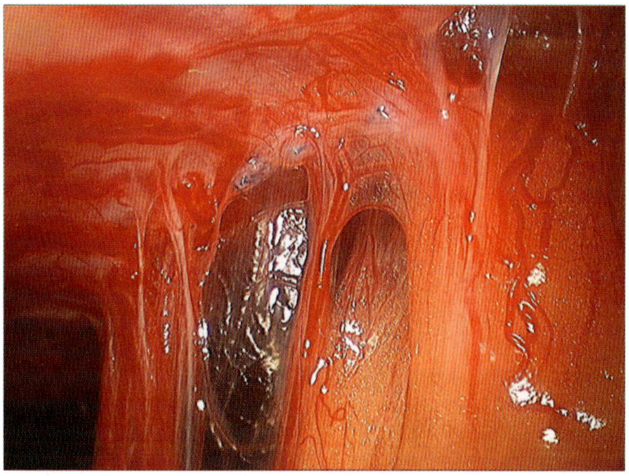

Fig. 14.13: Dense adhesions on lateral border of intra-abdominal mesh.

Repair of complex incisional wall hernia defects may involve the use of biologic grafts intra-abdominally or with an onlay over the anterior fascia. The biologic materials used currently consist of an acellular matrix of collagen and come in a variety of substances. The matrix is infiltrated with fibroblasts over time and the hosts' native collagen incorporated into the matrix, resulting in a thick scar. In complex hernia repairs, if a biologic graft is used internally, opening directly through the material is recommended with the same considerations and precautions being taken as recommended with opening through synthetic material for abdominal entry.

As discussed above, complex hernia repairs are being performed with primary closure and with combinations of onlay mesh, inlay (between the layers of the abdominal wall) and underlay mesh. It is strongly recommended for the surgeon to obtain prior operative notes in order to be familiar with the repair performed so entry into the abdomen can be accomplished safely. A prior knowledge of where the mesh was placed helps makes this possible.

Tips

- 2 cm or less defects: close primarily with nonabsorbable suture.
- 2–8 cm defects: Laparoscopic bridge repair with synthetic material with adhesive barrier. Anchor to the abdominal wall with tacking device and overlap fascial edges 5 cm.
- 2–8 cm defects: Open repair, reapproximate the fascial edges and incorporate synthetic mesh reinforcement either intra-abdominally, subfascial or overlay the midline closure.
- Defects larger than 8 cm usually require a more complex repair for closure of the midline fascia and should be performed in conjunction with surgeons familiar with these repair techniques.
- When entering the abdomen after prior incisional hernia repair with mesh, enter either through the center of the mesh with caution or at distant point and avoid the edges.
- Know beforehand what type of repair was performed on the patient prior to entry to help anticipate when the mesh will be encountered in opening.

Inguinal Hernias

Inguinal hernia defects, when seen during laparoscopy, are located in the pelvic side walls lateral to the obliterated umbilical veins. The two most common types of inguinal defects are direct and indirect hernias. Direct defects are medial to the inferior epigastric vessels and indirect defects are lateral to these vessels. The indirect defects can also be identified by the presence of the round ligament in or medial to the defect. Figure 14.14 is an example of a small asymptomatic indirect inguinal hernia and does not require repair.

Symptoms of inguinal hernia include swelling or bulge in the inguinal floor usually superior to the inguinal ligament. It may or may not be associated with pain. Pain in the area of the inguinal ligament may be the only symptom or sign of a hernia. Inguinal hernias are more difficult to diagnose in females as compared to males. The dilemma is when the hernia is identified at the time of surgery what needs to be done.

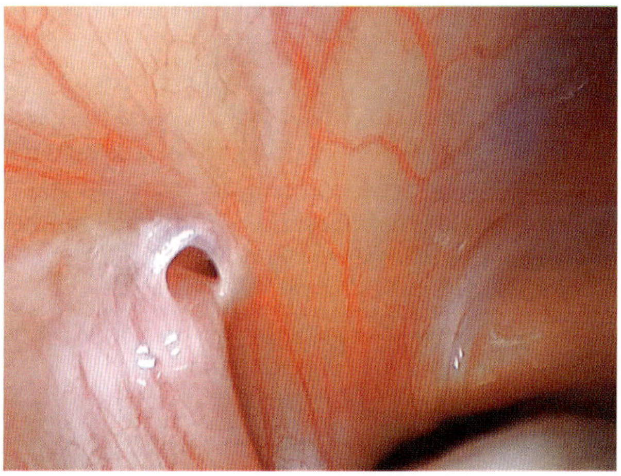

Fig. 14.14: Small left inguinal hernia defect next to round ligament.

Tip: If an inguinal defect is identified and the patient is asymptomatic, i.e., the patient does not have inguinal pain, then the defect is noted and the patient is informed but repair is not necessary.

When a single symptomatic inguinal hernia defect is discovered, the choice of repair technique is controversial among surgeons. Patients with a single inguinal hernia are still most commonly repaired using standard open technique. In single surgeon series, the recurrence rate with laparoscopic repair is comparable to open repair and pain scores much better.[5] In large studies, results with laparoscopic repair show slightly higher recurrence rate, but pain scores and return to normal activity was better in the laparoscopic group versus open.[6,7]

Cost must be taken into consideration when choosing a repair, but when evaluated, there is little difference in operating room costs but there can be large differences in facility reimbursement.[8]

The laparoscopic repair of inguinal hernias can be either performed entirely preperitoneal or transperitoneal. The principles of the repair and results are similar for both techniques. The anatomy of the inguinal canal and pelvic floor is constant, predictable and familiar to the gynecologic surgeon that performs anterior vaginal wall repairs or vesico-urethral neck suspensions such as Burch procedure. This is the same space routinely dissected and entered in a laparoscopic inguinal hernia repair.

In either repair, the peritoneum is dissected from the lower pelvic and inguinal floor exposing the inguinal canal, iliac vessels, pubic tubercle, femoral canal and lateral inguinal side wall. It is important to completely reduce the hernia contents into the preperitoneal space. Simply closing the peritoneal defect is inadequate for repair; the inguinal floor must be reinforced with synthetic materials (Video 14.1).

The mesh dimensions should be 10 by 15 cm in order to adequately cover the inguinal floor and all potential defects. If polypropylene mesh is used, then this material should be anchored to the inguinal floor. Care must be taken when anchoring the mesh to avoid the major vascular and neural structures that are in the dissection site as injury to these structures is possible.

Anchoring of mesh should only be performed medial to the inferior epigastric vessels on the anterior lower abdominal wall and into the symphysis pubis and Cooper's ligament. Tacking devices should not be utilized in the lateral pelvic side wall as the genitofemoral and ilioinguinal nerves are present and can be easily trapped, causing significant postoperative pain.

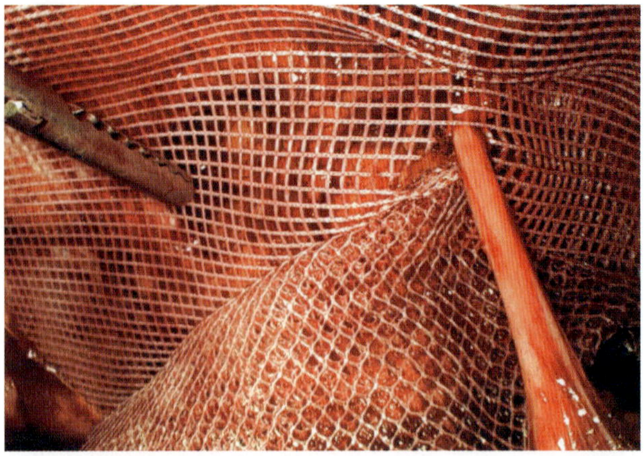

Fig. 14.15: Preperitoneal mesh placement right inguinal hernia.

If polyester mesh is used for repair, because of the hydrophilic nature of the material, the mesh adheres to the underlying tissues well and does not need to be tacked if the repair is performed in a preperitoneal fashion. Results with this type of repair are very good and as such problems with tacking are avoided. Figure 14.15 demonstrates coverage of the inguinal floor with mesh at the end of a repair.

Femoral hernias are more common in females than males and may be a source of chronic pelvic or lower abdominal pain.

Femoral hernia is difficult to diagnose preoperatively. Symptoms usually include pain radiating down the inner aspect of the thigh and or under the inguinal ligament with no palpable mass or bulge. Frequently the first sign that a femoral hernia is present is acute incarceration. The repair of femoral hernia defects can be accomplished either by open or laparoscopic techniques, but the laparoscopic approach affords excellent exposure and allows accurate placement of a single layer of mesh that adequately covers the femoral and inguinal canals creating a very good repair.

The contents of a femoral hernia must be carefully reduced into the preperitoneal space in order to adequately identify the femoral canal structures and complete the repair. Again, if polypropylene mesh is utilized it should be anchored to the pelvis taking precautions as noted previously to avoid major vascular or neural injuries (Video 14.2).

Special Considerations in Inguinal Hernias

Techniques for laparoscopic inguinal hernia repair have evolved over the past 15 years. In the 1990s plug

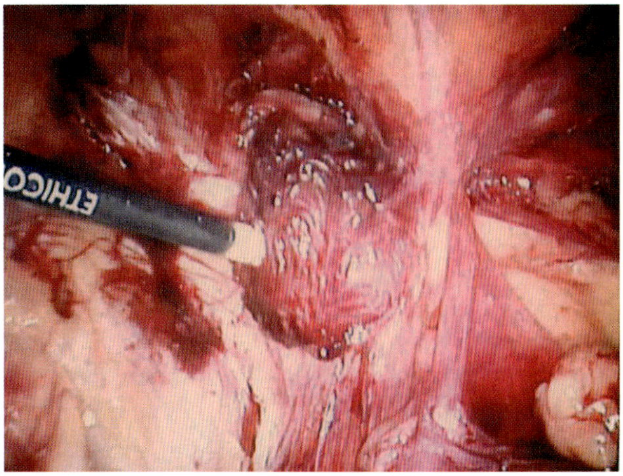

Fig. 14.16: Mesh plug in femoral canal.

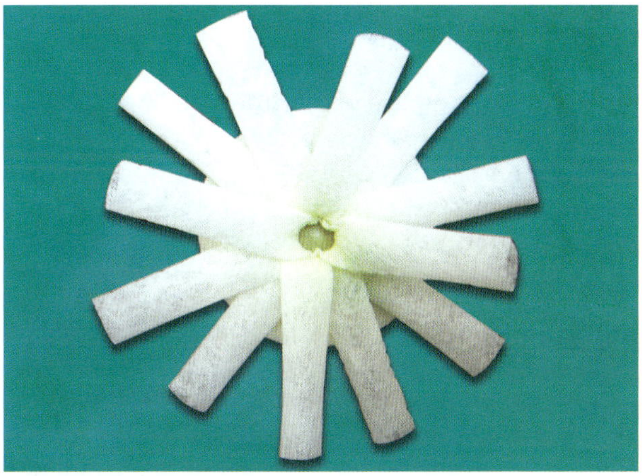

Fig. 14.17: Biomaterial absorbable mesh plug.

type repair was common, where a mesh plug usually consisting of polypropylene material was simply placed into the defect. This type of repair resulted in significant pain at the repair site because of scarring and contraction of the material and as a result, this procedure currently is rarely used. Patients who have had this type of repair may present with significant pain with no external palpable "mass" and removal of the mesh plug is usually required for relief. Figure 14.16 is an example of a plug-type repair in a patient who presented with pain several years later.

The plug repairs when performed currently utilize an absorbable material primarily or are in combination with open repair systems that utilize lower weight permanent synthetic materials. Figure 14.17 is an example of an absorbable material currently used in plug repairs. The material is Bio-A, manufactured by Gore corporation. This material provides a substrate for collagen deposition by the host, resulting in an adequate support for the repair.

Tips

- Asymptomatic inguinal hernias found at the time of surgery: Note and inform the patient of their presence but they do not require repair.
- Femoral hernias may be a source of pelvic pain: Symptoms are radiating pain to the inner thigh and pain in the groin below the inguinal ligament. If a femoral hernia is found, it should be repaired as incarceration is common.
- Previous repairs with plug-type materials may be a source of chronic pain: diagnosis can be made by prior history of surgery and imaging of the inguinal floor. Resolution of pain usually requires removal of the material.
- Single symptomatic inguinal hernias are usually repaired with open technique.
- Bilateral or recurrent inguinal hernias usually are repaired with laparoscopic technique.
- In patients who have had a prior laparoscopic inguinal hernia repair, the retropubic space will be very difficult to enter due to adherence of the mesh material to the underlying structures.

Internal Hernias

An internal hernia is an opening between any two adjacent structures in the abdominal cavity that has the potential for abdominal contents to protrude through creating a site for obstruction. These hernias are very difficult to diagnose preoperatively and can also be a source of chronic lower abdominal or pelvic pain. They most commonly present with incarceration and bowel obstruction as the first presenting symptom.

Internal hernias are usually the result of prior surgery and adhesive disease. When bowel resection with anastomosis or gastric bypass is performed and the mesenteric defect is not sufficiently closed then this site may be the location of an internal hernia.

Figure 14.18 demonstrates such an internal hernia where adhesions created a small defect and bowel became entrapped and obstructed. The prior operation that resulted in this defect was a cesarean section with scarring between the uterus, anterior abdominal wall and lateral pelvic side wall.

When an internal hernia is diagnosed it needs to be either fixed by primary closure of the defect or the

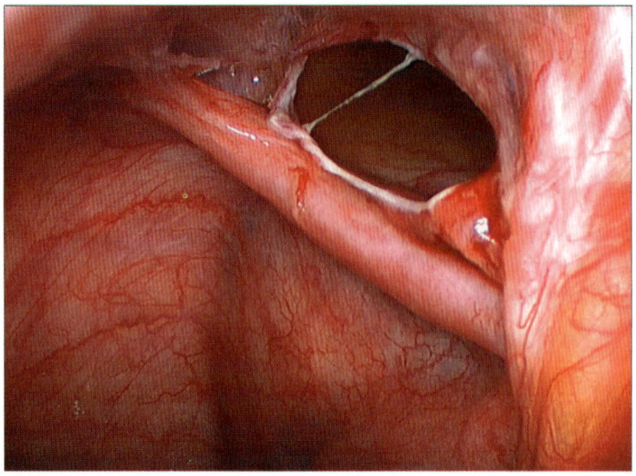

Fig. 14.18: Internal hernia right pelvic side wall.

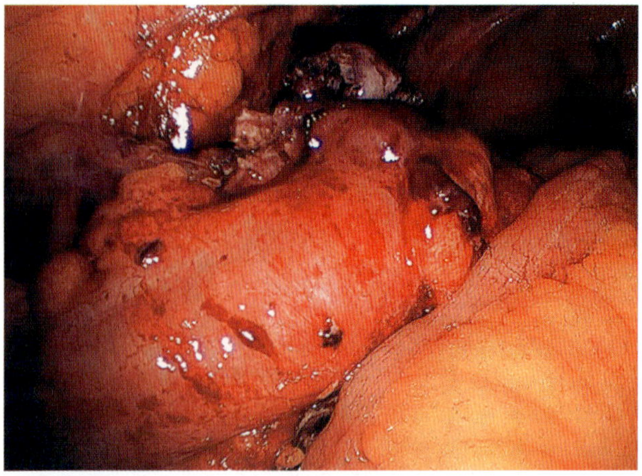

Fig. 14.19: Diverticulitis sigmoid colon.

defect opened widely so the bowel cannot become incarcerated because the potential for complications is high.

Tips

When an internal hernia defect is encountered, it should be either closed completely or opened completely to prevent incarceration of bowel.

VISCERAL PATHOLOGIES

In the true pelvis, the rectosigmoid and the appendix are common sources of pathology. It is important to be able to recognize common conditions affecting these structures that may mimic gynecologic conditions and be aware of the treatment for these processes. The small bowel also visits the pelvis and conditions that involve this organ may also mimic gynecologic pathologies.

Colon

The most common condition involving the colon in the West that may mimic gynecologic pathology is diverticular disease. Patients with acute hemorrhage or perforation as a result of their diverticular disease usually are referred directly to general surgery for care; however chronic pain from diverticulosis or low grade diverticulitis may be difficult to distinguish from a gynecologic etiology.

The sigmoid colon is the region of the colon that is most commonly involved with symptomatic diverticuli and the pain is usually present in the left lower quadrant, but may be suprapubic or even in the right lower quadrant.

On inspection and manipulation of the involved colon during laparoscopy, the bowel wall is usually thickened and has lost its normal pliability. In patients that have chronic diverticular disease there are usually adhesions adjacent to the involved segment as a result of repeated bouts of inflammation (Fig. 14.19).

Diverticuli may actually be seen protruding through the muscular wall of the colon aiding in diagnosis.

Once the GYN surgeon has ruled out any gynecologic pathology and the findings suggest diverticular disease whether it be chronic or acute, no further surgical intervention is necessary. Treatment consists of dietary fiber increase with or without intravenous or oral antibiotics depending on whether an acute process is present or not.

When a patient is explored for pelvic inflammatory disease or presumed tubo-ovarian abscess, one of the differentials is a contained diverticular perforation with abscess formation. When this is encountered, the segment of involved *colon does not require resection* (except in free perforation and peritonitis where a resection and diverting colostomy may be necessary). The abscess can be drained laparoscopically and a drain left in the abscess cavity.

Malignancies may also perforate; however, this is less common than in diverticular disease and these patients commonly manifest symptoms of bowel obstruction and as such are usually seen by general surgeons prior to this happening.

Frequently when operating in the pelvis, congenital "adhesions" are encountered between the sigmoid colon, cecum and the abdominal wall or pelvic side wall. When these structures are noted, if they do not interfere with the planned procedure they are usually left in place and not taken down. The potential problem with mobilizing these structures (sigmoid and cecum) too vigorously is the possibility of volvulus, or twisting of the bowel. So as a rule of thumb, if it is not interfering with the planned procedure leave these support bands in place.

Tips

- Diverticular disease of the sigmoid whether it is chronic or acute without perforation; does not require resection. Note and inform the patient.
- Perforation with abscess formation: drain the abscess; leave a drain in the cavity, no resection is required.

Appendix

The use of pelvic ultrasound and or CT scan to accurately diagnose appendicitis has been on the rise recently but these have sometimes been unreliable tools to include or exclude the diagnosis, so the use of laparoscopy particularly in the female patient is becoming more frequent when the diagnosis is uncertain. The benefits of laparoscopic appendectomy when compared to open appendectomy are still being hotly debated in the general surgery literature.[9] The majority of appendectomies performed in the United States are currently being done laparoscopically. The main advantage being reduction in wound infection rate when compared to open techniques.

The surgical technique used by gastrointestinal surgeons for appendectomy most commonly involves utilizing a linear stapling device. These instruments provide a quick simple technique for removal of the appendix; however, they are expensive and may not be readily available so other methods for dissection and removal should be in the surgeons' armamentarium. The technique for appendectomy will be described in stepwise detail.

Procedure Appendectomy

First the appendix must be mobilized from any retroperitoneal or lateral pelvic attachments. This step is important in order to have adequate access to the mesentery of the appendix and avoid injury to retroperitoneal structures, cecum or the ileocecal valve during removal.

Next, a small window is created in the mesoappendix at the base of the appendix. This can be done bluntly using dissectors or energy sources.

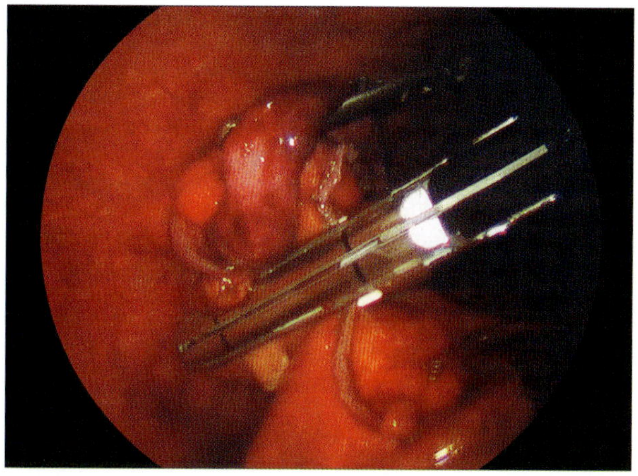

Fig. 14.20: Appendectomy utilizing laparoscopic GIA stapling device.

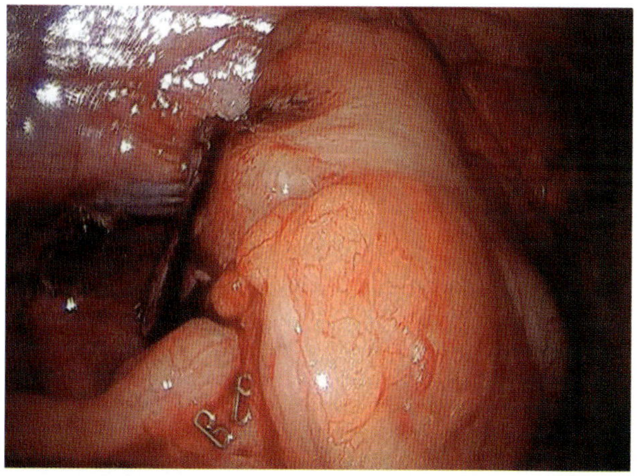

Fig. 14.21: Appendiceal stump after stapling.

Once this is accomplished, the third step is either ligation of the mesoappendix or appendix base. The choice of which one of these structures is to be ligated first is dependent on the anatomy and ease of visualization. Control can also be accomplished using a linear stapling device. The appendix base is usually transected using the 3.5 or 2.8 mm staple depth. The choice depends on whether the base of the appendix is inflamed or normal. The vascular pedicle is divided using the 2.8 mm staple load. Figure 14.20 shows placement of the stapling device and Figure 14.21 shows the appendix base after stapling.

Simple ligation of the appendix base or its vascular pedicle using 0-silk or other suture offers good control prior to transection of these structures. This method is much more cost effective when compared to stapling devices. Video 14.3 demonstrates ligation of the appendix base with suture.

After the base of the appendix or mesoappendix is ligated and transected, an Endoloop may be applied for extra security. Video 14.4 shows the transection of the appendix base after ligation.

In instances where the appendix is necrotic at its base, the stapler has its best utility. The proximal staple line should cross normal cecal wall in order to insure viable tissue is left in the staple line. Stapling across a necrotic appendix can result in delayed perforation and peritonitis since there is no viable tissue left in the staple line.

When the primary ligation method is utilized and the base of the appendix is necrotic, the appendix base should be inverted into the cecum utilizing either a Z stitch or purse string seromuscular stitch of 2-0 or 3-0 suture. Historically silk suture has been used however an absorbable suture may be utilized but the crucial point is that the tissue in question be closed and inverted with normal viable tissue overlying it.

Special Considerations

In instances where the appendix has perforated and an abscess is encountered, which may be the case in exploration for suspected tubo-ovarian abscess, then just as for diverticular abscess, the surgeon should drain the abscess, leave a drain in the abscess cavity and end the procedure. The appendix does not need to be removed at that time but this can be done at a later date usually several months later if indicated.

In patients with chronic lower abdominal or pelvic pain who are undergoing laparoscopy and the appendix is still present, it is recommended that the appendix be removed. In several studies, relief of pain after appendectomy even without obvious gross pathology shows benefit.[10,11]

Tips

- Appendectomy should be performed in patients with pelvic pain when the organ is still present and appears grossly normal.
- Appendectomy can easily be accomplished utilizing a stapling device, 3.5 or 2.8 mm load for the appendix base and 2.8 mm size for the mesentery.
- Suture ligation using 0-silk or other suture material is as effective as stapling and more cost-effective. Pretied loops can also be used to control the appendix base and mesentery base.
- In perforation and abscess formation, drain the abscess, do not remove the appendix and leave a drain in the cavity.

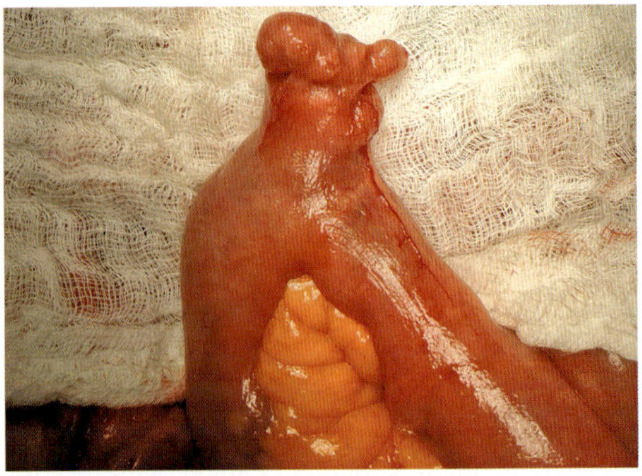

Fig. 14.22: Meckel's diverticulum.

Small Bowel

Small bowel pathology is much less common than either colon or appendix pathology; however, conditions do exist that may be found during exploration that mimic pelvic pathology.

Meckel's Diverticulum

Meckel's diverticulum is a true diverticulum that classically is located two feet from the ileocecal valve and can be a source of chronic pain. The appearance is typically that of an antimesenteric diverticulum with its own blood supply originating from the mesentery.

Figure 14.22 shows a typical Meckel's diverticulum.

The diverticulum can harbor gastric mucosa that can lead to gastrointestinal bleeding and also perforation. Bowel obstruction from intussusception also has been described. So when these structures are encountered they are usually removed.

Resection with a linear stapling device that is 3.5 mm size the staple load, placed at the base of the Meckel's diverticulum so as not to compromise the remaining bowel lumen, is recommended. Resection utilizing simple excision with two-layer suture closure may be used if the surgeon is adept with laparoscopic resection and suturing techniques.

Tips

When Meckel's diverticulum is found it should be removed.

Gastrointestinal Stromal Tumors

Gastrointestinal stromal tumors (GIST) can be found in the small bowel and have the same gross appear-

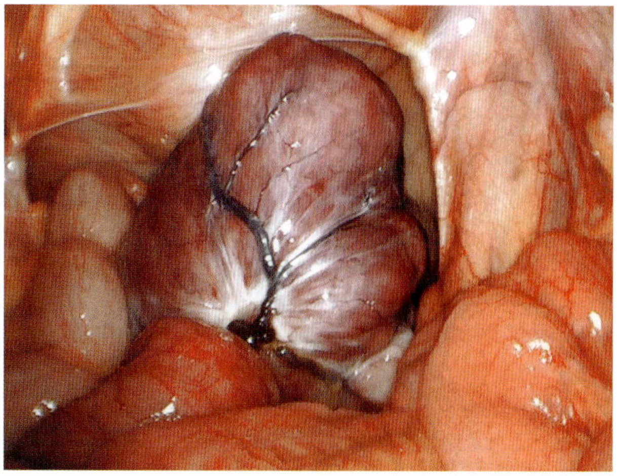

Fig. 14.23: Gastrointestinal stromal tumor of small bowel.

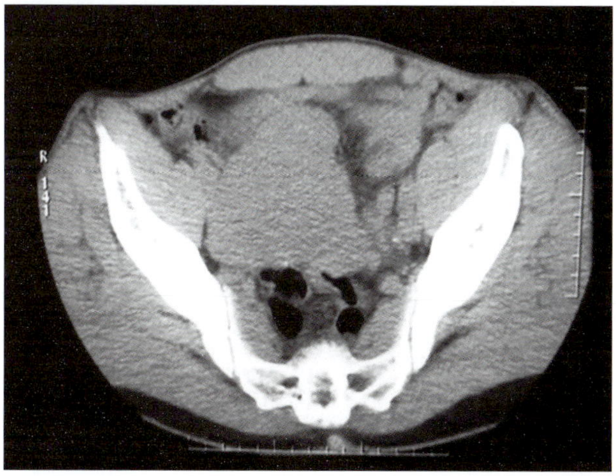

Fig. 14.24: CT scan of pelvis showing gastrointestinal stromal tumor.

ance as leiomyomas. Figure 14.23 is that of a small bowel GIST preoperatively mimicking a leiomyoma.

GIST tumors are most commonly found in the stomach 60% with 30% incidence in the large and small bowel. They can be intraluminal or extraluminal with a pedunculated base, which can lead to misdiagnosis via imaging as originating from the uterus or ovary. Figure 14.24 shows the appearance on CT of the lesion in Figure 14.23.

These tumors do have a malignant potential and so when encountered they should be removed. Despite their malignant potential, removal of GIST lesions requires only clear resection margins and a formal nodal dissection is not necessary. Lesions greater than 5 cm or with >5 mitoses per high power field should be referred for consideration for adjuvant chemotherapy.

Because these tumors resemble leiomyomas the urge to morcellate should be avoided when they are removed. They should be removed from the abdomen intact by extending the incision or utilizing a specimen retrieval bag device.

Tips

GIST tumors grossly resemble leiomyomas and as such may be mistaken for gynecologic pathology. When found, they should be removed intact, not morcellated and no formal cancer nodal dissection is necessary. The bowel margins should be clear.

Crohn's Disease

Regional enteritis or Crohn's disease can also cause pelvic or lower abdominal pain. The gross appearance is similar to that seen with chronic diverticular disease with marked thickening of the bowel wall, loss of pliability and the characteristic mesenteric creeping fat may be present.

Without any acute problems or complications of the patient's disease (perforation, obstruction), the involved segment does not need to be removed and in fact it is recommended that the involved bowel be left in place. Medical therapy is the mainstay of treatment with surgery being left only for complications such as perforation, stricture, obstruction or fistula formation.

Tips

Crohn's disease when encountered should be noted with no resection recommended except only for complications such as perforation, obstruction, stricture or fistula formation.

Special Considerations in Encountering Bowel Injuries

In the course of dissection particularly when adhesive disease is encountered, occasionally injury to the bowel wall is noted. Avoidance of injury is the key. The use of any energy source to release bowel from the abdominal wall is to be discouraged and when used, should be performed only with extreme caution.

Use of scissors without cautery is the preferred method. When very loose adhesions are encountered, the bowel may be gently pushed from the abdominal wall with the convex side of the instrument. Figure 14.25 demonstrates the recommended position of the scissors.

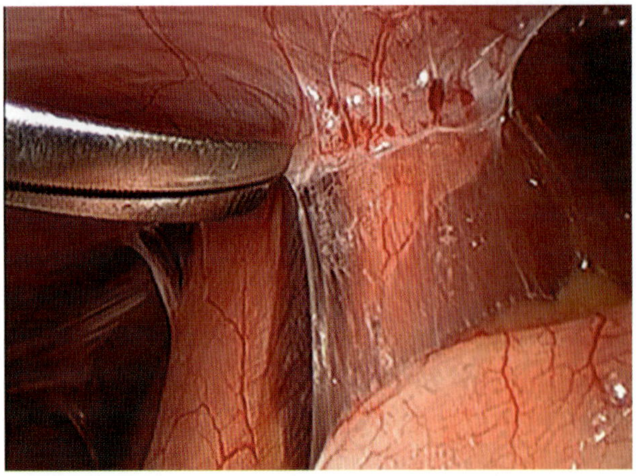

Fig. 14.25: Fibrinous adhesions.

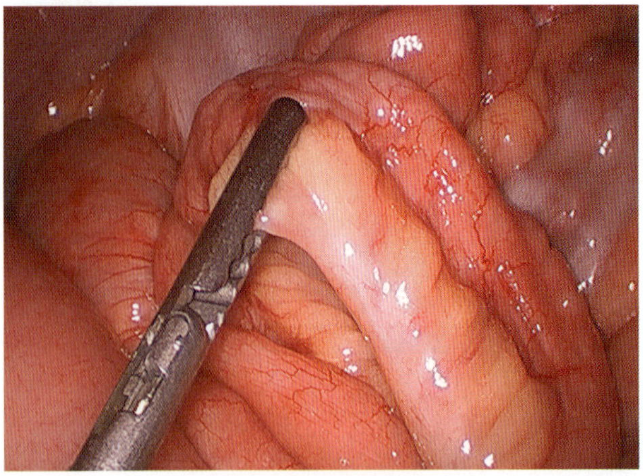

Fig. 14.27: Grasping mesentery of bowel.

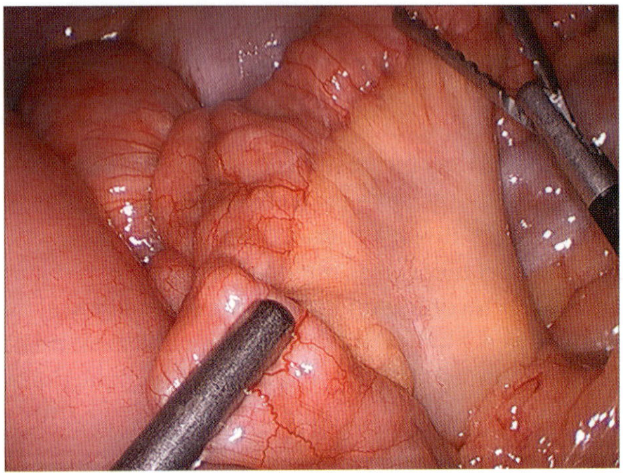

Fig. 14.26: Grasping of bowel at 0 degree angle.

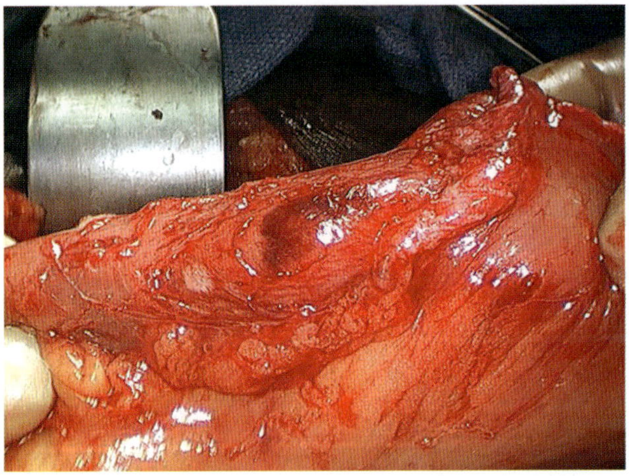

Fig. 14.28: Seromuscular tear of intestinal wall.

This helps reduce chance of an unseen injury by the tip of the scissors on the bowel.

Small bowel and colon are encountered frequently in the pelvis during surgery, despite placing the patient in Trendelenburg position. These structures must be mobilized from the pelvis in order to achieve adequate visualization. When grasping the bowel, a method recommended to help reduce the possibility of injury is that the bowel be grasped gently with an instrument with a large surface area and at an angle parallel to the mesentery (Fig. 14.26) or grasp the mesentery directly (Fig. 14.27).

The larger surfaced area grasper disperses the force generated by the grasper and by grasping the mesentery the bowel itself is avoided thus reducing the risk of injury. The amount of force generated at the tip of laparoscopic instruments has been measured at up to 1500 kPa, which is equal to a human bite so excessive force on the instrument can be transferred to the bowel and must be avoided.[12]

Extra care must be taken when the bowel is inflamed or diseased as this makes the possibility of injury more likely.

When to Repair Bowel Wall Injuries?

- If the mucosa is entered or visible, then primary repair is mandatory. Repair is accomplished either in one or two layers. Suture size used may be 4-0 or 3-0 and may be permanent or absorbable suture. The critical aspect of the repair is that the mucosa be completely inverted.
- When the muscular wall is damaged and mucosa is visible but not injured (Fig. 14.28), it is still recommended that the bowel wall be repaired. Again either a two- or one-layer closure is used.
- When muscular wall is damaged and no mucosa is visible, depending on the length of injury, the bowel wall may not need to be repaired. The decision is surgeon dependent but any injury over 1 cm in size should be reinforced.

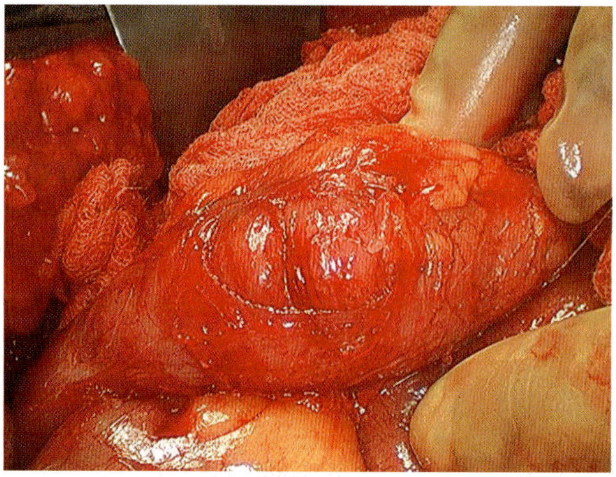

Fig. 14.29: Serosal tear intestinal wall.

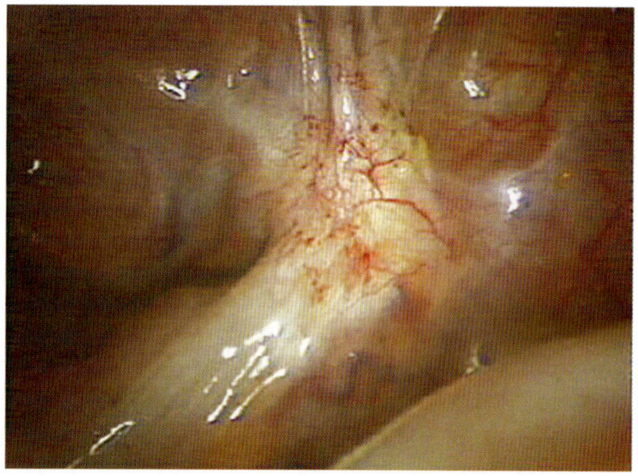

Fig. 14.30: Infiltrating endometriosis Pouch of Douglas.

- Serosal injuries do not need to be repaired (Fig. 14.29).

Tips

- Full thickness bowel wall injuries need to be repaired either with two- or one-layer technique making certain that mucosa is adequately inverted and or covered with viable tissue.
- Muscular wall injury should be repaired depending on degree and size. When in doubt, repair.
- Serosal injuries do not require repair.
- Grasp bowel carefully with large surface area instruments.

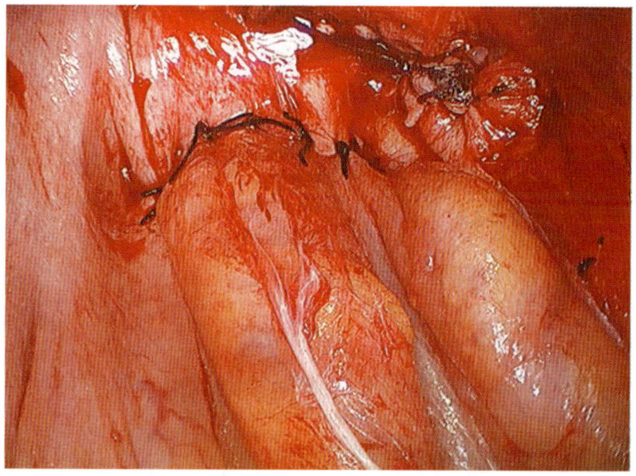

Fig. 14.31: Primary repair of distal sigmoid colon.

OTHER TOPICS

Endometriosis

Endometriosis may involve organs other than the uterus or ovaries and this can include bowel particularly the rectosigmoid. Figure 14.30 demonstrates an endometriotic plaque in the pouch of Douglas.

In order to adequately treat and relieve the patient from their symptoms, complete resection of the involved area is usually required.

When endometriosis involves the colon or rectum, the endometriotic nodule can usually be completely resected without having to perform a formal segmental resection.[13] Anticipation of the need to resect part of the large bowel is usually noted preoperatively and if necessary a general surgeon can be called to assist, however a well-trained laparoscopic surgeon competent in suturing can also treat the involved bowel.

If the nodule requires full thickness resection of the bowel wall and closure would not result in compromise of bowel lumen (usually 50% or less of the bowel wall circumference), then primary repair in a two-layer manner is appropriate. The first inverting layer is usually an absorbable suture (chromic or polyglactin) 4-0 or 3-0 in size. The injury should be closed so as not to compromise the lumen of the bowel so closure in a transverse fashion rather than longitudinal with interrupted suture is best (Fig. 14.31).

The second layer may be either absorbable or permanent and is usually either 4-0 or 3-0 size.

The ultimate success of closure depends on standard well recognized principals of general surgery. The first being a tension-free repair and the second being adequate blood supply.

If the rectum and not the sigmoid colon is involved, because of the lack of serosa, the anastomosis is at higher risk of leak since there is no serosa to aid in sealing of the anastomosis, so it is recommended that in these instances, the use of anti-adhesive agents be avoided. The successful sealing of an anastomosis in this circumstance is very dependent on adherence from surrounding tissues, so adhesions in this instance are crucial to good outcome.

Tips

- When endometriosis is encountered involving the bowel, it usually can be removed by local excision and primary closure.
- Two-layer closure without tension and adequate blood supply to the remaining tissues is standard.
- When rectum is involved, antiadhesive barrier products should be avoided.

Colon Injury

The same management principles apply in a situation where the distal colon or rectum is injured during surgery or entry. The injury is usually repaired in a two-layer fashion. If the defect is small, then a one-layer closure is adequate as long as the bowel mucosa is inverted. The need for creation of a colostomy is extremely rare when the injury is recognized early and closed primarily.

When bowel resection is anticipated preoperatively, usually the patients are placed on mechanical bowel prep. There is good evidence that when patients have not had bowel prep and subsequently underwent resection when compared to patients who did have a bowel prep and underwent resection with anastomosis, there was no difference in leak rate, abscess formation or complication such as wound infection.[14] The long-held notion that all patients that are to undergo bowel surgery need to be on a mechanical prep is now questioned.

In special cases where an entire segment of bowel needs to be removed, the availability of circular staplers has made creation of a low colonic anastomosis simpler. There are certain principles that need to be understood when using these devices. First is that there should be no tension on the anastomosis and staple line. The proximal bowel should easily reach into the pelvis without tension. The descending colon or splenic flexure may need to be mobilized in order to reach the distal sigmoid or rectal stump; if this is needed then care must be taken that the blood supply is not compromised in the process as this is the second important factor in a successful anastomosis.

Choosing staple size is very important. Lower colon anastomosis using a circular stapler should be performed with a 28 mm diameter stapler or larger.

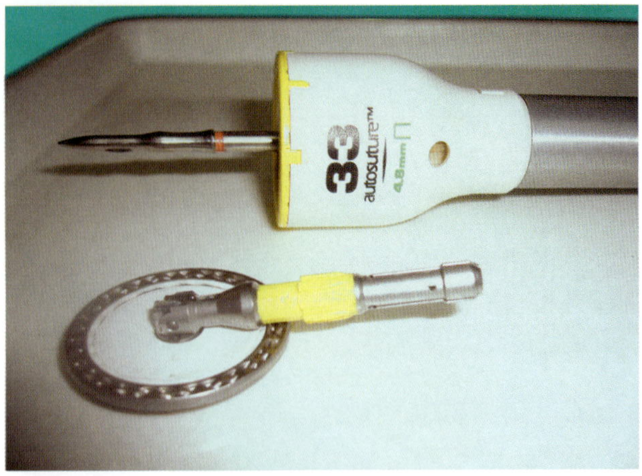

Fig. 14.32: EEA stapler by Covidien: Anvil and stapler.

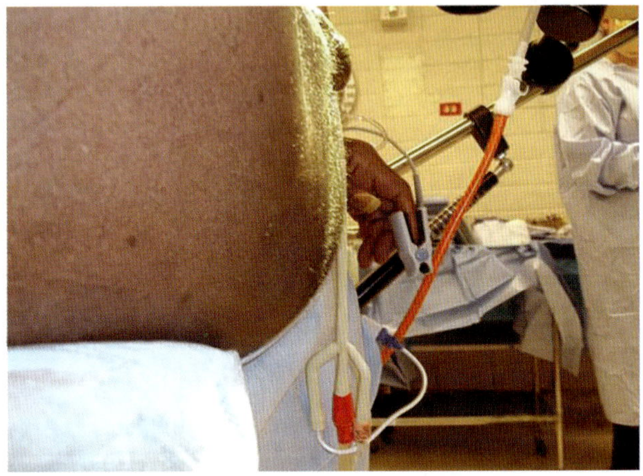

Fig. 14.33: Extension of buttocks over end of operating table in preparation for insertion of EEA stapler.

Figure 14.32 shows a stapling device manufactured by Covidien Corporation. The anvil and stapler are demonstrated.

Using a stapler smaller than 28 mm usually will lead to stricture. If the proximal bowel lumen is small the staple anvil may be placed in a side fashion forming an end-to-side anastomosis and thus creating an adequately large lumen.

In placing the anvil in the proximal bowel, the bowel should be closed firmly around the anvil post so that when the stapler is closed and fired no bowel wall is extruded from the side of the stapler, resulting in a compromised anastomosis.

In placing the stapling device transanally, it is very important that the patient's lower buttocks and perineum extend past the edge of the operating table. This allows adequate angling of the stapler into the rectum and first part of the sigmoid. This is absolutely crucial to successful docking and firing of the stapler (Fig. 14.33).

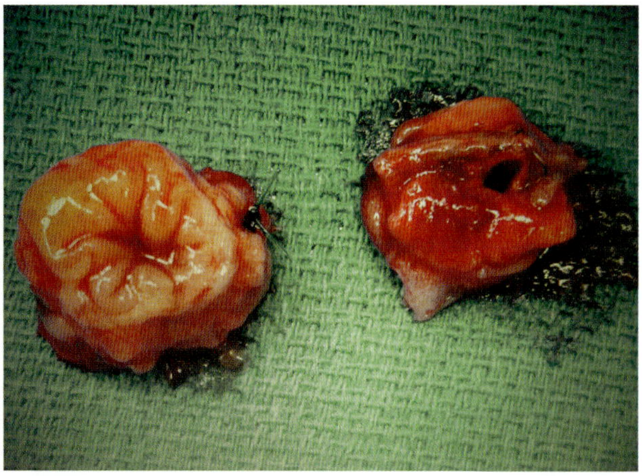

Fig. 14.34: Colon and rectal tissue donuts from EEA stapler.

Once the stapler and anvil are docked, the stapler fired and removed, the confirmation of two intact tissue "doughnuts" (Fig. 14.34) and a secure anastomosis via colonoscopy or insufflation using proctoscopy or other device with submersion leak testing should be performed. In the instance of a questionable staple line, the anastomosis site can be reinforced with an inverting stitch or redone. Drains are not usually placed.

Tips

- Mechanical bowel prep is not mandatory in colon surgery.
- Closure of colon after partial resection or injury should be in two-layer fashion.
- Circular stapling devices should be 28 mm or greater in diameter when used for anastomosis after segmental resection.
- In closure of rectal injury or resection, avoid anti-adhesive materials.
- Colostomies are rarely needed when the bowel is injured during surgery; primary repair is preferred.

General surgical conditions can mimic gynecologic disease and may be encountered in the course of surgery for gynecologic conditions. It is important to be able to recognize, diagnose and have knowledge of treatment for these conditions in order to have good surgical outcomes.

REFERENCES

1. Millennium Research Group. US Markets for Soft Tissue Repair 2009, Toronto, ON: Millennium Research Group, Inc; 2008.
2. Luijendijk RW, Hop WCJ, van den Tol MP, et.al. A comparison of suture repair with mesh repair of incisional hernia. N Engl J Med. 2000;343:392-8.
3. Jonas J. The problem with mesh shrinkage in laparoscopic incisional hernia repair. Zentralbl Chir. 2009; 134(3):209-13.
4. Olmi S, Scaini A, Cesana GC, et al. Laparoscopic versus open incisional hernia repair: an open randomized controlled study. Surg Endosc. 2007;21(4):555-9.
5. Morrison J, Jacobs VR. Laparoscopic preperitoneal inguinal hernia repair using preformed polyester mesh without fixation: prospective study with one year follow up results in a rural setting. Surg Laparosc Endosc Percutan Tech. 2008:18(1);33-9.
6. McCormack K, Scott NW, Go PM, et al. EU Hernia Trialists Collaboration. Laparoscopic techniques versus open techniques for inguinal hernia repairs. Cochrane Database Syst Rev. 2003;(1):CD001785.
7. Neumayer L, Giobbie-Hurder A, Jonasson O, et. al. Open mesh versus laparoscopic mesh repair of inguinal hernia. N Engl J Med. 2004;350(18):1819-27.
8. Jacobs VR, Morrison JE Jr. Comparison of institutional costs for laparoscopic preperitoneal inguinal hernia versus open repair and its reimbursement in an ambulatory surgery center. Surg Laparosc Endosc Percultan Tech. 2008:18(1):70-4.
9. Kathkouda N, Mason RJ, Towfigh S. Laparoscopic versus open appendectomy: a prospective randomized double-blind study. Ann Surg. 2005;242(3): 439-48;
10. Lyons T, Winer WK, Woo A. Appendectomy in patients undergoing laparoscopic surgery for pelvic pain. J Am Assoc Gynecol Laparosc. 2001;8(4): 542-4.
11. Agarwala N, Liu CY. Laparoscopic appendectomy. J Am Assoc Gynecol Laparosc. 2003;10(2):166-8.
12. Cartmill JA, Shakeshaft AJ, Walsh WR, et al. High pressures are generated at the tip of laparoscopic graspers. Aust NZJ Surg. 1999;69(2):127-30.
13. Roman H, Rozsnayi F, Puscasiu L, et.al. Complications associated with two laparoscopic procedures used in management of rectal endometriosis. JSLS. 2010; 14(2):169-77.
14. Zmora O, Mahajna A, Bar-Zakai B, et al. Colon and rectal surgery without mechanical bowel preparation: a randomized prospective trial. Ann Surg. 2003;237(3);363-7.

KIEL SCHOOL

15 of Gynaecological Endoscopy

Pneumoperitoneum

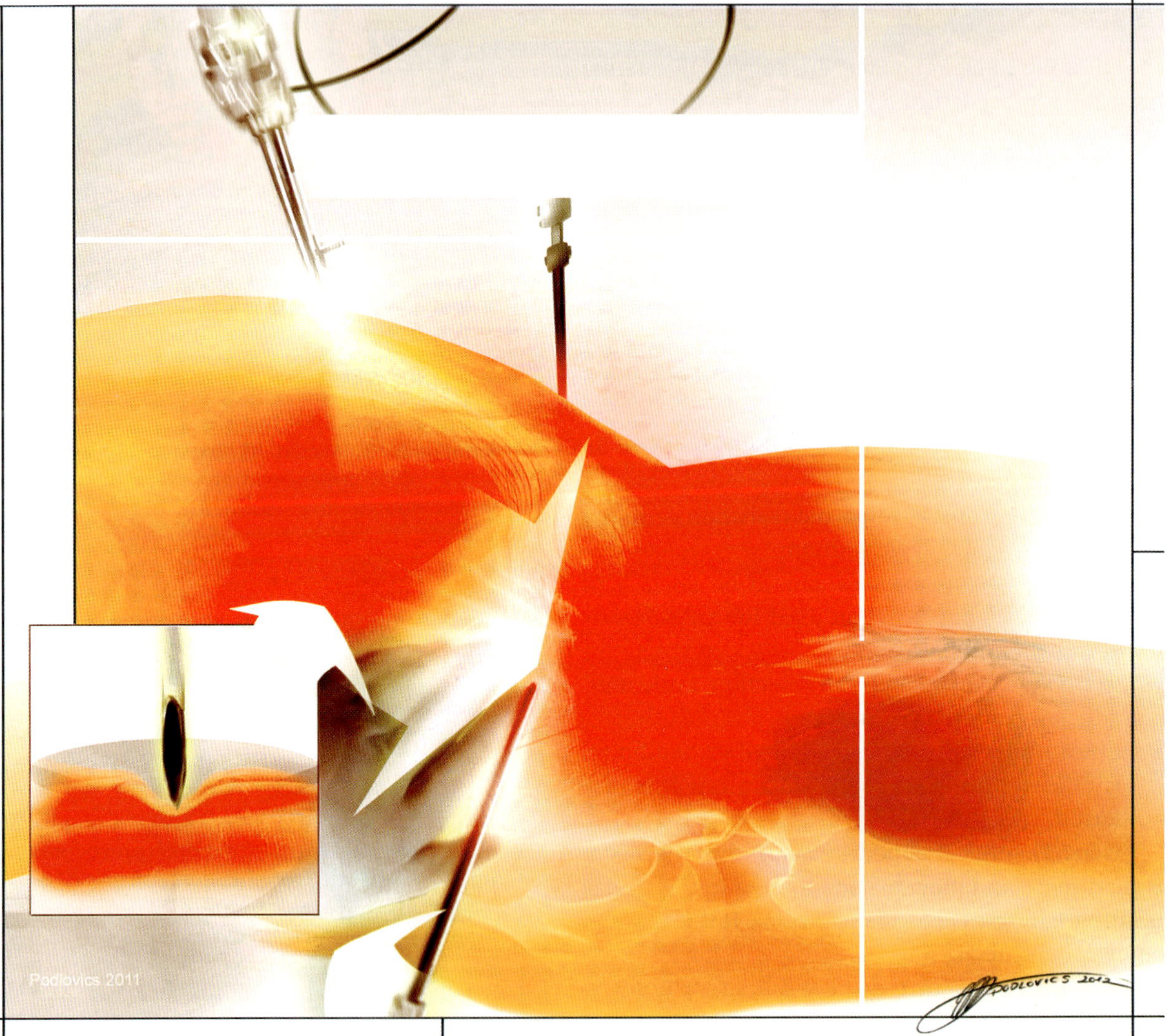

Chapter 15

Pneumoperitoneum: Known and Lesser-known Perspectives—Scope and Considerations

Douglas E Ott

INTRODUCTION

Laparoscopic pneumoperitoneum is the purposeful introduction of a gas or gases into the abdomen and is the focus of this chapter. The consequences of a laparoscopic pneumoperitoneum arise due to chemistry and physics influencing physiologic reactions and responses. It is not static but a dynamic, continuous and cumulative process with both intra- and postoperative effects and consequences.

Other than surgical appropriateness and skills of the surgeon laparoscopic pneumoperitoneum involves knowledge of the effects of a gas insufflator (a throttling-down pressure regulator), gas choice, abdominal access and entry, a working understanding of gas laws, physics, physiologic effects of gas chemistry and pressure, abdominal compliance, tissue effects and knowledge about preventions, handling and correction of complications.

Dynamics of the biologic surgical procedure and response to laparoscopy have cumulative effects on the outcome influenced by the interaction of all the components of the process. They are not passive or unimportant to the process. They should not be forgotten or disregarded once the pneumoperitoneum is created. Some are consequential some are not. Some depend on the patients' comorbidity status. Open laparotomy surgery is not without its consequences either. It is incumbent on the surgeon to understand these components and their interactions to mitigate untoward events and circumstances to control and reduce complications and subject patients to correct surgery for their problem with confidence that they are providing the best laparoscopic surgery and outcome. The ultimate goal is error elimination regardless of whether it is iatrogenic or committed by omission or commission.

SO IT BEGINS . . .

The gas used for a laparoscopic pneumoperitoneum is almost always carbon dioxide (CO_2). This is because it has the least undesirable consequences and effects on the patient. Chemistry, biochemistry and physiology make carbon dioxide (CO_2) the gas of choice[1] (Tables 15.1A to C). Carbon dioxide has a high diffusion coefficient (20:1 to oxygen and 25:1 to nitrogen) and is a normal metabolic end product rapidly cleared from the body by the lungs. It is highly soluble in blood and tissues and does not support combustion.

Government regulatory agencies mandate that the gas be extremely dry with less than 200 parts per million of water vapor, 0.02% relative humidity (RH).[2]

Table 15.1A: Physical, chemical and biological effects of CO_2 for pneumoperitoneum

Physical effects	Chemical effects	Biologic effects
Mechanical effects	Gas	Hypothermia
Abdominal compliance	Desiccation	Tissue disruption
Intra-abdominal pressure	Hypoxia	Increased peritoneal viscosity
Time	Acidosis	Acidosis
Patient position		Hypoxia

Table 15.1B: Factors affecting the pneumoperitoneum independent of the gas used

Intra-abdominal pressure	Patient position
Dryness of the gas	Volume of gas used
Acidosis	Hypoxia
Length of exposure	Abdominal compliance

Table 15.1C: Changes that occur due to a pneumoperitoneum regardless of the type of gas used

Increased		Decreased
Intra-abdominal pressure	Systemic blood pressure	Venous return
Neurohormonal vasoactivity	Mean arterial pressure	Cardiac output
Pulmonary vascular resistance	Heart rate	Splanchnic blood flow
Peripheral vascular resistance		Functional residual capacity

This makes it harsh and unphysiologic to the normal homeostatic condition of peritoneal tissue and abdominal cavity. Without modification in the raw state the gas goes into the abdomen at 20°C being 15°C below body temperature[3] (Flowchart 15.1). The gas is pressurized and flows at high velocities through constrictions from its path from the insufflator to the abdomen. The peritoneal surfaces are wet and the cavity high in moisture content (over 95% relative humidity (RH)). This circumstance of very dry cool gas rapidly flowing gas over wet warm tissue caused rapid evaporation, tissue hypothermia and tissue desiccation of the peritoneum. Correcting CO_2 to more physiologic parameters of 95% RH and within 7°C of normal body temperature reduces peritoneal desiccation and damage, inflammatory response, hypothermia and potential adhesion formation.[4,5] Carbon dioxide is listed in the United States.

In pharmacopeia and other countries in which carbon dioxide is used as a drug, it is sold with the following labeling: "WARNING! Administration of carbon dioxide may be hazardous or contraindicated. For use only by or under the supervision of a licensed practitioner who is experienced in the use and administration of carbon dioxide and is familiar with the indications, effects, dosages, methods and frequency and duration of administration and with the hazards, contraindications and side effects and the precautions to be taken."

The insufflator is a gas-throttling-down-pressure device regulating gas flow rate and pressure for creation and maintenance of a pneumoperitoneum.[6] As the very dry room temperature gas leaves the insufflator, it undergoes the Joule–Thompson effect decreasing the temperature further as the gas expands.[7] There are two settings on insufflators, gas flow rate and pressure. Flow occurs until the pre-set

Flowchart 15.1: Physiological effect of gas quality (water content and temperature) during laparoscopic procedures.

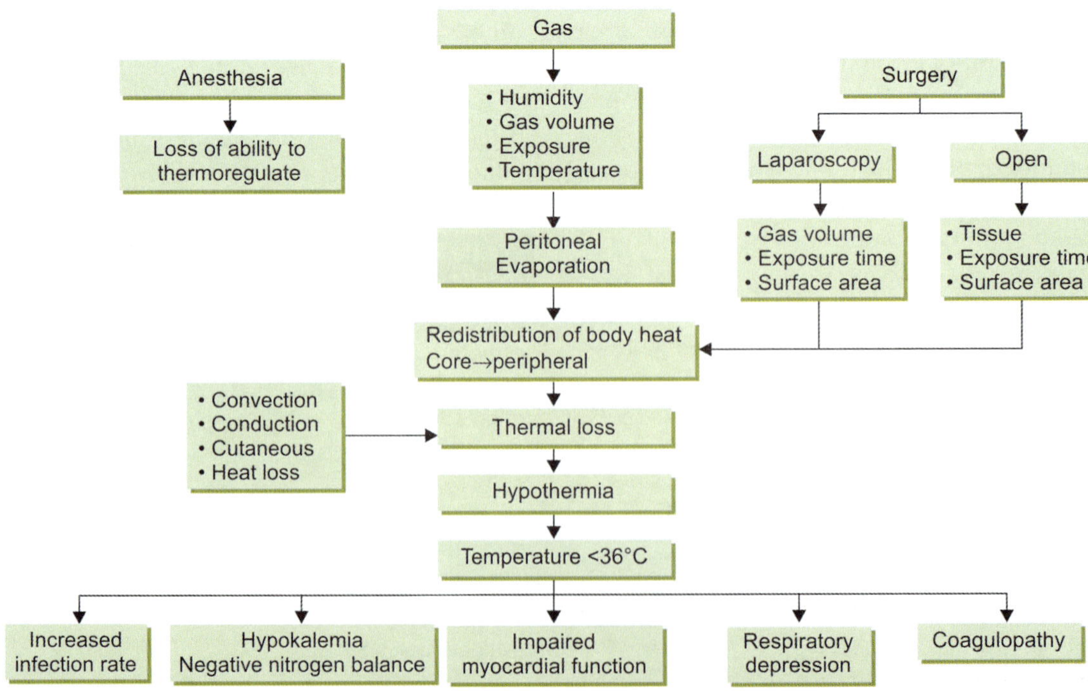

pressure is reached. Commercial insufflators comparatively do not have the same performance characteristics even at the same settings. A specific flow rate setting using the same setup and connections comparing performance does not result in the same fill rate or flow characteristics. They have different filling rates. What is set and visualized on the dials does not represent what is actually delivered to the abdomen and may be due to variances of gas flow and measuring components of the insufflator.

An insufflator set at 40 liters per minute (lpm) is not actually delivering 40 lpm to the abdomen. Why? Assuming the average adult abdomen has a 3 L capacity to reach full expansion beyond which more pressure does not expand the operating space, a setting of 3 lpm would take 1 min to fill at that set pressure. Set at 6 lpm would take 30 s, at 12 lpm 15 s, at 24 lpm 7.5 s and at 40 lpm would take about 4.5 s. Insufflators set at 40 lpm do not fill the abdomen in 4.5 s. This is not the real-world experience. If setting an insufflator at 40 lpm and seeing it at 40 lpm does not result in a pneumoperitoneum in 5 s either the delivery rate is really less than 40 lpm or the timing is incorrect. Seeing a dial showing a gas delivery rate of 40 lpm and getting something else does not make it so.

An abdomen will only stretch so much. The stretchability of the abdomen is its compliance. This is the change in volume per change in pressure. Insufflation volume into the abdominal cavity follows phases that overlap in occurrence: (1) a reshaping phase with minimal changes due to pressure, (2) the stretching phase that results in elastic expansion of the abdominal wall and (3) the pressure phase characterized by a pressure–volume relationship producing maximum stretch of the abdominal wall.[8]

A setting of 11 mm Hg may reach complete abdominal expansion in one person but not in another. When complete full abdominal compliance is reached adding even 1 mm Hg pressure of gas will not expand the abdominal wall any further. No more space is created in the pneumoperitoneum, but pressure is increased. This compromises capillary blood flow to the visceral splanchnic compartment and vessels under the abdominal fascia decreasing blood flow and increasing hypoxia and cellular inflammatory reactions.[9,10]

GAS CHEMISTRY: CO_2 EFFECTS

Despite the benefits of creating the operating space, a pneumoperitoneum is not without physiological consequences. Insufflation reduces blood flow to organs within the peritoneal space due to pressure and not chemistry of the gas. The reduction in blood flow promotes anaerobic metabolism leading to lactic acidosis, postoperative alteration in liver enzymes, subclinical hepatic dysfunction and increases in oxidative stress markers.[11] As a result, tissue ischemia and altered postoperative organ function contributes to laparoscopic-associated morbidity and mortality. The increase in intra-abdominal pressure (IAP) results in mechanical decrease of splanchnic blood flow. Release of vasoactive substances is also stimulated, including vasopressin, angiotensin, cortisol and adrenocorticotropin hormone (ACTH) attributable to CO_2 chemistry.[12]

Carbon dioxide causes vasodilatation and is counteracted by increased IAP-effecting changes in blood flow within the pneumoperitoneum. The regulation and net effect of the gas and pressure on tissues and organ blood flow is a combination of intrinsic and extrinsic mechanisms. Intrinsic factors include tissue metabolism, local reflexes, cell induced vasoactive chemicals that influence vasodilatation, hypoxia and flow regulation.[12] Extrinsic factors include systemic hemodynamics and circulating vasoactive chemicals including anesthetic agents and sympathetic nerve response. Increases in IAP cause hypoxia to abdominal organs as shown in Table 15.2.

The CO_2 or any gas used through an insufflator is very dry and cool compared to the patient and causes hypothermia, tissue desiccation and increased inflammatory responses compared to

Table 15.2: Percent decrease in blood flow causing hypoxia from 10 to 14 mm Hg, additional % decrease from 14 to 20 mm Hg and total % change with 20 mm Hg (IAP in parenthesis)

Initial opening (IAP = 0–3 mm Hg) baseline perfusion	% change (10–14 mm Hg)	(14–20 mm Hg) Additional % change and total % change
Peritoneum	55 ± 3	18 ± 2 (73)
Rectus sheath	26 ± 3	15 ± 3 (41)
Stomach	45 ± 2	12 ± 2 (57)
Duodenum	9 ± 1	3 ± 1 (12)
Jejunum	29 ± 1	5 ± 1 (34)
Liver	36 ± 2	6 ± 1 (42)
Mesenteric artery	40 ± 3	29 ± 2 (69)
Cecum	34 ± 2	7 ± 1 (41)
Colon	39 ± 2	9 ± 1 (48)
Ovary	14 ± 1	4 ± 1 (18)
Fallopian tube	47 ± 2	13 ± 2 (60)

pre-conditioned gas. When humidified warmed CO_2 is used there is less hypothermia, less peritoneal damage, less inflammatory response, less pain and shortened recovery time.[4]

PHYSICS: INTRA-ABDOMINAL PRESSURE

Decreasing operating IAP as much as possible is beneficial to a point. It is necessary that the pneumoperitoneal space be sufficient for the surgeon to do their best work without compromising their abilities and outcomes for the patient. Any gas put into a confined space will increase pressure. The usual operating IAP is 12–14 mm Hg with the effects of any gas related to pressure not the chemistry of the gas. The pressure caused by the gas is due to the limits of the space into which it is confined[13] (Flowchart 15.2). The chemical and biologic interactions of gas within the abdominal cavity are related to its surface characteristics, diffusion and local cellular and biochemical activities and global responses to pressure and chemical changes.[14,15] What matters is pressure, duration of pressure and total volume of gas used. Therefore, IAP should be kept just below the limit of complete abdominal compliance. This maintains sufficient operating space, improves perfusion and reduces hypoxia. There is no evidence that low-pressure pneumoperitoneum (6–10 mm Hg) offers any advantages.[16-19]

JET STREAMING

Gas velocity can reach 30 m/s becoming a "jet stream" flow when exiting a cannula during insufflation.[20] The gas jet stream touches peritoneal surfaces, causing a circular hydraulic deflection. If the gas is dry and cool it causes rapid evaporative cooling, peritoneal fluid viscosity thickening and constituent concentration changes and peritoneal tissue damage and disruption.[7,21] The thin layer of mesothelial cells of the peritoneum is damaged when dry gas is used destroying microvilli, retracting and bulging cells and exposing the basal lamina.[4,22-30] These conditions are reduced when humidified warmed gas is used.[4,23,24,29,30] Desiccation tissue damage is not possible if the gas is highly saturated with water vapor. When the gas is holding water at an elevated RH at the same temperature as the abdominal tissues.[4] Evaporative cooling, cell desiccation and peritoneal fluid viscosity changes do not take place when the gas is hydrated and warmed.[7,21,31] Heating gas without humidification has no beneficial and some detrimental effects.[32-35]

Whether the peritoneal cavity is open for laparotomy or closed during laparoscopy, tissues are exposed to gas or gases. Air is a mixture of gases for laparotomy and CO_2 with laparoscopy. Gas(es) have properties that effect the tissue locally and the organism globally. Operating room ambient air RH is usually between 45% and 55%. The RH of gases used for laparoscopy is less than 1%. During laparotomy gas flow is due to prevailing operating room conditions with air flow less than 2 m/s while during laparoscopy depending on insufflator setting and final orifice diameter gas flow can reach 30 m/s.[20]

CO_2 ABSORPTION

The rate of peritoneal gas absorption is determined by IAP and partial pressure gradients influenced by

Flowchart 15.2: Physiological effect of increased intra-abdominal pressure.

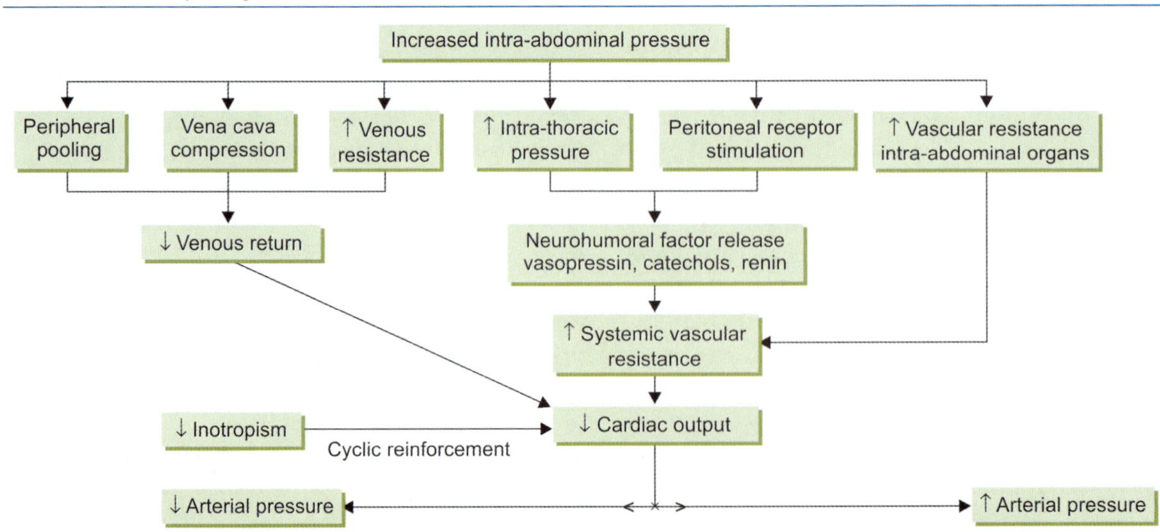

tissue/gas permeability, tissue absorptive capacity, temperature and surface area exposed. The amount of CO_2 absorption through the peritoneum during laparoscopy is between 14 and 48 mL/min[36] based on peritoneal cavity gas clearance estimates and peritoneal blood flow being between 2% and 7% of cardiac output or approximately 100 mL/min.[37,38] High-precision isotope-ratio mass spectrometry shows that 10–20% of CO_2 eliminated during laparoscopy is from peritoneal absorption variability due to different insufflation pressures. Carbon dioxide absorption reaches a plateau after 20–25 min of pneumoperitoneum and continues to be eliminated up to 30 min after desufflation.[39] Humidifying and warming CO_2 for insufflation leads to faster dissipation of residual gas after pneumoperitoneum desufflation.[40]

HYPOTHERMIA: VERY DRY GAS, TEMPERATURE DIFFERENTIAL AND EVAPORATIVE EFFECTS

In 1854 Claude Bernard recognized that the relative constancy of body temperature was integral to the regulation of the "milieu intérieur" required for health and proper functioning of cellular elements of warm-blooded animals.[41,42] He said the healthy man does not exist with an internal body temperature much outside the normal range of 36–38°C. Cannon used this internal stability concept to develop the idea of self-regulating homeostasis.[43]

The normal situation of patients having laparoscopy is a body temperature approximately 37°C with a peritoneal cavity high in humidity and a thin film of peritoneal fluid covering peritoneal tissues. Any gas used with an insufflator or external gas source is 15–17°C cooler and 100 times drier than the Sahara desert on purpose. Thinking this drastic difference will not matter or have no detrimental biologic or physiologic effects is wrong, illogical and incorrect. Hypothermia related to any surgical procedure multifactorial having many factors influencing the amount of temperature lost. These factors include patient age, sex, weight, anesthetic drugs, patients original temperature, room temperature, length of operation, temperature of infused or irrigation fluids, volume of fluids used, temperature of skin cleansing solutions and temperature and volume of irrigation left in the peritoneal cavity. Therefore infusion liquids, irrigation or cleansing solutions should be warmed prior to use.

Heat loss during surgery is due to radiation, convection, conduction and evaporation. Reducing or preventing thermal losses from these situations is preferred and beneficial. The difference between laparoscopy and laparotomy is an open peritoneal cavity compared to a closed cavity. The ambient environment for laparotomy is 20°C, 45–50% RH and mild air current of 1–3 m/s. For laparoscopy the ambient environment external to the peritoneal cavity is 20°C, 45–50% RH and mild air flow of 1–3 m/s on the patients surface and inside the peritoneal cavity intermittent gas flow of 20°C, 0.02% RH and up to 30 m/s flow and hundreds of liters gas consumed.[44-49]

The physiologic response to general anesthesia and anesthetic drugs is an increase in the threshold of warmth and a decrease in the threshold coldness. Anesthetic drugs cause a chemical disconnect between the hypothalamic pituitary axis suppressing control of both afferent and efferent thermoregulation. Therefore, the patient is at the mercy of their environment and what is done to them influencing the direction, rapidity and how far their temperature will trend. Mild hypothermia is defined as a core body temperature below 35°C.

Intraoperative hypothermia alters pharmacokinetics for each 0.1°C below 35°C (especially with inhalation agents as they are more soluble and many muscle relaxants having prolonged effect at lower internal temperatures causing patients taking longer to awaken), respiratory volume and frequency per minute decrease, decreases cerebral blood flow by 7% for each 1°C decrease in core temperature, increases coagulopathy, prolongs recovery time, increases oxygen consumption, increases discomfort due to chill and shivering, delays wound healing, increases infection rate, increases immunosuppression over euthermic patients and prolongs hospital stay. Despite other contributing factors, general anesthesia contributes to hypothermia through three phases. In phase one, central body heat is lost through thermal redistribution in the first 60 min with a temperature loss of 0.5–1.5°C. In phase two, peripheral and central heat loss leads to clinical mild hypothermia with a temperature below 35°C. In phase three, peripheral vasoconstriction causes core temperature to stay below 35°C. In addition to all these factors if dry cool gas is used for the pneumoperitoneum relative to core body temperature and wet tissue surfaces having rapid evaporation and local cooling and tissue desiccation, these physiologic reactions and responses add to the total hypothermia effect.

The best way to prevent problems of hypothermia is to prevent hypothermia. Conditioning CO_2 for laparoscopy to just below body core temperature and humidifying to 95% RH eliminates or reduces hypothermia, tissue desiccation, inflammation, adhesion formation, postoperative pain and has clinical benefits and utility.[4,24,50-63]

Local peritoneal hypothermia causes vasoconstriction disrupting gastrointestinal peristalsis and myoelectric conduction. Using a dry cool gas for a pneumoperitoneum induces a temperature gradient contributing to reduction in myoelectric activity. Paralytic ileus is a temporary dysmobility syndrome impairing peristalsis. Contributing factors include metabolic or electrical heterogeneities caused by regional ischemia, surgical trauma or physical stress changing electrical properties that maintain and regulate peristalsis. Induced temperature gradients create electrical instability caused by a generalized thermionic visceral response to temperature and mechanical manipulations. Thermal cooling ionic feedback response persistently deforms and destabilizes the physiological enteric electrical activity, leading to intestinal arrhythmias and paralytic ileus. The interruption in velocity propagation and dynamics of the electrophysiological wave propagation causes pain and paralytic ileus.[64] Intestinal hypothermia, disruption of gastrointestinal electrical activity and transit time and postoperative paralytic ileus are improved by pre-conditioning CO_2 gas.

FULCRUM EFFECT

Using a rigid rod (scope or instrument) through a cannula produces a lever rotating at a fixed point becoming a fulcrum. Applying force and angling whatever is in the cannula, the lever creates an output force, leverage, resulting in mechanical advantage of the lever. The distance from the fulcrum to the applied input force determines the power of the lever. The surgeon's intent is to direct the lever to a desired site for an action without using increased leverage to obtain the view. But leverage happens. The forces applied by the device at the fulcrum, the point where the trocar penetrates the abdominal fascia is resisted by the compliance and tensile strength of the tissues. Movement of the surgeon's hand on the scope or instrument, with straight stick non-robotic surgery, gives immediate resistance to tactile feedback. The user has the ability to know when the force is too large putting stress (force pressure) and strain (deformation) on tissues in the area of the fulcrum with the ability to reduce the force.[65]

With hands on straight-stick nonrobotic laparoscopy there is tactile haptic perceptive real-time instantaneous feedback. The ability to self-correct is present. During robotic surgery the surgeon is not holding the device, does not see the device, does not feel the device and does not know the movements or forces created by the device through the cannula. Prolonged angulation without knowledge of position or force increases hypoxia and anoxia to tissues in the immediate path of the levering device. The force of the fulcrum can additionally surpass the tissue strength of the fascia to maintain its original size and causes tearing and extension that may require suturing. Excessive instrument skin contact with the levering action can also cause irritation and abrasion. In an analysis of consequential surgical errors it was found that "the use of excessive force" was one of the errors contributing to the injuries and that "55% of the consequential errors were due to a step being done with too much force/distance."[66,67]

Performing surgery is more than an exercise of manipulating intra-abdominal tissues, remote and separate from the patient, having tunnel vision, non-haptic, non-contextual awareness of the dynamic activities that make up the total surgical episode for the patient. When a robot separates the surgeon from the patient and when the surgeon is unable to experience visual and nonverbal patient contact at operating table, the patient is put at risk. Proximity counts.

PERITONEAL FLUID

The first material the gas stream encounters during laparoscopy is peritoneal fluid. Peritoneal fluid is a thin film of approximately 60 µm covering the peritoneum having water content like serum. It contains cellular components, proteins, coagulation precursors and surface-active lipoproteins in specific quantities to maintain normal peritoneal health and homeostasis that respond to inflammation or cellular damage. Peritoneal fluid functions to maintain efficient hydrodynamic and boundary lubrication reducing surface wear and promoting protection of the peritoneal cells.[68] Peritoneal fluid covers the glycocalyx layer of the mesothelium.

A flow of very dry gas into the peritoneal cavity removes water by evaporation with the liquid peritoneal fluid moisture trying to equilibrate and maintain a homeostatic balance. As gas leaves the abdomen it carries away moisture rich gas and heat and new dry cool gas enters continuously repeating the drying evaporation process. The forceful rapid dry cool gas flow causes an 18°C temperature loss on contact with the peritoneum in less than 2 s. This changes local peritoneal fluid consistency and concentration, damaging peritoneal tissue in the path of the gas stream.[7] The dry gas alters peritoneal fluid viscosity and tribological interactions, diminishing its lubricating qualities of wear reduction from abrasion and friction, and increases solute concentration and alters normal inflammatory and fibrinolytic responses of peritoneal surfaces.[69] Surface evaporation and cooling decrease intestinal motility increasing the likelihood of ileus[70] (*see* hypothermia).

Peritoneum

When the peritoneum is penetrated to create and maintain a pneumoperitoneum it sets in motion a cascade of normal cellular responses to repair the peritoneal injury. This is normal. This normal process of healing and resurfacing may attach to or connect previously separated surfaces becoming intimately stuck to each other, tethering structures previously unattached, distorting anatomy, producing pain and interrupting, disrupting or blocking normal function. That is the abnormality not the process of healing, an important distinction.

The peritoneum is the largest serous membrane of the body with a surface area about equal to the integumentary system; 1.1–2.1 m^2.[2,12,71] The peritoneum consists of two layers: loose connective tissue and mesothelium. The peritoneal surface is a continuous sheet of mesothelial cells overlaying loose mesenchymal connective tissue, a basal lamina and basement membrane attached to the abdominal wall and viscera, and well supplied with blood vessels, capillaries, and lymphatics.[5,72] Peritoneal thickness ranges between 0.3 and 1.1 mm depending on the surface covered.[73] The peritoneal surface area covering the visceral peritoneum represents 81.89% and for the parietal peritoneal 18.11%. Peritoneal surfaces are not all the same with more importance related to the amount of area with microvilli, areas where vessels and microcirculation are prominent for exchange and volume of the intercellular matrix.[74]

Pneumoperitoneum affects the entire gas-exposed surface of the peritoneum-bearing portions of the basal lamina.[25,75] Characteristic alterations of the peritoneum caused by cold dry CO_2 pneumoperitoneum are mesothelial damage, desiccation, distorted and denuded peritoneal surfaces and exposed areas of basil lamina.[26,30,76-87] The authors plead that there is a need to "create a physiologic pneumoperitoneum." Pre-conditioning CO_2 for laparoscopy making the gas humidified and warmed enhances preservation of peritoneal integrity and has clinical benefits.[22,23,88-91]

Mesothelial cells and peritoneal fluid protect, promote and sustain peritoneal homeostasis. The apical surface of the mesothelium has a film on the surface, the glycocalyx, providing a slippery nonadhesive hydrodynamic boundary surface lubricant for the peritoneal viscera and protects the mesothelial surface from abrasions and adhesions. The glycocalyx is composed of lipoproteins, phospholipids, proteoglycans and hyaluronan. The glycocalyx plays an important role in cell-cell contact, tissue hydration, regulation of inflammation, tissue remodeling, and flow of nutrients and growth factors across the peritoneal membrane.[68,92-95] The mesothelial cells synthesize cytokines, growth factors and matrix protein components integral for induction and resolution of inflammation and tissue repair.

ADHESION FORMATION IS A MISNOMER: THE PERITONEAL HEALING PROCESS IS NORMAL

It is baffling to the scientific mind; acumen, facts and evidence garnered over the modern era of physiology and surgery that severely altering the homeostasis and normal conditions of the abdominal cavity during a procedure is a nonevent and should just be tolerated. Prevention is warranted when a known hazard is possible. Laparoscopy hardly avoids peritoneal drying as suggested by some authors "More important, laparoscopy avoids peritoneal drying. This reduces peritoneal trauma and potential for adhesion formation."[96] Not true.

The mesothelium repairs itself from peritoneal injury through a normal inflammatory response and regrowth of tissue by resurfacing the injury. This is a normal response not a departure from normal. If the repair response does not allow tissues to be in their original location or function properly as a result of normal tissue healing this is a departure from normal and is the abnormality. The response to peritoneal injury results in four outcomes: repair and resurfacing or the peritoneum with normal anatomic and functional location, and three "adhesion processes," locations with or without excess peritoneal attachments defined as "adhesion formation" (adhesions formed at operative sites); de novo adhesion formation (adhesions formed at nonoperative sites); and adhesion reformation (adhesions formed after lysis of previous adhesions).[98-100]

Regardless of how the insult occurred or its etiology, peritoneum reacts with the same cellular response. Initiation of repair occurs despite how the peritoneal injury happened, whether by a scalpel, instrument, gauze pad, drying, scissors, cautery, laser, harmonic scalpel, freezing or chemicals from bacteria or body fluids from the gallbladder, stomach, bowel, kidney, liver, ovary, uterus or pancreas is the same. Peritoneal drying as desiccation injury has long been recognized. It was reported on October 27, 1892 by George Hawkins-Ambler referencing Max Walthard that "exposure and desiccation of the peritoneum" is one of the greatest factors of postoperative complications.[101] In 1918, it was suspected that at laparotomy "the amount of peritoneal drying" detrimentally influenced postoperative recovery and it was recommended to "avoid peritoneal drying."[102] "Peritoneal drying causes mesothelial desquamation."[103] Others say "that the surgeon should try to avoid, peritoneal drying"[104] and that "adhesions may be due to peritoneal drying, injury"[105] with "insufflations with heated, humidified CO_2 are the least likely to induce mesothelial damage"[73,106] because "drying of tissue is a known cause of adhesion formation."[51,86,107] "Due to the high flow rates, warming and moistening of the insufflated CO_2 is necessary."[108] Pre-conditioning CO_2 with low concentrations of N_2O and O_2, humidification with warming, heparinized solution and dexamethasone has been shown to decrease adhesion formation and reduce the inflammatory process.[109]

Peritoneum is first damaged by abdominal wall penetration exposing surfaces to gas introduction and flow over time. One or multiple entry points, intermittent gas flow, instrument touching of tissue, suturing, coagulation, tissue manipulation for exposure or traction counter-traction and the quality of the gas all contribute to mesothelial damage and the initiation of the normal repair response. Gas flow does not have tactile or visual feedback letting the surgeon sense an observation due to this action. Gas flow is not seen or felt but the insufflator continuously attempts to maintain pressure and flow settings. The effects of gas introduction into the abdomen for the pneumoperitoneum are discussed in the jet-streaming section.[20] The only knowledge the surgeon has of gas flow and pressure effect is abdominal wall expansion. Gas replacement maintaining the pneumoperitoneum occurs automatically without surgeon's awareness of the process. Gas loss around abdominal wall entry points, leaks in the system at connections, instrument placement and removal and purposeful removal of smoke or aerosol creation are automatically replaced by the insufflator. If the gas is dry and cool, there is a constant loss of moisture and heat from the peritoneal surface and abdominal cavity being replaced with dry cool gas as long as the procedure lasts significantly influencing hypothermia, tissue damage and clinical outcome. Direct tissue damage by instrument or device touching is appreciated and understood by the surgeon but the unseen pressurized gas flow damage isn't but has just as much effect on the peritoneum and the tissue repair process. The first occurrence as a result of dry gas flow is a change in peritoneal fluid viscosity and direct tissue alteration due to desiccation and cell disruption depending on dwell time of gas flow but does not occur with humidified warmed gas.[4,7,21-30] Peritoneal desiccation damage is followed by a cascade of inflammatory, cellular, immunologic and repair tissue healing processes that are well documented.[4,5,23,28,68,72,76,88,94,95,97,106,108-124] When desiccation is prevented adhesion formation due to this cause is mitigated. The moderate adverse structural, metabolic and immune changes within the peritoneal cavity are dependent mostly on IAP, duration and volume of gas used except for transient potential of hydrogen (pH) changes due to CO_2. Laparoscopic surgery has more systemic and clinical outcome benefits when compared with open surgery.[121]

NORMAL CHANGES DUE TO A SURGICAL CO_2 PNEUMOPERITONEUM

Ceteris paribus (all other things being equal), any of the effects of creation and maintenance of the surgical pneumoperitoneum is mild, transient and reversible in healthy patients with no comorbidities and appropriate attention to detail and intra-operative surveillance by a skilled physician. Respiratory, cardiac, pH, intestinal, liver, hypoxia, blood flow, renal, oxidative stress and desufflation changes are all short lived and manageable.[87]

Because of CO_2 absorption, minute respiratory, end expiratory or end-tidal CO_2 levels ($EtCO_2$) should be maintained throughout the procedure with adjustments to maintain normocapnia. Increased levels of CO_2 may help in detecting a CO_2 embolism and should not exceed 25% of original $EtCO_2$. Pneumoperitoneum decreases thoraco-pulmonary compliance by 30–50% in healthy American Society of Anesthesia (ASA) class I patients.[125,126] Normal excretion of CO_2 is 100–200 mL/min and increased by 14–18 mL/min due to intra-peritoneal CO_2.[39,127-130]

Cardiovascular effects are due to hypercarbia, acidosis and increased IAP.[131]

Carbon dioxide causes reversible systemic and local acidosis and the effect of IAP on parietal peritoneal pH has minor significance.[132,133]

Renal effects due to a pneumoperitoneum are directly related to IAP and indirectly to CO_2 absorption, neuroendocrine factors and tissue damage from oxidative stress.[134] Transient oliguria is the most common renal effect due to activation of the renin-angiotensin-aldosterone system resulting from decreased renal perfusion.[127] During pneumoperitoneum IAP urine outflow decreases and creatinine increases. These normalized within 24 hours from a pneumoperitoneum less than 15 mm Hg.[20,21,135-137]

Surgical injury is associated with oxidative stress whether done open or by laparoscopy.[138] This is influenced by the surgery performed, IAP, length of time, ischemia, reperfusion and desufflation but is less severe with laparoscopy than open surgery.[139-141]

Surgical response and recovery are measured by inflammatory markers and the immune response.[124,142,143] These are cytokines, lymphokines and prostaglandins including tumor necrosis factor alpha, interleukin-6, IL-8, C-reactive protein and granulocyte colony-stimulating factor.[88,116,144] There is a decreased systemic immunologic response to laparoscopic surgery compared to open surgery.[145,146] Prolonged hypoxia due to IAP may be a co-factor of the inflammatory response.[147] Laparoscopic stress can be reduced further by making the distending gas more physiologic by being humidified and warmed.[111]

IAP decreases blood flow to intra-abdominal tissues during a pneumoperitoneum.[5,12] Increasing IAP from 10 to 15 mm Hg causes a reduction in blood flow by 40–54% to the stomach, 32% in jejunum, 44% in colon, 39% in liver and 60% to the peritoneum.[148,149] Operating at the lowest intra-abdominal pressure you are sure you will provide the patient the best operation and outcome is the correct pressure for you.

COMPLICATIONS

Abdominal Entry Technique is a Preference—all Different with the Same Outcomes

From the initiation of a purposeful pneumoperitoneum for laparoscopic surgery the potential complications exist. Since these are not unexpected it is wise and prudent to be prepared and have skills, methods and techniques to reduce their occurrence and severity and be knowledgeable about their treatment and consequences. Practice varies as to the method chosen to induce pneumoperitoneum, but there is no significant difference between the technique chosen and incidence of complications as supported by the literature.[65,127,150-154] No single technique or instrument has been proved to eliminate laparoscopic entry associated injury. Veress needle, blind, optical or open entry, they all can result in failed entry, extraperitoneal insufflation, vascular (abdominal wall and large vessel), omental, urologic and visceral injury. Attention to detail, vigilance, awareness, ability to check and correct, wisdom to convert to laparotomy and knowledge of anatomy are required skills. The determinant factor is what is safest in the hands of the surgeon based on judgment, training and experience, with opening pressure being the most reliable best indicator of correct placement to confirm peritoneal entry.

History of prior abdominal procedures or abdominal/pelvic infections influences trocar placement due to potential adhesions and altered anatomic relationships. There is a difference between preference and necessity of where, how and why a certain approach, procedure is required versus preferred and how its performance is accomplished. Preference means you are comfortable with the way you approach the problem and chosen to handle it as one method among choices. It is one way of many and is your preference. Other entry methods get the same result in another surgeon's hands. The choice of the entry preference does not matter. They result in the same type and frequency of complications. For a specific situation there may be only one option, not a preference since there is no choice. Knowing the difference is wisdom. Be open to alternative preferences and learn them as substitutes for specific circumstances. Know the mandatory no-options responses and alternatives to your preferences to minimize and/or correct a known, unexpected or unforeseen circumstance.

Irrigation

The viscera are covered by peritoneum and the cavity is created by the serosa of the parietal and visceral peritoneum making peritoneal fluid the only true content of the peritoneal cavity. Peritoneal fluid contains cells (white cells, macrophages, eosinophils), glycoproteins, glycosaminoglycans (hyaluronan) and phospholipids making a surfactant liquid that decreases frictional movements to maintain efficient hydrodynamic and boundary lubrication.

Peritoneal fluid volume and composition is affected by each lavage exchange during laparoscopy. The concentration, cellular components and mediators in the peritoneal fluid are influenced by the rate of production, degradation and by dilution. Four irrigation lavage cycles of 100 mL or more removes 99% of the normal resident cellular components and almost all of the soluble components of peritoneal fluid[15,155,156] (Box 15.1). Mediators produced by peritoneal fluid cellular components play an active role in mesothelial healing and modulation of the peritoneal inflammatory response. Replacement, recruitment and cellular activity and production of these mediators are patient specific. Gas desiccation and irrigation remove, dilute or damage peritoneal cells and remove hyaluronan protection.

Box 15.1: Soluble-modulating factors in peritoneal fluid associated with peritoneal adhesion formation induced by trauma and desiccation and diluted or removed by irrigation
Transforming growth factor-β (TGF-β)
Vascular endothelial growth factor (VEGF)
Metalloproteinases (MMP)
Tissue inhibitor of metalloproteinase (TIMP)
Tumor necrosis factor-α (TNF-α)
Interferon-γ (INF-γ)
Interleukin-1 (IL-1)
Interleukin-6 (IL-6)
Interleukin-8 (IL-8)
Interleukin-10 (IL-10)
Granulocyte-macrophage colony-stimulating factor (GM-CSF)
Monocyte chemotactic protein-1 (MCP-1)
Regulated on activation and normally T-cell expressed and presumably secreted (RANTES)
Plasminogen activator (PA)
Plasminogen activator inhibitor-1 (PAI-1)
Plasminogen activator inhibitor-2 (PAI-2)
Tissue plasminogen activator (tPA)
Urokinase-like plasminogen activator (uPA)
Cell adhesion molecules (CAM)
Intercellular adhesion molecule-1 (ICAM-1)
Vascular adhesion molecule-1 (VCAM-1)
Fibrin
Fibrin matrix
Plasmin

Surgical Aerosols and Smoke

Heated metal (cautery devices), vibrating apparatus (harmonic scalpels) or light optically amplified as stimulated emission of electromagnetic radiation (laser) are used to achieve a tissue effect for coagulation, vessel sealing or ablation. In addition to the desired effect there is creation of an aerosol due to partial tissue combustion creating smoke or plume. Smoke is a two-phase material having particulate and gaseous components. The particulates are carbonized tissue and other cellular material. Analysis of the gaseous portion of tissue combustion are shown in Box 15.2.[167] Many of these are toxic having mutagenic and carcinogenic potential. Many countries and health organizations have regulations concerning smoke removal and protection of health care workers.[158-165] Patients also have direct exposure from smoke due to peritoneal absorption of carbon monoxide causing carboxyhemoglobinemia and other gases from incomplete tissue combustion causing methemoglobinemia.[157,166] Intra-abdominal smoke should not be released into the operating room or recirculated in the patient but totally removed from the surgical suite.

SUBCUTANEOUS EMPHYSEMA, PNEUMOMEDIASTINUM AND PNEUMOTHORAX[68]

The potential for subcutaneous emphysema starts with the physician's preparation, knowledge and

Box 15.2: Gas chromatography evaluation of by products of human tissue combustion

Toxic chemical by products resulting from pyrolysis of protein and lipids		
Acrolein	Creosols	Phenol
Acetonitrile	Ethane	PAHs
Acrylonitrile	Ethene	Propene
Acetylene	Ethylene	Propylene
Alkyl benzenes	Formaldehyde	Pyridine
Benzene	Free radicals	Pyrrole
Butadiene	Hydrogen cyanide	Styrene
Butene	Isobutene	Toluene
Carbon monoxide	Methane	Xylene

experience. It is necessary to know where the gas goes during laparoscopy. Placing trocars through the abdominal wall requires more than skill. A planned approach to trocar placement for gas instillation requires a wide range of knowledge and consideration of the patients' topography and habitus, knowledge of the surgical procedure and modifications based on specific circumstances peculiar to the patient, number, placement, angle and trajectory of the trocars, understanding the instruments and devices being deployed, their intended uses, capabilities, and limitations, alternatives to routines, a plan B and ability to assess and handle adversity and complications.

Surgeons must know the 'why, what, where and who' of peritoneal cavity pneumoperitoneum and its potential and circumstances that lead to extension beyond this intended site and to increase awareness of the conditions that effect extravasation of gas beyond the intra-abdominal cavity during laparoscopy.

The incidence of subcutaneous emphysema varies from isolated and confined in a small space to extravasation outside the abdominal cavity extending into the labia, scrotum, legs, chest, head and neck. The literature range is 0.3–3.0%[127,167-169] for grossly detectable subcutaneous emphysema. Pneumothorax due to extension of insufflated gas through diaphragmatic congenital channels into the pleural cavities is reported as 0.03%.[170-172] Subcutaneous emphysema, pneumomediastinum and retroperitoneal extravasation without pneumothorax have also been described during laparoscopic surgery with CO_2 insufflation and may be associated with prolonged hypercarbia.[173] Recent use of a valveless trocar and dynamic pressure system have shown a 16.4% rate of subcutaneous emphysema, at least over five times greater incidence than reported with other systems, a 3.9% rate of pneumomediastinum two times the reported rate of 1.9% and a 0.94% complication rate of masked pneumothorax a rate 2.35 times the reported rate.[174-176]

Factors associated with subcutaneous emphysema during laparoscopic pneumoperitoneum are methods of laparoscopy (straight stick or robotic), insufflator settings for pressure and flow, actual IAP, actual flow rate, number of abdominal entry sites, size and geometry of fascial incision to trocar size of entry site, snugness of fit between trocar and fascia, number of times entry site is entered, amount of torqueing and pressure on entry sites, vectoring

Table 15.3: Physical + chemical + biological effects = Pneumoperitoneum

Physical effects	Chemical effects	Biologic effects
Mechanical effects	Gas	Hypothermia
Abdominal compliance	Desiccation	Tissue disruption
Intra-abdominal pressure	Hypoxia	Increased peritoneal viscosity
Time	Acidosis	Acidosis
Patient position		Hypoxia

of the laparoscope, fulcrum effect between laparoscope and fascia, length of procedure, volume of gas used, patients age, body mass index, co-existing metabolic diseases, tissue integrity, type of trocar used and purposeful extraperitoneal dissection (Table 15.3). Total amount of gas since it is a drug and a physician prescription the insufflator settings and total amount of gas used should be recorded in the operative record. The amount of gas used is not necessarily related to the length of time of the procedure and may be more important than the length of time of the procedure.[167,177-182]

The clinical significance of subcutaneous emphysema is hypercarbia and acidosis. A combination of factors contribute to increased arterial $PaCO_2$; rapid absorption of CO_2, reduced diaphragmatic movement, decreased residual functional capacity and decreased pulmonary CO_2 excretion causing ventilation-perfusion mismatch[183,184] (Box 15.3). Cardiovascular compromise is due to mechanical factors produced by increased IAP affecting ventilation and venous return, with circulatory accumulation of CO_2, leading to acidosis and cardiopulmonary system compromise[178] (Box 15.4). Hypercarbia increases heart rate, systemic blood pressure, central venous pressure, cardiac output, stroke volume and decreases peripheral vascular resistance and releases epinephrine and norepinephrine.[185-190]

To reduce the likelihood of subcutaneous emphysema the following are recommended: awareness of its potential, vigilance, attention to detail regarding abdominal entry, monitoring insufflator pressure settings and measurements, flow rate and volume of gas with alarm settings, being quick but not hurried during the procedure (since length of procedure and gas consumption relate to the condition), limit the number of attempts to enter the abdomen, have snug trocar skin interface, test for correct placement by initial IAP assessment and monitor $ETCO_2$.[191]

Box 15.3: Factors leading to subcutaneous emphysema

- Insufflator—high gas flow and high gas pressure setting
- Intra-abdominal pressure >15 mm Hg
- Multiple attempts at abdominal entry
- Veress needle or cannula not placed in peritoneal cavity
- Skin/fascial fit/seal around cannulas not snug
- Use of > 5 cannulas
- Laparoscope used as a lever
- Cannula acts as a fulcrum
- Long arm of laparoscope is a force multiplier
- Tissue integrity compromised by repetitive movements
- Structural weakness caused by repetitive movements
- Improper cannula placement causing stressed angulation
- Soft tissue dissection and fascial extension
- Gas dissection leads to more dissection
- Procedures lasting >3.5 h
- Positive end-tidal CO_2 >50 mm Hg

Box 15.4: Intraoperative causes and risk factors for hypercarbia during laparoscopy

- Integrity of anesthesia circuit
- Position and function of endotracheal tube
- Inadequate respiratory exchange
- Exclude causes other than CO_2 for acidosis
- Underlying obstructive lung disease
- Age > 65 years
- Type of surgery—Nissen fundoplication

Gas Embolism

Clinically significant CO_2 embolism is a rare but potentially fatal complication during laparoscopic surgery. Its most common cause is injection of CO_2 into a large vein, artery or solid organ. This usually occurs with insufflation of CO_2 into the suspected peritoneal space or is direct intravascular insufflation of CO_2 resulting in blockage of the right ventricle or pulmonary artery. The occurrence of clinically significant CO_2 embolism is rare with a reported incidence between 0.001% and 0.59%[127,192,193] with a mortality rate of 28%.[193-195] Transesophageal echocardiography (TEE) can be used to monitor for CO_2 embolism and shows it to be more common than thought ranging from mild to massive.[196]

Most cases of CO_2 embolism occur early in the procedure due to incorrect placement of gas directly in to a vessel but smaller amounts of gas can enter the circulation through injured vessels throughout the procedure. Prior to gas insufflation the tubing should be purged of air to assure that gas exiting the cannula is CO_2.[197] Compared to other gases, gas mixtures or air, CO_2 is highly soluble in blood and is absorbed rapidly with buffering making it comparatively more safe. For a 70 kg human it is estimated that a lethal dose of CO_2 gas emboli is between 600 and 1,750 mL.[198,199] Animal studies comparing the hemodynamic effects of CO_2 emboli to argon, helium or air emboli, found CO_2 safer because of its greater solubility in blood.[200-208] Suspicion of gas embolism should be managed quickly with the following steps: (1) deflate the pneumoperitoneum and stop insufflation, (2) position the patient in the left lateral position with head down, (3) increase minute ventilation with 100% oxygen, (4) discontinue nitrous oxide and (5) insertion of a central venous catheter for diagnosis and aspiration.[127,199-212]

ABDOMINAL WALL LIFTING—NO ADVANTAGES

Abdominal wall lift with or without pneumoperitoneum does not offer an advantage over pneumoperitoneum and therefore cannot be recommended routinely. The safety of abdominal wall lift is yet to be established. More research on the topic is needed because of the risk of bias in the included trials and type I and type II random errors due to the few participants in the trials and need for blinded assessment of outcomes.[213,214]

FACTS ABOUT THE PNEUMOPERITONEUM

Creating and maintaining a surgical pneumoperitoneum is not without consequences. Reducing these consequences to the least possible rate of occurrence and keeping conditions most like homeostatic physiologically normal is paramount to improved clinical outcomes. Knowledge of the concepts and laws of physics, chemistry and biology are necessary to understand the actions and reactions surrounding the surgical pneumoperitoneum. A keen awareness and attention to detail regarding anatomy, the surgical procedure, instrumentation, complications and dynamic responses to the surgical process interacting with the patient is necessary. When all things are considered and the effects of research, scientific and human camouflage techniques of biases (anchoring, availability, substitution, optimism and loss aversion, framing and sunk cost) are eliminated or reduced as much as possible the following recommendations are wise prudent and recommended.

Use CO_2 gas that is humidified and warmed insufflate the abdomen to the lowest IAP that the surgeon can do their best work without compromise, touch the peritoneum as little as possible, limit blood loss, judiciously irrigate and remove smoke beyond the operating room. Maintaining normal physiologic parameters are more beneficial, safer and have superior clinical outcomes than not maintaining them. This will reduce peritoneal damage due to desiccation, reduce adhesion formation, reduce hypothermia and pain and shorten postoperative recovery. Know that there are choices you make and decide on and that they have consequences. Expanding on and knowing the difference between choices and the decisions impacts the significance and magnitude of the action or lack of action taken.

REFERENCES

1. Ott DE. Pneumoperitoneum: production, management, effects and consequences. Prevention and Management of Laparoendoscopic Surgical Complications, 1st edition. SLS; 1999.
2. United States Pharmacopoeia and National Formulary and Supplements (1984) XXI-NF.
3. Ott DE. The Pneumoperitoneum. Prevention and Management of Laparoendoscopic Surgical Complications, 3rd edition. Society of Laparoscopic Surgeons.
4. Binda MM. Humidification during laparoscopic surgery: overview of the clinical benefits of using humidified gas during laparoscopic surgery. Arch Gynecol Obstet. 2015;292(5):955-71.
5. Ott DE. Laparoscopy and adhesion formation, adhesions and laparoscopy. Semin Repro Med. 2008;26(4):322-0.
6. Jacobs VR, Morrison JE Jr. The real intraabdominal pressure during laparoscopy: comparison of different insufflators. J Minim Invasive Gynecol. 2007;14(1):103-7.
7. Gray RI, Ott DE, Henderson AC, et al. Severe local hypothermia from laparoscopic gas evaporative jet-cooling; a mechanism to explain clinical observations. JSLS. 1999;3(3):171-7.
8. Blaser AR, Björck M, De Keulenaer B, et al. Abdominal compliance: a bench-to-bedside review. J Trauma Acute Care Surg. 2015;78(5):1044-53.
9. Balkin DM, Duh QY, Kind GM, et al. Failed pneumoperitoneum for laparoscopic surgery following autologous Deep Inferior Epigastric Perforator (DIEP) flap breast reconstruction: a case report. BMC Surg. 2016;16(1):28.
10. Goldman JM, Rose LS, Morgan MD, et al. Measurement of abdominal wall compliance in normal subjects and tetraplegic patients. Thorax. 1986;41(7):513-8.
11. Awonuga A, Belotte J, Abuanzeh S, et al. Advances in the pathogenesis of adhesion development. The role of oxidative stress. Reprod Sci. 2014;21(7):823-36.
12. Hatipoglu S, Akbulut S, Hatipoglu F, et al. Effect of laparoscopic abdominal surgery on splanchnic circulation: historical developments. World J Gastroenterol. 2014;20(48):18165-76.
13. Ishizaki Y, Bandai Y, Shimomura K, et al. Safe intraabdominal pressure of carbon dioxide pneumoperitoneum during laparoscopic surgery. Surgery. 1993;114(3):549-54.
14. Nguyen N, Wolfe BM. The physiologic effects of pneumoperitoneum in the morbidly obese. Ann Surg. 2005;241(2):219-26.
15. Srivastava A, Niranjan A. Secrets of safe laparoscopic surgery: anaesthetic and surgical considerations. J Minim Access Surg. 2010;6(4):91-4.
16. Özdemir-van Brunschot DM, van Laarhoven KC, Scheffer GJ, et al. What is the evidence for the use of low-pressure pneumoperitoneum? A systematic review. Surg Endosc. 2016;30(5):2049-65.
17. Gurusamy KS, Vaughan J, Davidson BR. Low pressure versus standard pressure pneumoperitoneum in laparoscopic cholecystectomy. Cochrane Database Syst Rev. 2014;18:CD006930.
18. Chok KS, Yuen WK, Lau H, et al. Prospective randomized trial on low-pressure versus standard-pressure pneumoperitoneum in outpatient laparoscopic cholecystectomy. Surg Laparosc Endosc Percutan Tech. 2006;16(6):383-6.
19. Kyle EB, Maheux-Lacroix S, Boutin A, et al. Low vs standard pressures in gynecologic laparoscopy: a systemic review. JSLS. 2016;20(1): pii: e2015.00113.
20. Lackey LW, Ott DE. Terminal gas velocity during laparoscopy. J Am Assoc Gynecol Laparosc. 2002;9(3):297-305.
21. Ott DE. Desertification of the peritoneum by thin-film evaporation during laparoscopy. JSLS. 2003;7(3):189-95.
22. Hazebroek EJ, Schreve MA, Visser P, et al. Impact of temperature and humidity of carbon dioxide pneumoperitoneum on body temperature and peritoneal morphology. J Laparoendosc Adv Surg Tech A. 2002;12(5):355-64.
23. Peng Y, Zheng M, Ye Q, et al. Heated and humidified CO_2 prevents hypothermia, peritoneal injury, and intra-abdominal adhesions during prolonged laparoscopic insufflations. J Surg Res. 2009;151(1):40-7.
24. Mouton WG, Bessell JR, Pfitzner J, et al. A randomized controlled trial to determine the effects of humidified carbon dioxide insufflation during thoracoscopy. Surg Endosc. 1999;13(4):382-5.
25. Volz J, Köster S, Spacek Z, et al. Characteristic alterations of the peritoneum after carbon dioxide pneumoperitoneum. Surg Endosc. 1999;13(6):611-4.
26. Suematsu T, Hirabayashi Y, Shiraishi N, et al. Morphology of the murine peritoneum after

pneumoperitoneum vs laparotomy. Surg Endosc. 2001;15(9):954-8.
27. Liu Y, Hou QX. Effect of carbon dioxide pneumoperitoneum during laparoscopic surgery on morphology of peritoneum. Zhonghua Yi Xue Za Zhi. 2006; 86(3):164-6.
28. Ryan GB, Grobéty J, Majno G. Mesothelial injury and recovery. Am J Pathol. 1973;71(1):93-112.
29. Davey AK, Hayward J, Marshall JK, et al. The effects of insufflation conditions on rat mesothelium. Int J Inflam. 2013;2013:816283.
30. Erikoglu M, Yol S, Avunduk MC, et al. Electron-microscopic alterations of the peritoneum after both cold and heated carbon dioxide pneumoperitoneum. J Surg Res. 2005;125(1):73-7.
31. Ott DE. Laparoscopy and tribology: the effect of laparoscopic gas on peritoneal fluid. J Am Assoc Gynecol Laparosc. 2001;8(1):117-23.
32. Jacobs, VR, Keichle M, Morrison JE Jr. Carbon dioxide gas heating inside laparoscopic insufflators has no effect. JSLS. 2005;9(2):208-12.
33. Slim K, Bousquet J, Kwiatkowski F, et al. Effect of CO_2 gas warming on pain after laparoscopic surgery: a randomized double-blind controlled trial. Surg Endosc. 1999;13(11):1110-4.
34. Saad S, Minor I, Mohri T, et al. The clinical impact of warmed insufflation carbon dioxide gas for laparoscopic cholecystectomy. Surg Endosc. 2000; 14(9):787-90.
35. Wills VL, Hunt DR, Armstrong A. A randomized controlled trial assessing the effect of heated carbon dioxide for insufflation on pain and recovery after laparoscopic fundoplication. Surg Endosc. 2001;15(2): 166-70.
36. Nunn J. Carbon dioxide. Applied Respiratory Physiology. London: Butterworth; 1987. pp. 207-34.
37. Grzegorzewska A, Antoniewicz K. Effective peritoneal blood flow and patient characteristics. In: Khanna R (Ed). Advances in Peritoneal Dialysis. Toronto: Peritoneal Dialysis Publications;1994;10:27-9.
38. Kim M, Lofthouse J, Flessner MF. A method to test blood flow limitation of peritoneal-blood solute transport. J Am Soc Nephrol. 1997;8(3):471-4.
39. Pacilli M, Pierro A, Kingsley C, et al. Absorption of carbon dioxide during laparoscopy in children measured using a novel mass spectrometric technique. Br J Anaesth. 2006;97(2):215-9.
40. Glew PA, Campher MJ, Pearson K, et al. The effect of warm humidified CO_2 on the dissipation of residual gas following laparoscopy in piglets. J Am Assoc Gynecol Laparosc. 2004;11(2):204-10.
41. Raffi A. Body temperature during surgery and anesthesia. MVC Quarterly. 1972;8(2):135-41.
42. Gross CG. Claude Bernard and the constancy of the internal environment. Neuroscientist. 1998;4(5): 380-5.
43. Cross S, Albury WR. Walter B, et al. Henderson and the organic analogy. OSIRIS. 1987;3:165-92.
44. Çam R, Yönem H, Özsoy H. Core body temperature changes during surgery and nursing management. Clin Med Res. 2016;5(2-1):1-5.
45. Whelan RL, Fleshman JW, Fowler DL (Eds). The SAGES Manual of Perioperative Care in Minimally Invasive Surgery. Berlin: Springer; 2006.
46. Rosenthal RJ, Friedman RL, Phillips EH. The pathophysiology of pneumoperitoneum. In: Bessell JR, Maddern GJ (Eds). Influence of Gas Temperature during Laparoscopic Procedures. Heidelberg: Springer; 1998. pp. 18-27.
47. Buhre W, Rossaint R. Perioperative management and monitoring in anaesthesia. Lancet. 2003;362(9398): 1839-46.
48. Sessler DI. Complications and treatment of mild hypothermia. Anesthesiology. 2001;95(2):531-43.
49. Jacobs VR, Morrison JE Jr, Mettler L, et al. Measurement of CO_2 hypothermia during laparoscopy and pelviscopy: how cold it gets and how to prevent it. J Am Assoc Gynecol Laparosc. 1999;6(3):289-95.
50. Binda MM, Molinas CR, Mailova K, et al. Effect of temperature upon adhesion formation in a laparoscopic mouse model. Hum Reprod. 2004; 19(11):2626-32.
51. Binda MM, Molinas CR, Hansen P, et al. Effect of desiccation and temperature during laparoscopy on adhesion formation in mice. Fertil Steril. 2006; 86(1):166-75.
52. Sajid MS, Mallick AS, Rimpel J, et al. Effect of heated and humidified carbon dioxide on patients after laparoscopic procedures: a meta-analysis. Surg Laparosc Endosc Percutan Tech. 2008;18(6):539-46.
53. Sammour T, Kahokehr A, Hill AG. Meta-analysis of the effect of warm humidified insufflation on pain after laparoscopy. Br J Surg. 2008;95(8):950-6.
54. Bessell JR, Ludbrook G, Millard SH, et al. Humidified gas prevents hypothermia induced by laparoscopic insufflation: a randomized controlled study in a pig model. Surg Endosc. 1999;13(2):101-5.
55. Bessell JR, Karatassas A, Patterson JR, et al. Hypothermia induced by laparoscopic insufflation. A randomized study in a pig model. Surg Endosc. 1995;9(7):791-6.
56. Ott DE, Reich H, Love B, et al. Reduction of laparoscopic-induced hypothermia, postoperative pain and recovery room length of stay by pre-conditioning gas with the Insuflow device: a prospective randomized controlled multi-center study. JSLS. 1998;2(4): 321-9.
57. Benavides R, Wong A, Nguyen H. Improved outcomes for lap-banding using the Insuflow device compared with heated-only gas. JSLS. 2009;13(3):302-5.
58. Beste TM, Daucher JA, Holbert D. Humidified compared with dry, heated carbon dioxide at laparoscopy to reduce pain. Obstet Gynecol. 2006; 107(2 Pt 1): 263-8.
59. Farley DR, Greenlee SM, Larson DR, et al. Double-blind, prospective, randomized study of warmed, humidified carbon dioxide insufflation vs standard carbon dioxide for patients undergoing laparoscopic cholecystectomy. Arch Surg. 2004;139(7):739-43; discussion 743-4.
60. Herrmann A, De Wilde RL. Insufflation with humidified and heated carbon dioxide in short-term

laparoscopy: a double-blinded randomized controlled trial. BioMed Res Int. 2015;412618.
61. Klugsberger B, Schreiner M, Rothe A, et al. Warmed, humidified carbon dioxide insufflation versus standard carbon dioxide in laparoscopic cholecystectomy: a double-blinded randomized controlled trial. Surg Endosc. 2014;28(9):2656-60.
62. Mouton WG, Bessell JR, Millard SH, et al. A randomized controlled trial assessing the benefit of humidified insufflation gas during laparoscopic surgery. Surg Endosc. 1999;13(2):106-8.
63. Hamza MA, Schneider BE, White PF, et al. Heated and humidified insufflation during laparoscopic gastric bypass surgery: effect on temperature, postoperative pain, and recovery outcomes. J Laparoendosc Adv Surg Tech A. 2005;15(1):6-12.
64. Gizzi A, Cherubini C, Migliori S, et al. On the electrical intestine turbulence induced by temperature changes. Phys Biol. 2010;7(1):16011.
65. Ott DE. Subcutaneous emphysema—beyond the pneumoperitoneum. JSLS. 2014;18(1):1-7.
66. Tang B, Hanna GB, Cuschieri A. Analysis of errors enacted by surgical trainees during skills training courses. Surgery. 2005;138(1):14-20.
67. Xin H, Zelek JS, Carnahan H. Laparoscopic surgery, perceptual limitations and force: a review. First Canadian Student Conference on Biomedical Computing. 2006;44-9. http://docplayer.net/15403785-Laparoscopic-surgery-perceptual-limitations-and-force-a-review-h-xin-a-j-s-zelek-a-h-carnahan-b.html.
68. Yung S, Chan TM. Pathophysiological changes to the peritoneal membrane during PD-related peritonitis: the role of mesothelial cells. Meditors Inflamm. 2012; 2012:484167.
69. Hills BA. Lubrication of visceral movement and gastric motility by peritoneal surfactant. J Gastroenterol Hepatol. 1996;11(9):797-803.
70. Tittel A, Schippers E, Grablowitz V, et al. Intra-abdominal humidity and electromyographic activity of the gastrointestinal tract. Laparoscopy versus laparotomy. Surg Endosc. 1995;9(7):786-90.
71. Hertzler AE. The Peritoneum, Vol. 1. St. Louis: CV Mosby Co.; 1919.
72. di Zerega G, Rogers K. The Peritoneum. New York: Springer-Verlag; 1992. pp.1–56.
73. Hanbidge A, Lynch D, Wilson S. Ultrasound of the peritoneum. Radiographics. 2003;23(3):663-84.
74. Albanese AM, Albanese EF, Miño JH, et al. Peritoneal surface area: measurements of 40 structures covered by peritoneum: correlation between total peritoneal surface area and the surface calculated by formulas. Surg Radiol Anat. 2009;31(5): 369-377.
75. Volz J, Köster S, Schaeff B, et al. Laparoscopic surgery: the effects of insufflation gas on tumor-induced lethality in nude mice. Am J Obstet Gynecol. 1998; 178(4):793-5.
76. Mutsaers SE, Birnie K, Lansley S, et al. Mesothelial cells in tissue repair and fibrosis. Front Pharmacol. 2015;6:113.
77. Ryan GB, Grobéty J, Majno F. Postoperative peritoneal adhesions: a study of the mechanisms. Am J Pathol. 1971;65(1):117-48.
78. Raftery AT. Regeneration of parietal and visceral peritoneum: an electron microscopical study. J Anat. 1973;115(Pt 3):375-92.
79. Raftery AT. Regeneration of parietal and visceral peritoneum. A light microscopical study. Br J Surg. 1973;60(4):293-9.
80. Volz J, Köster S, Weiss M, et al. Pathophysiologic features of a pneumoperitoneum at laparoscopy: a swine model. Am J Obstet Gynecol. 1996;174(1 Pt 1): 132-40.
81. Volz J, Köster S, Leweling H. Surgical trauma and metabolic changes induced by surgical laparoscopy versus laparotomy. Gynaecol Endosc. 1997;6(1):1-6.
82. Holmdahl L, Risberg B, Beck DE, et al. Adhesions: pathogenesis and prevention-panel discussion and summary. Eur J Surg Suppl. 1997;(577):56-62.
83. Rosario MT, Ribeiro U Jr, Corbett CE, et al. Does CO_2 pneumoperitoneum alter the ultra-structure of the mesothelium? J Surg Res. 2006;133(2):84-8.
84. Grabowski JE, Talamini MA. Physiological effects of pneumoperitoneum. J Gastrointest Surg. 2009;13(5): 1009-16.
85. Brokelman WJA, Lensvelt M, Borel Rinkes IHM, et al. Peritoneal changes due to laparoscopic surgery. Surg Endosc. 2011;25(1):1-9.
86. Papparella A, Nino F, Coppola S, et al. Peritoneal morphological changes due to pneumoperitoneum: the effect of intra-abdominal pressure. Eur J Pediatr Surg. 2014;24(4):322-7.
87. Mais V. Peritoneal adhesions after laparoscopic gastrointestinal surgery. World J Gastroenterol. 2014; 20(17):4917-25.
88. Ott DE. The peritoneum and laparoscopy. In: DiZerega GS (Ed). Peritoneal Surgery. New York: Springer-Verlag; 2000. pp. 175-81.
89. Wiseman D, Richardson J. Humidity and temperature of insufflation gas on intact peritoneum. J Am Assoc Gynecol Laparosc. 2002;9:552.
90. de Csepel J, Wilson E. Heating and humidifying carbon dioxide is indicated. Surg Endosc. 2007;21(2): 340-1.
91. Yung S, Chan TM. Mesothelial cells. Perit Dial Int. 2007;27(Suppl 2):S110-5.
92. Flessner MF. Endothelial glycocalyx and the peritoneal barrier. Perit Dial Int. 2008;28(1):6-12.
93. Anglani F, Forino M, Del Petre D, et al. Molecular biology of the peritoneal membrane: in between morphology and function. Contrib Nephrol. 2001; (131):61-73.
94. Molinas CR, Binda MM, Manavella GD, et al. Adhesion formation after laparoscopic surgery: what do we know about the role of the peritoneal environment? Facts Views Vis Obgyn. 2010;2(3):149-60.
95. Bird SD. Mesothelial primary cilia of peritoneal and other serosal surfaces. Cell Biol Int. 2004;28(2):151-9.
96. Nezhat CR, Berger GS, Nezhat F, et al. (Eds). Endometriosis: Advanced Management and Surgical Techniques. New York; Springer-Verlag; 1995. p. 93.

97. Pouly J, Seak-San S. Adhesions: laparoscopy versus laparotomy. In: DiZerega G (Ed). Surgery. New York: Springer-Verlag; 2000. pp. 183–192.
98. Arung W, Meurisse M, Detry O. Pathophysiology and prevention of postoperative peritoneal adhesions. World J Gastroenterol. 2011;17(41):4545-53.
99. Diamond M, Freeman M. Clinical implications of post-surgical adhesions. Hum Reprod Update. 2001; 7(6):567-76.
100. Ellis H. The clinical significance of adhesions: focus on intestinal obstruction. Eur J Surg Suppl. 1997; (577):5-9.
101. Hawkins-Ambler G. What makes for success in abdominal surgery? In: Shrady G (Ed). The British Gynaecological Society, 1892 Medical Record. New York: William Wood & Company.
102. Alvarez WC. The cause and prevention of postoperative gas pains. Cal State J Med. 1918;16(7): 338-41.
103. Nolph KD (Ed). Chapter 4, Peritoneal Dialysis. Boston, MA: Martinus Nijhoff Publishers; 1985.
104. Howard F. Approach to the patient with chronic pelvic pain. In: Howard F (Ed). Pelvic Pain, Diagnosis and Management. Philadelphia, PA: Lippincott Williams and Wilkins; 2000.
105. Diamond M, Manvinder S, Puscheck E. In: Vercellini P (Ed). Chronic Pelvic Pain and Adhesions. Chronic Pelvic Pain. Singapore: Wiley-Blackwell; 2011.
106. Davey AK, Maher PJ. Surgical adhesions: a timely update, a great challenge for the future. J Minim Invasive Gynecol. 2007;14(1):15-22.
107. Koninckx PR, Vandermeersch E. The persufflator: an insufflation device for laparoscopy and especially for CO_2-laser-endoscopic surgery. Hum Reprod. 1991;6(9):1288-90.
108. Koninckx PR, Corona R, Timmerman D, et al. Peritoneal full-conditioning reduces postoperative adhesions and pain: a randomized controlled trial in deep endometriosis surgery. J Ovarian Res. 2013;6(1): 90.
109. Brüggmann D, Tchartchian G, Wallwiener M, et al. Intra-abdominal adhesions: definition, origin, significance in surgical practice, and treatment options. Dtsch Arztebl Int. 2010;107(44):769-75.
110. Mutsaers SE, Prêle CM, Lansley SM, et al. The origin of regenerating mesothelium: a historical perspective. Int J Artif Organs. 2007;30(6):484-94.
111. Neuhaus SJ, Watson DI. Pneumoperitoneum and peritoneal surface changes: a review. Surg Endosc. 2004;18(9):1316-22.
112. di Zerega G. Pelvic Surgery: adhesion formation and prevention. New York: Springer-Verlag; 1996:1-25.
113. diZerega G. Biochemical events in peritoneal tissue repair. Eur J Surg Suppl. 1997;(577):10-6.
114. Van der Wal JB, Jeekel J. Biology of the peritoneum in normal homeostasis and after surgical trauma. Colorectal Dis. 2007;9 Suppl 2:9-13.
115. Duron JJ. Postoperative intraperitoneal adhesion pathophysiology. Colorectal Dis. 2007;9(Suppl 2): 14-24.
116. Chegini N. Peritoneal molecular environment, adhesion formation and clinical implication. Front Biosci. 2002;1;7:e91-115.
117. Saed GM, Diamond MP. Molecular characterization of postoperative adhesions: the adhesion phenotype. J Am Assoc Gynecol Laparosc. 2004;11(3):307-14.
118. Hellebrekers BW, Kooistra T. Pathogenesis of postoperative adhesion formation. Br J Surg. 2011; 98(11):1503-16.
119. diZerga GS, Campeau JD. Peritoneal repair and post-surgical adhesion formation. Hum Reprod Update. 2001;7(6):547-55.
120. Ellis H. Postoperative intra-abdominal adhesions: a personal view. Colorectal Dis. 2007;9(Suppl 2):3-8.
121. Koninckx PR, Gomel V, Ussia A, et al. Role of the peritoneal cavity in the prevention of postoperative adhesions, pain, and fatigue. Fertil Steril. 2016;106(5): 998-1010.
122. Blackburn SC, Stanton MP. Anatomy and physiology of the peritoneum. Semin Pediatr Surg. 2014;23(6): 326-30.
123. Van Baal JO, Van de Vijver KK, Nieuwland R, et al. The histophysiology and pathophysiology of the peritoneum. Tissue Cell. 2017;49(1):95-105.
124. Cheong YC, Laird SM, Li TC, et al. Peritoneal healing and adhesion formation/reformation. Hum Reprod Update. 2001;7(6):556-66.
125. Martín-Cancho MF, Celdrán D, Lima JR, et al. Anaesthetic considerations during laparoscopic surgery. In: Darwish A (Ed). Advanced Gynecologic Endoscopy. Rijeka, Croatia: Intech; 2011. Chapter 2.
126. Loring SH, Behazin N, Novero A, et al. Respiratory mechanical effects of surgical pneumoperitoneum in humans. J Appl Physiol. 2014;117(9):1074-9.
127. Veekash G, Wei LX, Su M. Carbon dioxide pneumoperitoneum, physiologic changes and anesthetic concerns. Ambulatory Surg. 2010;16:41-6.
128. Tan PL, Lee TL, Tweed WA. Carbon dioxide absorption and gas exchange during pelvic laparoscopy. Can J Anaesth. 1992;39(7):677-81.
129. Muelett CE, Viale JP, Sagnard PE, et al. Pulmonary CO_2 elimination during surgical procedures using intra- or extraperitoneal CO_2 insufflation. Anesth Analg. 1993;76(3):622-6.
130. Perrin M, Fletcher A. Laparoscopic abdominal surgery. Contin Educ Anaesth Crit Care Pain. 2004; 4(4):107-10.
131. Laureano B, Andrus C, Kaminski D. Cardiovascular changes during laparoscopy. In: Rosenthal R, Friedman R, Philips E (Eds). The Pathophysiology of Pneumoperitoneum. Berlin: Springer-Verlag; 1998.
132. Wildbrett P, Oh A, Naundorf D, et al. Impact of laparoscopic gases on peritoneal microenvironment and essential parameters of cell function. Surg Endosc. 2003;17(1):78-82.
133. Wong YT, Shah PC, Birkett DH, et al. Peritoneal pH during laparoscopy is dependent on ambient gas environment. Surg Endosc. 2005;19(1):60-4.
134. Sodha S, Nazarian S, Adshead JM, et al. Effect of pneumoperitoneum on renal function and physiology in patients undergoing robotic renal surgery. Curr Urol. 2016;9(1):1-4.
135. Wever KE, Bruintjes MH, Warlé MC, et al. Renal perfusion and function during pneumoperitoneum:

a systematic review and meta-analysis of animal studies. PLoS One 2016;11(9):e0163419.
136. Demyttenaere S, Feldman LS, Fried GM. Effect of pneumoperitoneum on renal perfusion and function: a systematic review. Surg Endosc. 2007;21(2): 152-60.
137. Taskin O, Buhur A, Birincioglu M, et al. The effects of duration of CO_2 insufflation and irrigation on peritoneal microcirculation assessed by free radical scavengers and total glutathione levels during operative laparoscopy. J Am Assoc Gynecol Laparosc. 1998;5(2):129-33.
138. Glantzounis GK, Tselepis AD, Tambaki AP, et al. Laparoscopic surgery-induced changes in oxidative stress markers in human plasma. Surg Endosc. 2001; 15(11):1315-9.
139. Arsalani-Zadeh R, Ullah S, Khan S, et al. Oxidative stress in laparoscopic versus open abdominal surgery: a systematic review. J Surg Res. 2011;169(1):e59-68.
140. Sammour T, Mittal A, Loveday BP, et al. Systematic review of oxidative stress associated with pneumoperitoneum. Br J Surg. 2009;96(8):836-50.
141. Yiannakopoulou ECh, Nikiteas, N, Perrea D, et al. Effect of laparoscopic surgery on oxidative stress response: systematic review. Surg Laparosc Endosc Percutan Tech. 2013;23(2):101-8.
142. Desborough JP. The stress response to trauma and surgery. Br J Anaesth. 2000;85(1):109-17.
143. Sammour T, Kahokehr A, Soop M, et al. Peritoneal damage: The inflammatory response and clinical implications of the neuro-immuno-humoral axis. World J Surg. 2010;34(4):704-20.
144. Cheong YS. Laird SM, Shelton JB, et al. The correlation of adhesions and peritoneal fluid cytokine concentrations: a pilot study. Hum Reprod. 2002; 17(4):1039-45.
145. Yahara N, Abe T, Morita K, et al. Comparison of interleukin-6, interleukin-8, and granulocyte colony-stimulating factor production by the peritoneum in laparoscopic and open surgery. Surg Endosc. 2002: 16(11);1615-9.
146. Luk JM, Tung PH, Wong KF, et al. Laparoscopic surgery induced inerleukin-6 levels in serum and gut mucosa: implications of peritoneum integrity and gas factors. Surg Endosc. 2009;23(2):370-6.
147. Schilling MK, Redaelli C, Krähenbühl L, et al. Splanchnic microcirculatory changes during CO_2 laparoscopy. J Am Coll Surg. 1997;184(4):378-82.
148. Yavuz Y, Rønning K, Lyng O, et al. Effect of carbon dioxide pneumoperitoneum on tissue blood flow in the peritoneum, rectus abdominus, and diaphragm muscles. Surg Endosc. 2003;17(10):1632-5
149. Molinas CR, Koninckx PR. Hypoxaemia induced by CO_2 or helium pneumoperitoneum is a co-factor in adhesion formation in rabbits. Hum Reprod. 2000; 15(8):1758-63.
150. Vilos GA, Ternamian A, Dempster J, et al. Laparoscopic entry: a review of techniques, technologies, and complications. J Obstet Gynaecol Can. 2007;29(5): 433-65.
151. Dunne N, Booth MI, Dehn TC. Establishing pneumoperitoneum: Verres or Hasson? The debate continues. Ann R Coll Surg Engl. 2011;93(1):22-4.
152. Cuss A, Bhatt M, Abbott J. Coming to terms with the fact that the evidence for laparoscopic entry is as good as it gets. J Minim Invasive Gynecol. 2015;22(3): 332-41.
153. Ahmad G, Gent D, Henderson D, et al. Laparoscopic entry techniques. Cochrane Database Syst Rev. 2015; 31;8:CD006583.
154. Krishnakumar S, Tambe P. Entry complications in laparoscopic surgery. J Gynecol Endosc Surg. 2009; 1(1):4-11.
155. Ott DE. Effect of irrigation on peritoneal fluid and cell count: dilutional effect of lavage. JAAGL. 2004; 11:33.
156. Dunn DL, Barke RA, Ahrenholz DH, et al. The adjuvant effect of peritoneal fluid in experimental peritonitis: Mechanism and clinical implications. Ann Surg. 1984:199(1):37-43.
157. Ott D. Smoke production and smoke reduction in endoscopic surgery: preliminary report. Endosc Surg Allied Technol. 1993;1(4):230-2.
158. Niosh Hazard Control (HC-11): https://www.cdc.gov/niosh/docs/hazardcontrol/pdfs/hc11.pdf. Recommendations for operating room ventilation and smoke evacuation measures: https://www.cdc.gov/niosh/docs/hazardcontrol/hc11.html.
159. OSHA. OSHA shelves plan to issue bulletin on surgical smoke. Hospital Employee Health. 2000;July;78-80.
160. Occupational Safety and Health Administration (OSHA 2011): http://www.osha.gov/SLTC/laserelectrosurgeryplume/index.html
161. Technische Regeln Fur Biologische Arbeitsstoffe (TRBA). 250. Anderung und Erganzung: GMB1 Nr. 4 v.
162. Mowbray N, Asnell J, Warren N, et al. Is surgical smoke harmful to theater staff? A systemic review. Surg Endosc. 2013;27(9):3100-7.
163. Bigony L. Risks Associated with exposure to surgical smoke plume: a review of the literature. AORN J. 2007;86(6):1013-20.
164. International Social Security Association (ISSA). Surgical Smoke: Risks and Preventive Measures. Hamburg: ISSA; 2011.
165. Weston R, Stepheson RN, Kutarski PW, et al. Chemical composition of gases surgeons are exposed to during endoscopic urologic resections. Urology. 2009;74(5):1152-4.
166. Ott DE. Carboxyhemoglobinemia due to peritoneal smoke absorption from laser tissue combustion at laparoscopy. J Clin Laser Med Surg. 1998;16(6): 309-15.
167. Murdock CM, Wolff AJ, Van Geem T. Risk factors for hypercarbia, subcutaneous emphysema, pneumothorax, and pneumomediastinum during laparoscopy. Obstet Gynecol. 2000;95(5):704-9.
168. Horak S, Blecharz A, Rzempoluch J, et al. Complications of endoscopy in gynecology. Ginekol Pol. 1992;63(12):619-22.

169. Niedzielski A, Gizewski J, Staraczewski A, et al. [Nineteen years of laparoscopy in the gynecology clinic IPG PAM]. Ginekol Pol. 1992;63(11):596-9.
170. Sharma KC, Kabinoff G, Ducherne Y. Laparoscopic surgery and its potential for medical complications. Heart Lung. 1977;26(1):52-64, quiz 65-7
171. Batra MS, Driscoll JJ, Coburn WA, et al. Evanescent nitrous oxide pneumothorax after laparoscopy Anesth Analg. 1983;62(12):1121-3.
172. Fitzgerald SD, Andrus CH, Baudendistel LJ, et al. Hypercarbia during carbon dioxide pneumoperitoneum. Am J Surg. 1992;163(1):186-90.
173. Rittenmeyer H. Carbon dioxide toxicity related to a laparoscopic procedure. J Post Anesth Care. 1994; 9(3):157-61.
174. Herati AS, Atalla MA, Rais-Bahrami S, et al. A new valve-less trocar for urologic laparoscopy: initial evaluation. J Endourlol. 2009:23(9);1535-9.
175. Herati AS, Andonian S, Rais-Bahrami S, et al. Use of the valveless trocar system reduces carbon dioxide absorption during laparoscopy when compared with standard trocars. Urology. 2011:77(5);1126-32.
176. Hillelsohn JH, Friedlander JI, Bagadiya N, et al. Masked pneumothorax: risk of valveless trocar systems. J Urol. 2013;189(3):955-9.
177. Kalhan SB, Reaney JA, Collins RL. Pneumomediastinum and subcutaneous emphysema during laparoscopy. Cleve Clin J Med. 1990;57(7):639-42.
178. Kent RB 3rd. Subcutaneous emphysema and hypercarbia following laparoscopic cholecystectomy. Arch Surg. 1991;126(9):1154-6.
179. Wolf JS Jr, Monk TG, McDougall EM, et al. The extraperitoneal approach and subcutaneous emphysema are associated with greater absorption of carbon dioxide during laparoscopic renal surgery. J Urol. 1995;154(3):959-63.
180. Waisbren SJ, Herz BL, Ducheine Y, et al. "Iatrogenic respiratory acidosis" during laparoscopic preperitoneal hernia repair. J Laparoendosc Surg. 1996;6(3):181-3.
181. Wolf JS Jr, Clayman RV, Monk TG, et al. Carbon dioxide absorption during laparoscopic pelvic operation. J Am Coll Surg. 1995;180(5):555-60.
182. Lee DW, Kim MJ, Lee, YK, et al. Does intraabdominal pressure affect development of subcutaneous emphysema at gynecologic laparoscopy? J Minim Invasive Gynecol. 2011:18(6);761-5.
183. Wittigen C, Andrus C, Fitzgerald SD, et al. Analysis of hemodynamics and ventilation during laparoscopic cholecystectomy. Arch Surg. 1991;126(8):997-1001.
184. Leighton T, Pianim N, Liu S, et al. Effectors of hypercarbia during experimental pneumoperitoneum. Am Surg. 1992;58(12):717-21.
185. Holzman M, Sharp K, Richards W. Hypercarbia during carbon dioxide gas insufflation for therapeutic laparoscopy: a note of caution. Surg Laparosc Endosc. 1992;2(1):11-4.
186. Hall D, Goldstein A, Tynan E. Profound hypercarbia late in the course of laparoscopic choleystectomy. Anesthesiology. 1993;79(1):173-4.
187. Marshall RL, Jebsen PJ, Davie IT, et al. Circulatory effect of carbon dioxide insufflation of the peritoneal cavity for laparoscopy. Br J Anaesth. 1972;44(7): 680-2.
188. Kelman G, Swapp G, Smith I. Cardiac output and arterial blood gas tension during laparoscopy. Br J Anesth. 1972;44(11):1155-62.
189. Pearce D. Respiratory acidosis and subcutaneous emphysema during laparoscopic cholecystectomy. Can J Anaesth. 1994;41(4):314-6.
190. Santana A, Crausman R, Dubin H. Late onset of subcutaneous emphysema and hypercarbia following laparoscopic cholecystectomy. Chest. 1999; 115(5):1468-71.
191. Ludwig K. Implications of subcutaneous emphysema and how to avoid and/or limit its development. The SAGES Manual. New York: Springer; 2006. pp 273-20.
192. Hynes SR, Marshall RL. Venous gas embolism during gynaecological laparoscopy. Can J Anaesth. 1992;39(7):748-9.
193. Bonjer HJ, Hazebroek EJ, Kazemier G, et al. Open versus closed establishment of pneumoperitoneum in laparoscopic surgery. Br J Surg. 1997;84(5): 599-602.
194. Cottin V, Delafosse B, Viale JP. Gas embolism during laparoscopy: a report of seven cases in patients with previous abdominal surgical history. Surg Endosc. 1996;10(2):166-9.
195. Magrina JF. Complications of laparoscopic surgery. Clin Obstet Gynecol. 2002;45(2):469-80.
196. Hong JY, Kim WO, Kil HK. Detection of subclinical CO_2 embolism by transesophageal echocardiography during laparoscopic radical prostatectomy. Urology. 2010;75(3):581-4.
197. Air embolism and CO_2 insufflators: the need for pre-use purging of tubing. Health Devices. 1996;25(5-6): 214-5.
198. Graff TD, Arbegast NR, Phillips OC, et al. Gas embolism: a comparative study of air and carbon dioxide as embolic agents in the systemic venous system. Am J Obstet Gynecol. 1959;78(2):259-65.
199. Mayer KL, Ho HS, Mathiesen KA, et al. Cardiopulmonary responses to experimental venous carbon dioxide embolism. Surg Endosc. 1998;12(8):1025-30.
200. Muth C, Shank ES. Gas embolism. New Engl J Med. 2000;342(7):476-82.
201. Menes T, Spivak H. Laparoscopy: searching for the proper insufflation gas. Surg Endosc. 2000;14(11): 1050-6.
202. Gutt CN, Oniu T, Mehrabi A, et al. Circulatory and respiratory complications of carbon dioxide insufflation. Dig Surg. 2004;21(2):95-105.
203. Groenman FA, Peers LW, Rademaker BM, et al. Embolism of air and gas in hysteroscopic procedures; pathophysiology and implication for daily practice. J Minim Invasive Gynecol. 2008;15(2):241-7.
204. Corson SL, Brooks PG, Soderstrom RM. Gynecologic endoscopic gas embolism. Fertil Steril. 1996;65(3): 529-33.
205. Corwin C. Pneumoperitoneum. In: Scott-Conner CEH (Ed). The SAGES Manual: Fundamentals of

Laparoscopy and GI Endoscopy. New York: Springer; 1999. pp 37-42.
206. Mann C, Boccara G, Grevy V, et al. Argon pneumoperitoneum is more dangerous than CO_2 pneumoperitoneum during venous gas embolism. Anesth Analg. 1997;85(6):1367-71.
207. Rudston-Brown B, Draper PN, Warriner B, et al. Venous gas embolism—a comparison of carbon dioxide and helium in pigs. Can J Anaesth. 1997; 44(10):1102-7.
208. Wolf JS Jr, Carrier S, Stoller ML. Gas embolism: helium is more lethal than carbon dioxide. J Laparoendosc Surg. 1994;4(3):173-7.
209. Park EY, Kwon JY, Kim KJ. Carbon dioxide embolism during laparoscopic surgery. Yonsei Med J. 2012;53(3): 459-66.
210. Souders JE. Pulmonary air embolism. J Clin Monit Comput. 2000;16(5-6):375-83.
211. Archer DP, Pash MP, MacRae ME. Successful management of venous air embolism with inotropic support. Can J Anaesth. 2001;48(2):204-8.
212. Haroun-Bizri S, ElRassi T. Successful resuscitation after catastrophic carbon dioxide embolism during laparoscopic cholecystectomy. Eur J Anaesthesiol. 2001;18(2):118-21.
213. Gurusamy KS, Koti R, Davidson BR. Abdominal lift for laparoscopic cholecystectomy. Cochrane Database Syst Rev. 2013;Aug 31;(8):CD006574.
214. Ren H, Tong Y, Ding XB, et al. Abdominal wall-lifting versus CO_2 pneumoperitoneum in laparoscopy: a review and meta-analysis. Int J Clin Exp Med. 2014; 7(6):1558-68.

Section 2

Specific Gynecological Laparoscopic Procedures

KIEL SCH•OL

16 of Gynaecological Endoscopy

Benign Ovarian Tumors

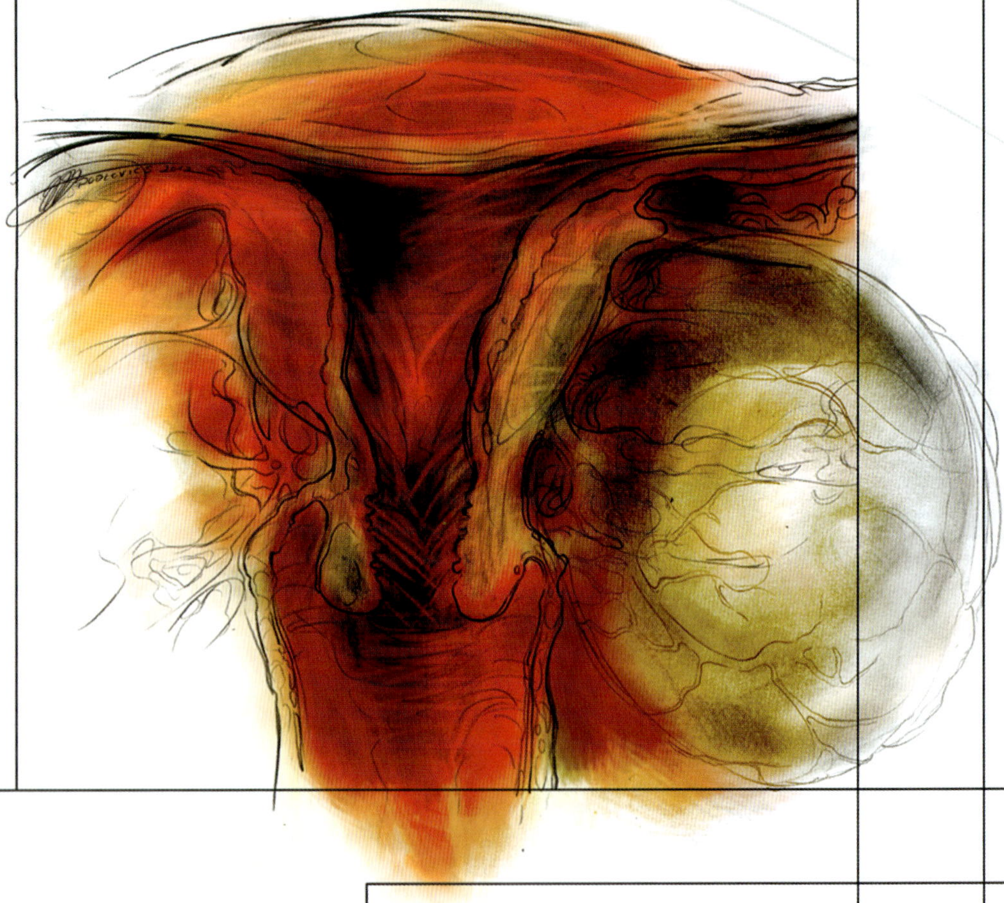

Chapter 16

Benign Ovarian Tumors

Saeed Alborzi, Bahareh Hamedi

INTRODUCTION

Laparoscopy is considered the approach of choice for treating benign ovarian tumors such as endometrioma, mature teratoma and cystadenoma.[1,2] The indications for visualization of an adnexal mass by surgery (laparoscopy or laparotomy) include suspicion of malignancy (size > 10 cm, thick septa, vegetation, heterogeneous content, low resistance index and persistence for more than 6 months), complicated tumors and chronic pelvic pain.[3]

The advantages of laparoscopy are reduction in postoperative pain, febrile morbidity, urinary tract infection, postoperative hospital admission, complications and total cost.[4,5]

PREOPERATIVE EVALUATION

History and Physical Examination

The first line in the evaluation of a patient with pelvic mass is history taking. She should be asked about menstrual irregularities, pelvic pain (pattern and severity), abdominal protrusion, urinary and bowel disturbances.[6]

Abdominopelvic and rectovaginal examination should be performed. Ovarian, uterine or other origins of pelvic masses may be detected by physical examination. The physician can evaluate the consistency, mobility, irregularity and tenderness of the mass. Any signs of malignancy such as adhesion to surrounding organs and presence of ascites may be detected.

Tumor Markers

Serum tumor markers play an important role in screening, diagnosis and follow-up of some gynecologic malignancies. The preoperative evaluation of serum biomarkers must be made before surgery in order to determine malignant disease.[7]

CA-125 is the most valuable marker to predict malignancy. A level of 35 IU/mL or higher is positive, but in some benign conditions (such as pregnancy, endometriosis and leiomyoma), elevated serum level of CA-125 is seen.[8] So, CA-125 is a specific and sensitive marker (97% and 78%) in postmenopausal women for predicting cancer.[9]

Human epididymis 4 (HE4) is another serum marker that is occasionally checked in combination with CA-125. Jacob et al.[10] reported that the major advantage of HE4 is due to its high specificity in borderline and early-stage ovarian cancer, but no benefit has been shown from combining CA-125 and HE4 together in routine practice.

Recent data suggests that serial tumor markers are more effective in distinguishing benign from malignant ovarian tumors.[11] Carcinoembryonic antigen (CEA), alpha-fetoprotein, LDH, inhibin, B-hCG and mesothelin are some of the other available tumor markers, which may predict the chance of malignant degeneration in ovarian masses.[8,12]

Ultrasound Examinations

Today, high-frequency ultrasound scans are considered as a routine gynecological assessment to detect ovarian tumors.[13,14] However, transvaginal sonography produces greater resolution and more detailed morphological pictures than transabdominal echography.[7] Transvaginal Doppler ultrasound is the other technique used for the evaluation of adnexal masses.[15,16] With tumor angiogenesis, there is an increase in the number and tortuosity of vascular supply, but because of absence of muscular intima, it has low impedance to flow.[11]

The pulsatility index (the difference between the peak systolic and the end-diastolic flow velocity divided by the mean flow velocity) lower than 1.0 is indicative of low impedance to flow and higher risk of malignancy.[11,16] However, preoperative color Doppler study is not a reliable indicator of malignancy because some benign lesions such as hemorrhagic, luteal and dermoid cysts and also inflammatory masses may show low impedance.[16,17]

Computed Tomographic Scan and Magnetic Resonance Imaging

Adjunctive imaging modalities are used to investigate the adnexal masses and improve diagnosis.[6] In patients with a confirmed ovarian tumor by transvaginal sonographic examination, computed tomographic (CT) scan is not necessary to perform except for R/O lymphadenopathy, omental disease and metastasis.[11] On the other hand, magnetic resonance imaging (MRI) is indicated to assess tumor infiltration and provides soft tissue contrast and clear pictures of pelvic organs.[6] But Satoh et al. showed that the best modality to supplement ultrasonography is still open to question and routine CT and MRI after sonographic scanning has little advantage,[13] except in case of suspected malignant lesions.[7]

SURGICAL APPROACH

As with the other surgical procedures, more surgical skills lead to better results and fewer complications of surgery. The surgeon should be experienced and understand the disease that is being treated.

Whether the plan is organ conservation or removal, it should be discussed with the patient before operation. Route and type of surgery, complications and possibility of conversion to laparotomy should be discussed and documented via an informed consent.

Those patients, in whom severe adhesion or malignancy might be detected, should have preoperative bowel preparation. All patients should receive preoperative prophylactic antibiotics and wear antithrombotic stocking and/or sequential compression devices.

The surgery routinely is performed under general anesthesia with tracheal intubation. Foley catheter should be placed to empty the bladder and reduce the risk of bladder injury.

Abdominal skin should be prepared from xiphoid process to mons pubis like an abdominal laparotomy preparation. If the patient has a uterus, uterine manipulator may be helpful to facilitate adnexal dissection. In the cases of previous hysterectomy, a vaginal-placed sponge-on-stick is helpful.

In a standard laparoscopic technique, after induction of general anesthesia, pneumoperitoneum is attained using a Veress needle. Then a 10 mm laparoscope is introduced though a 1 cm umbilical incision and on direct view two or three accessory 5–12 mm trocars are placed through lower abdominal incisions for the introduction of accessory instruments.

After initial diagnostic evaluation of the pelvis and abdomen by rotating the scope around, any sign of adhesion or malignancy should be evaluated. Adhesiolysis is performed when indicated to reestablish the normal anatomy. Any doubt of malignancy should be proved by biopsy and frozen sectioning. If a gynecologic malignancy is found either by initial evaluation by scope or on frozen section, management should be continued with the involvement of an oncology gynecologist who is expert in laparoscopy or can perform a laparotomy incision.

SPECIFIC CONSIDERATIONS

Endometrioma

Benign adnexal cysts such as endometrioma are seen frequently in young, infertile women, in whom residual ovarian function after surgery is important.[18] There are several modalities for the treatment of endometriotic cysts, which include medical and surgical treatment. The effects of danazol and GnRH-agonists on endometrioma have been compared in some studies[19–21] and about 40–57% decrease in the size of the cyst has been found. But, endometriomas equal to or larger than 3 cm are known not to respond well to medical therapy.[22]

The main surgical procedure for the treatment of endometrioma include the following:

- Ultrasound-guided or laparoscopy-guided aspiration
- Aspiration and sclerotherapy
- Laparoscopic surgery by means of cystectomy or fenestration and coagulation
- Radical treatment (oophorectomy or adnexectomy)

Because both laparoscopy and laparotomy provide the same results in terms of pregnancy and recurrence rates, laparoscopy can be considered to be the best approach for endometriotic cysts because blood loss during operation, length of hospitalization and need for analgesia are significantly lower in the laparoscopy group.[23-26]

Laparoscopic Drainage of Endometrioma

Nowadays it is accepted that simple aspiration by laparoscopy should not be used to treat endometrioma[19,27] because the recurrence rate is about 80–100%.[28,29]

Although giving GnRH-agonist after the drainage of endometrioma can reduce the size of the cyst up to 50%, it has no effect on recurrence rate[30,31] because the nature of the disease is persistent.

Laparoscopic Cystectomy

The first-line choice for conservative treatment of endometriotic cysts is laparoscopic cystectomy.[32] In this technique (Figs. 16.1 to 16.5), the inner lining of the cyst is dissected from the ovary by two atraumatic grasping forceps that are pulled in opposite directions.[32] Some studies reported that ovarian cystectomy may induce damage to ovarian reserve by removal of healthy ovarian tissue and this may cause reduction of follicular response in controlled ovarian hyperstimulation.[33,34]

Although Muzii et al.[35] reported that in 54% of cases of cystectomy ovarian tissue was detected with cyst pseudocapsule, the ovarian tissue did not show any follicular pattern, and it is suggested that post-cystectomy ovarian response to gonadotropin is comparable to the contralateral ovary.[36-38]

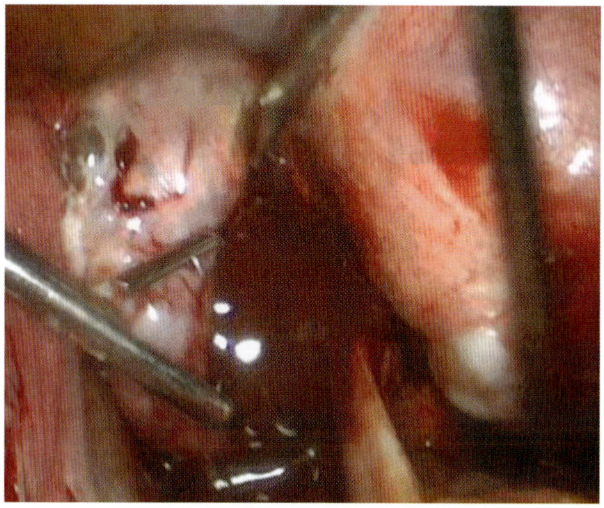

Fig. 16.2: Spillage of the cyst contents.

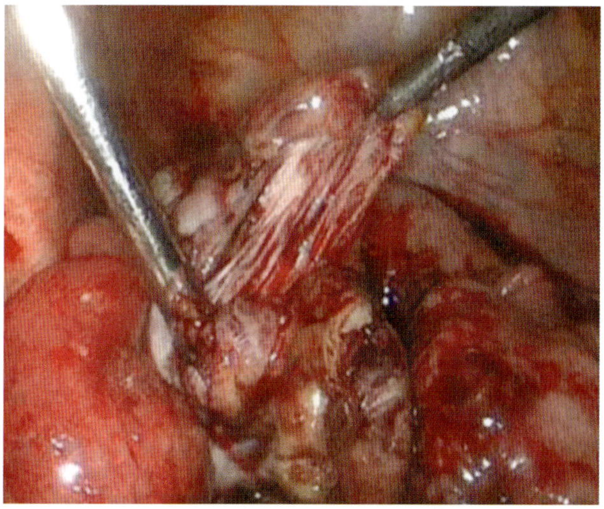

Fig. 16.3: Identification of proper cleavage plane for resection of endometrioma.

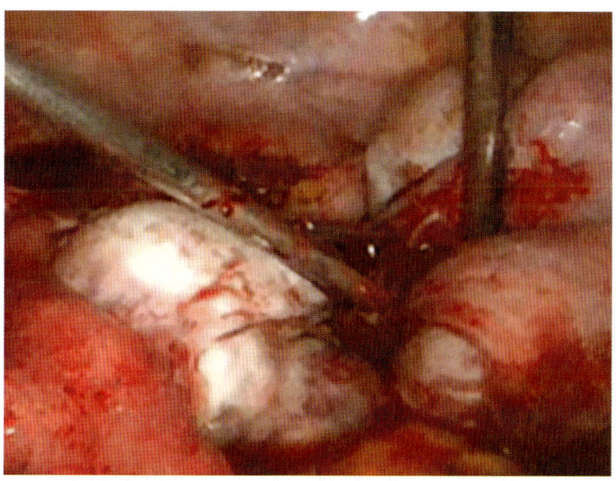

Fig. 16.1: Bilateral ovarian endometriomas with severe adhesion.

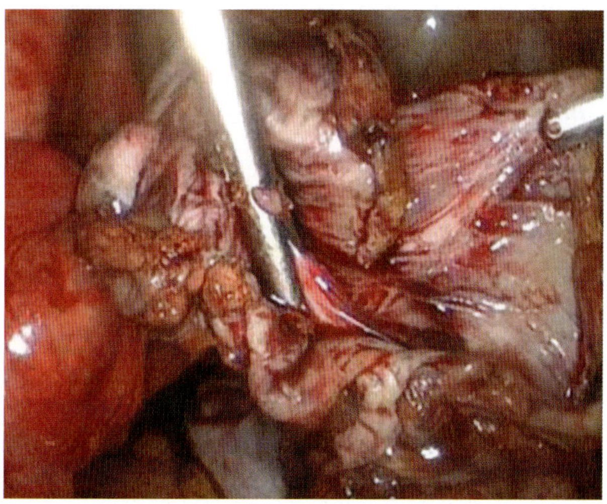

Fig. 16.4: Cystectomy with the stripping technique.

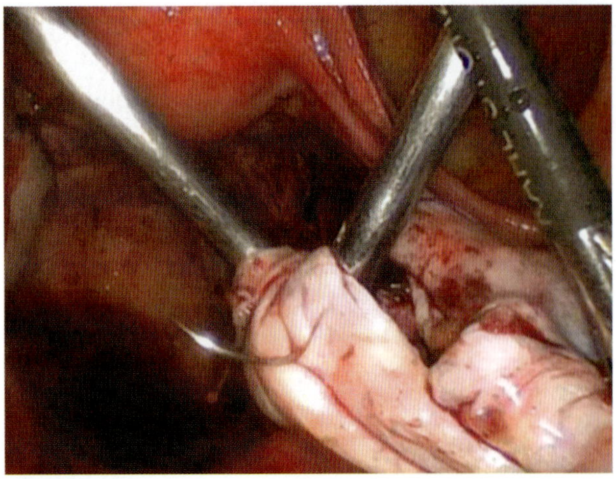

Fig. 16.5: Suturing the ovarian cortex.

Laparoscopic Fenestration, Drainage and Ablation of Cyst Wall

There are different techniques for performing fenestration and coagulation. In one method, fenestration and aspiration are done, a 1.5×1.5 cm biopsy is taken and followed by bipolar coagulation of the inner lining.[18,32]

Some authors perform fenestration and coagulation in two steps, using luteinizing hormone releasing hormone agonist before second laparoscopy.[34] Other groups use electrosurgery or laser for fenestration and coagulation of cyst wall in a single step.[32,39]

Combined Technique of Cystectomy and Ablative Surgery

In this technique, a large part of endometrioma wall is first excised according to the cystectomy technique. After the first step, CO_2 laser is used to vaporize the remaining wall (10–20%), close to the ovarian hilus. Donnez et al.[39] showed that this technique provides the best results by sparing the ovarian hilum from surgical damage.

Radical Treatment for Endometrioma

This technique includes adnexectomy and ovariectomy. According to a meta-analysis, which was performed by Alborzi et al., the excision of cyst wall in endometrioma is strongly recommended.[19]

Mature Teratoma

Mature cystic teratoma (dermoid cysts) are the most common ovarian neoplastic lesions found in adolescents and approximately 70% of benign ovarian tumors are seen in women below 30 years of age.[40–44] They are filled with all tissues derived from three embryonic layers (ectoderm, mesoderm and endoderm) and filled with fatty, semisolid, sebaceous materials with bone, hair and cartilage.[6]

Many gynecologic and pediatric surgeons agree that large dermoid cyst (larger than 5 cm in diameter, due to higher risk of torsion) and symptomatic teratomas need surgical operation.[41,45] When surgery is indicated, a minimally invasive approach by laparoscopy offers many benefits. However, when very large, bilateral dermoids suspicious of malignancy are present, some surgeons prefer laparotomy for surgical staging.[41]

On the other hand, spillage of the cyst contents during laparoscopy may lead to adhesion formation and peritonitis, but in the hand of an expert surgeon, laparoscopic approach with preserving the ovary in young women is the method of choice (Figs. 16.6 to 16.9).

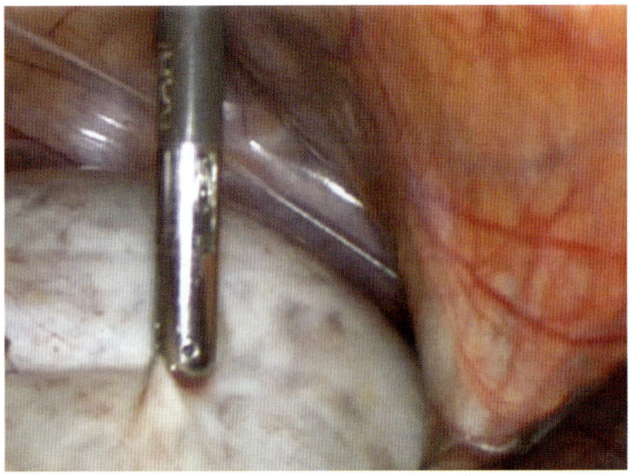

Fig. 16.6: Ovarian dermoid cyst.

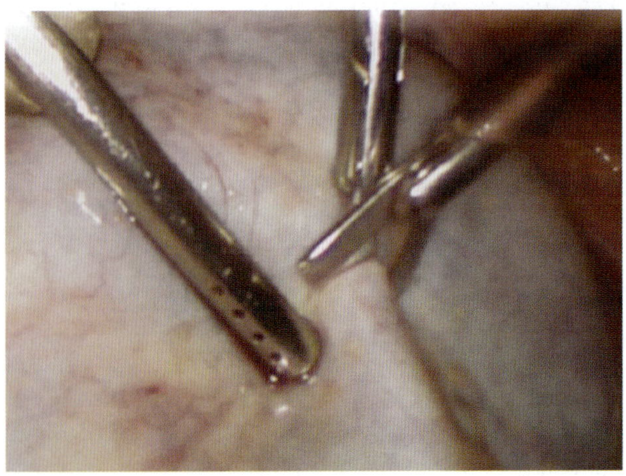

Fig. 16.7: Sharp dissection of the ovarian cortex to find cleavage plane.

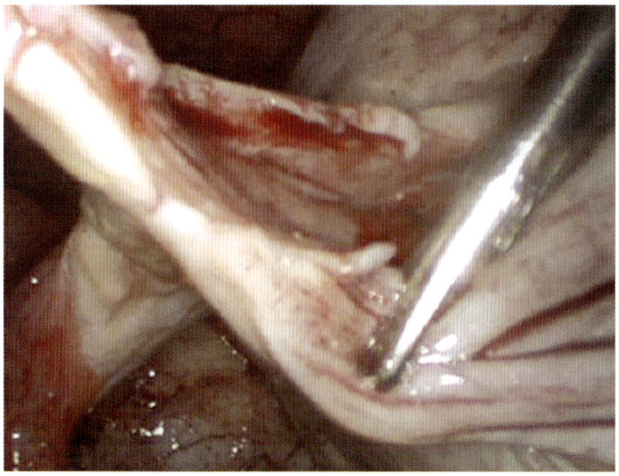

Fig. 16.8: Dissection of fibrous adhesion between the ovary and the cyst capsule.

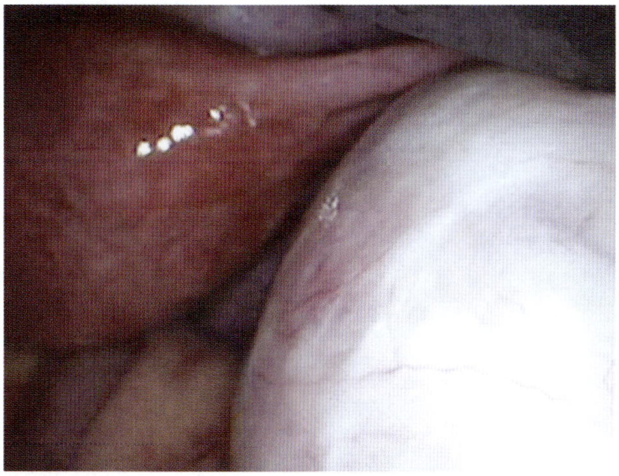

Fig. 16.9: Tearing of the cyst wall during excision.

Serous and Mucinous Cystadenoma

Serous cystadenoma is common in women aged between 30 and 40 years. Their diameter is usually less than 15 cm. They may have smooth internal surface or papillary projection in the internal wall. Mucinous cystadenomas are commonly unilateral and may reach 30–50 cm or even more in diameter.[6]

Cystectomy: After an incision is made on antimesenteric surface of the cyst, two atraumatic grasping forceps are used to pull the cyst wall and the normal ovarian parenchyma in opposite directions, so that the cyst wall is stripped from the bed of normal ovarian tissue (Figs. 16.10 to 16.13). At the ovarian hilus, the dissection is often more difficult, but nevertheless, dissection should continue until the cyst is completely removed from the ovary. Hemostasis is achieved by bipolar coagulation.

Oophorectomy: The indications for laparoscopic oophorectomy usually include large endometriotic

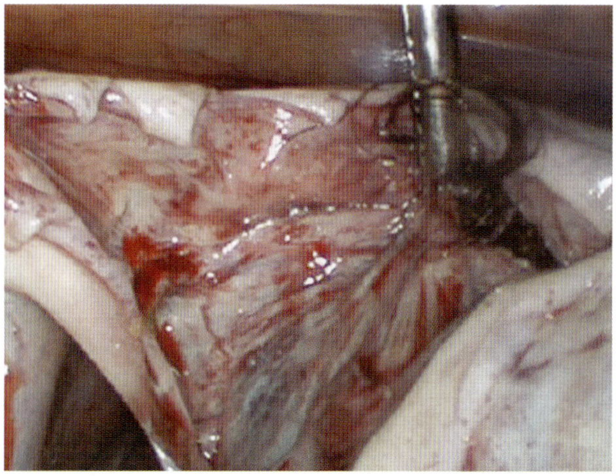

Fig. 16.10: Right ovarian serous cyst adenoma.

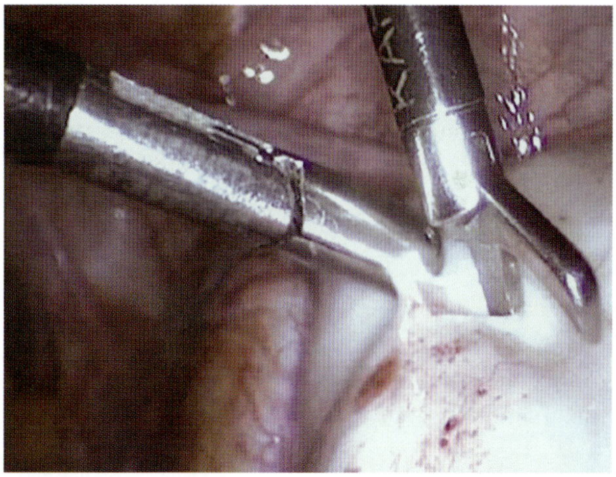

Fig. 16.11: Incision on ovarian cortex.

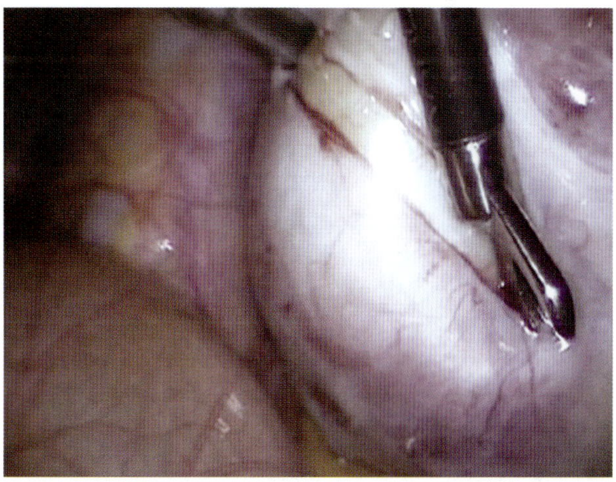

Fig. 16.12: Dissection of ovarian cortex to separate it from underlying cyst.

cysts and benign ovarian cysts in patients older than 40 years. Properly placed uterine manipulator is important to get a good exposure of ovary and tubes.

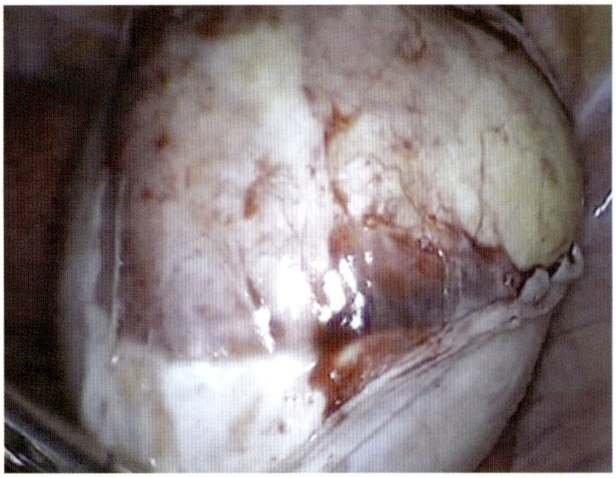

Fig. 16.13: Adequate incision on the ovarian cortex to allow removal of the cyst.

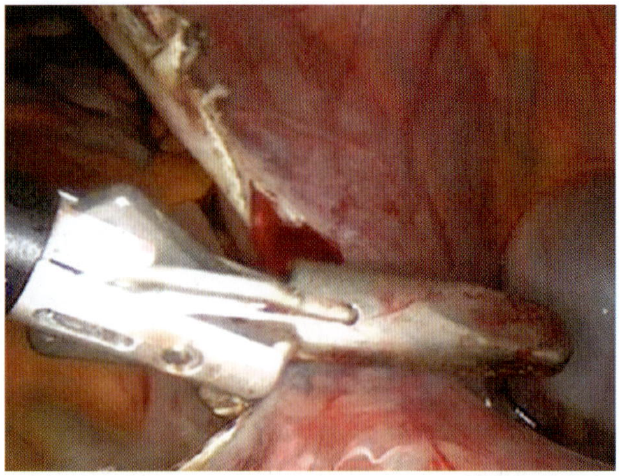

Fig. 16.15: Dissection continued to remove adhesion.

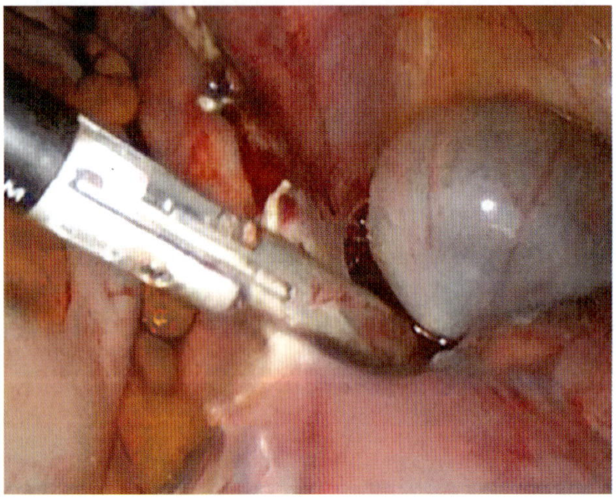

Fig. 16.14: Left adnexectomy. Bipolar coagulation of the infundibulopelvic ligament.

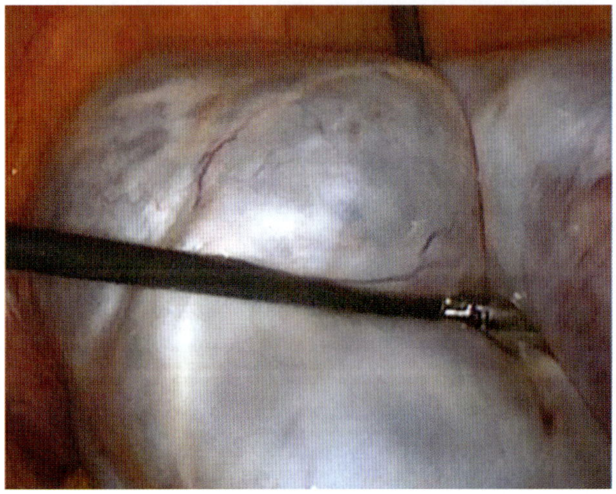

Fig. 16.16: Aspiration of ovarian cyst using a 5 mm aspiration device.

Three techniques have been described for managing the infundibulopelvic ligament: bipolar electrodessication, suture ligation with pretied loop and stapling. A bipolar coagulation forceps is used to coagulate the ovarian pedicle (Figs. 16.14 to 16.17). After total desiccation of the tissue, 5 mm scissors or the CO_2 laser was used for excision. Before starting the procedure, it is important to observe the course of the ureter as it crosses the external iliac artery near the bifurcation of the common iliac artery at the pelvic brim.

OVARIAN TORSION

The common complaint of patients who come to emergency gynecological room in acute pelvic pain is adnexal torsion.[46-48] It is defined by Huchon et al.[44]

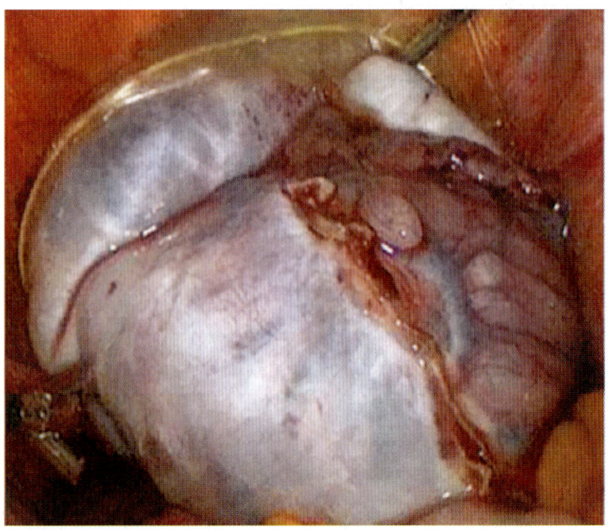

Fig. 16.17: Cyst is put in the endobag.

as the twisting by at least one complete turn of the adnexa, ovary or more rarely the tube, around a centerline. Its frequency is about 2.5–7.4%.[49,50]

Early detection of torsion is very important because most of the patients are very young and nearly all of them desire future fertility.[51,52] The quality of pain may be different. Sudden onset pain is usual, but half of the patients do not experience it. Occasionally, the pain is felt on just one side.[53] Other signs and symptoms include nausea, vomiting, vagal reflex, leukocytosis, peritoneal irritation and fever.[53-55]

Doppler imaging is a modality to diagnose, but according to Pena et al.,[47] 60% of the cases of torsion have normal Doppler, but its positive predictive value is 100%. A sure and certain diagnosis of adnexal torsion can be made only by laparoscopy.[46-51]

The technique of surgery (Figs. 16.18 to 16.20) consists of untwisting the adnexa, even when necrosed and resection of cyst ± ligamentopexy.[54,56] To prevent delayed diagnosis, a high index of suspicion throughout pregnancy is recommended to rule out torsion.

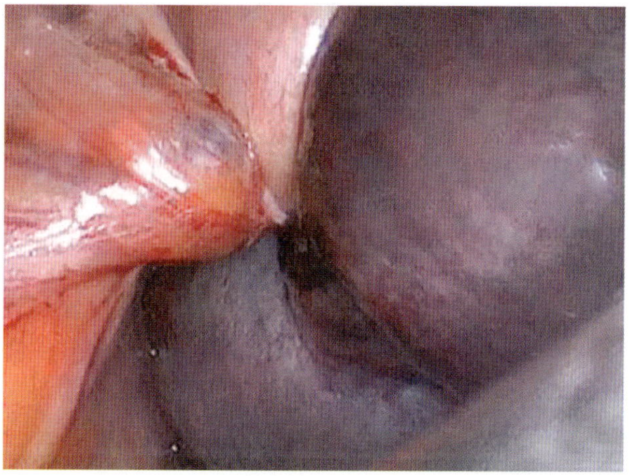

Fig. 16.18: Right ovarian torsion.

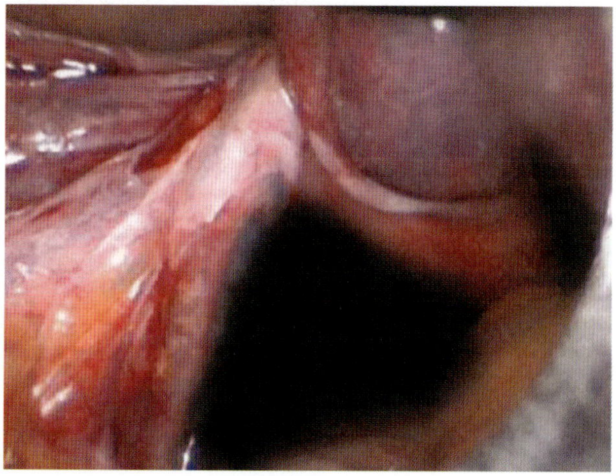

Fig. 16.19: Right ovarian torsion.

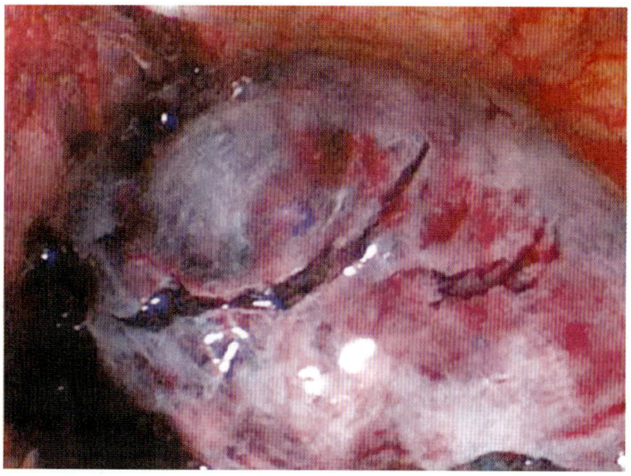

Fig. 16.20: Black discoloration of the adnexa due to torsion and necrosis.

BORDERLINE AND MALIGNANT OVARIAN TUMORS

The preoperative evaluation of an adnexal mass involves radiologic and serum tumor marker evaluation.[57] Regardless of the index of suspicion for malignancy, laparoscopic evaluation of adnexal masses is appropriate in the hands of a skillful surgeon.[58]

Approximately 10% of all ovarian serous tumors are borderline, and 50% occur before the age of 40 years.[59] If borderline and malignant tumors were detected, complete surgical staging should be performed by laparoscopy or laparotomy. An early stage ovarian cancer is rarely diagnosed preoperatively and occasionally is found incidentally during laparoscopy for benign ovarian tumors.[59-61]

Some advantages of laparoscopic surgery for ovarian cancer include less traumatic surgery, faster recovery and earlier possibility for chemotherapy administration. On the other hand, some disadvantages of the surgery are rupture of cyst and spillage of cyst contents, difficulty to remove large ovarian masses, inability to palpate lymph nodes and possibility of trocar metastasis.[60-62]

In conclusion, laparoscopic management of ovarian cancer, especially in advanced stages, is still controversial.

OVARIAN TUMORS IN PREGNANCY

The use of laparoscopic technique has become common for diagnosis and management of a number of surgical disorders in pregnancy. With established pregnancy, the most usage of laparoscopy has been for the evaluation and management of adnexal masses.[63]

Occasionally, pregnant women are young; therefore, borderline and malignant ovarian tumors are uncommon during pregnancy.[63] As Leiserowitz et al. reported, incidences of ovarian masses are 1% in pregnancy.[64] The most common pregnancy-associated ovarian tumors are luteomas, hyperreactio luteinalis, benign cystic teratoma and ovarian hyperstimulation syndrome (OHSS).[65,66]

Indications for exploration (by laparotomy or laparoscopy) in pregnancy are suspicion of torsion or rupture, tumor size more than 10 cm, tumors obstructing labor and presence of signs in favor of malignancy such as nodule, papillary projection or solid component.[51,67] High-resolution sonography and color Doppler sonography has been used for better evaluation of adnexal masses.[68,69]

Elective surgery should be avoided in first trimester, because many lesions resolve spontaneously. Then sonography should be repeated after 6 weeks to detect the persistent cysts.[63,67] If the origin is not known, MRI may be helpful. Tumor markers such as CA-125, AFP and β-hCG are not specific in pregnancy because their levels change in this period.[51,68]

Laparoscopy is a safe and efficient method in pregnancy and should be considered in second trimester if the operation is elective and the mass has no signs of malignancy.[63,64]

General anesthesia is the choice for pregnancy but the surgeon and anesthesiologist should be aware of delayed gastric emptying, esophageal reflux and IVC and aortic compression.[62,64]

The technique of laparoscopy is the same for nonpregnant women except for no intracervical instrument for the mobilization of uterus.

SUTURING IN OVARIAN SURGERY

Laparoscopic surgery is an important skill for the minimally invasive surgeon. There are various types of sutures including endoloop, intracorporeal and extracorporeal knots and it is always necessary to select the ideal stitch (Figs. 16.21 to 16.23).

In ovarian cystectomy and oophorectomy, suturing is used for hemostasis when bipolar is not efficient. On the other hand, suturing may be helpful to prevent adhesion formation in a gapped ovary after removal of a large ovarian tumor.

LAPAROSCOPY COMPLICATIONS

General Complications

Cardiopulmonary complications, reflux of gastric contents, and electrosurgical, hemorrhagic and gastrointestinal complications may occur during laparoscopy. Infection, incisional hernia of trocar place, nerve injury and ureter and bladder injury may occur.[70]

Special Complications

Spillage

When cystectomy is performed, rupture of cyst during surgery may occur. Rupture and spillage of cyst contents is especially important in mature teratoma, which may create chemical peritonitis and adhesion. In malignant lesions, seeding of tumoral cells also may occur.[71,72]

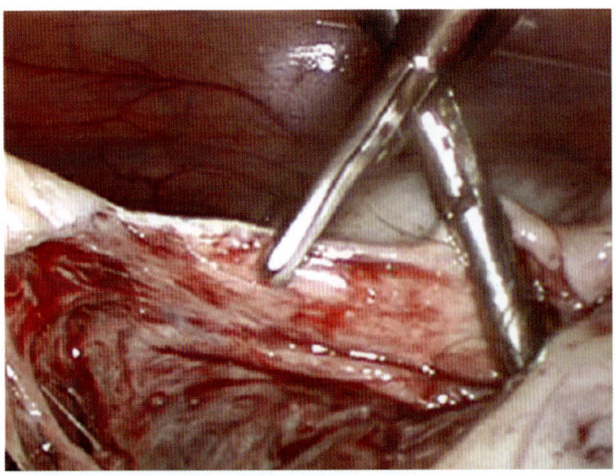

Fig. 16.21: Dissection of left ovarian cyst.

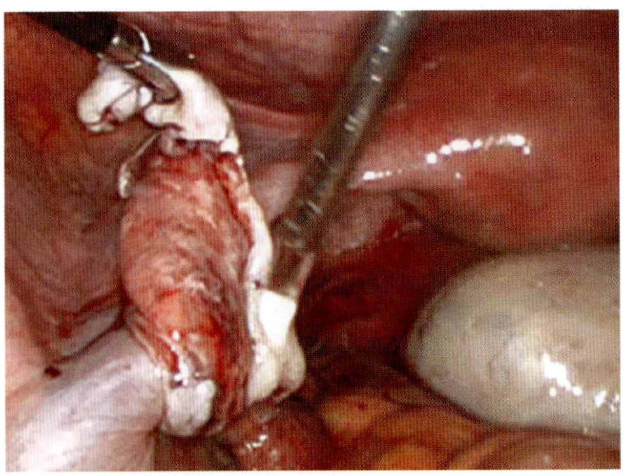

Fig. 16.22: Ovary after removal of the cyst.

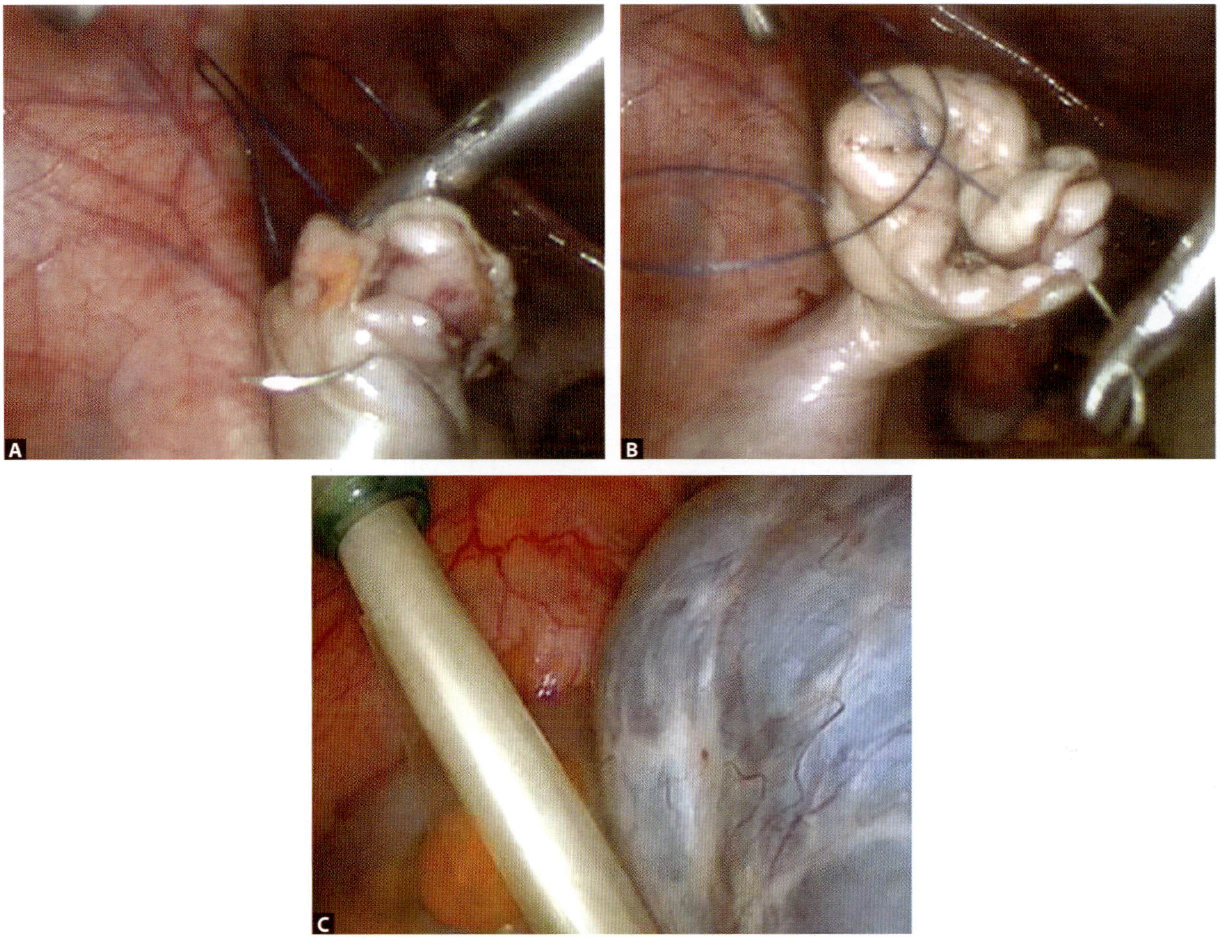

Figs. 16.23A to C: Suturing of the ovarian cortex.

All efforts are made to avert rupture of cysts including limited manipulation of tumors, use of atraumatic graspers and good hemostasis to see cleavage plane.[73] Also, spillage can be avoided by using endoscopic bags.

To introduce the endobag, the parietal port is removed and skin incision is extended to 10 mm and the bag cannula is introduced. After placing the mass in the bag, the edges of bag are pulled outside the wall and clamped (Figs. 16.24 to 16.28). It is sometimes necessary to aspirate the cyst contents before pulling the endobag out of the abdominal wall.

If spillage occurs, the patients position should change to reverse Trendelenburg and abdominopelvic cavity lavage should be performed by several liters of Ringer's lactate solution.[73]

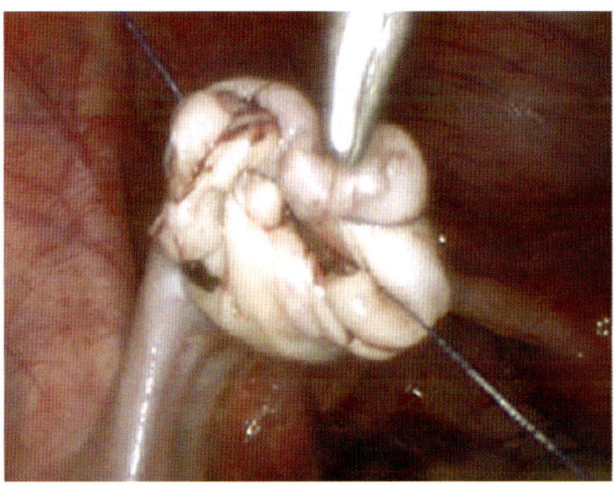

Fig. 16.24: Removed ovarian cyst and entering the endobag into the peritoneal cavity.

Adhesion

Adhesion formation after abdominal operations causes significant morbidity. Many studies show that adhesion formation is less after laparoscopy versus laparotomy.[74]

Although endoscopic approach has been shown to be less adhesiogenic than traditional laparotomy,

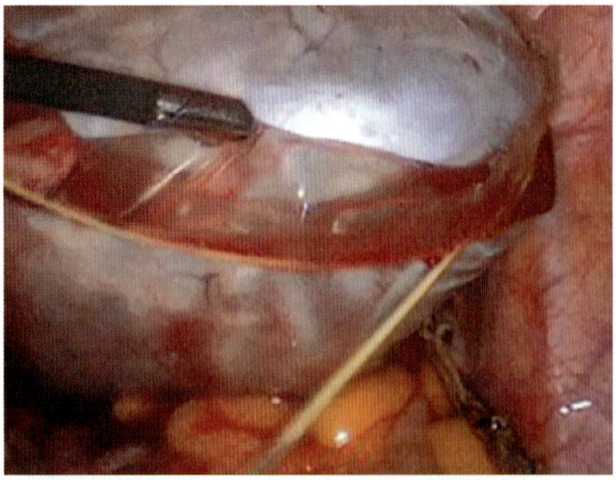

Fig. 16.25: Putting the ovarian cyst in an endobag.

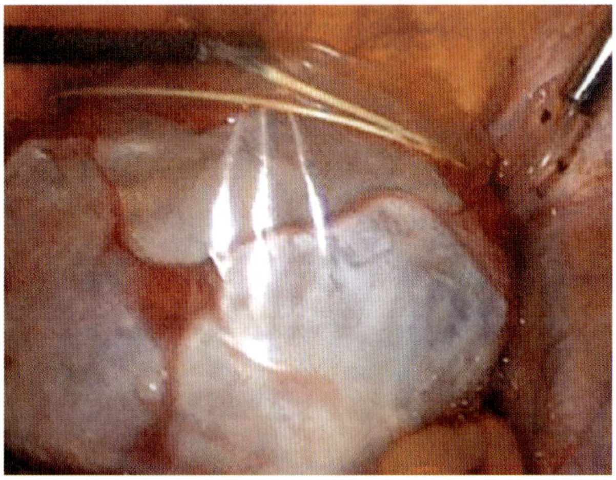

Fig. 16.26: Closing the endobag.

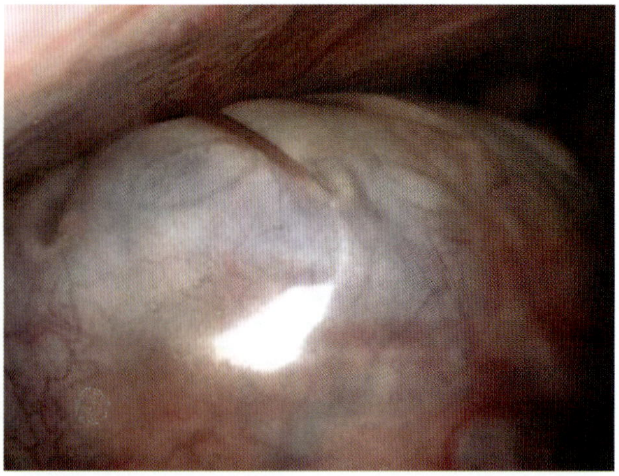

Fig. 16.27: Taking the endobag toward the abdominal wall.

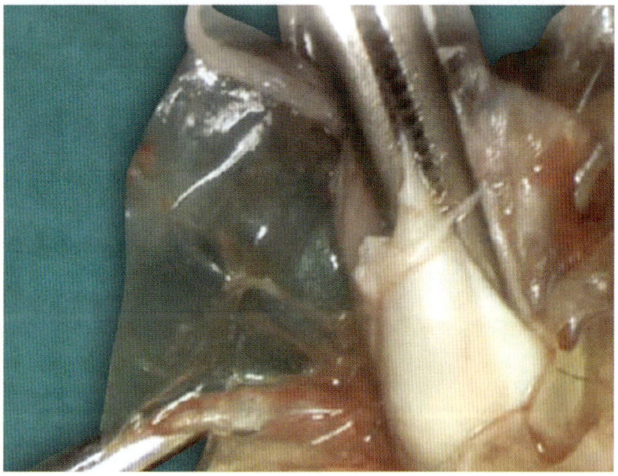

Fig. 16.28: Extraction of the cyst wall after drainage of the cyst contents from the abdominal wall.

at least with regard to selected procedures, it does not totally eliminate the problem. Consequently, many attempts have been made to further reduce adhesion formation and a wide variety of strategies, including surgical techniques, pharmacological agents and mechanical barriers, have been advocated to address this issue.[75-77]

TIPS AND TRICKS

- If there is a large enough area after ovarian cystectomy, reapproximation of ovarian incision in two layers with fine nonreactive sutures with good technique is the best way to avoid adhesion formation.
- Extensive cauterization of ovarian tissue in patients with endometrioma can lead to a rise in FSH levels postoperatively and should be avoided. Fine hemostasis under irrigation with microbipolar and use of sutures to approximate the bed of ovary is the best option to avoid premature ovarian failure in patients with bilateral endometrioma.
- Small endometriomas less than 1 cm in size may effectively be treated by fenestration and coagulation of the inner lining. However, for larger endometriomas, cystectomy is the best technique in terms of chance of recurrence of symptoms and signs, reoperation rate and cumulative pregnancy rate.
- Deep infiltrating endometrioses (DIEs) in ovarian fossa should be excised to avoid recurrence of endometrioma at the time of cystectomy. Covering deperitonealized and operated areas by absorbable barriers significantly reduces the incidence, extent and severity of postsurgical adhesions.

- Operative laparoscopy could be performed in patients with unilateral borderline or malignant tumors and for staging the disease. For more advances ovarian malignant neoplasms, laparotomy is the better option.
- Preparation is essential in laparoscopic surgery for patients with adnexal cyst or mass.
- Assessing ovarian reserve by hormonal profiles or antral follicles count before surgery should be performed in patients with endometriomas or bilateral ovarian cysts or tumors. These assays should be repeated after surgery. Also tumor markers should be checked before operation in those patients suspicious to have borderline or malignant tumors.
- Transvaginal ultrasound is the best and cheapest way for imaging the ovarian cysts or adnexal masses, in addition, one may benefit from spiral CT or MRI imaging.[78]
- In patients with benign cysts such as serous, mucinous or dermoid neoplasms, every attempt should be done to avoid rupturing the cyst wall; however, if accidentally leakage occurs, pelvic and abdominal cavity should be thoroughly washed. Chance of chemical peritonitis is not high as previously thought.
- Adverent tissues removed after removing endometrioma is much higher than other benign cysts such as serous, mucinous or dermoid cysts.[79]

REFERENCES

1. Maris V, Ajossa S, Piras B, et al. Treatment of nonendometriotic benign adnexal cyst: a randomized comparison of laparoscopy and laparotomy. Obstet Gynecol. 1995;86:770-4.
2. Yuen PM, Yu KM, Yip SK, et al. A randomized prospective study of laparoscopy and laparotomy in the management of benign ovarian masses. Am J Obstet Gynecol. 1997;177:109-14.
3. Doret M, Raudrant D. Functional ovarian cysts and the need to remove them. Eur J Obstet Gynecol. 2001; 100:1-4.
4. Mederios LR, Rosa DD, Bozzetti MC, et al. Laparoscopy versus laparotomy for benign ovarian tumours. Chochrane Database Syst Rev. 2009;(2):CD004751.
5. Medeiros LR, Fachel JM, Garry R, Stein AT, Furness S. Laparoscopy versus laparotomy for benign ovarian tumours. Chochrane Database Syst Rev. 2005;(3): CD004751.
6. Malzoni M, Imperato F. Laparoscopic treatment of adnexal masses. In: Mencaglia L, Minelli L, Wattiez A (Eds). Manual of gynecological laparoscopic surgery. 11th ed. Tuttlingen: Straub Druck+Medien AG; 2009. p. 152-63.
7. Donnez J, Squifflet J, Jadoul P. Laparoscopic management of ovarian cysts. In: Donnez L (Ed). Atlas of operative laparoscopy and Hystroscopy. 3rd ed. Boca Raton, FL: Taylor & Francis; 2008. p. 195-210.
8. Husseinzadeh N. Status of tumor markers in epithelial ovarian cancer has there been any progress? A review. Gynecol Oncol. 2011;120:152-7.
9. Malkasian GD, Knapp RC, Lavin PT, et al. Preoperative evaluation of serum CA-125 levels in premenopausal and postmenopausal patients with pelvic masses: discrimination of benign from malignant disease. Am J Obstet Gynecol. 1988:159:341-6.
10. Jacob F, Meier M, Caduff R, et al. No benefit from combining HE4 and CA125 as ovarian tumor markers in a clinical setting. Gynecol Oncol. 2011;121:487-91.
11. Van Nagell JR, Gershenson DM. Ovarian cancer: etiology, screening and surgery. In: Rock JA, Jones III HW (Eds). Telinde's operative Gynecology. 10th ed. Philadelphia, PA: Wolters Kluwer/Lippincott-Williams and Wilkins; 2008. p. 1307-39.
12. Aggarwal P, Kehoe S. Serum tumor markers in gynecological cancers. Maturitas. 2010;67:46-53.
13. Satoh S, Takashima T, Nakano H. Role of imaging modalities in ovarian tumors. Int J Obstet Gynecol. 2002;76:195-7.
14. Campbell S, Bhan V, Royston P, et al. Transabdominal ultrasound screening for early ovarian cancer. Br Med J. 1989;299:1363-7.
15. Kurjak A, Schulman H, Sosic A, et al. Transvaginal ultrasound, color flow, and Doppler waveform of the postmenopausal adnexal mass. Obstet Gynecol. 1992;80:917-21.
16. Kawai M, Kano T, Kikkawa F, et al. Transvaginal Doppler ultrasound with color flow imaging in the diagnosis of ovarian cancer. Obstet Gynecol. 1997; 79:163-7.
17. Helm CW, Pasic R. Laparoscopic management of the adnexal mass. In: Pasic RP, Levine RL (Eds). A practical manual of laparoscopy and minimally invasive gynecology. 2nd edn. Boca Raton, FL: Taylor & Francis/ Thomsong; 2007. p. 179-90.
18. Alborzi S, Momtahan M, Parsanezhad ME, et al. A prospective, randomized study comparing laparoscopic cystectomy versus fenestration and coagulation in patients with endometriomas. Fertil Steril. 2004;82:1633-7.
19. Alborzi S, Zarei A, Alborzi S, Alborzi M. Management of ovarian endometrioma. Clin Obstet Gynecol. 2006; 49:480-91.
20. Crikel U, Ochs H, Schneider HP. A randomized comparative trial of triptorelin depot and danazol in the treatment of endometriosis. Eur J Obstet Gynecol Reprod Biol. 1995;59:61-9.
21. Dmowski WP, Tummon I, Pepping P, et al. Ovarian suppression induces with buseralin or danazol in the management of endometriosis: a randomized comparative study. Fertil Steril. 1989;51:395-400.
22. Rena N, Thomas S, Rotman C, et al. Decrease in the size of ovarian endometrioma during ovarian suppression in stage IV endometriosis, role of

pre-operative medical treatment. J Reprod Med. 1996;41: 384-92.
23. Donnez J, Smets M, Jadoul P, et al. Laparoscopic management of peritoneal endometriosis, endometriotic cyst and rectovaginal adenomyosis. Ann N Y Acad Sci. 2003;997:274-81.
24. Bateman BG, Kolp LA, Mills S. Endoscopic versus laparotomy management of endometriomas. Fertil Steril. 1994;62:690-5.
25. Catalano GF, Marana R, Carvana P, et al. Laparoscopy versus microsurgery by laparotomy for excision of ovarian cysts in patients with moderate to severe endometriosis. J Am Assoc Gynecol Laparosc. 1996;3: 267-70.
26. Milingos S, Loutradis D, Kallipolitis G, et al. Comparison of laparoscopy with laparotomy for the treatment of extensive endometriomata with large endometrioma. Fertil Steril J Gynecol Surg. 1999;15: 131-6.
27. Sawada T, Satoshi O, Kawakami S, et al. Laparoscopic surgery versus laparotomy management of infertile patients with ovarian endometriomas. J Gynecol Endosc. 1999;8:17-9.
28. Marana R, Carvana P, Muzzi L, et al. Operative laparoscopy for ovarian cysts excision vs aspiration. J Reprod Med. 1996;41:435-8.
29. Saleh A, Tulandi T. Reoperation after laparoscopic treatment of ovarian endometriomas by excision and fenestration. Fertile Steril. 1999;72:322-4.
30. Donnez J, Nisolle M, Goillerot S, et al. Ovarian endometrial cysts: the role of gonadotropin-releasing hormone agonist and/or drainage. Fertil Steril. 1994; 62:63-6.
31. Vercellini P, Vendola N, Bocciolone L, et al. Laparoscopic aspiration of ovarian endometriomas effect with postoperative gonadotropin releasing hormone agonist treatment. J Reprod Med. 1992;37: 577-85.
32. Beretta P, Franchi M, Ghezzi F, et al. Randomized clinical trial of two laparoscopic treatment of endometrioma cystectomy versus drainage and coagulation. Fertil Steril. 1998;70:1176-80.
33. Brosens I, Van Ballaer P, Puttemans P, et al. Reconstruction of the ovary containing large endometrioma by an extraovarian endosurgical technique. Fertil Steril. 1996;66:517-21.
34. Donnez J, Nisolle M, Gillet N, et al. Large ovarian endometrioma. Hum Reprod. 1996;11:641-6.
35. Muzii L, Bianchi A, Croce C, et al. Laparoscopic excision of ovarian cysts: is the stripping technique a tissue sparing procedure? Fertil Steril. 2002;77: 609-14.
36. Loh FH, Tan AL, Kumar J, et al. Ovarian response after laparoscopic ovarian cystectomy for endometriotic cysts in 132 monitored cycles. Fertil Steril. 1999; 72:316-21.
37. Alborzi S, Foroughinia L, Kumar PV, et al. A comparison of histopathologic finding of ovarian tissue inadvertently excised with endometrioma and other kinds of benign ovarian cyst in patients undergoing laparoscopy vs laparotomy. Fertil Steril. 2009;92:2004-7.
38. Alborzi S, Ravanbakhsh R, Parsanezhad ME, et al. A comparison of follicular response of ovaries to ovulation induction after laparoscopic ovarian cystectomy or fenestration and coagulation versus normal ovaries in patients with endometriosis. Fertil Steril. 2007;88:507-9.
39. Donnez J, Lousse JC, Jadoul P, et al. Laparoscopic management of endometriomas using a combined technique of excisional (cystectomy) and ablative surgery. Fertil Steril. 2010;94:28-32.
40. O'Neill KE, Cooper AR. The approach to ovarian dermoids in adolescents and young women. North Am Soc Pediatr Adolesc Gynecol. 2011;24(3):176-80.
41. Ayhan A, Bukulmez O, Genc C, et al. Mature cystic teratomas of the ovary: case series from one institution over 34 years. Eur J Obstet Gynecol Reprod Biol. 2000;33:153.
42. Templeman CL, Fallat M, Lam AM, et al. Managing mature cystic teratomas of the ovary. Obstet Gynecol Surv. 2000;55:738.
43. Borgfeldt C, Andolf E. Transvaginal sonographic ovarian findings in a random sample of women 25–40 years old. Ultrasound Obstet Gynecol. 1999;13:345.
44. Huchon C, Favconnier A. Adnexal torsion: a literature review. Eur J Obstet Gynecol Reprod Biol. 2010;150: 8-12.
45. Kontorovdis A, Chryssikopoulos A, Hassiakos D, et al. The diagnostic value of laparoscopy in 2365 patients with acute and chronic pelvic pain. Int J Gynecol Obstet. 1996;52:243-8.
46. Walker JW. Abdominal and pelvic pain. Emerg Med Clin N Am. 1987;5:425-8.
47. Pena JE, Ufberg D, Cooney N, et al. Usefulness of Doppler sonography in the diagnosis of ovarian torsion. Fertile Steril. 2000;73:1047-50.
48. Oelsner G, Shashar D. Adnexal torsion. Clin Obstet Gynecol. 2006;49(3):459-63.
49. Ozcan C, Celik A, Ozok G, Erdener A, Balik E. Adnexal torsion in children may have a catastrophic sequel: asynchronous bilateral torsion. J Pediatr Surg. 2002;37(11):1617-20.
50. Bar-On Sh, Mashiach R, Stockheim D, et al. Laparoscopy for suspected ovarian torsion: are we too hasty to operate? Fertil Steril. 2010;93: 2012-15.
51. Sanfilippo JS, Rock JA. Surgery for benign disease of the ovary. In: Rock JA, Jones III HW (Eds). Telinde's Operative Gynecology. 10th edn. Philadelphia, PA: Wolters Kluwer/Lippincott-Williams and Wilkins; 2008. p. 629-47.
52. Lomano JM, Trelford JD, Ullery JC. Torsion of the uterine adnexa causing an acute abdomen. Obstet Gynecol. 1970;35:221-5.
53. Houry D, Abott JT. Ovarian torsion: a fifteen year review. Ann Emerg Med. 2001;38(2):156-90.
54. McWilliams GD, Hill MJ, Dietrich 3rd CS. Gynecologic emergencies. Surg Clin North Am. 2008;88(2): 265-83.

55. Tsafrir Z, Azem F, Hasson J, et al. Risk factors, symptoms, and treatment of ovarian torsion in children: the twelve-year experience of one center. J Minimal Invas Gynecol. 2012;19(1):29-33.
56. Adams Hillard PJ. Benign diseases of female reproductive tract. In: Berek JS (Ed). Berek and Novak's gynecology. 14th ed. Philadelphia, PA: Lippincott-Williams and Wilkins; 2007. p.432-500.
57. Nezhat F, Nezhat C, Welander CE, Benigno B. Four ovarian cancers diagnosed during laparoscopic management of 1011 women with adnexal masses. Am J Obstet Gynecol. 1992;167:790-6.
58. Liu CS, Nagarsheth NP, Nezhat FR. Laparoscopy and ovarian cancer: a paradigm change in the management of ovarian cancer? J Minim Invasive Gynecol. 2009;16:250-62.
59. Berek JS, Natarajan S. Ovarian and fallopian tube cancer. In: Berek JS (Ed). Berek and Novak's gynecology. 14th ed. Philadelphia, PA: Lippincott-Williams and Wilkins; 2007. p. 1458-547.
60. Katz VL, Lentz GM, Lobo RA, Gershenson DM. Comprehensive Gynecology. 5th edn. Philadelphia, PA: Mosby Elsevier; 2007.
61. Chi DS, Abu-Rustum NR, Sonoda Y, et al. The safety and efficacy of laparoscopic surgical staging of apparent stage I ovarian and fallopian tube cancers. Am J Obstet Gynecol. 2005;192:1614-9.
62. Amara DP, Nezhat C, Teng NN, et al. Operative laparoscopy in the management of ovarian cancer. Surg Laparosc Endosc. 1996;6:38-45.
63. Whitecar P, Turner S, Higby K. Adnexal masses in pregnancy: a review of 130 cases undergoing surgical management. Am J Obstet Gynecol. 1999;181:19-24.
64. Leiserowitz GS. Managing ovarian masses during pregnancy. Obstet Gynecol. 2006;61:463-70.
65. Mazza V, Di Monte I, Ceccarelli PL, et al. Prenatal diagnosis of female pseudohermaphroditism associated with bilateral luteoma of pregnancy. Hum Reprod. 2002;17:821-4.
66. Kaiser UB. The pathogenesis of the ovarian hyperstimulation syndrome. N Engl J Med. 2003;349: 729-32.
67. Schmeler KM, Mayo-Smith WW, Peipert JF, et al. Adnexal masses in pregnancy: surgery compared with observation. Obstet Gynecol. 2005;105:1098-103.
68. Sherard GB III, Hodson CA, Williams HJ, et al. Adnexal masses and pregnancy: a 12-year experience. Am J Obstet Gynecol. 2003;189:358-62.
69. Zanetta G, Mariani E, Lissoni A, et al. A prospective study of the role of ultrasound in the management of adnexal masses in pregnancy. Br J Obstet Gynaecol. 2003;110:578-83.
70. Soper DE. Gynecolodic endoscopy. In: Berek JS. Berek and Novak's gynecology. 14th edn. Philadelphia, PA: Lippincott-Williams and Wilkins; 2007. p. 432-500.
71. Mecke H, Savvas V. Laparoscopic surgery of dermoid cysts—intraoperative spillage and complications. Eur J Obstet Gynecol. 2001;96:80-4.
72. Lee Ch-L, Kay N, Chen H-L, et al. The role of laparoscopy in treating ovarian cancer. Taiwan J Obstet Gynecol. 2009;48:9-15.
73. Perutelli A, Garibaldi S, Basile S, et al. Laparoscopic adnexectomy of suspect ovarian masses: surgical technique used to avert spillage. J Minim Invasive Gynecol. 2011;18:372-7.
74. Garrard C L, Clements RH, Nanney L, et al. Adhesion formation is reduced after laparoscopic surgery. Surg Endosc. 1999;13:10-3.
75. Sekiba K. Use of Interceed (TC7) absorbable adhesion barrier to reduce post-operative adhesion reformation in infertility and endometriosis surgery. Obstet Gynecol. 1992;79:518-22.
76. Haney AF, Hesla J, Hurst BS, et al. Expanded polytetrafluoroethylene (Gore-Tex Surgical Membrane) is superior to oxidized regenerated cellulose (Interceed TC7+) in preventing adhesions. Fertil Steril. 1995;63:1021-6.
77. Wiseman DM, Trout JR, Diamond MP. The rates of adhesion development and the effects of crystalloid solutions on adhesion development in pelvic surgery. Fertil Steril. 1998;70:702-11.
78. Alborzi S, Rasekhi A, Shomali Z, et al. Diagnostic accuracy of magnetic resonance imaging, transvaginal and transrectal ultrasonography in deep infiltrating endometriosis. Medicine (Baltimore). 2018;97(8):e9536.
79. Mettler L, Alkatout I, Keckstein J, Meinhold-Heerlein I. Endometriosis: a concise practical guide to current diagnosis and treatment. Tuttlingen, Germany: Endo Press; 2017. p. 1-478.

KIEL SCH•OL

17 of Gynaecological Endoscopy

Ectopic Pregnancy

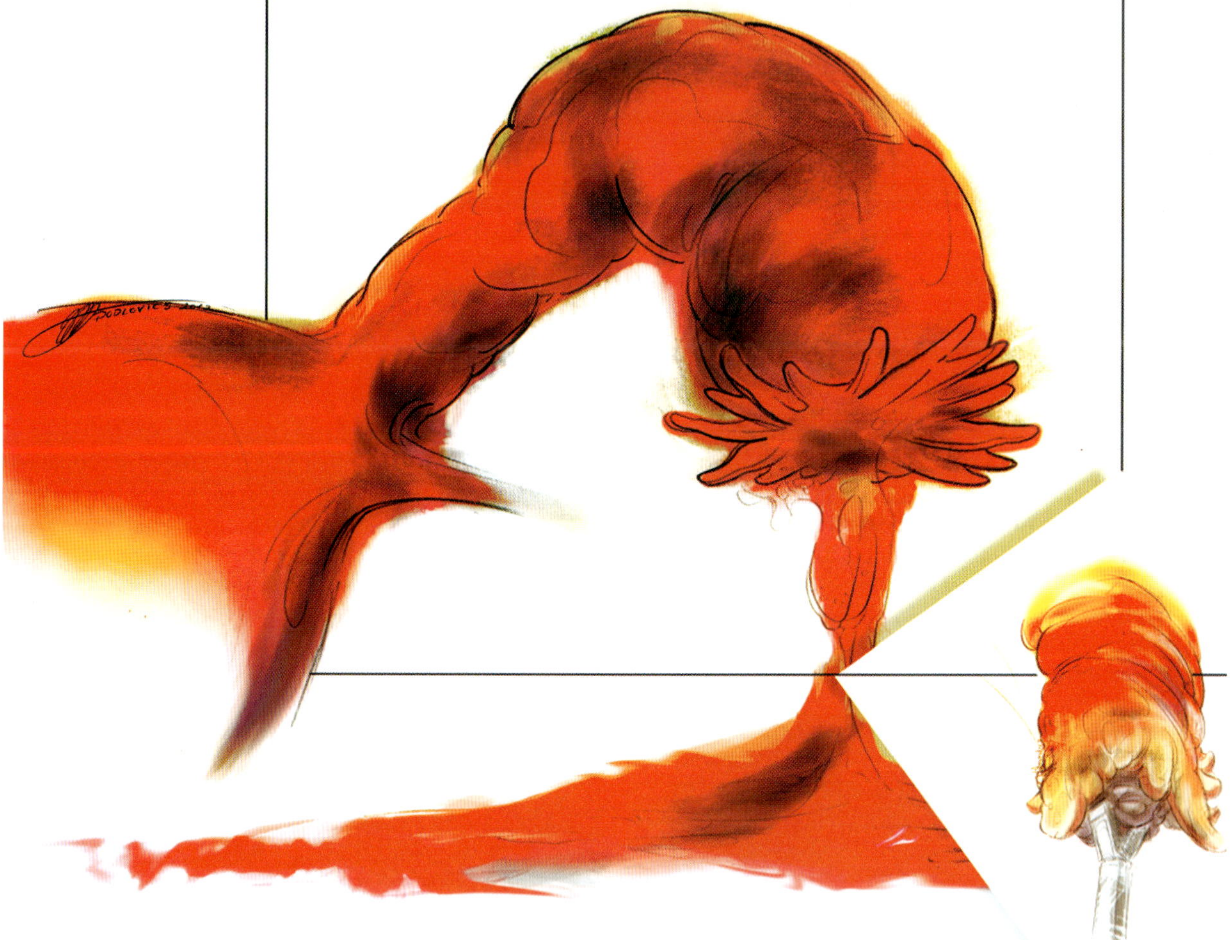

Chapter 17

Ectopic Pregnancy

Ibrahim Alkatout, Liselotte Mettler

INTRODUCTION

Usually the oocyte and the sperm meet in the ampullary part of the fallopian tube and impregnation takes place. The growing morula moves slowly toward the uterus cavity while differentiating into embryoblast and trophoblast. Implantation in the uterine cavity usually takes place after 6 or 7 days.

Implantation of the zygote outside the uterine cavity occurs in about 2% of all pregnancies. Pregnancy outside the uterine cavity has been described for the last hundreds of years. Today, intraoperatively the product of conception and its surroundings can be removed safely and submitted for histological examination (Figs. 17.1 to 17.3). The rate of ectopic pregnancies has increased from 0.5% in 1970 to 2% today. Although the incidence is low, the prevalence of ectopic pregnancy in all women presenting with first-trimester bleeding, lower abdominal pain or a combination of the two to an emergency department is between 6% and 16%.[1] These numbers justify a more intensive diagnosis due to the persistent suspicion of ectopic pregnancy and a lower threshold for operative investigation.

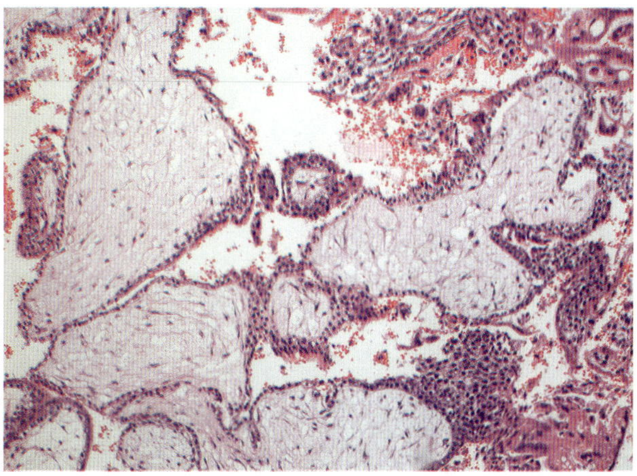

Fig. 17.2: Trophoblastic giant cells next to regressive altered villous stroma, trophoblast, and decidual stroma.

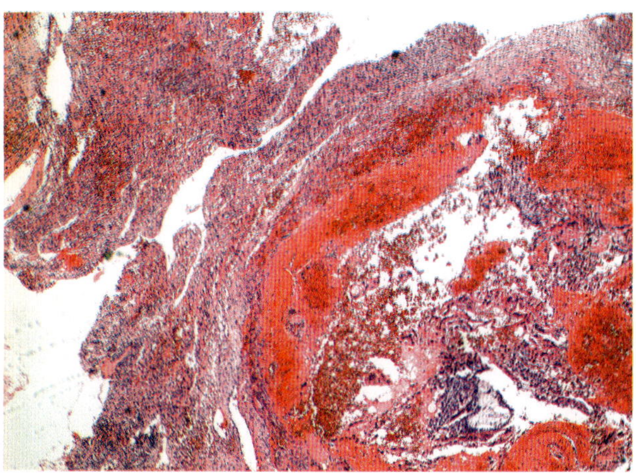

Fig. 17.1: Gestational material next to hemorrhage and fibrin exudation as well as regressive altered villi.

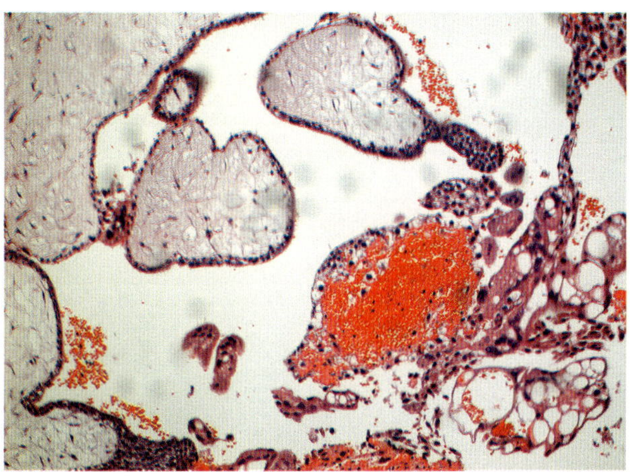

Fig. 17.3: Regressive altered villous stroma, trophoblast, hemorrhage and fibrin, trophoblastic giant cells.

The majority of ectopic pregnancies are located in the fallopian tube (approximately 97%): ampulla, isthmus and fimbria, in descending order. This might be accounted for by the narrowing of the tubal diameter from ampullary to isthmic region and the fact that fertilization begins in the ampulla. On the other hand, the ampullary region is the most distal place where ascending infections can cause phymosis and therefore either infertility or an increased risk for motility disorder. Ectopic pregnancy is often mentioned synonymously with tubal pregnancy due to the location of majority of the cases. Nevertheless, one must be aware of the unusual sites of ectopic pregnancies. About 3% are located in the rudimental uterine horn, ovary, abdominal cavity, broad ligament, cervix and vagina or are simultaneously intra- and extrauterine (Figs. 17.4A and B and Box 17.1).[2]

Two hundred years ago, the mortality rate of ectopic pregnancies was over 60%. Today, it has decreased to 9% of pregnancy-related mortality and less than 1% of overall mortality in women. Despite a fivefold increase in the incidence of ectopic pregnancy from 1970 to 1992, its mortality could be reduced by more than 90%. Until 1970, over 80% of ectopic pregnancies were not diagnosed before rupture, leading to a high rate of morbidity and mortality. Owing to the advances made in transvaginal ultrasound and radio immunoassays for serum β-hCG levels and an increased vigilance by clinicians with more experience of diagnostic laparoscopy, more than 80% of ectopic pregnancies are now diagnosed intact. This allows a more conservative management and is responsible for the decline from 35.5 deaths to 3.8 per 1,000 ectopics. The decrease of mortality is due to early diagnosis before the occurrence of hemoperitoneum and/or hypovolemic shock.[2,3]

Nevertheless, as ruptured ectopic pregnancies are responsible for 10–15% of all pregnancy-related deaths, the further improvement of earlier diagnosis is desirable. Earlier diagnosis is made by sensitive and specific radioimmunoassays for human chorionic gonadotropin (β-hCG), high-resolution transvaginal ultrasonography (TVS) and, most importantly, laparoscopy. Before the improvement of

Box 17.1: Different localizations of ectopic pregnancies and the associated percentages

Localizations of ectopic pregnancy	
• Fallopian tube	97%
• Rudimental uterine horn	
• Ovary	
• Abdominal	
• Intraligamental gravidity	3%
• Cervical gravidity	
• Vaginal gravidity	
• Simultaneous intra- and extrauterine	

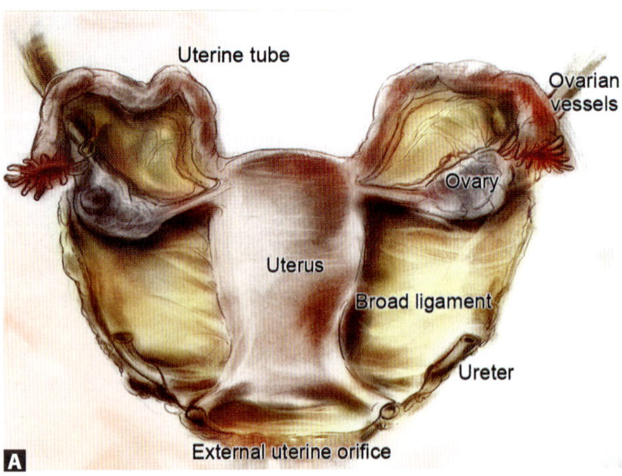

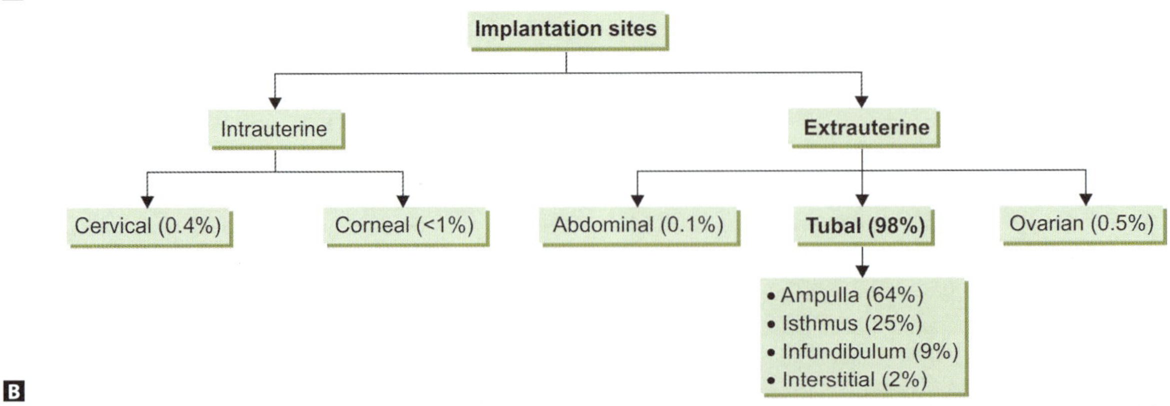

Figs. 17.4A and B: (A) Female inner genital organ. Illustration of the possible implantation sites of ectopic pregnancies; (B) Anatomical overview of the interior inner female genital with the potential sites of ectopic pregnancies and their percentage distribution.

these diagnostic methods majority of ectopic pregnancies were only detected after rupture and a life-threatening emergency.[1,4]

The great advances in diagnostic methods and the decrease of their side effects over the last 25 years has enabled the diagnosis of mildly symptomatic or even asymptomatic patients with ectopic pregnancy. As a consequence more than 80% of women with an ectopic pregnancy are treated correctly before tubal rupture or severe intra-abdominal bleeding in most of the developed countries where the above-mentioned capabilities are available. The gain in knowledge and the advancing operative experience of ectopic pregnancies lead to a high rate of fertility-preserving operating methods. Despite all diagnostic and therapeutical progress and the decline in the invasiveness of laparoscopic procedures, in 50% of all women with ectopic pregnancy presenting to an emergency department, the condition is not detected at the initial medical assessment.[1,5]

ETIOLOGY AND RISK FACTORS

The incidence of ectopic pregnancies is independent of maternal age and ethnic origin. Moreover, there is no accumulation at a certain place outside the uterus.[1]

Theoretically, anything that impedes migration of the conceptus to the uterine cavity may predispose woman to develop an ectopic gestation (Box 17.2).

Box 17.2: Major contributing factors (Risk factors) for ectopic pregnancy

- Previous tubal surgery
- History of ectopic pregnancy
- Sexually transmitted disease
- Pelvic inflammatory disease
- *In utero* diethylstilbestrol exposure
- History of infertility
- Anatomical uterine /tubal abnormality
- Previous tubal ligation
- Previous or current IUD use
- Assisted reproductive technologies
- Current smoking
- Nonwhite (all races other than white)
- Age between 35 and 44 (compared to those from 15 to 24)
- Induced abortion
- T-shaped uterus
- Myomata
- Progestin-only contraceptives

These may be intrinsic anatomic defects in the tubal epithelium, hormonal factors that interfere with normal transport of the conceptus, or pathologic conditions that affect normal tubal functioning. The hormonal interference is explained by the different effect that estrogen and gestagen show on the growth and the motility of the epithelial cilia. A dysbalance of the hormonal concentration can lead to a longer stay of the developing morula in the fallopian tube. Other maternal reasons can be explained by a dysfunction of the epithelial cilia that can be caused by smoking.[4,6,7]

DIAGNOSTICS

Preoperative Assessment

The aim of professional and target-aiming diagnostics is the early diagnosis and adequate treatment of an ectopic pregnancy as well as minimizing the amount of unnecessary laparoscopies.

The suspicion of an extrauterine gravidity has to be excluded if a woman of reproductive age presents with abdominal pain and vaginal bleeding approximately 5–7 weeks after her last period and has a positive pregnancy test. Although these symptoms are common in women with early physiologic intrauterine pregnancy, extrauterine pregnancy and women who may miscarry, they are nonspecific with a negative pregnancy test.[8]

After a positive pregnancy test additional unspecific parameters are a normal or slightly enlarged uterus, vaginal bleeding or spotting, pelvic pain triggered by manipulation of the cervix and a palpable adnexal mass. Although these parameters increase the risk of a prevalent ectopic pregnancy and significant abdominal tenderness, guarding and rebound tenderness together with hypotension or syncopes can suggest a ruptured ectopic pregnancy, these clinical parameters remain unspecific. Consequently, no clinical examination alone can reliably exclude ectopic pregnancy. Apart from mimicking the symptoms of other gynecological and even nongynecological diseases, ectopic pregnancies come in many variations often causing no pain at vaginal examination. Severe pain can also be experienced in a normal pregnancy.

Usually the earliest appearance of symptoms occurs in the 6th week after the last period. Patients with ectopic pregnancy can show all symptoms of a normal early pregnancy, such as interruption of the normal menstrual period, nausea, vomiting, breast fullness and fatigue. Beyond that, typical symptoms of ectopic pregnancies are lower abdominal pain and abnormal uterine bleeding, ranging from spotting to severe bleeding. Muscular defense and peritonism are indicative of intraperitoneal blood flowing. Severe hemorrhage leading to hypovolemia can cause syncopes or tachycardia. There may be tenderness on cervical motion. On examination the uterus is enlarged and soft in consistency. In some cases an adnexal mass can be palpated.[1]

Lower abdominal pain is caused by the distension of the peritoneum due to the swelling of the affected tube or free blood in the abdominal cavity. Usually the pain is alternating and spasmodic, followed by intervals free of complaints. In general, the intensity and frequency of pain increases.[4]

Another leading symptom is vaginal bleeding. An extrauterine gravidity can be associated with a complete amenorrhea, recurrent bleedings or persistent bleedings or even a normal menstrual cycle. As most extrauterine gravidities produce only decreased hCG, the uterus is not able to sustain the decidually transformed endometrium. Therefore, it often comes to breakthrough bleedings appearing as spotting.[4]

Hence, additional diagnostic tests are necessary to exclude an ectopic pregnancy. These include repeated monitoring of β-hCG serum level, transvaginal ultrasonography and in some cases even diagnostic curettage or measurement of serum progesterone level.

The two diagnostic parameters that have to be monitored are β-hCG serum levels and repeated transvaginal ultrasonography.

β-hCG Serum Level

The first diagnostic step is the assurance of an existing pregnancy, which can be detected about 10 days following ovulation using a sensitive β-hCG serum array. hCG is a glycoprotein produced by the syncytiotrophoblast starting with secretion on day 5 to day 8. A serum array detects levels as low as 5 mIU/ml while the detection limit in urine is 20–50 mIU/ml. After diagnosis of an existing pregnancy β-hCG level can be used as a follow-up titer and its change can be recognized and monitored. The β-hCG levels double every 1.5 days in the first 5 weeks of a regular gestation. After 7 weeks the sequence for double titers is 3.5 days.

In comparison, only 30% of ectopic pregnancies show a normal β-hCG course. In 70% of ectopic pregnancies β-hCG levels rise more slowly and reach a plateau or even show a decrease in serum levels. An abnormal β-hCG pattern is highly suspicious for an ectopic gestation or a no longer intact gestation. Besides the unconventional rise of β-hCG level compared to normal pregnancies, ectopic pregnancy can be differentiated from a spontaneous abortion by a slower decrease of serum titer. Therefore, ectopic pregnancies and intrauterine pregnancies have a considerable overlap. Accordingly, a single measurement is insufficient and only a serial measurement can give the necessary additional information for the location of gestational sac.

Although ectopic pregnancies can have normal as well as rising, falling or plateau β-hCG levels, the serial measurements of β-hCG levels are most useful to confirm or to prove false the fetal viability instead of giving straight evidence for an ectopic pregnancy.

Taken together, an extrauterine pregnancy often presents with β-hCG levels below the expected value and the increase is delayed. The trend can be stagnating or decreasing.[7,9-11]

Ultrasound Imaging

The development of transvaginal ultrasonography has enormously improved identification and visualization of both normally developing embryos and abnormalities. With a gestational age of about 5 weeks a normally developing gestational sac can be visualized showing an ovoid collection of fluid clinging to the endometrium stripe as well as a yolk sac of 8 mm or more in diameter. However, a pseudogestational sac can mimic a gestational sac at an early stage. The pseudogestational sac is often situated in the center of uterine cavity. Its margin is homogenous and round but it is difficult to define its boundary to the outside tissue. By contrast, a physiologic gestational sac is asymmetric and contains two concentric rings, separated by a thin echogenic layer. At a gestational age of 6 to 6.5 weeks the embryonic structures measure 4 to 5 mm and cardiac activity might already be detected.

The threshold value of β-hCG serum reliably showing sonographic signs of an intrauterine growing pregnancy lies between 1,000 and 2,000 mIU/mL, depending on the ultrasound unit and the experience of the examiner. Even though β-hCG levels of women with ectopic pregnancy are often less than 2,000 mIU/mL at presentation, an empty uterus does not allow a clear differentiation between an early undetected intrauterine pregnancy and an ectopic pregnancy. The regular or irregular increase of β-hCG level is the assisting factor interpreting the ultrasound signals but again, β-hCG levels alone do not allow discrimination between a regular, an irregular and an ectopic pregnancy.

The identification of an intrauterine gestational sac plus a yolk sac or additional embryonic signs minimizes the doubt of an ectopic pregnancy. However, it is important to consider the rare possibility of a heterotopic pregnancy whose total number is growing with the increase of assisted reproduction.

Verifying an ectopic pregnancy by the means of an ultrasound scan is burdened with a high false-negative rate. The infrequent identification of an extrauterine gestational sac containing a yolk sac and possibly an embryo with cardiac activity confirms the suspected diagnosis. Supporting the diagnosis of an extrauterine gestation is an empty uterus, a cystic or solid extrauterine mass adjacent to the fallopian tube or the ovary (including the tubal ring sign, representing a tubal gestational sac), and echogenic or sonolucent free fluid in the cul-de-sac (Figs. 17.5 and 17.6).

The combination of transvaginal ultrasonography and serial quantitative β-hCG serum levels detects with a sensitivity of 96% and a specificity of

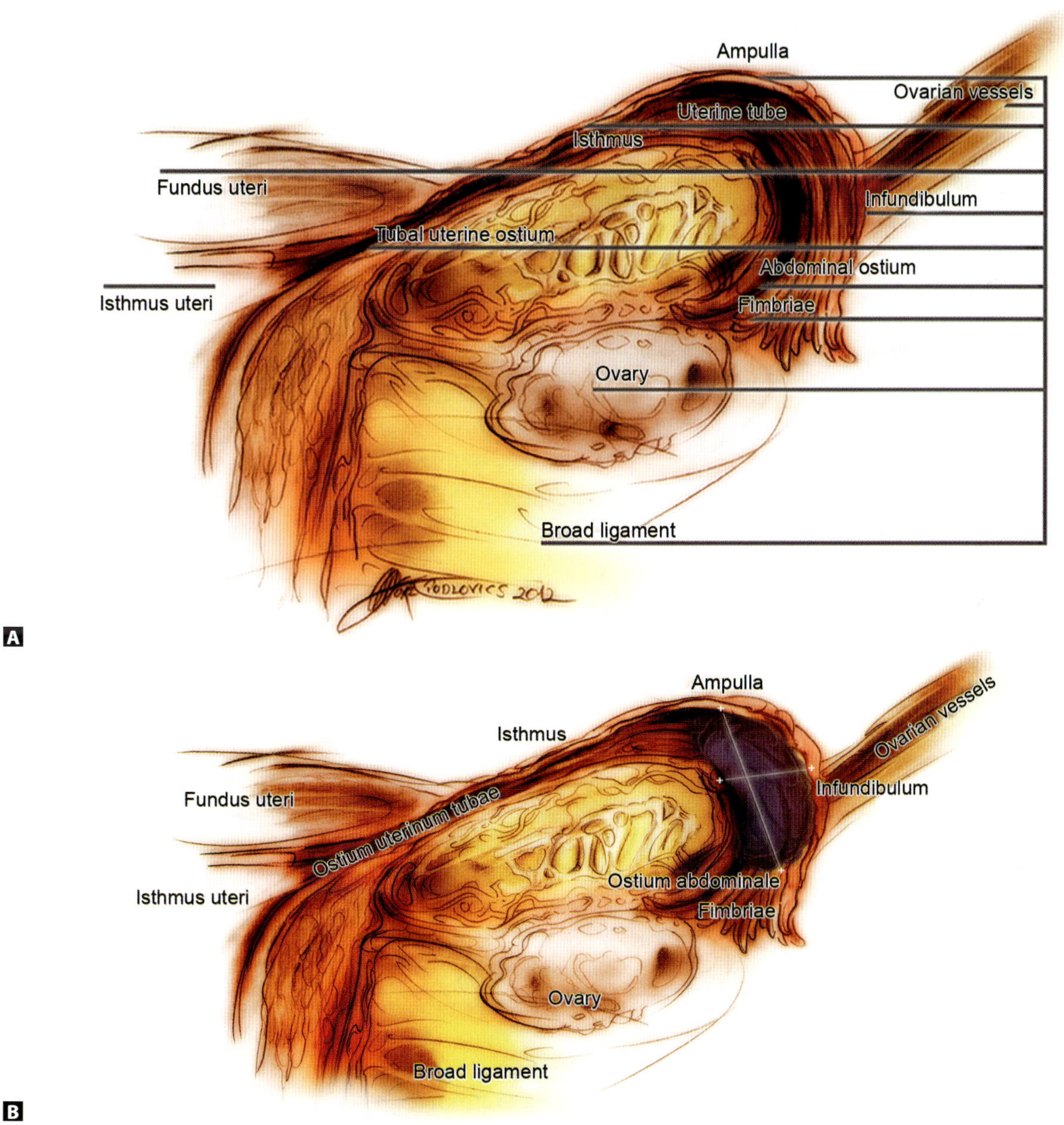

Figs. 17.5A and B: (A) Schematic drawing of the expected ultrasound layer. Ovary, fallopian tube and the transition to the uterus are clear beside the surrounding meso; (B) Corresponding to the schematic drawing of the expected ultrasound layer, the ultrasound detected ectopic pregnancy is visualized.

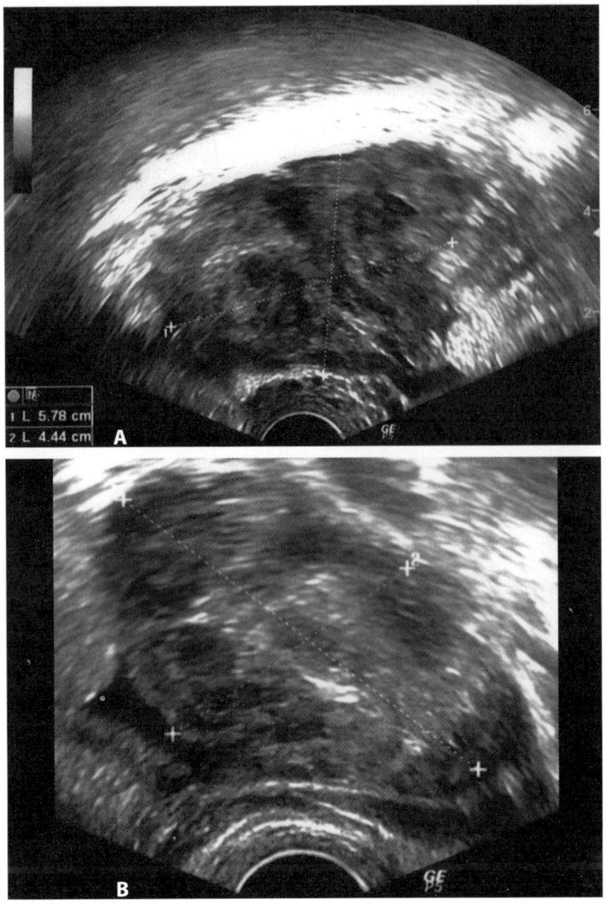

Figs. 17.6A and B: (A) Transvaginal ultrasound with an ectopic pregnancy measuring more than 5 cm in diameter; (B) Transvaginal ultrasound showing magnification in the inhomogenic structures and free fluid in the pouch of Douglas. The capsula and the boundary of the fallopian tube are visualized.

97% in an ectopic pregnancy and remains the gold standard as well as the most cost-effective strategy for diagnosing ectopic pregnancy.

A positive fetal heart beat is often absent because extrauterine pregnancies seldom develop vitally and only display an agglomeration of trophoblast tissue and a surrounding hematoma.[8,12,13]

Progesterone Serum Level

Progesterone levels can be useful in the substantiation of a suspected ectopic pregnancy and in the identification of women at risk for ectopic pregnancy. However, the progesterone serum level only has a sensitivity of 15% to detect pregnancy failure. As a stable marker in the first trimester, a serum level above 22 ng/mL speaks for a viable intrauterine pregnancy whereas levels under 5 ng/mL are indicative of a nonviable pregnancy. Nevertheless, the progesterone level cannot positively differentiate between ectopic pregnancy and intrauterine pregnancy. Furthermore, values in between the limiting values are more common and they make the progesterone serum level inconclusive.

In conclusion, progesterone as a supplemental factor for identifying ectopic pregnancies has not proved itself and can therefore be disregarded.[2,8,14]

Uterine Diagnostic Curettage

Uterine diagnostic curettage can detect gestational material in the form of chorionic villi. If they are not detected, the suspicion of an ectopic pregnancy is hardened. Nevertheless, a diagnostic curettage could abort an early and desired physiological pregnancy and therefore its indication has to be taken carefully. Diagnostic curettage provides additional information when β-hCG levels are falling or when β-hCG levels are elevated and there is no ultrasound confirmation of an intrauterine pregnancy.[8]

Puncture of the Pouch of Douglas

Puncture of the pouch of Douglas has become obsolete. Before the establishment of ultrasonography and β-hCG blood examination, the puncture of blood in the pouch of Douglas was an additional indicator leading to the clinical but indefinite diagnosis of extrauterine gravidity.[4]

Diagnosis of ectopic pregnancy can be challenging as its symptoms are often similar to normal early pregnancies or early miscarriages and therefore confusing. Women suffering from ectopic pregnancy can present with one-sided pelvic pain and variable bleeding. However, 20% of women with first trimester bleeding deliver a healthy baby even though bleeding might be the only sign of an ectopic pregnancy.

The awareness of the eventuality of an ectopic pregnancy is most crucial for early detection. Doubling of the β-hCG serum levels every 2–3 days should be registered in a normal gestation. Nevertheless, about 10% of normal pregnancies vary in this regime as well as up to 60% of ectopic pregnancies demonstrate and imitate this doubling time. Transvaginal sonography has a reliable, sensitive predictive value if β-hCG levels are higher than 1,000 mIU/ml. The detection rate is then 98%, depending on the quality of the ultrasound unit and the experience of the examiner. An additional sign of an ectopic pregnancy that might assist in an early diagnosis once an extrauterine pregnancy is suspected is culdocentesis. This used to be a more prognostic feature

Flowchart 17.1: The three pillars that substantiate an early suspicion of ectopic pregnancy.

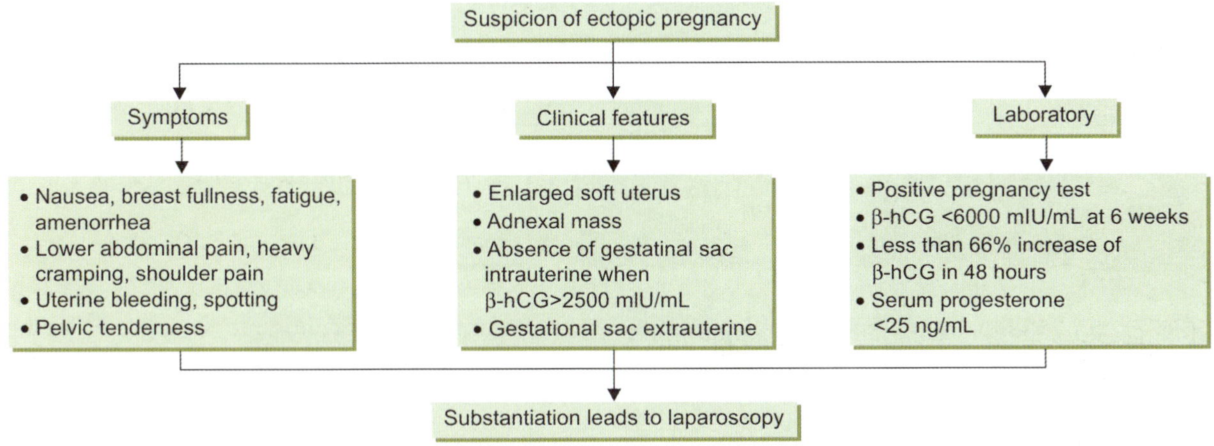

in times when β-hCG monitoring and transvaginal ultrasound scan were not available presenting non-clotting blood after aspiration of the free fluid in the pouch of Douglas.[2]

In summary, the straightforward diagnosis of ectopic pregnancy is based on three pillars: symptoms that can be determined during physical examination, clinical features that appear in ultrasound scan and laboratory tests that can substantiate a primary suspicion (Flowchart 17.1).

After the suspicion of ectopic pregnancy has hardened, the next steps should be routine. If the necessary clinical and laboratory investigations are carried out and the diagnosis of ectopic pregnancy is made early, the risk for severe hemorrhage and rupture is minimal (Flowchart 17.2).

DIFFERENTIAL DIAGNOSIS

The symptoms of patients suffering from ectopic pregnancy show a great variety. This explains the many possibilities of differential diagnosis. Symptoms are dependent on the progress of the ectopic pregnancy and its effect on the peritoneum once haemorrhage has occurred. The possibility of dynamic clinical changes is responsible for the great variability of differential diagnosis. It is not possible to follow up all possible differential diagnoses and exclude them before the diagnosis of ectopic pregnancy can definitely be made. Ectopic pregnancy can imitate a great variety of other precarious and harmless diseases. However, it is crucial not to miss the point of time where the correct treatment is associated with a minimal morbidity and mortality of the patient. For possible differential diagnosis of ectopic pregnancy, see Table 17.1.

The therapeutic regimen chosen for treatment of a suspected ectopic pregnancy should ensure for each individual patient the lowest morbidity and maximum safety. The aim, beyond preventing an emergency case, is to preserve the greatest potential for reproductive function.

TREATMENT

In view of the high incidence of ectopic pregnancies among pregnant women with first-trimester bleeding, further investigation must be undertaken to exclude an ectopic pregnancy. Once an ectopic pregnancy has been confirmed, a treatment plan has to be created. The treatment decision includes operative management and medical treatment as well as the option not to treat and follow up with clinical and laboratory tests. It is known that many early ectopic pregnancies result in spontaneous abortion and re-absorption and this might make aggressive treatment unnecessary. Medical treatment with methotrexate is restricted to a few limited indications. There is no general policy of treating suspected ectopic pregnancies and each patient requires individual assessment.

The indication for a primary laparotomy is given for patients with circulatory instability and a massive hemoperitoneum when the medical team is not trained for immediate and emergency laparoscopy or contraindications for laparoscopy exist. The other indication for primary laparotomy can be an isthmic location with a high intramural proportion and a severe risk for uncontrollable intraoperative bleeding. In all other circumstances the operative management should be laparoscopy.

Flowchart 17.2: Diagnostic and operative processing in case of potential ectopic pregnancy.

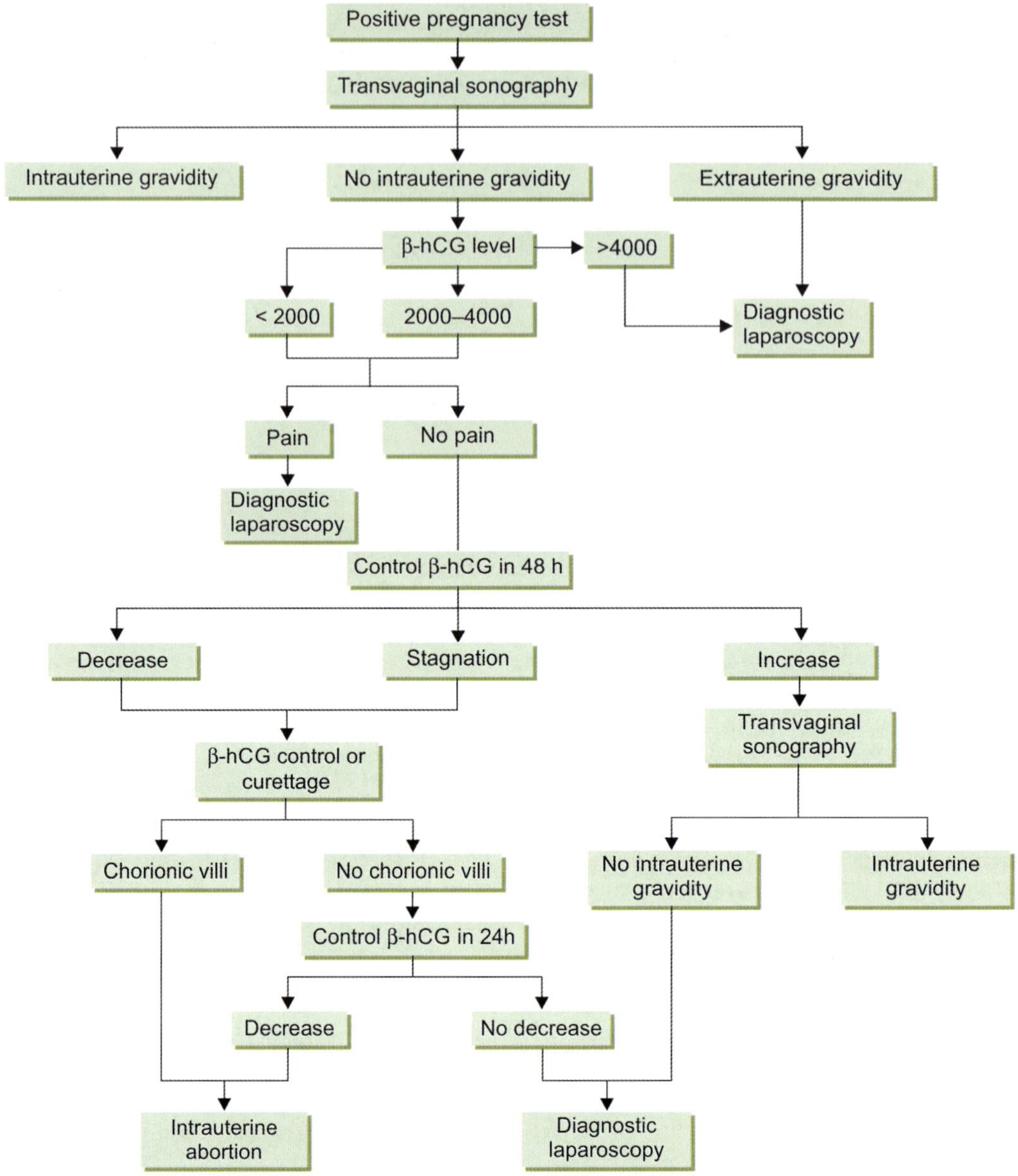

Table 17.1: Differential clinical diagnosis of ectopic pregnancy separated in gynecological and nongynecological origin

Gynecological	Nongynecological
Early stage of normal pregnancy	Acute appendicitis
Miscarriage	Cystitis
Intrauterine abortion	Pyelonephritis
Torsion of ovary or fallopian tube	Nephrolithiasis
Ovarian cyst	Perforation of stomach, bowel, gallbladder (hollow organs)
Ruptured corpus luteum cyst or follicle	Obstruction of hollow organs
Necrotic myoma	Intra-abdominal inflammation (peritoneum, all abdominal organs, diverticulum)
Pelvic inflammatory disease (salpingitis)	Rupture of parenchymatous organs (liver, spleen, kidney)
Tubo-ovarian abscess	Vascular ischemic disease (bowel, mesenterium)
	Vascular hemorrhagic disease (aorta, all abdominal vessels)

PREOPERATIVE MANAGEMENT

Once the diagnosis of ectopic pregnancy has been made, therapeutic management has to be planned. Thus, the treatment can be 'wait and see' (expectant management), medical treatment (preferably with methotrexate) or surgical treatment.[8]

Wait-and-see Attitude

Before operative investigation is planned, it has to be realized that in some cases ectopic pregnancy can resolve spontaneously through regression and resolution. Positive prognostic parameters are lack of clinical symptoms, a sonographic adnexal tumor below 4 cm with a decreasing tendency, less than 50 mL of free fluid and an initial β-hCG level of below 2000 mU/mL with a decreasing tendency after a 48-h interval. However, more than 90% of all affected women with ectopic pregnancies develop increasing and endangering symptoms that lead to an operative intervention.[4] Although methotrexate therapy might be effective in some cases, it is not suitable for first-line treatment of ectopic pregnancy in the majority of cases. Diagnostic laparoscopy and simultaneously operative pelviscopy is the gold standard for the diagnosis and therapy of ectopic pregnancies. It is prompt, minimally invasive, takes less operative time, has a lower blood loss, is cost-effective, is associated with a reduced hospital stay, a limited postoperative analgesia requirement, a lower risk of adhesions, a better visualization of the operative field and has no medical side effects. Even hemodynamic instability is not an absolute contraindication to primary laparoscopy.[15-19]

Positioning of the Patient

The patient is positioned in the classic gynecological lithotomy position. A Foley bladder catheter should be used and an intrauterine manipulator should be at hand for certain circumstances.[3]

Instrumentation

Table 17.2 provides a detailed list of all instruments that are necessary or at least desirable for laparoscopic treatment.

Table 17.2: Instruments necessary for operating on expected ectopic pregnancy

Laparoscope, diameter 5 mm or 10 mm	**Atraumatic grasping forceps**
Video camera	Scissors
Microprocessor-controlled insufflations system	Suction and irrigation system
Electrosurgical unit	Monopolar hook electrode
Xenon cold light source	Bipolar forceps
Trocars, diameter 6 or 11 mm	Disposable extraction bag
Veress needle	Uterine manipulator

GENERAL OPERATIVE BEGINNING

After creating pneumoperitoneum, a 5 mm and after dilatation and 11 mm optic trocar is introduced into the abdominal cavity through an umbilical Z-track incision using a conical trocar. Two 5 mm instrument trocars are introduced through small left and right lateral suprapubic incisions. In cases of severe hemoperitoneum the Veress needle is placed into the accumulation of blood. Therefore, a higher initial insufflation pressure might be of advantage since the tip of the needle may be immersed in blood.[2,3,20]

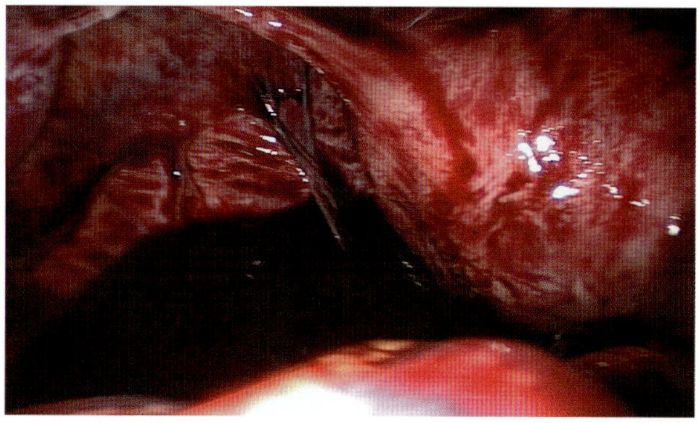

Fig. 17.7: Severe hemoperitoneum with the volume of 1200 mL blood in the pouch of Douglas.

Diagnostic Laparoscopy: Evacuation of Hemoperitoneum

At laparoscopy, the location, size and nature of ectopic pregnancy are ascertained. If there is hemoperitoneum (Figs. 17.7 and 17.8), this can complicate the whole operation. Dependent on the degree of bleeding a primarily inserted grasper localizes the ruptured tube and tamponades the bleeding site. After safe compression of the bleeding source, blood and blood clots can be removed by suction and irrigation.

The 5 mm suction cannula is usually sufficient for this purpose. In emergency cases, such as hemoperitoneal shock or large hemoperitoneum, a 11 mm

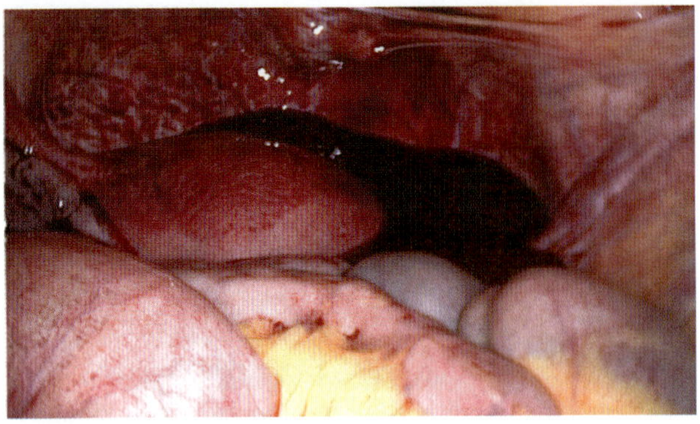

Fig. 17.8: Hemoperitoneum of a ruptured tubal pregnancy. Visualization after insertion of the optic trocar.

cannula with the appropriate suction tube can be preferable. Even organized blood clots can be removed with only the suction instrument. Under constant suction with the suction device, blood clots are aspirated and broken by pulling the suction tip just behind the trocar end. By this means bigger blood clots are broken and can more easily be evacuated through the suction aspirator. Excessive irrigation lifts the bowel and worsens the overview.[2]

Once bleeding is controlled, the remaining blood clots and the product of conception can be removed from abdominal cavity. The suction instrument and the use of forced irrigation will cleanse abdominal cavity quickly with minimal trauma to these structures. Forced irrigation with physiological saline or Ringer's lactate solution will dislodge clots and trophoblastic tissue from the serosa of the peritoneal organs with minimal trauma to these structures as they are irrigated.[3,4,21,22]

SURGICAL TREATMENT OF TUBAL PREGNANCY

Several different conservative techniques have been developed to preserve tubal function. These include salpingotomy, partial salpingectomy followed by anastomosis, salpingectomy and extirpation of the tubal pregnancy through the fimbrial end by milking it from the distant ampulla. Independent of the type of surgery, the existence of tubal abnormalities on the contralateral site predispose the patient to recurrence.[7]

Salpingostomy

Before incising the fallopian tube one has to recall that the tube is composed of the tunica mucosa and two muscular layers. The inner layer is oriented in a circular fashion and the outer layer is oriented in a longitudinal fashion to the axis of the tube. The surrounding blood vessels originate from uterine and ovarian blood supply and often lay in the thick longitudinal muscle layer. This branching is located in the mesosalpinx between the fallopian tube and the ovary.[2]

The lumen of the fallopian tube is paved with ciliated secretory cells that might be damaged after ascending infection, previous ectopic pregnancy or any other circumstances, which might disrupt morula transport, as listed in Box 17.2.[2]

Preservation of the tube should be attempted in all patients without contraindications or explicit wish for salpingectomy. By preserving the tube, fertility can be maintained. Precondition for a tubal-preserving procedure is hemodynamic stability and evidence that the tube is not ruptured. The ectopic pregnancy should be less than 5 cm in diameter, the gestational sac must be located in the ampulla, infundibulum or isthmic portion of the tube and there should be no pathology of the contralateral tube (Fig. 17.9). Nevertheless, majority of ectopic pregnancies located in infundibulum have to be operated either by salpingectomy or by segmental tubectomy and secondary reanastomosis after a certain interval.[3,4] Whenever feasible, salpingostomy is preferred to salpingectomy. However, approximately 8% of patients have persistent ectopic pregnancy after salpingostomy. This has to be kept in mind and be part of the preoperational discussion.[1]

After careful inspection and identification of tubal pregnancy, the tubal part is mobilized with one or two forceps.

Vasopressin: Before preparation of the tube and the ectopic pregnancy vasopressin, 20 IU diluted in

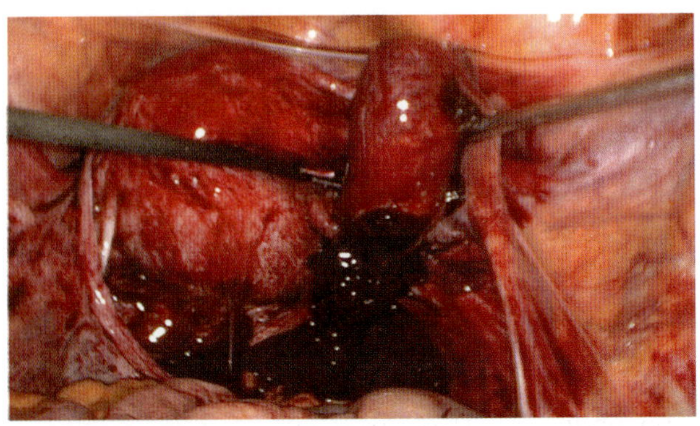

Fig. 17.9: Tubal pregnancy already protruding of the fimbrial end into the abdominal cavity.

100 mL of normal saline, is injected into mesosalpinx. A syringe with a 22-gauge injection needle can be placed either through one of the working trocars under sight or the outer sheath of a Veress needle can be placed directly through the abdominal wall under sight, lateral to the deep inferior epigastric vessels. Alternatively, vasopressin is inserted by a 22-gauge spinal needle through the sheath. Close attention must be given because of the good vascularization of the mesosalpinx and risk of laceration. After gently grasping the serosa, 10–20 mL of the solution is injected and controlled by a visible swelling of mesosalpinx just below the ectopic pregnancy and over the antimesenteric surface of tubal segment containing gestational products. Hemostatic effect lasts for about 2 h permitting a safer preparation. Vasopressin must not be allowed to infiltrate into a blood vessel as this can lead to acute arterial hypertension, bradycardia and even death.[3,7]

Besides the better operative management vasopressin has a positive side effect on prognosis. As trophoblast has a high cell division, its metabolic rate is equivalently high. The iatrogenic anoxia reduces the oxygen supply for about 2 h and thereby reduces the persistence risk by a factor of 5. The use of vasopressin is contraindicated in patients with chronic vascular diseases (e.g. ischemic heart disease).[3]

Evacuation by Aquadissection or Aspiration, Luxation and Preparation

Incision and evacuation: A unipolar needle electrocautery (cutting current of 10 W), scissors or a knife electrode is introduced through the 6 mm port. Alternatively, a CO_2 laser with a power density of 10,000 W/cm^2 can be used. A 1–2 cm longitudinal incision is made on the most distended part of the antimesenteric tubal wall, which is often of bluish discoloration, using a cutting or blended current (20 or 70 W). Usually it is possible to identify the different tubal wall layers: serosa, muscularis externa and interna and the mucosa. It is important to cut through all layers for the whole length of the incision. If the product of conception cannot be identified after the primary incision, it is necessary to advance deeper as the muscularis externa, interna and/or the mucosa might be still intact. Once the lumen is open, the friable gestational sac bulges out of the wound and can be evacuated by aspiration. If the product of conception is surrounded by coagel clotting, it must be extracted through tubal incision with alternating pressurized suction and irrigation or with the aid of grasping or biopsy forceps. The site of implantation is then irrigated extensively. The irrigation fluid must drain from both sites, salpingotomy and fimbrial end.[3]

Using a high-pressure irrigating solution the gestational sac can be flushed out of the salpingostomy as forceful irrigation in the salpingostomy can dislodge the gestation from its implantation. Combining hydrodissection and gentle blunt dissection with a suction irrigator, product remnants are removed from the tube. If possible, this technique is preferable to extraction in pieces as products of conception can then adhere to the implantation site by a ligamentous structure containing blood vessels. Minimal bleeding from the tubal bed is normal and ceases in most cases spontaneously.[2]

To remove the product of gestation, it can be cut and taken out in small pieces but generally it is safer to extract the material with a spoon after dilating one of the working trocars to 11 mm. In most cases it is advisable to use an endobag for safe extraction of the gestational product.

Suturing of the salpingostomy incision is controversial. Usually the incision does not require suturing. The tubal incision is supposed to heal by secondary intention. Only if the defect is very wide and its edges do not come together spontaneously or the mucosa everts, might suturing be recommended. If the defect has to be closed, a continual suture or single knots approximating the edges with single 4-0 resorbable sutures excepting the mucosa are made. The follow-up and prognosis for recurrent extrauterine gravidities is not improved after suturing.[2,3,22]

Hemostasis: Oozing from the tube is common and usually ceases spontaneously. Slight bleeding from mucosal bed or from incisions of the tubal walls can be treated conservatively in a majority of cases. Bleeding can appear from the incision margins or the site of implantation. The bleeding situation can best be observed by inspection of the tube "underwater." The first hemostatic option should be a hemostatic tamponade applied with grasping forceps. Compression of bleeding location for 5 min is sufficient in most cases. Alternatively, for conservative bleeding management adnexa can be elevated out of pelvis for an indirect compression of the vessels of mesosalpinx. Continuous bleeding points can be detected and coagulated with bipolar coagulation in a tissue-saving method. Stronger venous or even arterial bleeding can be controlled effectively and safe by using electrocoagulation with bipolar forceps, particularly if combined with continuous irrigation, especially in the muscle layer. A superficial eschar, not involving the tubal mucosa, heals normally.

With uncontrolled bleeding and bleeding that cannot be localized, mesosalpingeal vessels can be coagulated selectively until bleeding stops. Ultima ratio is the tubectomy.[1,3,7]

Before terminating the operation another "underwater" examination is done by the introduction of 500–1000 mL of solution. The abdominal cavity and the pelvic organs are once again inspected carefully.[22]

Partial Salpingectomy

If salpingostomy cannot resolve the problem, partial salpingectomy can be tried before salpingectomy is performed. Indications for a partial salpingectomy are tubal rupture, pregnancy located in the isthmus or a recurrent tubal pregnancy. In most cases of isthmic pregnancy linear salpingostomy is unsuccessful as these gestations grow through lumen of the tube and into tunica muscularis; therefore, segmental resection is recommended.

After evacuation of hemoperitoneum and possibly infiltration of vasopressin in the corresponding mesosalpinx, coagulation of the tubal part is done by bipolar forceps on both ends of the affected part including the corresponding mesosalpinx. The proximal and distal boundaries of affected tubal segment are grasped with forceps and thoroughly coagulated from antimesenteric surface to mesosalpinx. The segment is then cut with little risk for bleeding. After resecting the affected part of the tube mesosalpinx is cauterized stepwise. Particular attention is given to arcuate anastomosing branches of the ovarian and uterine vessels. In the next step mesosalpinx is cut. The tubal segment is taken out after dilation of one of the working trocars to 11 mm. If the piece is too big or unstable, the use of an endobag should be preferred. Hemostasis is achieved by bipolar coagulation of any bleeding parts.

If the surgeon is experienced in such procedures, partial salpingectomy can be completed by reanastomosis. Otherwise the reanastomosis is postponed to a later date.[2]

Salpingectomy

Salpingectomy, where the tube is removed from its anatomical attachments, is the alternative procedure to salpingostomy. This may be a safer method for persistent bleeding or tubal rupture. The indications for salpingectomy include no desire for future pregnancies, recurrent tubal pregnancies and the occurrence of extrauterine pregnancy after a failed sterilization or a previously reconstructed tube. Other indications for salpingectomy are made intraoperatively, e.g., severe adhesions, hydrosalpinx, tubal rupture, persistent bleeding after a safe tubal procedure or if the tubal pregnancy is over 5 cm in diameter.

After evacuation of hematoperitoneum the proximal isthmus of the tube and mesosalpinx are coagulated and dissected stepwise, beginning with the proximal isthmic portion and progressing to fimbriated end of the tube. The tube is immobilized with one or two grasping forceps. Coagulation of the segments to be excised is performed with bipolar cautery and cut either with laser, electrocautery or scissors. Alternative methods include stapling devices, harmonic energy or endoloops. After preparation of the tube containing gestational sac, the tube is removed from peritoneal cavity in an endobag through one of the instrument trocars that has been dilated to 10 mm.

Afterward, a final inspection is made to coagulate any bleeding caused by grasping the tube and the mesosalpinx and to make sure that the product of conception has not slipped out of the tube unnoticed.[22]

Extirpation of Tubal Pregnancy through Fimbrial End

If the product of conception is located at the outer region of fallopian tube or fimbrial end, it can be removed by grasping tubal segment and stepwise milking the gestational product out of fimbriae of the tube (Figs. 17.10A and B). The product of conception is gently pushed until it is extruded. The stepwise movements begin in the proximal part and gently push the product into abdominal cavity. Alternatively, small ectopic pregnancies located at the very outside of fimbriae can be extracted by aspiration. Then, however, there is no histologic confirmation of an ectopic pregnancy.

After removal of trophoblast, suction tip should be placed in the tubal end and the tube cleaned by suction and irrigation. Remnants are washed out of the tube without damage to the tubal wall.

Although this type of operation is gentle and organ saving, it has a higher rate of incomplete

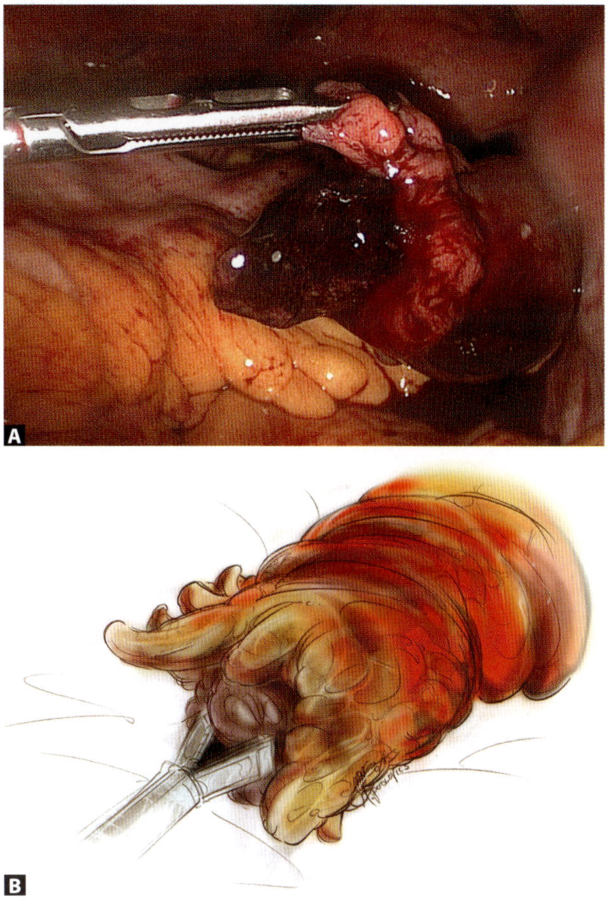

Figs. 17.10A and B: (A) Protruding ectopic pregnancy of the fimbrial end with the option of extirpation without incising the tube; (B) Schematic drawing of the protruding ectopic pregnancy out of the fimbrial end with the option of extirpation without incising the tube. Nevertheless, this operation technique is only feasible, if the total extraction of the ectopic pregnancy is assured.

removal and therefore a higher risk of recurrence and of trophoblast residuals. This is because many ectopic pregnancies are not implanted in the intraluminal tubal portion and therefore cannot be completely removed in a gentle way without severe damage to the tubal wall. In addition, an eventual extraluminal pregnancy, implanted between serosa and tunica muscularis, would be treated more mildly by salpingostomy. Therefore, the indication for this operative technique should be made reluctantly. For cases of intraluminal ectopic pregnancies that are not yet visible and where it is postulated that the tubal wall has not yet been invaded, irrigation and suction of the tube might dislodge and expel the product of conception into peritoneal cavity and thereby avoid an incision of the tubal wall. Postoperative examination of β-hCG levels below the detectable limit must be carried out twice.[4]

SURGICAL TECHNIQUE FOR NONTUBAL ECTOPIC PREGNANCY

Ovarian Pregnancy

Localization of primary ovarian gravidity can be separated into a superficial and an intrafollicular type due to their pathogenesis. Ninety percent of ovarian gravidities are located intrafollicularly. The unusual site and rarity of ovarian pregnancies lead to a more complex clinical course, beginning with the difficulty in making an early and accurate diagnosis, an inconsistent therapeutic approach, leading to an unpredictable outcome and a life-threatening status if the ovary ruptures.

(a) *Superficial pattern*: The implantation takes place in an ovarian focus of endometriosis.
(b) *Intrafollicular pattern*:
  - *Primary*—insemination of an ovum that has not yet ovulated.
  - *Secondary*—after regular ovulation implantation of the inseminated ovum in the follicle or corpus luteum.

The exact etiology is still unclear. It is postulated that the superficial form is correlated to endometriosis genitalis externa. The presumption is that fertilization occurs extraovarian and abundant granulosa cells of the zygote adhere to the ruptured follicle. The intrafollicular pattern allows the division into two subunits. The subcortical or cortical place of development is associated with insemination in an unruptured follicle and is called primary, whereas juxtafollicular or secondary implantation postulates that inseminated ovum after regular ovulation is placed in deeper parts of the ovary in a second step.

Preoperative diagnosis of ovarian pregnancy is difficult as the clinical findings are similar to those of tubal pregnancy, hemorrhagic ovarian cyst, endometrioma and other pelvic diseases (Table 17.1).

The defined diagnosis of an ovarian gravity is still bound to the four anatomical and histopathological criteria suggested by Spiegelberg in 1878.[23]

- The fallopian tube and the infundibulum with its fimbriae of the affected site are intact. There is no connection between the fallopian tube and the ovary.
- The gestation should occupy the normal position of ovary.
- The gestation should be connected to uterus by uterine ligament.
- Ovarian tissue must be present in the specimen attached to gestation sac.

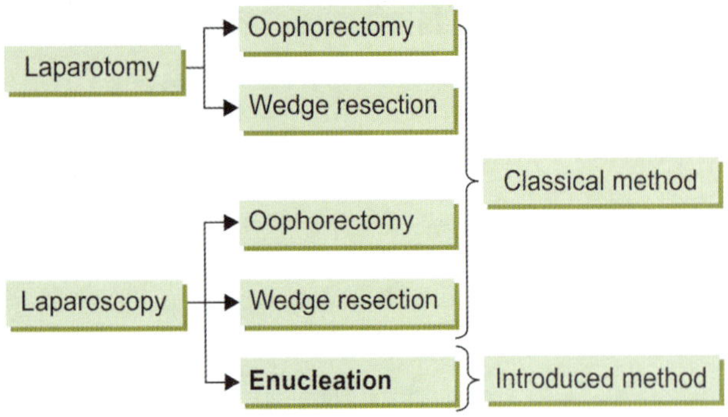

Fig. 17.11: Introduction of a new method on laparoscopic management of ovarian pregnancies.

The Spiegelberg criteria can be extended to include the follow-up of the serum β-hCG levels. Criteria number[4] is no longer compulsory in view of the improved operative methods described here.[20]

The traditional operative treatment for ovarian pregnancies has been oophorectomy. However, the desire to maintain reproductive capability and improvements in laparoscopy have more recently led to the ovarian-preserving operational technique.

The first operative steps are the same as for tubal pregnancy. Once the ectopic pregnancy has been localized and bleeding is under control, an operative plan has to be decided upon. This is either oophorectomy, wedge resection (in both cases by laparotomy or by laparoscopy) or laparoscopic enucleation of the ovarian pregnancy (Fig. 17.11). Laparoscopic enucleation of the gestational product is gentlest type of operation for ovarian pregnancy. By enucleating gestational sac bluntly from ovary, the surrounding ovarian tissue is protected to the greatest possible extent. Careful surgical extraction of the trophoblast tissue from the place of nidation under optical magnification is an essential precondition.

Gestational sac is enucleated with no more than the outer margins of the functional ovary. In the overview, hemorrhage from the ruptured ectopic pregnancy was identified. In the background, a soft slightly enlarged uterus was found (Fig. 17.12A). The left and right fallopian tubes were normal without dilation or bleeding from fimbrial end; however, the left ovary was enlarged to approximately 6.5 × 7.0 cm in diameter with a central bleeding defect. The right ovary showed a fresh corpus luteum cyst without bleeding. Manipulation of the left ovary led to bleeding and rupture of the cyst, and for management after suction (Fig. 17.12B) 10 mL of diluted POR 8® solution (5 I.U. ornipressin in 100 ml saline) was injected into the infundibulo pelvic ligament to achieve vasoconstriction (Fig. 17.12C). The product of conception was bluntly prepared and enucleated from the orthotopic ovarian tissue (Figs. 17.12D and E) and removed from left ovary using microscissors and spoon forceps (Fig. 17.12F). After complete separation of the trophoblast from the left ovary, it could be easily removed from abdominal cavity through a 20 mm trocar in the midline using the 10 mm spoon forceps. Adequate hemostasis on the ovarian tissue was maintained with the use of endocoagulation.[20]

Histopathological examination of the tissues removed from the left ovary showed signs of diffuse bleeding alongside chorion villi, decidual cells and decidual changed stroma with normal ovarian cortical tissue in the outer margins (Figs. 17.13A to D).

The problem of leaving behind remaining trophoblast material or disseminated trophoblast tissue is mentioned in context with tubal pregnancy. After performing laparoscopic enucleation technique, an adequate follow-up of the β-hCG serum level decrease is a necessary part of the postoperative monitoring regime.

Operative laparoscopy has the benefit of reduced morbidity, reduced hospitalization and rapid recovery of the patient. Because it has the advantage of reducing postoperative adhesions compared to laparotomy, it is the preferable technique for treatment of ovarian gestation after laparoscopic diagnosis, especially for women who wish to preserve their fertility potential. With more extensive use of pelviscopy to evaluate abnormal quantitative β-hCG values, intact ovarian pregnancy can be diagnosed at an early stage and hemorrhage or hypovolemic shock can be avoided.[20]

Extraluminal Ectopic Pregnancy

Ectopic pregnancy is defined as extraluminal when the gestational product is situated between muscularis externa and serosa. Etiology is a fast growing tubal pregnancy with early infiltration of the tubal wall.

Incision with monopolar needle or hook over the point of maximum distention results in the product of conception slipping out without the need of a long incision. Irrigation of the wound does not lead to liquid flowing out of the fimbrial end as there is no connection to the tubal lumina and its opening should be avoided if possible.

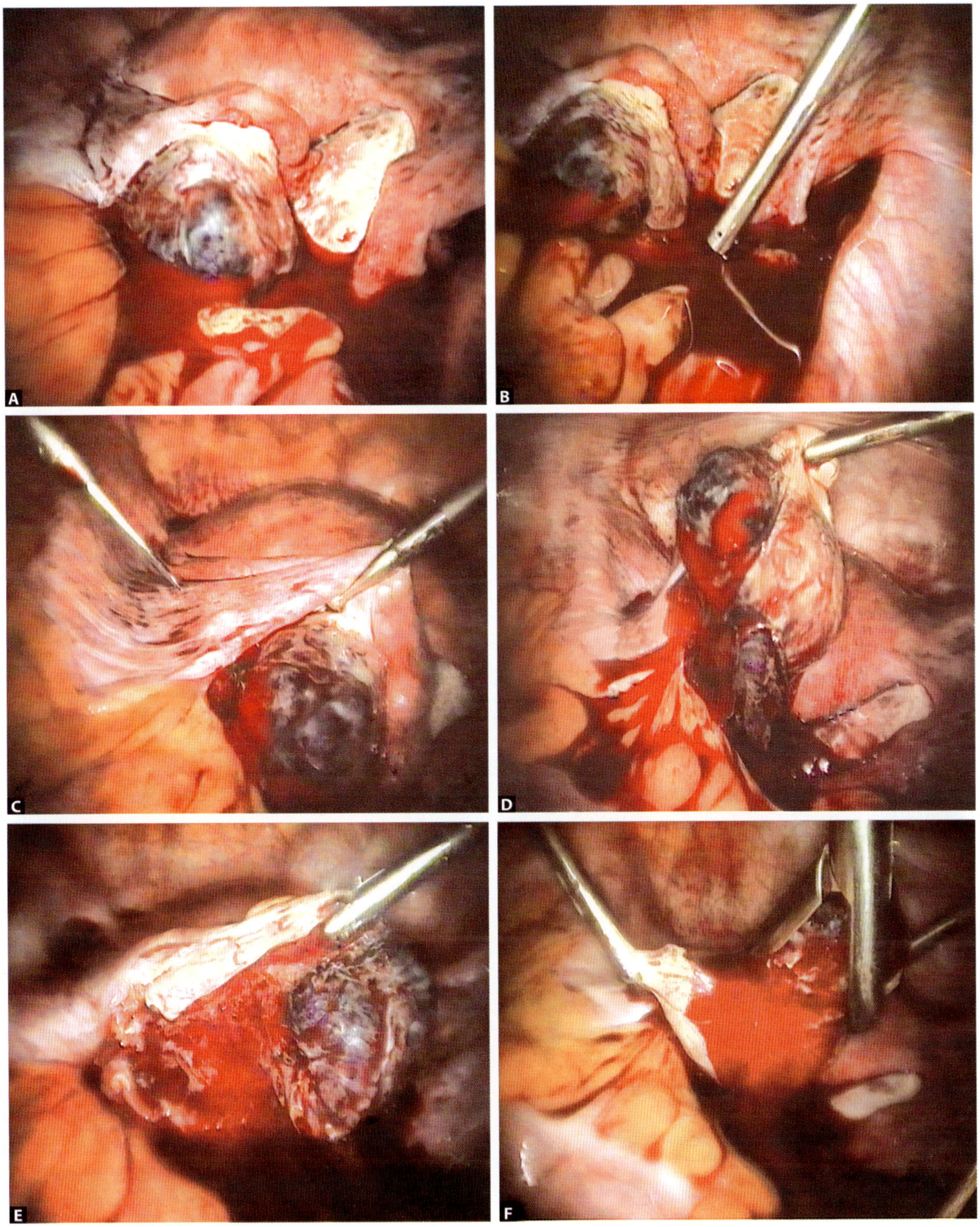

Figs. 17.12A to F: (A) Overview after creating a pneumoperitoneum for diagnostic laparoscopy. Bleeding from the ruptured ectopic pregnancy of the left ovary. In the background, the slightly enlarged uterus and the right ovary with the corpus luteum cyst; (B) Suction of the blood out of the cul-de-sac; (C) Preparation of the left ovary and injection of ornipressin into the infundibulopelvic ligament; (D) Blunt preparation and enucleation of the gestational sac from the orthotopic ovarian tissue. Removal of the product of conception by (E) enucleation. Healthy ovarian tissue can be seen on the left; (F) Removal after complete separation of the trophoblast from the ovary.[20]

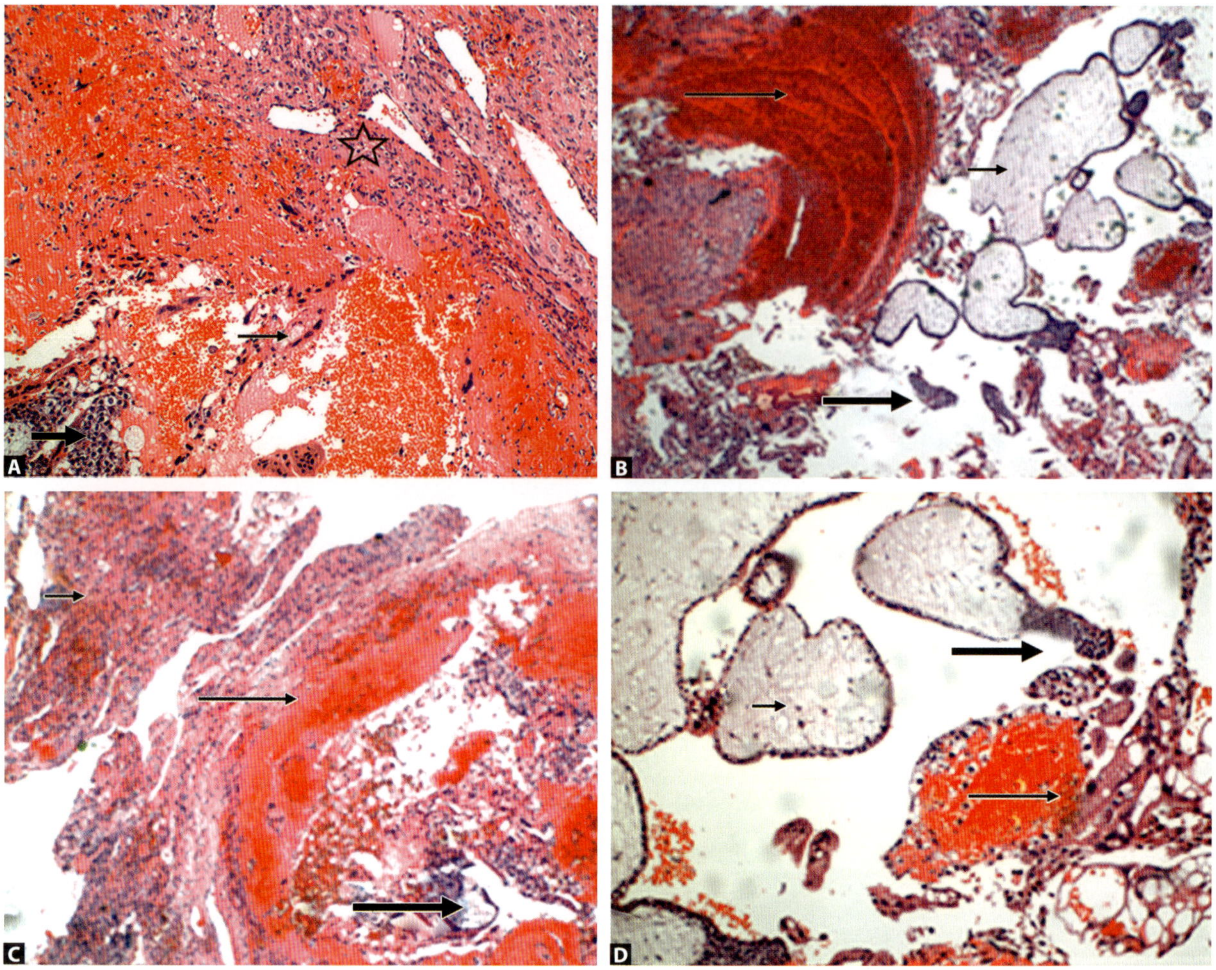

Figs. 17.13A to D: (A) Histological examination of the material shows hemorrhage into the gestational sac and orthotopic normal ovarian cortical tissue (star) next to decidualized stroma (thick arrow) at low magnification. Alongside, trophoblastic giant cells (thin arrow); (B) Hemorrhage (thin arrow) and regressive villous stroma (small arrow) in addition to decidualized stroma (thick arrow); (C) Gestational material (small arrow) and regressive villous stroma (thick arrow), in between hemorrhage and fibrin (thin arrow); (D) Regressive villous stroma (small arrow) next to trophoblast tissue (thick arrow) trophoblastic giant cells (thin arrow) at higher magnification.[20]

The patient's β-hCG levels have to be controlled carefully after discharge and methotrexate can be considered as a possible adjuvant treatment or as treatment of choice in case of recurrence.

Ectopic Abdominal Pregnancy

Ectopic abdominal pregnancy can either be primary or secondary if a tubal pregnancy ruptures and implants abdominally. This rare localization occurs in only about 1% of all ectopic pregnancies. Nevertheless, it has a high morbidity and mortality rate and makes detection by ultrasound or magnetic resonance imaging (MRI) necessary.

Laparoscopic removal is possible if the tumor is detected early and does not involve vessels that can cause uncontrollable bleeding. Due to comparatively few symptoms abdominal gravidity is often recognized very late. The usual clinical features, such as persistent diffuse abdominal pain, nausea and vomiting often appear at a late stadium, and sometimes only painful fetal movements in the upper abdomen are recognized. Treatment of an advanced abdominal pregnancy is associated with an enormous risk for life-threatening maternal bleeding. Removal of placenta is dependent on its localization as it can be implanted on any organ in the abdominal cavity. Sometimes placenta is better left intra-abdominally to be calcified and reabsorbed or embolized by an interventional radiologist prior to removal at a second intervention. Its management is strictly by laparotomy.[4]

Interstitial or Cornual Pregnancy/ Rudimental Uterine Horn

The intramural or interstitial part of fallopian tube is about 1 cm long and begins with the tubal ostium.

It then permeates the myometrium leading to the fallopian tube. This highly vascularized area has to be forded by the sperm on its way to fertilization and backward by the embryo before nidation takes place in the uterine cavity. Anatomy of this area makes conservative operating procedures difficult.

This rare type of tubal pregnancy occurs in 1 of 5,000 live births (2–4% of all ectopic pregnancies) and has an increased risk of traumatic rupture with hemorrhagic shock and maternal death. Its mortality rate is about 2%. This is due to the high vascularity of this area where the uterine and ovarian vessels join together. This localization is a great challenge even for experienced surgeons. The classical treatment methods are laparotomy, uterine horn resection or even hysterectomy. Laparotomy can be necessary if expert laparoscopic knowledge is not available.

Intramural or interstitial pregnancy lies deep in the myometrium and therefore has to be treated conservatively or by laparoscopy with the possibility to convert quickly to laparotomy in combination with hysteroscopy.

Cornual pregnancy, by contrast, implants in the same anatomical area of the tube but opens to the uterine cavity. Therefore, the operative method of choice can be hysteroscopy. True cornual gestations can be resected by hysteroscopy using electrosurgery. Alternatively laparoscopy can be combined with a hysteroscopic approach. If the overlying myometrium is thick and intact, removal can be completely performed by hysteroscopy. To avoid uterine perforation, larger pregnancies can be removed by curettage under laparoscopic guidance. Intraoperatively it has to be decided whether the overlaying myometrium is thin enough to resect the gestational product by laparoscopy.[2]

In most cases the corresponding part has to be resected. Major part of the tube can be saved in this way but end-to-end anastomosis has only a low success rate as the interstitial part is completely destroyed.

If pregnancy has eroded through myometrium, depending on the experience of the surgeon, it may be better to perform laparotomy to evacuate pregnancy. No matter what solution is taken, it should always be possible to perform an immediate laparotomy.[3,7]

Vasopressin is used in the same way and in the same concentration as for tubal pregnancy at any other site. The thinnest portion of the interstitium has to be coagulated properly with bipolar forceps before the lumen is incised. Once the lumen is open, the gestational product is removed in the same way as for tubal pregnancy at a more distal location. Hemostasis is performed with bipolar forceps and the uterus has to be reconstructed. Reconstruction can be performed by extracorporeal or intracorporeal knotting techniques. The best anatomic reconstructing effect is given by inverted single knots in one layer.[24]

Resection of the cornu is done step by step using cutting or blend current. Local hemostasis should be achieved with bipolar coagulation. Severe bleeding can lead to coagulation of the ascending branch of the uterine artery as well as the utero-ovarian arteries.[3]

The risk of acute and severe bleeding leads to preoperative preparation of several blood units of packed red blood cells. Prior consent of the patient should be obtained for a possible laparotomy.

Intraligamental Gravidity

This entity is very rare and occurs in about one of 250 ectopic pregnancies. For intraligamental development the gestational sac must split the oviduct precisely between the leaves of the broad ligament. Amnion, at least, must remain intact to permit the fetus to continue to develop in its extraperitoneal sac. Rupture must occur early enough so that the villi are capable of expanding their areas of nidation.

Anatomically intraligamental gravidity is bordered anteriorily and posteriorly by the two leaves of the broad ligament. Uterus is located medially, side pelvic wall laterally and the levator muscle inferiorly. The growing placenta is able to infiltrate any of the abovementioned anatomical neighboring structures and can pose a dangerous threat, as described under abdominal pregnancy.[25]

Cervical and Vaginal Pregnancy

The criteria for a cervical pregnancy have been described by Rubin in 1911:

- Cervical glands must be present opposite the placental attachment.
- The attachment of placenta to cervix must be intimate.
- Placenta must be below the peritoneal reflection of the anterior and posterior surfaces of uterus.
- Fetal elements must not be within the uterine cavity.[26]

Cervical and vaginal pregnancies are threatening localizations for the patient. Due to their anatomic closeness to the uterine artery they connect early to corresponding drainage. Damage to uterine artery during any operative procedure can lead to massive, unslakable bleeding. Diagnostic detection of cervical pregnancy should implicate a local or systemic medical treatment with methotrexate when possible to avoid blood loss and hysterectomy and to preserve the patient's fertility options for future. Medical treatment can be accompanied by selective uterine artery embolization. An operative alternative is the hysteroscopic resection of gestational product although there is a risk of severe haemorrhage and hypovolemic shock even when carried out by experienced surgeons. For this reason the indication for operative management has to be taken very cautiously.[4]

Simultaneous Intra- and Extrauterine Gravidity

The incidence of a simultaneous intra- and extrauterine gravidity has become a remarkable differential diagnosis with the increase of reproductive methods. Having detected an intrauterine gravidity, a simultaneous extrauterine pregnancy is not usually expected.

In majority of the cases simultaneous pregnancy is an incidental finding. Persistent abdominal pain or other clinical features alongside an irregular rise in the β-hCG level can lead to this infrequent diagnosis. Once a simultaneous pregnancy has been discovered, the operative method of choice is laparoscopic salpingectomy. Alternative methods to preserve the fallopian tube do not allow postoperative β-hCG measurements due to the existing intrauterine gestation and therefore cannot be used as a therapeutic option.[4]

GENERAL OPERATIVE STEPS AFTER THE REMOVAL OF ECTOPIC PREGNANCY

Hemostasis and Extended Operation

Adhesions or other pathologic processes such as endometriosis can be treated simultaneously during removal of the ectopic pregnancy without significantly prolonging the operation in most of the cases. If the operative sidelines demand long and complex operative procedures their treatment has to be made dependent on circulatory stability of the patient and urgency of the redress of the secondary problem.

Complications

The major complication of tubal pregnancy is tubal rupture. Precedent bleedings are caused by the invasion of trophoblast tissue into the local vascular system leading to intraluminal hematoma and bleeding of the fimbrial end. If the stretching capacity of the tube is exceeded, this results in tubal rupture.

The possibility of leaving behind products of conception is the same after laparoscopy as after laparotomy (5–15%). Careful attention must be given to medial portion of the tube as this is the preferential site where trophoblastic tissue can outlast and be responsible for elevated serum β-hCG levels in the follow-up. The reoperative assessment as well as the adjuvant use of methotrexate should be kept in mind.

The risk for postoperative hemorrhage is low. If postoperative hemorrhage occurs, surgical revision is necessary in most cases.[1-5,7,8,21,24,27-29]

MEDICAL TREATMENT

The predominant drug is methotrexate, but other systemic drugs can also be used to treat ectopic pregnancy, e.g., actinomycin D, prostaglandins and RU 486. In view of the uncertainty of treatment success and possible adverse side effects, the indication for a conservative treatment has to be weighed up carefully.

Methotrexate is a well-studied folic acid antagonist. It deactivates dihydrofolate reductase that can inhibit the synthesis of deoxyribonucleic and ribonucleic acid. Methotrexate can therefore disrupt the rapidly dividing trophoblastic cells. The expected time to resolution of the ectopic pregnancy is 3 to 7 weeks after methotrexate application.

The selective use of methotrexate can be as effective as surgery although adverse side effects are possible, such as bone marrow suppression, elevated liver enzymes, rash, alopecia, stomatitis, nausea, diarrhea and to a lesser extent pleuritis, dermatitis, conjunctivitis, gastritis and enteritis. The success rate of methotrexate is up to 94%. Nevertheless, this depends on the β-hCG level. The lower the serum level at the beginning of the therapy, the higher the success rate is.

The use of medical treatment for extrauterine gravidity is only indicated if the invasiveness of treatment can be diminished (Flowchart 17.3). The indication for methotrexate treatment has to be recommended carefully and reserved for special situations.

Flowchart 17.3: Algorithm of methotrexate therapy.

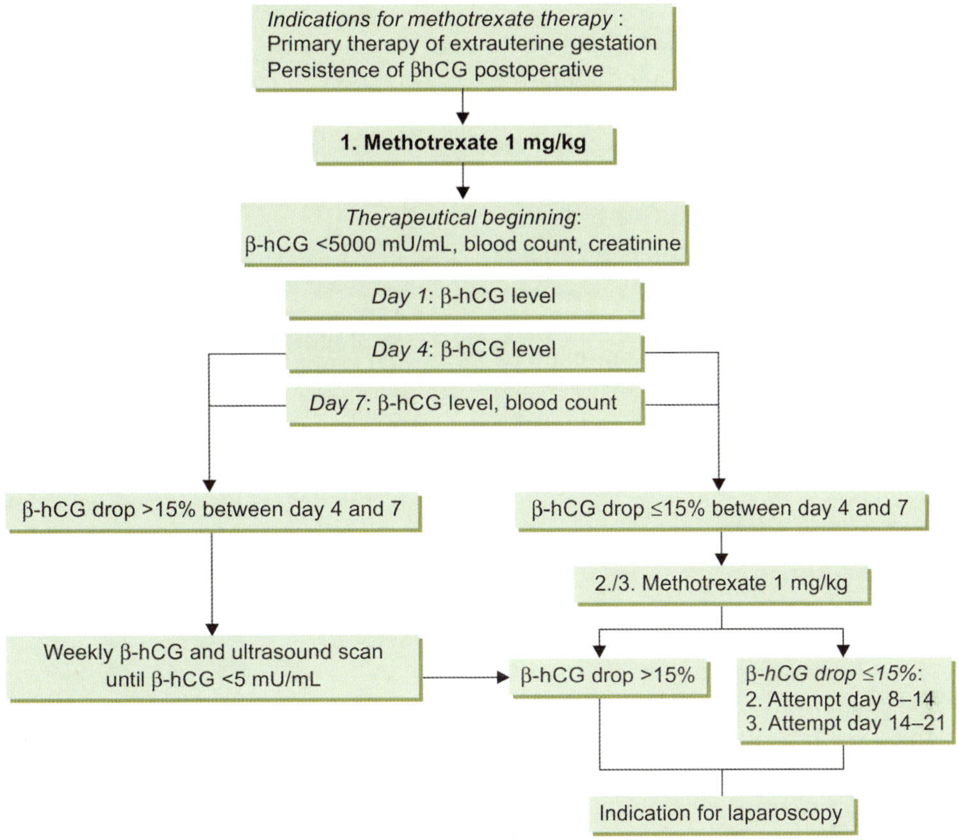

The use of methotrexate to destroy an ectopic pregnancy has been advocated for women with an atypical localization in the cervix, interstitially, cornual or in the abdominal cavity, an incomplete resolution of surgically treated ectopic gestation, residual trophoblast tissue or persisting low β-hCG levels after curettage with no evidence of trophoblast material in the histological examination. Furthermore, patients with a high operative risk and contraindications to anesthesia, e.g., after induced ovarian hyperstimulation syndrome and patients who are expected to have extensive intraperitoneal abdominal adhesions might be optimal candidates for a preliminary medical treatment if they are hemodynamically stable. The use of methotrexate for the treatment of extrauterine pregnancy can only be considered if the diameter of the tumor is less than 4 cm, there is no sonographic evidence of fetal cardiac activity and the β-hCG level is below 5000 mIU/mL.

Methotrexate can be given locally or systemically by intramuscular injection of 1 mg/kg or 50 mg/m^2. Patients with a hematocrit below 35% should take 325 mg ferrous sulfate twice daily. Before recruiting patients for a conservative treatment method, the absence of fetal cardiac activity must be confirmed and the patients have to agree to comply with the follow-up requirements.

If the β-hCG level does not decline over 15% after 7 days, a second dose of methotrexate has to be given. The weekly follow-up includes monitoring of the β-hCG decrease and transvaginal ultrasonography. If clinical symptoms persist or ultrasonography reveals more than 100 mL of free fluid in the cul-de-sac, a laparoscopy has to be performed.

During and after methotrexate therapy, reliable contraception is necessary.[2,4,8,17,21,30]

FOLLOW-UP AND PROGNOSIS

After the operative procedure the removed gestational material is examined histologically (Figs. 17.1 to 17.3 and 17.13) for clinical and forensic safety by a pathologist. The bladder catheter is removed at the end of the operation. The patient should be admitted overnight in case of postoperative bleeding and the need of emotional support.

To prevent Rhesus factor incompatibility in the next pregnancy, a prophylactic dose of anti-D-prophylaxis has to be administered to patients with Rhesus factor negative.

Reduction of the β-hCG level correlates with treatment success. The β-hCG level after operative treatment should be reduced by 70% after 2 days and another 70% after 7 days. To ascertain the resolution of ectopic pregnancy, β-hCG level must be either undetectable or very low. Persistence of β-hCG suggests the persistence of trophoblast tissue. The test is repeated after another 2-week interval. In case of an inadequate decrease, the patient has to undergo medical treatment with methotrexate or renewed surgical treatment, especially if β-hCG levels increase. A secure sign for treatment success is a repeated β-hCG serum level below the detection line.

FUTURE FERTILITY AND RISK OF RECURRENCE

Laparoscopy and medical therapy have similar future fertility rates. About 30% of women with a previous ectopic pregnancy have difficulty in conceiving. The conception rate is about 77%, no matter what kind of therapy they received.

The incidence of recurrence is between 5% and 20% and rises up to 32% following two ectopic pregnancies.[4,8,28]

The desire to maintain reproductive capability has led to the organ-preserving operational technique whenever possible. Operative laparoscopy has the benefits of reduced morbidity, reduced hospitalization and rapid recovery, and because it has the advantage of reducing postoperative adhesions compared to laparotomy, it is the preferable technique for treatment of ectopic gestation after laparoscopic diagnosis, especially for women who wish to preserve their fertility potential. With the more extensive use of pelviscopy to evaluate abnormal quantitative β-hCG values, intact ectopic pregnancy can be diagnosed at an early stage and hemorrhage or hypovolemic shock can be avoided. Local excision, accomplished without open exploratory surgery or organ harvesting, is possible.

The limiting factor in the treatment of ectopic pregnancy is difficulty in diagnosing the condition at the right moment before rupture. Repeated ultrasound examination in cases of menstrual irregularities, pelvic pain, palpable adnexal masses and positive serum β-hCG levels raises the probability of preoperative diagnosis of this entity.

The question arises whether it is useful to perform routine early ultrasound scans of all women with positive pregnancy tests to check the location of the gestation so that earlier and more conservative treatment options are possible in cases of ectopic pregnancies. Nevertheless, the presence of an intrauterine pregnancy does not exclude the possibility of heterotopic pregnancy (coexistence of an intrauterine with an ectopic pregnancy).

TIPS OF THE EXPERTS

Tip 1: Prior to any surgical performance in the abdomen, careful cleaning of the situs.

Tip 2: Attempt to preserve the affected organ whenever possible and indicated.

Tip 3: Always extract the pregnancy product within an endobag for histological confirmation.

Tip 4: If uterine and abdominal cavities do not contain any specimen, always incise the tube at the distended site antimesenterially in a longitudinal incision.

REFERENCES

1. Murray H, Baakdah H, Bardell T, et al. Diagnosis and treatment of ectopic pregnancy. CMAJ. 2005;173(8): 905-12.
2. Luciano D, Roy G, Luciano A. Ectopic pregnancy. In: Pasic R, Levine R (Eds). A Practical Manual of Laparoscopy: A Clinical Cookbook. Andover, UK: Informa Healthcare; 2007. pp. 155-68.
3. Barbosa C, Mencaglia L. Laparoscopic management of ectopic pregnancy. In: Mencaglia L, Minelle L, Wattiez A, editors. Manual of Gynecological Laparoscopic Surgery. 11th ed. Schramberg, Germany: Endo Press; 2010. pp. 115-23.
4. Hucke J, Füllers U. Extrauterine Schwangerschaft. Der Gynäkologe. 2005;6(38):535-52.
5. Carson SA, Buster JE. Ectopic pregnancy. N Engl J Med. 1993;329(16):1174-81.
6. Marchbanks PA, Annegers JF, Coulam CB, et al. Risk factors for ectopic pregnancy. A population-based study. JAMA. 1988;259(12):1823-7.
7. Nezhat C, Nezhat F, Luciano A, et al. Ectopic pregnancy. In: Nezhat C, Nezhat F, Luciano A, et al., editors. Operative Gynecologic Laparoscopy: Principles and Techniques. New York: McGraw-Hill; 1995. pp. 107-20.
8. Lozeau AM, Potter B. Diagnosis and management of ectopic pregnancy. Am Fam Physician. 2005;72(9): 1707-14.
9. Kadar N, Romero R. Serial human chorionic gonadotropin measurements in ectopic pregnancy. Am J Obstet Gynecol. 1988;158(5):1239-40.
10. Fritz MA, Guo SM. Doubling time of human chorionic gonadotropin (hCG) in early normal pregnancy: relationship to hCG concentration and gestational age. Fertil Steril. 1987;47(4):584-9.

11. Brennan DF. Ectopic pregnancy—Part I: Clinical and laboratory diagnosis. Acad Emerg Med. 1995; 2(12):1081-9.
12. Mehta TS, Levine D, Beckwith B. Treatment of ectopic pregnancy: is a human chorionic gonadotropin level of 2,000 mIU/mL a reasonable threshold? Radiology. 1997;205(2):569-73.
13. Ardaens Y, Guerin B, Perrot N, et al. [Contribution of ultrasonography in the diagnosis of ectopic pregnancy]. J Gynecol Obstet Biol Reprod (Paris). 2003;32(7 Suppl):S28-38.
14. Mol BW, Lijmer JG, Ankum WM, et al. The accuracy of single serum progesterone measurement in the diagnosis of ectopic pregnancy: a meta-analysis. Hum Reprod. 1998;13(11):3220-7.
15. Koike H, Chuganji Y, Watanabe H, et al. Conservative treatment of ovarian pregnancy by local prostaglandin F2 alpha injection. Am J Obstet Gynecol. 1990;163(2):696.
16. Lang PF, Weiss PA, Mayer HO, et al. Conservative treatment of ectopic pregnancy with local injection of hyperosmolar glucose solution or prostaglandin-F2 alpha: a prospective randomised study. Lancet. 1990; 336(8707):78-81.
17. Lipscomb GH, Stovall TG, Ling FW. Nonsurgical treatment of ectopic pregnancy. N Engl J Med. 2000; 343(18):1325-9.
18. Shamma FN, Schwartz LB. Primary ovarian pregnancy successfully treated with methotrexate. Am J Obstet Gynecol. 1992;167(5):1307-8.
19. Chelmow D, Gates E, Penzias AS. Laparoscopic diagnosis and methotrexate treatment of an ovarian pregnancy: a case report. Fertil Steril. 1994;62(4): 879-81.
20. Alkatout I, Stuhlmann-Laeisz C, Mettler L, et al. Organ-preserving management of ovarian pregnancies by laparoscopic approach. Fertil Steril. 2011; 95(8): 2467-70.
21. Hoover KW, Tao G, Kent CK. Trends in the diagnosis and treatment of ectopic pregnancy in the United States. Obstet Gynecol. 2010;115(3):495-502.
22. Tulandi T. Tubal ectopic pregnancy: salpingostomy and salpingectomy. In: Tulandi T, editor. Atlas of Laparoscopic Technique for Gynecologists. London: W. B. Saunders; 1994. pp. 33-42.
23. Spiegelberg O. Zur Kasuistik der Ovarialschwangerschaft. Arch Gynecol Obstet. 1878;13:73-9.
24. Vogler A, Ribic-Pucelj M. Ectopic pregnancy. In: Ribi-Pucelj M, editor. Endoscopic Surgery in Gynecology. Ljubljana, Slovenia: Didakta; 2007. pp. 115-20.
25. Ziel HK, Miyazaki FS, Baker TH, et al. Advanced intraligamentary pregnancy. Report of a case with survey to date. Obstet Gynecol. 1968;31(5): 643-8.
26. Chelli D, Dimassi K, Bouaziz M, et al. [Early diagnosis and management of cervical ectopic pregnancy]. Tunis Med. 2009;87(9):616-20.
27. Bonatz G, Lehmann-Willenbrock E, Hedderich J, et al. Follow-up of beta-hCG after pelviscopic linear salpingotomy for therapy of tubal pregnancy. Geburtshilfe Frauenheilkd. 1995;55(1):37-40.
28. Tay JI, Moore J, Walker JJ. Ectopic pregnancy. BMJ. 2000;320(7239):916-9.
29. Zockler R, Dressler F, Raatz D, et al. Risk of recurrence and rate of intrauterine pregnancy after endoscopic therapy of extrauterine pregnancies. 10 years experiences with the treatment of 709 extrauterine pregnancies. Geburtshilfe Frauenheilkd. 1995;55(1): 32-6.
30. Yao M, Tulandi T. Surgical and medical management of tubal and non-tubal ectopic pregnancies. Curr Opin Obstet Gynecol. 1998;10(5):371-4.

KIEL SCH•OL

18 of Gynaecological Endoscopy

Laparoscopic Surgery in Pregnancy

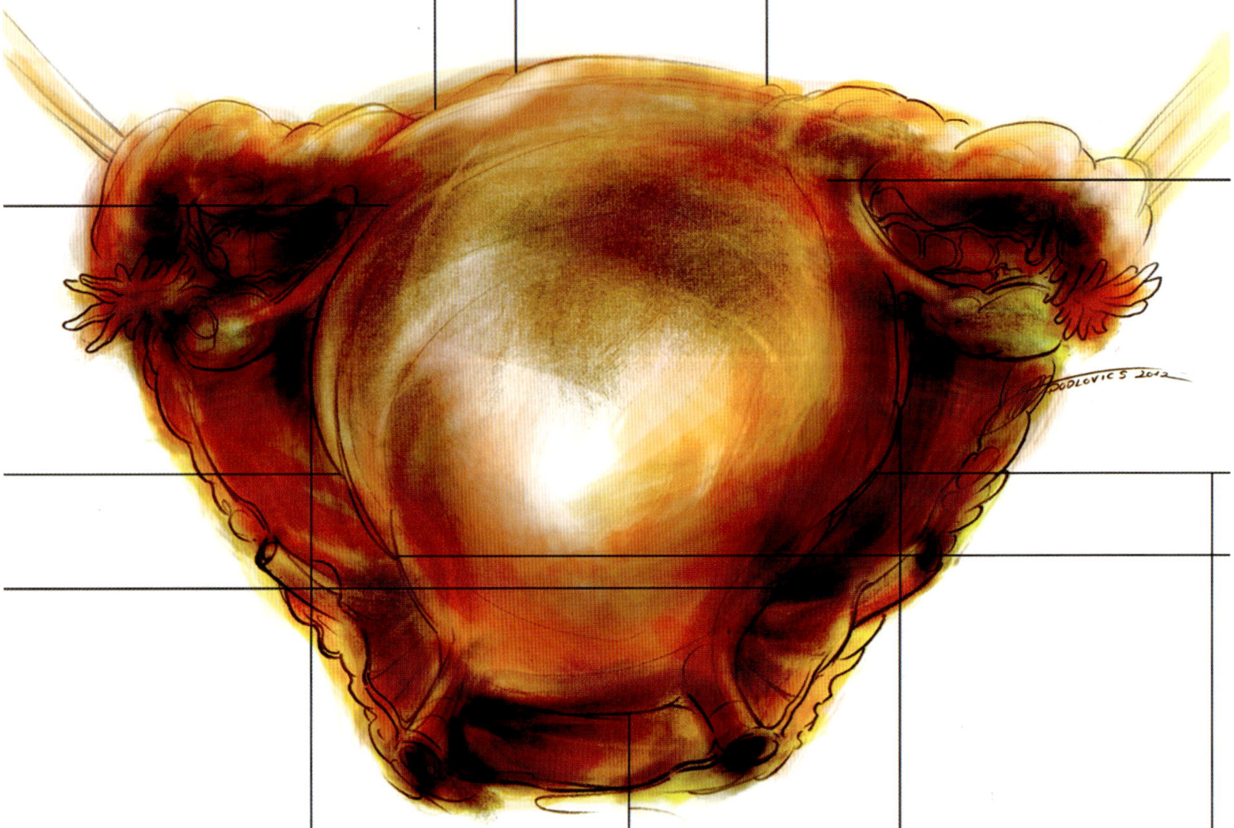

Chapter 18

Laparoscopic Surgery in Pregnancy

Wael Sammur, Liselotte Mettler

INTRODUCTION

Before taking the decision to perform laparoscopic surgery during pregnancy, it is important to keep in mind that the surgeon has two persons to care for: the patient and her fetus. The concern of potential obstetric complications for both of them and potential harm to the fetus due to laparoscopic surgery are important factors that have to be taken into consideration. It has been reported that the benefits of laparoscopic surgery during pregnancy appear similar to the benefits for nonpregnant patients. These include less post-operative pain, decreased hospital stay, fast recovery and less post-operative ileus.[1-5] There are also many other advantages of laparoscopy for pregnant patients: decreased fetal respiratory depression due to diminished postoperative narcotic requirements, lower risk of wound complications, diminished post-operative hypoventilation[6-10] and decreased risk of thromboembolic events. The improved visualization in laparoscopy may reduce the risk of uterine irritability by decreasing the need for uterine manipulation.[11] Postponing a necessary operation until after delivery may, in some cases, increase the rate of complications for both mother and fetus.[12-15] One recent study evaluated 11 children from 1 to 8 years and found no growth or development delay.[16]

INDICATIONS FOR LAPAROSCOPIC SURGERY DURING PREGNANCY

Gynecological Indications

Complicated Ovarian and Adnexal Masses

These conditions require immediate laparoscopic surgery and management according to the findings. Diagnostic laparoscopy is safe in the workup and treatment of acute abdominal diseases in pregnancy.[17]

- *Torsion*: This is a surgical emergency. Treatment is the same as for nonpregnant women.
- *Ruptured ovarian cyst*: This could involve intraperitoneal bleeding or just leakage of ovarian cystic fluid. This is also a surgical emergency and treatment is the same as for nonpregnant women.
- *Intra-abdominal bleeding*: This requires emergency laparoscopic surgery to stop the bleeding and treat the main lesion according to the findings.
- *Ectopic pregnancy (heterotopic pregnancy)*: Classically, the incidence of naturally occurring heterotopic pregnancy has been reported as 1 in 30,000 pregnancies.[18] Nowadays, it is encountered more often than before for many reasons, e.g., the increase in ovulation induction and assisted reproduction techniques. Patients treated with clomiphene citrate have been reported to have a heterotopic rate of 1 in 120 to 1 in 3,000 pregnancies, while the use of menotropins for ovulation induction and intravenous fluid (IVF) increase the rate up to 1 in 100 pregnancies.[19] Laparoscopic management is the same as for nonpregnant patients. It is important to minimize manipulation of the pelvic organs, especially the uterus (Fig. 18.1).
- *Ovarian hyperstimulation syndrome (OHSS)*: The surgical approach must be avoided in cases of OHSS, with only three exceptions: ruptured ovarian cyst, ovarian torsion and ectopic pregnancy. In these cases a conservative surgical procedure is indicated, whereby the laparoscopic technique is by far the most appropriate for OHSS.[20]
- Road accident.

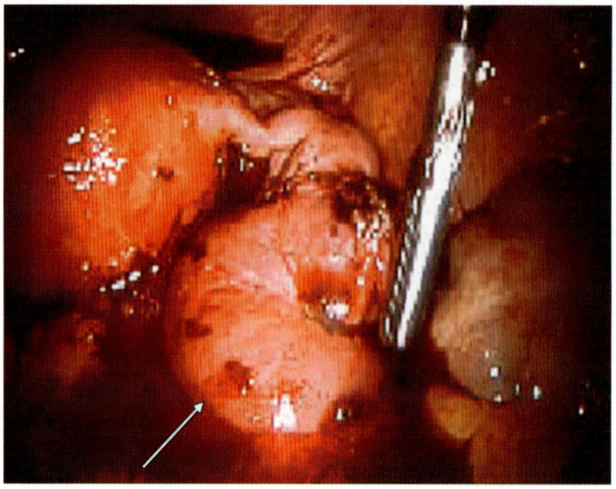

Fig. 18.1: Ectopic pregnancy (7 weeks).

Persistent Adnexal Masses

The management of ovarian tumors in pregnancy is crucial because of various complications that may develop, such as pelvic impaction, obstructed labor, torsion of ovarian pedicle, hemorrhage into the tumor, rupture of the cyst, infection and malignancy changes.[21] Surgery may be indicated if the lesion has not resolved after 14–16 gestational weeks, is larger than 6 cm, has a solid or complex ultrasound appearance and shows bilateral adnexal abnormalities.[22] However, recent literature supports the safety of close observation in these patients if ultrasound findings indicate no malignancy, tumor markers (CA-125, LDH) are normal and the patient is asymptomatic.[23-26] In the event that surgery is indicated, various case reports support the use of laparoscopy in the management of adnexal masses in all trimesters.[27-39] An informative and retrospective review of 88 pregnant women demonstrated equivalent maternal and fetal outcomes in adnexal masses managed laparoscopically and by laparotomy.[11]

- The frequency of adnexal masses in pregnancy may be as low as 1 in 190 pregnancies[40] or as high as 2%.[41]
- Persistent adnexal masses are most commonly functional cysts or mature cystic teratomas with incidence of malignancy reported at 2–6%.[42]
- Most of the functional, physiological cysts resolved spontaneously by the end of the first trimester.[22]
- The most common ovarian germ cell tumor is dysgerminoma, followed by endodermal sinus tumor.[22]
- The risk of malignancy in pregnant women with adnexal mass is 5%. Most of them are borderline tumors or germ cell tumors.[21]
- Careful differentiation between benign and malignant masses is important. The sonographic appearance may be helpful.[22]
- Doppler and magnetic resonance imaging (MRI) could be helpful in the diagnosis of those cases in which ultrasound alone is not clear in the final diagnosis. Regardless of the size, adnexal masses with the blood flow characterized by high resistant index appear to carry little risk.[22]
- In the case of ovarian cancer, complete surgical staging must be done exactly the same as with nonpregnant patients. However, if both ovaries have malignant infiltrates in the second trimester, a bilateral salpingectomy should be performed as the pregnancy no longer requires hormonal support for corpus luteum.[22]

Non-gynecological Indications

It has been estimated that 0.2% of pregnancies require nongynecological surgery.[43]

Laparoscopic treatment of acute abdominal disease has the same indications in pregnant and nonpregnant patients.[1]

- *Gallbladder disease:*
  - The cholecystectomy is the most common general surgical procedure performed during pregnancy.[44,45]
  - Nonoperative treatment of pregnant women with biliary disease results in 12% with spontaneous abortion and in 30% with cholecystectomy.[46]
  - A delay in the surgical management of gravid patients with symptomatic gallstones results in increased rates of hospitalization, spontaneous abortion, pre-term labor and delivery compared to those undergoing cholecystectomy.[1,3,47-51]
  - There have been no reports of fetal demise for laparoscopic cholecystectomy performed during the first and second trimesters.[52]
  - Decreased rates of spontaneous abortion and preterm labor have been reported after laparoscopic cholecystectomy compared to laparotomy.[53]
- *Appendicitis (Fig. 18.2):*
  - Approximately 0.05–0.1% of pregnant women will have acute appendicitis.[43,54]

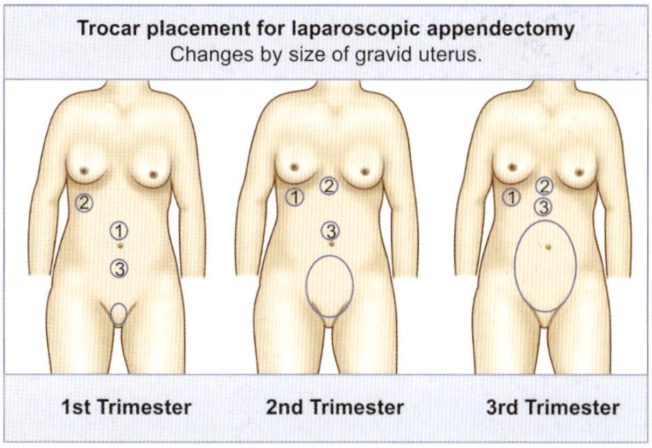

Fig. 18.2: Trocar placement in various pregnancy stages for laparoscopic appendectomy.
Source: Rollins MD, Price RR. Laparoscopic surgery during pregnancy. In: Inderbir SG (Ed). Textbook of Laparoscopic Urology. New York: Informa Healthcare USA, Inc., 2006:983-6.

- The most common general surgery emergencies during pregnancy are appendicitis, intestinal obstruction, cholecystitis and peritonitis.[54]
- The rate of fetal loss is 1.5% with uncomplicated appendicitis and increased to 35% with perforated appendicitis.[55]
- The presence of leukocytosis, nausea, vomiting and abdominal pain in pregnant patients can make the diagnosis of acute appendicitis difficult.[56]
- Laparoscopic appendectomy is the preferred treatment for pregnant patients with appendicitis.[57]
- Retrospective studies of laparoscopic appendectomy have shown very low rates of preterm delivery and, in most series, no reports of fetal demise.[58-66]

- *Solid organ resection:*
  - Laparoscopic adrenelectomy, nephrectomy and splenectomy are safe procedures in pregnant patients.[17]

PRACTICAL CONSIDERATIONS

General

- In the past, recommendations have been given when to perform surgery in the second trimester, in order to reduce the rates of spontaneous abortion and preterm labor.[67,68] Recent literature has shown that pregnant patients may undergo laparoscopic surgery safely during any trimester without any increased risk to the mother or fetus.[1,5,12,51,58,59,69,70]
- Informed consent of spontaneous abortion and pre-term delivery must be obtained.
- Pre- and postoperative fetal heart activity should be documented.
- Low-pressure pneumoperitoneum should be used in pregnant patients at 8–12 mm Hg, to minimize any adverse effect on the fetal perfusion.[71] Pressure of 15 mm Hg has been used by other authors during laparoscopy in pregnant patients without increasing adverse outcomes to the patient or her fetus.[58,59] There are no data showing detrimental effects to the human fetuses from CO_2 pneumoperitoneum.[71]
- Trocar placement should be adjusted depending on the size of the pregnant uterus and the lesion to be treated. During the first trimester, umbilical access is safe for placement of the first trocar; however, later in pregnancy, left, right upper quadrants and mid-clavicular line should be used.[71]
- Initial abdominal access with open Hasson technique,[46,71] and Veress technique in the upper abdomen could be used.[44,72]
- Because of the increased risk of thrombosis, useful prophylaxes for deep venous thrombosis are encouraging early postoperative mobilization, subcutaneous heparin injection and using intra- and post-operative sequential pneumatic compression devices.[73]
- Gravid patients should be placed in a left-side-down position to minimize compression of the vena cava and to minimize a reverse Trendelenburg position.[74]
- Several studies have documented the safety and efficacy of end-tidal carbon dioxide ($EtCO_2$) measurement in pregnant women, making routine blood gas monitoring unnecessary.[58,59,71]

LAPAROSCOPIC MANAGEMENT OF BENIGN ADNEXAL MASS

- Under general anesthesia
- Insertion of Foley's catheter
- Placement of primary and secondary trocars, taking into consideration the gestational age and height of the gravid uterus as mentioned above
- Inspection of the upper abdomen and pelvis. Cell washings are obtained from the pelvis and the abdomen if suspected masses have been seen.
- Careful aspiration of cystic fluid to avoid any leakage or spill into the pelvis or abdominal

cavity. This can be achieved by using an 18-gauge laparoscopic aspiration needle or a 5-mm trocar.

- A window should be opened in the cyst wall. The cavity of the cyst wall is carefully inspected. Suspicious lesions are biopsied and are sent for frozen section.
- Careful complete excision of the cyst wall, followed by hemostasis using bipolar coagulation or any other suitable hemostatic tool. Minimal damage to healthy ovarian tissue must be observed. Usually sutures are not used to avoid adhesions.
- Removal of the cyst wall by using an endobag.
- Retract instruments and secondary trocars under vision. Deflate the peritoneal cavity from CO_2 gas. Suture the skin incisions with suitable stitches.
- Fetal heart activity should be monitored at the end of the laparoscopic surgery.
- No need for prophylactic tocolytics.
- Titers of tumor markers, AFP, hCG and CA-125, are elevated in pregnancy for reasons not related to malignancy.[23] Therefore, these markers are of little significance.
- To decrease the likelihood of pregnancy loss, supplementary progesterone should be administered if ovarian cystectomy is performed in the first trimester. The efficacy of this treatment, however, remains unproven.[22]

COMPLICATIONS AND BENEFITS OF LAPAROSCOPIC PROCEDURES IN PREGNANCY

In addition to the complications that can occur during any laparoscopic procedure, for example, a penetrating injury from the Veress needle or the trocar to the bowel, blood vessels and urinary bladder or diathermy damage to any pelvi-abdominal structure, the following complications must be considered when pregnant women undergo laparoscopic surgery. Let us also keep in mind that there are certain benefits which definitely indicate laparoscopic procedures in pregnancy.

Complications

- At laparoscopic appendectomy the rate of preterm delivery is 21.4%, statistically significant higher than the rate for those not undergoing surgery. No fetal or maternal mortality.[45]
- No abnormal fetal organogenesis in laparoscopic appendectomies during first trimester.[75]
- In laparoscopic cholecystectomy no fetal losses, no birth defects and no uterine injuries.[73] Others reported IUFD and incomplete abortions.[76]
- The risk of trocar injuries to the uterus increase with increased gestational age.[21]
- Abdominal surgery in the first trimester is associated with a 12% spontaneous abortion rate.[22]
- Preterm labor in 30–40% of pregnant patients who underwent abdominal surgery in the third trimester.[22]

Benefits:

In a national cohort study conducted in the United States from 2003 to 2012, published in May 2017, 19,926 women undergone appendectomy and cholecystectomy during pregnancy. When compared to laparoscopy, laparotomy was associated with threefold increased risk of both postoperative obstetric complications, including preterm delivery, preterm labor without preterm delivery and miscarriages.[77]

CONCLUSION

In cases of surgical or gynecological emergency, laparoscopic treatment has the same indications in pregnant as in nonpregnant patients. The laparoscopic procedure can be safely done during any trimester of pregnancy.

Adnexal masses present challenging problems in diagnosis and management during pregnancy. Most of the adnexal masses resolve by the end of the first trimester. If they persist, accurate diagnosis and follow-up is mandatory. If cysts are asymptomatic and nonsuspicious, observation is acceptable. For all other cystic lesions laparoscopic cystectomy is safe and effective. There are different reports on laparoscopic treatment of abdominal diseases; however, all of them showed no maternal mortality and very few reported fetal demise. None reported abnormal fetal organogenesis. Obstetric complications with laparoscopic surgery are less than that with laparotomy. Some reports mentioned an increase in spontaneous abortions and preterm deliveries after abdominal surgery.

TIPS AND TRICKS

- Only perform a surgical intervention if absolutely necessary.
- Use the same safety steps as in a normal laparoscopy.

- Be prepared for higher placement of optic trocar and secondary trocars.
- Use the left side position whenever possible.
- Be aware of thrombosis prophylaxis.

REFERENCES

1. Reedy MB, Galan HL, Richards WE, et al. Laparoscopy during pregnancy. A survey of laparoendoscopic surgeons. J Reprod Med. 1997;42(1):33-8.
2. Curet MJ, Allen D, Josloff RK, et al. Laparoscopy during pregnancy. Arch Surg. 1996;131(5):546-50; discussion 550-1.
3. Andreoli M, Servakov M, Meyers P, et al. Laparoscopic surgery during pregnancy. J Am Assoc Gynecol Laparosc. 1999;6(2):229-33.
4. Shay DC, Bhavani-Shankar K, Datta S. Laparoscopic surgery during pregnancy. Anesthesiol Clin North Am. 2001;19(1):57-67.
5. Oelsner G, Stockheim D, Soriano D, et al. Pregnancy outcome after laparoscopy or laparotomy in pregnancy. J Am Assoc Gynecol Laparosc. 2003;10(2): 200-4.
6. Pucci RO, Seed RW. Case report of laparoscopic cholecystectomy in the third trimester of pregnancy. Am J Obstet Gynecol. 1991;165(2):401-2.
7. Weber AM, Bloom GP, Allan TR, et al. Laparoscopic cholecystectomy during pregnancy. Obstet Gynecol. 1991;78(5 Pt 2):958-9.
8. Williams JK, Rosemurgy AS, Albrink MH, et al. Laparoscopic cholecystectomy in pregnancy. A case report. J Reprod Med. 1995;40(3):243-5.
9. Arvidsson D, Gerdin E. Laparoscopic cholecystectomy during pregnancy. Surg Laparosc Endosc. 1991;1(3): 193-4.
10. Costantino GN, Vincent GJ, Mukalian GG, et al. Laparoscopic cholecystectomy in pregnancy. J Laparoendosc Surg. 1994;4(2):161-4.
11. Soriano D, Yefet Y, Seidman DS, et al. Laparoscopy versus laparotomy in the management of adnexal masses during pregnancy. Fertil Steril. 1999;71(5): 955-60.
12. Glasgow RE, Visser BC, Harris HW, et al. Changing management of gallstone disease during pregnancy. Surg Endosc. 1998;12(3):241-6.
13. Davis A, Katz VL, Cox R. Gallbladder disease in pregnancy. J Reprod Med. 1995;40(11):759-62.
14. Muench J, Albrink M, Serafini F, et al. Delay in treatment of biliary disease during pregnancy increases morbidity and can be avoided with safe laparoscopic cholecystectomy. Am Surg. 2001;67(6): 539-42; discussion 542-3.
15. Visser BC, Glasgow RE, Mulvihill KK, et al. Safety and timing of nonobstetric abdominal surgery in pregnancy. Dig Surg. 2001;18(5):409-17.
16. Rizzo AG. Laparoscopic surgery in pregnancy: long-term follow-up. J Laparoendosc Adv Surg Tech A. 2003;13(1):11-5.
17. Practice/Clinical Guidelines published on 01/2011 by the Society of American Gastrointestinal and Endoscopic Surgeons (SAGES).
18. De Voe RW, Pratt JH. Simultaneous intrauterine and extrauterine pregnancy. Am J Obstet Gynecol. 1948;56(6):1119.
19. Tal J, Haddad S, Gordon N, et al. Heterotopic pregnancy after ovulation induction and assisted reproductive technologies: a literature review from 1971 to 1993. Fertil Steril. 1996;66(1):1-12.
20. Gianaroli L, Ferraretti AP, Fiorentino A. The ovarian hyperstimulation syndrome. Reproduc Med Rev. 1996;5(3):169-84.
21. Disala PJ, Creasman WT. Cancer in pregnancy. Clinical Gynecologic Oncology, 6th edition. St. Louis, MO: Mosby; Vol. 202, pp. 439-72.
22. Sophia R, Pejovic T, Nezhat F. Management of adnexal masses. Nezhat's Operative Gynecologic Laparoscopy and Hysteroscopy, 3rd edition. New York: Cambridge University Press; 2008. pp. 179-86.
23. Schmeler KM, Mayo-Smith WW, Peipert JF, et al. Adnexal masses in pregnancy: surgery compared with observation. Obstet Gynecol. 2005;105(5 Pt 1): 1098-103.
24. Zanetta G, Mariani E, Lissoni A, et al. A prospective study of the role of ultrasound in the management of adnexal masses in pregnancy. BJOG. 2003;110(6): 578-83.
25. Condous G, Khalid A, Okaro E, et al. Should we be examining the ovaries in pregnancy? Prevalence and natural history of adnexal pathology detected at first-trimester sonography. Ultrasound Obstet Gynecol. 2004;24(1):62-6.
26. ACOG Practice Bulletin. Management of adnexal masses. Obstet Gynecol. 2007;110(1):201-14.
27. Nezhat F, Nezhat C, Silfen SL, et al. Laparoscopic ovarian cystectomy during pregnancy. J Laparoendosc Surg. 1991;1(3):161-4.
28. Parker WH, Levine RL, Howard FM, et al. A multicenter study of laparoscopic management of selected cystic adnexal masses in postmenopausal women. J Am Coll Surg. 1994;179(6):733-7.
29. Tazuke SI, Nezhat FR, Nezhat CH, et al. Laparoscopic management of pelvic pathology during pregnancy. J Am Assoc Gynecol Laparosc. 1997;4(5):605-8.
30. Chung MK, Chung RP. Laparoscopic extracorporeal oophorectomy and ovarian cystectomy in second trimester pregnant obese patients. JSLS 2001;5(3): 273-7.
31. Yuen PM, Chang AM. Laparoscopic management of adnexal mass during pregnancy. Acta Obstet Gynecol Scand. 1997;76(2):173-6.
32. Loh FH, Chua SP, Khalil R, et al. Case report of ruptured endometriotic cyst in pregnancy treated by laparoscopic ovarian cystectomy. Singapore Med J. 1998;39(8):368-9.
33. Stepp KJ, Tulikangas PK, Goldberg JM, et al. Laparoscopy for adnexal masses in the second

trimester of pregnancy. J Am Assoc Gynecol Laparosc. 2003;10(1):55-9.

34. Neiswender LL, Toub DB. Laparoscopic excision of pelvic masses during pregnancy. J Am Assoc Gynecol Laparosc. 1997;4(2):269-72.
35. Yuen PM, Ng PS, Leung PL, et al. Outcome in laparoscopic management of persistent adnexal mass during the second trimester of pregnancy. Surg Endosc. 2004;18(9):1354-7.
36. Parker J, Watkins W, Robinson H, et al. Laparoscopic adnexal surgery during pregnancy: a case of heterotopic tubal pregnancy treated by laparoscopic salpingectomy. Aust N Z J Obstet Gynaecol. 1995; 35(2):208-10.
37. Moore RD, Smith WG. Laparoscopic management of adnexal masses in pregnant women. J Reprod Med. 1999;44(2):97-100.
38. Lin YH, Hwang JL, Huang LW, et al. Successful laparoscopic management of a huge ovarian tumor in the 27th week of pregnancy. A case report. J Reprod Med. 2003;48(10):834-6.
39. Mathevet P, Nessah K, Dargent D, et al. Laparoscopic management of adnexal masses in pregnancy: a case series. Eur J Obstet Gynecol Reprod Biol. 2003; 108(2):217-22.
40. Whitecar MP, Turner S, Higby MK. Adnexal masses in pregnancy: a review of 130 cases undergoing surgical management. Am J Obstet Gynecol. 1999;181(1): 19-24.
41. Bozzo M, Buscaglia M, Ferrazzi E. The management of persistent adnexal masses in pregnancy. Am J Obstet Gynecol. 1997;177(4):981-2.
42. Sherard GB, 3rd, Hodson CA, Williams HJ, et al. Adnexal masses and pregnancy: a 12-year experience. Am J Obstet Gynecol. 2003;189(2):358-62; discussion 362-3.
43. Koonings PP, Campbell DR, Mishell JR, et al. Relative frequency of primary ovarian neoplasms: a 10-year review. Obstet Gynecol. 1989;74(6):921-6.
44. Grab D, Flock F, Stohr I. Classification of asymptomatic adnexal masses by ultrasound, magnetic resonance imaging, and positron emission tomography. Gynecol Oncol. 2000;77(3):454-9.
45. Brooks SE. Preoperative evaluation of patients with suspicious ovarian cancer. Gynecol Oncol. 1994;55(3 Pt 2):80-90.
46. Jacobs I, Davies AP, Bridges J, et al. Prevalence screening for ovarian cancer in postmenopausal women by CA125 measurement and ultrasonography. BMJ. 1993;306(6884):1030-4.
47. Oguri H, Taniguchi K, Fukaya T. Gasless laparoscopic management of ovarian cysts during pregnancy. Int J Gynaecol Obstet. 2005;91:258-9.
48. Iafrati MD, Yarnell R, Schwaitzberg SD. Gasless laparoscopic cholecystectomy in pregnancy. J Laparoendosc Surg. 1995;5(2):127-30.
49. Hume RF, Killiam AP. Maternal physiology. In: Scott JR, KiSaia J, Hammon DB (Eds), Obstetrics and Gynecology. Philadelphia, PA: Lippincott; 1990. pp. 93-100.
50. Guidelines for laparoscopic surgery during pregnancy. Society of American Gastrointestinal Endo-scopic Surgeons (SAGES). Surg Endosc. 1998;12(2):189-90.
51. Reedy MB, Kallen B, Kuehl TJ. Laparoscopy during pregnancy: a study of five fetal outcome parameters with use of the Swedish Health Registry. Am J Obstet Gynecol. 1997;177(3):673-9.
52. Jelin EB, Smink DS, Vernon AH, et al. Management of biliary tract disease during pregnancy: a decision analysis. Surg Endosc. 2008;22(1):54-60.
53. Graham G, Baxi L, Tharakan T. Laparoscopic cholecystectomy during pregnancy: a case series and review of the literature. Obstet Gynecol Surg. 1998; 53(9):566-74.
54. Dorum A, Blom GP, Ekerhovd E, et al. Prevalence and histologic diagnosis of adnexal cysts in post-menopausal women: an autopsy study. Am J Obstet Gynecol. 2005;192(1):48-54.
55. Sassone A, Timor-Tritch I, Artner A, et al. Transvaginal sonographic characterization of ovarian disease: evaluation of a new scoring system to predict ovarian malignancy. Obstet Gynecol. 1991;78:7-11.
56. Shalev E, Eliyahu S, Peleg D, et al. Laparoscopic management of adnexal cystic masses in post-menopausal women. Obstet Gynecol. 1994;83(4): 594-6.
57. Korndorffer JR Jr, Fellinger E, Reed W. SAGES guideline for laparoscopic appendectomy. Surg Endosc. 2010;24(4):757-61.
58. Affleck DG, Handrahan DL, Egger MJ. The laparo-scopic management of appendicitis and cholelithiasis during pregnancy. Am J Surg. 1999;178(6):523-9.
59. Rollins MD, Chan KJ, Price RR. Laparoscopy for appendicitis and cholelithiasis during pregnancy: a new standard of care. Surg Endosc. 2004;18(2): 237-41.
60. Schwartzberg BS, Conyers JA, Moore JA. First trimester of pregnancy laparoscopic procedures. Surg Endosc. 1997;11(12):1216-7.
61. Thomas SJ, Brisson P. Laparoscopic appendectomy and cholecystectomy during pregnancy: six case reports. JSLS 1998;2(1):41-6.
62. Barnes SL, Shane MD, Schoemann MB, et al. Laparoscopic appendectomy after 30 weeks pregnancy: report of two cases and description of technique. Am Surg. 2004;70(8):733-6.
63. de Perrot M, Jenny A, Morales M, et al. Laparoscopic appendectomy during pregnancy. Surg Laparosc Endosc Percutan Tech. 2000;10(6):368-71.
64. Schreiber JH. Laparoscopic appendectomy in pregnancy. Surg Endosc. 1990;4(2):100-2.
65. Sadot E, Telem DA, Arora M, et al. Laparoscopy: a safe approach to appendicitis during pregnancy. Surg Endosc. 2010;24(2):383-9.
66. Lemieux P, Rheaume P, Levesque I, et al. Laparoscopic appendectomy in pregnant patients: a review of 45 cases. Surg Endosc. 2009;23(8):1701-5.
67. McKellar DP, Anderson CT, Boynton CJ, et al. Cholecystectomy during pregnancy without fetal loss. Surg Gynecol Obstet. 1992;174(6):465-8.
68. McKenna DA, Meehan CP, Alhajeri AN, et al. The use of MRI to demonstrate small bowel obstruction

during pregnancy. Br J Radiol. 2007;80(949): e11-4.
69. Barone JE, Bears S, Chen S, et al. Outcome study of cholecystectomy during pregnancy. Am J Surg. 1999;177(3):232-6.
70. Alcazar JL, Jurado M. Prospective evaluation of a logistic model based on sonographic morphologic and color Doppler findings developed to predict adnexal malignancy. J Ultrasound Med. 1999;18(12): 837-43.
71. Fatum M, Rojansky N. Laparoscopic surgery during pregnancy. Obstet Gynecol Surg. 2001;56(1):50-9.
72. Dottino PR, Levine DA, Ripley DL, et al. Laparoscopic management of adnexal masses in premenopausal and postmenopausal women. Obstet Gynecol. 1999;93(2):223-8.
73. Davison J, Park W, Penney L. Comparative study of operative laparoscopy vs. laparotomy: analysis of financial impact. J Reprod Med. 1993;38(5):357-60.
74. Ehren IM, Mahour GH, Isaacs H. Benign and malignant ovarian tumors in children and adolescents. A review of 63 cases. Cancer. 1984;147(3):339-43.
75. Mais V, Ajossa S, Piras B, et al. Treatment of nonendometriotic benign adnexal cyst. A randomized trial to evaluate benefits in early outcome. Am J Obstet Gynecol. 1996;174(2):654-8.
76. Curtin JP. Management of the adnexal mass. Gynecol Oncol. 1994;55(3 Pt 2):S42-6.
77. Sachs A, Guglielminotti J, Miller R, et al. Risk factors and risk stratification for adverse obstetrical outcomes after appendectomy or cholecystectomy during pregnancy. JAMA Surg. 2017;152(5):436-41.

KIEL SCHOOL

19 of Gynaecological Endoscopy

Extragenital Findings in Gynecological Laparoscopy

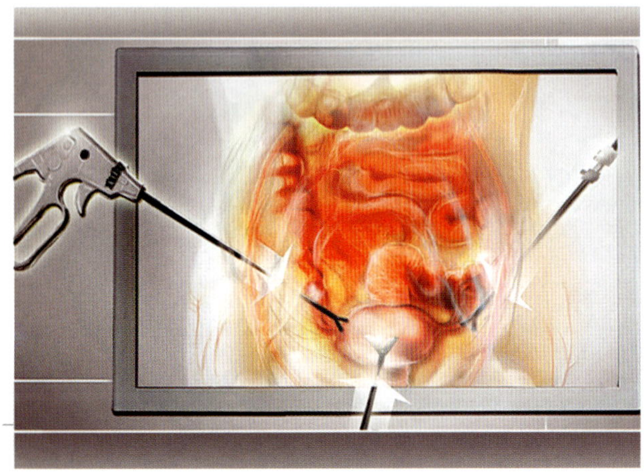

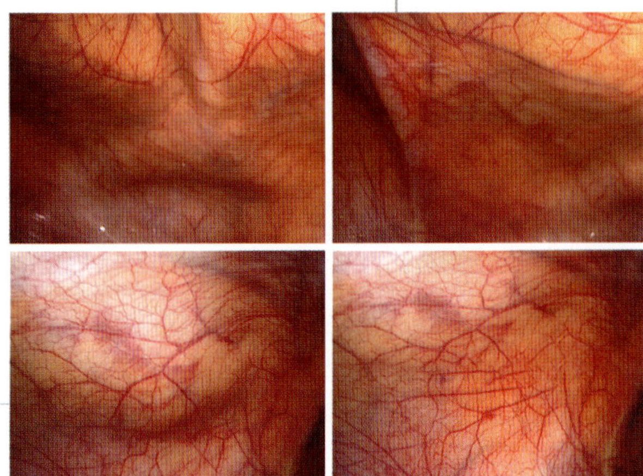

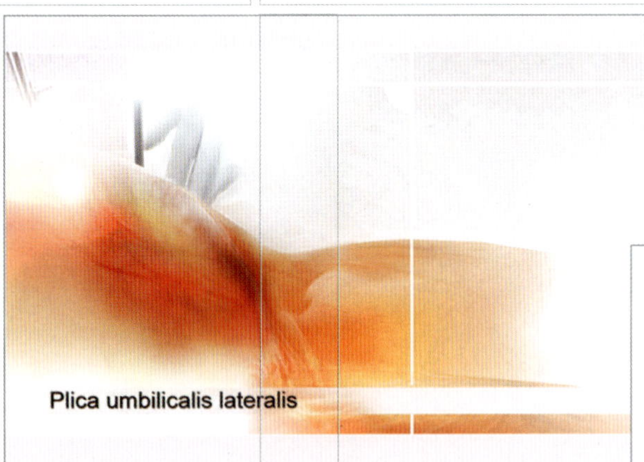

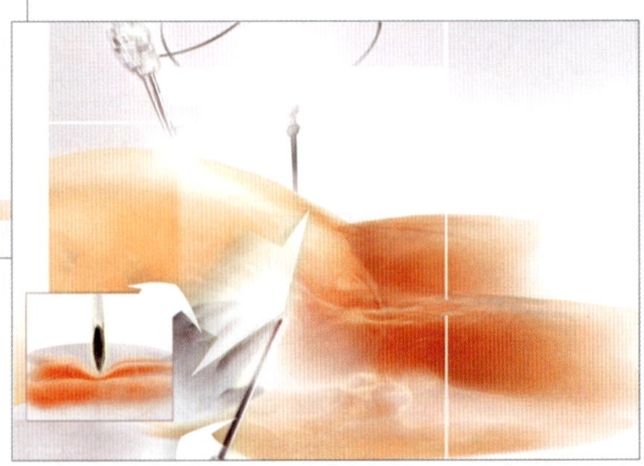

Chapter 19

Extragenital Findings in Gynecological Laparoscopy

Ibrahim Alkatout, Frederike Egberts, Manfred Schollmeyer, Liselotte Mettler

INTRODUCTION

Although the anatomy of the human being has not changed, technical developments in operating materials and methods demand a simultaneous development in operative management. Developments in electronic and optical technologies permit many gynecological operations to be performed laparoscopically. One fundamental distinction between any other operating method and laparoscopy is the hurdle that the initial entry, whether with a needle, cannula, or trocar, is mostly performed as a blind entry. Blind entry may result in vascular or organ damage. One of the difficulties associated with entry complications is that any damage may not be immediately recognized, leading to major abdominal reparative surgery and at worst a temporary colostomy. Therefore, the technical and operative quality of laparoscopic surgery begins with port placement and trocars. Visual access systems are available but are not yet widely used.

Against the backdrop of the rapid development in endoscopic instruments, equipment, optic systems and documentation techniques, the story of laparoscopy in the last decade is characterized by its change from a diagnostic to an operative procedure. This development has been accompanied by the improvement of laparoscopic skills and its use in almost every operating unit. The further development of laparoscopic operative methods which started in the 1980s, particularly in oncology, has unfortunately curbed interest in comprehensive intra-abdominal laparoscopic diagnosis and its interdisciplinary value. Moreover, the continuous specialization of operating units inhibits the simple interdisciplinary contact and reciprocal demonstration of suspect intraoperative findings. It also has to be kept in mind that medical politics with, e.g., special settlements makes friendly cooperation through unofficial channels nearly impossible.

In contrast to laparotomy, where the mid and upper abdomen cannot be significantly assessed by the Pfannenstiel incision or by a lower abdominal median incision, with the laparoscope, under optimal anesthesia and positioning and use of optical magnification, it is possible to display the genital and intra-abdominal organs very well. The live demonstration of the findings is of particular value to the internists and visceral surgeons. A video or still picture documentation should be a matter of course. Furthermore, training and education is possible for those attending the operation and through later discourse of the crucial pictures.

The aim of this chapter is to introduce physiological anatomical regions that do not belong directly to the gynecological field. Furthermore, extragenital pathologies are mentioned that should be thought of and dealt with by gynecological surgeons.

STEP 1

Preoperative Assessment

Patients undergoing a laparoscopic procedure should be informed of the risks and potential complications as well as the alternative operating methods. Counseling before laparoscopy should include discussion of the entry technique used and the different risks associated with laparoscopic entry: injury of the bowel, urinary tract, blood vessels, omentum and other surrounding organs and, at a later date, wound infection, adhesion-associated pain, and hernia formation. Counseling should also integrate the intraoperative procedure once extragenital pathologies are found.

Counseling needs to integrate the individual risk dependent on the body mass index (BMI) and obesity or significant underweight of the patient. Depending on the medical history, it is important to consider anatomical malformations, midline abdominal incisions, a history of peritonitis or inflammatory bowel disease.[1]

STEP 2

Preoperative Relevant Skin Findings

Before the gynecological operative procedure begins, the whole body of the patient needs to be inspected carefully. This can either be done during preoperative diagnostics or more discreetly while the patient is narcotized. The whole body is examined closely for physiological and pathological findings. All pathological or suspect skin findings must be demonstrated to a dermatologist, whenever available. Detailed and extensive counseling before surgery allows the surgeon to take biopsies or even perform skin surgery simultaneously in one narcosis procedure. If a dermatologist is not available, careful photo documentation is necessary.

Most incidental skin findings appear to be multiple and are of benign origin. Nevertheless, some can transform into cutaneous carcinoma if left untreated. Others are already malignant when diagnosed and need a complex and heterogeneous treatment. The definite treatment indication can only be performed by an experienced dermatologist. All nondermatologists can only generate a delicate sense for extra-ordinary and possibly even dangerous skin lesions (Figs. 19.1 to 19.8).

Dependent on the patient's history, e.g., previous operations and/or chronic diseases, skin lesions can be residual or new and responsible for the patient's symptoms or determine the patient's prognosis (Figs. 19.9 to 19.12).

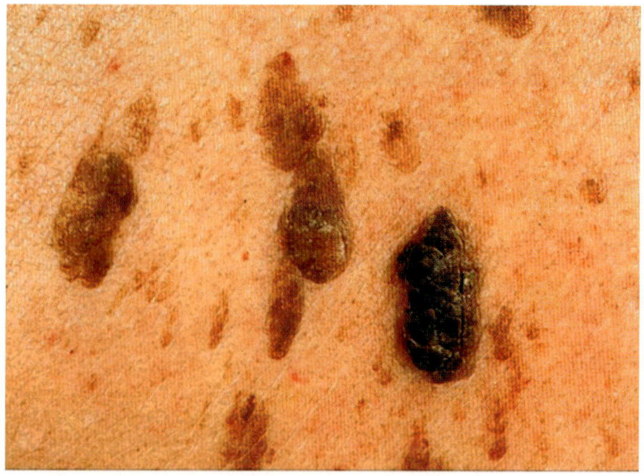

Fig. 19.1: Seborrheic keratoses (senile warts, basal cell papillomas) often multiple, benign lesions.
Clinical appearance: Sharply demarcated, gray to dark brown, hyperkeratotic macules and plaques, sometimes covered with greasy scales, mainly on the chest wall, interscapular region, and forehead. Sometimes arranged along lines of cleavage or in a linear "raindrop" pattern.

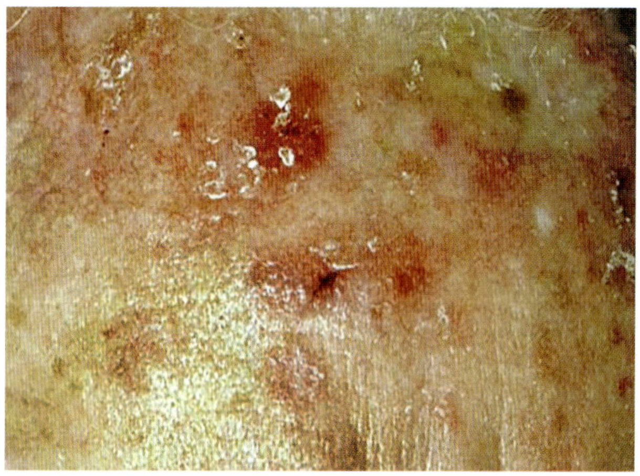

Fig. 19.2: Actinic keratoses (solar keratoses).
Keratinocytic intraepidermal neoplasia, 8–20% can transform into cutaneous squamous cell carcinoma (cSCC) if left untreated.
Clinical appearance: Often multiple, poorly circumscribed scaly erythematous lesions on sun-exposed skin of elderly patients.

STEP 3

Extra-abdominal Relevant Anatomy

The anterior abdominal wall has four muscles, which are penetrated at all entries: rectus abdominis, external obliquus abdominis, internal obliquus abdominis, and transversus abdominis. At laparotomy the incision possibilities are transversal with the conventional "Pfannenstiel" incision in the lower abdomen, a little higher the fascial opening called "Misgav Ladach cesarean section incision" and the longitudinal incision up to the umbilicus or around it.

Although at laparoscopy the penetrating areas are variable, the normal trocar placement uses similar inserting areas. Therefore, it is obligatory for any surgeon to be experienced in the anatomy of the abdominal wall and its consecutive relevant anatomical structures.

There are no significant vascular structures that need to be respected on insertion of the subumbili-

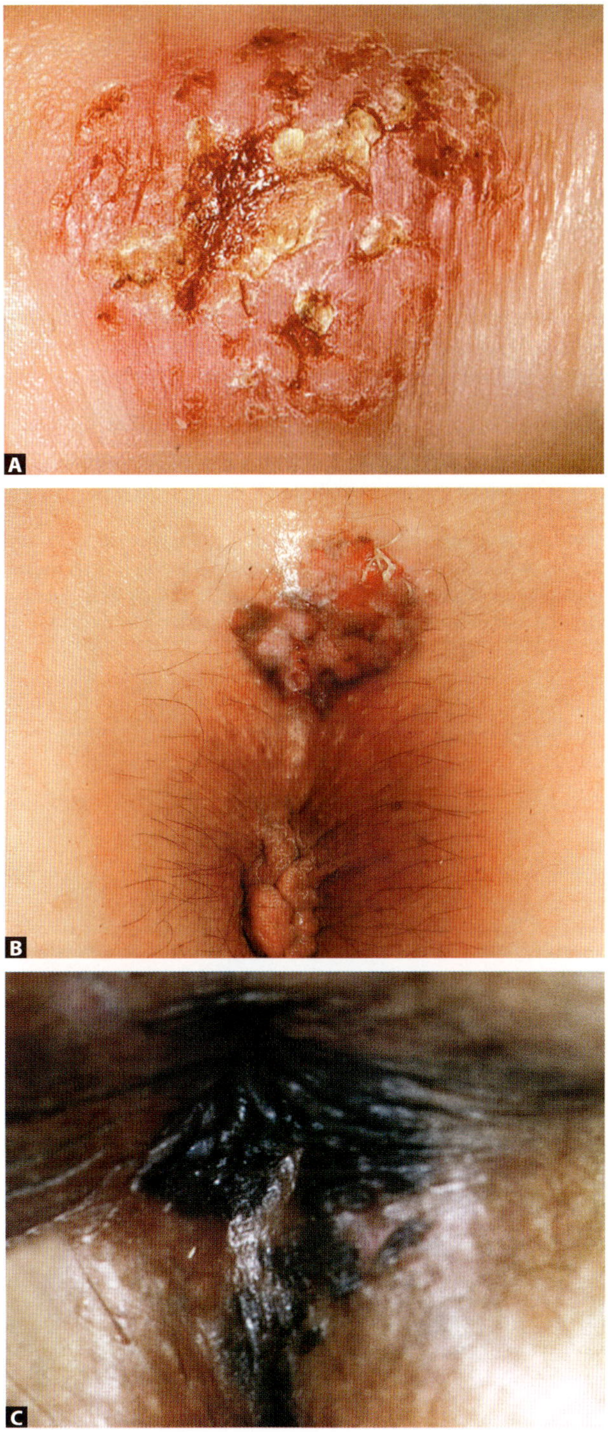

Figs. 19.3A to C: Bowen's disease.
Clinical variant of intraepidermal squamous cell carcinoma (SCC in situ) with distinct histopathologic changes.
Clinical appearance:
(A) Well-circumscribed erythematous scaly plaque, sometimes nodular or eroded variants.
(B) Pigmented variant in the anogenital area.
(C) Bowenoid papulosis. Mainly multiple, brownish macules and plaques with verrucous appearance in the genital area with close histological resemblance to Bowen's disease (vulvar lesions often bilateral and pigmented). Most cases are related to HPV-16 and -18.

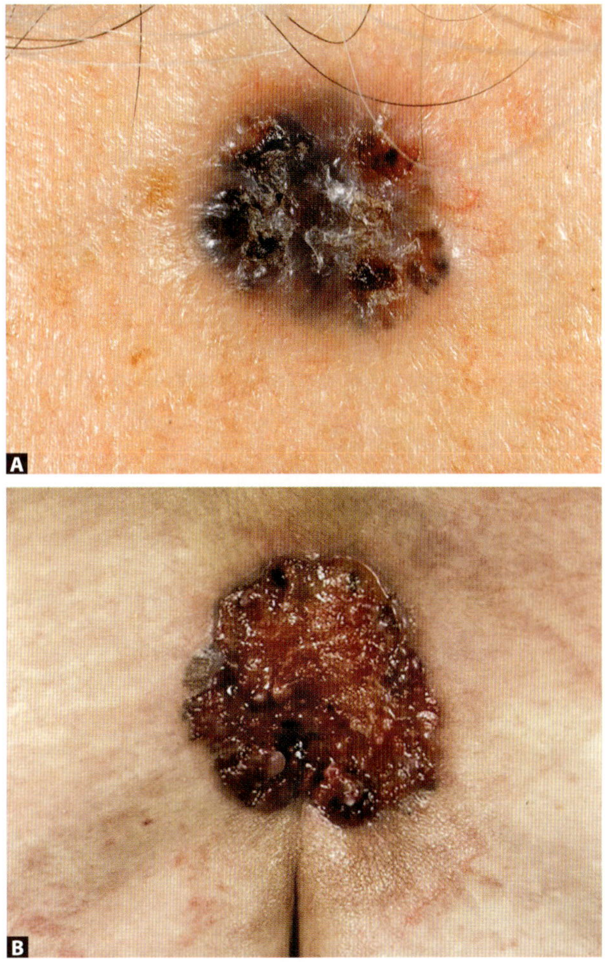

Figs. 19.4A and B: Basal cell carcinoma (BCC).
Most common malignant tumor in Caucasians, increasing incidence, accounts for more than 90% of all skin malignancies.
Clinical appearance: Mainly on sun-exposed skin of elderly patients (80% head and neck, 15% shoulders/chest, 5% others). Erythematous, sometimes pigmented (A), papulonodular plaques with telangiectasias and an ulcerated central part. *Clinical variants:* Solid, cystic, superficial, infiltrating (morpheic) type.

cal trocar. Solely, strict attention has to be given to holding to the median line to avoid any accidental damage to paramedian structures.

There are two arteries in the superficial abdominal wall that should be visualized. Damage to these arteries should be avoided as even superficial incisions can lead to severe bleedings that require the conversion from laparoscopy to laparotomy. Both vessels can be visualized by diaphanoscopy (Fig. 19.13). Trocar placement is performed, dependent on the corresponding internal site, at a 90 degrees angle to the abdominal wall once the aiming point has been located. The superficial epigastric artery arises from the femoral artery about 1 cm below the inguinal ligament through the fascia cribrosa,

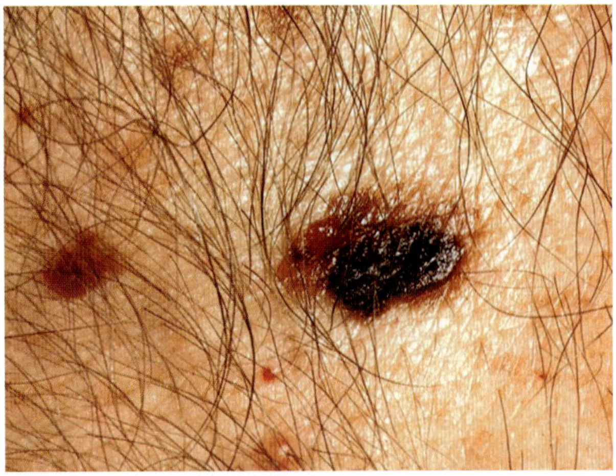

Fig. 19.5: Malignant melanoma (MM) in a patient with "dysplastic (atypic) nevus syndrome."
Third most common malignant skin tumor in Caucasians with increasing incidence worldwide.
Clinical appearance: Poorly circumscribed, asymmetric light-brown to black plaque and an erythematous, eroded nodule in the left upper part (secondary nodular superficial spreading melanoma) found in a patient with multiple asymmetric, multicolored nevi.

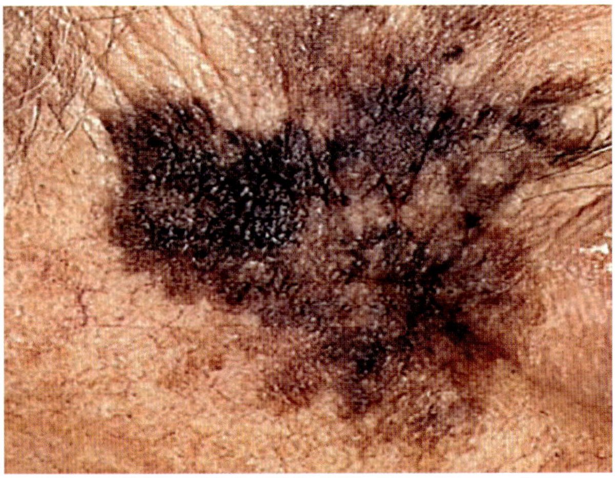

Fig. 19.6: Lentigo malignant melanoma.
Variant of malignant melanoma with clinically and histopathologically distinct features.
Clinical appearance: Most commonly on the face and sun-exposed skin of elderly patients. Poorly circumscribed, asymmetric, brown to black macule, which expands centrifugally.

turns upward in front of the inguinal ligament, and ascends while spreading out between the two layers of the superficial fascia of the abdominal wall, nearly as far as the umbilicus. The circumflex iliac superficial artery originates from the femoral artery close to the superficial epigastric artery. After perforating the fascia lata it runs parallel to the inguinal ligament and laterally to the iliac crest while spreading into smaller branches.

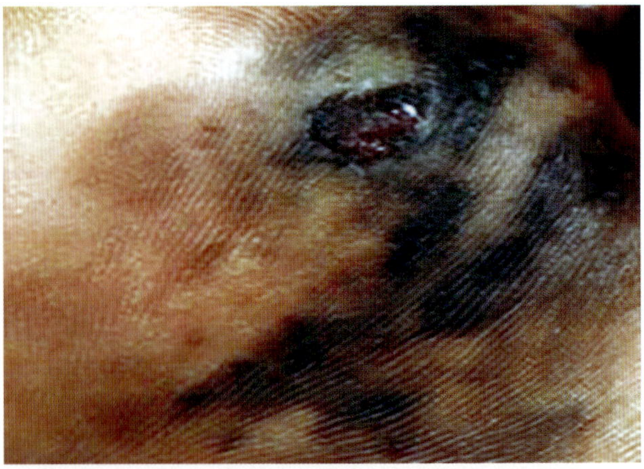

Fig. 19.7: Acral lentiginous malignant melanoma (ALM).
Malignant melanoma developing on palmar, plantar, and subungual skin.
Clinical appearance: Poorly circumscribed, asymmetric, brown to black plaque, sometimes nodular or eroded. Subungual melanomas often present as an amelanotic variant or as a longitudinal melanonychia (melanonychia striata).

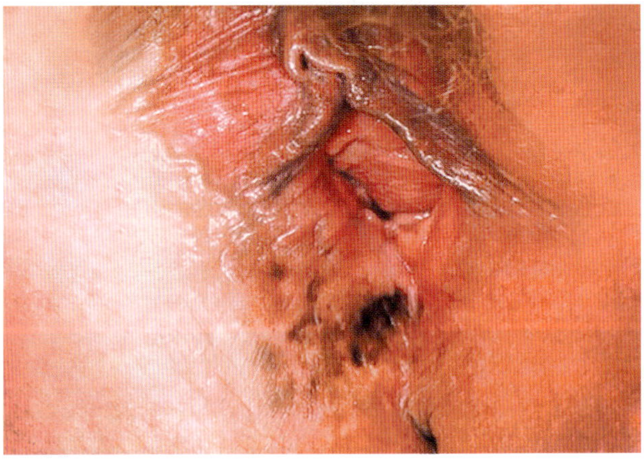

Fig. 19.8: Vulvar melanoma.
Can develop on the basis of a benign labial lentigo. Clinically aggressive type of malignant melanoma.
Clinical appearance: Poorly circumscribed, asymmetric, brown to black macule, which expands centrifugally.

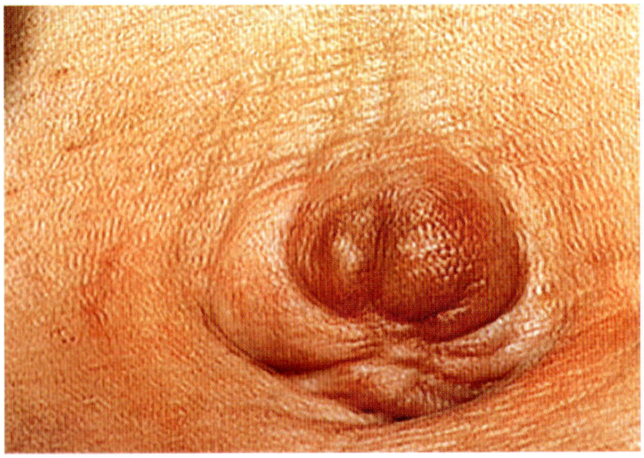

Fig. 19.9: Endometriosis extragenitalis in the umbilicus. This patient had previously undergone endometriosis resection by laparoscopy.

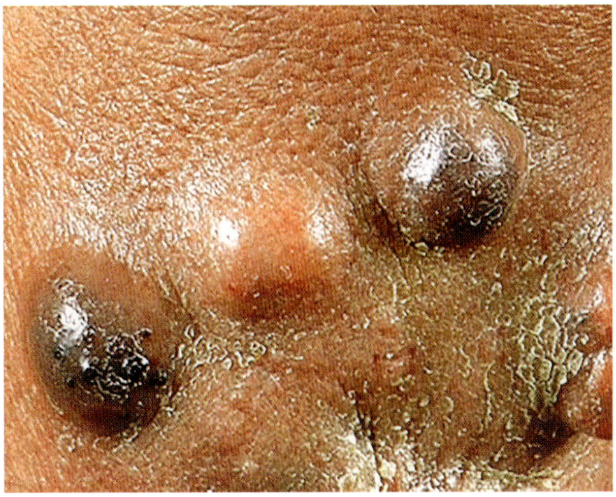

Fig. 19.10: Skin metastasis of the thorax after breast cancer.

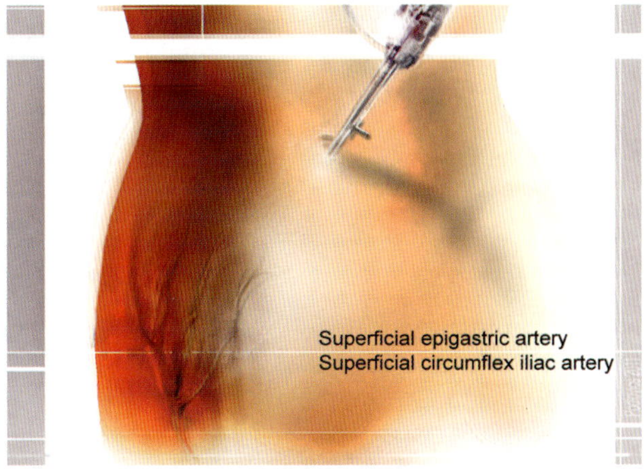

Fig. 19.13: Diaphanoscopy illuminates the region of insertion of the ancillary trocars while demarcating the superficial epigastric artery and the circumflex iliac superficial artery.

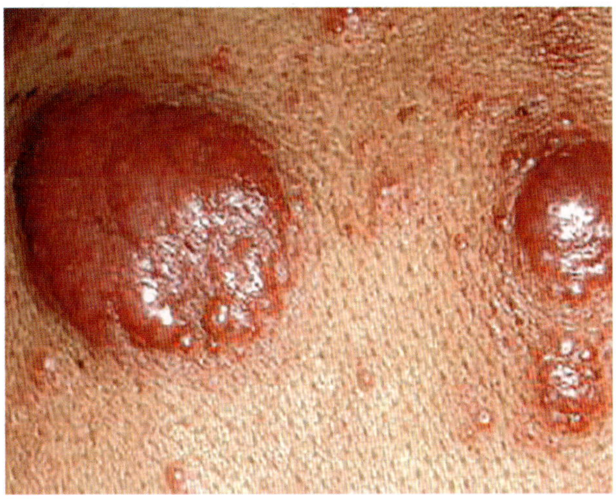

Fig. 19.11: Primary cutaneous follicular B-cell lymphoma. Papules and nodules of the lower leg.

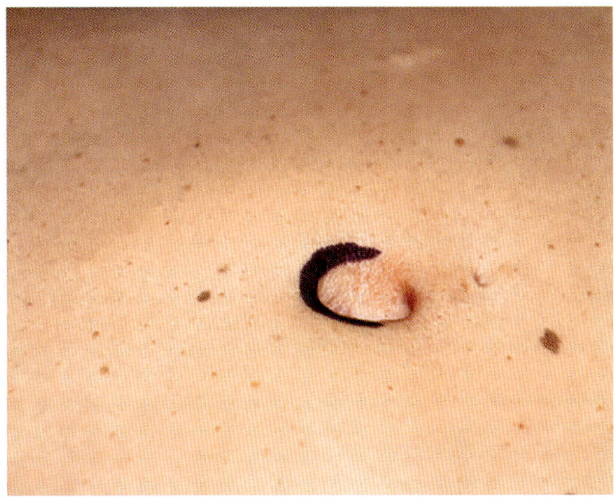

Fig. 19.14: Subumbilical incision and local palpation demonstrate the short distance from the skin to the spine. The retroperitoneal vessels are visible.

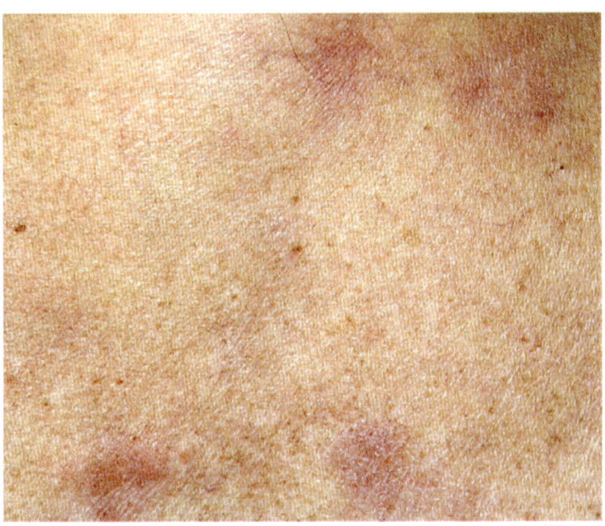

Fig. 19.12: Primary cutaneous T-cell lymphoma of the back. Can easily be overseen if not suspected and not examined carefully.

Places for Trocar Insertion

The laparoscope and optic trocar should be inserted, whenever possible, in the subumbilical region using a semilunar or straight incision (Fig. 19.14). Only if trocar placement is not possible, due to severe adhesions or large intra-abdominal tumors, are alternative entry sites negotiated, e.g., above the umbilicus or Palmer's point (Figs. 19.15A and B) as a precursor entry site.

Subcostal Insufflation Technique (Palmer's Point)

For all patients with a significantly increased risk for adhesions, with a history of abdominal surgery including cesarean section, a large fibroid uterus, an umbilical hernia, large ovarian cysts, preperi-

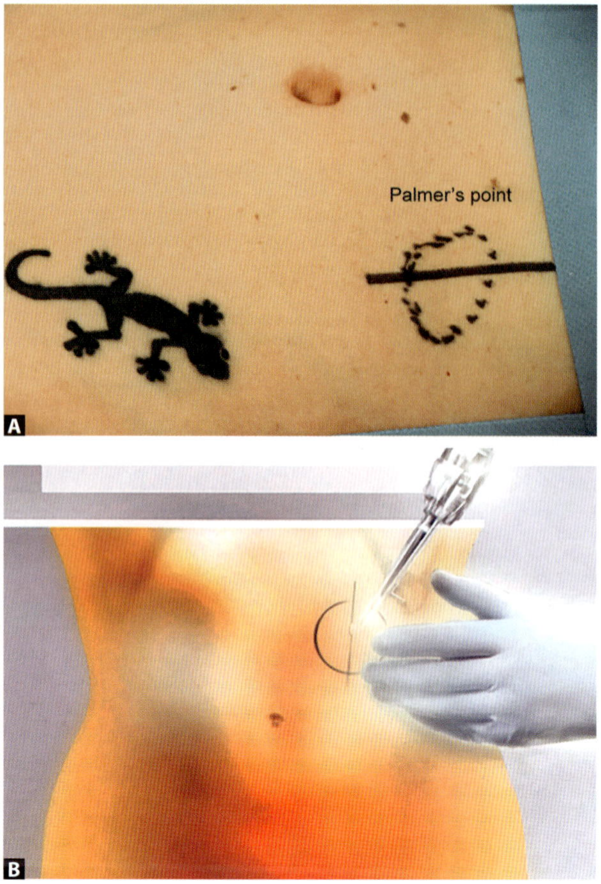

Figs. 19.15A and B: (A) Palmer's point is situated in the midclavicular line about 3 cm below the costal margin; (B) Palmer's Point is situated in the midclavicular line about 3 cm below the costal margin.

toneal gas insufflation, or failed umbilical entry, Palmer described in 1974 an abdominal entry point in the midclavicular line about 3 cm below the costal margin. Palmer's point can be used for Veress needle entry as well as for small trocars. No entry technique can completely eliminate the risk of entry-related injury of the vascular, intestinal, and urinary tract and gas embolism. Palmer's point is the safest laparoscopic entry point as this place is known to be the least likely to be affected by adhesions (Figs. 19.15A and B).

The left upper quadrant is easily accessible and is mostly free of intra-abdominal adhesions. The rigid rib cage provides high tension and prevents the downward placement of the abdominal wall.

Indications for the use of Palmer's point are:

- after two failed attempts of subumbilical insufflation;
- primarily in selected very obese patients;
- primarily in selected patients with previous abdominal surgeries and suspicion of intra-abdominal adhesions; and
- in patients with previous longitudinal abdominal incisions.

When using this entry site, there is the risk of puncture of the left lobe of the liver, the spleen, the stomach, and the transverse colon although this can be prevented by inserting the needle at an angle slightly less than 90°. Creating a subcutaneous emphysema is awkward as the insertion is straight and unambiguous.

Any auxiliary trocar can be placed in the midline suprasymphysically.

STEP 4

Intra-abdominal Relevant Anatomy through the Eye of the Trocar

Before any additional trocar to the optic trocar is inserted, the area of insertion has to be examined carefully with the laparoscope. Assuming a standard operation, the placement of two additional working trocars in the lower abdomen alongside an auxiliary trocar in the midline can be performed. Apart from the obliterated urachus and the bladder in the lower region, no remarkable anatomical structures are to be found (Fig. 19.16A).

It is important to identify the different landmarks of the abdominal wall (Fig. 19.16B). Beginning in the midline, the plica umbilicalis mediana contains the obliterated urachus and requires no further attention besides a hoisted bladder, e.g., after cesarean section. Moving laterally, the paired plica umbilicalis medialis contains the obliterated umbilicalis artery in the medial umbilical ligamentum that carries fetal blood through the umbilical cord to the placenta before it obliterates after birth and is therefore hazard-free, too. The next step leads to the plica umbilicalis lateralis with the integrated vasa epigastrica inferiors. The inferior epigastric artery originates at the inguinal ligament of the external iliac artery. It cuts along the subperitoneal tissue ventrally and then moves upwards oblique—alongside the medial edge of the annulus inguinalis profundus. Afterward, it perforates the fascia of the musculus transversus abdominis and climbs upward between the musculus rectus abdominis and the rectus wall, thereby moving ventrally of the linea arcuata. Above the umbilicus it divides into many small branches that anastomose with the superior epigastric artery. In contrast to the superficially spreading vascular branches, the inferior epigastric artery cannot be visualized by diaphanoscopy.

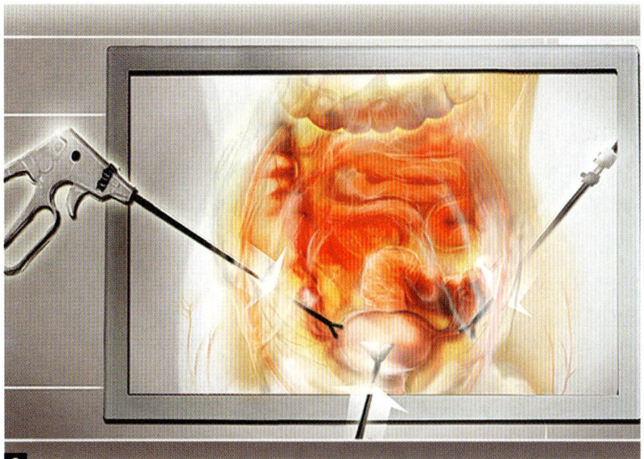

A

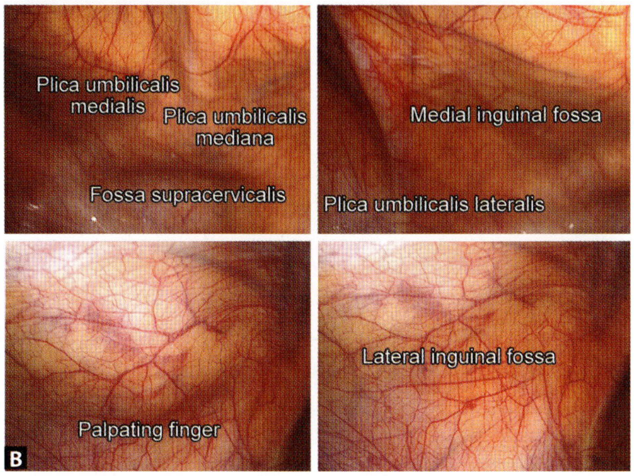

B

Figs. 19.16A and B: (A) Overview after insertion of the laparoscope and 3 ancillary trocars; (B) Abdominal wall inside view demonstrating the plica umbilicalis lateralis containing the epigastric vessels. The point of insertion needs to be lateral to this structure.

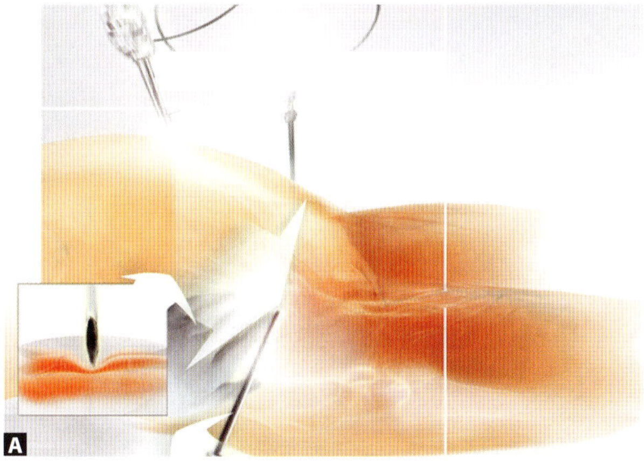

A

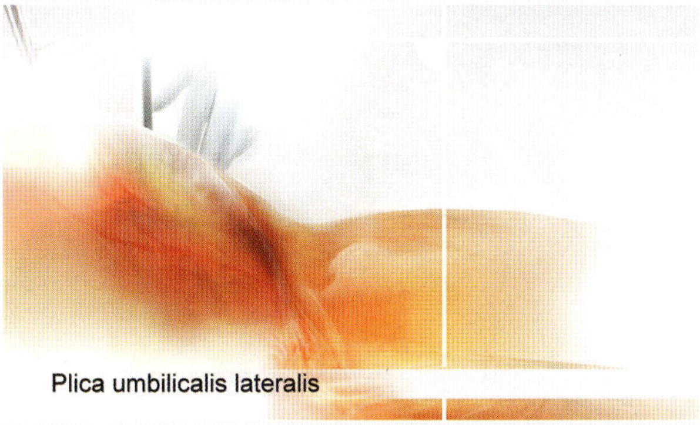

B

Figs. 19.17A and B: (A) Abdominal wall inside view demonstrating the plica umbilicalis lateralis containing the epigastric vessels. The point of insertion needs to be lateral to this structure.; (B) Abdominal wall inside view demonstrating the plica umbilicalis lateralis containing the epigastric vessels. The point of insertion needs to be lateral to this structure.

Places for Trocar Insertion

Once the cutaneous region has been determined from the outside with the aid of diaphanoscopy, the safe distance to the plica umbilicalis lateralis can be verified by palpation (Figs. 19.17A and B). The correct point of insertion is usually about two thumbs medial of the spina iliac anterior superior (Fig. 19.18). Being distant to the plica, the trocar is placed at a 90 degrees angle and pushed forward until the tip of the trocar can be seen with the laparoscope (Figs. 19.19A and B).

STEP 5

Risk Management

Abdominal access and the creation of a pneumoperitoneum carry a significant risk of bowel injuries. Such injuries are more frequent in laparoscopic surgery and are often avoided in open surgery. Although these injuries are uncommon, they represent a major reason for mortality from laparoscopic procedures, and a significant source of the morbidity associated with any laparoscopic procedure.

Many intraoperative bowel lesions can be sutured; a partial excision and suturing as well as resections of lacerated areas can be necessary, including end-to-end anastomosis and temporary ileostomy. Unlike major vascular injuries where the risk and presentation are immediate, many bowel injuries go unrecognized at the time of the procedure. Consequently, patients present postoperatively, often after discharge, with specific or unspecific symptoms of peritonitis. Persistent pyrexia, tachycardia, or ileus in the postoperative period should raise the index of suspicion for bowel injuries. This delay makes it a significant cause of morbidity and mortality.

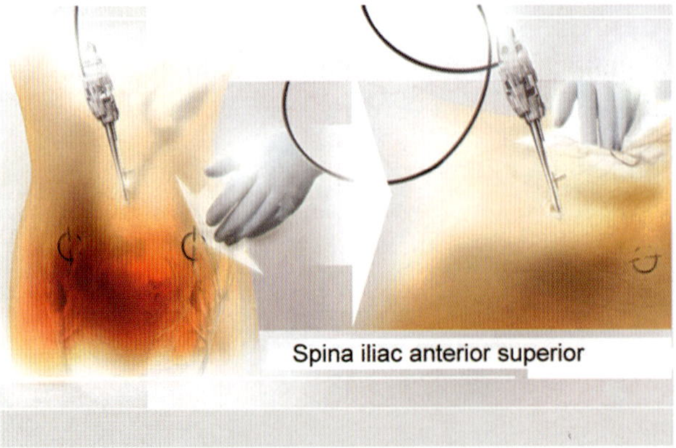

Fig. 19.18: Point of insertion from the outside (two thumbs medial of the anterior superior spine), at a 90° angle to the surface with penetration of all abdominal wall layers.

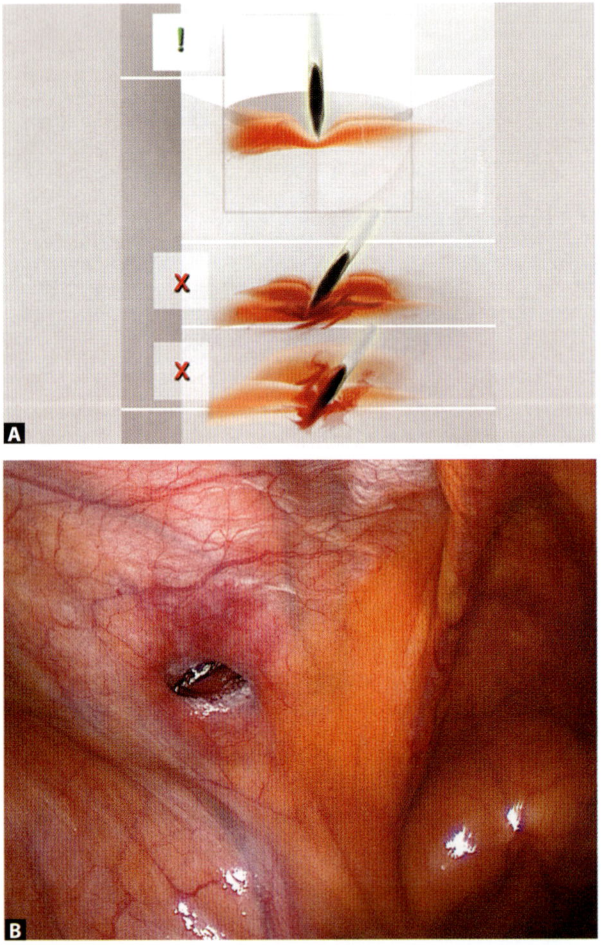

Figs. 19.19A and B: (A) Trocar insertion site lateral to the plica umbilicalis lateralis; (B) Trocar insertion site lateral to the plica umbilicalis lateralis.

The experience of the surgeon is an important factor in the overall complication rate and in the incidence of intestinal injury. A sound knowledge of laparoscopic anatomy is essential to understand the distorted anatomy often present in the disease. Failure to keep to tissue planes, blunt dissection, diathermy in close proximity to the intestine, excessive traction, and poor visualization account for most injuries. Previous surgery, endometriosis, chronic pelvic inflammatory disease, malignancy, or radiotherapy may distort anatomy and obliterate tissue planes. Bowel preparation is no longer advisable before major pelvic surgery.

Injuries with healthy edges can be repaired primarily using tension-free, single-layer, interrupted sero-submucosal 3-0 vicryl or 4-0 PDS sutures. For more extensive injuries, resection and primary anastomoses are required.

STEP 6

Preoperative Management

Diagnostic laparoscopy and simultaneously operative pelviscopy is the gold standard for a number of gynecological, urological, general surgical, and interdisciplinary operations. It is prompt, minimally invasive, takes less operative time, has a lower blood loss, is cost-effective, is associated with a reduced hospital stay, a limited postoperative analgesia requirement, a lower risk of adhesions, a better visualization of the operative field and has no medical side effects. Even hemodynamic instability is not an absolute contraindication to primary laparoscopy.[2-6]

Instrumentation

Box 19.1 provides a detailed list of all instruments that are necessary or at least desirable for laparoscopic treatment.

Box 19.1: Instruments necessary for operating on expected ectopic pregnancy.

Laparoscope, diameter 5 or 10 mm	Atraumatic grasping forceps
Video camera	Scissors
Microprocessor-controlled insufflations system	Suction and irrigation system
Electrosurgical unit	Monopolar hook electrode
Xenon cold light source	Bipolar forceps
Trocars, diameter 6 or 11 mm	Disposable extraction bag
Veress needle	Uterine manipulator

STEP 7

General Operative Beginning

After creating a pneumoperitoneum, a 5 mm and after dilatation an 11 mm optic trocar is introduced into the abdominal cavity through an umbilical Z-track incision using a conical trocar. Two 5-mm instrument trocars are introduced through small left and right lateral suprapubic incisions. In cases of severe hemoperitoneum the Veress needle is placed into the accumulation of blood. Therefore, a higher initial insufflation pressure might be of advantage since the tip of the needle may be immersed in blood.[7-9]

STEP 8

Intraoperative Management

For diagnostic purposes, it is recommended to proceed in a systematic way and to evaluate the findings in the mid and upper abdomen before examining the lower pelvis. After creating the pneumoperitoneum and insertion of the optic trocar subject to precautionary measures, a panoramic viewing is carried out to exclude any injury by the Veress needle or trocar. Attention must be paid to free blood, intestinal secretions or retroperitoneal hematoma. Similarly, suspected umbilical adhesions in this area are to be immediately assessed, if necessary by suprapubic access.

During diagnosis, due to the created pneumoperitoneum, attention is first drawn to very impressive adhesions of different genesis and localization. The greater omentum, ileum, and the colon are particularly affected. These adhesions are mostly found in patients with a history of previous abdominal surgery, after intra-abdominal infections and also after blunt abdominal trauma (Figs. 19.20A to C).

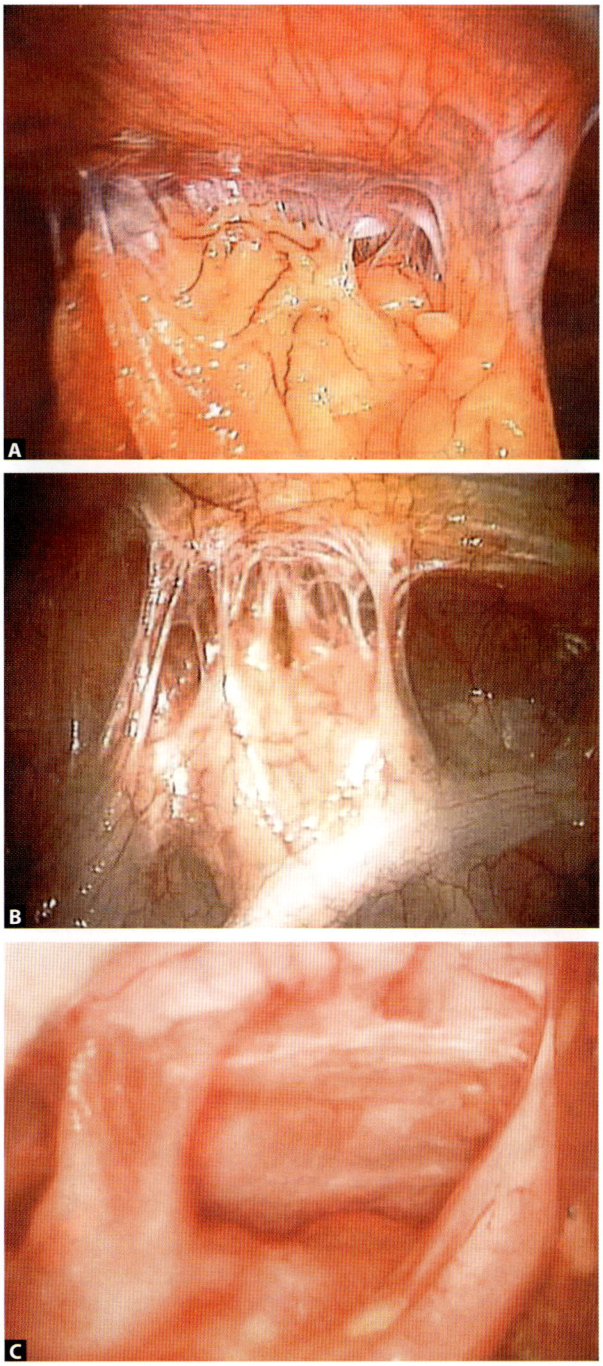

Figs. 19.20A to C: (A) Adhesions between the greater omentum and the appendectomy scar; (B) Adhesions between the ascending colon and the appendectomy scar; (C) Adhesions between the ileum and the anterior abdominal wall after peritonitis.

Further laparoscopic diagnosis should include examination of the vermiform appendix (Figs. 19.21A to F), cecum, colon (Fig. 19.22) and ileum (Fig. 19.23). Even with a previous history of appendectomy it is advisable to inspect the operated ileocecal region (Figs. 19.24A and B).

The inspection of gallbladder and liver follows and often yields pathological findings unsuspected till then. Anatomical anomalies (Fig. 19.25), asymptomatic cholelithiasis (Fig. 19.26), focal nodal hyperplasia (Figs. 19.27A and B), adenomas (Fig. 19.28), hemangiomas (Fig. 19.29), abscesses (Figs. 19.30A and B) and cysts of the liver (Figs. 19.31A to C) as well as primary carcinoma of liver (Fig. 19.32) or liver metastasis are very easy to diagnose (Figs. 19.33A and B). Systemic disorders, such as steatosis hepatitis (Figs. 19.34A to D) or cirrhosis (Fig. 19.35), can also be recognized easily. Adhesions of the liver and diaphragm give the impression, in a sense, of past perihepatitis as a possible consequence of gonococcal or chlamydial infection (Fig. 19.36).

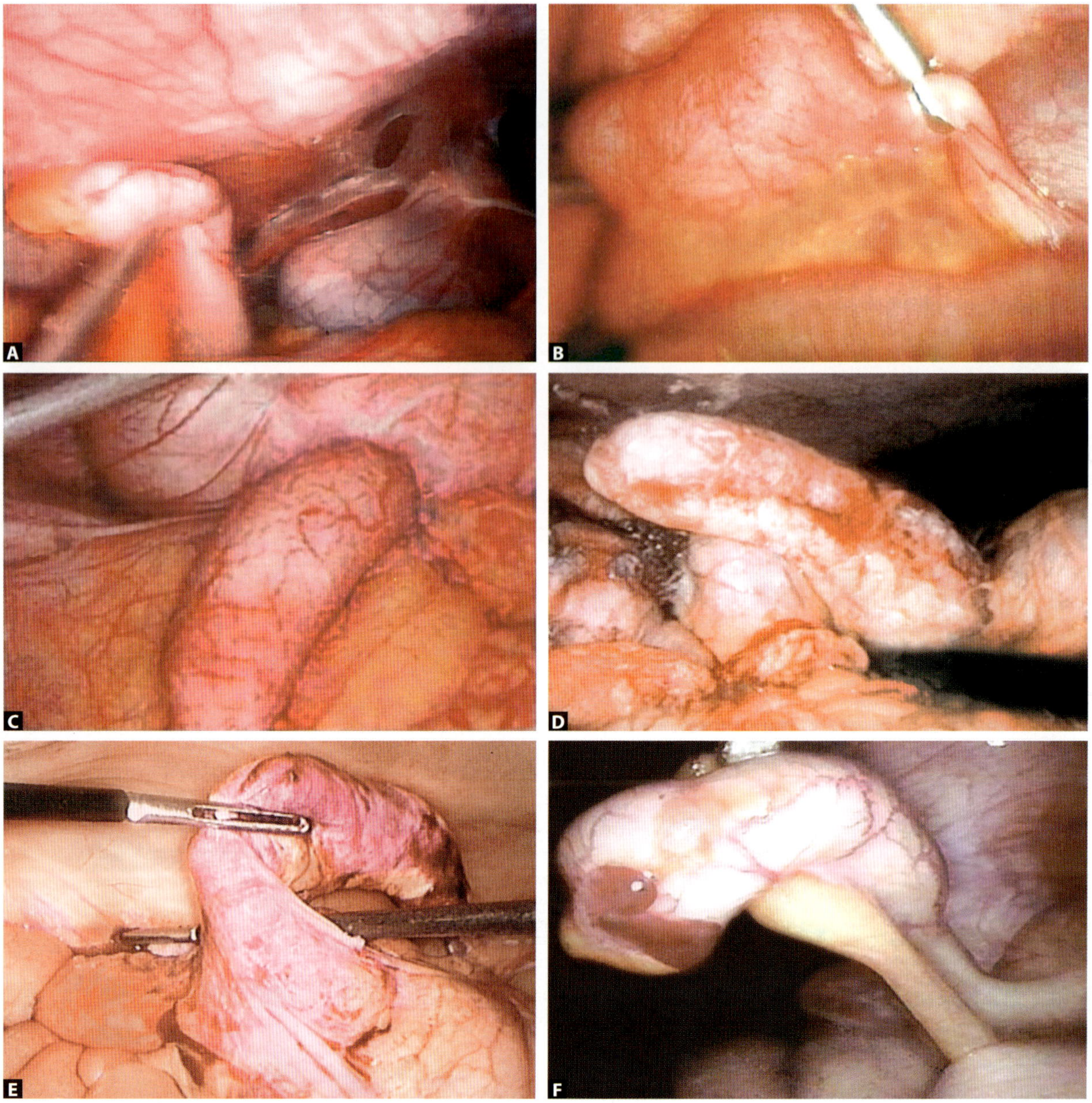

Figs. 19.21A to F: (A) Dislodged vermiform appendix lying near the gallbladder; (B) Vermiform appendix with mucocele; (C) Chronic appendicitis in Crohn's disease; (D) Acute appendicitis with peritoneal involvement; (E) Acute perforated appendicitis with local peritonitis; (F) Endometriosis of the appendix vermiformis.

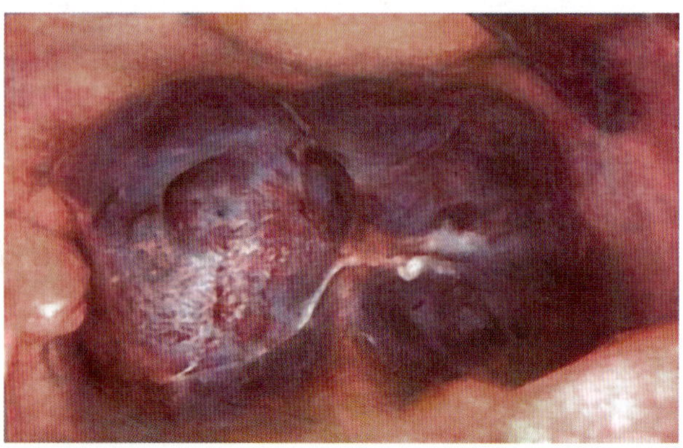

Fig. 19.22: Chronic diverticulosis of the sigma colon.

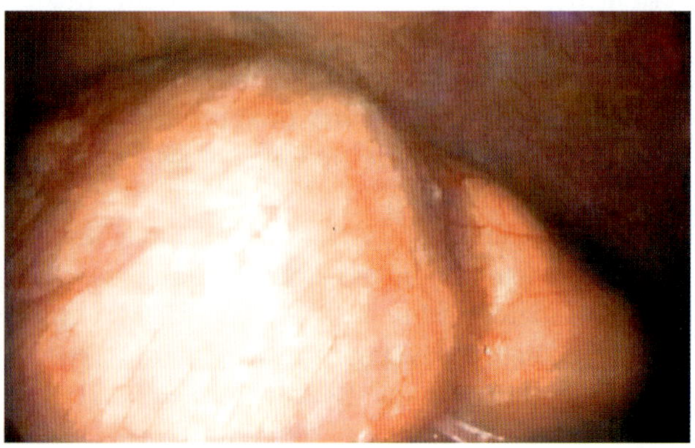

Fig. 19.23: Tumor of the ileum, histologically encrusted gallstones (8.5 × 5.5 × 5 cm).

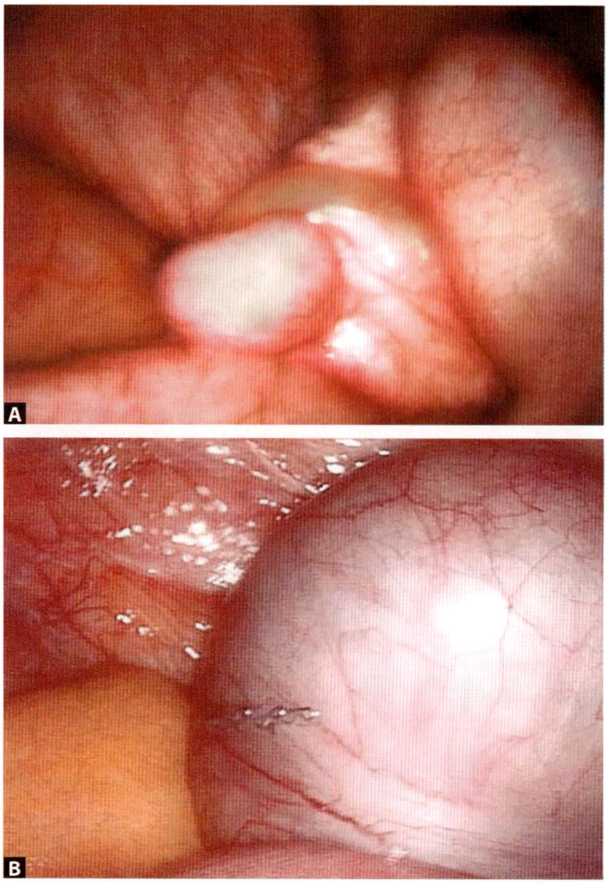

Figs. 19.24A and B: (A) Situation after appendectomy with residual appendix and continuous infection; (B) Situation after appendectomy with residual titan clips at the cecum end.

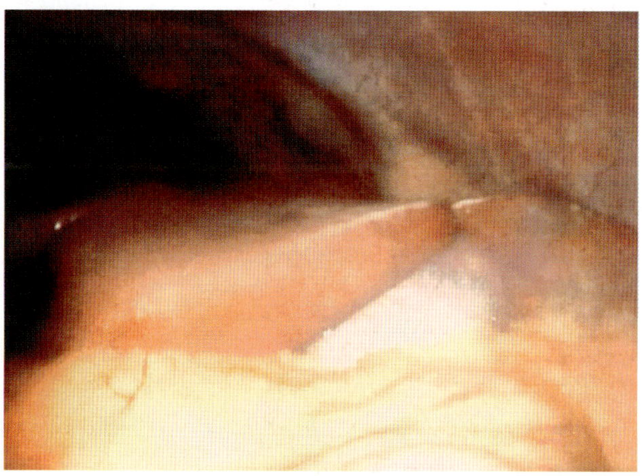

Fig. 19.25: Situs inversus showing the liver and gallbladder on the left hand side of the patient.

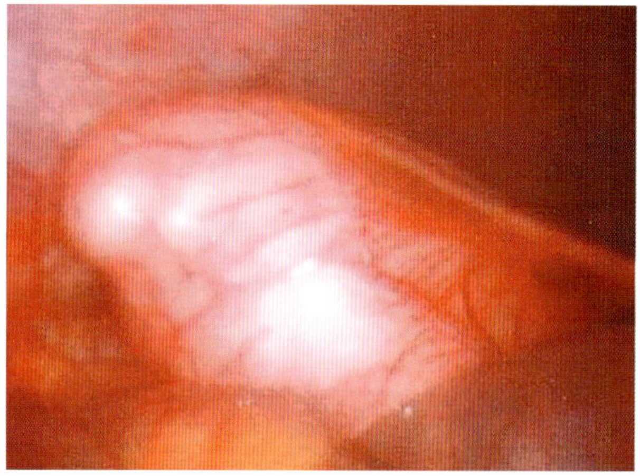

Fig. 19.26: Asymptomatic cholelithiasis.

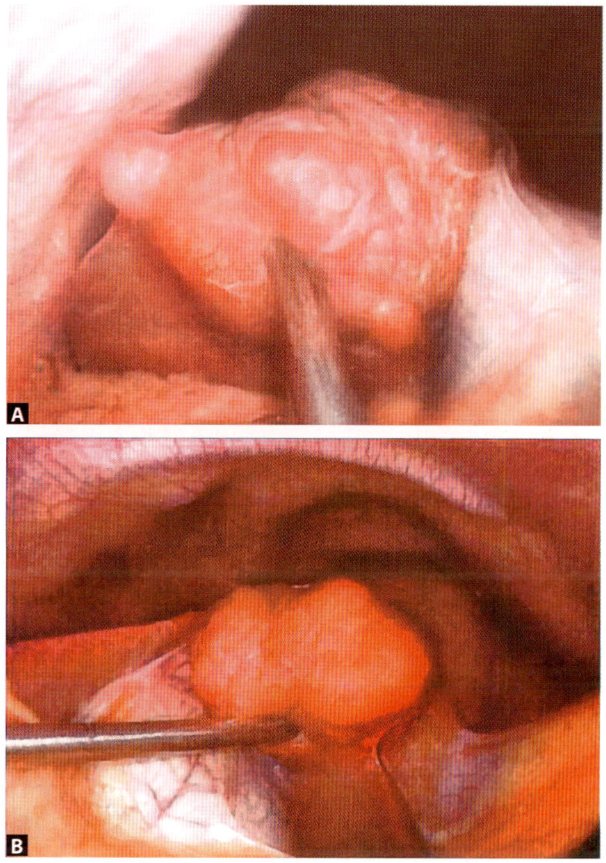

Figs. 19.27A and B: (A) Focal nodular hyperplasia; (B) Focal nodular hyperplasia.

Whereas diseases of the stomach and pancreas can hardly be recognized laparoscopically, changes in the spleen can be found in the maximum right lateral position of the patient (Fig. 19.37). Next follows examination of the peritoneum. Peritoneal residua (Fig. 19.38), peritoneal cysts (Figs. 19.39A to C), peritoneal tumors (Fig. 19.40), inflammatory infiltrates and foreign body reactions as

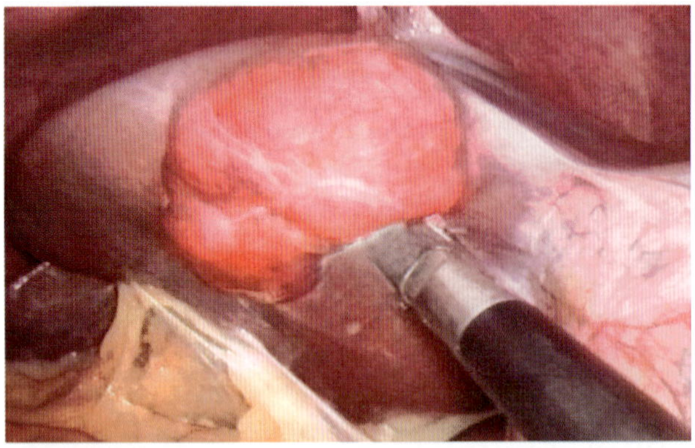

Fig. 19.28: Solitary adenoma of the liver next to the gallbladder.

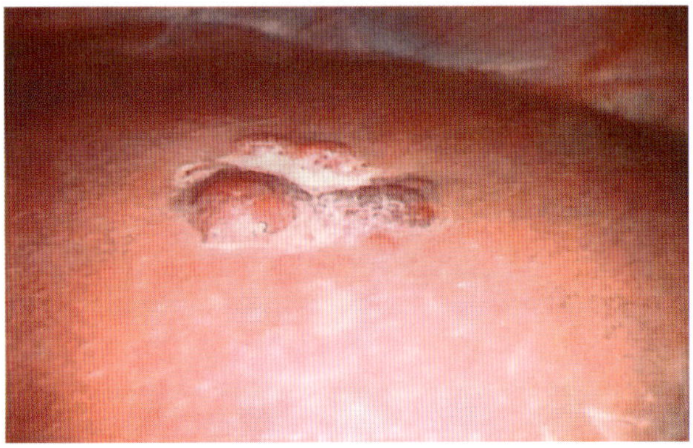

Fig. 19.29: Hemangioma of the liver.

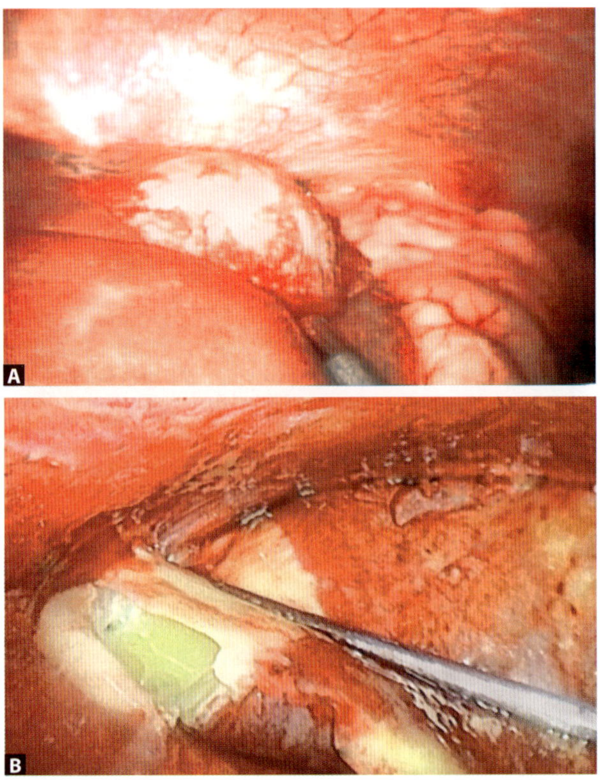

Figs. 19.30A and B: (A) Asymptomatic abscess of the liver; (B) Appendicular abscess of the liver.

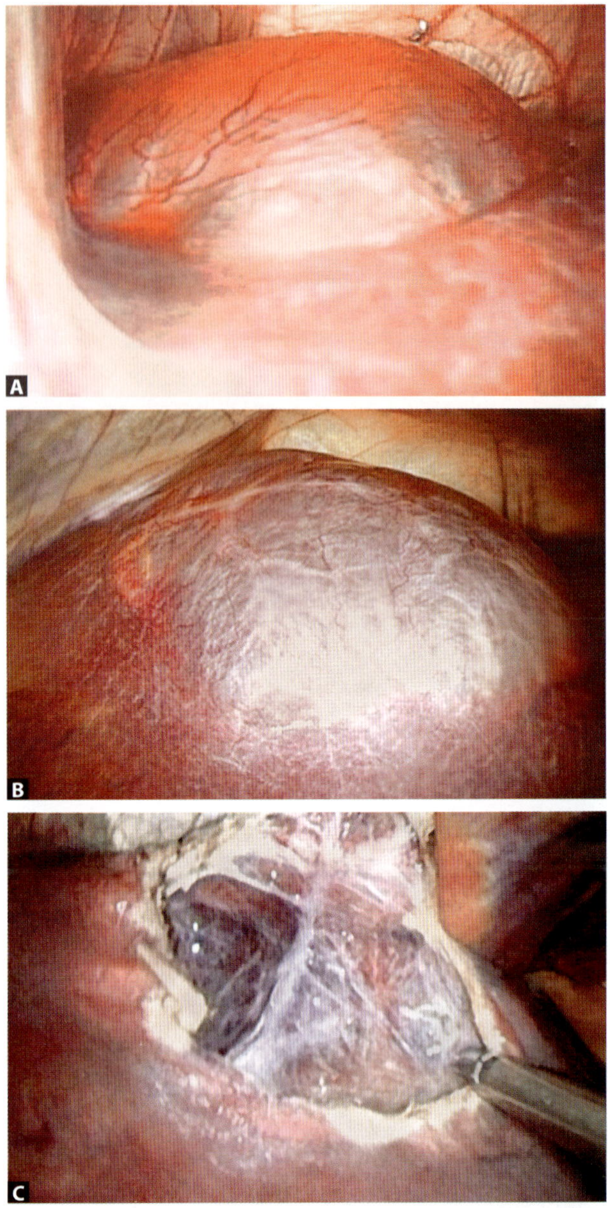

Figs. 19.31A to C: (A) Liver cyst of the left liver lobe; (B) Huge multichambered liver cyst; (C) Huge multi-chambered liver cyst (opened).

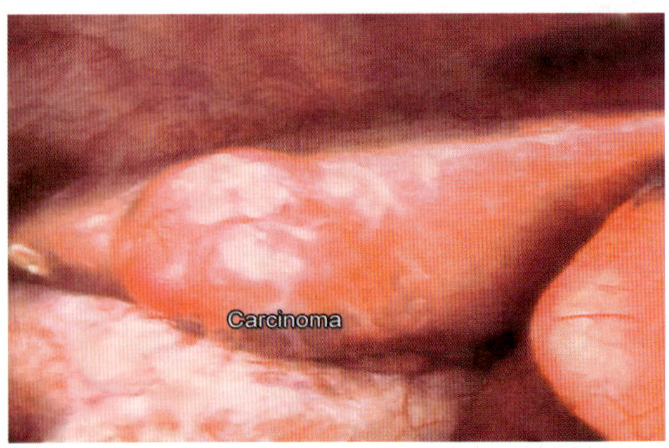

Figs. 19.32: Hepatocellular carcinoma.

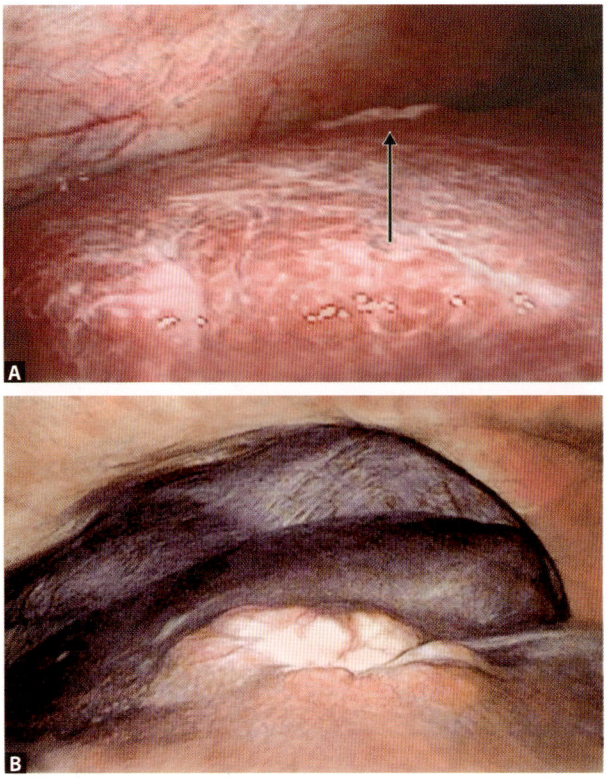

Figs. 19.33A and B: (A) Liver metastasis; (B) Liver metastasis with superficial ulcer.

manifestation of past surgeries and also primary diseases of the peritoneum (Figs. 19.41A and B) can be detected as well as incisional and congenital hernias (Figs 19.42A to C). An overview and examination of the omentum majus and mesenterium of jejunum, ileum and colon can offer important findings playing a role in differential diagnosis of imaging or chronic symptoms (Figs. 19.43 and 19.44). By patient examination and good localization, it is sometimes possible to pick up retroperitoneal pathological findings (Figs. 19.45 to 19.47). After previous laparotomy, any foreign materials introduced are located and removed, when necessary (Fig. 19.48). Additional bacteriological, cytological, and histological tests can further verify the clinical picture. After finishing the mid or upper abdominal diagnosis, examination of the internal reproductive organs is usually carried out.

Gynecological findings that can be misinterpreted as extragenital findings are found ubiquitous (Figs. 19.49 to 19.52). Congenital abnormalities must only be registered (Figs. 19.53 and 19.54). Unusual findings might appear with or without clinical symptoms (Figs. 19.55A and B).

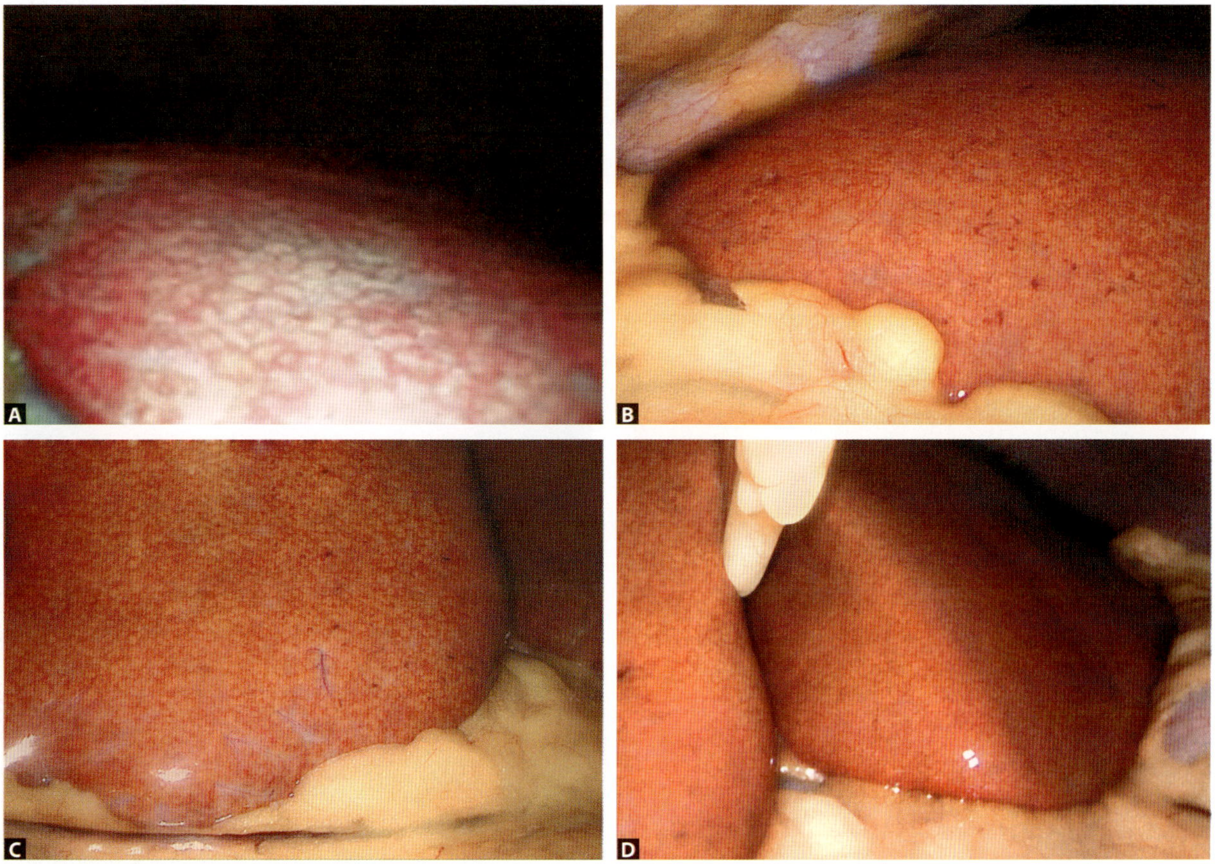

Figs. 19.34A to D: Steatosis hepatitis.

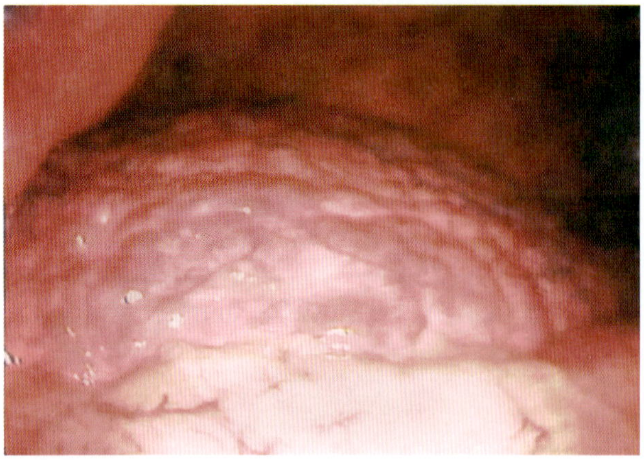

Fig. 19.35: Cirrhosis of the liver.

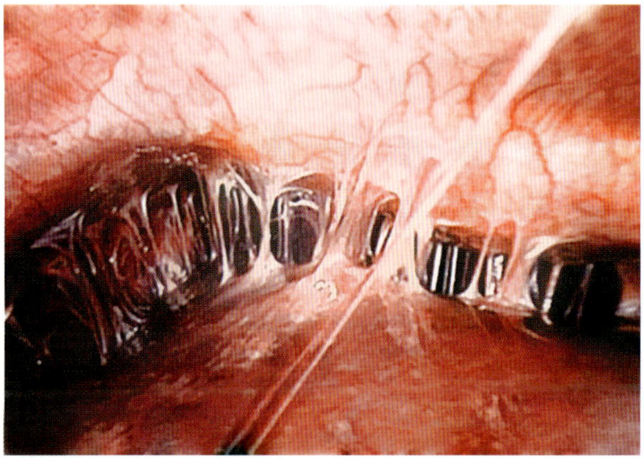

Fig. 19.36: Fitz–Hugh–Curtis syndrome in the region of the right lobe of the liver.

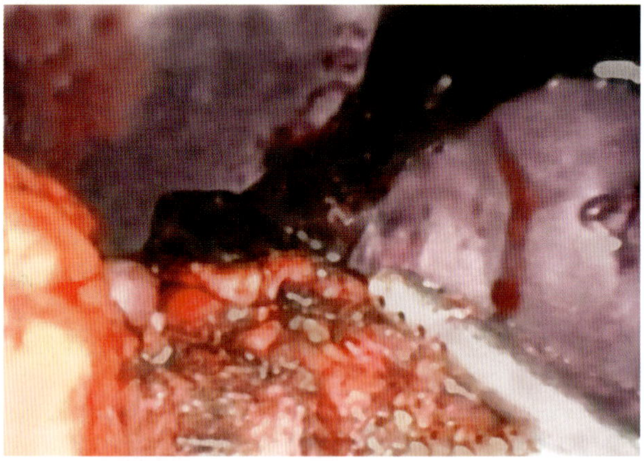

Fig. 19.37: Splenic injury after myomectomy due to anatomical variety of the omentum majus.

STEP 9

Hemostasis and Extended Operation

Adhesions or other pathologic processes, such as biopsy of other organs or endometriosis resection,

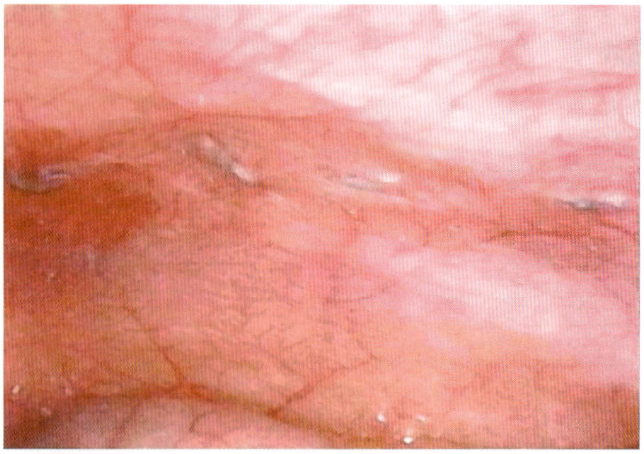

Fig. 19.38: Nonresorbable sutures after appendectomy.

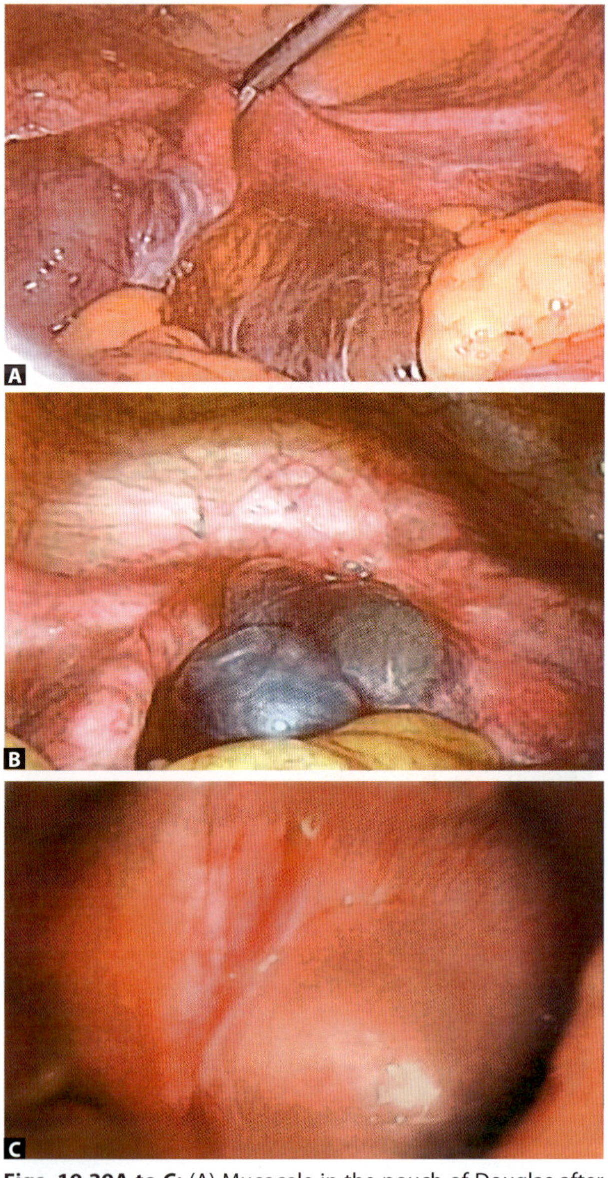

Figs. 19.39A to C: (A) Mucocele in the pouch of Douglas after hysterectomy; (B) Mucocele in the pouch of Douglas after hysterectomy; (C) Mucocele in the pouch of Douglas after hysterectomy.

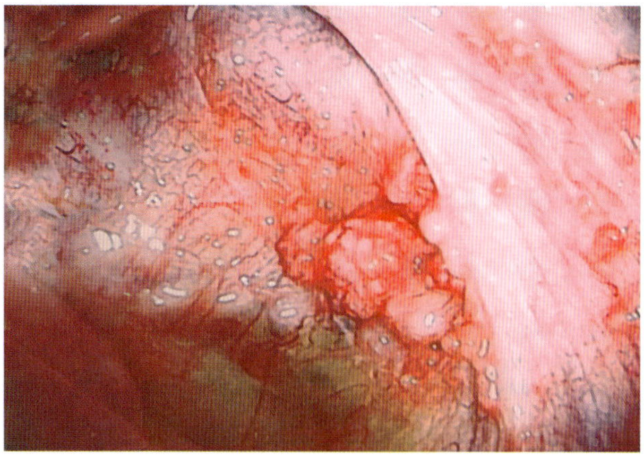

Fig. 19.40: Leiomyomatosis peritonei disseminate in the pouch of Douglas.

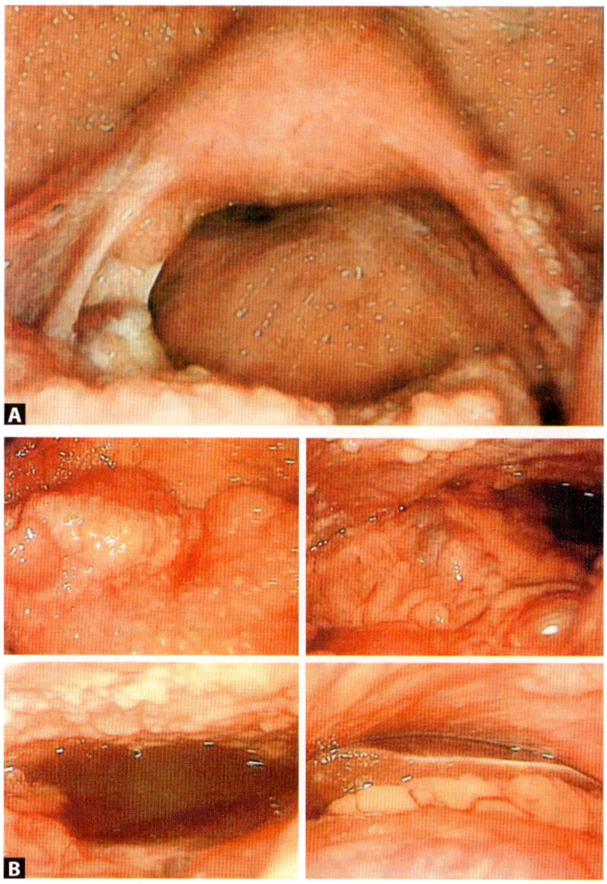

Figs. 19.41A and B: (A) Malignant mesothelioma of the peritoneum; (B) Malignant mesothelioma of the peritoneum.

can be treated simultaneously without significantly prolonging the operation in most cases. If the operative sidelines demand long and complex operative procedures, their treatment has to be made dependent on the circulatory stability of the patient and the urgency of the redress of the secondary problem.

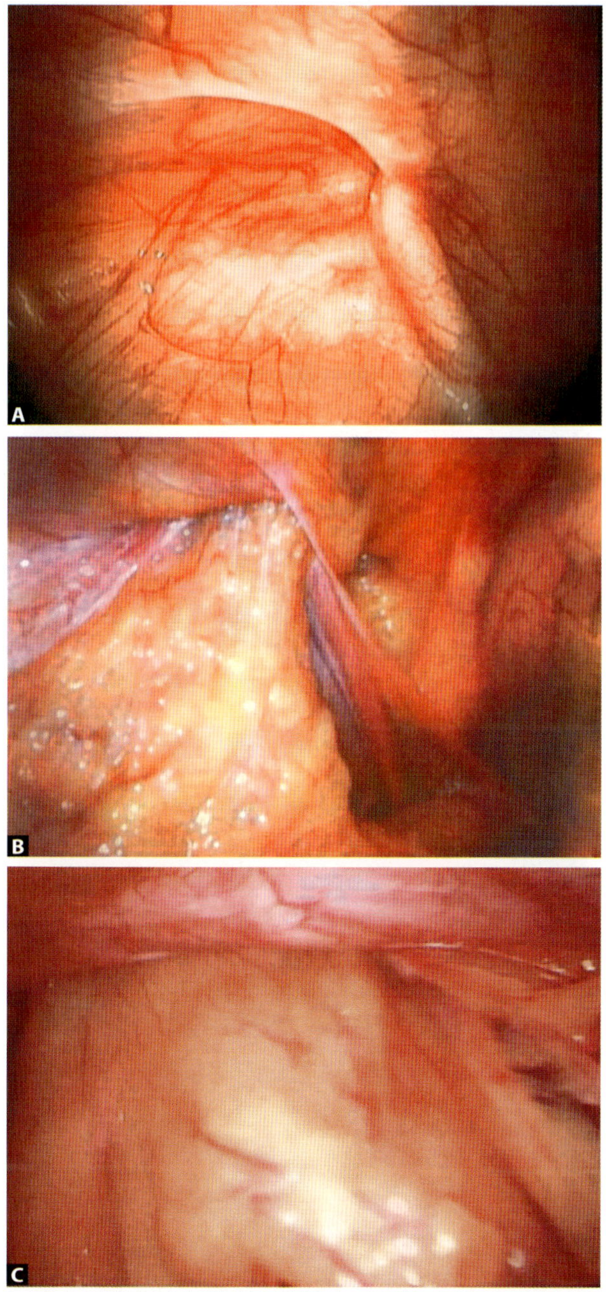

Figs. 19.42A to C: (A) Left side located congenital inguinal hernia; (B) Left side located inguinal hernia with incarcerated omentum majus; (C) Incisional hernia with incarcerated greater omentum.

CONCLUSION

The gynecological laparoscopic view should not be restricted only to the female pelvis. Compared with laparotomy, apart from the known merits of laparoscopy, the opportunity to inspect the entire abdomen is an advantage not to be underestimated; it unearths many extragenital findings and sets the course for more specific treatment. In the

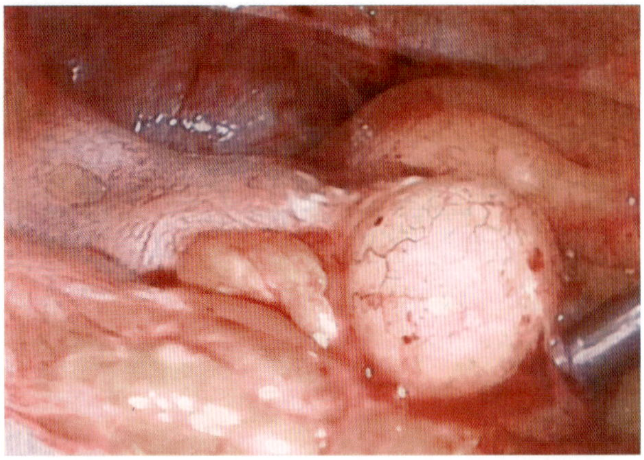

Fig. 19.43: Benign mesothelial cyst of the sigmoid colon.

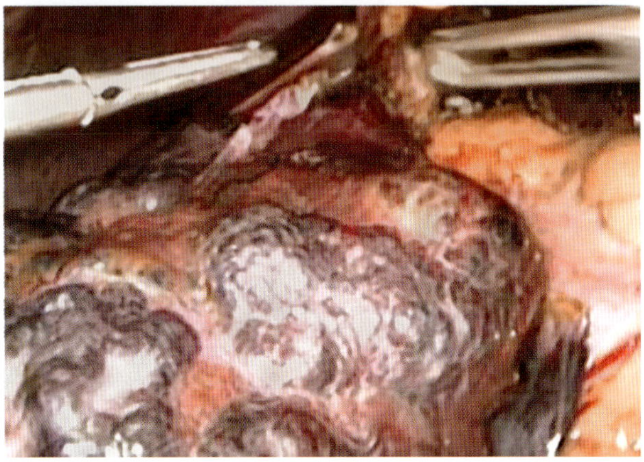

Fig. 19.44: Mesenteric multi-chambered cyst.

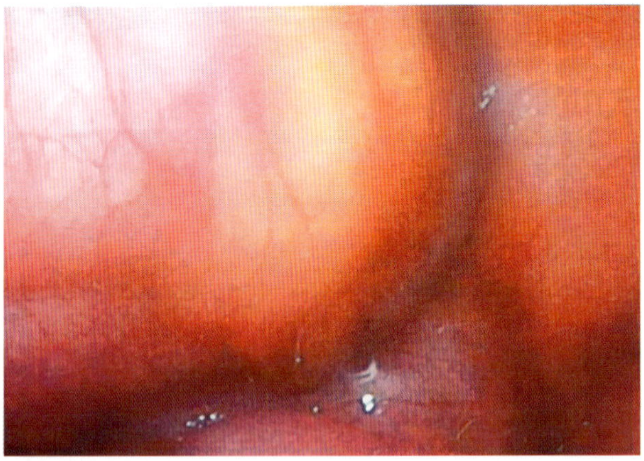

Fig. 19.45: Retroperitoneal lipoma on the anterior abdominal wall.

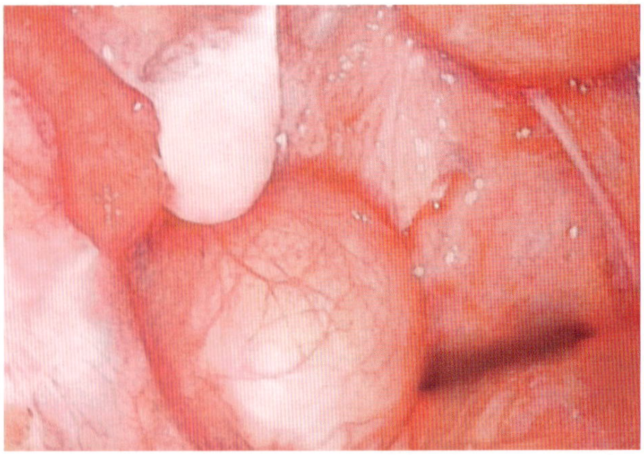

Fig. 19.46: Retroperitoneal lymphangioma.

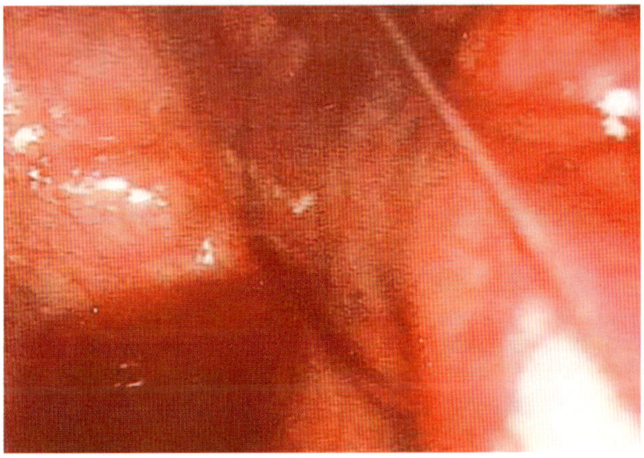

Fig. 19.47: Megaloureter right.

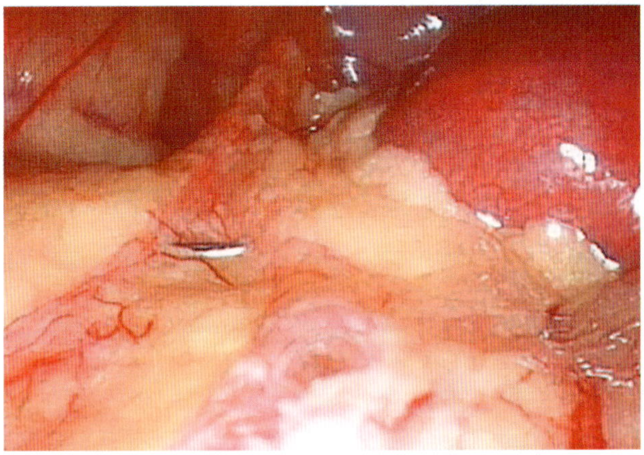

Fig. 19.48: Titanium clip on the greater omentum after cholecystectomy.

interests of more relevant diagnosis and differential diagnosis, the extragenital findings should be demonstrated live to the respective colleagues, documented photographically and written down precisely in the operative notes. Whenever useful and possible, excisions for histological examinations should be taken.

TIPS OF THE EXPERTS

Tip 1: Prior to any surgical performance in the abdomen, a careful cleaning of the situs and a careful overview of all skin predilection sites should be carried out. Whatever seems abnormal or suspicious, show it to the dermatologist.

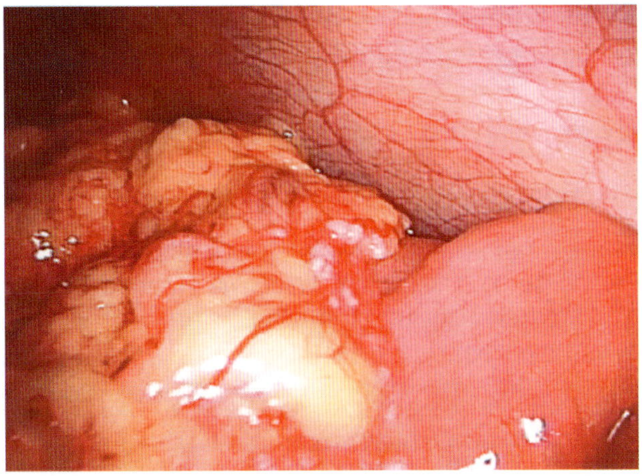

Fig. 19.49: Leiomyomatosis peritonei disseminate in the greater omentum.

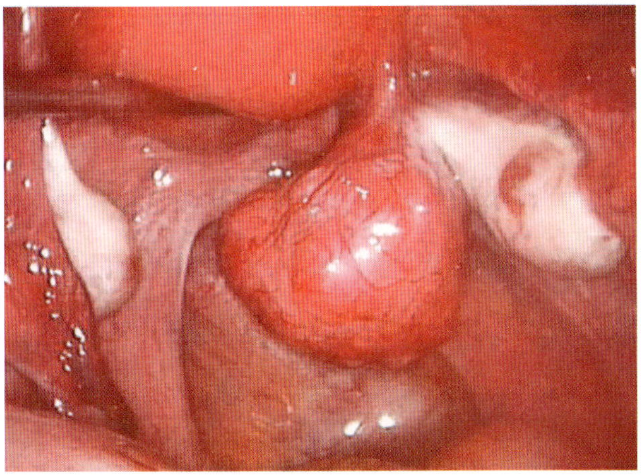

Fig. 19.50: Pedunculated myoma of the left ligamentum ovarium proprium.

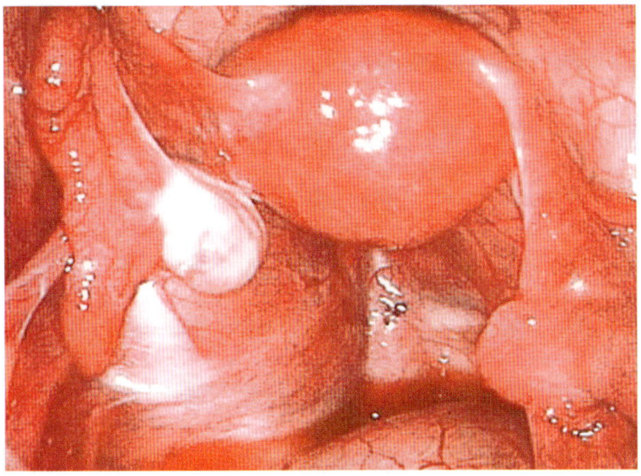

Fig. 19.51: Retroperitoneal myoma of the cervix.

Tip 2: Once pneumoperitoneum has been completed, a careful and systematic overview of the whole abdominal cavity should be performed. Always follow the same procedure to avoid any possibility of neglect.

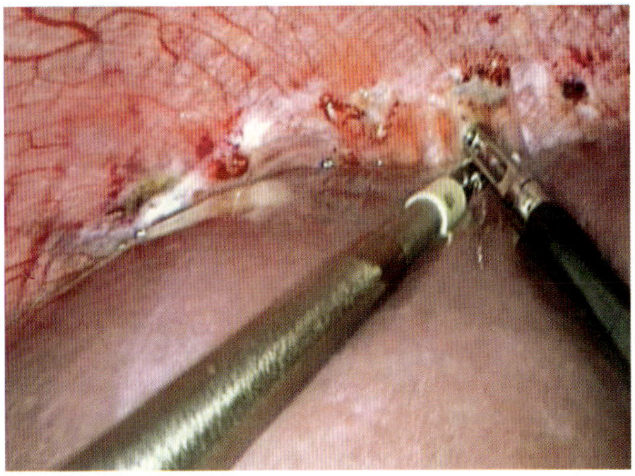

Fig. 19.52: Endometriosis extragenitalis located on the liver diaphragm.

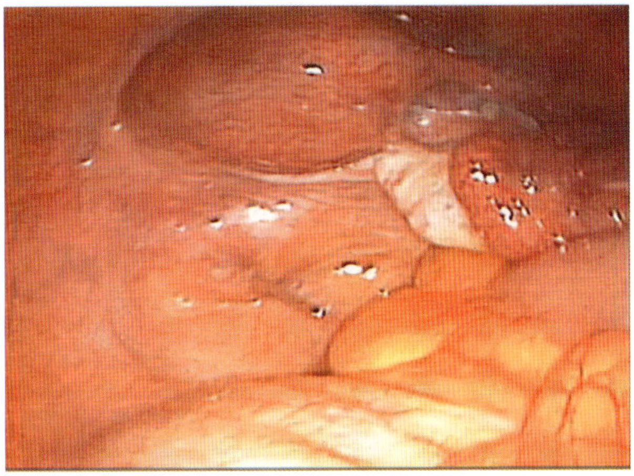

Fig. 19.53: Aplasia of the left adnexa.

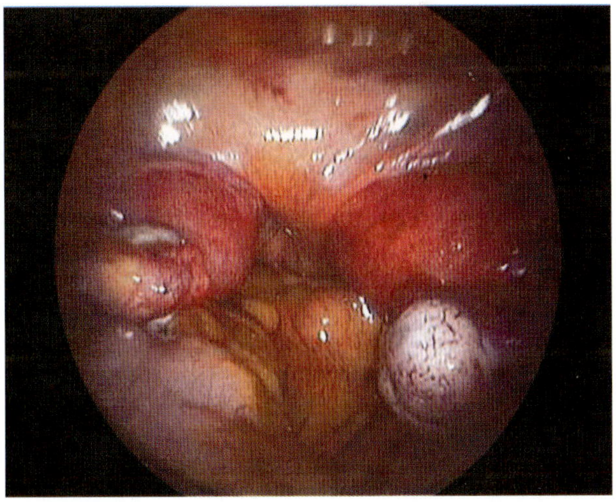

Fig. 19.54: Uterus duplex unicollis.

Tip 3: Do not forget to look on the ventral abdominal wall, on top of the liver and spleen and to lift up omentum, small bowel and uterus to survey possible hidden pathologies.

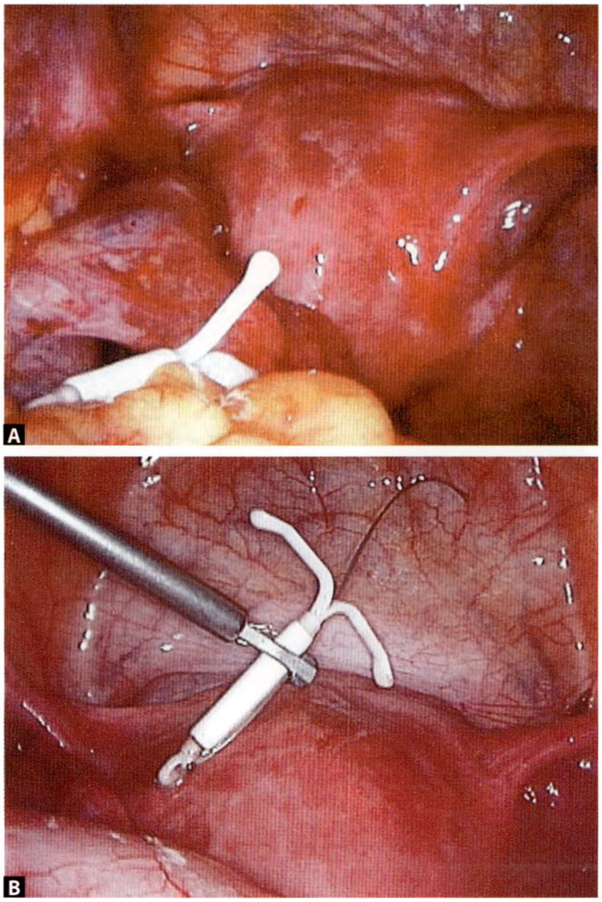

Figs. 19.55A and B: (A) Lost IUD (Mirena); (B) Lost IUD (Mirena).

Tip 4: Always take photos and, whenever possible, demonstrate the appropriate findings to a general surgeon or urologist.

Tip 5: Only a biopsy and histological examination can give an exact diagnosis. Therefore, all possible findings and operative consequences should be discussed before the operation.

REFERENCES

1. Gynecologists, RCOG Preventing entry-related gynaecological laparoscopic injuries. RCOG Green-top Guideline 2008;No.49:1-10.
2. Koike, H, Chuganji Y, Watanabe H, et al. Conservative treatment of ovarian pregnancy by local prostaglandin F2 alpha injection. Am J Obstet Gynecol. 1990;163(2):696.
3. Lang, PF, Weiss PA, Mayer HO, et al. Conservative treatment of ectopic pregnancy with local injection of hyperosmolar glucose solution or prostaglandin-F2 alpha: a prospective randomised study. Lancet. 1990; 336(8707):78-81.
4. Shamma FN, Schwartz LB. Primary ovarian pregnancy successfully treated with methotrexate. Am J Obstet Gynecol. 1992;167(5):1307-8.
5. Chelmow D, Gates E, Penzias AS. Laparoscopic diagnosis and methotrexate treatment of an ovarian pregnancy: a case report. Fertil Steril. 1994;62(4):879-81.
6. Lipscomb, GH, Stovall TG, Ling FW. Nonsurgical treatment of ectopic pregnancy. N Engl J Med. 2000; 343(18):1325-9.
7. Alkatout I, Stuhlmann-Laeisz C, Mettler L, et al. Organ-preserving management of ovarian pregnancies by laparoscopic approach. Fertil Steril. 2011; 95(8):2467-70.
8. Luciano D, Roy G, Luciano A. Ectopic pregnancy. In: Pasic R, Levine R (Eds), A Practical Manual of Laparoscopy: A Clinical Cookbook. Andover, UK: Informa Healthcare; 2007. pp. 155-68.
9. Barbosa C, Mencaglia L. In: Mencaglia L, Minelle L, Wattiez A (Eds). Laparoscopic Management of Ectopic Pregnancy. Manual of Gynecological Laparoscopic Surgery. Schramberg, Germany: Endo Press; 2010. pp. 115-23.

KIEL SCH•OL

20 of Gynaecological Endoscopy

Tubal Surgery

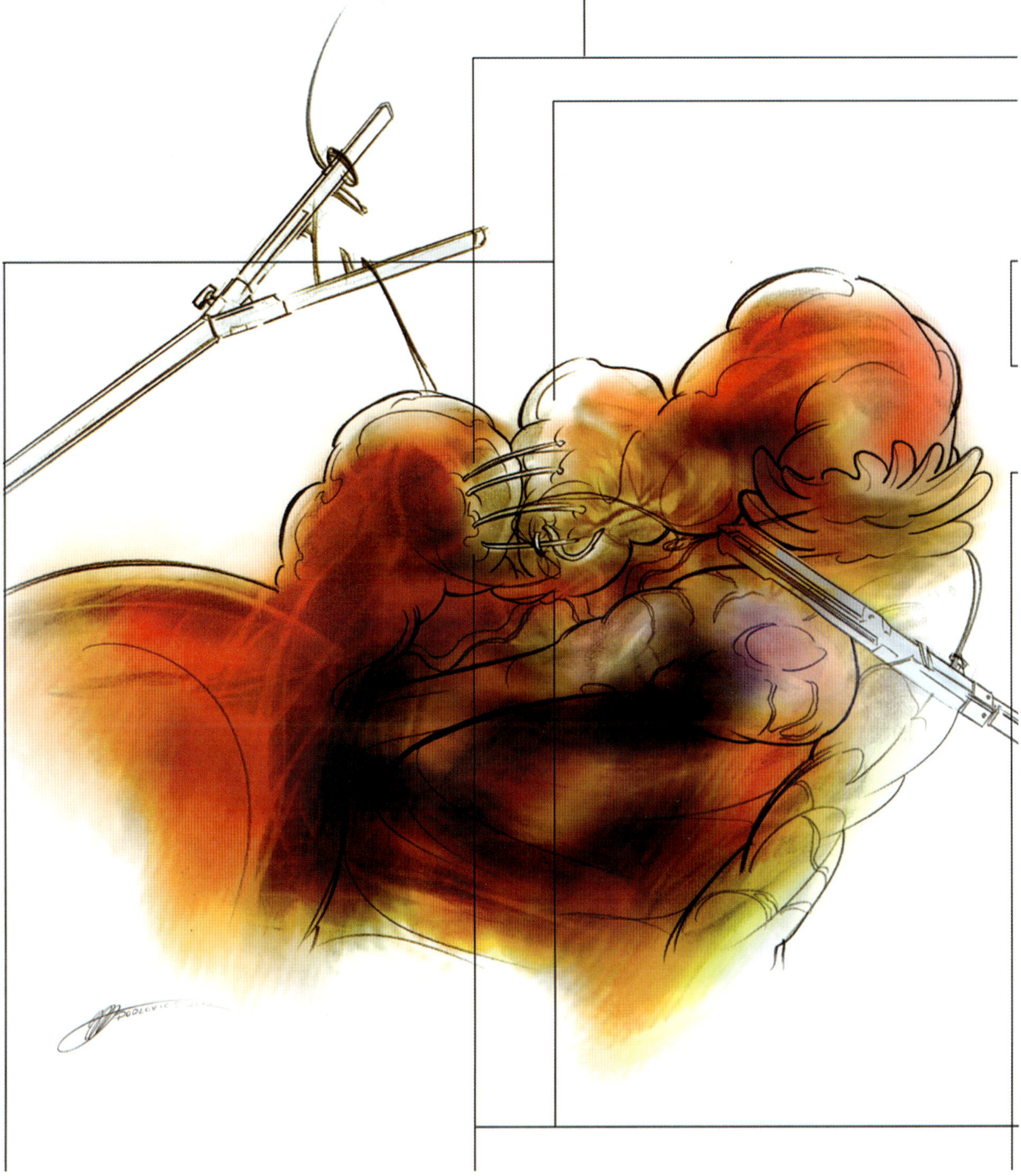

Chapter 20

Tubal Surgery

Sanjay Patel

Approximately 25–30% of infertility in women is the result of tubal disease.

TYPES OF TUBAL SURGERY

- Hysteroscopic tubal cannulation
- Laparoscopic tubal microsurgery
- Laparoscopic salpingo-ovariolysis and fimbrioplasty.

HYSTEROSCOPIC TUBAL CANNULATION

Patients having proximal tubal occlusion (PTO) are candidates for hysteroscopic tubal cannulation. PTO accounts for 10–25% of tubal disease as found on hysterosalpingograms. The causes of PTO are as follows:

Noninfectious causes	Infectious causes
1. Obstruction due to tubal spasm	1. Salpingitis isthmica nodosa (SIN)
2. Plugging by mucus and amorphous material	2. Pelvic inflammatory disease (PID)
3. Occlusion from fibrosis or endometriosis	3. Tuberculosis

These infections may damage other areas of the tube, which will affect the prognosis of the treatment.

Technique

We prefer to do hysteroscopic tubal cannulation under general anesthesia and laparoscopic guidance. 5F catheter along with obturator is inserted into the operating channel of the hysteroscope (Figs. 20.1 and 20.2). The obturator is then removed and tip of this catheter is curved and wedged against the tubal ostium. Then dilute methylene blue dye is injected. If the dye is seen coming from the tube, patency is confirmed and the procedure is finished. If no dye is seen, then guidewire is introduced inside the catheter. The guidewire is advanced slowly through the uterotubal junction into the intramural portion of the tube into the isthmic portion. The guidewire is

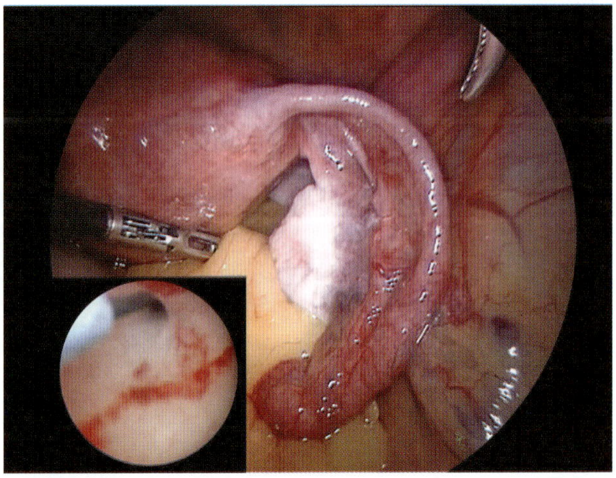

Fig. 20.1: Terumo guidewire.

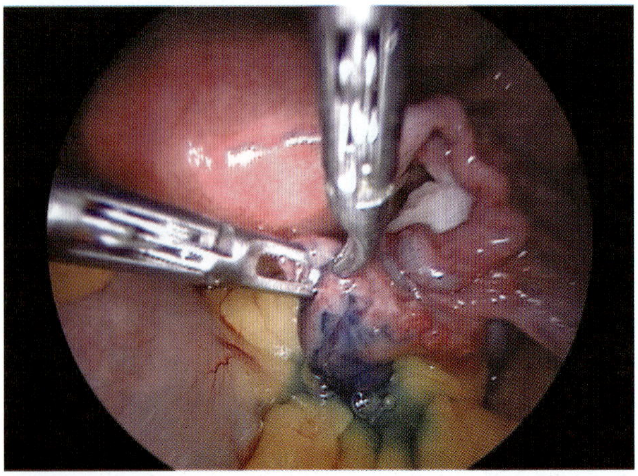

Fig. 20.2: Spill after hysteroscopic tubal cannulation.

removed and the dilute dye is again injected under laparoscopic observation. If dye is observed, the procedure is finished. If there is resistance to passage of the guidewire or catheter, an attempt is made to mobilize the tube laparoscopically. If unsuccessful, the procedure is terminated. If the cause of the obstruction is not apparent, the next step is to counsel the patient regarding tubal surgery or IVF.

Contraindications to hysteroscopic tubal cannulation include active infection, heavy uterine bleeding, potential pregnancy and uterine malignancy. Adverse effects of hysteroscopic tubal cannulation include damage to normal tube, which may be either dissection or perforation and other is ectopic pregnancy.

LAPAROSCOPIC TUBAL MICROSURGERY

Laparoscopic microsurgery is a new discipline that synergizes the potential of classical microsurgery and laparoscopy. It can overcome the deficiencies in each of the techniques. The advent of microsurgical technique is attributed to Swolin in 1967. The first microsurgical reversal of the sterilization was done by Gomel and Winston in 1977.

Around 25–30% of the subfertile females have tubal damage and quite a few of them seek tubal microreconstruction for fertility enhancement. Also those with tubal sterilization procedure seeking reversal for further childbearing are better candidates. This can now be achieved with principles of laparoscopic microsurgery.[1-13]

Advantages

- All microsurgical principles are well maintained like magnification, tissue handling, hemostasis and lavage.
- Avoids laparotomy and tissue trauma associated with packing and retractors.
- Minimal tissue handling and trauma
- Adhesions are minimal
- Cosmetically far better
- Faster recovery
- Single-step procedure as compared to IVF where multiple sittings may be required.

Preoperative Workup

- Semen analysis to rule out male factor.
- Day 3 serum follicle-stimulating hormone (FSH) level to know the ovarian reserve
- Hysterosalpingogram (HSG) to know the length and condition of the proximal tube
- Saline infusion sonography and hysterosalpingography may be helpful.

Indications

- Reversal of tubal sterilization procedure
- Mid-tubal block secondary to various pathologies
- Tubal occlusion secondary to ectopic pregnancy treatment
- Salpingitis isthmica nodosa
- Failed tubal cannulation for proximal tubal block
- Failed previous macrosurgical sterilization reversal.

Contraindications

Absolute contraindications:

- Aged 40 years or older
- Decreased ovarian reserve or ovarian failure
- Tubal infertility not amenable to tubal reconstruction
- Extensive tubal damage
- Hydrosalpinx with a diameter of more than 3 cm
- Inadequate proximal or distal tubal segment for reanastomosis
- Projected tubal length of less than 3 cm after the reconstruction procedure
- Extensive pelvic/peritubal adhesions
- Abnormal uterine cavity
- Any contraindication to pregnancy or surgery
- Severe male factor infertility or male sterility.

Equipment and Instruments

Magnification, resolution and digital enhancement

- 25–40 X magnification is essential to identify healthy mucosa of the fallopian tube. 10–15 X magnification is adequate for microsuturing.
- Use of endoscope, digital three-chip camera (image 1) with monitor has a "multiplier effect" and the magnification can be achieved up to 20–25 X.

Micro-instrumentation

- It is collectively known as "Koh ultramicro series" (Fig. 20.3).
- Terminal serration of the jaw is especially treated so that microsuture material does not get crushed.
- Handle design should be such that least friction and maximum transmission of hand movement

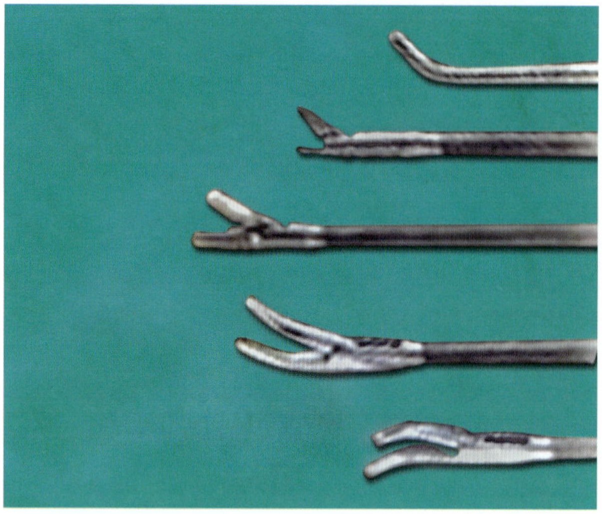

Fig. 20.3: KOH ultramicro series.

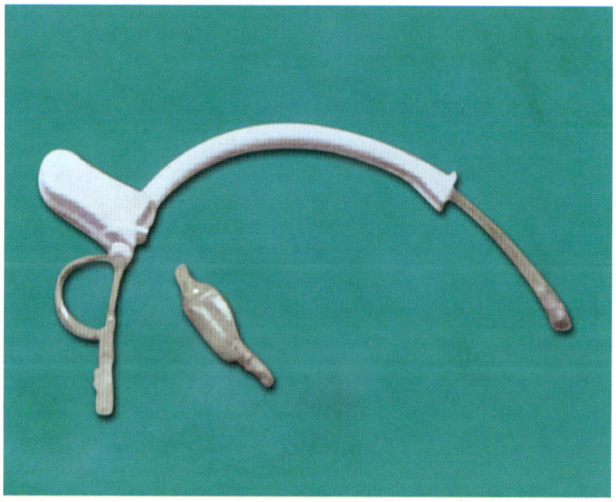

Fig. 20.4: Handlin's uterine manipulator.

occur to the instrument tip. An angle of 130° between handle and shaft of the instruments provides better movements.

Sutures, Needles and Energy

- More rigid needles are better for microendosuturing.
- The suture material should be 6-0 to 8-0 polypropylene, depending upon the surgeon's experience of material handling and preference.
- *Electrosurgery:* 15–20 W for cutting and 15 W for fulguration, use minimum cautery to preserve sub-tubal vasculature (Fig. 20.4).
- Handlin's uterine manipulator is a fine disposable instrument (Fig. 20.4), which allows administration of the dye and manipulation of the uterus without causing any significant trauma.

Selection of Cases

Length of Tubal Damage in Various Methods of Ligation

Type of TL	Length of damage	Case type
Monopolar diathermy	50 mm	Unfavorable
Falope Ring TL (Fig. 20.5)	40 mm	Unfavorable
Pomeroy's method	30 mm	Intermediate
Bipolar diathermy (Fig. 20.6)	30 mm	Intermediate
Hulka clip	7 mm	Favorable
Filshie clip (Fig. 20.7)	4 mm	Most favorable

Other nonsuitable cases are pathological tubes with PID, salpingitis isthmica nodosa and failed tubal cannulation.

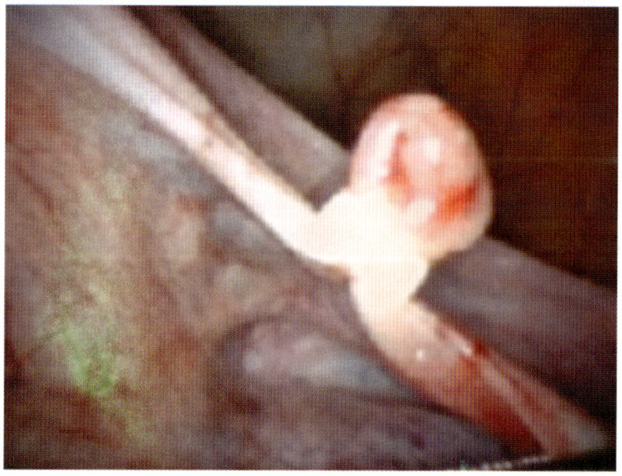

Fig. 20.5: Falope ring tubal ligation.

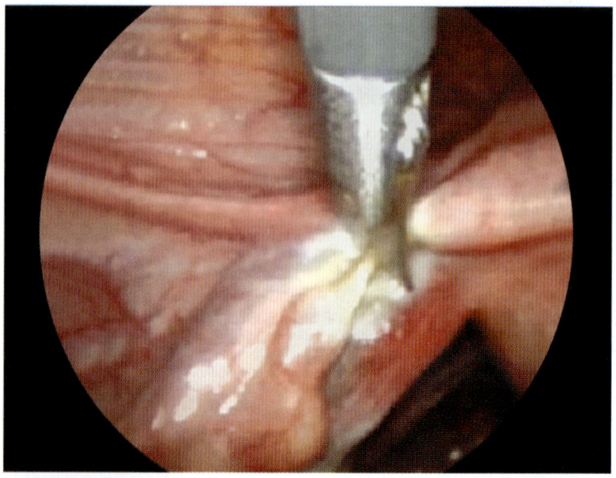

Fig. 20.6: Bipolar diathermy.

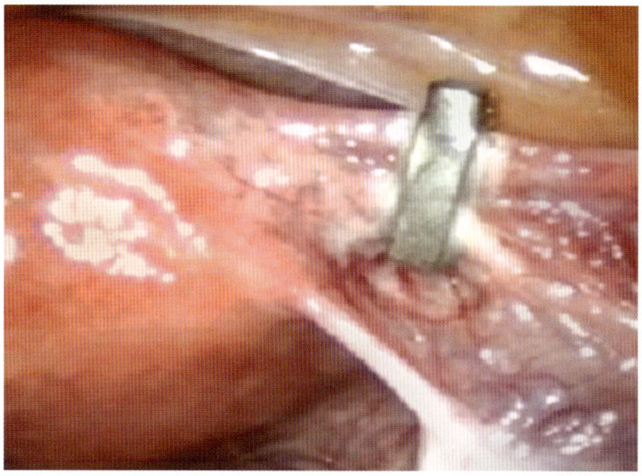

Fig. 20.7: Filshie's clip.

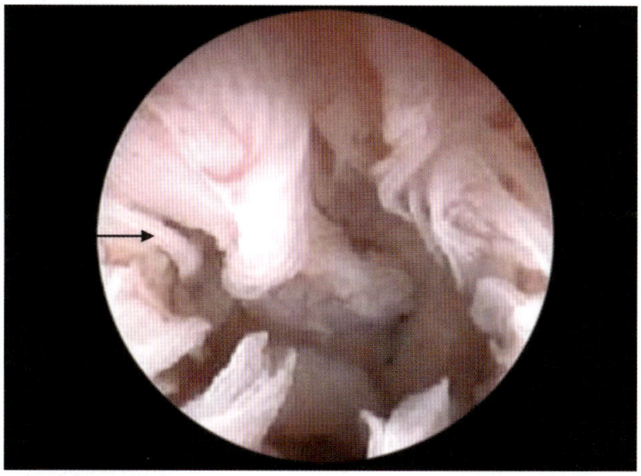

Fig. 20.8: Salpingoscopy Grade 1.

Intraoperative Evaluation

Before proceeding for the tubal reconstruction, one must evaluate the inside of the tube, so as to be confirmed that the anastomosis is going to be fruitful or not at all worthwhile. This involves salpingoscopy and falloposcopy.

- Salpingoscopy allows direct inspection of tubal mucosa in the ampullary part.
- The degree of tubal mucosal damage is probably the major factor in establishing the prognosis for tubal surgery (Figs. 20.5 to 20.7).
- Brosen's classification is useful for evaluation according to degree of mucosal atrophy and mucosal adhesions.

Salpingoscopy Grade 1 (Fig. 20.8): Normal intraluminal findings with healthy major (primary) and minor (secondary) folds.

Salpingoscopy Grade 2 (Fig. 20.9): Mucosal nuclear staining with methylene blue dye.

Salpingoscopy Grade 3 (Fig. 20.10): Minimal flattening and minimal adhesion of endosalpinx.

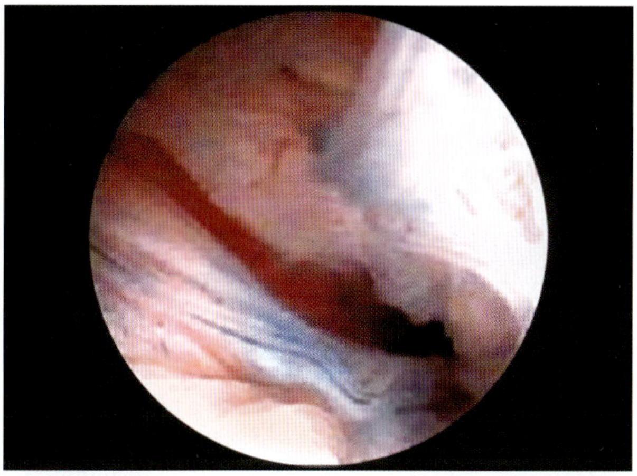

Fig. 20.9: Salpingoscopy Grade 2.

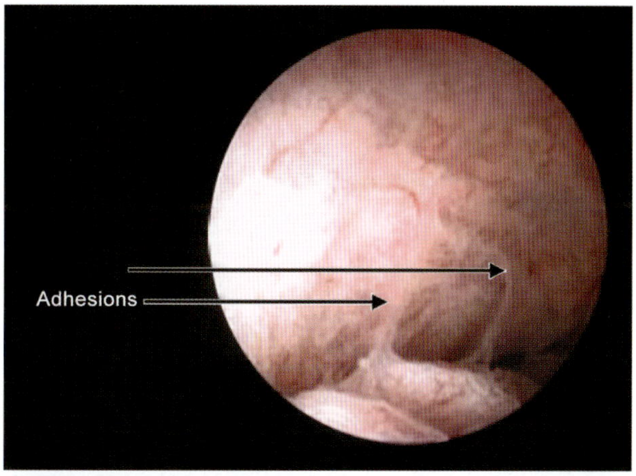

Fig. 20.10: Salpingoscopy Grade 3.

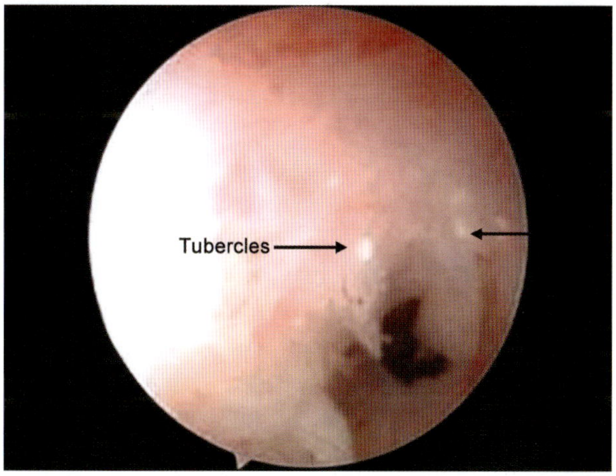

Fig. 20.11: Salpingoscopy, grade 4.

Salpingoscopy Grade 4 (Fig. 20.11): Moderate flattening of endosalpinx with intraluminal adhesion.

Salpingoscopy Grade 5 (Fig. 20.12): Severe flattening of mucosa with severe intraluminal adhesions.

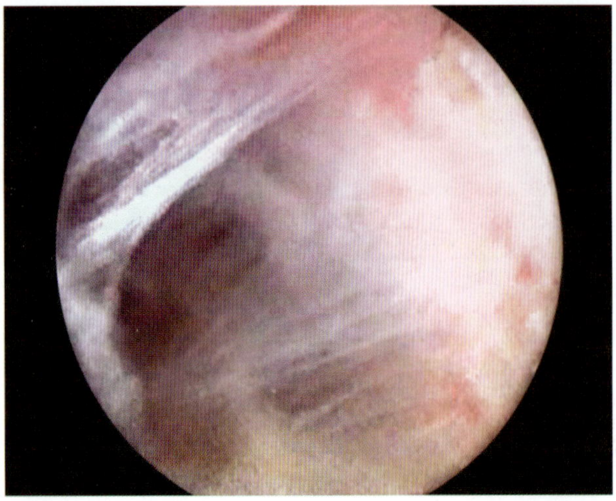

Fig. 20.12: Salpingoscopy Grade 5.

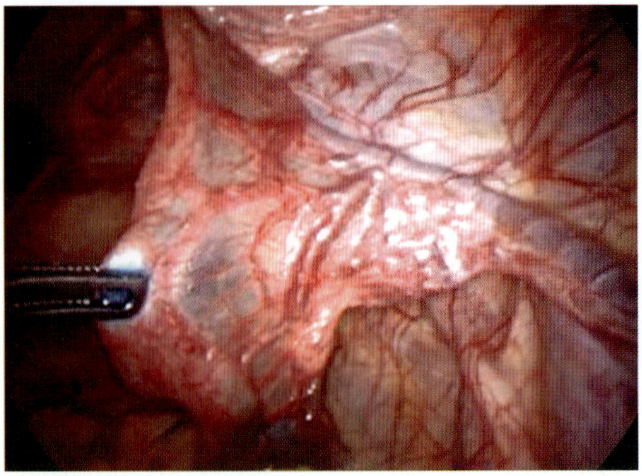

Fig. 20.14: Sub-tubal vessels.

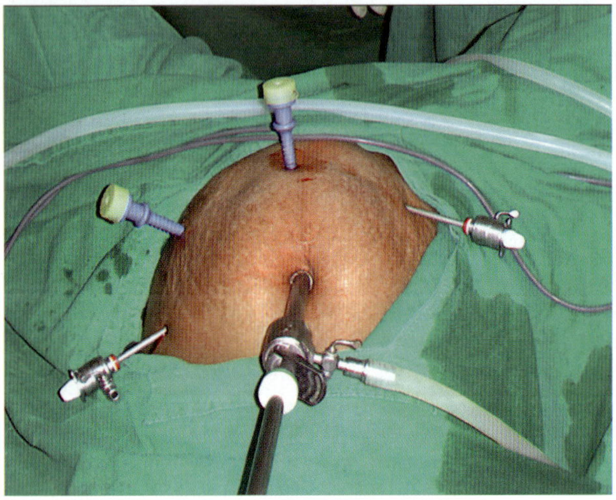

Fig. 20.13: Port positioning.

Surgical Technique

A total of five ports are used (Figs. 20.13 and 20.14)

- 10 mm laparoscope through the primary umbilical port.
- Four ancillary ports: two 5 mm and two 3 mm.
- The lower pelvic port of 5 mm is placed 4 cm medial and above the anterior superior iliac spine, i.e. ipsilateral port.
- Contralateral port of 3 mm size placed exactly opposite to ipsilateral port.
- Another ipsilateral port of 3 mm is para-umbilical and laterally in the anterior axillary line.
- One 5 mm central port, 2–3 cm above the pubic symphysis.

The position of the ports is critical in enabling fluent two-handed operating as well as suturing. The so-called fulcrum effect is virtually eliminated by adopting specific port positions.

Important Surgical Steps

- Distension of the proximal segment of the tube by transcervical chromoperturbation to know the exact site of the block
- Excision of pathological segment of the tube
- Make sure that the incision does not extend beyond the mesosalpinx.
- Ensure the right-angled cut of the tubal ends for better alignment and approximation
- Free spillage of the dye
- Mesosalpinx is sutured first, using 6 '0' polypropylene.

The most difficult and important step is end-to-end anastomosis in two layers. The first layer is the mucosal-muscularis layer.

- Most important is 6 o'clock position stitch.
- To keep the knot outside the lumen, stitches are taken from outer to inner side on proximal end and vice versa on distal end.
- Rests of the stitches are taken at 12, 3, and 9 o'clock positions in the similar manner.

The second layer, the sero-muscularis layer, is sutured with 6-0 polypropylene.

- Thorough peritoneal irrigation with Ringer's lactate solution throughout the operation.

Types of Anastomosis

Isthmo-isthmic Anastomosis

- Lumen size is 500 μm to 1 mm.
- Equal lumen size and thick muscularis allows technically easier and better anastomosis (Figs. 20.15A to H).

Isthmo-ampullary Anastomosis

Luminal disparity is the potential problem which can be adjusted by cutting the isthmic end (Figs. 20.16A to D).

Ampullo-ampullary Anastomosis

Technically difficult anastomosis due to thin muscularis and tendency for mucosal folds prolapse (Figs. 20.17A to C).

Tubo-cornual Anastomosis

Wedge excision in the cornual end mobilises good length of interstitial tube (Figs. 20.18A to G).

Our Experience

Pregnancy rates were comparable with open tubal recanalization. Average surgical duration was 2 h and 30 min. The average hospital stay was 2 days.

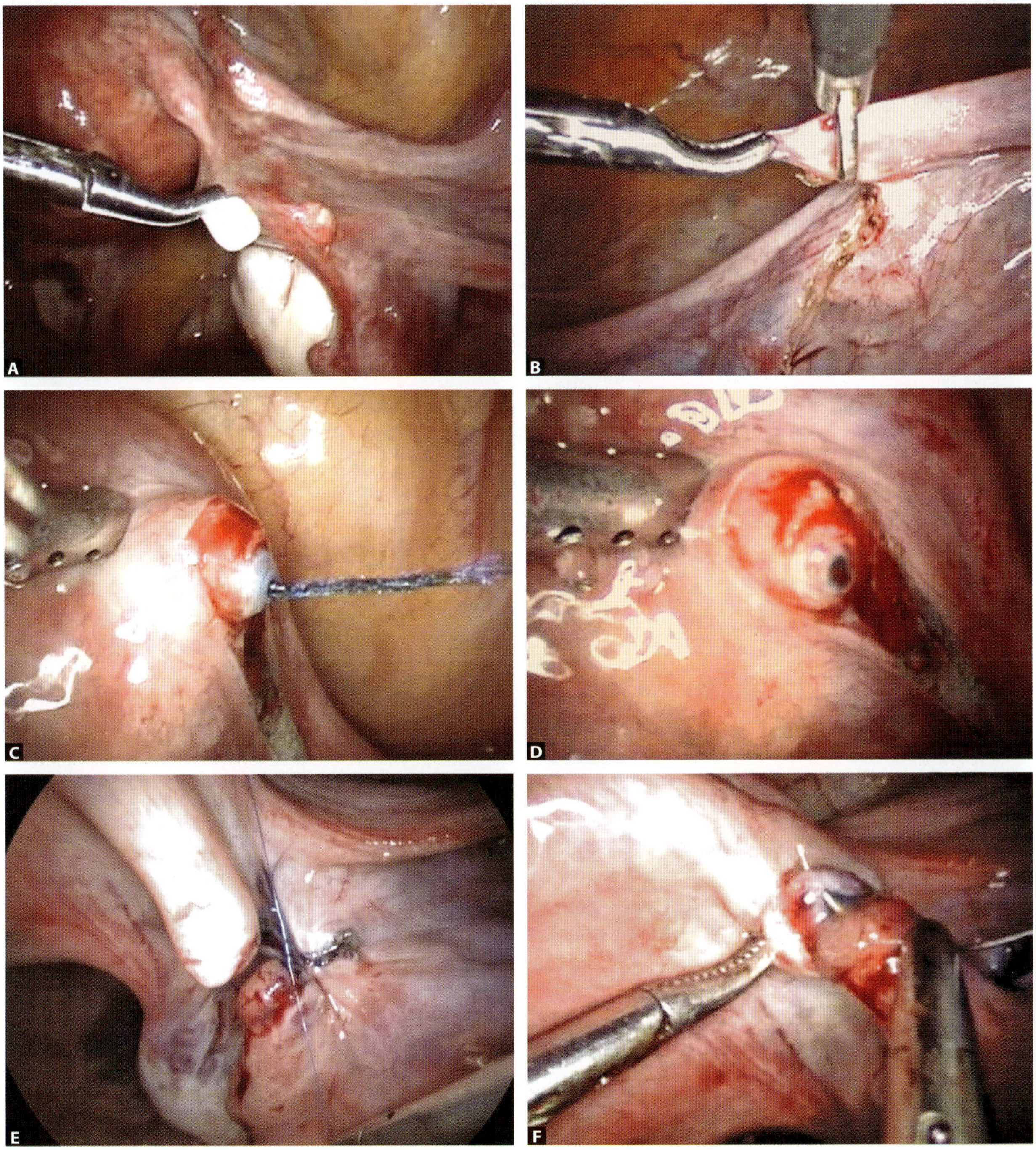

Figs. 20.15A to F

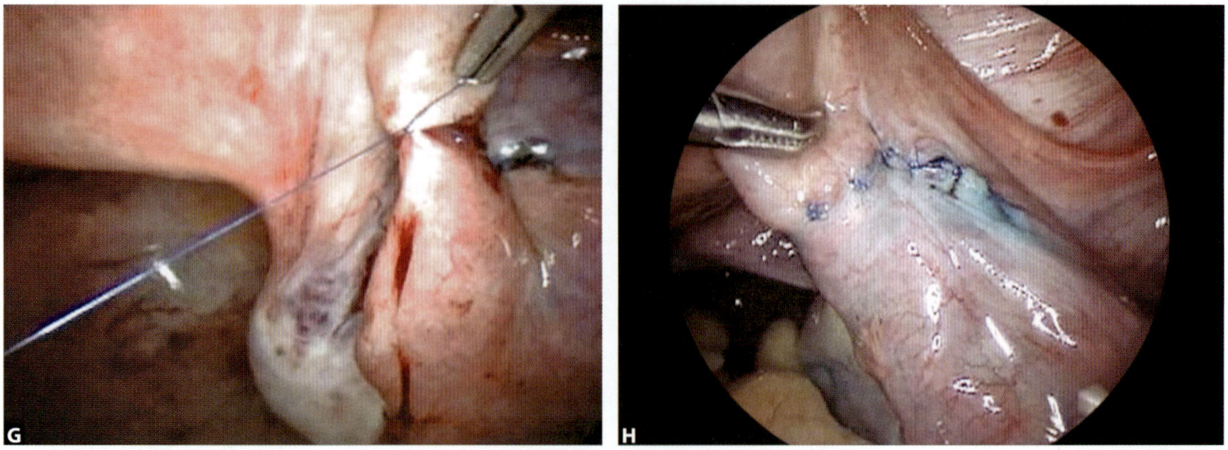

Figs. 20.15G and H

Figs. 20.15A to H: (A) Falope ring excision; (B) Refreshening of edges; (C) Free dye flow; (D) Magnified view; (E) Mesosalpinx stitch; (F) 12 o' clock; (G) Second layer; (H) End result.

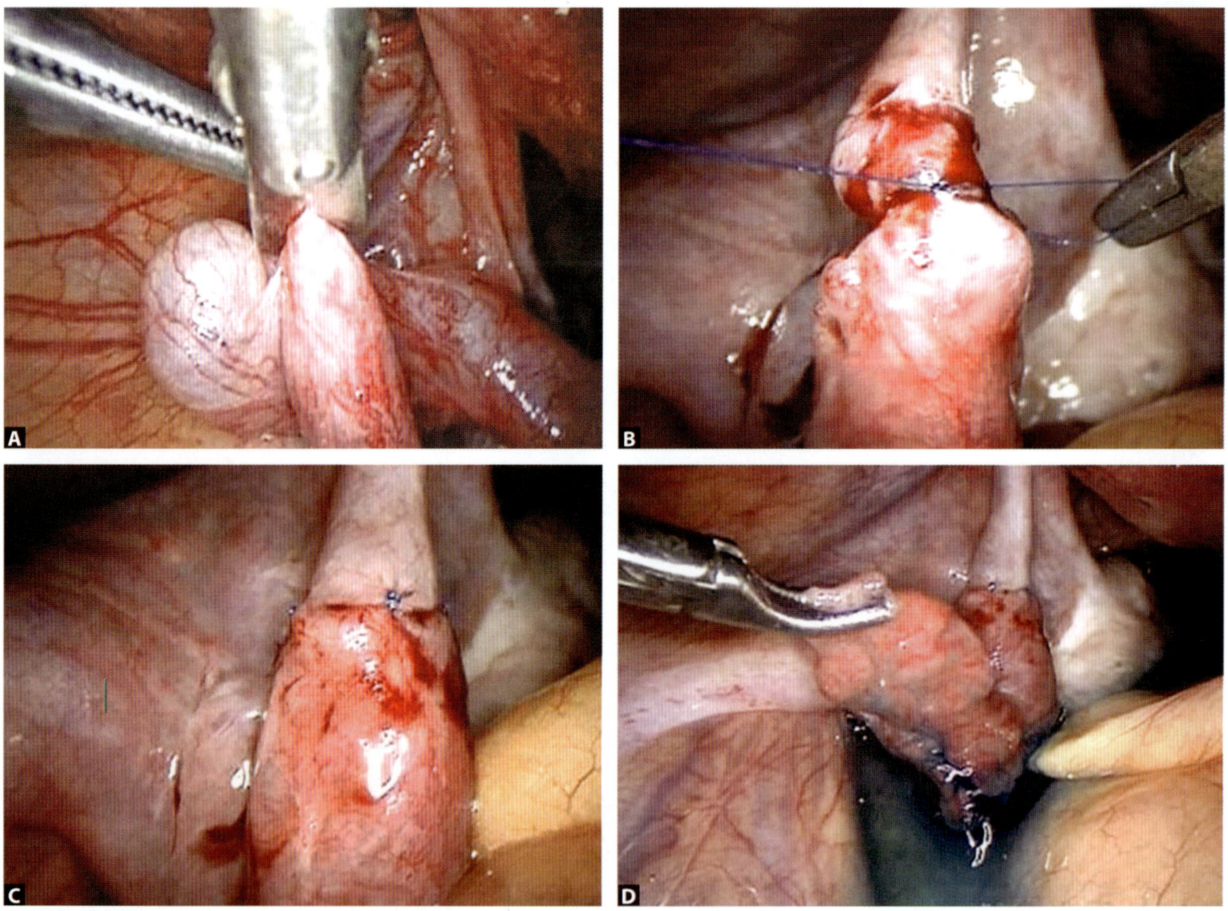

Figs. 20.16A to D: (A) Refreshening ends; (B) First layer; (C) Second layer; (D) Free spill.

Study between 1996 and 2006

TL reversal	Tubal block due to PID	Tubal block secondary to ectopic pregnancy	Failed tubal cannulation for proximal block	Total
299 (68.57%)	90 (20.64%)	16 (3.66%)	31 (7.11%)	436 cases

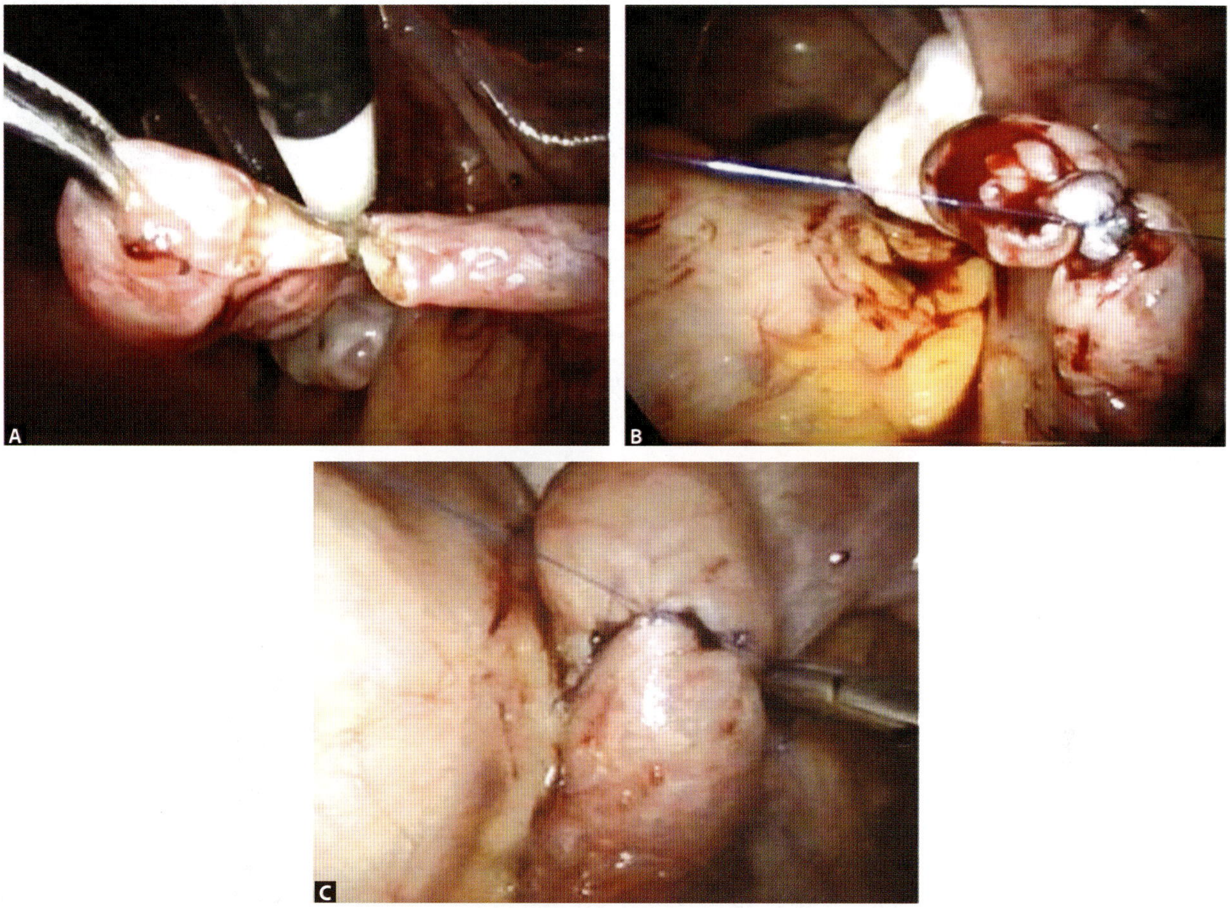

Figs. 20.17A to C: (A) Refreshening ends; (B) First layer; (C) Second layer.

Types of Anastomosis

Bilateral	Unilateral	Incomplete (due to multiple blocks)	Total
324 (74.31%)	92 (21.1%)	20 (4.58%)	436 cases

Types of Anastomosis and Its Results

Types of anastomosis	Isthmo-isthmic	Isthmo-ampullary	Ampullo-ampullary	Juxtamural-isthmic	Juxtauterine-isthmic	Intramural-isthmic	Total
Total No.	186 (42.66%)	137 (31.42%)	57 (13.0%)	26 (5.96%)	12 (2.75%)	18 (4.13%)	436
Cases conceived	165 (88.7%)	119 (86.86%)	26 (45.61%)	13 (50%)	03 (25%)	5 (27.77%)	331 (75.92%)

Case Type vs Result

Out of the 436 successful surgeries, 331 (75.92%) conceived, including 14 cases of ectopic pregnancy (4.2%).

Type of cases	TL reversal (N=299)	Pathological tubes (N=137)	Total (N = 436)
Cases conceived	266 (88.96%)	65 (47.45%)	331 (75.92%)

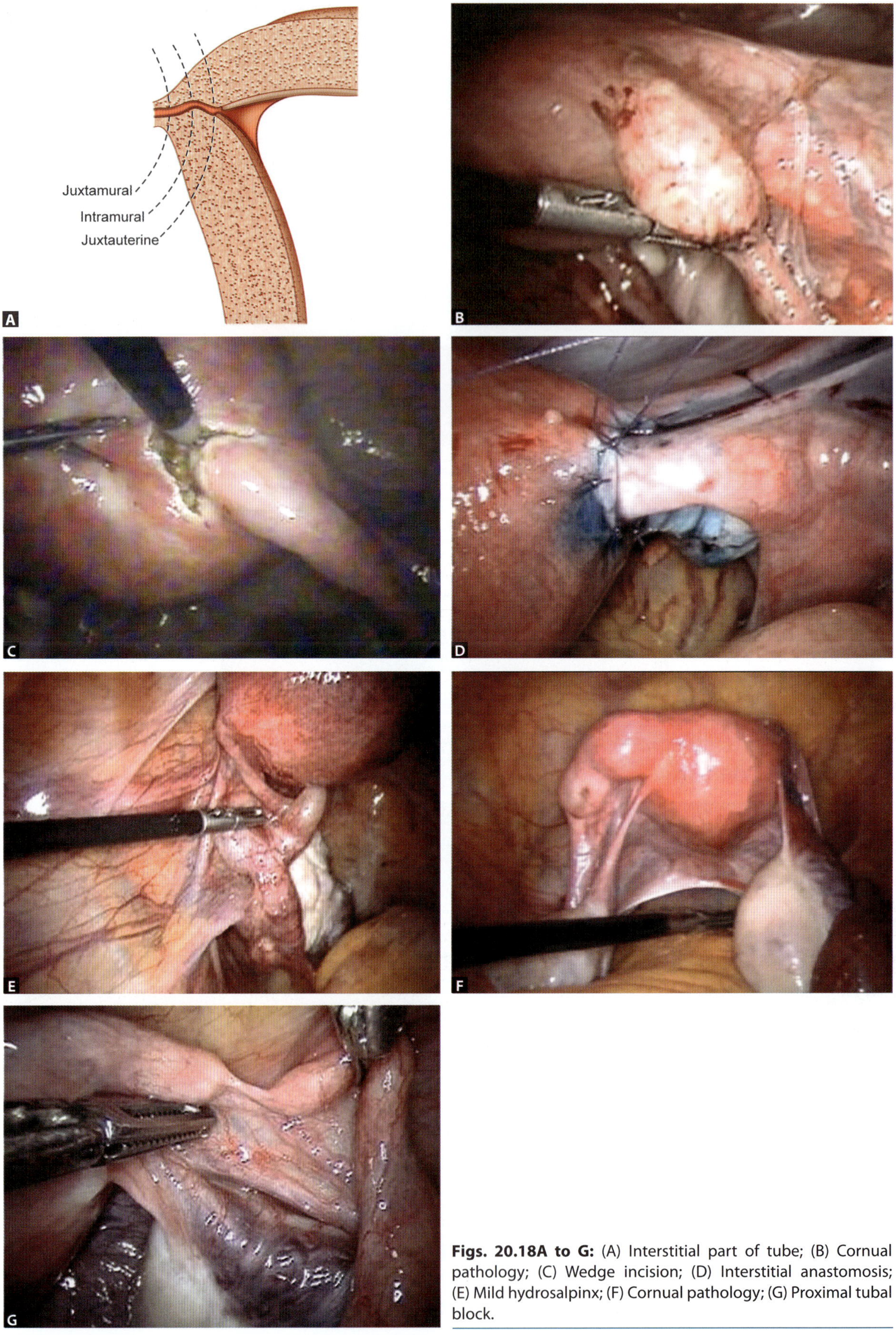

Figs. 20.18A to G: (A) Interstitial part of tube; (B) Cornual pathology; (C) Wedge incision; (D) Interstitial anastomosis; (E) Mild hydrosalpinx; (F) Cornual pathology; (G) Proximal tubal block.

LAPAROSCOPIC SALPINGO-OVARIOLYSIS AND FIMBRIOPLASTY

The risk factors for pelvic adhesions include a history of pelvic inflammatory disease (PID), prior surgery, perforated appendix, endometriosis, inflammatory bowel diseases, bacterial peritonitis, tuberculosis, chemical peritonitis, foreign body reaction and long-term continuous peritoneal dialysis. Adhesions may result in infertility by causing mechanical blockage to the fallopian tubes, thus preventing oocyte retrieval. Para-ovarian peritubal adhesions inhibit follicular growth by possible ovarian entrapment from adhesions around the ovaries. Peritubal as well as intratubal adhesions may affect tubal motility and ovum transport. The slowing or prevention of the embryo's arrival in the uterus may lead to either infertility or an ectopic pregnancy. Infertility may be caused not only by tubal dysfunction but also by adhesion formation following treatment of an ectopic gestation either by laparotomy or laparoscopy.

Technique

Before adhesiolysis is attempted, the surgeon should consider whether (1) lysis of the adhesions would benefit the patient, (2) whether a sharp or blunt dissection should be used and (3) which side of the adhesion should be excised to reduce the risk of injury to vital organs.

Adhesions are cut close to the affected organ at both ends and, if possible, removed from the abdomen. Vascular adhesions are coagulated with microelectrodes. When scissors are used, filmy and avascular adhesions are stretched and then cut. Thick, vascular adhesions must be coagulated before being cut.

Whenever possible, either the adhesions or the ovarian ligaments are grasped instead of the ovarian cortex to reduce trauma. Once the ovaries are lifted from the cul-de-sac and mobilized, the peritubal adhesions are removed.

Once the pelvic structures are freed and hemostasis is achieved, the cul-de-sac is filled with lactated Ringer's solution and the adnexa are allowed to float in the clear fluid. Filmy adhesions that are difficult to identify on the surface of the ovary become visible as they float from the ovarian cortex. These adhesions are grasped with the forceps, cut and removed from their attachments, using laparoscopic microscissors. They are filmy and avascular, and so coagulation is not required.

Agglutinated fimbrial folds are caused by fine avascular adhesions. As the fimbrial folds float and disperse in the fluid, the adhesions become visible; they are grasped, stretched, and sharply cut with fine scissor (Figs. 20.19A to H).

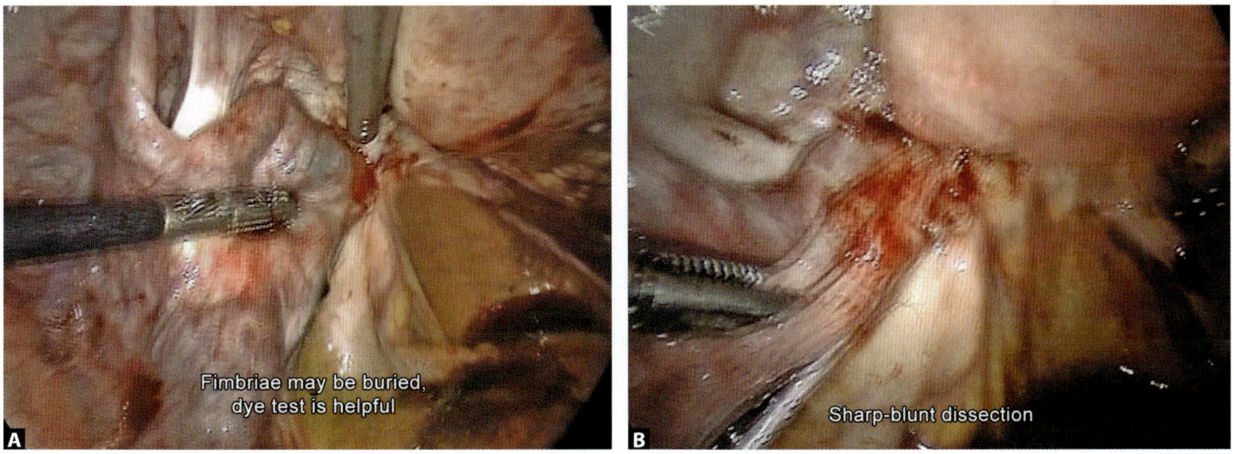

Figs. 20.19A and B

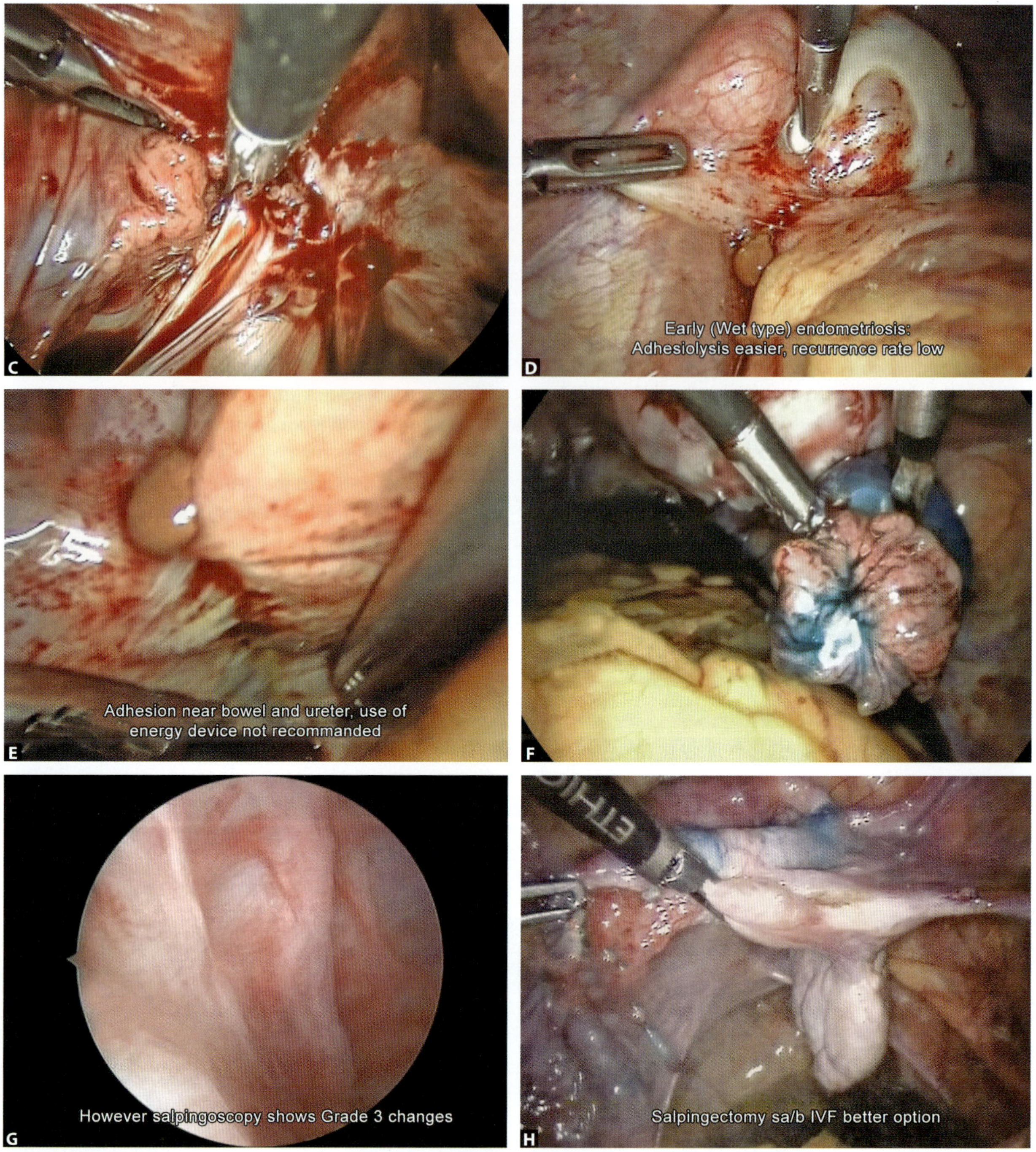

Figs. 20.19C to H

Figs. 20.19A to H: (A) Fimbriae may be buried, dye test is helpful; (B) Sharp blunt dissection; (C) Sharp dissection; (D) Fimbrial adhesions in endometriosis; (E) Do not use energy near bowel, ureter and urinary bladder; (F) Hydrosalpinx: fimbrioplasty performed and patency restored; (G) Salpingoscopy of hydrosalpinx tube shows Grade III findings; (H) Salpingectomy followed by in vitro fertilization is better option.

CONCLUSION

- Establishment of tubal patency is most important task in fertility enhancement.[1-13]
- There is no role of tubal implantation, instead interstitial anastomosis is preferred.
- For ectopic pregnancy, segmental excision is better option than salpingostomy or total salpingectomy, if the sac is <2 cm in size.
- Salpingoscopy appears to have good prognostic and predictive value. It is very helpful in presence of pathological block.

- Significant rise in pregnancy rate in infertile women after laparoscopic adhesiolysis.
- The aim is to restore near normal anatomy.
- Follow microsurgical principles.
- Hydrosalpinx, tuberculosis and endometriosis have poor prognosis.
- Salpingectomy for hydrosalpinx doubles the chances of pregnancy in in vitro fertilization (IVF).
- However, in presence of extensive adhesions, consider proximal ligation and distal fenestration.
- Tubal surgery is more cost-effective than IVF in the long run. It is a single-step treatment as compare with IVF which requires multiple steps in each cycle.
- IVF should be considered when fertility prognosis is likely to be poor with tubal surgery.

REFERENCES

1. Dubuisson JB, Chaperon C, Nos C, et al. Sterilization reversal: fertility results. Hum Reprod. 1995;10(5):1145-51.
2. Gomel V. Microsurgical reversal of female sterilization: a reappraisal. Fertil Steril. 1980;33(6):587-97.
3. Reich H, McGlynn F, Parente C, et al. Laparoscopic tubal anastomosis. J Am Assoc Gynecol Laparosc. 1993;(1):16-9.
4. Swolin K: [50 fertility operations. I. Literature and methods]. Acta Obstet Gynecol Scand. 1967;46(2):234-50.
5. American College of Obstetricians and Gynecologists: ACOG technical bulletin. Sterilization. Number 222—April 1996 (replaces no. 113, February 1998). Int J Gynaecol Obstet. 1996;53(3):281-8.
6. Cetin MT, Demir SC, Toksoz L, et al. the effect of laparoscopic reversal of tubal sterilization on pregnancy rate. Fertil Steril. 1985;43:351-2.
7. Bateman BG, Nunley WC. Jr, Kitchin JD. Fertil Steril. 1987;48:523-42.
8. Mage G, Pouly JL, Bouquet de Jolinière J, et al. Fertil Steril. 1986;46:807-10.
9. Reich HJ. Reprod. Med. 1987;32:736-42.
10. Sauer MV. In: Mishell DR, Davajan V, Lobo RA (Eds). Infertility, Contraception and Reproductive Endocrinology, 3rd ed. Boston, MA: Blackwell; 1991. pp. 682-707.
11. Williams TJ. Obstet Gynecol Clin North Am. 1987;14:1037-48.
12. Van Voorhis BJ. Comparison of tubal ligation reversal procedures. Clin Obstet Gynecol. 2000;43(3):641-9.
13. Nezhat C, Nezhat F, Nezhat C. Nezhat's Operative Gynecologic Laparoscopy and Hysteroscopy. 3rd ed. Cambridge: Cambridge University Press; 2008.

21 of Gynaecological Endoscopy

Endoscopy Techniques for Tubal Sterilization

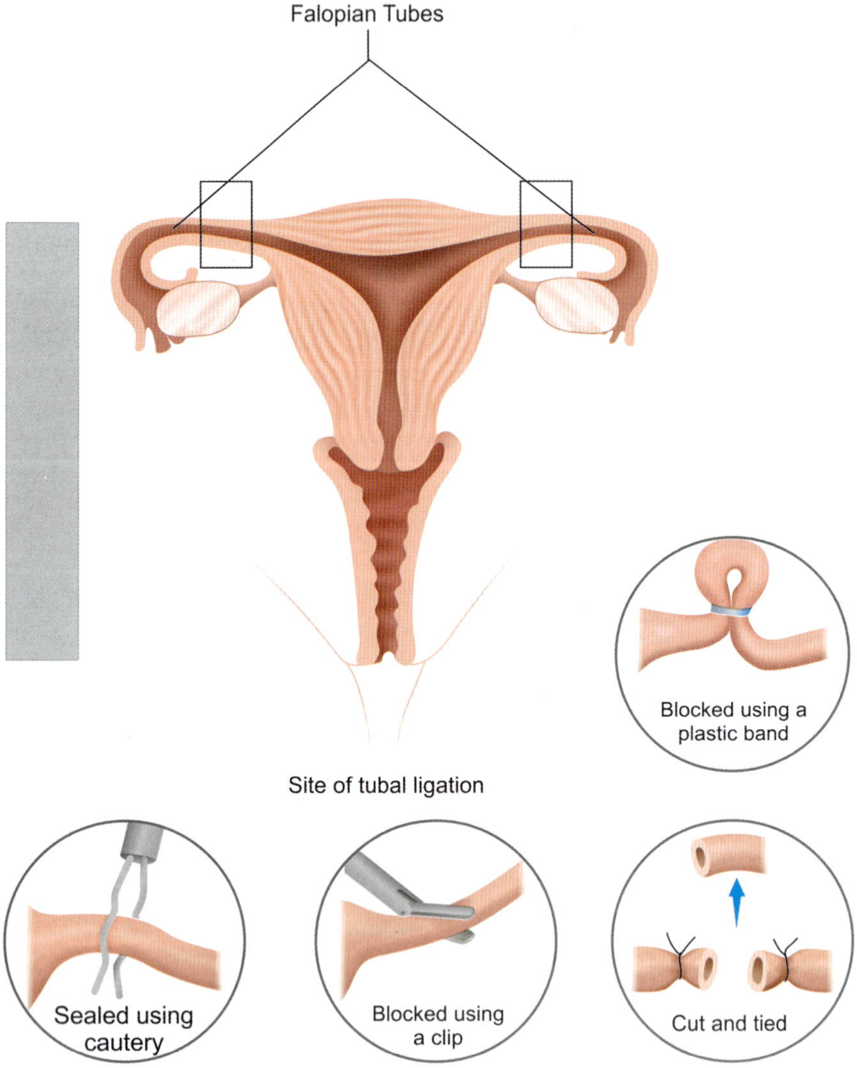

Chapter 21

Endoscopy Techniques for Tubal Sterilization

Parul Kotdawala, Janesh Gupta, Munjal Pandya

INTRODUCTION

Despite extensive research and multiple options available to prevent unwanted pregnancy, even as of today, the most popular and prevalent method of contraception is female sterilization. The World Health Organization (WHO) and United Nations data published recently confirm this fact globally. India is topping the list with almost 40% women having opted for sterilization among all contraceptive users. The advent of laparoscopy in late 1960s led to great shift from mini-laparotomy to laparoscopic sterilization, which remains the method of choice even today. Although it required sophisticated equipment and special training, the minimal access approach led to quick surgery with very high success rates, quick recovery and minimal post-op problems like pain and infection.

LAPAROSCOPIC ROUTE

The laparoscopic sterilization can be performed by blocking the fallopian tubes, transecting them or excising them.

- *Blocking the tube:*
  - With bipolar coagulation at one or multiple sites
  - Applying the silastic Falope ring (Yoon band)
- *Applying clips like Hulka or Filshie:*
  - Bipolar coagulation and cutting the tube (transaction)
  - Salpingectomy

TRANSCERVICAL OR TRANSUTERINE ROUTE

Achieving blockage of the fallopian tubes through transcervical route in a bid to avoid access to the peritoneal cavity was explored by intrauterine placement of quinacrine gel and pallets to achieve chemical inflammation and adhesions leading to blockage of cornual openings. This was a blind technique and became unpopular due to side effects and possible teratogenicity in the event of pregnancy.[1,2]

Recently a new approach of blocking the tubes through trans-uterine route under vision via hysteroscopy has been explored by following techniques:

- Hysteroscopic injection of liquid silicone into each cornual openings (plugs)
- Insertion of coils (Essure)
- Insertion of chemical granule to produce inflammatory blockage (Adiana).

Minimal access to achieve female sterilization seems to be the most acceptable and accurate methods of contraception. This chapter delineates the details of the techniques and their current status.

LAPAROSCOPIC TECHNIQUES

Generally performed under general anesthesia and the technique can be performed as single puncture (needs specially made device) or a double puncture technique. Band/clip technique can be performed under sedation and local trocar site infiltration, but these are usually single puncture.

- Bipolar coagulation
- Coagulation and transaction
- Salpingectomy
- Silicone band (Falope ring) application: The technique is most popular in India, as it has been used as single puncture technique under sedation and local infiltration, as a quick method in a camp setting to enable multiple cases on a single day.
- Clips (Hulka, Filshie): These clips obviate the need to create a loop and hence are less painful. The length of tube is not reduced much.

Counseling

A detailed counseling of the woman and her husband or partner is very important to avoid regrets later on. A complete knowledge of the procedure to be carried out, all the alternatives of contraception, the failure rate and complications needs to be conveyed. The women also need to be counseled about the fact that this procedure causes permanent sterility. In current societies newer alliances following a divorce or separation, or untimely demise of male partner are distinct possibilities. Desire to have another child under such circumstances is very likely. Although a recanalization of the fallopian tubes or recourse to in vitro fertilization (IVF) embryo transfer (ET) is a possibility, the woman must be made aware of this before she embarks on sterilization procedure. Generally the menstruation and the sexuality are not affected. A possibility of the failure of the procedure in spite of appropriate surgical technique also needs to be impressed upon. The quoted failure rates are low, 5–10/1000 procedures, and approximately one-third of these pregnancies after tubal sterilization are ectopic pregnancies.[3] Although the complications are rare, surgical and anesthetic complications may occur. Sterilization does not give protection against sexually transmitted diseases. The procedure does not affect ability to perform day-to-day activity.

Clinical Assessment

A detailed clinical assessment before any surgical procedure requiring general anesthesia is necessary. Allergies and history of any reactions need to be enquired about. Routine history taking, physical examination and necessary investigations along with an informed consent are in order. The WHO has developed eligibility criteria for a woman desiring sterilization operation. There are five major groups A, B, C, D, S under which the client is categorized.[4]

Instruments

Mainly two approaches to enter peritoneal cavity are employed; a single puncture technique where the scope and operating instruments are sheathed in a single sleeve of 11–13 mm diameter and are inserted in to abdomen by a single puncture of 12–14 mm, and the double puncture technique, where the two incisions of 5–7 mm are used for insertion of viewing channel and operating channel separately. A 5 mm laparoscope suffices for the double puncture procedure and angled vision is not very vital for tubal sterilization. When using double puncture technique, the operating channel will be of 5 mm for coagulation technique and 7 mm for using either the silastic rings or the Filshie clip. A fiber-optic cable and either halogen or a xenon light source is used for illumination. Mechanized, electronic gas insufflation system is used for controlled and accurate pneumo-peritoneum and CO_2 is the preferred gas for this. However, nitrous oxide or even air may be used when silastic ring or clip is applied. A 2 mm Veress needle with spring-loaded blunt ended obturator is used to create pneumoperitoneum. Needed trocars for the instrument to be used are kept handy. Speculum, tenaculum and suitable uterine manipulator to manipulate the uterus are required.

Techniques

A semi-Trendelenburg position with thighs abducted is necessary. Abdomen and perineum are painted with antiseptic solution and draped. Vagina is swabbed with antiseptic, followed by vaginal bimanual examination to evaluate uterine size and adnexa. The anterior cervix is caught with vulsellum and the uterine manipulator is introduced in the cavity of the uterus. An infraumbilical semilunar incision on the inferior verge of the umbilicus is the preferred site due to technical and aesthetic aspects. The insufflation with Veress needle followed by trocar insertion, or a direct trocar insertion may be carried out. As the procedure is carried out in the anterior part of pelvis, the insufflation pressure may be kept lower (< 10 mm Hg) than other operative laparoscopy, to reduce postop pain. The entire pelvis is scanned with the scope for concomitant pathologies and for the presence of adhesions.

In the precamera era, laparoscopy surgery was performed by the surgeon bending medially toward the scope to look through. Since the right eye was used for looking through the microscope in younger age, by default the operator was more comfortable using the right eye to look through the scope and keeping the left eye closed or idle. This required standing on the left side of the patient. This also made him or her use the right hand to hold the scope and to use the left hand, being the caudally placed, for performing the procedures. Many senior right-handed surgeons used to find this very uncomfortable. With advent of camera system all these are now unnecessary and the surgeon can stand on the right side of the patient equally well. But with the old habits, most surgeons still continue to stand on the left side. For a general surgeon operating on appendix and gall bladder, the left side gives better callisthenic positioning. If Veress needle is used, an initial flow of 2 L/min is used for insufflation, and once confirming that the needle is in peritoneal cavity, the flow is increased to 10–15 L/min. A pressure of 20 is desirable before the trocar is inserted. But if the procedure is performed under sedation and local infiltration, a quantity of 1.5–2 L of gas is adequate. Since a woman would generally have borne children before opting for the sterilization operation, the stretching of abdominal muscles during pregnancy makes the abdominal wall is fairly lax. Lifting up such a wall is easier and hence trocar insertion is easier.

The head low position along with pneumoperitoneum produces an air (CO_2) filled empty space in front of the pelvis, and lifting up the uterus by manipulation brings it in to this space along with lateral cornual structures. One should carefully identify the fallopian tube, which is in the middle with the round ligament in the front and the ovarian ligament behind.

Silastic bands (Figs 21.1 to 21.3): The Falope ring, also known as the silastic band or the Yoon band, was developed in 1973 by In Bae Yoon and other researchers of the Johns Hopkins School of Medicine.[5-9] Falope ring is made up of silicone rubber with 5% barium sulfate with outer diameter of 3.6 mm, inner diameter 1 mm and thickness of 2.2 mm. The rings have elastic memory when stretched, but only for a few minutes. Blanching and necrosis of the loop occur with immediate effect.

The ring applicator is usually pre-loaded with two Falope rings and is set on ring no. 1 to allow discharge of one ring only (Figs. 21.4 to 21.8). Once the tube is identified, the tongs of the ring applicator are brought out in vacant place in the middle, and the longer tong is rotated to inferior position, with shorter tong on the superior position. The longer tong is guided—in open position—below the fallopian tube, and the

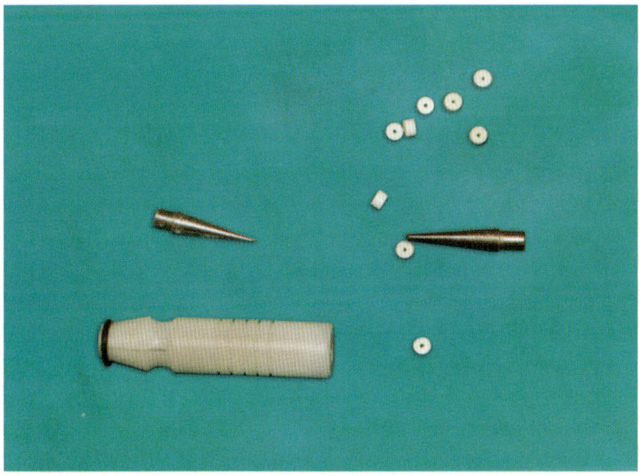

Fig. 21.1: Fallope rings (Yoon Bands), with loader (metal cone) and Applicator (white tube).

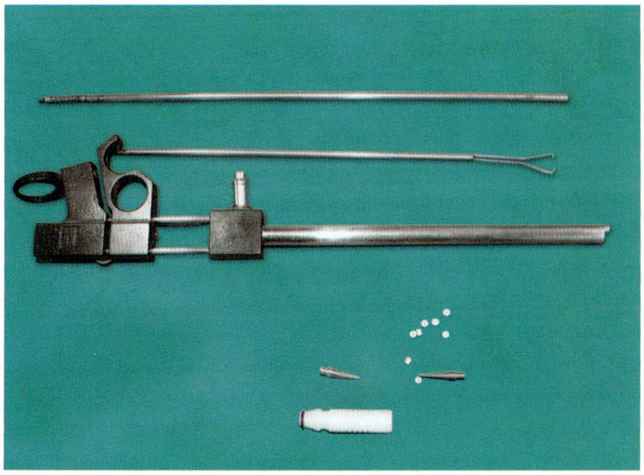

Fig. 21.2: Single puncture TL, Laparocator (KLI make) Scope + Ring applicator.

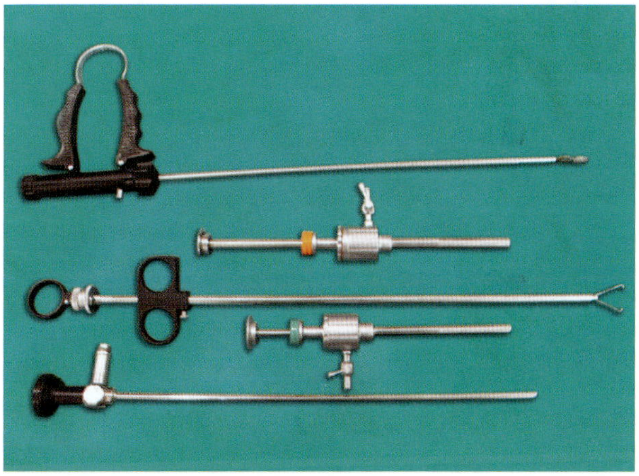

Fig. 21.3: Double puncture TL, Bipolar coagulator, Ring Applicator, and trocars (7 mm for ring applicator and 5 mm for scope).

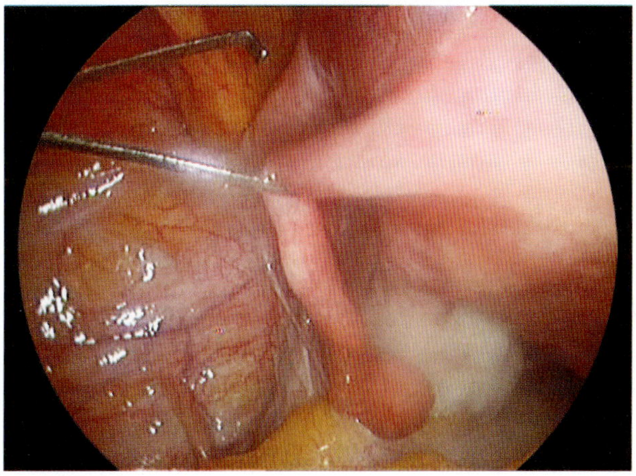

Fig. 21.4: Double puncture TL, Tong lifting and isolating the left fallopian tube.

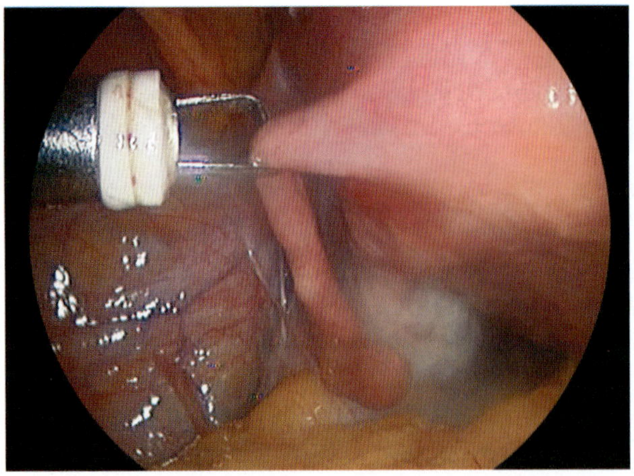

Fig. 21.5: Double puncture TL, closing the tongs.

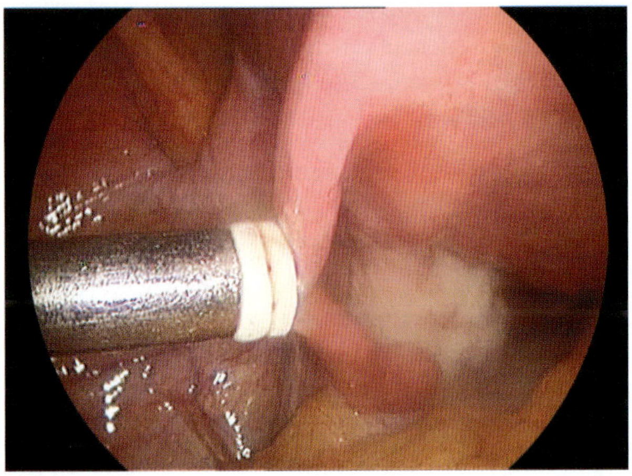

Fig. 21.6: Double puncture TL, pulling the tongs in the sheath to make a loof of the tube.

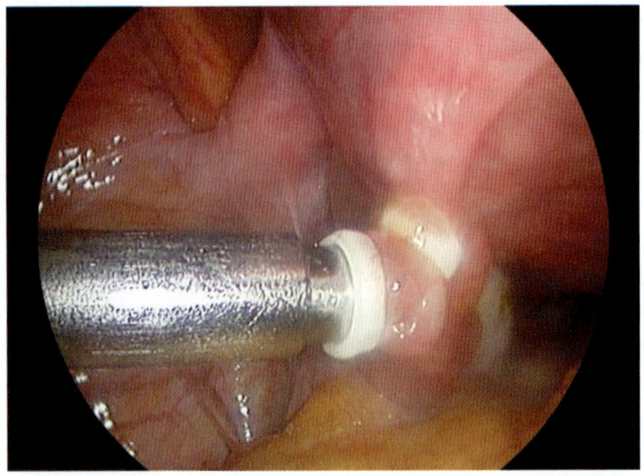

Fig. 21.7: Double puncture TL, discharging the ring on the loop of the left tube.

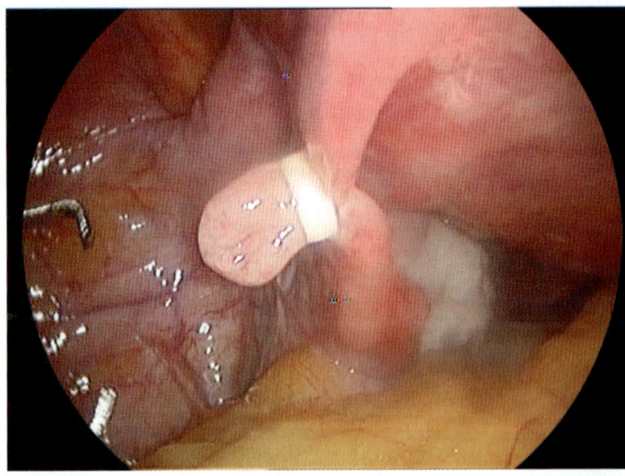

Fig. 21.8: Double puncture TL, releasing the loop, and confirming the correct application.

tube is lifted up in empty space to isolate it from all other structures and let the tubal artery fall away from the tube. This then is held firm and the outer sleeve of the applicator is pushed in, resulting in overlapping approximation of the tongs, holding the tube between them. Further push of outer tube brings the tube inside forming a loop of the tube. A further push releases the ring on to the base of the loop, blocking it twice. Now the outer tube is withdrawn, and the tongs are gently pushed out, releasing the tube in open space. A good loop is 1–1.5 cm long. A shorter loop may lead to partial blockage or displacement of the ring. The loop is checked on both, the upper and the lower margin to see that it covers both surfaces of the tube, to avoid partial application. Now the applicator is set on ring no. 2 to allow discharge of the second ring, and the same procedure is repeated on the opposite tube. The best location for ring application is just proximal to the isthmo-ampullary junction, as that is one of the thinnest area of the tube, and is the most mobile part, to allow good loop formation. Medial to this area brings the loop too close to the tubal cornu, a relatively immobile area, making a smaller loop or ending in tearing of the tube. Too lateral to this the tube is wider making the loop formation difficult. The scope is withdrawn from the cavity then after confirming proper placement, and confirming that there are no complications like tearing, bleeding or trauma to other viscera. CO_2 is removed as much as possible. All equipment are disengaged, and the trocar is withdrawn. A stitch or a stapler is used to close the wound. A careful inclusion of rectus sheath in the stitch is important to avoid scar site hernia whenever the incision is more than 7 mm in length. Falope ring leads to destruction of about 1–3 cm of the tube.[10] Restoring fertility is more likely than with electrocoagulation or the more complex ligation techniques. The rings are easy to apply unless there are pelvic adhesions or edematous enlarged tubes. Transection or tearing of the tubes and short-term postoperative pain are the most common complications.

Clips: The use of clips for female sterilization was reported first in 1953 in the United States.[11] The current spring-loaded silicone-titanium clips, are very safe, effective and easy to apply. The clip is placed on the isthmus of each tube, 2–3 cm from the cornu, with a special applicator. The clips can be used with minilaparotomy and vaginal route also in addition to laparoscopic approach. Among all sterilization techniques the clips cause minimum damage to the tubes, < 1 cm of the tube getting destroyed, compared with approximately 1–3 cm with rings, 3–4 cm with Pomeroy technique and 3–6 cm with electrocoagulation.[12-14] Hence the results of reversing clip sterilization are much better. The original spring-loaded clip was designed by JF Hulka and G. Clemens in 1972. Filshie clip was designed by GM Filshie in 1973 (Figs. 21.9 to 21.17). The clip is made of titanium with inner surfaces lined by silicone. When the clip is closed, the upper jaw closes over the tube and hooks in the lower jaw. The silicone is compressed. As the

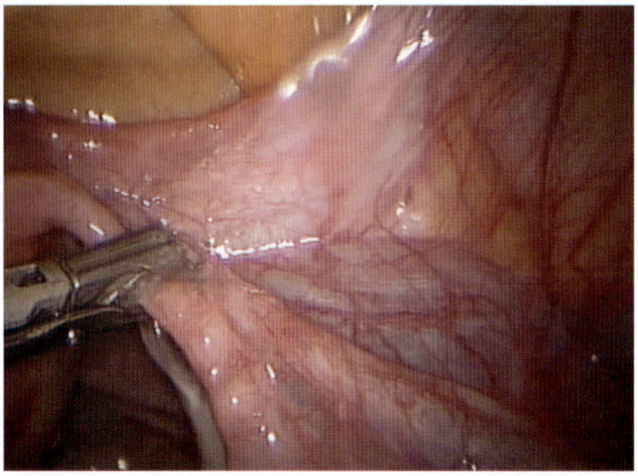

Fig. 21.11: Filshie clip, Clip applied on isthmoampullary junction, and locked.

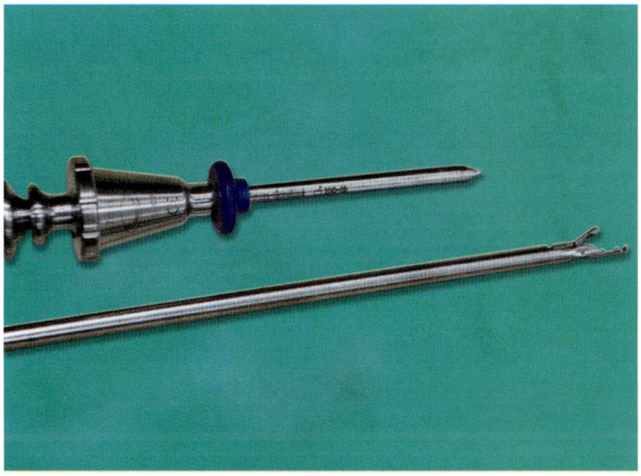

Fig. 21.9: Trocar and Filshie Clip applicator.

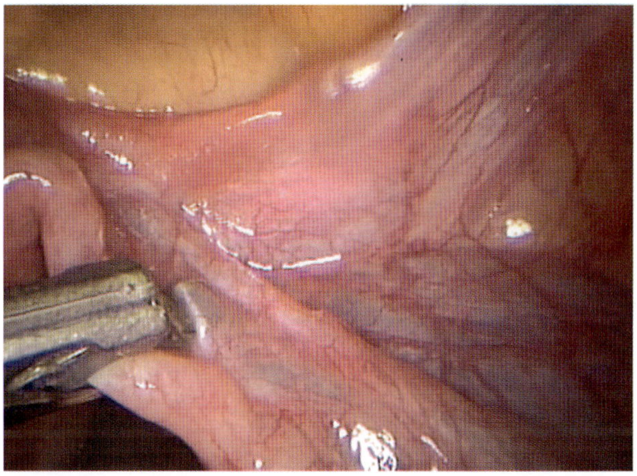

Fig. 21.12: Filshie clip, Clip applied on isthmoampullary junction, and locked.

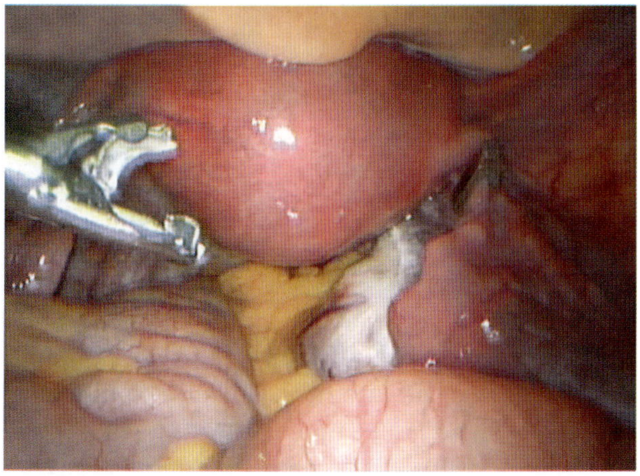

Fig. 21.10: Filshie clip, Clip loaded on applicator.

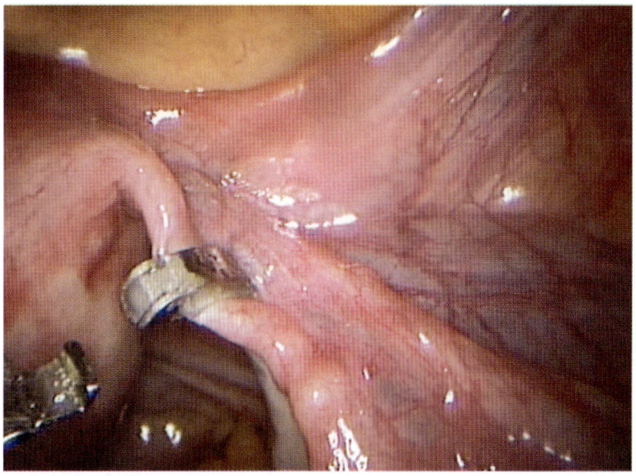

Fig. 21.13: Filshie Clip, Checking the correct application.

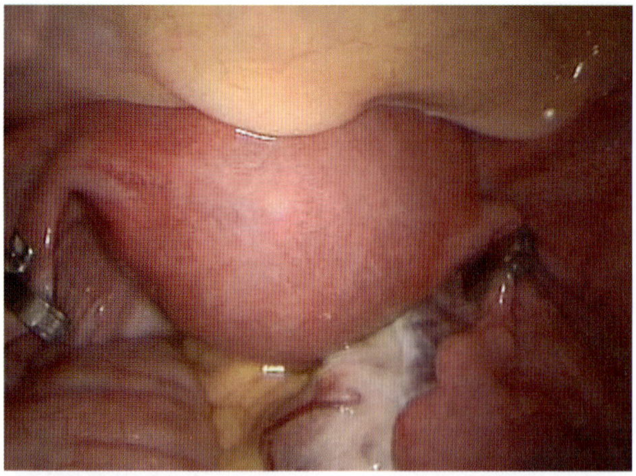

Fig. 21.14: Filshie clip, Final look, both tubes blocked.

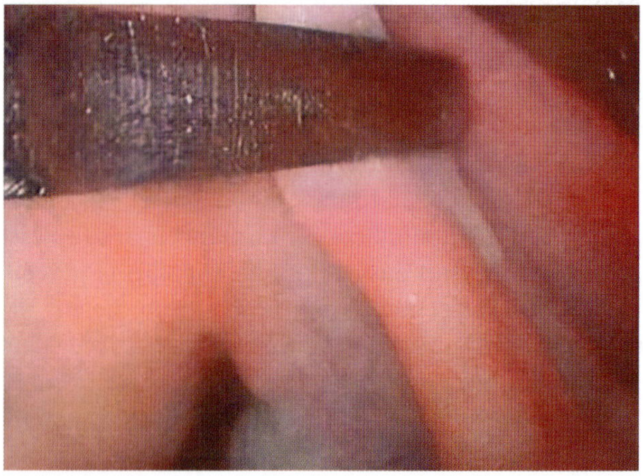

Fig. 21.16: Bipolar coagulation of right fallopian tube at isthmo-ampullary junction.

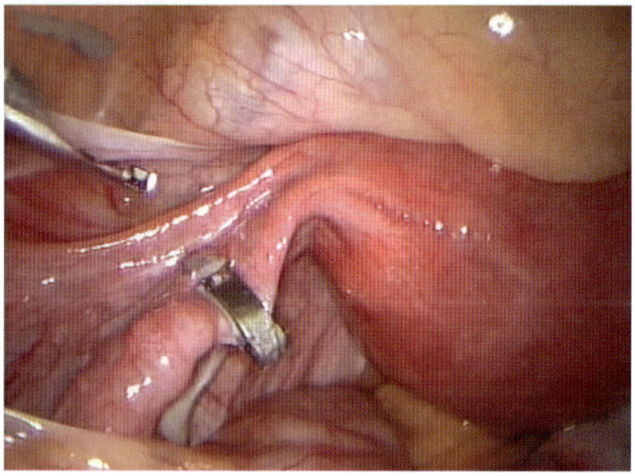

Fig. 21.15: Filshie clip, checking the correct application, left tube.

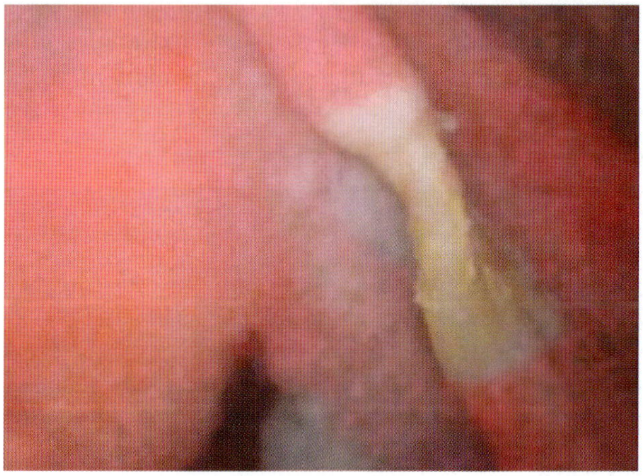

Fig. 21.17: *Bipolar coagulation:* Adequacy of coagulation (1–1.5 cm) checked.

enclosed tubal tissue atrophies, the silicone expands, keeping the tube blocked. The latest models have hinged jaws that open and close easily, allowing the surgeon to remove incorrectly placed clips and reposition them easily. The Filshie clip is big enough to occlude tubes that are enlarged or edematous after pregnancy or pelvic infection.[12,13,15]

Electrocoagulation (Figs. 21.18 to 21.20): Electrocoagulation uses high-frequency electrical current to coagulate and block the tubes. The first technique available, unipolar coagulation, was developed in early 1960s. Electric current passes from the end of forceps through the woman's body to the ground plate placed under her buttocks or thighs. Unipolar coagulation damages 20–50% fallopian tube.[16-18] It is very effective, but after it a reversal is unlikely. As the body is part of the electrical circuit, burns to other organs like the bowel can occur.[19,20] Although rare it is a serious complication. Concerns about bowel burns led to a development of bipolar coagulation in the early 1970s as well as the clips and rings. In bipolar coagulation, electric current passes between the two jaws of the forceps, and a very small portion of the tube is exposed to the current.[21] Accidental burns can occur only if the forceps tongs touch bowel or other organs. Bipolar coagulation destroys lesser tubal tissue than unipolar coagulation does. Using the bipolar coagulation at three to four places on each tube was employed to be sure of complete occlusion.[22-24] With electrocoagulation the tube is occluded by coagulation only, by coagulation and cutting the tube or by coagulation along with removal of a segment of tube. After putting in a laparoscope the tubes are isolated by lifting the uterus up and anterior through vaginally placed uterine manipulator. The tubes are blocked by the passage of electric current via bipolar electrodes. This can be done by a single-puncture device, or a double-puncture device.

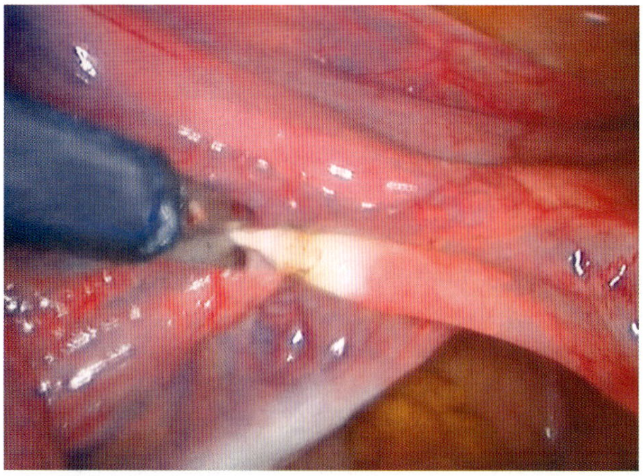

Fig. 21.18: Applying scissors on the centre of coagulation, to divide the fallopian tube.

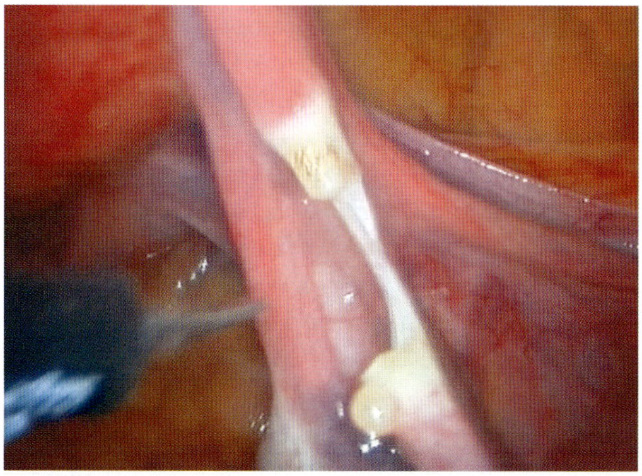

Fig. 21.19: Checking the adequate depth of the cut and falling apart of both ends.

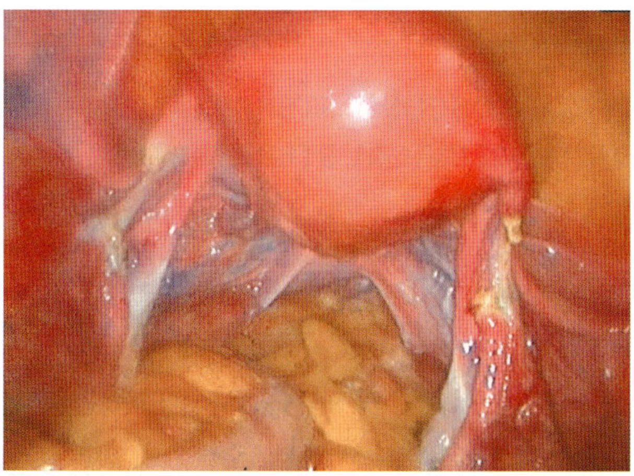

Fig. 21.20: Final picture of both tubes.

Efficacy

Laparoscopic sterilization is effective, more convenient method as compared to conventional laparotomy methods (Table 21.1). Proper history taking and patient workup reduces the failure rates. Failure rate in the United States is reported at 0.4% at the end of the first year, whereas in India, it is reported to be 0.2–1.3% (Table 21.2).

Table 21.1: Female tubal sterilization methods 10-year cumulative failure rates.[25]

Method	Failure rate
Unipolar coagulation	0.75%
Postpartum tubal excision	0.75%
Silastic (Falope or Yoon) ring	1.77%
Interval tubal excision	2.01%
Bipolar coagulation	2.48%
Hulka-Clemens clip	3.65%

Table 21.2: Filshie vs Falope—interval sterilization.

Interval sterilization	Success rate	Failure rate
Filshie clip	99.73%	2.7/1000[a]
Bipolar diathermy	97.52%	24.8/1000[b]
Falope ring	98.23%	17.7/1000[b]
Hulka clip	96.35%	36.5/1000[b]
Unipolar diathermy		7.5/1000[b]
Partial salpingectomy/ Pomeroy*		20.1/1000[b]
Essure	99.74%	2.6/1000[c]

[a]FDA: Food and Drug Administration. The Filshie Clip System. summary of safety and effectiveness. FDA Rep. 1990; 134:1-4.

[b]Peterson, et al. CREST Study, 1990 (NB: Filshie clip not included in the CREST Study as the product was not FDA approved at that time).

[c]Essure Clinical Data (5 years follow-up PMMA supplement, 2005) (NB: Essure, have not included in their statistics those that were unable to be inserted in the tubes).

*Partial salpingectomy is defined as "including modified Pomeroy-type ligation, other types of partial salpingectomy, and total salpingectomy performed by laparotomy" (CREST, 1996)

Complications

Pain: Postop pain is a common complaint. It is more with Falope ring, as the loop swells after ring application. The longitudinal muscles go in to a spasm and cause pain. Infiltration of the tubes with local anesthetic Lignocaine has been tried at the time of procedure to reduce the post op pain. But this has not been very popular as it causes edematous tube. Routine use of analgesic and anti-inflammatory medications for 2–3 days suffice.

Pregnancy after sterilization occurs for various reasons, primarily because the woman is already pregnant at the time of the operation, surgical errors are made, usually by confusing another pelvic structure with the fallopian tube, equipment fails, the ends of the fallopian tube reconnect spontaneously (anastomosis), fistulous (abnormal openings) develop in the tube allowing the sperm and ovum to meet. Unrecognized pregnancies at the time of surgery account for 8–45% of reported failure. Often called "luteal phase pregnancies," these are most likely when sterilization is performed in the postovulatory phase of the menstrual cycle after fertilization has already occurred. Careful questioning all clients about the timing of their last menses and coitus and about their use of contraception can reduce the rate of such pregnancies. Timing sterilization with the preovulatory phase of the menstrual cycle would also help but is not always possible. Surgical errors also cause pregnancies to occur 30–50% of later pregnancies.[6,13,26-32] Most often the round ligament or ovarian suspensory ligament is mistaken for the fallopian tube.[33,34] In an unpublished data in our own department we found that 70% of 18 failed sterilization operations had surgical errors as the cause of the failure of the procedure. If the surgeon identifies the fimbria first, and then applies the rings/clips, the error can be minimized significantly. Other possible mistakes include applying a clip or ring to the wrong part of the tube, not locking a clip properly, and with electrocoagulation failing to coagulate the inner layer of the tube. Surgical mistakes are most frequent when a doctor is in learning phase. One study found that if the surgeon has performed less than 100 cases, the failure rate was three times higher.[35] Other factors like equipment failures; the malfunction of the spring in a clip, breakage of ring/clip even when properly applied, leave the tube patent. Clips and rings can slip off the tube, especially if it is unusually thick. Spontaneous recanalization of the tubes can also happen. F Hulka and colleagues reported one recanalization among 25 pregnancies in 1,079 sterilizations with the spring loaded clips.[30] In another study of 47 sterilization failures, 12 were caused by recanalization of the tubes.[36] The formation of fistulas in the tubal wall at operation site also leads to both intrauterine and ectopic pregnancies.

Ectopic pregnancy is an infrequent complication of tubal sterilization. The reported incidence of ectopic pregnancy within 2 years after sterilization ranged from 0.02–0.31/100 operations. Ectopic pregnancies are more likely to occur after bipolar coagulation of the tubal segment, possibly due to sperm traversing through the peritoneal cavity into the fistula of coagulated segment.[3,35,37]

Procedure-related complications: Depending upon the surgical expertise and functioning of instrument units, complications like vasovagal shock, wound sepsis, abdominal wall hematoma, uterine perforation, surgical emphysema, intestinal injury, large vessel injury and gastrointestinal tract burns may occur. incisional hernia and even death may occur. Few patients may face regret following procedure, especially those who are of young age and have low parity.[38]

Anesthesia-related complications: Anesthetic complications, cardiorespiratory embarrassment, hypoventilation, sepsis.

Death: Female sterilization causes very few deaths. Most recent large surveys around the world report 3–19 deaths/100,000 procedures. Mortality is not common, but may occur due to anesthetic complications, infection or hemorrhage. Reported US mortality rate is around 1.5/1,00,000 procedures and from India, it varies from 10 to 60/1,00,000 procedures.

Contraindications

Laparoscopic sterilization is contraindicated in patients with severe respiratory dysfunction, uncompensated heart disease and large abdominal mass. It should not be performed in postpartum phase and in patients with pregnancy over 12 weeks size.

HYSTEROSCOPIC STERILIZATION OR TRANSCERVICAL STERILIZATION

The minimally invasive laparoscopic tubal sterilization procedure is very safe. And yet it still carries the risk of anesthesia and some major complications. To obviate these by bypassing the transperitoneal route, by reaching the fallopian tubes via uterine cavity was explored. A new innovation along these lines was introduced in 2002 by the name of Essure. This was a hysteroscopic approach to plug the medial end of tube namely the cornual opening. This procedure could be carried out with minimum anesthesia and could be performed as an office procedure. Later on, in 2009, another such device in form of "Adiana" device was introduced in the market for a hysteroscopic sterilization.

Various techniques have been employed for hysteroscopic sterilization.

- Destructive methods: Electrocoagulation, cryocoagulation, bipolar radiofrequency ablation (Adiana), laser, quinacrine.
- Occlusive methods: Silicone, nylon + elastic loop, tubal screw, Essure device.

Essure

Mechanism of Action

The device or system consists of inner coil of stainless steel and polyethylene terephthalate fibers and an outer coil of nickel-titanium. This microinsert is of 3.85 cm in length, which is placed approximately 3–3.5 cm into the intramural part of the fallopian tube via hysteroscopic approach. Once it is placed in the tube, tissue inflammatory response is initiated, by invasion of inflammatory cells including macrophages, foreign body giant cells, plasma cells and fibroblasts, occluding the tubal lumen.[39] Complete tubal occlusion takes usually around 12 weeks, till which time other alternative contraceptive method needs to be used. The confirmation is achieved by hysterosalpingography. Pelvic X-ray can be used for confirming its placement.

Procedure

Hysteroscope is introduced under local paracervical infiltration. The uterine cavity & both tubal ostia are observed and the introducer guide is passed through to the working channel of the scope. The device is introduced into the ostium up to the black mark followed by anti-clockwise rotation of the thumbwheel on handle. The guide catheter is retracted, followed by uncoiling of the filament in the tube. Further anti-clockwise rotation of the thumbwheel will release coil from the device. Three to seven coils should be visible in the uterine cavity (Figs. 21.21 to 21.24).

Placement might be unsuccessful in cases of blocked or stenosed fallopian tubes.

Efficacy

The procedure is more successful if performed during proliferative phase of menstrual cycle. An accurate reporting of postsurgical hysterosalpingography and use of alternative contraceptive methods till confirmed tubal occlusion after 12 weeks is very vital.[40] There was no pregnancy due to method failure for Essure. This method of female sterilization is reported to be the most effective of all the sterilization techniques.[41]

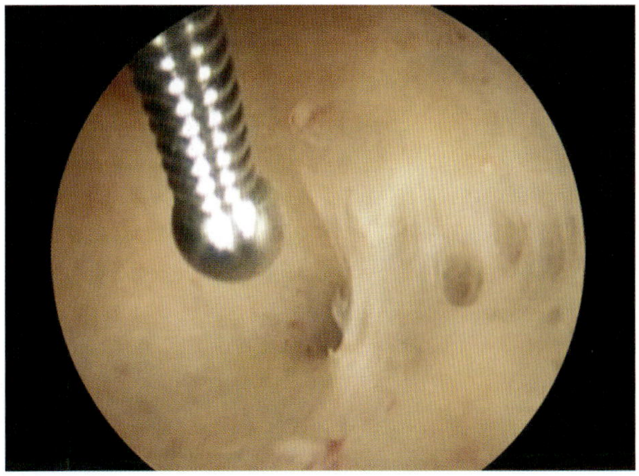

Fig. 21.21: Essure; Aligning to the left cornual opening.

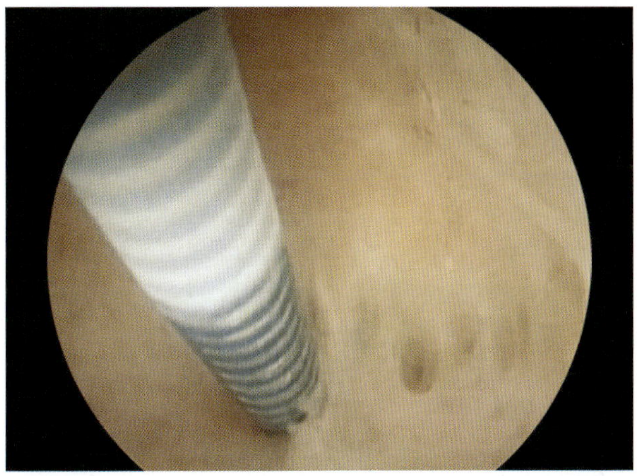

Fig. 21.22: Essure; Inserting the device tip into left cornu.

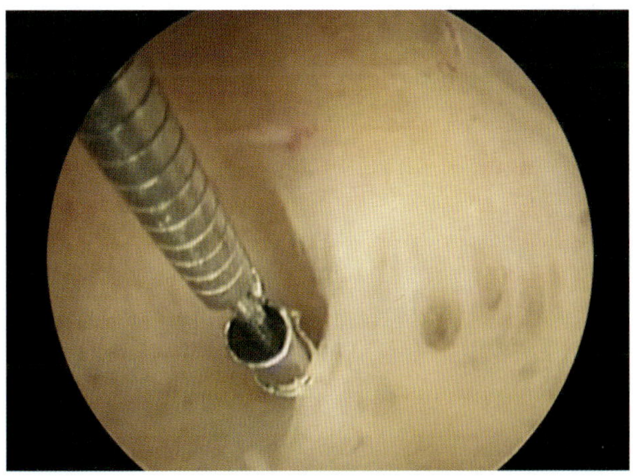

Fig. 21.23: Essure; Disengaging the device from the insert.

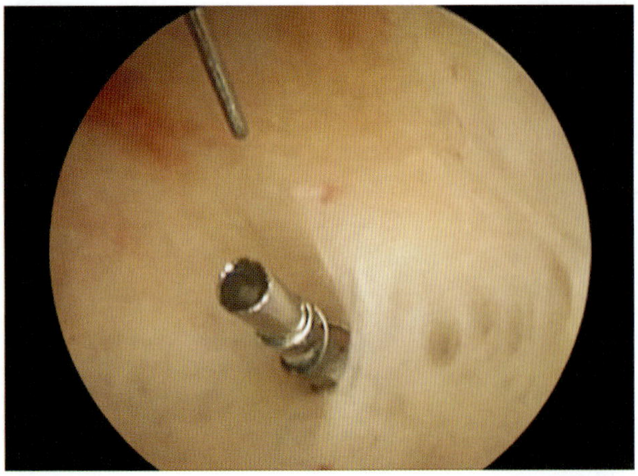

Fig. 21.24: Essure; Final look at the insert.

Table 21.3: Comparison of cumulative risk of pregnancy in CREST study vs Essure sterilization.[44]

Method	5-year follow-up
Bipolar	16.5
Unipolar	2.3
Silicone band	10.0
Spring clip	31.7
Interval salpingectomy	15.1
Postpartum salpingectomy	6.3
All CREST average	13.1
Essure, posterior mean	2.6

As the procedure is performed under local anesthesia, recovery of patient is faster with marked reduction in postprocedure pain. More than 90% patients return to daily routine within 24 h after insertion.[42] In a study comparing Essure with Lap TL, 82% of patients from Essure group had excellent to good tolerance, as compared to only 41% of patients from Lap TL group (Table 21.3).[43]

Safety

Studies conducted showed fewer complications, i.e., perforation, postprocedure pain, ectopic pregnancy, incorrect placement of Essure.[24,45]

Patient can undergo MRI without any problem with Essure device in situ.

Severe cardiac patients with considerable surgical risk has Essure as the best option in form of permanent contraception.[46]

The Essure device is being withdrawn from UK and possibly European markets from September 1, 2017: https://www.fsrh.org/news/fsrh-and-rcog-joint-statement-on-bayers-decision-to-discontinue/.

Adiana

Mechanism of Action

The system works on dual mechanism of thermal damage and insertion of an implant under hysteroscopic guidance. The microinsert is of 3.5 mm length and is made up of nonabsorbable, biocompatible silicone elastomer matrix. The device has position detection array (PDA), which consists of four sensors, which are designed to monitor uniform tissue contact during the step of ablation.

The delivery catheter is soft and pliable, making it flexible. Catheter shaft can bend and buckle in case of resistance.

A delivery catheter is introduced via hysteroscopy approximately 1.4 cm into the intramural part of tube, followed by bipolar radiofrequency energy delivery of 3 W from the tip, creating temperature of 64°C for around 1 min. The generator is equipped with liquid crystal display (LCD), which indicates surgeon of completion of radiofrequency energy delivery.[47] The thermal damage caused creates approximately 5 mm lesion in the tube, within which the matrix of 3.5 mm is placed. Fibroblast invasion into the matrix leads to complete tubal occlusion, which can be confirmed by hysterosalpingography after 12 weeks.[48] Adiana is not visible in X-ray, but visible on ultrasound scans.

Proper placement of the device is usually guided by black mark reaching tubal ostium. Caution needs to be taken not to allow any movement of hands while applying radiofrequency energy and implanting matrix. As the matrix is placed in the ablated area, no part of the device protrudes in the uterine cavity. Blocked/stenosed fallopian tubes may pose difficulty in introducing the device in the fallopian tube.

While introducing the matrix, excessive pressure may dilate the tube or it may dislodge the implant beyond the ablated area.

During HSG, excessive pressure of dye needs to be avoided.

Efficacy

The cumulative failure rate at 1 year was 1.08% and at 2 years, it was 1.82%.[49] Majority of the cases were attributed to method failure and misinterpretation of HSG. In a study of efficacy of various contraceptive methods, failure rate of Adiana was found to be higher and was better only than spring clip application.[50] Adiana system was very well tolerated by patients, with only 9.2% of the patients describing it as very uncomfortable.[49] Adiana matrix is made up of cured silicone and no nickel is used, thus making allergic response unlikely. Nickel allergy may be seen in 10–30% of the women.[51,52]

No major complication was noted in various studies conducted.

Advantage over Essure

As Adiana device does not protrude through into the uterine cavity, the women with Adiana device can undergo future gynecological procedures safely, i.e., hysteroscopy, dilation and curettage, in vitro fertilization, endometrial ablation and endometrial biopsy.

Patient Preparation

Adiana device is best placed when the endometrial lining is atrophic, which is usually better at proliferative phase. Additional preparation can be done by giving progesterone for 6 weeks prior to the placement.

Quinacrine

Quinacrine was initially introduced as slurry with dilutions of 125 mg/mL and 250 mg/mL, but was abandoned due to deaths attributed to absorption of slurry into endometrial capillaries.[53] Pellet-based system was introduced in form of 7 pellets of 36 mg of quinacrine per pellet, using CuT intrauterine device like inserter, and pellets were placed into the uterus for two to three doses, 1 month apart. Anti-inflammatory medication is given on the days of insertion.

Alternative contraceptive methods (oral contraceptives) are advised for next 3 months from the time of first insertion.

Mechanism of Action

Exact mechanism is not known, but it is believed that quinacrine forms quinacrine–DNA complexes, leading to fibrosis of proximal tubal endothelial lining.

Efficacy

Cumulative pregnancy rate of 4.3–4.6% is noted with this method.

Safety

Quinacrine is a mutagen, though no in vivo study has found increase in cancer rate, nor any teratogenesis in fetus born out of failure of this method. Studies confirmed that it was mutagenic in vitro and carried a potential risk due to intrauterine exposure.[1]

On this basis, WHO (Department of Reproductive Health and Research) stated quinacrine as "genotoxic."[54] Patients experienced cramp, like pain, salpingitis, menstrual disorders and dysmenorrhea.[54]

OTHER METHODS OF HISTORICAL IMPORTANCE

- *Electrocautery*: Blind attempts were made at uterotubal junction by using electrocautery under hysteroscopic guidance, but almost one in four cases reported to have tubal patency after the procedure, along with potential risk of uterine perforation and bowel injury.[55]
- *Nd:YAG laser*: Laser was delivered through quartz fiber applying thermal injury to tissues, but around three in four cases reported tubal patency after the procedure, making the procedure obsolete.[56]
- *Ovabloc*: Introduced in 1970s, this system delivers liquid silicone into tubes via hysteroscopic approach, forming plugs, which occlude ostia and tubes. It was not approved by the Food and Drug Administration (FDA).

REFERENCES

1. Clarke JJ, Sokal DC, Cancel AM et al. Re-evaluation of the mutagenic potential of quinacrine dihydrochloride dehydrate. Mutat Res. 2001;494(1-2):41-53.
2. World Health Organization, Department of Reproductive Health and Research. The safety of quinacrine when used as a method of non-surgical sterilization in women. WHO/RHR/09.21;http://www.who.intreproductivehealth/publications/family_planning/en/index.html.2009
3. Peterson HB, Xia Z, Hughes JM, et al. The risk of ectopic pregnancy after tubal sterilization. New Engl J Med. 1997;336(11):762.
4. World Health Organization. Medical Eligibility criteria for contraceptive use. 5th edition, 2015.
5. Lay CL. The new improved silastic band for ligation of fallopian tubes. Fertility and Sterility. 1977;28(12): 1301-5.
6. Poliakoff SR, Yoon IB, King TM. A four-year experience with the Yoon ring. In: Phillips JM, editor. Endoscopy in Gynecology: Proceedings of the Third International Congress on Gynecologic Endoscopy, San Francisco, California. American Association of Gynecologic Laparoscopists, 1978. p. 197-208.
7. Yoon LB. Silicone ring. In: Phillips JM, editor. Laparoscopy. Baltimore, MD: Williams & Wilkins, 1977. p. 174-8.

8. Yoon LB, King TM. A preliminary and intermediate report on a new laparoscopic tubal ring procedure. J Reproduct Med. 1975;15(2):54-6.
9. Yoon LB, Wheelers CR Jr, King TM. A preliminary report on a new laparoscopic sterilization approach: the silicone rubber band technique. Am J Obstet Gynecol. 1974;120(1):132-6.
10. Kleinman RL. Female sterilization. London: International Planned Parenthood Federation (IPPF) (IPPF Medical Publications); 1982. 44 p.
11. Evans TN. Simplified method for sterilization of the female. Am J Obstet Gynecol. 1953;66(2):393-5.
12. Filshie GM. The Filshie clip. In: Van Lith DAF, Keith LG, Van Hall EV (Eds). New Trends in Female Sterilization. Chicago, IL: Year Book Medical Publishers, 1983; pp. 115-23.
13. Filshie GM, Casey D, Pogmore JR, et al. The titanium/silicone rubber clip for female sterilization. Br J Obstet Gynaecol. 1981;86(6):655-62.
14. Sciarra JJ. Surgical female sterilization techniques. In: Goldsmith A, Toppozada M (Eds). Long acting contraception. (Presented at the Symposium on Long-acting Contraception, Alexandria, Egypt, November 3-4, 1983.) Chicago, IL: Northwestern University, Program for Applied Research in Fertility Regulation; 1983. pp. 191-201.
15. Filshie GM. The Filshie clip for female sterilization and its reversal. Presented at the 112th Annual Meeting of the American Public Health Association. Anaheim, CA: November 11-15,1984. p. 126.
16. Loffer FD, Pent D. Risks of laparoscopic fulguration and transection of the fallopian tube. Obstet Gynecol. 1977;49(2):218-22.
17. Sciarra JJ. Survey of tubal sterilization procedures. In: Sciarra JJ, Zatuchni GI, Speidel JJ, editors. Reversal of Sterilization. Hagerstown, MD: Harper & Row; 1978. pp. 117-33.
18. Yuzpe AA, Rioux JE, Loffer FD, et al. Laparoscopic tubal sterilization by the "burn only" technique. Obstet Gynecol. 1977;49(1):106-9.
19. Loffer FD, Pent D. Indications, contraindications and complications of laparoscopy. Obstet Gynecol Surv 1975;30(7):407-27.
20. Peterson HB, Ory HW, Greenspan IR, et al. Deaths associated with laparoscopic sterilization by unipolar electrocoagulating devices, 1978 and 1979. Am J Obstet Gynecol. 1981;139(2):141-3.
21. Rioux JE, Cloutier D. A new bipolar instrument for laparoscopic tubal sterilization. Am J Obstet Gynecol. 1974;119(6):737-9.
22. Peterson HB, Xia Z, Wilcox LS et al. Pregnancy after tubal sterilization with bipolar electrocoagulation. Obstet Gynecol. 1999;94(2):163-7.
23. Hirsch HA, Nesser E. Bipolar high frequency coagulation. In: Van Lith DAF, Keith IG, Van Hall EV, editors. New Trends in Female Sterilization. Chicago, IL: Year Book Medical Publishers; 1983. pp. 83-90.
24. Roy S, Mishell DR Jr. The optimal method of female sterilization. In: Zuspan, FP, Christian CD, editors. Reid's Controversies in Obstetrics and Gynecology. Vol. 3. Philadelphia, PA: WB Saunders; 1983. pp. 528-35.
25. Peterson HB, Xia Z, Hughes M et al. The risk of pregnancy after tubal sterilization: findings from the US Collaborative Review of sterilization. J Obstet Gynecol. 1996;174(4):1161-70.
26. Burkman RT. The Johns Hopkins experience with laparoscopic Falope ring sterilization. In: Hingorani V, Randit RD, Bhargava VL, editors. Proceedings of the Third International Seminar on Maternal and Perinatal Mortality Pregnancy Termination and Sterilization, New Delhi. India, October 3-5. New Delhi; New Roxy Press; 1980. pp. 423-4.
27. Chi IC, Garddner SD, Laufe LE. The history of pregnancies that occur following female sterilization. Int J Gynecol Obstet. 1979;17(3):265-7.
28. Devilliers VP. Sterilization failure: an analysis of 27 pregnancies after a previous sterilization procedure. South African Med J. 1982;61(16):589-90.
29. Hughes GJ. Sterilisation failure. Br Med J. 1977; 2(6098):1337-9.
30. Hulka JF, Mercer JP, Fishburne JI et al. Spring clip sterilization: one-year follow-up of 1,079 cases. Am J Obstet Gynecol. 1976;125(8):1039-43.
31. Tadjerouni A, Flici O, Wauters G. et al. Failure of laparoscopic sterilization by Hulka-Clemens clips. Eur J Obstet Gynecol Reproduct Biol. 1983;14(6):393-8.
32. Trias M. Preliminary data from sterilization failure study. [Memorandum]. Atlanta, GA: Centers for Disease Control, Department of Health and Human Services; 1984 (Unpublished).
33. Loffer FD, Pent D. Pregnancy after laparoscopic sterilization. Obstet Gynecol. 1980;55(5):643-8.
34. World Health Organization (WHO). Female Sterilization: Guidelines for the Development of Services. 2nd ed. Geneva: WHO; 1980. (WHO Offset Publication No. 26). 47 p.
35. Chi IC, Laufe LE, Gardner SD, et al. An epidemiologic study of risk factors associated with pregnancy following female sterilization. Am J Obstet Gynecol. 1980;136(6):768-73.
36. Soderstrom RM. Sterilization failures and their causes. Am J Obstet Gynecol. 1985;152(4):395-403.
37. McCausland A. High rate of ectopic pregnancy following laparoscopic tubal coagulation failure. Am J Obstet Gynecol. 1980;136:977.
38. Royal College of Obstetricians and Gynecologists. Male and Female Sterilization: Evidence-based Clinical Guideline Number 4, January 2004.
39. Valle RF, Carigan CS, Wright TC et al. Tissue response to the STOP microcoil transcervical permanent contraceptive device: results from a prehysterectomy study. Fertil Steril. 2001;76(5):974-80.
40. Kerin JF. Pregnancies in women who have the Essure hysteroscopic sterilization procedure: a summary of 37 cases. J Minim Invasive Gynecol. 2005;12(suppl):28. Abstract 67.
41. Adiana Transcervical Sterilization System PMA P070022 Panel Package (pp. 47-48). US Food and

Drug Administration Obstetrics and Gynecology Devices Panel Web site. http://www.fda.gov/ohrms/dockets/ac/07/breifing/2007-4334b 100-index.html. Updated December 11, 2007.

42. Scarabin C, Dhainaut C. The ESHYME study. Women's satisfaction after hysteroscopic sterilization (Essure micro-insert). A retrospective multicenter survey. Gynecol Obstet Fertil. 2007;35(11):1123-8.
43. Duffy S, Marsh F, Rogerson L et al. Female sterilization: a cohort controlled comparative study of ESSURE versus laparoscopic sterilization. BJOG. 2005;112(11):1522-8.
44. Levy B, Levie MD, Childers ME. A summary of reported pregnancies after hysteroscopic sterilization. J Minim Invasive Gynecol. 2007;14(3):271-4.
45. MAUDE database. US Food and Drug Administration Center for Devices and Radiological Health Web site. http://www.accessdata.fda.gov/scripts/cdrh/cfdocs/cfMAUDE/search.CFM
46. Famuyide AO, Hopkins MR, El-Nashar SA et al. Hysteroscopic sterilization in women with severe cardian disease: experience at a tertiary center. Mayo Clin Prac. 2008;83(4):431-8.
47. Hologic, Inc. Adiana Permanent Contraception Instructions for Use and Radiofrequency (RF) Generator Operator's Manual. Marlborough. MA: Hologic; 2009.
48. Adiana Transcervical Sterilization System PMA P070022 Panel Package. US Food and Drug Administration Obstetrics and Gynecology Devices Panel Web site. http://www.fda.gov/ohrms/dockets/ac/07/briefing/2007-4334b 100-9ndex.html. Updated December 11, 2007. pp. 13-5.
49. Vancaillie TG, Anderson TL, Johns DA. A 12-month prospective evaluation of transcervical sterilization using implantable polymer matrices. Obstet Gynecol. 2008;112(6):1270-7.
50. Ory EM, Hines RS, Cleland WH et al. Pregnancy after microinsert sterilization with tubal occlusion confirmed by hysterosalpingogram. Obstet Gynecol. 2008;111(2 Pt 2):508-10.
51. Lassere J. Nikel induced allergic dermatitis and Essure device. J Nouvelles Dermatol. 2010;29: 142-3.
52. Peltonen L. Nickel sensitivity in the general population. Contact Dermat. 1979;5(1):27-32.
53. Zipper J, Medel M, Goldsmith A et al. the clinical efficacy of the repeated transcervical instillation of quinacrine for female sterilization. Int J Gynaecol Obstet. 1976;14(6):499-502.
54. Sokal DC, Hieu do T, Laon ND, et al. Safety of quinacrine contraceptive pellets: results from 10-year follow-up in Vietnam. Contraception. 2008;78(1): 66-72.
55. Greenberg JA. Hysteroscopic sterilization: history and current methods. Rev Obstet Gynecol. 2008;1(3): 113-21.
56. Brumsted JR, Shirk G, Soderling MJ et al. Attempted transcervical occlusion of the fallopian tube with Nd:YAG laser. Obstet Gynecol. 1991;77(2):327-8.

KIEL SCH•OL

22 of Gynaecological Endoscopy

Tubal **Torsion**

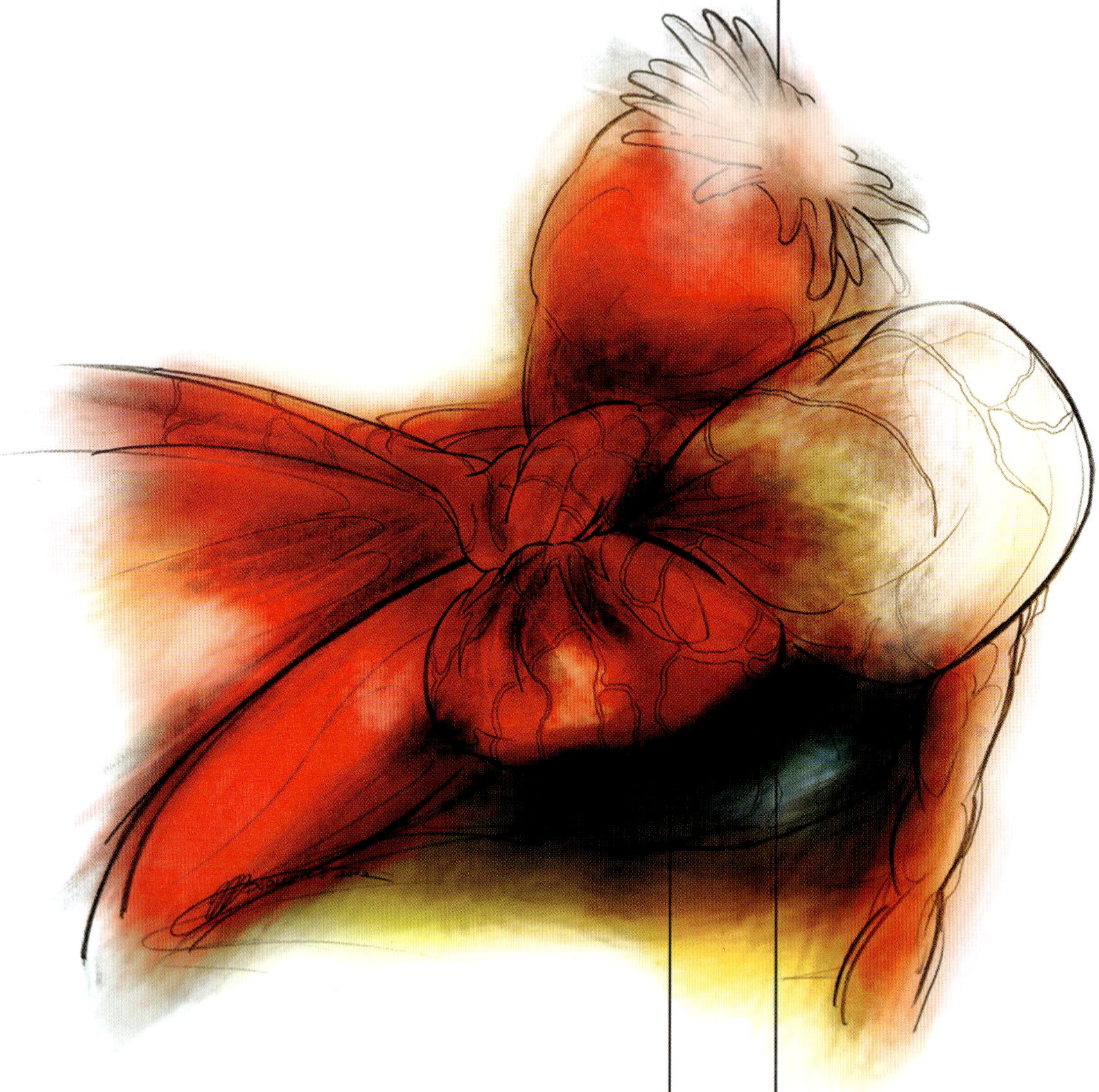

Chapter 22

Tubal Torsion: The Diagnostic Dilemma

Ibrahim Alkatout, Ivo Meinhold-Heerlein, Liselotte Mettler

INTRODUCTION

Acute fallopian tube torsion is a very rare event and occurs in both normal and pathological fallopian tubes. There are intrinsic and extrinsic causes of fallopian tube torsion (Table 22.1).

Usually the torsion of the fallopian tube is accompanied by torsion of the ovary. An ovarian mass contributes to 50–60% of the cases of fallopian tube torsion.

Fallopian tube torsion is a cause for acute low abdominal pain, which is quite difficult to diagnose. The purpose of this chapter is to review the available data on tubal torsion and update its diagnosis and treatment in the era of laparoscopic surgery.

Table 22.1: Intrinsic and extrinsic causes of fallopian tubal torsion.

Intrinsic
• Congenital anomalies
• Excessive length of tube or spiral course
• Acquired pathology
• Hydrosalpinx
• Hematosalpinx
• Neoplasm
• Previous surgery
• Autonomic dysfunction and abnormal peristalsis
Extrinsic
• Disease (chronic or acute) of the neighboring structures
• Neoplasm
• Adhesions
• Pregnancy
• Mechanical factors
• Movement or trauma to the pelvic organs
• Pelvic congestion

In literature several hundred cases have been reported since the original description by Bland-Sutton in 1890.[1] The lack of pathognomonic symptoms, clinical findings on physical examination, and specific imaging or laboratory characteristics makes this entity difficult to diagnose preoperatively, which can cause surgical intervention to be postponed. Today, surgical repair is definitely performed by laparoscopy. The introduction of laparoscopy for routine use in gynecology has changed the approach to both the diagnosis and treatment of fallopian tube torsion.

Isolated torsion of the fallopian tube is a rare entity with an incidence of 1 in 1.5 million women.[2] Here we report on an adolescent patient with chronic torsion of the left fallopian tube and the necessary surgical steps, which, in this case, were performed very late after recognition of the disease.[3]

The differential diagnosis of tubal torsion is given in Table 22.2.

A 15-year-old nulligravid girl was referred to the outpatient gynecology clinic with a history of intermittent left iliac fossa colicky pain of 18-month duration, which was not related to her menstrual cycle. She had neither developed pyrexia nor presented any signs of inflammation such as leukocytosis at any time. She had undergone abdominal ultrasonographic examination at the beginning of her complaint which diagnosed a left simple ovarian cyst of 2 × 3 cm in diameter. She had received combined oral contraceptive pills for 3 months but without any improvement. Over a period of 18 months, she underwent many examinations requested by different physicians in different centers. She had been admitted to emergency units six times and received various treatments (Table 22.3). Attendance at school was also irregular due to her symptoms.

Table 22.2: Differential clinical diagnosis of tubal torsion separated in gynecological and nongynecological origin.

Gynecological	Nongynecological
	Acute appendicitis
	Cystitis
Ectopic pregnancy	Pyelonephritis
Torsion of ovary	Nephrolithiasis
Ovarian cyst	Perforation of (Hollow organ) stomach, bowel, gallbladder
Ruptured corpus luteum cyst or follicle	Obstruction of Hollow organ
Necrotic myoma	Intra-abdominal inflammation (peritoneum, all abdominal organs, diverticulum)
Pelvic inflammatory disease (salpingitis)	Rupture of parenchymatous organs (liver, spleen, kidney)
Tubo-ovarian abscess	Vascular ischemic disease (bowel, mesenterium)
	Vascular hemorrhagic disease (aorta, all abdominal vessels)

On presentation to our center, the patient was asymptomatic. She was on the third day of her menstrual cycle and had been using combined oral contraceptive pills for 9 months prior to presentation. Menarche was at the age of 13. Her previous medical, surgical, gynecological histories were otherwise uneventful. There were no abnormalities on physical examination. Transvaginal ultrasonographic scan revealed normal uterus and ovaries and evidenced the presence of a round, thick-walled, cystic structure measuring 4.7 × 3.2 cm adjacent to the left ovary and mild fluid collection in the pouch of Douglas (POD). Furthermore, magnetic resonance imaging (MRI) revealed a well-circumscribed mass with thickened wall and contrast enhancement adjacent to the left ovary (Fig. 22.1).

In view of the long debilitating history of pain and the psychological impact on the patient, coupled with the ultrasound and MRI findings, she was counseled and scheduled for diagnostic laparoscopy with the possibility of surgical intervention as deemed necessary, despite the fact that she was at this point symptomless.

On laparoscopy, there was mild fluid collection in POD. The left tube was observed to have two twists at its middle part and a thick-walled cystic dilation at its distal portion that was adherent to the POD and the left lateral pelvic wall (Figs. 22.2A to C). The uterus, both ovaries and the right tube, were normal. There were no other abnormal findings on laparoscopic abdominal inspection.

Fluid from the POD was aspirated and preserved for cytological examination. The left tube was freed by blunt dissection. After detorsion of the tube, a chord-like, obliterated segment at the site of twisting was observed. After rinsing of the tube with warm Ringers solution and observation for 15 min, there were obviously no signs of reperfusion of the distal portion.

Left salpingectomy was performed using bipolar coagulation forceps and scissors. The postoperative course was uneventful and the patient was discharged home on the next day. Histopathological examination showed the presence of hematosalpinx and hemorrhagic infarctions of the tubal wall. Cytological examination of the cul-de-sac aspirate also revealed the presence of chronic inflammatory cells.

OPERATIVE STEPS

1. Diagnosis via ultrasound or MR (for this technique see also the chapter on 'Ectopic Pregnancy'). The development of transvaginal ultrasonography has enormously improved the early detection of female inner genital pathologies such as tubal torsion.
2. Diagnostic laparoscopy, even if the patient at that moment has no symptoms (for the technique see also the detailed description in the chapter 'Ectopic Pregnancy').

   At laparoscopy, the location, size, and nature of the pathology are ascertained. If there is hemoperitoneum, this can complicate the whole operation. Dependent on the degree of bleeding, a primarily inserted grasper localizes the ruptured tube and tamponades the bleeding site. After safe compression of the bleeding source, blood and blood clots can be removed by suction and irrigation.

   The 5-mm suction cannula is usually sufficient for this purpose. In emergency cases, such as hemoperitoneal shock or large hemoperitoneum, an 11 mm cannula with the appropriate suction tube can be preferable. Even organized blood clots can be removed with only the suction instrument. Under constant suction with the suction device, blood clots are aspirated and broken

Table 22.3: Timetable of preoperative consultations.

Date	Presenting symptoms	Location	Examination	Diagnosis	Treatment
04 Feb 2004	Severe lower abd. pain	Emergency Unit, Kiel	Abd. US	Ovarian cyst (2 × 3 cm)	Analgesics
04 March 2004	Consultation visit	Gynecologist (private clinic)	TVUS	IDEM (Intradural extramedullary)	Combined OC pills
03 June 2004	Follow-up visit	Gynecologist (private clinic)	TVUS	IDEM (Intradural extramedullary)	
05 March 2005	Severe lower abd. pain	Emergency Unit, Kiel	TVUS	IDEM (Intradural extramedullary)	
07 March 2005	Followup visit	Gynecologist (private clinic)	TVUS	IDEM (Intradural extramedullary)	Reassurance
03 May 2005	Left loin pain				Analgesics
04 May 2005	Left loin pain	Family practitioner (PC)	Abd. + back examination	Low back pain	Analgesics
28 May 2005	Severe lower abd. pain	Emergency Doctor home visit	Bedside blood glucose testing, urine analysis	Mild hypoglycemia	Analgesic injection and psychological counseling
31 May 2005	Followup visit	Same Emergency Doctor (PC)	Laboratory blood tests	-	-
04 July 2005	Severe lower abd. pain	Emergency Doctor. Hotel visit Mallorca	Abd. + back examination, Bedside urine test	-	Analgesic supp., Referral to hospital for X-ray
04 July 2005	-	Hospital Manacor	Clinical examination, Laboratory blood tests	Lower abd. colics	Spasmolytic injection
05 July 2005	Followup visit	Polyclinic, Cala Agulla	Abd. and back examination	Suspicion of rupture of abd. muscles	Referral to hospital for X-ray examination
05 July 2005	-	Hospital Alcudia	X-ray examination	Suspicion of intestinal, muscle troubles	Recommendation to perform Abd. US examination
06 July 2005	Followup visit	Polyclinic, Cala Agulla	Abd. and back examination	Suspicion of rupture of abd. muscles	Counseling, analgesic cream
14 July 2005	Followup visit	Family practitioner (private clinic)	Abd. US	Suspicion of abd. lymphadenopathy and intestinal polyps	Referral to hospital for CT scan and MRI
24 July 2005	Lower abd. pain and vomiting	Emergency Unit, UKSH	Abd. US	-	Analgesic injection
28 July 2005	-		CT, MRI	Abd. Flatulence	Herbal therapy
03 Aug 2005	Severe, acute lower abdominal pain and vomiting	Pediatric Surgery Unit, UKSH	Abd. US	Constipation	Admission for 2 days, analgesic infusion.
05 Aug. 2005	Lower abdominal pain	General Surgery Unit, UKSH	Colonoscopy	No abnormal findings	Exclusion of the cyst as a source of pain
11 Aug 2005	Gynecological consultation	Gynecology Clinic, UKSH	TVUS	Left cystic adnexal mass	Recommendation for laparoscopy

Abd., abdominal; TVUS, transvaginal ultrasound; OC, oral contraceptive; UKSH, Universitätsklinikum Schleswig Holstein Campus Kiel; PC, private clinic

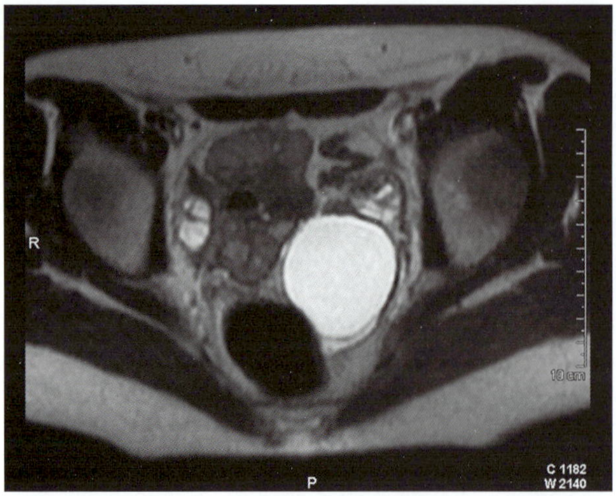

Fig. 22.1: MRI evaluation of the pelvis. Axial MRI view of the pelvis shows a contrast-enhanced roundish structure adjacent to left pelvic sidewall and an echolucent pool of fluid in the pouch of Douglas.

by pulling the suction tip just behind the trocar end. By this means the bigger blood clots are broken and can more easily be evacuated through the suction aspirator. Excessive irrigation lifts the bowel and worsens the overview.

Once bleeding is controlled, the remaining blood clots be removed from the abdominal cavity. The suction instrument and the use of forced irrigation will cleanse the abdominal cavity quickly with minimal trauma to these structures.

After evacuation of the cul de sac and movement of the bowel upward the whole tube must be presented beginning with the proximal isthmic portion and progressing to the fimbriated end of the tube. The tube is primarily held with one or two grasping forceps trying to proceed with the detorsion bluntly.

Afterward, a final inspection is made to coagulate any bleeding caused by grasping the tube and the mesosalpinx.

3. *Detorsion of the tube:* The tube is untwisted, to allow revascularization to occur. This is performed by grasping the tube at its proximal and distal part and simply turning the tube with atraumatic forceps.
4. *Look for reperfusion of the tube:* The enlarged and blood-filled tube, with a diameter of up to 5 cm, is dark blue to black and partly necrotic. If after detorsion and within 15 min the tube does not show any signs of reperfusion with a slight change of color toward the pinkish appearance, it must be considered as definitely necrotic

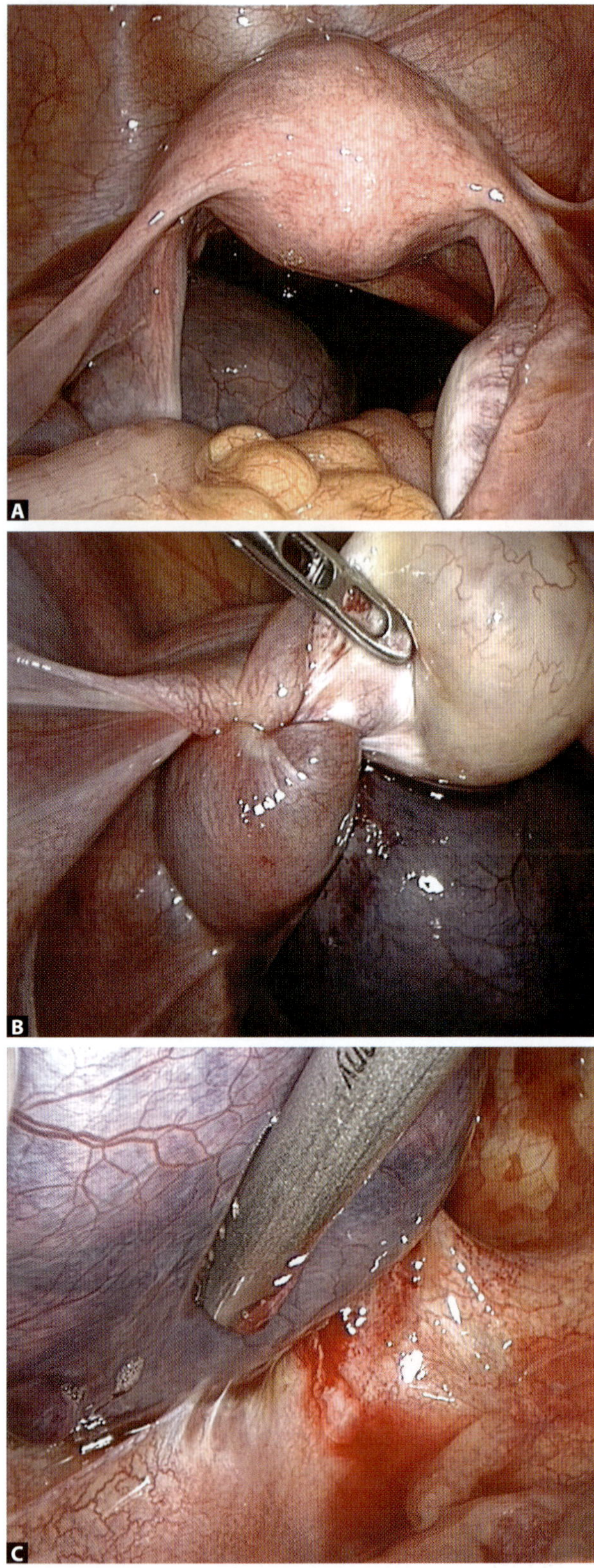

Figs. 22.2A to C: Laparoscopic views. (A) Laparoscopic pelvic overview shows a normal uterus and right adnexa, a cystic mass attached to the left pelvic sidewall and fluid in the pouch of Douglas; (B) The region of torsion of the left fallopian tube is displayed; (C) Adhesions of the torted fallopian tube with the pelvic sidewall are presented.

without any chance of successful functional preservation.
5. If reperfusion occurs, fix the tube to the pelvic side wall or mesosalpinx with a stitch to hinder future torsion. A stitch with a nonresorbable suture connecting the mesosalpinx to the pelvic side wall, but still leaving a good connection from the tube to the ovary for fertilization, will hinder a secondary torsion of the tube on that side. If the contralateral side shows a similar free movement of the tube, a prophylactic stitch on that side to avoid future tubal torsion is also advisable.
6. If reperfusion does not reoccur after 30 min, salpingectomy should be performed. Only the tube then has to be removed with a sharp dissection into the myometrium, in order to avoid ectopic pregnancy in a consecutive in vitro fertilization (IVF) cycle.

   After evacuation the cul de sac and movement of the bowel upward the whole tube must be presented beginning with the proximal isthmic portion and progressing to the fimbriated end of the tube. Tube and the mesosalpinx are coagulated and dissected stepwise, beginning with the proximal isthmic portion and progressing to the fimbriated end of the tube. The tube is immobilized with one or two grasping forceps. Coagulation of the segments to be excised is performed with bipolar cautery and cut either with laser, electrocautery, or scissors. Alternative methods include stapling devices, harmonic energy, or endoloops. After preparation of the tube it is removed from the peritoneal cavity in an endobag through one of the instrument trocars that has been dilated to 10 mm.

   Afterward, a final inspection is made to coagulate any bleeding caused by grasping the tube and the mesosalpinx.

Isolated fallopian tube torsion is a rare cause of lower abdominal pain. Differential diagnosis can involve gynecological conditions such as acute appendicitis, ectopic pregnancy, pelvic inflammatory disease, ovarian accidents, degenerative leiomyoma and other gastrointestinal and urinary conditions.[4]

The lack of pathognomonic symptoms, specific findings on physical examination and specific imaging or laboratory characteristics makes this entity difficult to diagnose, as witnessed by the long list of consultations that this patient had. There is often a delay in suspecting tubal torsion as a cause of lower abdominal pain with a subsequent delay of timely intervention that may result in failure to save tubal function.[5]

Although some intrinsic and extrinsic factors have been documented, the exact mechanisms underlying torsion of the fallopian tube are not well understood. Proposed etiologies include anatomical abnormalities such as hydrosalpinx, hematosalpinx, long mesosalpinx, hydatids of Morgagni, tubal malformations, etc., and physiological abnormalities such as hypermotility, tubal spasms and abnormal peristalsis. Others include hemodynamic abnormalities such as venous congestion in the mesosalpinx, the Sellheim theory relating to sudden body position changes, trauma, previous surgery such as tubal ligation and even a gravid uterus.[6]

Theoretically, torsion may undergo spontaneous detorsion. Undiagnosed torsion may undergo alternative states of mild torsion–detorsion that finally bring the condition to chronicity. Raziel et al.[7] reported a case of recurrent isolated primary tubal torsion 2 years after successful laparoscopic detorsion. However, in this case, recurrence was preoperatively suspected due to the previous history of tubal torsion. Also, many reports indicate that torsion of the fallopian tube is predominantly in the reproductive age group and more on the right than on the left side, possibly attributable to the presence of sigmoid colon on the left side, the relatively less venous flow on the right side and to the increase index of suspicion for appendicitis and thus more frequent operations in episodes of right-sided lower abdominal pain.[4] Our reported case is peculiar because the presentation was on the left and the symptomatology had a chronic course of about 18 months that dates back to her perimenarcheal period.

Imaging findings in torsion of the fallopian tube are nonspecific and should therefore be correlated with clinical impression. Some have reported using ultrasound for preoperative diagnosis of torsion.[8] Sonographic features are usually that of an elongated, convoluted cystic mass tapering as it nears the uterine cornu, and the demonstration of the ipsilateral ovary separate from the mass. This may lead to timely laparoscopy, which can for all intents and purposes be regarded as the gold standard of diagnosis. Doppler evaluation can also be indicative of diagnosis if available on presentation.[8]

The management of tubal torsion is laparoscopy or laparotomy and the emphasis is on early surgery.[4] The latter is more favored when it occurs in mid-pregnancy upward. Plausible options include detorsion and/or operative fixation of the tube to prevent a recurrence. Pregnancy has been reported after detorsion of the tube.[9] Tubal preservation should be the rule especially in nulligravids. Our patient however had a salpingectomy because that segment of the tube was necrotic and beyond salvage.

SUMMARY AND COMPLICATIONS

Isolated fallopian tube torsion is a rare cause of lower abdominal pain. The lack of pathognomonic symptoms, specific findings on physical examination and specific imaging or laboratory characteristics makes this entity difficult to diagnose; however, a history of current or previous pelvic pathologic conditions or surgery, as well as pregnancy, should draw the attention of the attending physician to its occurrence.[5] Early laparoscopy is the reference standard for the management of tubal torsion.

As for complications, many patients with tubal torsion receive laparotomic treatment and even an adnexectomy, which we consider to be a severe complication of treatment if it is performed in centers where laparoscopy is established. If a laparoscopy cannot be performed, then a laparotomy must be performed as transvaginal treatment is not possible. Adnexectomy in cases of tubal torsion has to be considered an overtreatment. Common laparoscopic complications, such as vascular, bowel and entry complications, can of course occur in this pathological entity.

TIPS AND TRICKS

- Listen to your patient's symptoms.
- The decision whether to preserve the tube or not has to be taken at the first laparoscopic inspection.
- Use modern imaging technology (transvaginal ultrasound with Doppler mode, MRI).
- Make a quick decision for laparoscopy and cystic mass resection if there is a suspicious abnormal ovarian cyst.
- At laparoscopy release torsion and observe revascularization.
- Resect tube only when absolutely necessary.
- Consider fixation of the tube to prevent retorsion.

REFERENCES

1. Bland-Sutton B. Salpingitis and some of its effects. Lancet. 1890;2:1146.
2. Hansen OH. Isolated torsion of the Fallopian tube. Acta Obstet Gynecol Scand. 1970;49(1):3-6.
3. Schollmeyer T, Soyinka AS, Mabrouk M, et al. Chronic isolated torsion of the left fallopian tube: a diagnostic dilemma. Arch Gynecol Obstet. 2008;277(1):87-90.
4. Gross M, Blumstein SL, Chow LC. Isolated fallopian tube torsion: a rare twist on a common theme. Am J Radiol. 2005;185(6):1590-2.
5. Krissi H, Shalev J, Bar-Hava I, et al. Fallopian tube torsion: laparoscopic evaluation and treatment of a rare gynecological entity. J Am Board Fam Pract. 2001;14(4):274-7.
6. Bernardus RE, Van der Slikke JW, Roex AJ, et al. Torsion of the fallopian tube: some considerations on its etiology. Obstet Gynecol. 1984;64(5):675-8.
7. Raziel A, Mordechai E, Friedler S, et al. Isolated recurrent torsion of the fallopian tube: case report. Hum Reprod. 1999;14(12):3000-1.
8. Baumgartel PB, Fleischer AC, Cullinan JA, et al. Color Doppler sonography of tubal torsion. Ultrasound Obstet Gynecol. 1996;7(5):367-70.
9. Blair CR. Torsion of the fallopian tube. Surg Gynecol Obstet. 1962;114:727-30.

23 of Gynaecological Endoscopy

Endometriosis

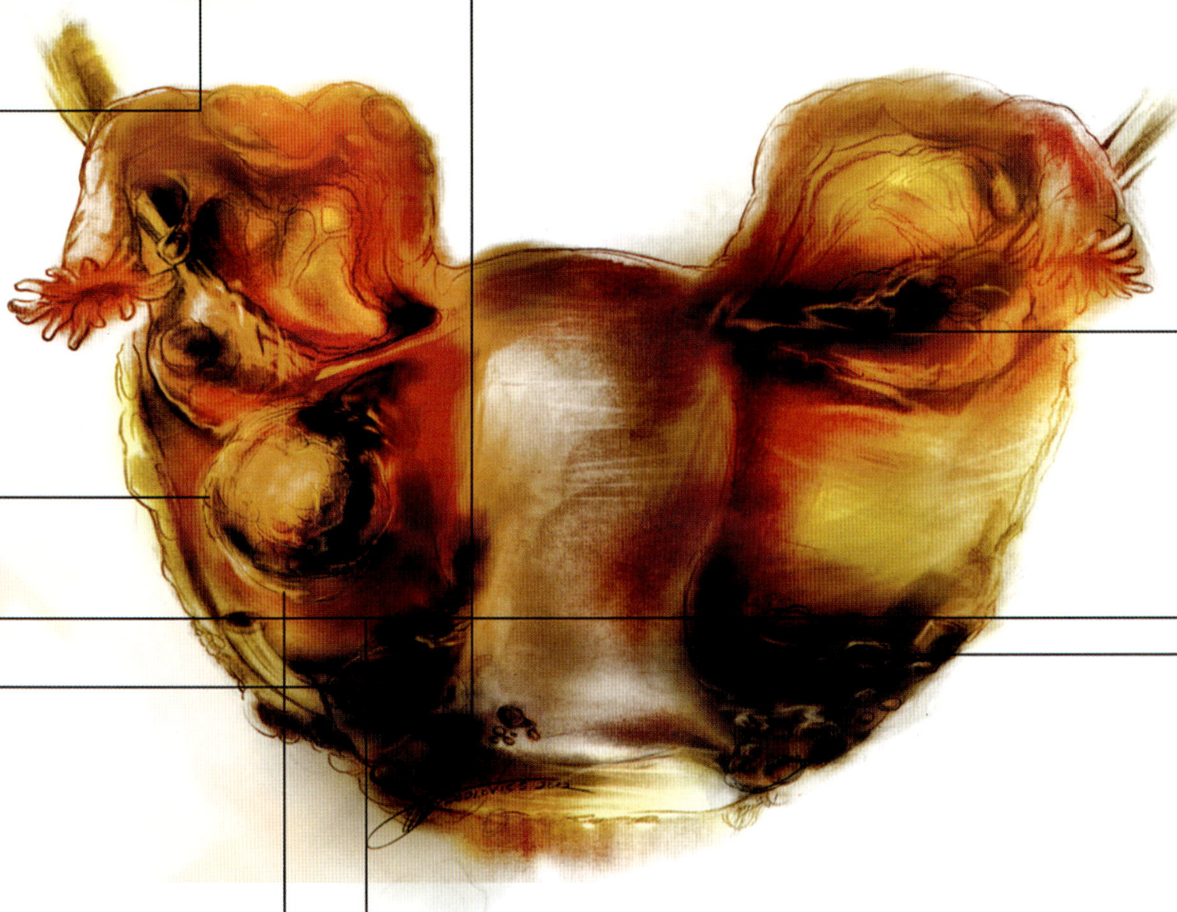

Chapter 23

Endometriosis

Maria Fernanda Brancalion, Ibrahim Alkatout, Liselotte Mettler

INTRODUCTION

Endometriosis is considered one of the most important benign gynecological diseases in view of its high prevalence, which is probably underestimated, and the degree to which the disease affects patients' quality of life as a result of the often incapacitating pain and of its negative effect on women's reproductive capacity.[1] It is defined as the presence of endometrial glands and/or stroma outside the uterine cavity, which provokes a chronic inflammatory process.[2]

Although this disease was described for the first time over a century ago, its precise etiopathogenesis remains unknown to the present day.[3] Some theories merit particular mention and include retrograde menstruation, coelomic metaplasia, vascular dissemination and immunological causes as being the principal triggers of this clinical condition.[4] It is estimated that 10% of women worldwide suffer from endometriosis and that endometriosis is the cause of infertility in 40% of infertile women. The great majority of patients present with pain and infertility; however, 10% of patients with deep endometriosis are asymptomatic, which cannot exactly be considered an advantage in view of the risk, albeit rare, of stenosis and obstruction of the bowel or urinary tract.[5]

Endometriosis presents as superficial or deep peritoneal lesions and its morphological characteristics may range from black lesions, considered typical, to red and white lesions, deemed atypical.[6] According to the definition of Cornillie et al.,[7] deep endometriosis infiltrates the peritoneum to a depth of 5-mm or more and is considered to be more aggressive. It is often associated with extremely intense pelvic pain and infertility as a result of the higher risk of neuronal involvement, adhesions and the anatomical distortions caused by the lesions.[7]

Endometriotic implants can be found more commonly in the pelvic peritoneum, ovaries, uterine ligaments (uterosacral, round and broad ligaments), retrocervical region, vagina, rectovaginal septum, rectosigmoid, cecal appendix, ileum, ureter and bladder. They have also been described in the umbilicus, abdominal wall (cesarean scar and episiotomy), in the pleural and pericardial cavities, diaphragm, lung, nasal cavity and brain.[8]

In our opinion, an early and precise diagnosis is the most important component in planning the optimal therapeutic management of the patient, whether treatment is clinical or surgical, or assisted reproductive techniques in cases of infertility. In addition, attention should be paid to the patient's clinical history, taking into consideration any complaints of dysmenorrhea, deep dyspareunia, chronic acyclic pelvic pain, cyclic dyschezia (tenesmus and constipation), cyclic dysuria and infertility, all of which constitute typical symptoms of endometriosis.[8]

Painful nodules in the retrocervical region, bowel, rectovaginal septum, vagina and bladder are detectable at physical examination, as well as any indirect signs such as reduced uterine mobility and pain at mobilization.[9]

With respect to supplementary tests, many studies have been conducted to define the most favorable noninvasive method for diagnosing the presence and depth of lesions. Of these, barium enema, echoendoscopy, multislice computed tomography and magnetic resonance imaging deserve particular mention, since they all constitute methods capable of identifying lesions, albeit each with its own specific applicability. However, the best specificity and sensitivity rates and the best cost-benefit ratio have been found with transvaginal and transabdominal ultrasonography, performed following prior bowel preparation.[9-12]

In view of the multiplicity of symptoms, clinical treatment may be the first choice in cases in which the patient complains of pain and has no interest in becoming pregnant, since all the therapeutic options involve inhibiting ovarian endocrine and ovulatory function.[13] Also in asymptomatic or oligosymptomatic patients with intestinal endometriosis, whose lesions are diagnosed incidentally, clinical treatment may be offered. However, in cases where clinical treatment is chosen, vigilance is mandatory. Surgical approach should be considered to stop progression of the disease, inferred by evaluation of imaging tests, worsening of symptoms or nodules invading the rectum wall or sigmoid that may compromise intestinal transit.[14]

In cases of infertility, no advantage is gained by treating the patient clinically prior to the initiation of fertility treatment and may, indeed, be viewed by the patient as a delay. Assisted reproductive techniques (ART) should be considered as the first option for asymptomatic patients with ovarian endometriomas of less than 4.0 cm in diameter. ART is also indicated for patients with a history of previous ovarian surgery when tubal obstruction or male factor infertility are present.[15]

The objective of surgical treatment is to relieve pain, restore pelvic anatomy and improve the patient's reproductive capacity. It is indicated for symptomatic patients with AVS > 7 (dysmenorrhea, dyspareunia, chronic acyclic pelvic pain, dyschezia or dysuria) with negative impact on quality of life in infertile patients with two or more in vitro fertilization (IVF) cycles. In patients who did not respond to hormonal treatment, and patients with signs of intestinal subocclusion.[14]

Optimal therapeutic management consists of resecting all possible endometriosis lesions, thus avoiding persistence of the disease and minimizing recurrence rates. Nevertheless, this involves advanced surgical techniques and the surgeon should have adequate experience in navigating the retroperitoneal space and a good knowledge of pelvic anatomy.[16,17] Laparoscopy is better than laparotomy since it provides amplification of the image, permitting better visualization of the lesions and enabling structures such as the ureter, pelvic vessels and nerves of the hypogastric plexus to be more finely dissected.[18]

This chapter provides technical guidelines for performing these surgeries safely and reproducibly.

GENERAL CONSIDERATIONS

Preoperative

Once the disease has been diagnosed and the affected sites defined, the surgical indication is discussed with the patient, who is counseled with respect to the advantages of the treatment and the inherent risks of the anesthesia and of the proposed surgery. Once the patient's questions have been answered, she is asked to sign an informed consent form confirming that she agrees with the planned surgical treatment and that she is aware of the potential risks and complications.

Bowel Preparation

Irrespective of the procedure proposed, all patients who are to be submitted to video-laparoscopy for the treatment of endometriosis are instructed to follow a light diet on the two days preceding the date of the surgery. Cooked, unseasoned, fiber-free food is recommended.

In cases of bowel surgery, 667 mg of lactulose, a 10-g envelope, is prescribed and should be taken approximately 16 h prior to the procedure. A 100-mL sodium phosphate enema is given rectally three hours prior to surgery.[19] Complete fasting for 8 h before surgery is required.

Precautions with Hygiene

As part of the preoperative preparation on the eve of surgery, the patient is asked to remove her pubic hair from the suprapubic region (using any hair removal method) and to use a cotton bud to carefully clean inside her navel using chlorhexidine.

Anesthesia

The type of anesthesia recommended for laparoscopic surgery is general anesthesia with orotracheal intubation. In cases in which bowel resection (rectosigmoidectomy) is recommended, we suggest the additional use of intradural anesthesia with 60 μg of morphine sulfate and 15 μg of fentanyl, since this provides a long-lasting analgesic effect, greatly reducing discomfort in the immediate postoperative period. In addition, a nasogastric tube is inserted to remove the stomach contents and to distend the

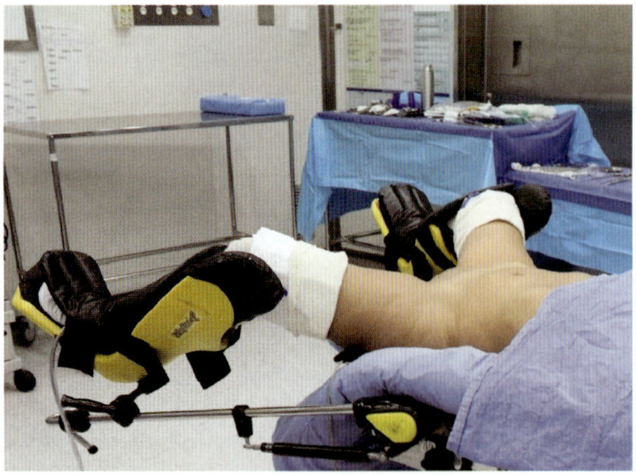

Fig. 23.1: Position of the patient.

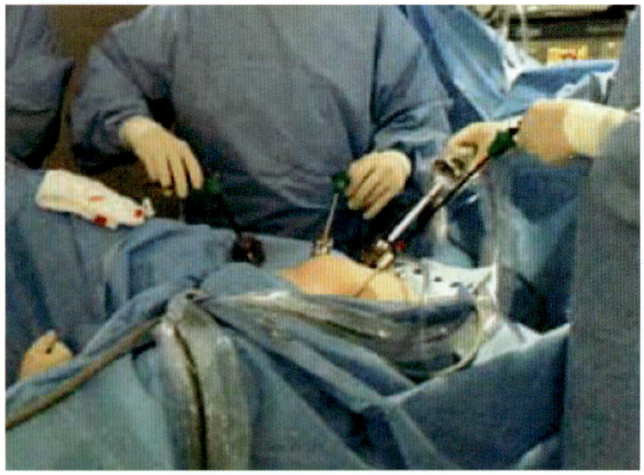

Fig. 23.2: Position of the team.

stomach, thus reducing the risks of complications resulting from puncture.[20]

Position of the Patient

The patient is operated in a semi-gynecological position, with her arms stretched alongside her body (Fig. 23.1). The use of anti-embolism stockings is recommended, and an intermittent pneumatic compression device should be installed as prophylaxis against deep vein thrombosis.[21]

Position of the Team

With respect to the surgical team, the chief surgeon should be in position on the patient's left side and the first assistant on her right side. The second assistant stands between the patient's legs, controlling the uterine manipulator. The surgical technologist should be standing beside the surgeon (Fig. 23.2).

Placement of the Uterine Manipulator and Bladder Catheter

The uterine manipulator is used in all laparoscopic procedures performed to treat endometriosis and represents an extremely important tool for this procedure since the great majority of lesions are found in the posterior pelvic compartment, in the Douglas pouch. It is simple to use; however, care should be taken to choose a manipulator device that permits adequate anteversion of the uterus. The second surgical assistant, who is in-charge of positioning the uterus throughout the entire surgical procedure, is responsible for inserting the manipulator and for bladder catheterization.[22]

Creation of Pneumoperitoneum

The procedure is initiated by making a 1.2-cm umbilical skin incision, after which the subcutaneous cell tissue is lightly dissected until the aponeurosis is seen. Next, the aponeurosis is firmly grasped using two straight Kocher forceps and the anterior abdominal wall is elevated sufficiently to enable it to be punctured using a Veress needle.

Veress needle puncture is performed toward the pelvis, at a 45 degrees angle in the case of thin patients and at an angle of up to 90 degrees in obese patients. Following Veress needle puncture, safety tests are performed to confirm the position of the needle prior to initiating CO_2 infusion. The test is performed by connecting a 20 mL syringe containing 5 mL of saline solution to the external tip of the Veress needle and instilling the entire contents of the syringe in order to eliminate any fragment of tissue that could have entered the needle when the puncture was made. When the piston of the syringe is pulled back, resistance should be felt as a result of the negative pressure, confirming that the peritoneal cavity has been reached.[23]

The insufflation tubing that transports CO_2 in the Veress needle is adapted according to the following pre-established parameters:

- CO_2 pressure: 20 mm Hg
- Infusion speed: 3 L/min

Puncture with Primary Trocar

When the established pressure is achieved, the Veress needle is removed and the surgeon inserts the 11-mm trocar, exerting slight pressure with his/her left hand on the patient's upper abdomen and positioning the trocar towards the pelvis at a 45 degrees angle. Disposable trocars are preferable, as they improve the safety of the procedure.[24]

Parameters for the Control of Pneumoperitoneum

Following puncture with the primary trocar and after the lens has been introduced into the peritoneal cavity, the pre-established parameters are changed to:

- CO_2 pressure: 12 mm Hg
- Infusion speed: 30 L/min.[24]

Once this change has been implemented, these parameters are maintained for the remainder of the laparoscopic procedure.

Inventory of the Abdominal Cavity

The optics chosen for all video-laparoscopies for the treatment of endometriosis is 0 degree lens, which is 10-mm in diameter.

The lens selected for all laparoscopies performed for the treatment of endometriosis, irrespective of which organ is affected, is the 0 degree lens with a diameter of 10-mm. After the lens has been inserted, the region immediately below the umbilical port is examined to confirm the integrity of the mesogastric structures. At this time, an inventory is made of the entire abdominal cavity and pelvis.

Position of the Patient on the Operating Table

To facilitate access to the pelvic organs and reduce the risk of trauma to adjacent organs such as the bowel, all laparoscopies for the treatment of endometriosis should be performed with the patient in the Trendelenburg position.

Auxiliary Ports

Auxiliary ports are extremely important in optimizing the access of the surgeon performing the laparoscopy and improving physical ergonomics, particularly in the case of lengthy procedures and when the retroperitoneum has to be dissected. In the great majority of laparoscopic procedures for the treatment of deep endometriosis, the recommended position of the auxiliary ports is as follows: one port in right iliac fossa region, one in the suprapubic region and one in the region of the left iliac fossa. This arrangement will depend on the type of surgery proposed and its complexity[25] (Fig. 23.3).

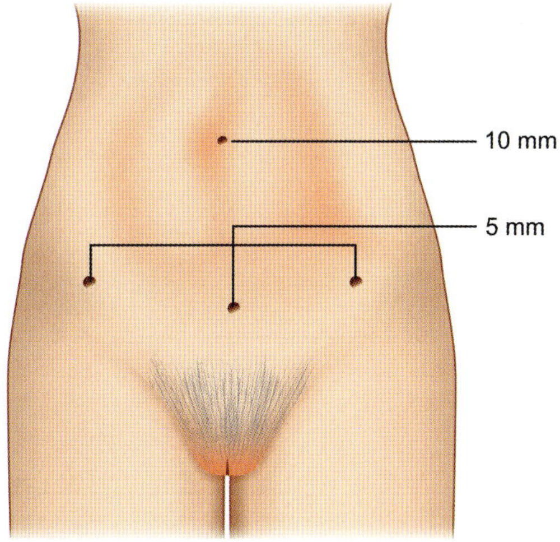

Fig. 23.3: Position of the auxiliary ports.

To facilitate comprehension of this chapter, description of the surgical techniques and their individual specifications has been separated into the following divisions and subdivisions:.

- *Peritoneal endometriosis:*
  - Superficial endometriosis
  - Deep endometriosis
- *Endometriosis of the reproductive tract:*
  - Ovarian endometriosis
  - Tubal endometriosis
- *Endometriosis of the urinary tract:*
  - Bladder and ureteral endometriosis
- *Bowel endometriosis:*
  - Endometriosis of the vermiform appendix
  - Endometriosis of the ileum
  - Endometriosis of the rectosigmoid
- *Extragenital endometriosis:*
  - Diaphragmatic endometriosis
  - Abdominal wall endometriosis

SURGICAL TECHNIQUE

Peritoneal Endometriosis

In our opinion, every laparoscopic surgery for the treatment of endometriosis should begin by identifying the course of the ureters, which are often situated very close to peritoneal endometriotic lesions.[4] Identification of the ureters is simpler if they are detected at their mid-point at the entrance of the pelvis minor, close to the bifurcation of the iliac arteries (Fig. 23.4). It is possible to stimulate peristalsis of the ureter using an atraumatic forceps, thus facilitating its localization.

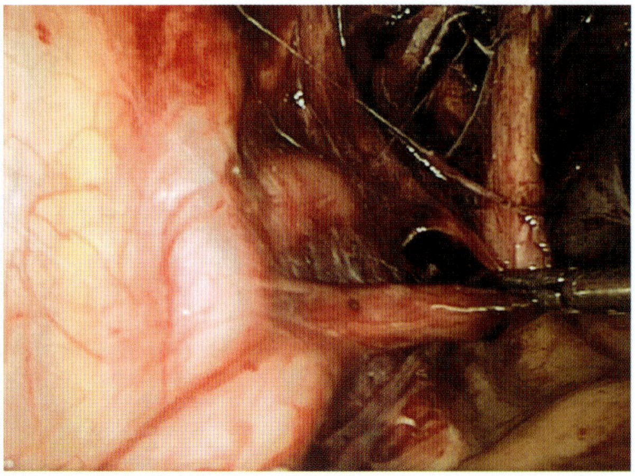

Fig. 23.4: Identification of the ureter at the entrance to the pelvis, crossing the bifurcation of the common iliac artery.

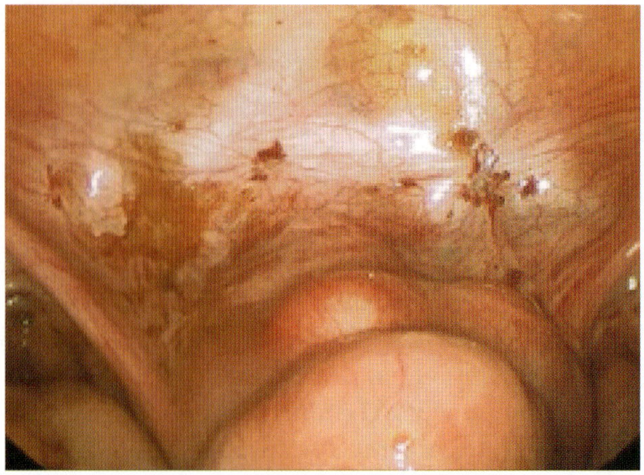

Fig. 23.5: Superficial peritoneal endometriotic lesion (left) and deep peritoneal endometriosis lesion (right). Vesicouterine reflection. Uterus with subserous myomas in the anterior corpus.

Peritoneal endometriosis may be superficial or deep. The need for diagnostic laparoscopy is currently questioned; therefore, superficial lesions are generally treated when they are found during laparoscopic procedures performed to treat deep endometriosis.[26]

We consider that, in the presence of superficial peritoneal endometriosis, the surgical treatment may be only through the coagulation of the scissors or hook lesions connected to the monopolar current or preferably with the bipolar forceps.

In our opinion, when peritoneal endometriosis is superficial, the most adequate surgical treatment is to resect the lesions using monopolar scissors or a monopolar hook or with the use of a CO_2 laser. Likewise, in the case of deep peritoneal lesions, our treatment of choice is complete resection of the lesions, which definitively extinguishes the foci and greatly reduces the likelihood of recurrence (Fig. 23.5).

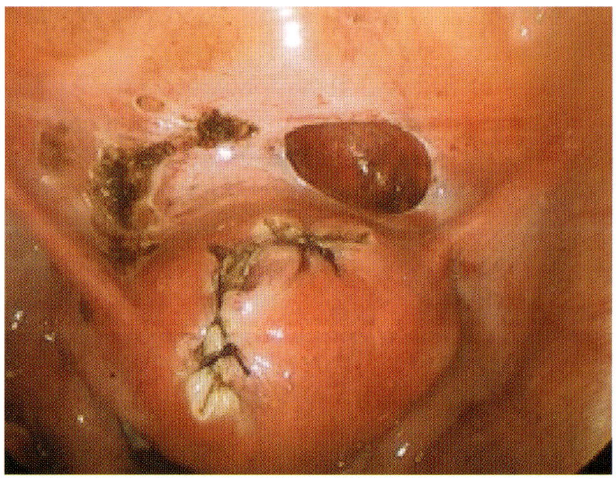

Fig. 23.6: Following treatment: Bipolar coagulation of a superficial lesion (left); resection of a deep lesion (right) and myomectomies.

We recommend the use of three auxiliary punctures, where the surgeon will have a bipolar forceps in his left hand (left iliac fossa trocar) and with laparoscopic scissors with monopolar function in the right hand (suprapubic trocar). In the hands of the first assistant will be the optics in his left hand (umbilical trocar) and an atraumatic grasping forceps or aspirator / irrigator in the right hand (right iliac fossa trocar)(Fig. 23.6). The use of the harmonic scalpel has been widely used by surgeons operating endometriosis. In this case, it should be replaced by the laparoscopic scissors and handled by the surgeon's right hand in a suprapubic puncture.

Deep endometriotic lesions merit particular attention and the surgical procedures required to completely resect these lesions often represent a challenge, even for surgeons with advanced laparoscopic skills. The surgeon must have a solid knowledge of the anatomical relationships, considering that deep lesions often adhere firmly to retroperitoneal structures such as the arteries, veins and nerves that cross the lateral wall of the pelvis, in addition to the ureters (Figs. 23.7 and 23.8).

As a technical recommendation, we suggest that the ureter should always be dissected in cases of pelvic wall lesions, initiating at the point at which the ureters cross the iliac vessels (Fig. 23.4). We also recommend that this be performed initially through the healthy tissue surrounding the endometriosis lesion so that the lesion can be safely removed after adequate identification of the retroperitoneal structures.

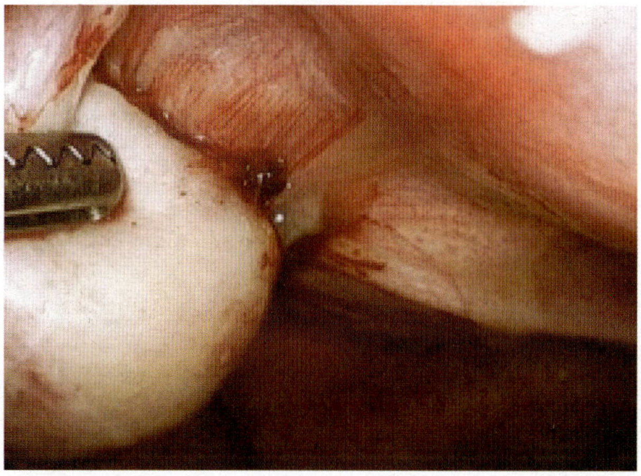

Fig. 23.7: Deep peritoneal endometriosis lesion in the left uterosacral ligament and left ovarian fossa, causing the ovary to adhere firmly to the posterior wall of the uterus in the paracervical region.

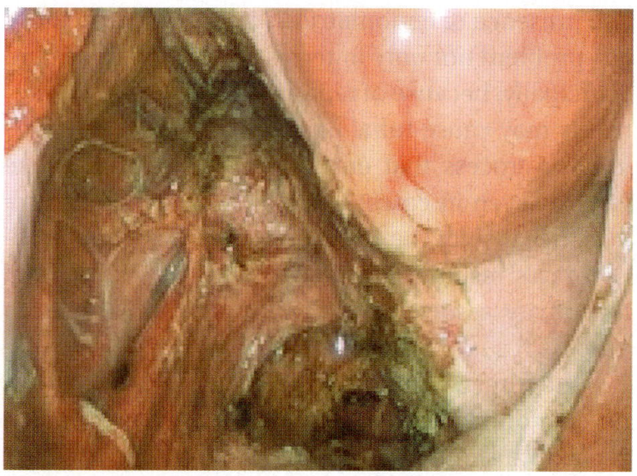

Fig. 23.8: Image taken postoperatively, showing the retroperitoneal structures and resection of the entire lesion.

In cases of lesions on the pelvic wall in which the retroperitoneum has to be dissected, the ovary is first held by temporary suturing, which is extremely advantageous in terms of exposing the region to be operated. These sutures are removed at the end of the procedure.

Endometriosis of the Reproductive Tract

Ovarian Endometriosis

There is no doubt that this surgical procedure continues to generate controversy among surgeons and fertility specialists in view of the damage it causes to the healthy ovarian tissue adjacent to the pseudocapsule of the endometrioma. Since, unlike ovarian cysts of other etiologies, ovarian endometriomas adhere firmly to the ovarian parenchyma, their extraction may be traumatic, removing healthy follicles, causing bleeding and requiring hemostasis by bipolar coagulation, which may damage the ovarian parenchyma.[13]

Emptying the contents of the cyst followed by coagulation or vaporization of the internal surface of the capsule using monopolar or bipolar energy or CO_2 laser is known to be associated with a recurrence of endometriomas. Removing ovarian cysts should be avoided in the case of patients with endometriomas of 3 cm or less in diameter. Bearing in mind that ovarian endometriomas may be associated with the presence of deep endometriosis, particular attention should be paid when patients present with a clinical complaint of pelvic pain.[13,27]

From a technical point of view, our recommendation is to provoke as little trauma as possible when manipulating the ovary. Furthermore, the surgeon should ensure that the pseudocapsule is completely resected so as to avoid recurrences, since repeat ovarian surgeries are known to be harmful to ovarian reserve and consequently to the patient's reproductive capacity.

Care should be taken to aspirate the intracystic contents prior to resection so as to avoid the chocolate-like fluid from the endometrioma spreading throughout the peritoneal cavity (Fig. 23.9).

An atraumatic laparoscopic forceps is used to extract the pseudocapsule from the endometrioma using the traction-countertraction technique so as to cause as little damage as possible to the adjacent healthy ovarian tissue, thus minimizing the need for power output to control hemostasis (Fig. 23.10).

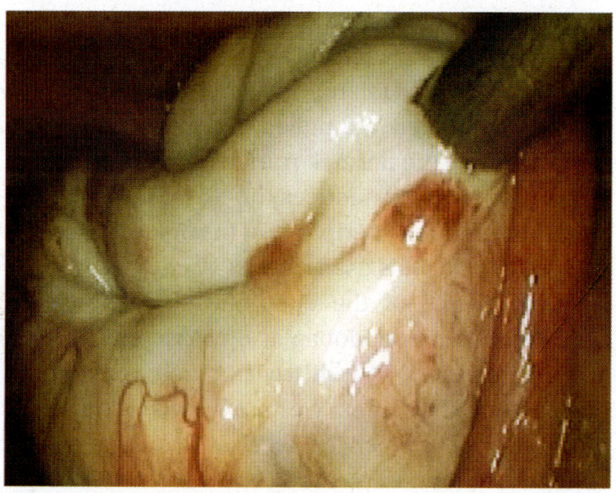

Fig. 23.9: Prior aspiration of intracystic contents.

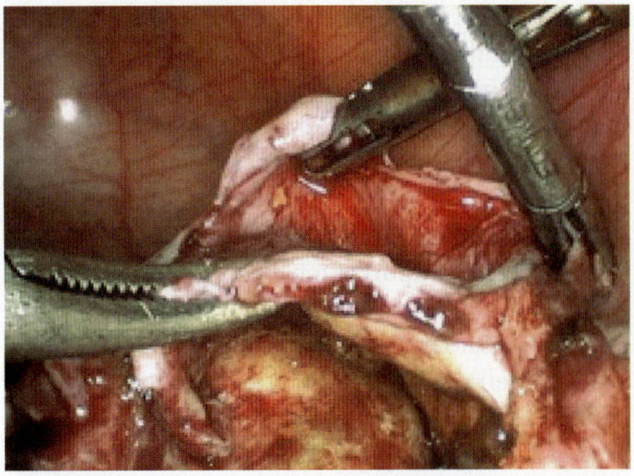

Fig. 23.10: Extraction of the pseudocapsule of an ovarian endometrioma using traction–countertraction, with an atraumatic forceps.

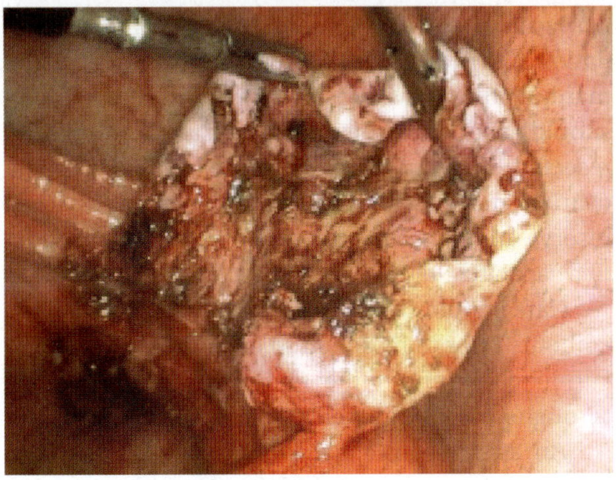

Fig. 23.11: Coagulation of the ovarian parenchyma using a bipolar energy source.

Following removal of the capsule, controlled hemostasis of the healthy ovarian parenchyma is achieved with bipolar coagulation, the power output being set to 20 W (Fig. 23.11).

Following coagulation of the ovarian parenchyma, the borders are pulled together and sutured to reconstitute the normal ovarian anatomy, since, in our experience, this reduces the likelihood of adhesions forming at the periphery of the organ. A braided suture (Vicryl 3-0) is used (Fig. 23.12).

The capsule of the endometrioma should be removed using an endobag or by passing it through the interior of an 11-mm trocar, since this method ensures that there is no contact between the endometrioma and the pelvic wall, thus avoiding the risk of endometriotic implants in the subcutaneous tissue of the laparoscopy scar.

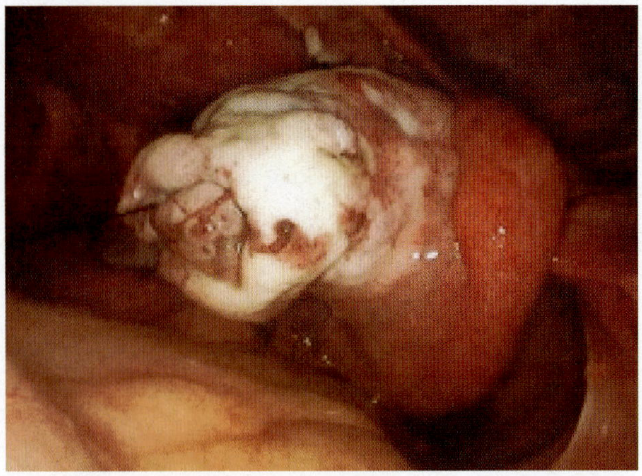

Fig. 23.12: Image of the ovary following resection of an endometrioma and suturing using Vicryl 3-0.

Tubal Endometriosis

The presence of endometriosis in the fallopian tubes is a problem not only in terms of pain, but also, and principally, because of reproductive issues. Endometriosis may cause tubal obstruction, but the inflammatory process that ensues may also compromise fertility, even in cases in which there is no obstruction, because of the reduction in embryo implantation rates resulting from alterations in endometrial receptivity associated with the tubal inflammatory process.[28]

The surgical treatment indicated for patients with tubal endometriosis is salpingectomy; however, this procedure should be thoroughly discussed with the patient and her consent should be duly documented in view of the complexity of the question of removing a fallopian tube from a patient who wishes to become pregnant. Preoperative imaging tests often fail to provide an adequate picture of the status of the tube, and it may only be possible to confirm its pathological status at laparoscopy, making the decision to operate even more difficult.

Technically, the procedure first involves lysing any adhesions, since the fimbrial end of the tube may be adhered to the posterior wall of the uterus, to the ovary or to the bowel (Fig. 23.13). For this type of procedure, use of the bipolar forceps with grasping capacity and scissors is recommended, thus ensuring a blunt, precise dissection.

After performing lysis of adhesion and anatomical restitution, we used bipolar forceps for clotting of the tubal artery near the infundibulopelvic ligament and also for clotting previously the section of the tube with scissors in the isthmic portion, close to its

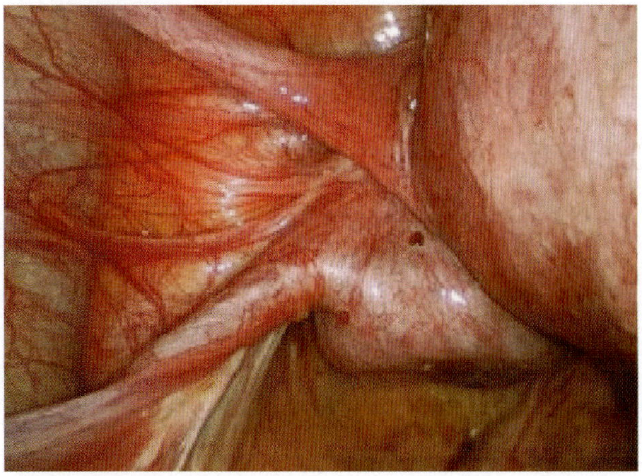

Fig. 23.13: Fimbrial end of the left fallopian tube totally adhered to the left ovary and left uterosacral ligament.

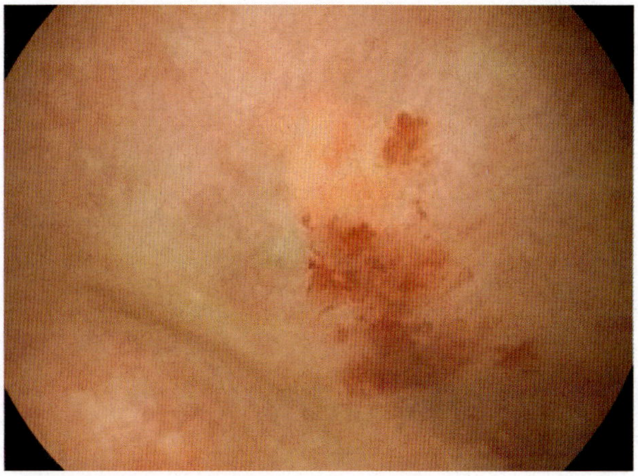

Fig. 23.14: Cystoscopic view of an endometriotic lesion on the anterior wall of the bladder.

insertion into the uterine wall. With the aid of these two tools, bipolar and scissors, we finished the salpingectomy with the coagulation and cut of the ligament mesosalpinges. The harmonic scalpel may also be useful for this type of procedure, reducing the surgical time and the smoke normally released by bipolar coagulation.

After salpingectomy is complete, the tube should be removed from the abdominal cavity, as described previously for cystectomy, using an endobag or passing it through the interior of an 11-mm trocar to avoid contact with the subcutaneous tissue.

Endometriosis of the Urinary Tract

Endometriosis of the bladder and ureter are found in 3.8% and 3.4% respectively of our population of patients with deep endometriosis and, in our experience, the bladder may be affected irrespective of whether or not the ureter is affected, despite the fact that they are part of the same system. Ureteral lesions are extrinsic in the vast majority of cases and are often associated with bowel and retrocervical lesions.[29]

For the treatment of endometriosis lesions on organs such as the urinary tract and bowel, that do not form part of the reproductive system, having a multidisciplinary team offers advantages with respect to the safety of the procedure and, consequently, to the safety of the patient.

Bladder Endometriosis

Bladder endometriosis generally affects the posterior wall, a region that is distant from the ureteral meatus and vesical trigone. Involvement is extrinsic and it may affect the serous, muscular and mucosal layers. Symptoms associated with bladder involvement range from chronic pelvic pain in the hypogastric region to cyclic hematuria that occurs concomitantly with menstruation, dysuria, urinary urgency and recurrent urinary infections.[29]

Cystoscopy must always precede surgical treatment and, if the lesion is close to the ureteral meatuses, double J stents are inserted to improve visualization at resection (Fig. 23.14). However, as mentioned previously, the lesions are usually distant from the meatuses.

During laparoscopy for partial cystectomy, lysis of the adhesions is initially performed on all the structures affixed to the bladder lesion in order to individualize the nodule of endometriosis invading the posterior wall of the bladder. The ideal strategy is to begin with the healthy adjacent tissue surrounding the entire periphery of the lesion so as to release the healthy bladder muscle tissue adhered to the nodule, thereby minimizing the area of the bladder to be resected (Fig. 23.15).

After the adhesions have been lysed, resection of the nodule is initiated. In cases in which the mucosal layer of the bladder is affected, the organ will be opened, and it will be possible to see the Foley balloon (Fig. 23.16). After the lesion has been completely resected, the interior of the bladder is inspected laparoscopically and the ureteral meatuses are evaluated. Suturing then begins and it is performed on two planes, initially closing the mucosal layer using continuous nonanchored suture with Vicryl 3-0 and then suturing the seromuscular layer with continuous anchor suture using Vicryl 2-0.

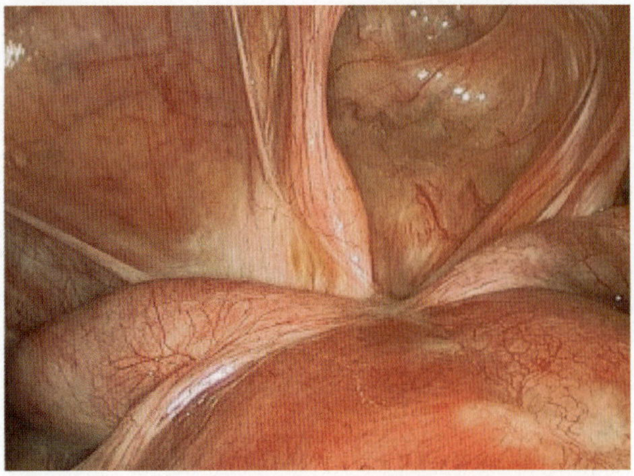

Fig. 23.15: Bladder lesion with retraction of the peritoneum and round ligaments on the nodule of endometriosis.

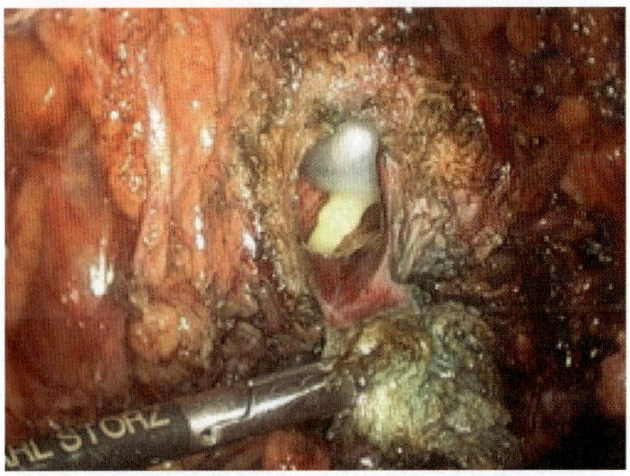

Fig. 23.16: Individualization of the nodule of endometriosis in the bladder. Note the presence of the Foley catheter.

Suture dehiscence is treated prophylactically by leaving the #16 Foley catheter in the patient for 7–10 days following surgery. Urinary tract infections are treated prophylactically with 500 mg cefadroxil every 12 h during the entire period of catheterization.

Ureteral Endometriosis

In general, ureteral endometriosis is associated with the presence of deep peritoneal lesions on the pelvic wall, affecting the ureter externally, exerting extrinsic compression and possibly leading to obstruction, progressing to hydronephrosis and kidney failure, as reported in the literature.[30]

Although rare, intrinsic involvement of the ureter is a more serious condition and may be associated with loss of kidney function when diagnosis is delayed as a result of the nonspecific symptomatology.[31] Ureteral involvement is often unilateral, the left side being most often affected. In rare cases, involvement may be bilateral, a situation that is associated with the severity of endometriosis, principally in cases in which the posterior cul de sac is totally obliterated.[29]

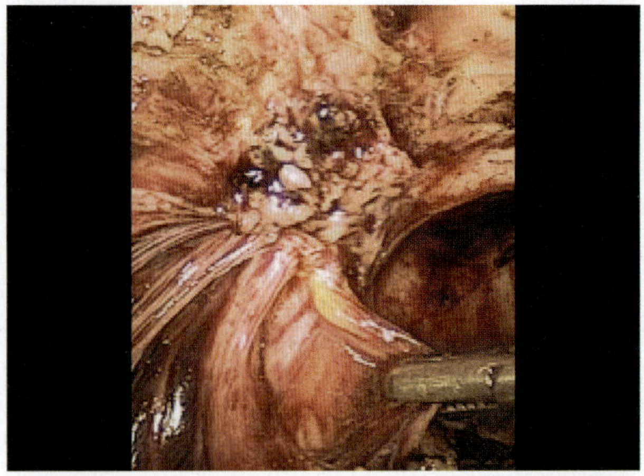

Fig. 23.17: Nodule of endometriosis on the left ureter in the pelvic region close to where the left uterine artery crosses over the ureter.

The region of the ureter most commonly affected is the intrapelvic area in its distal third, close to its crossing with the uterine artery. In cases of extrinsic involvement (75% of cases), the layers involved are the adventitia and the conjunctive tissue adjacent to the ureter[32] (Fig. 23.17).

The most commonly used surgical treatment is ureterolysis, which consists of completely releasing the ureter from the nodule of endometriosis without, however, opening the lumen. Dissection should then be performed from the pelvic border, under the infundibulopelvic ligament, exposing the adjacent structures and the ureter itself, preferentially at a site in which the peritoneum is not affected by endometriosis.

With the aid of a 30-W bipolar forceps in the left hand, with a tissue-holding capacity, and in the right hand, laparoscopic energy-less scissors, which may eventually be replaced by the monopolar hook, in a pure 30 Watt cut or the harmonic scalpel, the surgeon will perform a delicate dissection in order to release the ureter from the endometriosis lesion. The surgical assistant has a fundamental importance in presenting the previously individualized peritoneal sheath and maintaining the traction required for the surgeon to be able to cut with precision. Devascularization of the ureter during dissection should be avoided.

Inserting a double-J stent prior to surgery is not obligatory and it should only be left in place following surgery when there are signs of ureteral stenosis at urethrocystoscopy or in cases in which surgical manipulation was extensive.

Endometriosis of the Bowel

In recent years, many studies have been carried out in an attempt to acquire further knowledge on bowel endometriosis in view of the high incidence of this disease, its painful symptomatology and the risks of obstruction of the digestive tract, which could potentially lead to a condition of acute abdomen. Intestinal endometriosis can be found in 6–30% of women with deep endometriosis and among these patients the most frequent symptoms are dysmenorrhea, acyclic abdominal pain, deep dyspareunia, constipation, pain at evacuation, cyclic rectal bleeding, or symptoms associated with stenosis and obstruction, as well as infertility.[14,33] Although it is a cause of severe symptoms, up to 10% of patients with intestinal endometriosis may be asymptomatic.[14]

Diagnosis by imaging is crucial, not only for deciding whether surgical treatment is necessary but also for defining the strategy to be used during surgery and providing the patient with information prior to the operation. Transvaginal and transabdominal ultrasonography with prior bowel preparation, performed by a specialist with experience in the disease, is highly accurate in diagnosing the presence of bowel endometriosis, in evaluating whether a single lesion or multiple lesions are present, the bowel layers that are affected by the lesions, the distance from the anal border, in measuring the circumference of the affected segment of the bowel and in establishing whether lesions are present in the ileum and vermiform appendix.[12,14]

With this information, the gynecologist will then be able to assemble a multidisciplinary team, define the equipment required for the chosen procedure and prepare the bowel adequately. The current options of surgical treatment range from shaving in the case of superficial lesions to discoid resection for deep lesions of less than 3.0 cm in diameter and segmental resection for large, multiple lesions.[12,14]

Endometriosis of the Vermiform Appendix

In most cases of endometriosis of the appendix, deep endometriosis is usually also present concomitantly at other sites, principally the bladder, rectosigmoid and retrocervical region. The incidence of involvement of the appendix by endometriosis is approximately 5%[34] (Fig. 23.18).

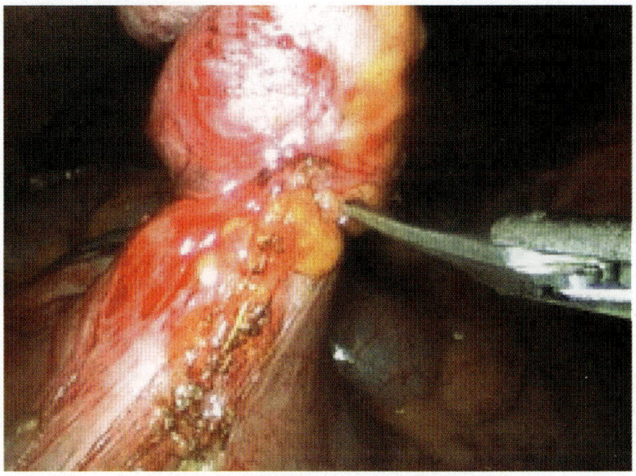

Fig. 23.18: Endometriosis of the appendix.

Surgical treatment consists of performing laparoscopic appendectomy. The procedure should begin by releasing and opening the mesoappendix, and immediately afterwards ligating the appendicular artery with the bipolar forceps or harmonic scalpel, releasing the appendix up to base of the cecum. The appendix may be amputated either with the 45-mm laparoscopic linear stapler or by doubly ligating the appendix stump with a nonabsorbable multifilament thread, using Roeder extracorporeal knot technique. In our opinion, there is no need for invagination of the remaining stump to the cecum. After checking hemostasis, the piece is removed through the interior of a trocar of 11- or 12-mm.

Endometriosis of the Ileum

Although cases of endometriosis have already been documented in the jejunum, proximal and medial ileum, they are extremely rare and their exact incidence is unknown. In cases of endometriosis of the small bowel, the principal region affected is the distal ileum, with an incidence of 1–7% of all cases. It is rare for the small bowel alone to be affected and this form of involvement is usually associated with the presence of deep endometriosis at other sites in the pelvis. The true incidence of bowel obstruction is unknown, although it is estimated that complete obstruction occurs in less than 1% of patients, and in 7-23% of these cases the obstruction occurs in the small bowel[35] (Fig. 23.19).

The surgical treatment of endometriosis of the ileum is performed by laparoscopy during resection of lesions at other sites or even in cases in which

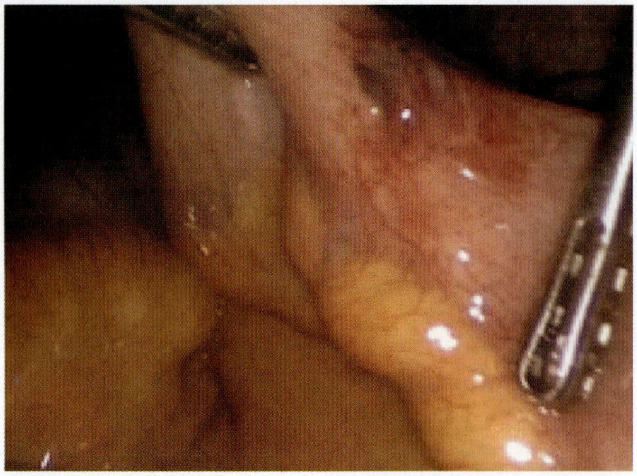

Fig. 23.19: Lesion of endometriosis in the small bowel close to the ileocecal valve.

there is a single ileal lesion. Initially, the lesion is identified by meticulously inspecting the loop of the small bowel to verify whether it consists of a single lesion or whether there are other lesions close by. Any adhesions found are lysed and the mesoileum is released. At this time, a small 3-4 cm incision is made in the skin in the right iliac fossa region and the segment of the loop is exteriorized. Once the loop is exteriorized and the segment to be resected has been identified, the peritoneum is opened manually, preserving the irrigation as much as possible, with a small safety margin in the loop. The affected segment is resected and manual end-to-end anastomosis is performed on two separate planes using Vicryl 3-0 or Prolene 3-0 sutures. Hemostasis is reviewed and the loop is reinserted into the cavity.

We consider it more appropriate to perform external manual resection, since the lesions are usually very close to the ileocecal valve and the use of staplers can considerably increase the surgical time.

Rectosigmoid Endometriosis

Rectosigmoid endometriosis has been a subject of investigation for over twenty years, with the result that new techniques based on meticulous follow-up have been incorporated as part of its surgical treatment. Due to the high complexity of the surgery, fibrous adhesions and obliteration of the posterior pouch, resection is known to be often incomplete, with consequent persistence of symptomatology and a need for the patient to undergo further surgery. Based on the need to guarantee complete resection, thus ensuring that treatment of the disease is definitive, some criteria such as the size and quantity of the lesions, the distance from the anal border, the circumference of the affected loop and the layers affected by the disease have been taken into consideration.

The techniques used are shaving, performed exclusively on serosa or external muscularis layer lesions of the rectum or sigmoid, discoidal resection with transanal circular stapler performed when, regardless of the depth of the lesion, it has an estimated measurement of approximately 3.0 cm. In our opinion, this type of resection is ideal for very low lesions, i.e. those situated less than 6 cm from the anal border (rectovaginal septum) because of the increased risk of an iatrogenic lesion of the pelvic splanchnic nerves responsible for bladder and bowel voiding and which are located bilaterally at this position in the mesorectum.

For larger lesions or multiple lesions in the rectosigmoid, we prefer laparoscopic segmental resection using linear or circular staplers for end-to-end reanastomosis. The respective techniques are as follows.

Shaving

The shaving technique, indicated for external muscularis layer and serous lesions, begins with lysis of adhesions, since this lesion is usually adhered to another peritoneal endometriosis, more frequently in the retrocervical, retrovaginal or ovarian regions. After individualizing the segment of the rectosigmoid containing the lesion, the assistant surgeon uses a grasping forceps in the right iliac fossa port, which will then be used to firmly grip the central area of the lesion to be resected. Another atraumatic laparoscopic forceps held in the surgeon's left hand in the left iliac fossa port will be used to provide slight countertraction in the opposite direction. In a suprapubic port, the surgeon uses laparoscopic scissors held in his/her right hand to perform the resection through a cold cut of a thin layer of the bowel serosa. A small area of the external muscle layer may also be sectioned.

After revision of hemostasis, we performed a "U" suture of the seromuscularis layer with Vicryl 3-0 or Prolene 3-0, in the longitudinal direction (perpendicular to the lumen of the loop) to avoid postoperative stenosis.[14]

At the end of the procedure, the integrity of the wall of the loop is tested by instilling 120 mL of saline solution with diluted methylene blue through a 60 mL syringe with a beak into the anus, the segment of the bowel above the sutured area being occluded using an atraumatic laparoscopic forceps.

Transanal Discoid Resection using a Circular Stapler

For performing discoid resection using a transanal circular stapler, first the adhesions are lysed and all other lesions of concomitant deep endometriosis are resected. After releasing the rectosigmoidal lesion from the retrocervical region or the posterior wall of the vagina, care should be taken to leave a free bowel margin of approximately 2.0 cm under the lesion. The nodule is individualized on the anterior wall of the rectum, taking care to release the entire surrounding area of the lesion from the mesorectum and ensuring adequate hemostasis, to leave the area free for stapling (Fig. 23.20).

A suture is performed over the lesion, including the rectal wall to be resected. The surgical thread remains without the needle so that it can be used for repair (Fig. 23.21).

Next, a 33-mm circular stapler is inserted into the rectum and opened so that the anvil points away from the uterine manipulator, creating a free space between the two. With the help of the threads, the lesion is positioned inside the space created by opening the stapler and we then begin to close it.

The stapler is then slowly closed, using pressure to ensure that the lesion remains inside the space, positioning the stapler at a forward angle so that there is no risk of stapling the posterior wall of the rectum and ensuring that the entire lesion is inside the space.

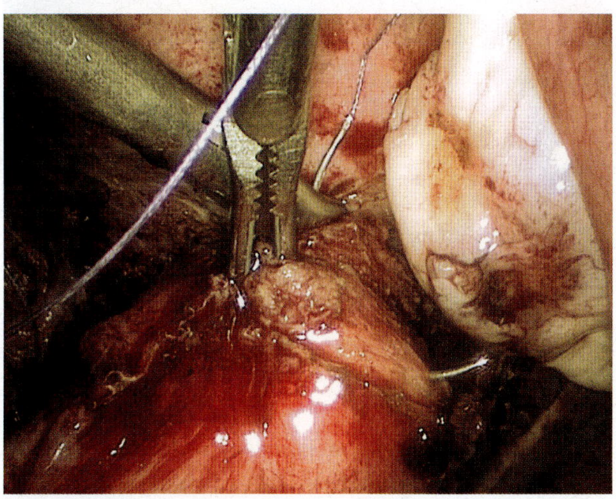

Fig. 23.20: Nodule on the rectum and isolated area surrounding the lesion.

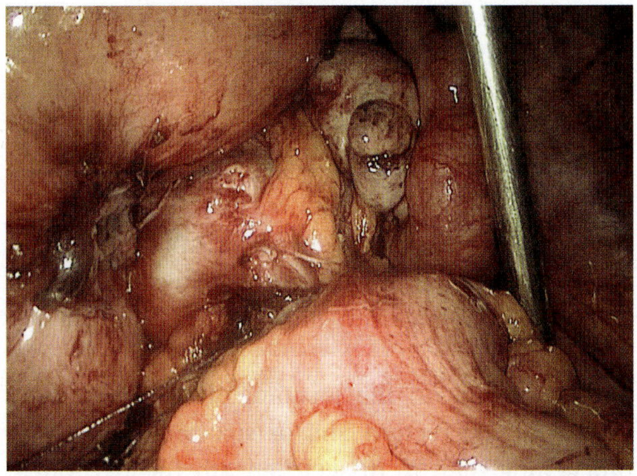

Fig. 23.21: Suture on the rectal wall over the lesion, with the thread maintained for repair.

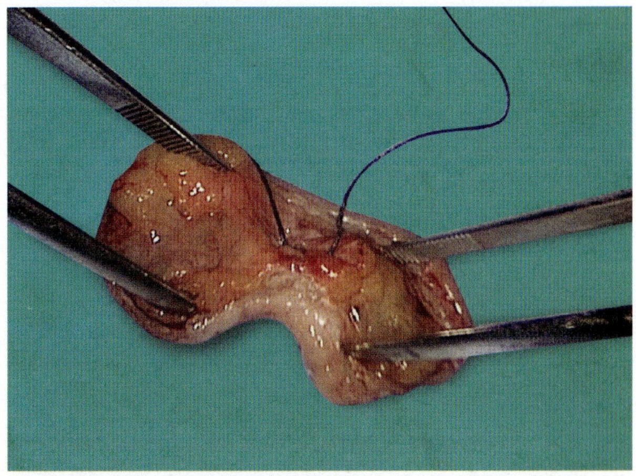

Fig. 23.22: Disc following resection.

After completely closing the circular stapler and certifying that the entire lesion is inside, the stapler is fired and then removed through the rectum using a twisting motion to avoid any trauma that could be caused if it were removed abruptly[36] (Fig. 23.22).

The oval-shaped resected area is then inspected to ensure that the margins are free of the disease.

The safety test described in the previous section is then performed. If bleeding occurs following resection, the bleeding vessel is coagulated during a colonoscopy.

This procedure is limited to the rectum, since the length of the stapler does not allow to reach nodules above the rectosigmoid junction.[14]

Laparoscopic Rectosigmoidectomy with End-to-end Anastomosis

To perform laparoscopic rectosigmoidectomy, we prefer an umbilical port for the 0 degree and 10-mm lens, a port in the left iliac fossa region for the 5-mm trocar, a 5-mm port in the midclavicular line between the right iliac crest and right hypochondrium and a 12-mm port in the right iliac fossa region.

First, the sigmoid colon is released through the medial mesentery followed by the left parietocolic gutter, after which the left ureter and vessels are identified, as well as the point at which the sacral plexus and hypogastric nerve emerge. These are preserved.

Depending on the location of the lesion, the vessels of the rectum and/or sigmoid are ligated, proceeding then to dissect beneath the peritoneal reflection or the lesion, leaving a margin of at least 2 cm of disease-free rectum. The lesion is then resected using the 60-mm linear stapler. At this time, all the other deep endometriosis lesions found in the pelvis are treated, as well as the ovarian endometriomas.

The 12-mm trocar situated in the right iliac fossa is removed and the incision is increased to 3–4 cm in length to exteriorize the previously sectioned and stapled proximal rectum. The endometriosis lesion is identified manually and rectosigmoidectomy is performed, leaving a 2.0 cm free margin above the lesion and we made its section with a linear 60-mm stapler (Fig. 23.23).

Following resection of the bowel segment affected by deep endometriosis, the anvil of the 33-mm circular stapler is fixed for end-to-end anastomosis, the bowel is reinserted into the cavity and the abdominal wall is closed to recreate the pneumoperitoneum (Fig. 23.24).

After resection of all peritoneal lesions and ovarian endometriomas, we removed the 12-mm trocar placed in the right iliac fossa and enlarged the skin incision to 4 cm in length for the exteriorization of the precut proximal pre sectioned and stapled. We manually identified the endometriosis lesion and performed a rectosigmoidectomy leaving a free margin of 2.0 cm above the lesion.

After resecting the intestinal segment with deep endometriosis, we fixed the 33-mm circular stapler's ogive for end-to-end anastomosis, reintroduced the intestine into the cavity and closed the abdominal wall to redo the pneumoperitoneum (Fig. 23.25).

The two edges are gently brought together and a check is made to ensure that no tissue (ovary, tube or vagina) has been left between the two stumps within the 369 degrees of the anastomosis. The position of the longitudinal tena is also checked before the stapler is fired (Fig. 23.26).

After it has been fired, the circular stapler is gently removed with a twisting motion. A safety test is

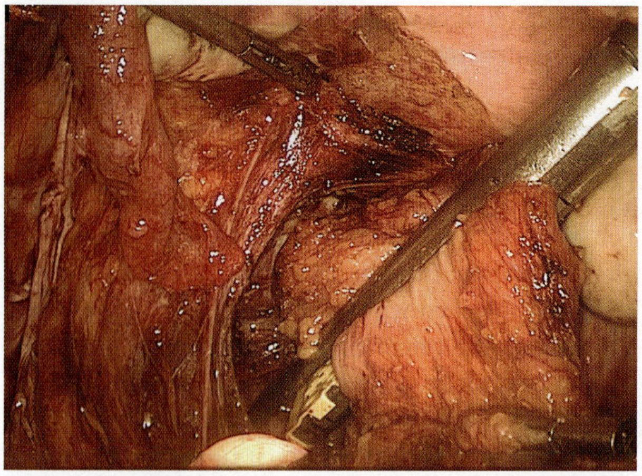

Fig. 23.23: Stapling and sectioning of the rectosigmoid using the 60-mm linear stapler.

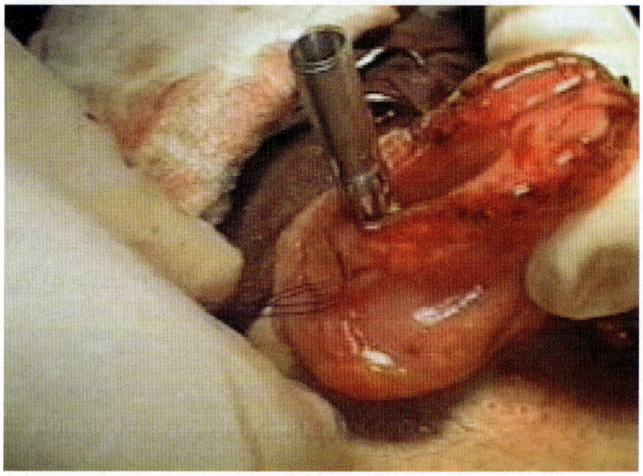

Fig. 23.24: Fixing the anvil of the 33-mm with a 60-mm linear stapler.

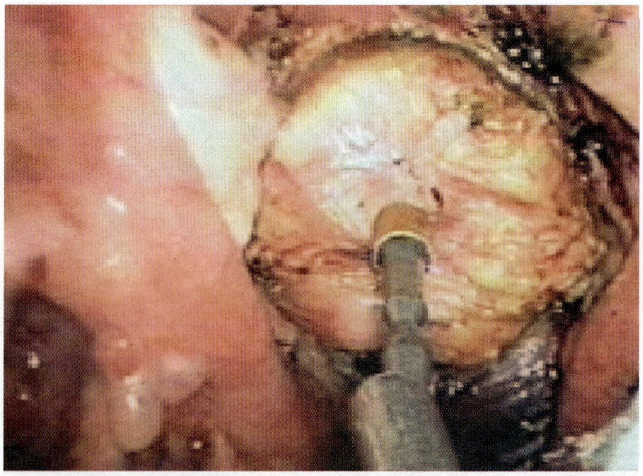

Fig. 23.25: Connecting the anvil to the plug of the circular stapler.

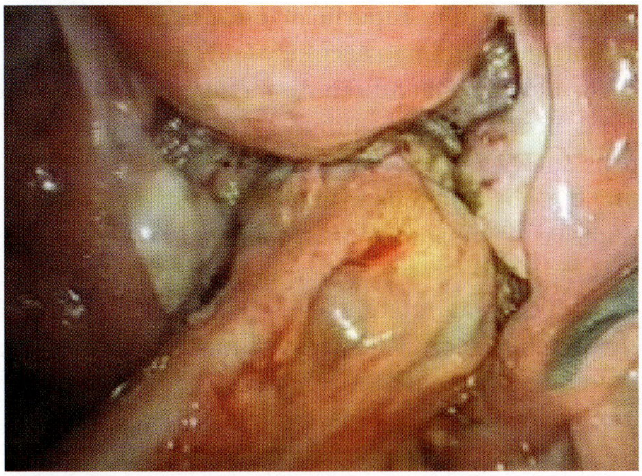

Fig. 23.26: Moment at which the stapler was fired.

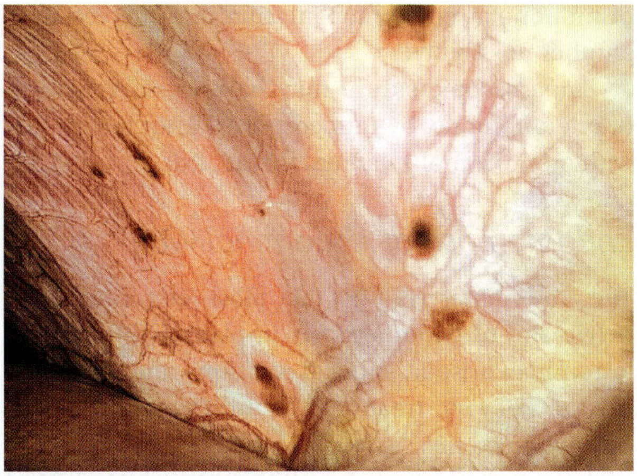

Fig. 23.27: Diaphragm lesion—foci.

then performed and, finally, the peritoneal cavity is drained using a vacuum drain.

Extragenital Endometriosis

Endometriosis of Diaphragm

Scioscia et al. in 2011[37] reported a prevalence of 0.19% of diaphragmatic lesions in a series of 1548 cases of ASRM IV deep stage endometriosis. Ceccaroni et al in 2013[38] found a prevalence of 1.5%. Diaphragmatic disease is higher in cases of severe endometriosis and 100% of women with diaphragmatic disease had pelvic disease, of which 93.4% were in stages III and IV.[38]

Laparoscopy is the gold standard approach for radical treatment of pelvic endometriosis, with the advantage of properly investigating the surfaces of the diaphragm without completely mobilizing the liver. Three different types of lesions: "foci," thin and superficial, with a diameter usually less than 1 cm; solid and three-dimensional "nodules," with diameters usually greater than 1 cm; "plaques," two-dimensional lesions responsible for dense adhesions between the diaphragm and the liver, usually with diameters larger than 3 cm[38] (Figs. 23.27 and 23.28).

In order to approach diaphragmatic lesions, a transumbilical puncture with a 10-mm trocar should be performed for 30 degrees optic placement,[38] three 5-mm trocars (two lateral to 2 cm cranial to the iliac spine and one in the suprapubic region). For a better visualization of the diaphragm, the Trendelenburg position should be used.[38,39] For access of the upper right abdomen, a 5-mm trocar is placed in the subcostal region to the right in the hemiclavicular line.

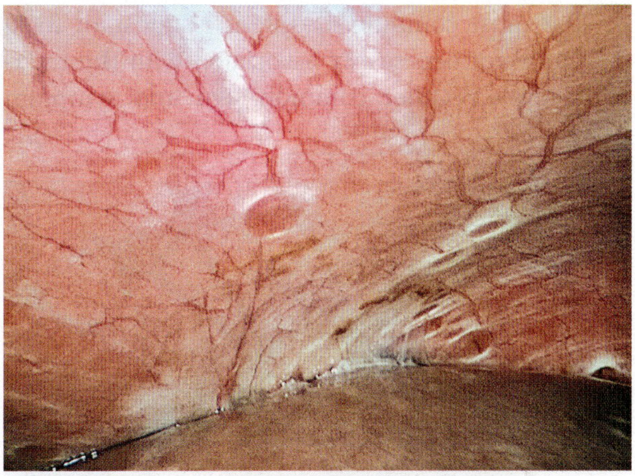

Fig. 23.28: Diaphragm lesion—plaque.

Dissecting the falciform ligament is performed with bipolar forceps and scissors while the assistant draws the liver down with intestinal clamp.[39] This technique improves the exposure of the posterior diaphragmatic peritoneum. Another 10-mm trocar can be placed just below the left costal border immediately to the left of the falciform ligament. So, to approach the upper abdomen, the surgeon is positioned between the legs of the patient.[38,39]

Superficial lesions less than 5-mm should be vaporized with argon laser to avoid ischemia. The deep lesions should be removed by dissection and hemostasis should be performed with bipolar coagulation. The lesions with free peritoneal margin are tractioned with gripping forceps. Bipolar scissors can be used to make an incision around the disease to initiate disease-free area dissection and separate the diaphragmatic peritoneum underlying the muscle. The technique of peritonectomy with the use of monopolar energy for incision and dissection is another possibility.

Laparoscopic suture may be necessary in case of pneumothorax by intracorporeal knot technique, with mono or multifilament thread, 2-0.

Endometriosis of Abdominal Wall

The abdominal wall is the most common extra pelvic site of endometriosis implants. This type of lesion may arise in surgical incisions after cesarean section delivery, treatment of pelvic endometriosis or myomectomy, when it reaches the endometrial cavity.[40] Khan et al. in 2017[41] found 34 (1.34%) patients with endometriosis of the wall of a total of 2539 of women with endometriosis, of these 59% presented the lesion in a cesarean section (Fig. 23.29).

The most common symptom is constant focal pain and not necessarily associated with the menstrual cycle.[40] Other common sign and symptom are bleeding from superficial lesions.[42] Independent risk factors, with high accuracy for the diagnosis, are cyclic pelvic pain without dysmenorrhea and a previous history of laparotomy[41] (Fig. 23.30). Imaging tests such as ultrasonography, computed tomography (CT) or magnetic resonance imaging (MRI) can improve diagnostic accuracy[40] and help with surgical planning.

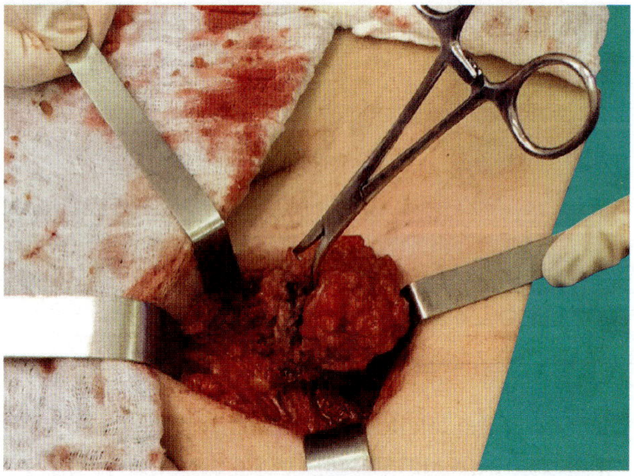

Fig. 23.29: Cesarean section lesion of multiparous woman.

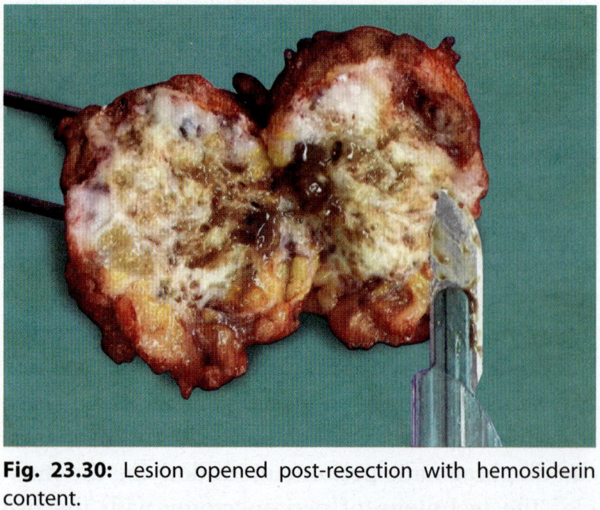

Fig. 23.30: Lesion opened post-resection with hemosiderin content.

The treatment of choice is the broad local excision of the lesion with negative margins. When the lesion incorporates the abdominal wall musculature, it requires block resection of adjacent myofascial elements. Surgeons need to be prepared for the coexistence of hernia and the need for mesh placement. The recurrence rate is low if the lesions are adequately removed in their entirety.[43]

TIPS AND TRICKS

- Dissection of the retroperitoneum always begins close to the entrance of the pelvis minor, next to the ureter, in an area of healthy tissue, proceeding in the direction of the deep endometriotic lesion, as this allows better individualization of the nodules to be removed.
- We use atraumatic grasping forceps to carefully remove the capsule of the endometrioma, thus minimizing bleeding and consequently reducing the need for coagulation and trauma to the ovarian parenchyma. This prevents the occurrence of a drastic reduction in the ovarian follicular reserve.
- In cases of resection of deep endometriotic lesions, both retrocervical lesions and those in the posterior vaginal fornix, we recommend simultaneously performing a digital vaginal examination to help identify the presence of the nodule, improve its exposure and also confirm whether resection was complete.
- We temporarily lift the ovaries during surgery, following removal of the capsule of the endometrioma, and suture them to facilitate access to the ovarian fossa, a peritoneal site often affected by endometriosis, thus making it easier to perform ureterolysis and to resect endometriotic nodules from the uterosacral ligaments.
- When endometriotic lesions have to be resected in the bowel and/or in cases of deep paracervical lesions, if bilateral, particular care should be taken to preserve pelvic innervation in order to prevent functional damage. As anatomical safety limits, we dissect along the medial surface of the uterosacral ligaments and above the middle rec-

tal arteries, thus avoiding lesions to the hypogastric nerve, lower hypogastric plexus and pelvic splanchnic nerves.

CONCLUSION

The surgical treatment of deep endometriosis represents a major challenge to the gynecologist in view of the high degree of anatomical distortion caused by fibrous adhesions in the pelvic peritoneum and involvement of adjacent organs such as the bowel, bladder and ureter. Knowledge of the retroperitoneal anatomy of the region is crucial in order to minimize the risks of unintentionally damaging nerves or blood vessels. A multidisciplinary team is strongly recommended in cases of lesions to nongynecological organs as a strategy for reducing the risks of surgery and avoiding persistence of the disease. We also recommend the use of laparoscopy, which permits better visibility of the lesions.

REFERENCES

1. Viganò P, Parazzini F, Somigliana E, et al. Endometriosis: epidemiology and etiological factors. Best Pract Res Clin Obstet Gynaecolol. 2004;18(2): 177-200.
2. Farquhar CM. Extracts from the "clinical evidence." Endometriosis. BMJ. 2000; 320(7247):1449-52.
3. Benagiano G, Brosens I. Who identified endometriosis? Fertil. Steril. 2011;95(1):13-6.
4. Falcone T, Golgberg JM, Park AJ. Indications and techniques for the laparoscopic management of endometriosis. In: Karram M (Series Ed), Female Pelvic Surgery Video Atlas Series, 1st edn. Basic, Advanced and Robotic Laparoscopic Surgery. Amsterdam; Elsevier; 2010.
5. Yildirim S, Nursal TZ, Tarim A, et al. Colonic obstruction due to rectal endometriosis: report of a case. Turkish J Gastroenterol. 2005;16(1):48-51.
6. Jansen RP, Russell P. Nonpigmented endometriosis: clinical, laparoscopic, and pathologic definition. Am J Obstet Gynecol. 1986;155(6):1154-9.
7. Cornillie FJ, Oosterlynck D, Lauweryns JM, et al. Deeply infiltrating pelvic endometriosis: histology and clinical significance. Fertil. Steril. 1990;53(6): 978-83.
8. Bellelis P, Dias JA Jr, Podgaec S, et al. Epidemiological and clinical aspects of pelvic endometriosis—a case series. Revista Assoc Med Brasileira 2010;56(4): 467-71.
9. Abrao MS, Gonçalves MO, Dias JA Jr, et al. Comparison between clinical examination, transvaginal sonography and magnetic resonance imaging for the diagnosis of deep endometriosis. Hum Reproduct. 2007;22(12):3092-7.
10. Abrao MS, Podgaec S, Dias JA Jr, et al. Diagnosis of rectovaginal endometriosis. Hum Reproduct. 2008; 23:2386.
11. Goncalves MO, Dias JA Jr, Podgaec S, et al. Transvaginal ultrasound for diagnosis of deeply infiltrating endometriosis. Int J Gynaecol Obstet. 2009;104(2): 156-60.
12. Goncalves MO, Podgaec S, Dias JA Jr, et al. Transvaginal ultrasonography with bowel preparation is able to predict the number of lesions and rectosigmoid layers affected in cases of deep endometriosis, defining surgical strategy. Hum Reproduct. 2010;25(3):665-71.
13. Bulletti C, Coccia ME, Battistoni S, et al. Endometriosis and infertility. J Assis Reproduc Genetics. 2010;27(8):441-7.
14. Abrao MS, Borelli GMB, Clarizia R, et al. Strategies for management of colorectal endometriosis. Sem Reproduc Med. 2017;35(1):65-71.
15. Abrão MS, Petraglia F, Falcone T, et al. Deep endometriosis infiltrating the recto-sigmoid: critical factors to consider before management. Hum Reproduct Update. 2015;21(3):329-39.
16. Taylor E, Williams C. Surgical treatment of endometriosis: location and patterns of disease at reoperation. Fertil Steril. 2010;93(1):57-61.
17. Nassif J, Trompoukis P, Barata S, et al. Management of deep endometriosis Reproduc BioMed Online. 2011;23(1):25-33.
18. Schollmeyer T, Pandit K, Schmutzler A, et al. Correlation of endoscopic interpretation of endometriosis with histological verification. Clin Exp Obstet Gynecol. 2004;31(2):107-9.
19. Yang LC, Arden D, Lee TT, et al. Mechanical bowel preparation for gynecologic laparoscopy: a prospective randomized trial of oral sodium phosphate solution vs single sodium phosphate enema. J Minim Invasive Gynecol. 2011;18(2):149-56.
20. Gerges FJ, Kanazi GE, Jabbour-Khoury SI. Anesthesia for laparoscopy: a review. J Clin Anesthesia. 2006;18(1):67-78.
21. Shveiky D, Aseff JN, Iglesia CB. Brachial plexus injury after laparoscopic and robotic surgery. J Minim Invasive Gynecol. 2010;17(4):414-20.
22. Corson SL. Two new laparoscopic instruments: bipolar sterilizing forceps and uterine manipulator. Med Instrument. 1977;11(1):7-8.
23. Ahmad G, Gent D, Henderson D, et al. Laparoscopic entry techniques. Cochrane Database Syst Rev. 2015;8:CD006583.
24. Vilos GA, Ternamian A, Dempster J, et al. Laparoscopic entry: a review of techniques, technologies, and complications. J Obstet Gynaecol Canada. 2007;29(5):433-65.
25. Supe AN, Kulkarni GV, Supe PA. Ergonomics in laparoscopic surgery. J Minim Access Surg. 2010;6(2):31-6.
26. Badawy A, Khiary M, Ragab A, et al. Laparoscopy—or not—for management of unexplained infertility. J Obstet Gynaecol. 2010;30(7):712-5.

27. Chapron C, Pietin-Vialle C, Borghese B, et al. Associated ovarian endometrioma is a marker for greater severity of deeply infiltrating endometriosis. Fertil Steril. 2009;92(2):453-7.
28. Strandell A. Treatment of hydrosalpinx in the patient undergoing assisted reproduction. Curr Opin Obstet Gynecol. 2007;19(4):360-5.
29. Abrao MS, Dias JA Jr, Bellelis P, et al. Endometriosis of the ureter and bladder are not associated diseases Fertil Steril. 2009;91(5):1662-7.
30. Smith IA, Cooper M. Management of ureteric endometriosis associated with hydronephrosis: An Australian case series of 13 patients. BMC Res Notes. 2010;25(3):45.
31. Takeuchi S, Minoura H, Toyoda N, et al. Intrinsic ureteric involvement by endometriosis: a case report. J Obstet Gynaecol Res. 1997;23(3):273-6.
32. Frenna V, Santos L, Ohana E, et al. Laparoscopic management of ureteral endometriosis: our experience. J Minim Invasive Gynecol. 2007;14(2): 169-71.
33. Abrao MS, Podgaec S, Dias JA, Jr et al. Endometriosis lesions that compromise the rectum deeper than the inner muscularis layer have more than 40% of the circumference of the rectum affected by the disease. J Minim Invasive Gynecol. 2008;15:280-5.
34. Abrão MS, Dias JA Jr, Rodini GP, et al. Endometriosis at several sites, cyclic bowel symptoms, and the likelihood of the appendix being affected. Fertil Steril. 2010;94(3):1099-101.
35. De Ceglie A, Bilardi C, Blanchi S, et al. Acute small bowel obstruction caused by endometriosis: a case report and review of the literature. World J Gastroenterol. 2008;14(21):3430-4.
36. Woods RJ, Heriot AG, Chen FC. Anterior rectal wall excision for endometriosis using the circular stapler. ANZ J Surg. 2003;73(8):647-8.
37. Scioscia M, Bruni F, Ceccaroni M, et al. Distribution of endometriotic lesions stage IV supports the menstrual reflux theory and requires specific preoperative assessment and therapy. Acta Obstet Gynecol Scand. 2011;(90):126-39.
38. Ceccaroni M, Roviglione G, Giampaolino P, et al. Laparoscopic surgical treatment of diaphragmatic endometriosis: a 7-year single-institution restrospective review. Surg Endosc. 2013;27:625-32.
39. Chiantera V, Dessole M, Petrillo M, et al. Laparoscopic en bloc right diaphragmatic peritonectomy for diaphragmatic endometriosis according to the Sugarbaker technique. J Minim Invasive Gynecol. 2016;23(2):198-205.
40. Davis AC, Goldberg JM. Extrapelvic endometriosis. Semin Reproduc Med. 2017;35(1):98-101.
41. Khan Z, Zanfagnin V, El-Nashar SA, et al. Risk factors, clinical presentation, and outcomes for abdominal wall endometriosis. J Minim Invasive Gynecol. 2017;24(3):478-84.
42. Horton JD, Dezee KJ, Ahnfeldt EP, et al. Abdominal wall endometriosis: a surgeon's perspective and review of 445 cases. Am J Surg. 2008;196 (2):207-12.
43. Rindos NB, Mansuria S. Diagnosis and Management of abdominal wall endometriosis: a systematic review and clinical recommendations. Obstet Gynecol Surv. 2017;72(2):116-22.

Adenomyosis Treatment

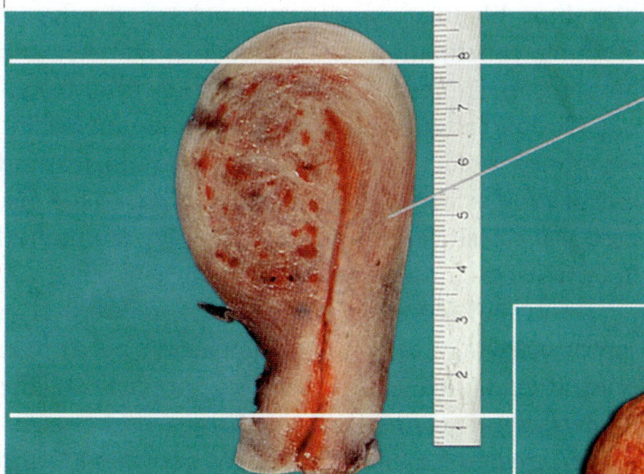

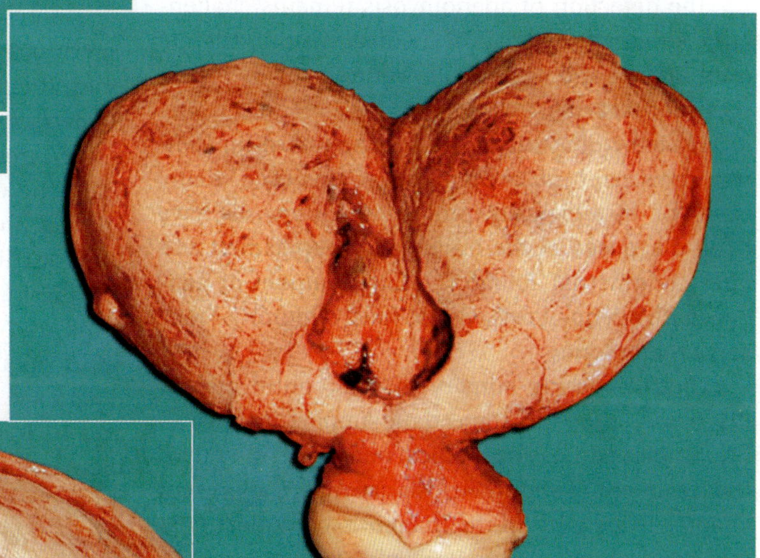

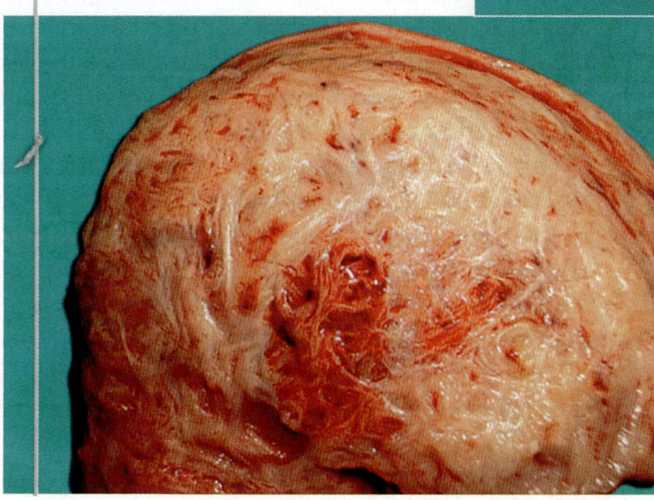

Chapter 24

Adenomyosis Treatment

Ibrahim Alkatout, Liselotte Mettler

GENERAL

Adenomyosis is defined as the presence of heterotopic endometrial glands and stroma within myometrial tissue; the condition is known to cause globular and cystic enlargement of the uterus. Some of the cysts are filled with extravasated, hemolyzed red blood cells and siderophages.

The detection of adenomyosis remains challenging, although the triad of medical history, vaginal examination and vaginal ultrasound provide extensive information.

Hysterectomy still is the gold standard for definite treatment of adenomyosis. However, many cases of histologically proven adenomyosis have been diagnosed in the hysterectomy specimen and after endometrial ablation. A large number of patients with adenomyosis wish to have children or preserve their uterus.

Uterine-sparing surgery is still controversially discussed, although some data support its feasibility. Studies addressing medical treatment other than the treatment of endometriosis are rare. The present chapter is focused on the diagnosis of clinical data and research on adenomyosis of the uterus, and its definite surgical treatment as a step-by-step procedure. Hysterectomy is the treatment of choice for women with significant symptoms who have completed their families.

INTRODUCTION

Endometriosis is the second most common benign genital disease in women after uterine myoma. It is defined as the presence of endometrial glands and stroma outside the internal epithelial lining of the uterine cavity. The symptoms include chronic pelvic pain, dysmenorrhea, deep dyspareunia, cyclical bowel or bladder symptoms (such as dyschezia, bloating, constipation, rectal bleeding, diarrhea and hematuria), subfertility, abnormal menstrual bleeding, chronic fatigue or low back pain. The unspecific symptoms reflect the diversity of pathologies and localization as well as individual reactions to the disease. All classifications suggested so far are limited in terms of their predictive value.[1]

About 50% of teenagers and 32% of women of reproductive age, operated on for chronic pelvic pain or dysmenorrhea, suffer from endometriosis. The percentage of women with confirmed endometriosis and treated for infertility ranges between 9% and 50%. The exact prevalence of endometriosis in the general population is unknown because the symptoms are diverse and non-specific.[2,3]

The interval between the first unspecific symptoms and the medical diagnosis of endometriosis is about seven years. The condition is usually diagnosed for the first time between the ages of 20 and 40. In cases of secondary sterility, the frequency increases parallel to the time elapsed since the last pregnancy: less than 5 years 7%, 5–10 years 19% and longer than 10 years 26%.[4]

As the pathogenesis of endometriosis is not clear, its causal treatment remains impossible. The treatment options include expectant management, analgesia, hormonal therapy, surgical intervention and a combination of medical treatment before and/or after surgery. As it has been shown that the growth of endometriosis is promoted by estrogen, various medical treatments can be used to address the condition.[5,6]

Adenomyosis of the uterus can be distinguished from endometriosis in that adenomyosis is marked by the appearance of endometrial glands and endometrial stroma within the myometrium. The spread

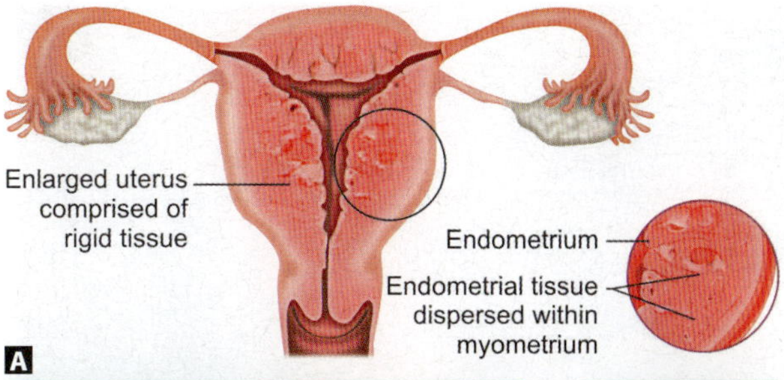

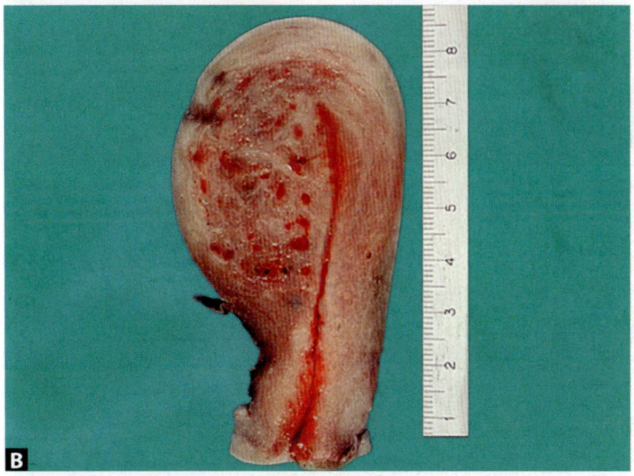

Figs. 24.1A and B: (A) Schematic drawing of an enlarged uterus with adenomyosis. Endometrial glands are dispersed within the myometrium; (B) Anatomical specimen in a sagittal cut. The posterior wall is much thicker than the anterior wall, with endometrial glands spread diffusely in the wall of the myometrium.

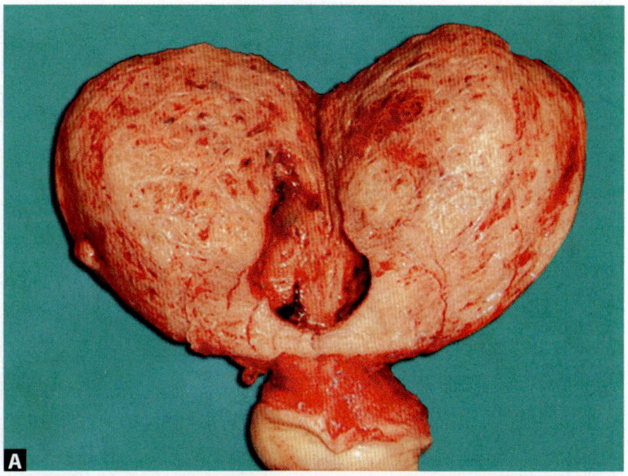

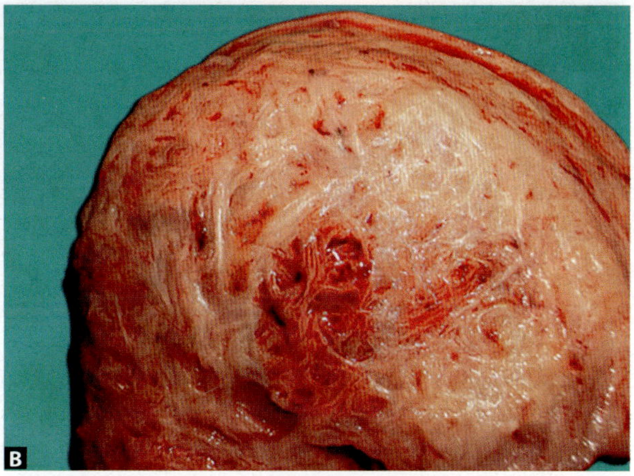

Figs. 24.2A and B: (A) Pathological specimen in a sagittal cut; (B) Magnification of (A) showing the infiltration of small endometriosis islands deep into the myometrium.

of endometrial tissue induces hypertrophy and hyperplasia of the surrounding tissue. This leads to an enlarged, occasionally softened, and sometimes rigid uterus. Adenomyosis can be identified very clearly by imaging procedures. Nevertheless, focal adenomyosis can be easily mistaken for a leiomyoma (Figs. 24.1 to 24.5).

EPIDEMIOLOGY AND PATHOLOGY

According to estimates, adenomyosis occurs in about 20% of women. However, the frequency of the actual diagnosis and published data on the subject are very diverse (5–70%). In the majority of cases the diagnosis is established after histopathological examination of the hysterectomy specimen. In terms of epidemiology, our understanding of adenomyosis is hindered by the fact that it tends to coexist along with endometriosis and/or fibroids. In some investigations, histopathological investigation of the specimen obtained from hysterectomy suggested adenomyosis, independent of symptoms, and was the reason for performing surgery. In yet other studies, women with adenomyosis—as compared to those with endometriosis—had higher parity, early menarche and shorter menstrual cycles. However, more numerous pregnancies do not increase the risk of developing adenomyosis.[7] Another study showed that women with adenomyosis were subject to a higher risk of dysmenorrhea, pelvic pain and depression, and had undergone previous surgery more frequently.[8]

Adenomyosis of the uterus is an estrogen-dependent disease. Most likely, the endometrial–myometrial interface or the uterine junction zone are involved in the disease as anatomical and functional entities.[9]

The pathogenesis of adenomyosis is similar to that of endometriosis. Three theories of pathogenesis have been proposed:

1. Adenomyosis de novo is induced by metaplastic transformation of embryologic pluripotent Müllerian remnants.
2. Adenomyosis grows by invagination of the basal endometrium into the myometrium through an altered or absent junctional zone.

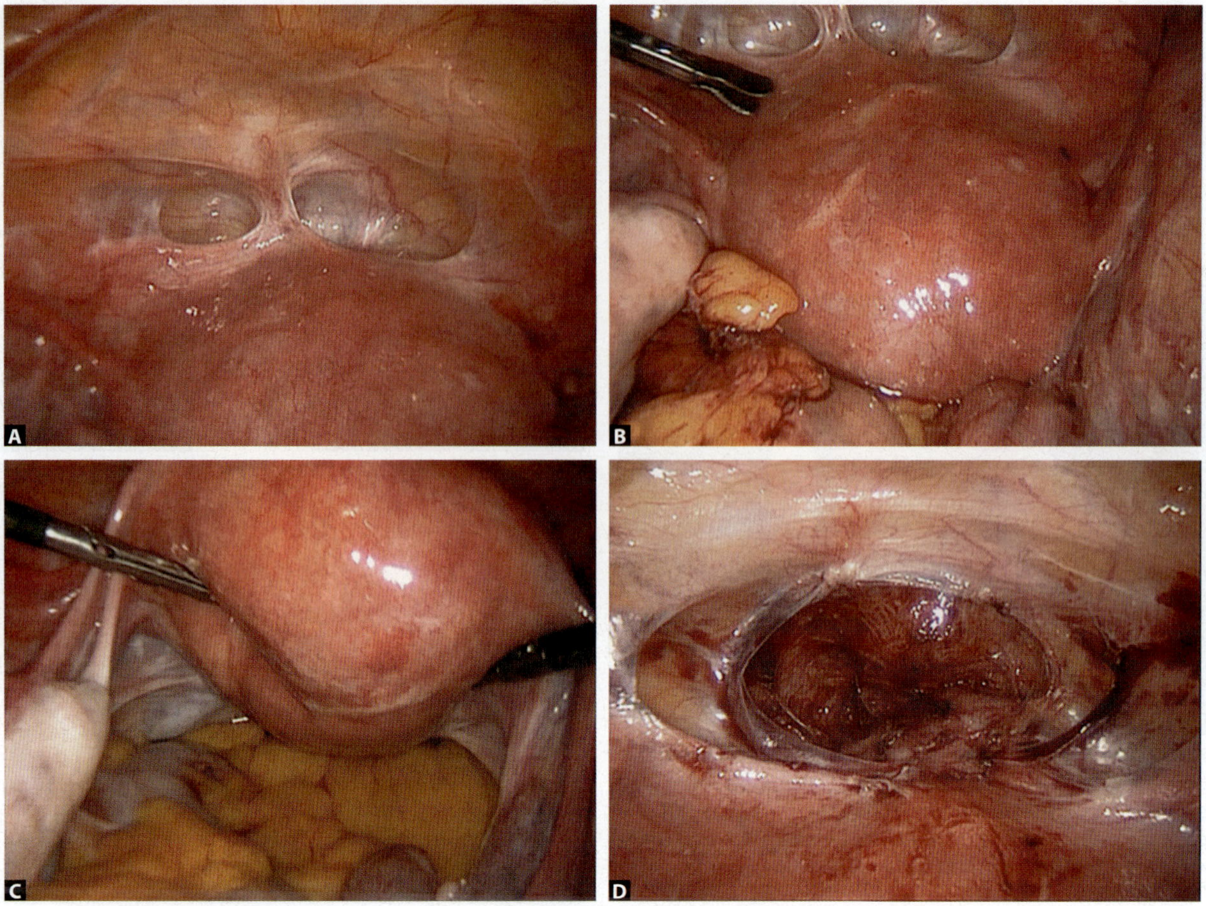

Figs. 24.3A to D: (A to C) Laparoscopic view of a patient with severe dysmenorrhea. The uterus is enlarged and soft. The anterior wall is connected to the bladder peritoneum through multiple adhesions; (D) After adhesiolysis, it appears that the adenomyosis has grown through the uterine wall into the neighboring bladder.

3. Adenomyosis is a consequence of tissue injury and repair, stimulated by the hypersecretion of estrogen.[9]

Adenomyosis may exist diffusely throughout the myometrium, or as a focal entity or adenomyoma. The pathological specimen shows chocolate-colored areas, representing endometriotic islands. Adenomyomas are difficult to differentiate from leiomyomas on clinical investigation, have no plane and cannot be excised as easily as fibroids. Closure of the uterine wall is rendered difficult by the fragile and unstable myometrium. Sutures are therefore a challenging step. Adenomyosis is frequently accompanied by endometriosis (Figs. 24.6 and 24.7).

On microscopic investigation the endometrial tissue is located within the myometrium, at a significant distance from it. Usually a zone of myometrial hypertrophy and hyperplasia surrounds the adenomatous tissue. The spread of endometrial tissue occurs as a response to fluctuations in estrogen and progesterone levels during the menstrual cycle (Figs. 24.8A and B).

CLINICAL MANIFESTATIONS AND DIAGNOSIS

The principal symptoms of adenomyosis are severe dysmenorrhea (25%) and heavy menstrual bleeding (60%). Chronic pelvic pain, as in the presence of endometriosis, may also occur. Many of these symptoms do not appear before the age of 40 or 50 years. One-third of the women tend to be asymptomatic. The impact of adenomyosis on infertility is still controversially discussed because most women have concomitant leiomyomas, endometriosis and endometrial polyps.

Histological examination of a hysterectomy specimen is essential before adenomyosis can be established with certainty and its causal treatment initiated. The preoperative diagnosis is based on the patient's medical history (menorrhagia, dysmenorrhea, dyspareunia), bimanual examination, transvaginal ultrasound and magnetic resonance imaging (especially T2-weighted). In a meta-analysis of 23 articles, the sensitivity and specificity of MRI

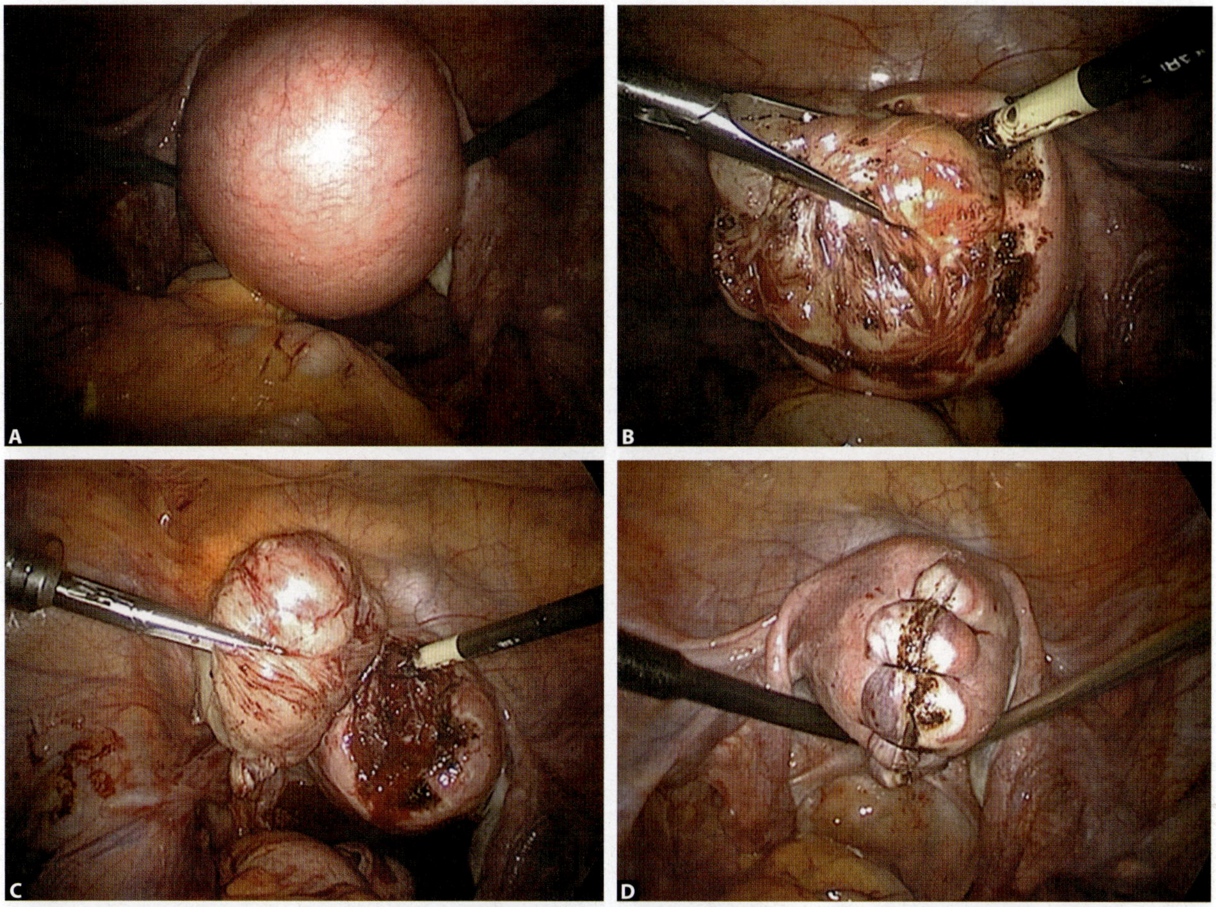

Figs. 24.4A to D: (A) Enlarged uterus due to a transmyometrial myoma; (B to D) Laparoscopic enucleation of the myoma and reconstruction of the uterine wall. The uterine myometrium still appears dense and hypervascularized. Clinically adenomyosis may look soft or tightened and rigid.

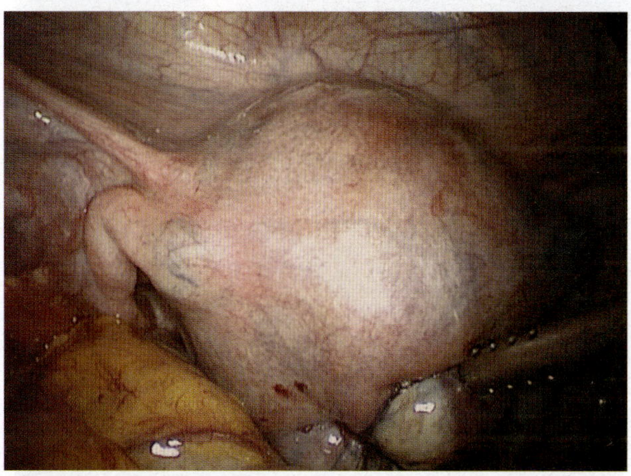

Fig. 24.5: Same patient as in Fig. 24.3 after chromopertubation. The injection of blue dye reveals the intramural vessels, which appear to be massively increased. This appearance is also characteristic of adenomyosis of the uterus.

in revealing adenomyosis was 77% and 89%, respectively, as compared to 72% and 81% for ultrasound (Figs. 24.9 to 24.11).[10] Visible signs of adenomyosis include the following:

- Asymmetrical thickening of the anterior and posterior myometrium (especially the posterior myometrium)
- Intramyometrial cysts
- Linear striations extending from the endometrium
- Loss of a clear endomyometrial margin
- Greater myometrial heterogeneity.[11,12]

The differential diagnosis of adenomyosis is summarized in Box 24.1.

Especially dysmenorrhea in the patient's medical history is indicative of adenomyosis; the exact etiology of dysmenorrhea must be established. Causes of secondary dysmenorrhea are given in Table 24.1.

ADENOMYOSIS AND INFERTILITY

General endometriosis is associated with infertility, which can be addressed by medication and/or surgery. Surgery enhances the likelihood of natural conception.

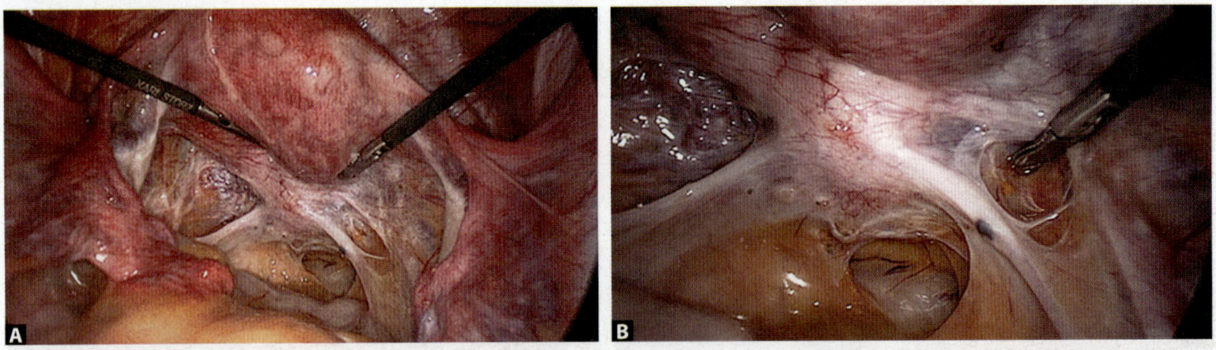

Figs. 24.6A and B: Patient with severe adenomyosis, multiple signs of external genital endometriosis and suspected fibroid on ultrasound.

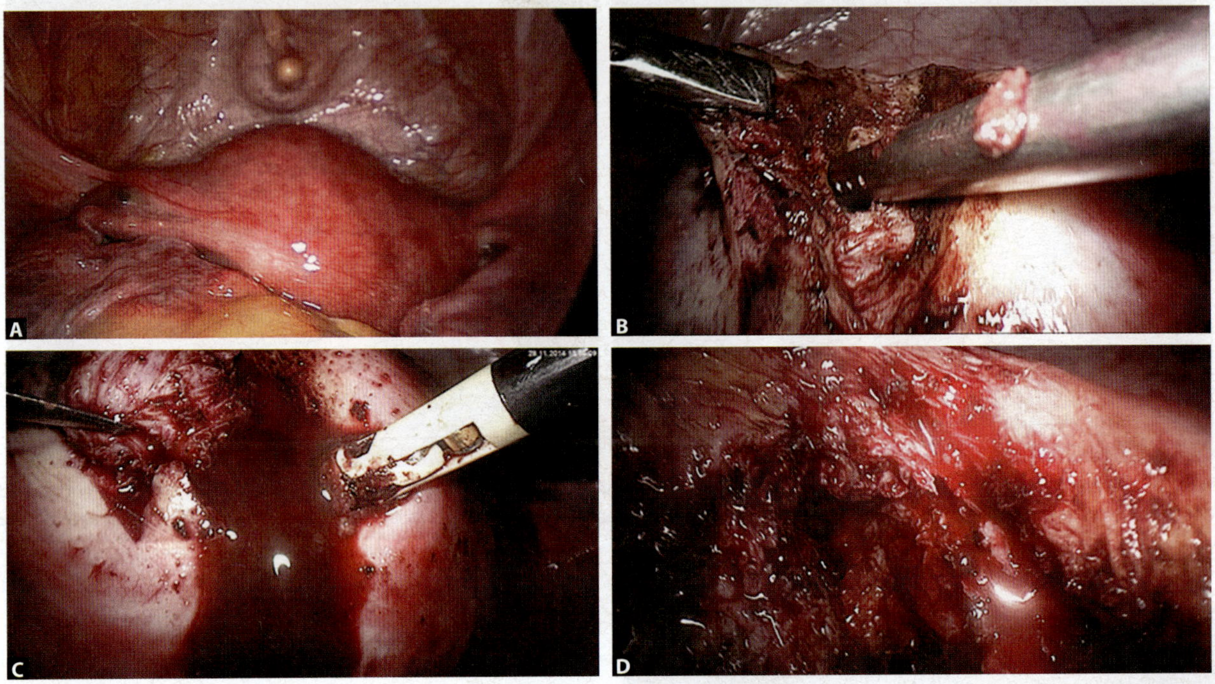

Figs. 24.7A to D: Same patient as in Fig. 24.5. (A) An asymmetrical uterus with suspected endometriosis at the left tube and a central space-consuming lesion; (B) Opening of the central intramural lesion that was suspected to be a fibroid; (C) Chocolate-like fluid after entering the adenomyoma; (D) The middle layers of endometrium wall can be seen in the magnification.

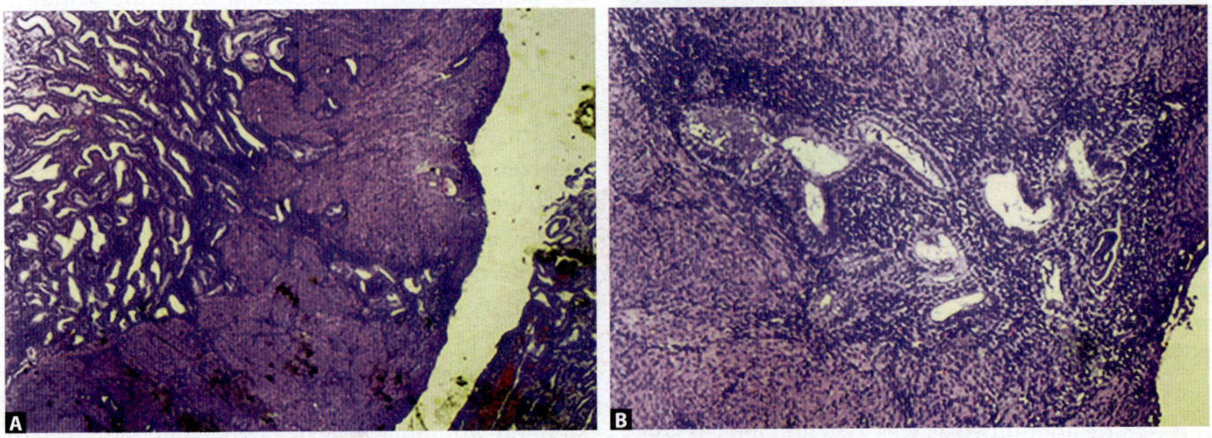

Figs. 24.8A and B: (A) Low magnification of a piece of endometrial tissue obtained by ablation, with the connecting myometrium tissue in the early secretion phase; (B) Islets of endometrial glands in the myometrium stroma with no connection to the uterine cavity. The endometrium shows clear signs of being involved in the endocrine cycle.

Courtesy: Professor Martin Anlauf, Institute of Pathology and Cytology, Limburg, Germany.

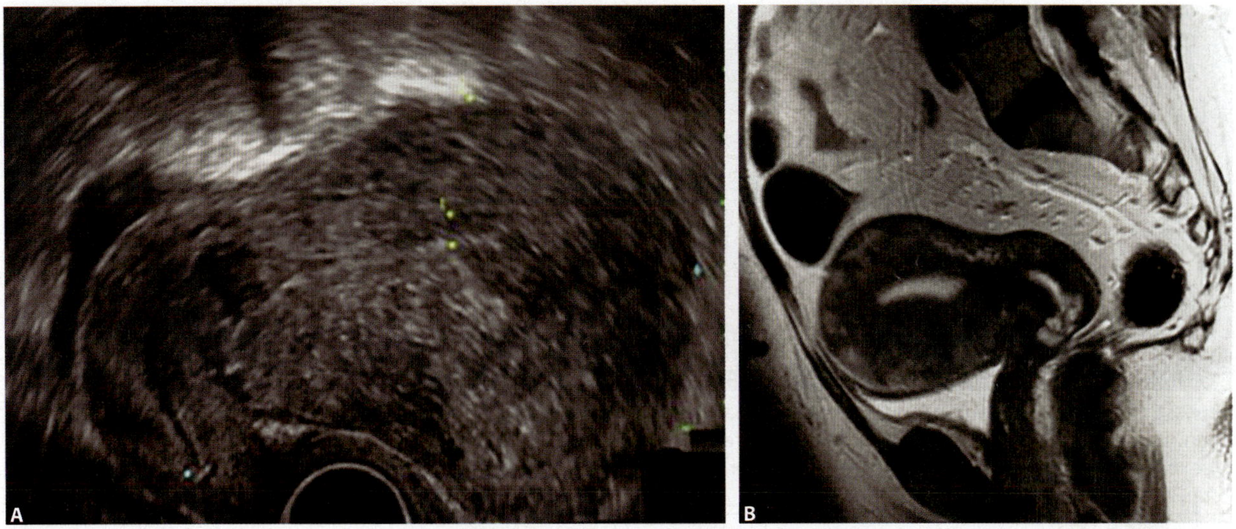

Figs. 24.9A and B: (A) Irregular anterior wall with a heterogeneous appearance on ultrasound. The wall is thickened and the affected area cannot be clearly demarcated. Nevertheless, focal adenomyosis can be easily mistaken for a myoma; (B) MRI scan confirms the clinical diagnosis of adenomyosis. The T2-weighted image shows irregular vascularization and clearly confirms the presence of adenomyosis rather than a myoma.
Courtesy: Dr Werner Dürr.

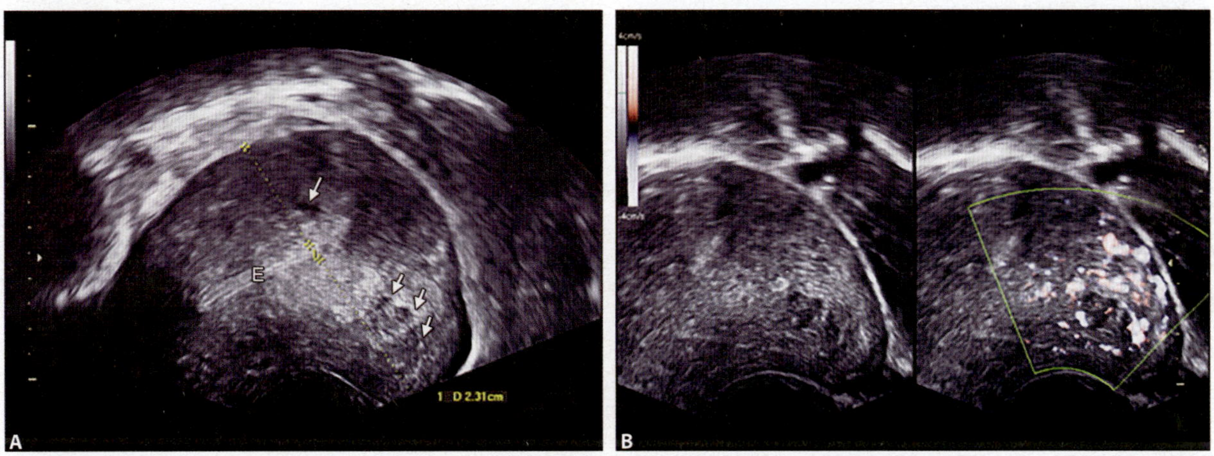

Figs. 24.10A and B: (A) A different patient: Cystic structures surrounded by an echogenic endometrium-like margin; (B) Color Doppler shows very marked and diffuse neovascularization in the cystic area as a sign of adenomyosis prone to progression. Streaky shadows indicate older processes while cystic entities are a more recent manifestation of adenomyosis.
Courtesy: Dr Werner Dürr.

The detrimental effects of adenomyosis on fertility may be due to the impairment of sperm transport, hyperperistaltic or dysperistaltic uterotubal transport. The eutopic and heterotopic endometrium of these patients might be associated with biochemical and functional alterations, leading to poor receptivity. The high spontaneous abortion rate may be due to a dysfunctional junctional zone. Adenomyosis is also known to influence the outcome of in vitro fertilization (IVF) and intracytoplasmic sperm injection (ICSI) adversely: lower rates of clinical pregnancy and implantation as well as higher rates of early pregnancy loss have been reported. The long downregulation protocol appears to exert a protective effect (Figs. 24.12 and 24.13).[13,14]

TREATMENT

Causal treatment of adenomyosis is difficult. Conservative medical therapy is identical to that of endometriosis. In many cases, adenomyosis of the uterus and endometriosis exist simultaneously.[15]

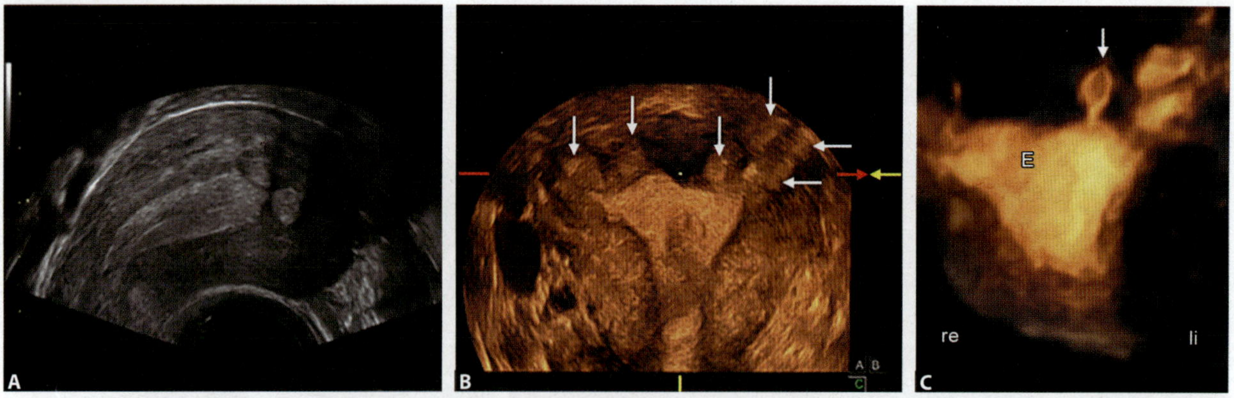

Figs. 24.11A to C: (A) Ultrasound in this patient demarcates focal intramural, and rather homogeneous areas; (B and C) More pronounced and irregular vascularization of the area affected by adenomyosis compared to the regular vascularization achieved by preexisting vessels can only be seen on 3D and power Doppler.
Courtesy: Dr Werner Dürr.

Box 24.1: Differential diagnosis of adenomyosis of the uterus.

- Pregnancy
- Polyps
- Submucosal myoma
- Endometrial hyperplasia
- Synechiae
- Adenocarcinoma
- Infection (endometritis)

Table 24.1: Causes of secondary dysmenorrhea.

Gynecologic	• Endometriosis • Adenomyosis • Fibroids • Ovarian cysts • Intrauterine or pelvic adhesions • Chronic pelvic inflammatory disease • Obstructive endometrial polyps • Congenital obstructive Müllerian malformations • Cervical stenosis • Use of an intrauterine contraceptive device • Pelvic congestion syndrome
Nongynecologic	• Inflammatory bowel disease • Irritable bowel syndrome • Uteropelvic junction obstruction • Psychogenic disorders

General Treatment of Endometriosis Combined with Adenomyosis of the Uterus

As the pathogenesis of endometriosis is not clearly understood, no causal treatment other than hysterectomy is available at the present time. The treatment options include expectant management, analgesia, hormonal medical therapy, surgical intervention and a combination of medical treatment before and/or after surgery. The therapeutic procedures may be divided into three groups: medical, surgical and combined treatment. The fact that the growth of endometriosis is assisted by estrogen has led to a variety of medical treatments.[5,6,16] The first structured therapy was introduced by Mettler and Semm. It involves diagnostic laparoscopy, removing all visible endometriosis foci as far as possible, 3–6 months of endocrine therapy and a subsequent second-look laparoscopy with resection of residual foci, removal of adhesions and reconstruction of organs. If the patient desires children, the gynecologist is advised to use assisted reproductive treatment.[17]

Medical treatment: In the past, the main strategy consisted of the induction of a pseudopregnancy, the application of gestagens, and later danazol and GnRH analogs.[5] This approach was long regarded as the gold standard, but has now been supplemented by add-back therapy and progesterone (Visanne).[18] A serum estradiol level of approximately 60 pg/mL is needed to prevent side effects of the GnRH agonist, such as bone demineralization, vasomotor symptoms, or mood swings.[5,18-20] Levonorgestrel-releasing intrauterine contraception may be effective in reducing menorrhagia and dysmenorrhea. Nevertheless, the symptoms may recur within 6 months after cessation of therapy.[21]

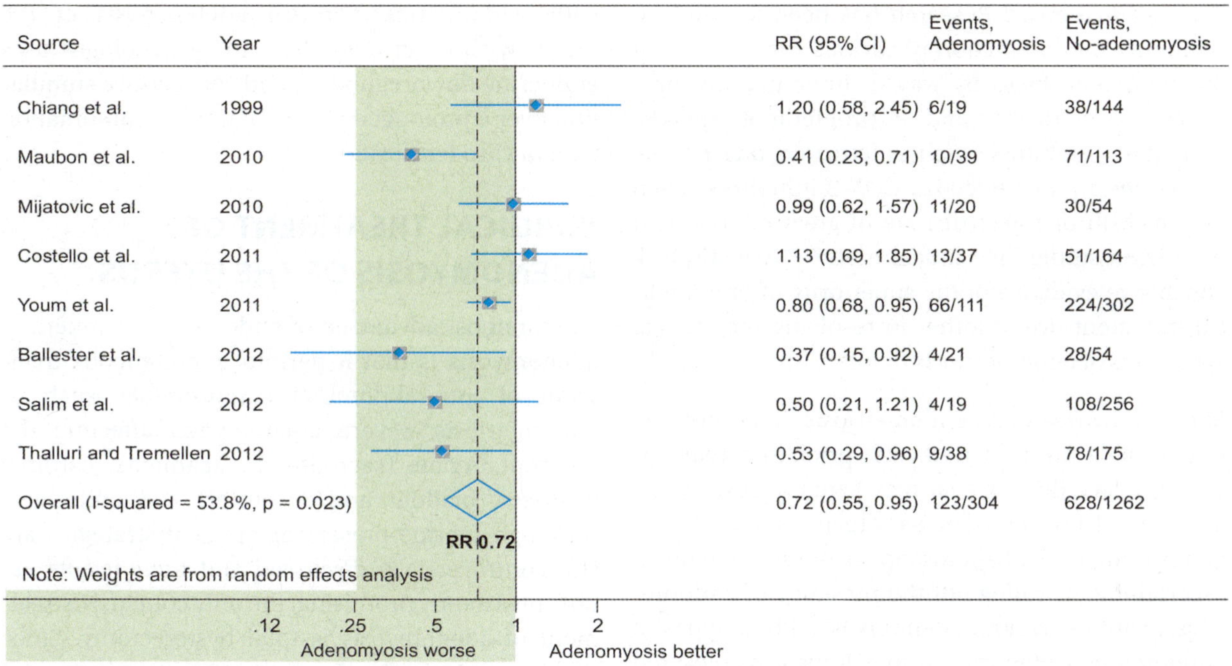

Fig. 24.12: Forest plot showing individual and combined effect size estimates and 95% confidence intervals (CIs) in studies addressing the likelihood of clinical pregnancy in infertile women with or without adenomyosis undergoing IVF/ICSI. Horizontal lines indicate 95% CIs, boxes show the study-specific weight, the diamond represents the combined effect size, and the dashed line indicates the overall estimate.
(*Source:* Adapted from Vercellini P, Consonni D, Dridi D, et al. Uterine adenomyosis and in vitro fertilization outcome: a systematic review and meta-analysis. Hum Reprod. 2014;29(5):964-77)

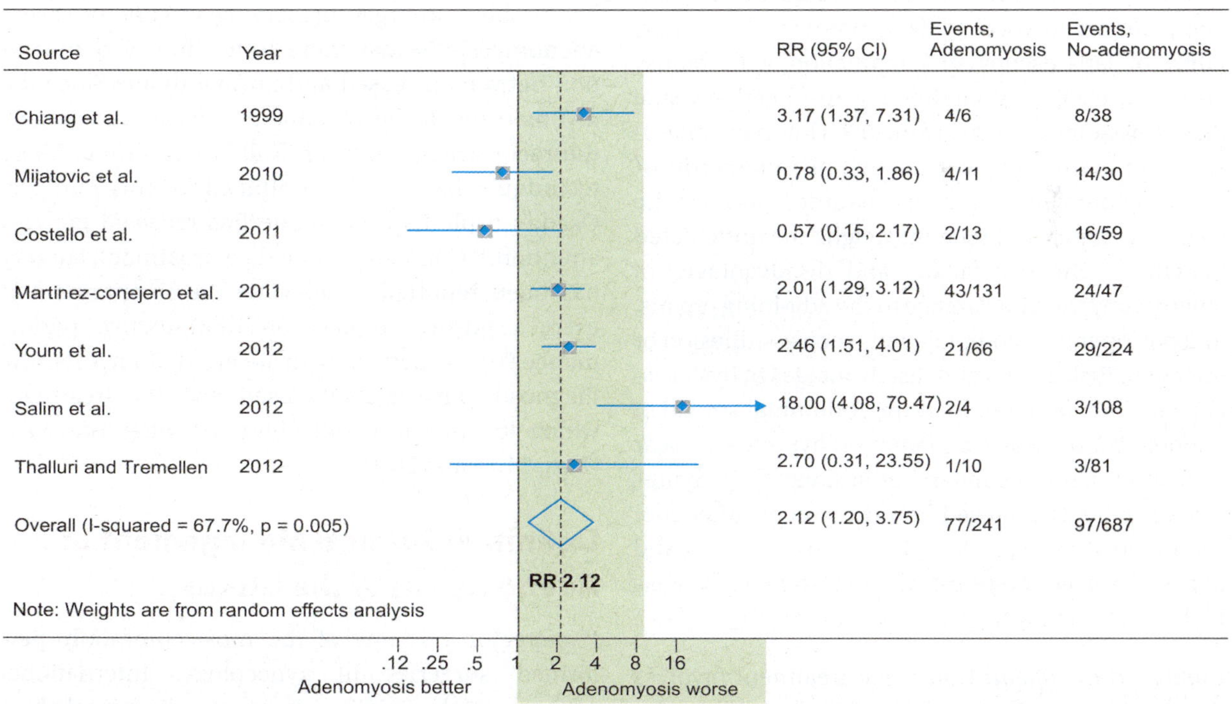

Fig. 24.13: Forest plot showing individual and combined effect size estimates and 95% confidence intervals (CIs) in studies addressing the risk of miscarriage in clinical pregnancies achieved after IVF/ICSI in women with or without adenomyosis. Horizontal lines indicate 95% CIs, boxes show the study-specific weight, the diamond represents the combined effect size and the dashed line indicates the overall estimate.
(*Source*: Adapted from Vercellini P, Consonni D, Dridi D, et al. Uterine adenomyosis and in vitro fertilization outcome: a systematic review and meta-analysis. Hum Reprod. 2014;29(5):964-77)

Targeted treatment: Research has been focused on inhibiting the interaction of various mediators that maintain the illness by way of inflammatory processes, vascularization and cell proliferation. Specific aromatase inhibitors (such as letrozole, anastrozole or exemestane) or selective COX-2 inhibitors (such as celecoxib or rofecoxib) are of great interest and have been studied in clinical trials.[22-24] We still lack conclusive evidence of the superiority of one medical treatment over another in resolving the clinical symptoms of endometriosis or infertility.

Surgical treatment: As endometriosis, often not distinguishable from adenomyosis prior to surgery, is a progressive disease that may actually destroy the anatomy of the reproductive organs, surgery plays an important role. Laparoscopy is the sole means of ascertaining or ruling out the presence of endometriosis with or without adenomyosis. Phenotypes of endometriosis may vary: it may appear as elevated flame-like patches, whitish opacifications, yellowish-brown discolorations, translucent blebs or reddish irregularly shaped spots.[2,25] In advanced stages, pain and sterility are predominantly caused by organ damage, fibrosis and adhesions, thus constituting a clear indication for surgical intervention. Early laparoscopy may help in timely detection of the disease and delay the progression of its symptoms. The importance of laparoscopy in conjunction with biopsy and/or resection is underlined by the fact that visual diagnosis alone may be erroneous. However, laparoscopic or hysteroscopic extraction of endometrium/myometrium chips has been discarded because the traumatic injury of tissue outweighs the anticipated benefit.[26,27] The risk factors and disadvantages of laparoscopy include damage to the adjoining organs, and postoperative complications such as adhesion or infection. Risk factors and disadvantages of hysteroscopy include perforation, intra-abdominal spread of endometrium tissue (implantation hypothesis), scar formation, and secondary adhesions.[16,28-31] Symptomatic relief is achieved in most patients after successful ablation/resection of the endometriosis and adhesiolysis. Nevertheless, the recurrence rate is as high as 40% after a 10-year follow-up.[30,32-34]

Combined treatment: Combined treatment involves diagnostic laparoscopy, removal of all visible endometriosis foci as far as possible, 3–6 months of endocrine therapy and a subsequent second-look laparoscopy with resection of residual foci, adhesiolysis and reconstruction of organs. When women with endometriosis and/or adenomyosis of the uterus wish to have children, the gynecologist uses endocrine downregulation and consecutive stimulation over a prolonged period of time in combination with in vitro fertilization.[33-38]

SURGICAL TREATMENT OF ADENOMYOSIS OF THE UTERUS

The foremost advantage of endoscopic treatment of adenomyosis is that it permits simultaneous treatment of intra-abdominal comorbidities such as endometriosis, severe adenomyosis affecting the adjacent organs (sacrouterine ligaments, cardinal ligament, bladder and/or bowel) and adhesions. Although uterine-preserving surgical strategies are still controversially discussed and their results are not consistently promising, the only conclusive treatment of adenomyosis is total hysterectomy. Since the disease is confined to the uterus, the ovaries can be preserved.

Organ-Preserving Surgical Management of Adenomyosis of the Uterus

The problem in organ-preserving surgery for severe adenomyosis is that there is no line of demarcation between diseased and normal tissue. Since the myometrium to be readapted is weak and fragile, the reconstructed uterine wall is not strong. Many techniques have been introduced for this purpose; Osada's triple-flap technique has received greatest attention.[39] Compared to medical treatment, surgery has been reported to alleviate the symptoms and exert a positive impact on reproductive performance.[40] In a patient with focal adenomyosis, the diagnostic investigations used and the treatment which led to successful childbirth after one year (Figs. 24.14 and 24.15).

Definitive Surgical Management of Adenomyosis of the Uterus

Hysterectomy is one of the most commonly performed surgeries in gynecology. International gynecological societies recommend vaginal hysterectomy as the most acceptable technique. However, operative endoscopic methods have gained importance over the last two decades and are now given preference over the traditional approaches

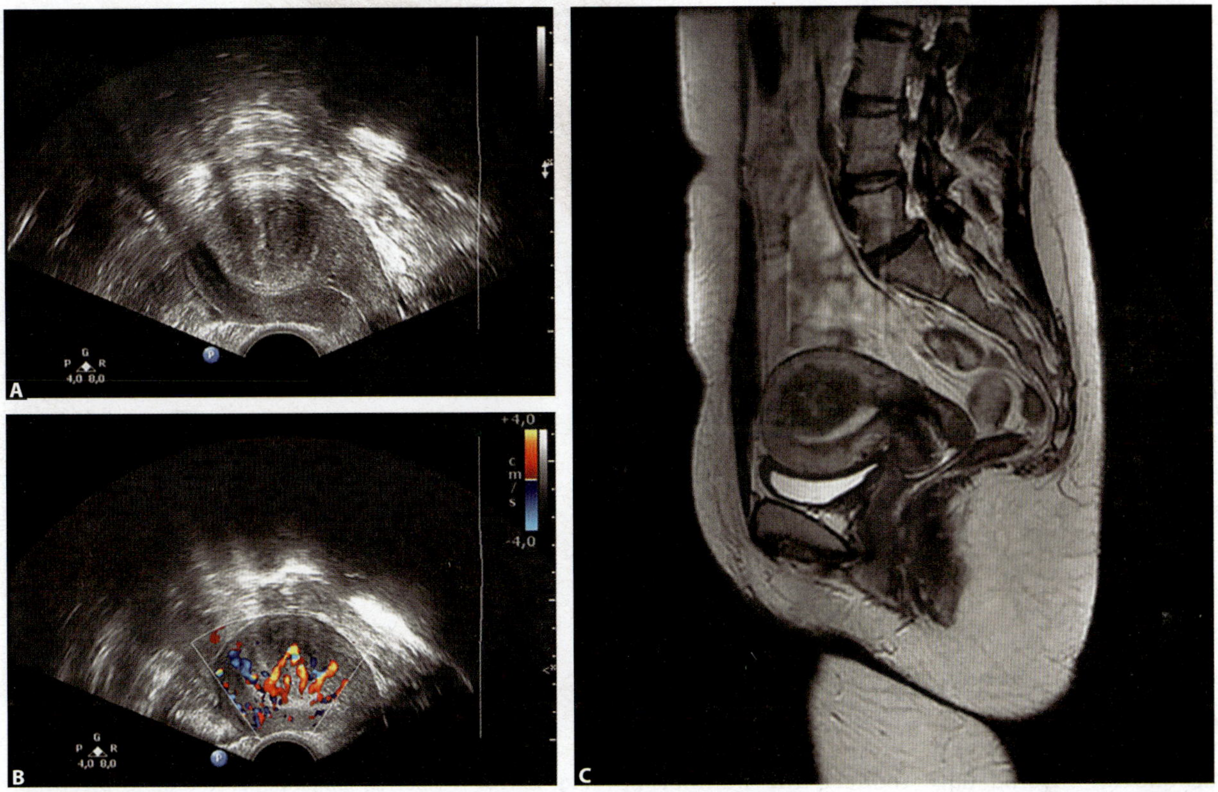

Figs. 24.14A to C: (A and B) Vaginal ultrasound and; (C) MRI scan showing focal adenomyosis of the uterus, located in the back wall; Doppler scan showing diffuse vascularization.

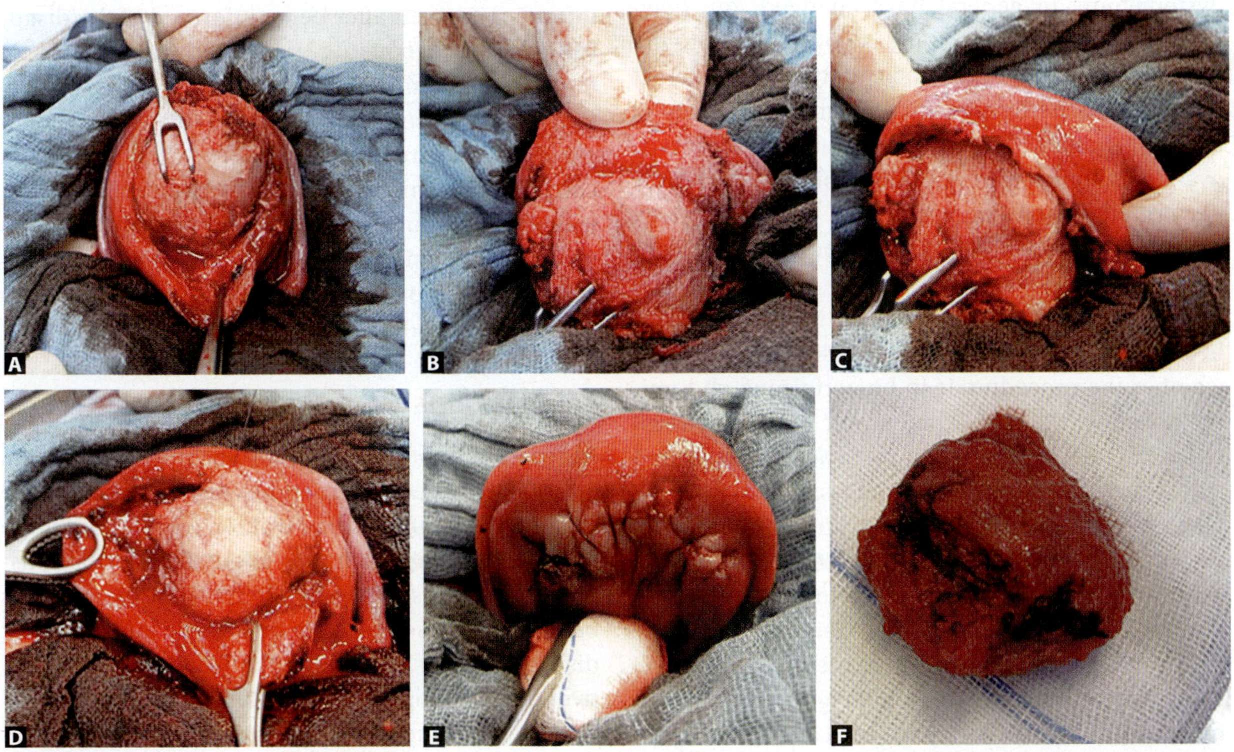

Figs. 24.15A to F: Intraoperative setting of organ preserving (A to D) enucleation of focal adenomyosis; (E) The uterus has been reconstructed in multiple layers; (F) The specimen is stony and porous.

of abdominal and vaginal hysterectomy. Among hysterectomies performed for benign disease, the number of abdominal hysterectomies is decreasing. The frequency of vaginal hysterectomies varies, but laparoscopic and robot-assisted laparoscopic procedures are on the increase.[41] This trend is observable throughout the world.[42] The problem in vaginal hysterectomy, but less so in abdominal hysterectomy, is that it is impossible to remove all lesions. Endoscopic techniques, including conventional laparoscopic and robotic-assisted ones, permit more extensive and exact resection of the lesions.

Currently the most frequent indications for hysterectomy are uterine leiomyomas, adenomyosis, diffuse endometriosis, uterine prolapse and therapy-resistant idiopathic bleeding. These constitute up to 60% and more of the indications for hysterectomy.[43] Alternative therapeutic strategies, such as uterine artery embolization or focused ultrasound scan, have been developed in Germany[44] and other countries[45] over the last 10 years. Conservative surgical management and the introduction of ulipristal acetate for myoma have reduced the number of hysterectomies. Hysterectomy rates depend not only on the indication but also the age group, family planning, and the centers at which the patients are treated. The indication and performance of hysterectomy in general have changed; the decision to perform hysterectomy is now adapted to the patients' desire to retain their uterus.[46,47] Hysterectomy is also performed for malignant diseases of the inner genital organs (endometrium or cervix, ovary or fallopian tubes). Endoscopic surgery is only performed for endometrium and cervical cancer. Box 24.2 provides a summary of the indications for hysterectomy.

Once the decision in favor of hysterectomy has been made, the physician and patient must decide whether the procedure is to be performed abdominally, vaginally or with laparoscopic or robotic assistance.[5,31,48] Each of these approaches is associated with advantages and disadvantages, which must be taken into account when counseling the individual patient (Fig. 24.16). The surgeon's familiarity with the surgical technique and the economic resources of the hospital are also important considerations.[49]

In many cases, conservative medical or conservative surgical treatment would signify undertreatment of the patient's condition and call for additional surgery later on.[40] Subtotal hysterectomy, the least invasive hysterectomy approach, is a compromise that meets the requirements of patients, society and doctors. However, the patient must provide her informed consent after being informed of the disadvantages of the remaining cervix. Only a laparoscopic total hysterectomy (LTH) provides complete protection from renewed fibroids, avoids subsequent cervical cancer or sarcoma, cell spilling when cutting the corpus and during morcellation, uncontrolled menstrual bleeding and other problems arising from the uterus. The persistence or recurrence of adenomyosis-related symptoms after subtotal hysterectomy is still controversially discussed.

Box 24.2: Indications for performing hysterectomy.

- Uterine leiomyomas
- Endometriosis and adenomyosis of the uterus
- Pelvic organ prolapse
- *Pelvic pain or infection (other than endometriosis):* Pelvic inflammatory disease, adhesions
- Abnormal uterine bleeding of known and unknown origin
- Malignant and premalignant diseases

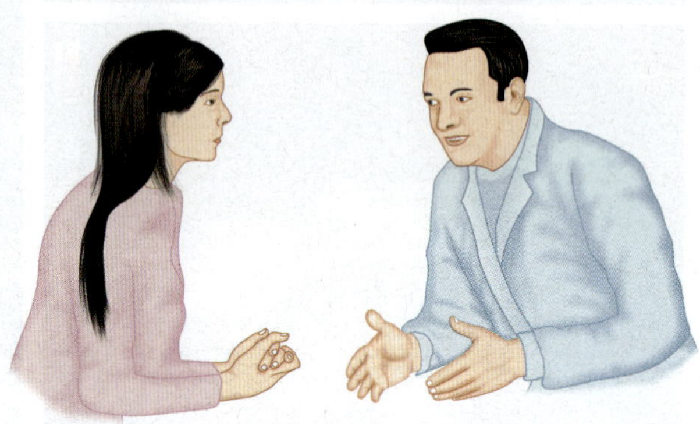

Fig. 24.16: A sincerely empathetic attitude in preoperative counseling includes the elements of congruence and esteem.

Total Versus Subtotal (Supracervical)

Independent of the surgical technique (subtotal or total hysterectomy), endoscopic surgery is the approach of choice. Some women wish to retain the cervix, believing that it may affect their sexual satisfaction after hysterectomy. Removal of the cervix is believed to cause excessive neurologic and anatomic disruption, thus increasing the likelihood of operative and postoperative morbidity, vaginal shortening, subsequent vault prolapse, abnormal cuff granulations and fallopian tube prolapse. These issues were addressed in a systematic review of three randomized trials on total versus subtotal hysterectomy for benign gynecological conditions.[50]

- No difference was observed in rates of incontinence, constipation or measures of sexual function (sexual satisfaction, dyspareunia).
- The duration of surgery and the quantity of blood loss during surgery were significantly less during subtotal hysterectomy than total hysterectomy, but there was no difference in the need for transfusion.
- Febrile morbidity was less likely and ongoing cyclical vaginal bleeding one year after surgery more likely after subtotal hysterectomy.
- The rates of other complications, recovery from surgery or readmission rates did not differ.

In the short term, randomized trials have shown that preservation or removal of the cervix does not affect the rate of subsequent pelvic organ prolapse.

The anatomical and therefore functional advantage of preserving the cervix is that the cardinal and uterosacral ligaments remain in place.

The advantages of supracervical hysterectomy include shorter operating times compared to total abdominal hysterectomy, and a shorter length of hospital stay when the procedure is performed by the laparoscopic approach. Furthermore, women who undergo subtotal hysterectomy are able to withstand physical loads earlier because there is no risk of vaginal cuff dehiscence.[51] Some authors have reported a shorter recovery period following subtotal hysterectomy, but randomized trials do not support this statement. In a prospective cohort study, supracervical hysterectomy was associated with greater improvement in short-term quality of life scores than total hysterectomy, but no difference was registered in regard of postoperative pain or return to activities of daily living.[52] There may also be fewer injuries to the urinary tract because dissection is not performed as close to the cervix or as deep into the pelvis as in total hysterectomy. However, clinical trials designed to demonstrate this clinical observation have not been performed yet.

Other differences include posthysterectomy body image and health status. Women who had undergone subtotal versus total hysterectomy reported a significantly better body image and health-related quality of life. Both groups experienced greater sexual satisfaction.[53]

The only absolute contraindication for subtotal hysterectomy is a malignant or premalignant condition of the uterine corpus or cervix.

Extensive endometriosis is a relative contraindication because the patient may experience persistent dyspareunia when the cervix is retained. The significance of adenomyosis has been underestimated so far. The uterus is morcellated in the abdomen. If the morcellated uterus is not collected in a bag, adenomyosis may spread into the abdominal cavity (theory three, see above). Besides, the patient may experience persistent pain in the central segment of the lower abdomen. In laparoscopic supracervical hysterectomy (LSH), the involvement of the cervix or the retrocervical/precervical space is ignored. Very often the sacrouterine ligaments or the lateral cardinal ligaments leading to the ovarian fossa are also affected. In these cases, either the adenomyosis has grown through the uterine wall into the adjacent organs or there is concomitant endometriosis. To rule out all causes of symptoms, it would be advisable to remove all visible endometriosis-associated pathologies. LTH, if performed correctly, is associated with very few additional risks or side effects. Therefore, in cases of adenomyosis of the uterus we explain the situation to the patient in detail and advise LTH [personal statement]. Arguments in favor of LTH include fewer cases of urinary incontinence, less prolapse and cervical stump problems. However, subtotal hysterectomy is performed faster in most cases and seems to be associated with fewer intraoperative and postoperative complications. We lack convincing data concerning the advantages of simultaneous removal of the cervix; the cervix is very rarely involved in the disease.[54-56]

Elective supracervical hysterectomy should be preceded by cervical cytology to confirm the absence of cervical intraepithelial neoplasia (PAP smear). Women who have had a supracervical hysterectomy should be screened for cervical cancer according to standard guidelines for their age and risk status. In women with abnormal uterine bleeding (especially metrorrhagia), endometrial cancer or any sort of sarcoma should be excluded prior to performing a supracervical hysterectomy.

Sometimes the cervix needs to be removed later as a separate procedure. This approach is associated with frequent damage to the bowel and the bladder because the anatomical spaces cannot be exposed clearly and adhesions are common. However, the approach is readily accepted because primary surgery is associated with fewer risks than subsequent procedures. Patients who wish to minimize the likelihood of subsequent surgery may prefer an LTH.[57]

Total laparoscopic hysterectomy involves removal of the uterus and the cervix. The entire procedure is performed laparoscopically. The specimen can usually be removed through the vaginal vault. Laparoscopic-assisted vaginal hysterectomy (LAVH) has been entirely replaced by the endoscopic technique, which has become a standard procedure since the learning curve for laparoscopic suturing is now favorable. Taking into account the advantages of endoscopic surgery (shorter hospital stay, faster recovery, better cosmetic result and fewer infections), the question arises as to whether the risk of posthysterectomy prolapse during LSH can be reduced by preserving the existing structures of the pelvic floor in the middle compartment or reconstructing them. In cases of preexisting defects, LTH provides sufficient fixation of the pelvic floor and thus minimizes the risk of a posthysterectomy prolapse. Mesh implants such as those used for sacrocolpopexy may be employed in both procedures simultaneously.

Our multimodality concept of laparoscopic intrafascial hysterectomy for the treatment of adenomyosis is aimed at total removal of all visible endometriotic spots and reducing the risk of posthysterectomy prolapse:

- Removal of all endometriosis spots and demarcating the extent of adenomyosis
- Intrafascial hysterectomy with preservation of existing ligaments, yet opening the medial compartment when performing total laparoscopic hysterectomy
- A technique of stable fixation of the vaginal stump

Development of Laparoscopic Hysterectomy Techniques and Instruments

The popularity of laparoscopic hysterectomy rose gradually after Harry Reich's initial publication of the procedure.[58,59] A number of approaches evolved, such as LAVH, LSH, total laparoscopic hysterectomy and LTH. LTH had a steep learning curve and was initially associated with rather high complication rates.[45] The development of new instruments and consistent training improved the situation. The introduction of the intrauterine manipulator helped to develop the classic intrafascial concept, which today is the aim of every gynecological surgeon performing total laparoscopic hysterectomy. Hohl used Kurt Semm's procedure of classic intrafascial supracervical hysterectomy (CISH)[60] and developed it further with the use of his manipulator.[61] The majority of the available manipulators are well accepted because they are easy to handle, reusable and durable. The uterus can be moved in all directions while the elliptical long tip of the manipulator eases out vaginal and paravaginal tissue intra-abdominally. The manipulator can be pushed straight toward the field of operation field, especially when cutting the uterus off the vagina with the monopolar hook and targeting the tip of the manipulator.

The large majority of manipulators are provided with a ceramic cap that creates a flat surface to work on. Consequently, there is very little or virtually no need for dissection of the bladder. It should be noted that the use of the manipulator for bladder dissection is useful and safe even after a cesarean section. The application of the manipulator imitates the classical movements during abdominal hysterectomy; the ureters are kept out of the field of operation. The cap allows intrafascial hysterectomy, which preserves the ligaments and avoids vaginal shortening. The smooth cutting edge is useful for vaginal occlusion.

Points to be considered:

- Monopolar electricity can be used on the ceramic cap. Bipolar current causes a larger defect, bearing the risk of subsequent wound healing problems and vaginal cuff dehiscence. The fact that ultrasound is liable to destroy this apparatus must be taken into account when using ultrasound for dissection during hysterectomy.
- Intrafascial hysterectomy involves a much smaller opening to the vagina and preserves the circular ligaments. Large uteruses may need to be morcellated. Extended endometriosis or adenomyosis may involve the circular ligaments, which then have to be removed.[61]

The other instruments may be of the disposable or reusable type. Disposable tissue sealing instruments are faster and dispense with the need to replace the instrument frequently. However, the instruments are costly and fusion of the layers of tissue results in a less clear overview of the anatomical structures. Bipolar forceps are essential. Extracorporeal sutures (PDS 1.0) are helpful, although intracorporeal sutures (Vicryl) are sufficient for vaginal closure. The monopolar hook facilitates the removal of endometriotic spots and the uterus from the manipulator, but can be replaced by bipolar forceps and scissors. In cases of a large uterus, the tenaculum can be used to lift out the uterus; a morcellator avoids troublesome comminution of the uterus.

Preoperative Considerations and Preparation

When severe endometriosis (Figs. 24.17A to D) is suspected on vaginal examination (Figs. 24.18A and B) and the ultrasound scan is correlated with the patient's medical history, it will be necessary to perform furtherdiagnostic investigations such as MRI, cystoscopy, rectoscopy or endosonography (Figs. 24.19 and 24.20). Radical interdisciplinary surgery can then be planned and performed (Figs. 24.21 to 24.23).

A hysterectomy must always be accompanied by antibiotic protection, such as a second-generation cephalosporin. In cases of suspected bowel involvement, a single shot of metronidazole is also essential. The antibiotic should be applied about 30 min before the start of the operation.

The instruments consist of trocars, a uterine manipulator (for LTH only), needle holders and sutures. Additionally, one needs an instrument for coagulation, graspers, scissors, window forceps and a suction irrigation unit. If a robotic setup is available, the instruments must be adjusted accordingly. A thermofusion device with an integrated knife is optional.

Prerequisites

Obesity or comorbidities, a large uterus or a uterus with multiple myomas is no contraindication for a laparoscopic procedure. However, in these cases the preoperative assessment and the anesthesia procedure must be discussed with the patient in advance. The trocars may need to be placed higher in the abdominal wall and the surgeon may need more than the usual two ancillary trocars. In cases of a large uterus, the need for morcellation and its risks must be explained to the patient.

INTRAFASCIAL HYSTERECTOMY WITH PRESERVATION OF EXISTING STRUCTURES

Operative Steps of Total Laparoscopic Hysterectomy

Step 1: A vaginal examination in anesthesia is performed before using the manipulator. When no

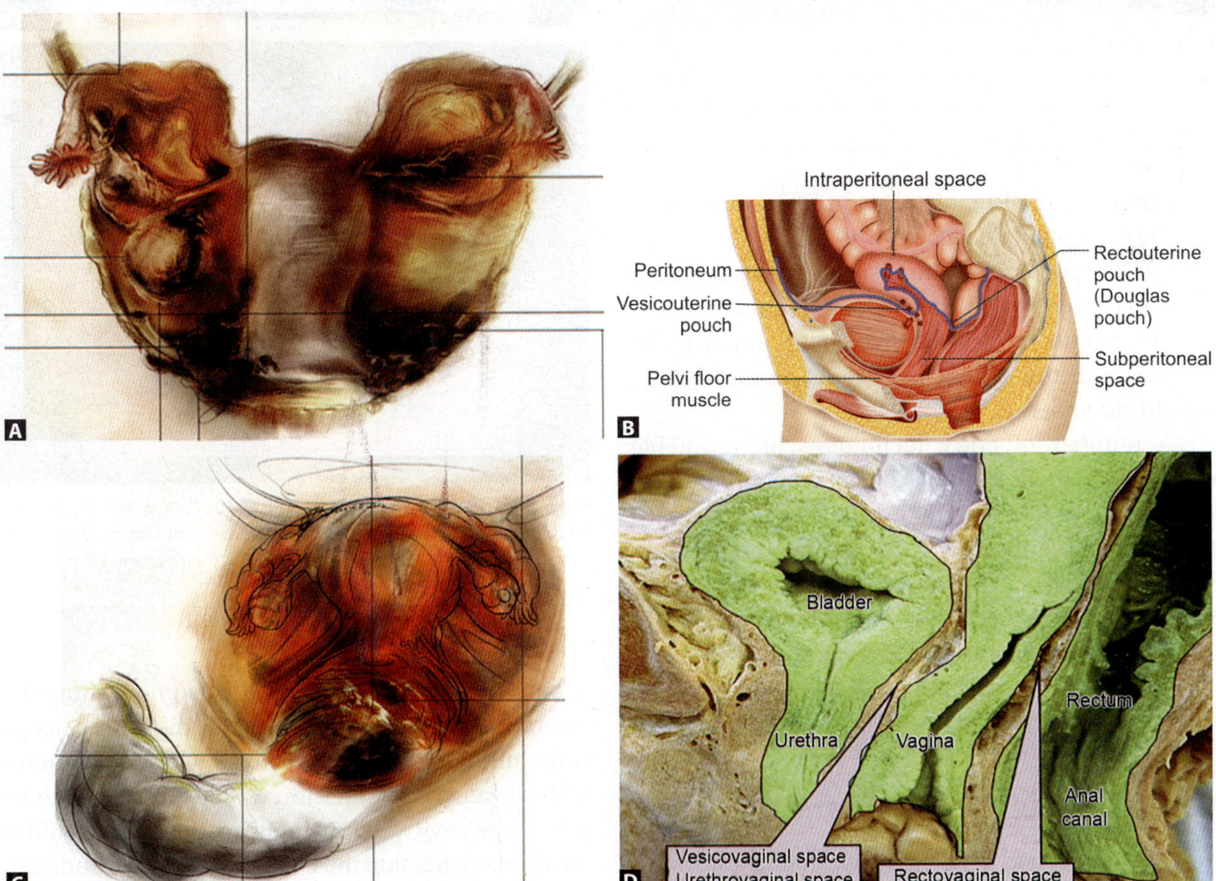

Figs. 24.17A to D: (A) Severe endometriosis and correlation with anatomical landmarks (B to D).

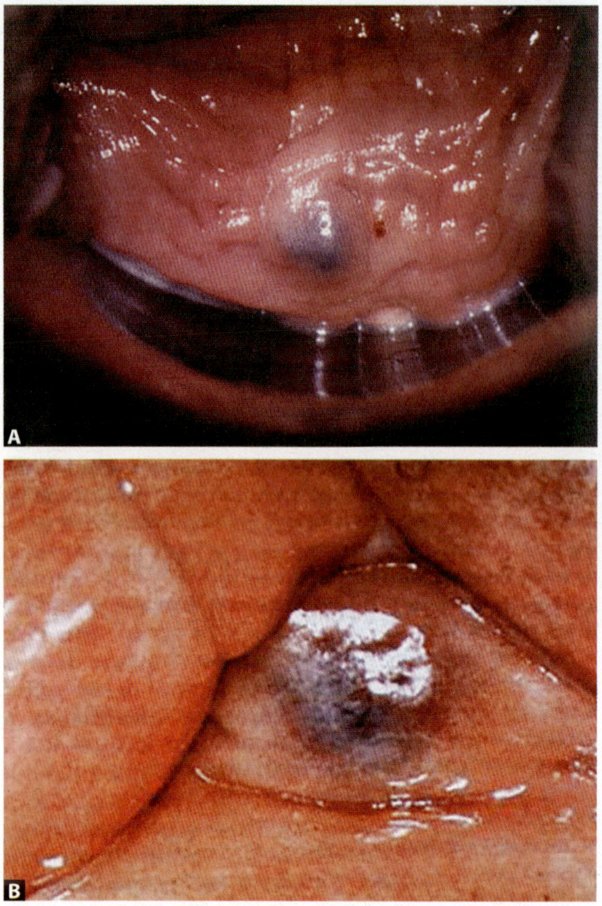

Figs. 24.18A and B: Vaginal photograph of a small endometriotic nodule in the dorsal vaginal wall and another patient with vaginal involvement of severe deep infiltrating endometriosis.

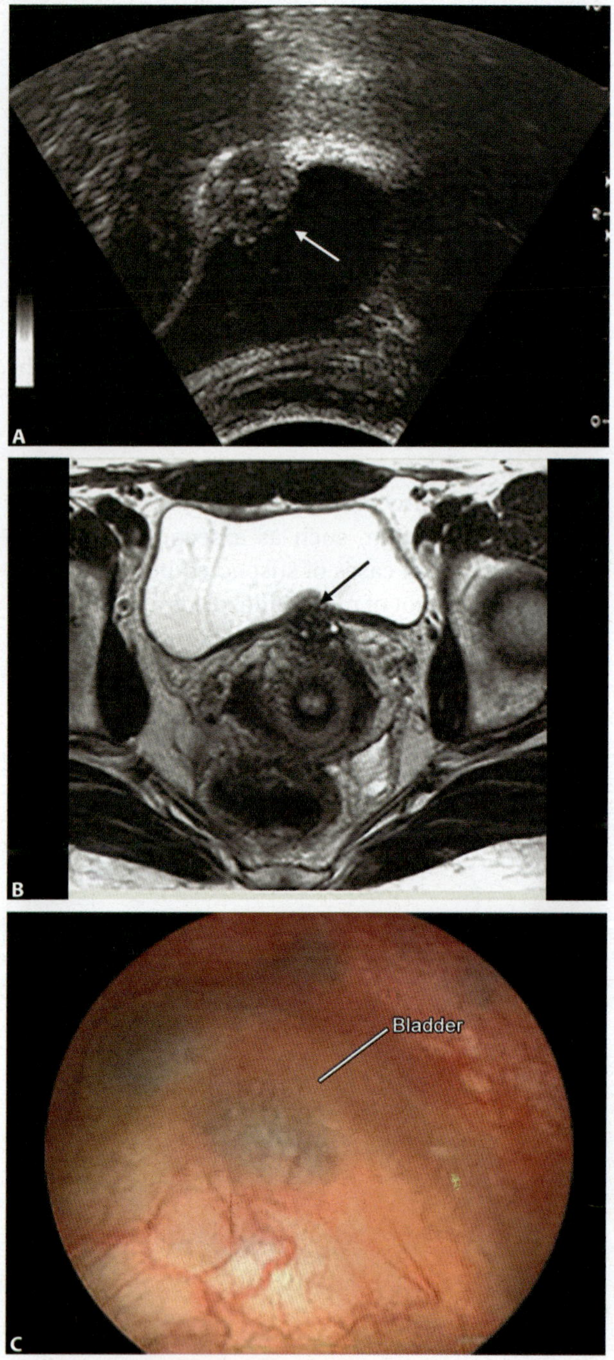

Figs. 24.19A to C: (A) Vaginal ultrasound of a solitary nodule between the anterior wall of the uterus and the bladder (vesicovaginal space); (B) MRI scan and; (C) Cystoscopy of the same patient.

further vaginal or rectal pathologies are found, the manipulator is inserted.

Step 2: *Port placement*: The first step of the operation is placement of the uterine manipulator.[62]

The points of trocar placement are selected according to the size of the uterus along with the fibroid elements.

A number of entry techniques are available; direct entry under sight has become very popular in the last few years. Nevertheless, the traditional entry technique described by Kurt Semm and Liselotte Mettler from the University Hospitals Schleswig-Holstein, Kiel, in the 1980s, and still used at the Kiel School of Gynecological Endoscopy is shown here.

Optical Trocar

Veress Needle Technique and CO_2 Gas

To insert the Veress needle, the operating table needs to be in horizontal position. The Trendelenburg tilt is carried out after creating a pneumoperitoneum. The most common site of entry for the Veress needle is the umbilical area. As the wall layers are thinnest at this level, a deep incision will ensure access to the peritoneal cavity. Before incising the skin it would be advisable to palpate the course of the aorta and identify the iliac bifurcation. This will permit inspection

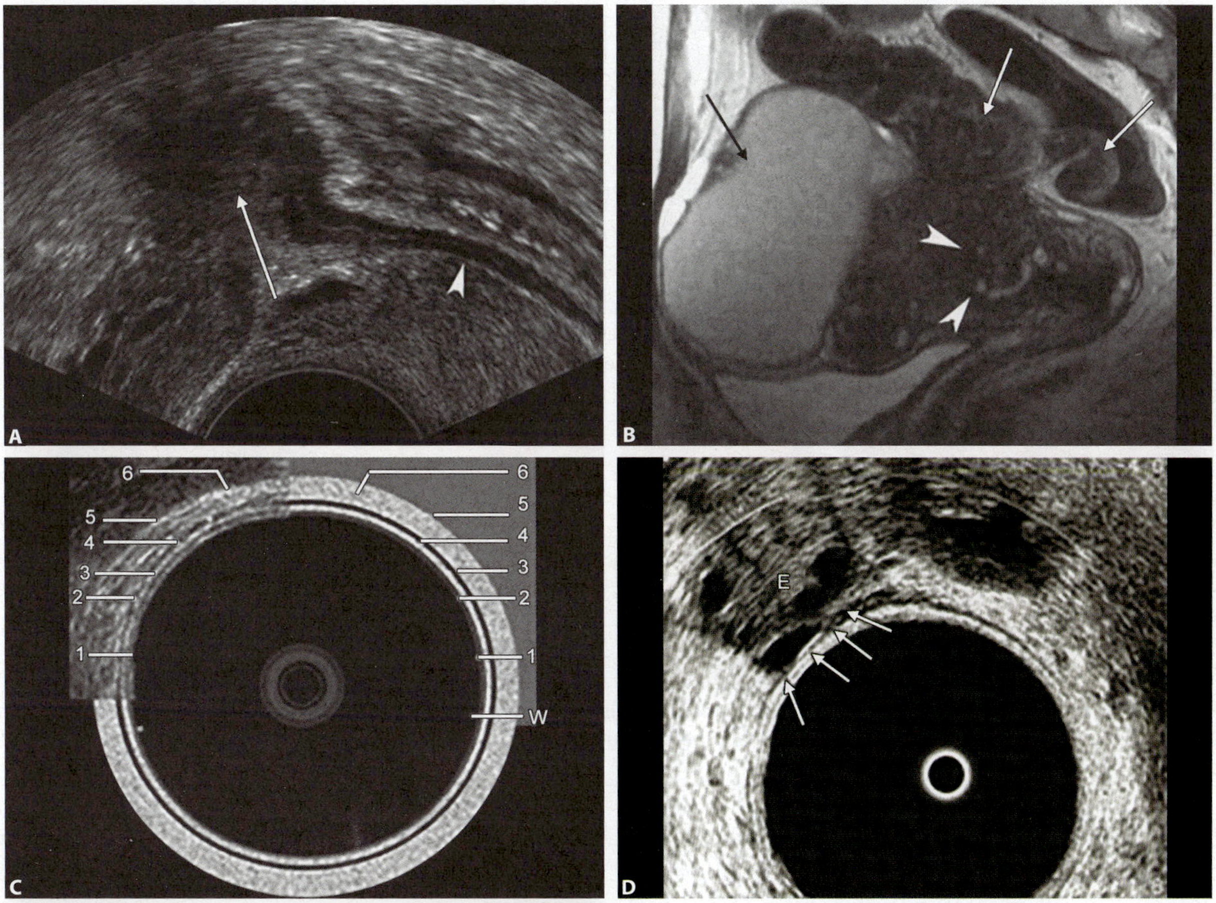

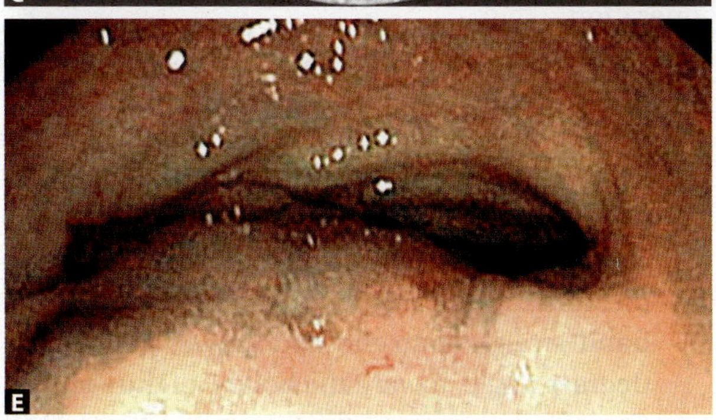

Figs. 24.20A to E: (A) Vaginal ultrasound of a solitary nodule between the lower back wall of the uterus/cervix and the rectum (rectovaginal space); (B) MRI scan; (C and D) Endosonography and; (E) Rectoscopy.

and palpation of the abdomen in order to detect any unusual masses (Figs. 24.24 to 24.26).[63]

The Veress needle must be tested to ensure that the valve springs, and that gas flow is between 6 and 8 mm Hg. In this position the insertion of the primary instrument at a 45° angle toward the uterus involves the least risk of damaging the major vessels coursing downward retroperitoneally. The abdominal wall should be lifted before inserting the instrument. In obese patients the insertion angle is close to 90 degrees, whereas in slim patients the angle is close to 45 degrees. If the first attempt fails, a second attempt is made before selecting an alternative entry site. Before placing the Veress needle, a number of safety checks should be performed in order to minimize the risk of complications:

Usually *two clicks* are heard: the first after perforation of the muscle fascia and the second after perforation of the peritoneum. Proper needle placement is ensured by keeping the Veress needle between the thumb and the index finger.

Aspiration test: Injection of 5–10 mL of normal saline solution results in negative aspiration when the Veress needle is correctly placed and yields a blood-tinged aspirate, or one with intestinal contents when the needle is placed in a blood vessel or the intestine.

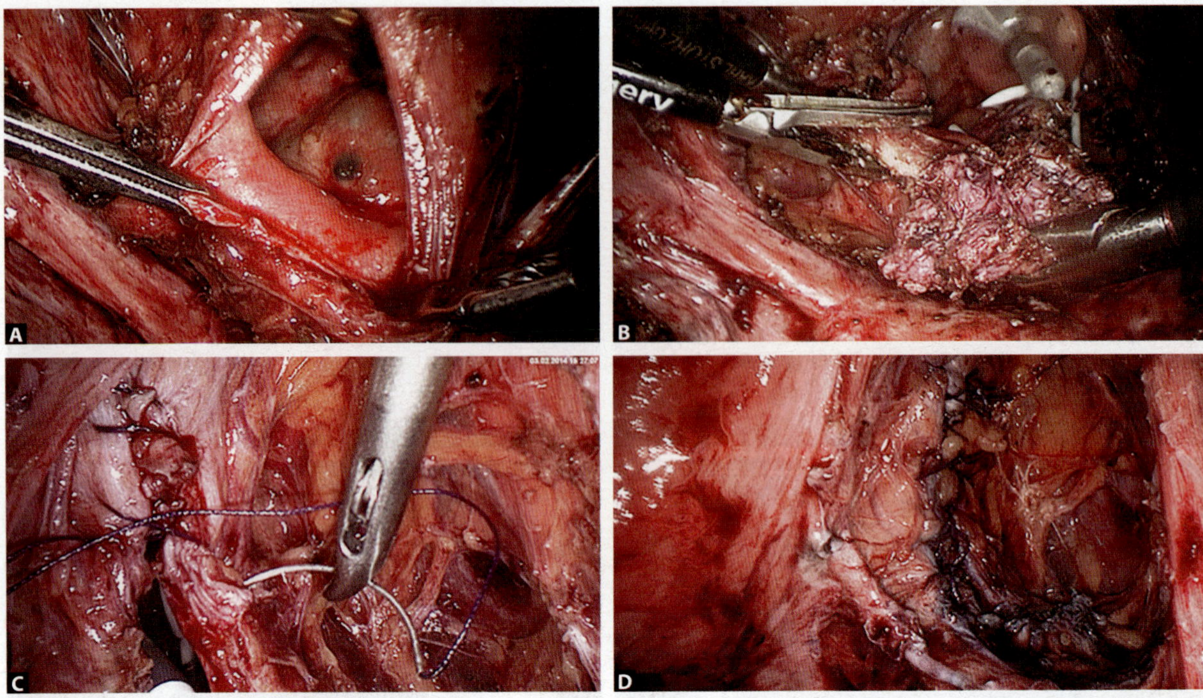

Figs. 24.21A to D: Resection of a solitary bladder endometriosis nodule. (A) The nodule is seen after opening the bladder. Two double J-catheters are placed in both ureters so that (B) the nodule can be cut out with an energy device; (C and D) Closure of the bladder in two layers.

Hanging drop test and fluid in flow: With the Veress needle placed in the abdominal cavity, lifting the abdominal wall creates negative intra-abdominal pressure. A drop of water is then placed on the open end of the Veress needle. If the needle is correctly positioned, the water will move down the shaft.

Any movement of the needle after placement must be avoided, as this may convert a small needlepoint injury into a complex and threatening tear. After ensuring that the Veress needle has been positioned correctly, the insufflation is started. Once adequate gas flow and pressure have been achieved the influx may be raised so that 2–3 L of CO_2 gas can be insufflated per minute until 3–6 L have been insufflated, depending on the patient's size and obesity. After an insufflation volume of about 300 mL, percussion of the liver region will confirm the *loss of liver dullness*, which is a reliable sign of proper positioning of the Veress needle and the creation of a pneumoperitoneum. Abdominal pressure should then be increased to 20–25 mm Hg before inserting the primary trocar because this maximizes distension of the abdominal wall from all underlying structures (Figs. 24.17A to C).[60]

The optic trocar is inserted in two steps. In the first step, a 5-mm optic trocar and the laparoscope are inserted to confirm the pneumoperitoneum and the absence of local adhesions. Dilation to 10 mm is achieved in the second step, either under sight or blindly, thus ensuring optimum visibility during the operation.

Step 1: Entry is performed by the *Z-technique* in the following manner: After proceeding forward horizontally with the trocar to about 1.5 cm, the tip is moved to about 1.5 cm to the right at a 90 degree angle. The abdominal wall is lifted in the same manner as when inserting the Veress needle, and the trocar is screwed with the dominant hand straight into the abdominal wall at a 90 degrees angle, toward the hollow of the sacrum. Correct placement of the trocar is indicated by a hissing sound when gas escapes through the open valve of the trocar. The obturator is then removed and the trocar held in place. Before dilating to 10 mm, a 5-mm laparoscope is introduced and rotated through 360 degrees to check visually for any bleeding, intra-abdominal abnormality, or adherent bowel loops. If the surgeon suspects adherence of the bowel in the umbilical region, the primary trocar site must be visualized from a secondary port site, such as the lower abdominal wall, with a 5-mm laparoscope.

Step 2: A blunt palpation probe is placed in the 5-mm trocar; the shaft is pulled over the palpation probe and taken out. A 10-mm trocar is then screwed into the abdominal cavity.[60]

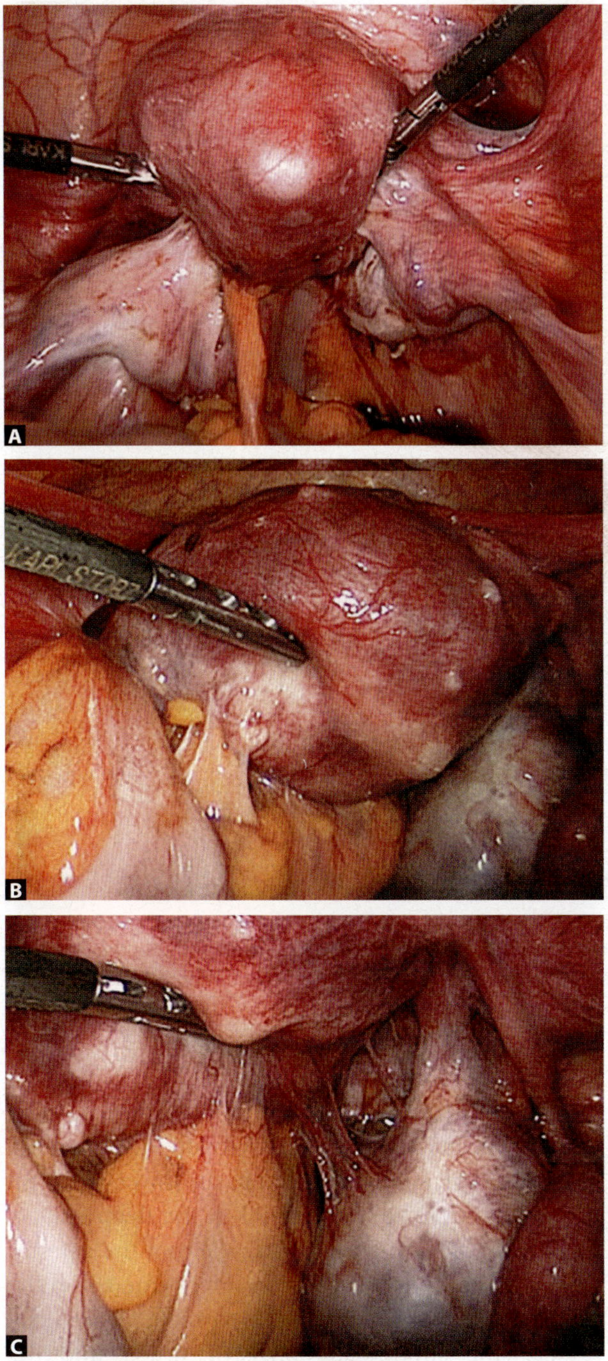

Figs. 24.22A to C: Severe deep infiltrating endometriosis associated with adenomyosis of the uterus, affecting the lower sigma/rectum.

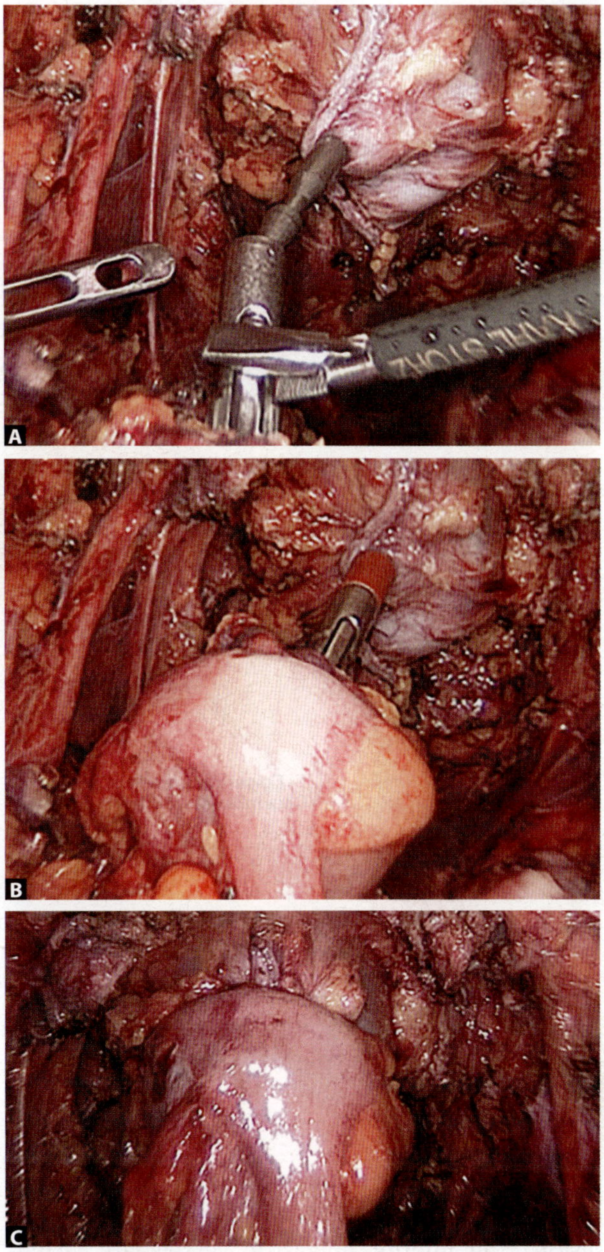

Figs. 24.23A to C: Endoscopic re-anastomosis can be achieved after partial bowel resection.

Subcostal Insufflation Technique (Palmer's Point or Lee Huang Point)

No entry technique is entirely devoid of the risk of gas embolism or injury to vessels, intestines or the urinary tract. Palmer's point is the safest laparoscopic entry point because it is least likely to be affected by adhesions.

For all patients with a significantly higher risk of adhesion, a history of abdominal surgery including cesarean section, a large fibroid uterus, umbilical hernia, large ovarian cysts, preperitoneal gas insufflation or failed umbilical entry, Palmer described in 1974 an abdominal entry point in the midclavicular line, about 3 cm below the costal margin. Palmer's point can be used for the Veress needle as well as for small trocars. In case adhesions are suspected in the subcostal region on the left side, the Lee Huang point in the midline is a suitable alternative (Fig. 24.26).[60]

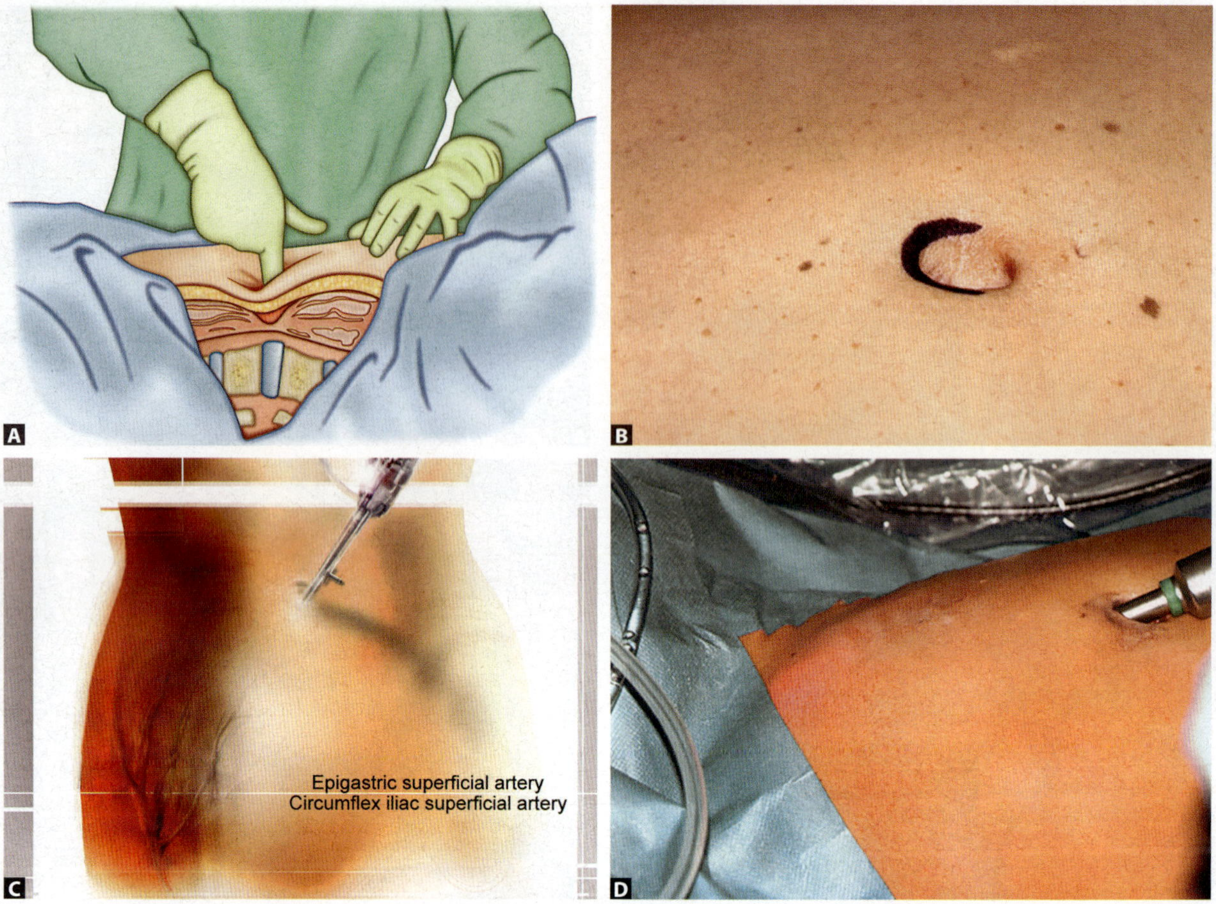

Figs. 24.24A to D: (A) Typical palpation point in the subumbilical region. The fingertip is pointing to the promontory. Subumbilical incision and local palpation demonstrate the short distance from the skin to the spine; (B to D) Diaphanoscopy shows the region of insertion of the ancillary trocars while demarcating the superficial epigastric artery and the superficial circumflex iliac artery.

Ancillary Trocars

All ancillary trocars must be inserted with an intra-abdominal pressure of 15-20 mm Hg under direct vision. The inferior epigastric vessels are visualized laparoscopically, whereas the superficial vessels can be visualized by diaphanoscopy (Figs. 24.28 and 24.29).

Once the tip of the trocar has pierced the peritoneum, it should be angulated in the direction of the uterine fundus under visual control until the port is placed correctly and the sharp tip can be removed.

Before inserting any ancillary trocars, the patient should be moved into the Trendelenburg position. Premature Trendelenburg positioning may increase the risk of retroperitoneal vascular injury because the iliac vessels are located exactly in the axis of a preconceived 45 degrees insertion angle, especially in slim patients with minimal retroperitoneal fat. The number of ancillary trocars is variable; all of them must be inserted under direct vision. If two working trocars are needed, they should be placed in the lower quadrant above the pubic hairline lateral to the deep epigastric vessels from the interior view. From the exterior view the trocars are placed two fingers medial to the anterior superior iliac spine. Two major superficial vessels—the superficial epigastric artery and the superficial circumflex iliac artery—must be avoided. These vessels can be visualized by diaphanoscopy. When a third ancillary trocar is required, the suprapubic midline is the most common site. Diaphanoscopy cannot be relied upon to locate the deep vessels, especially in obese patients (Figs. 24.24 and 24.25).

Finger-tapping from the outside can be used to verify correct positioning of the trocar. A small skin incision should be performed before the trocar sleeve is inserted. The trocars must be inserted by the shortest route at a 90 degrees angle to the skin surface so

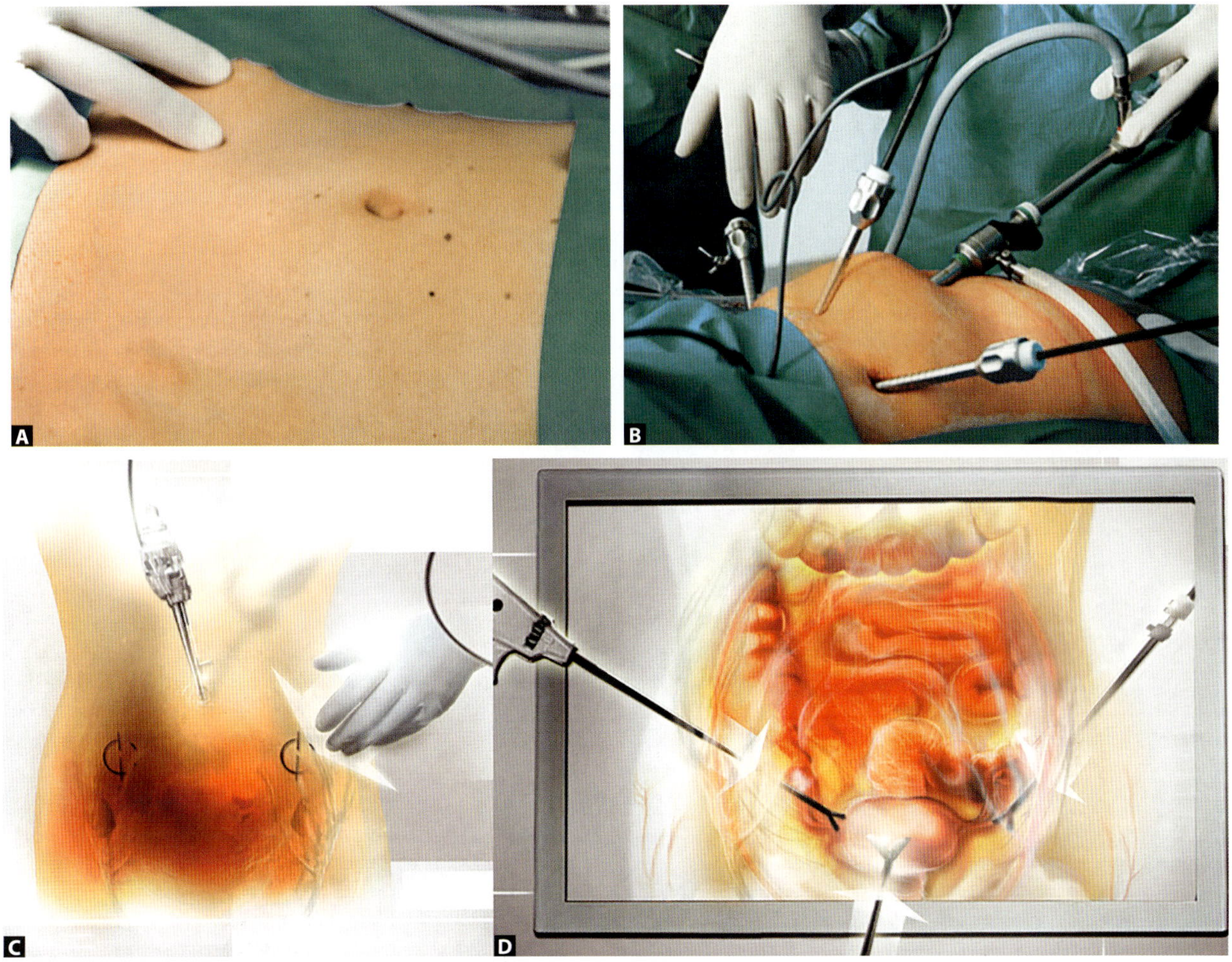

Figs. 24.25A to D: (A and C) Point of insertion from the outside (two thumbs medial of the anterior superior spine), at a 90 degrees angle to the surface with penetration of all layers of the abdominal wall. Trocar insertion site lateral to the lateral umbilical plica; (B and D) Overview after insertion of the laparoscope and three ancillary trocars.

that the risk of injuring structures on the way to the abdominal wall is minimized. When inserting a trocar in the midline, the Foley catheter must be identified in order to avoid accidental bladder perforation[60,64] (Figs. 24.27A to C).

Step 3: *Resection of Endometriosis:* The primary step in hysterectomy is removal of all visible endometriosis spots. These may be superficial and easy to excise (Figs. 24.29 to 24.32), or adherent to more delicate structures and difficult to eliminate (Figs. 24.33 and 24.34).

Laparoscopic Total Hysterectomy

In patients being operated on for surgical staging, the surgeon will be able to assess the abdomen, pelvis, obtain pelvic washings, perform salpingo-oophorectomy, lymph node dissection, tissue biopsies and omentectomy in addition to laparoscopic hysterectomy (Figs. 24.35A and B).

Classic Intrafascial Hysterectomy

Surgical Steps

3.1 Inspection of the pelvis, tracing the ureters and planning the operation (Figs. 24.29, 24.30, 24.36 to 24.38)

3.2 Start on the right side. Push the uterus in the opposite direction when separating the adnexa or the ligaments from the pelvic sidewall, with the assistance of the intrauterine manipulator or by traction (Figs. 24.39A to D).

3.3 Separation of the infundibulopelvic ligament and round ligament from the pelvic sidewall or, when the adnexa are retained, separation of the adnexa from the uterus (Figs. 24.40A to D).

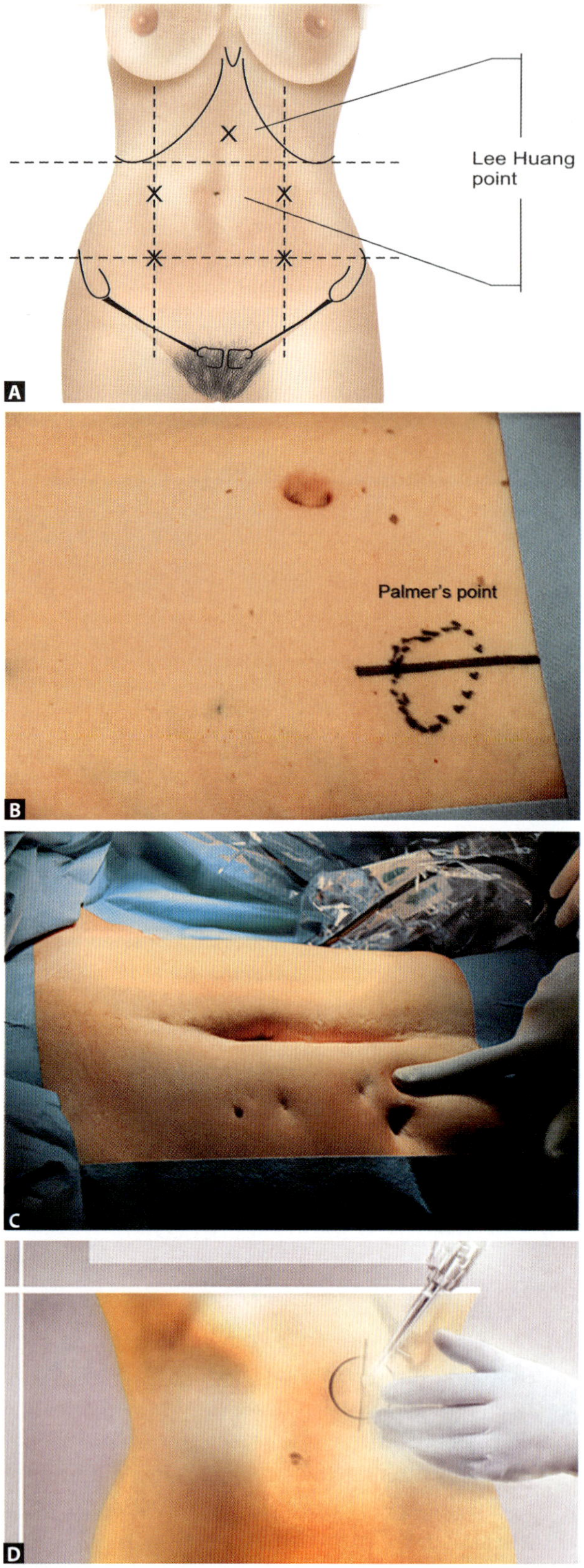

Figs. 24.26A to D: Alternative entry sites: (A) In cases of a large uterus, especially one extending to or beyond the umbilicus, the Lee–Huang point is recommended for video-assisted laparoscopy. In case adhesions are anticipated in the region of Palmer's point (C), (B to D) this point is used. Palmer's point is located in the midclavicular line, about 3 cm below the costal margin.

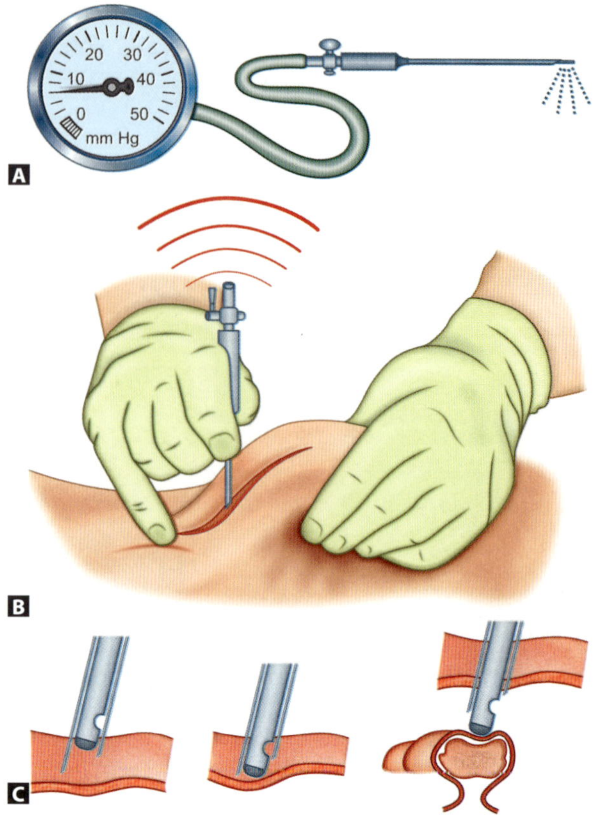

Figs. 24.27A to C: Veress needle and its insertion. The safety mechanism avoids damage or injury to the bowel or vessels.

3.4 *Dissection of the broad ligament:* The broad ligament is opened and each leaf coagulated separately (Figs. 24.41A to D). This is not possible when a sealing and cutting instrument is used, because the two leaves of the broad ligament are sealed together. The direction of exposure is as close to the uterus as possible but as distant as necessary, thus avoiding exposure close to the sidewall and the ureter (Fig. 24.36).

3.5 Separation of the bladder from the uterus by opening the vesicouterine ligament and pushing the bladder downward by about 1–2 cm (Fig. 24.41).

3.6 Presentation of the ascending branch of the uterine artery and separation of the uterine pedicles (Fig. 24.41).

3.7 Identical stepwise dissection of the left adnexa (Figs. 24.42 and 24.43), opening the bladder peritoneum and broad ligament (Figs. 24.44A to D), and dissection of the uterine vessels (Figs. 24.45 and 24.46) on the left side. A thorough inspection of the cervix is performed.

3.8 After separation of the bladder from the uterus, the bladder is pushed and dissected down by

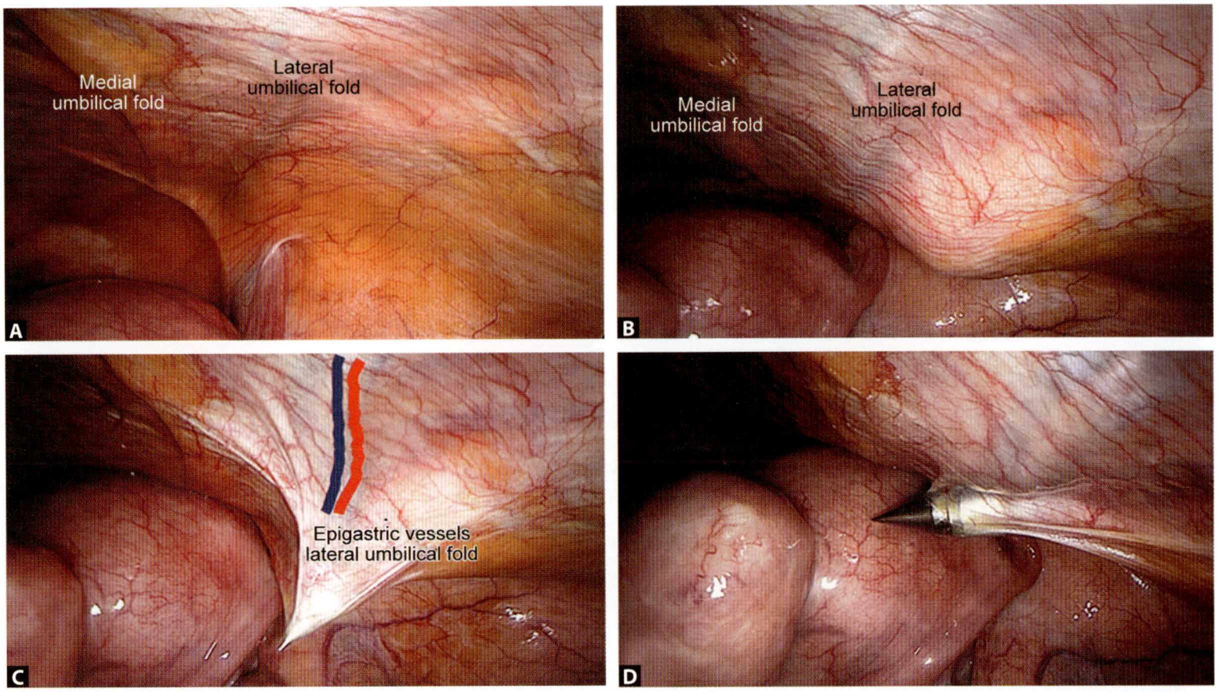

Figs. 24.28A to D: Secondary trocar placement, left lower abdominal entry. (A) The three different plicae are visualized; (B) The palpating finger indicates the area lateral to the lateral umbilical fold; (C) Entry of the sharp ancillary trocar lateral to the lateral umbilical fold; (D) Once the peritoneum has been penetrated, the trocar points towards the fundus of the uterus to avoid injury to the major vessels and the bowel.

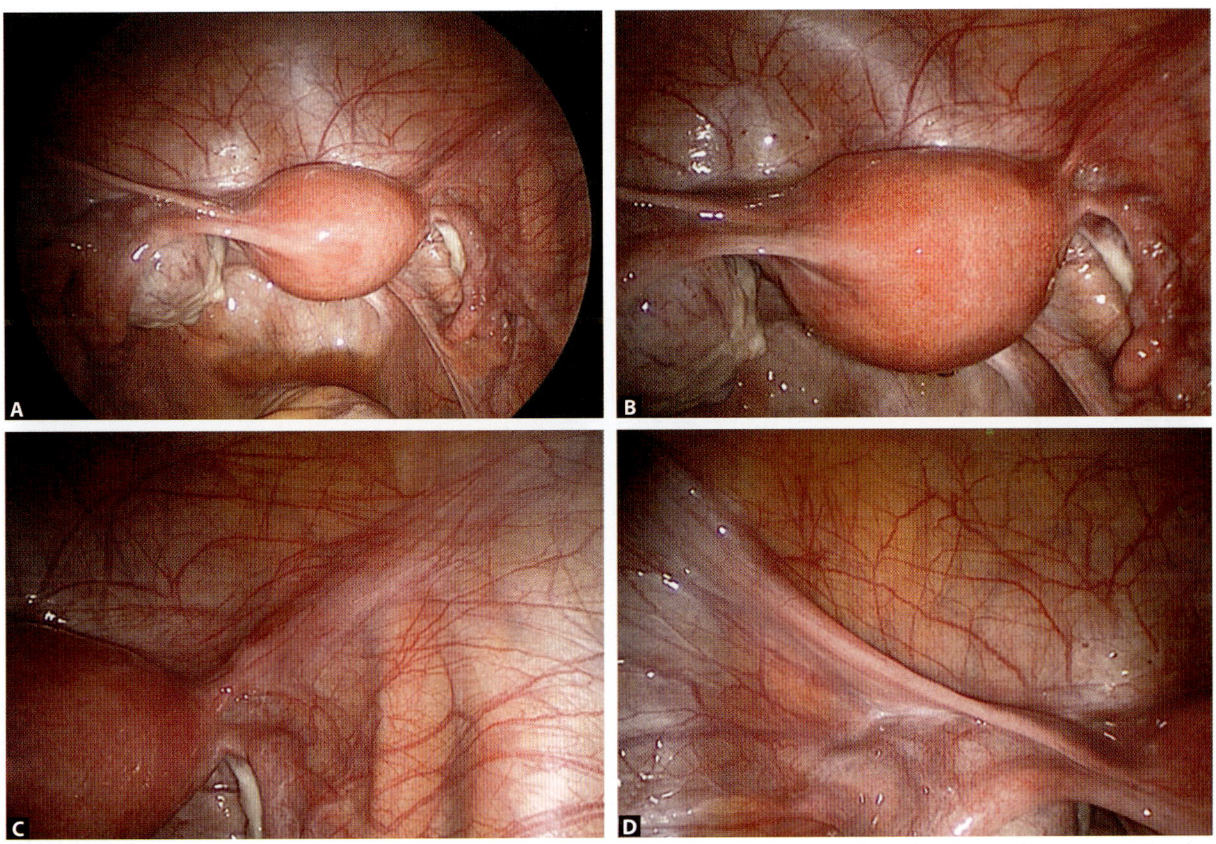

Figs. 24.29A to D: Laparoscopic overview of a patient with dysmenorrhea. (A and B) An enlarged and irregular uterus and serosal hypervascularization. The chronic disease has caused asymmetry of the round ligaments; (C) The right side is much shorter than (D) the left side.

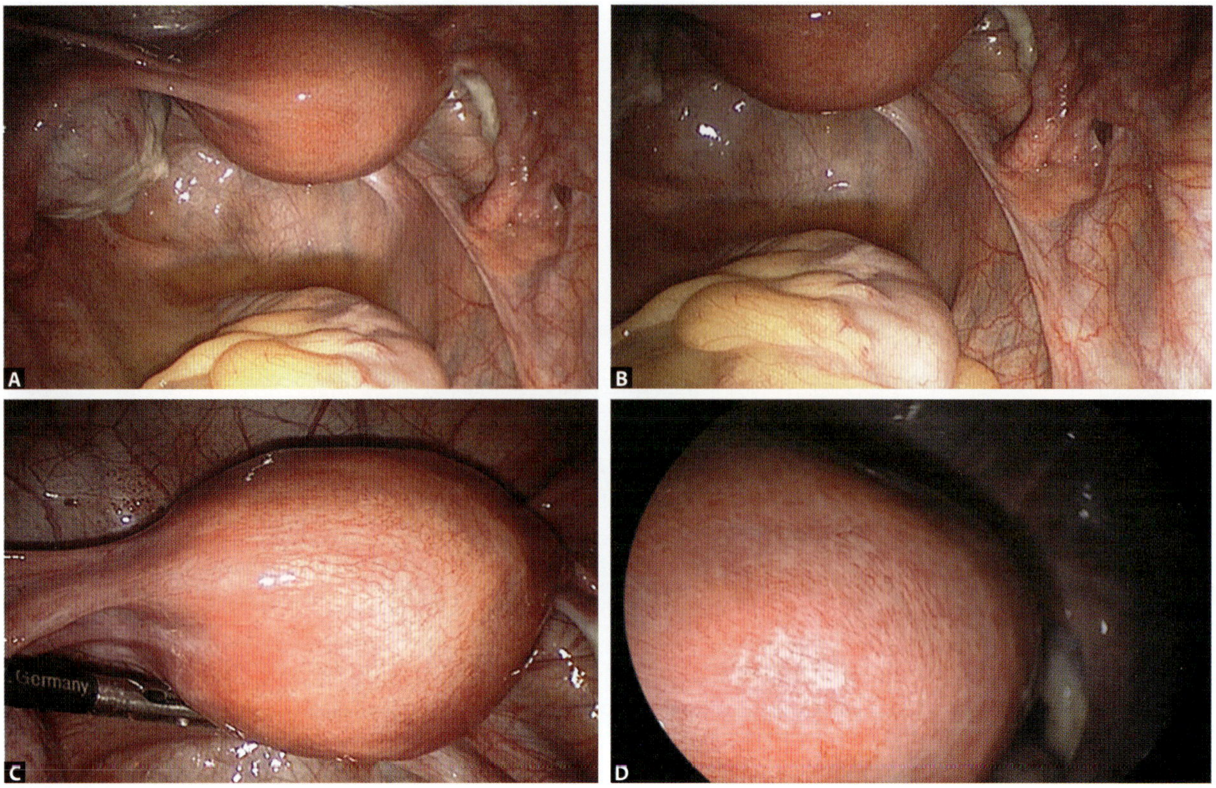

Figs. 24.30A to D: (A and C) The uterus appears to be less mobile but is fixed in the pelvis; (B) The ureteral portion of the peritoneum along its course to the bladder is under tension and can be demarcated from the sacrouterine ligament; (C and D) The surface of the uterus is hypervascularized; the efferent portion of the tubes appears to be steep.

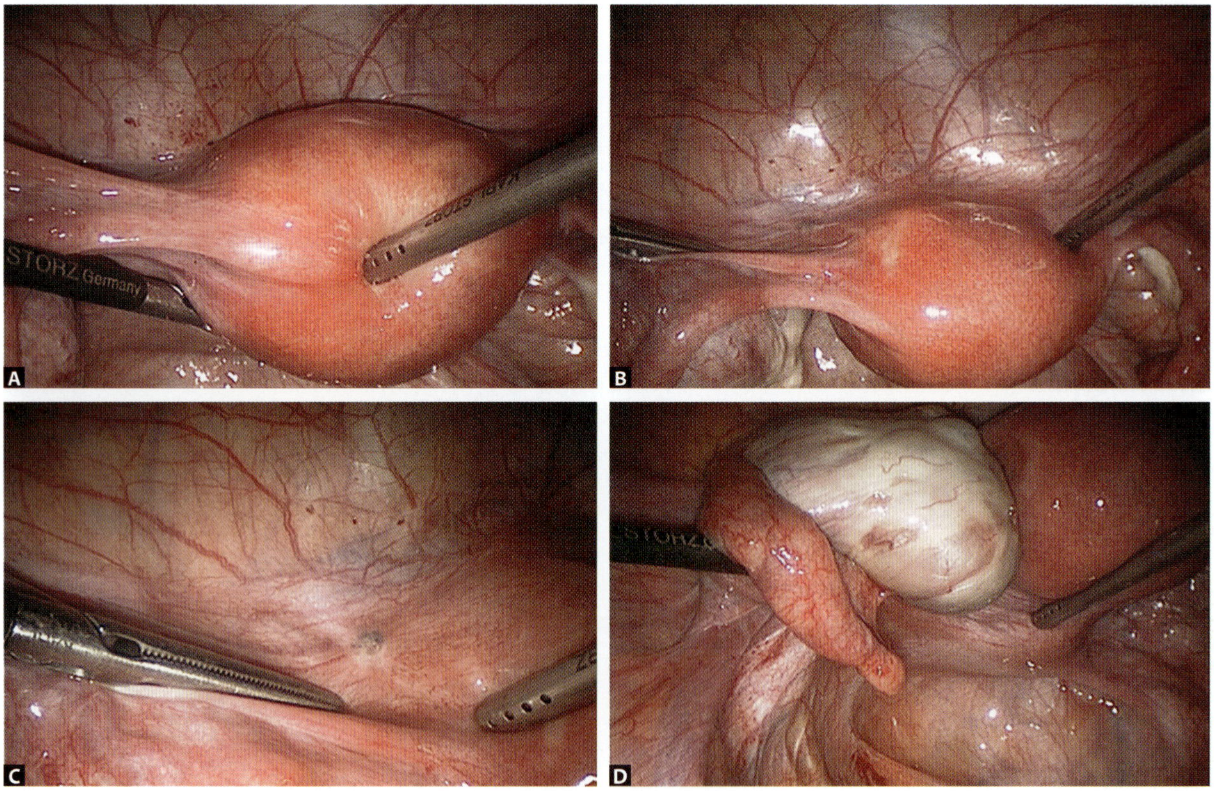

Figs. 24.31A to D: (A and B) Palpation of the uterus with a blunt instrument shows that it is less soft rather tight, but hypervascularized; (C) Endometriotic nodule on the lower uterine anterior wall; (D) Enlarged cystic left ovary fixed to the ovarian fossa. The ureter can be demarcated behind the peritoneum and is lifted to the fixed area.

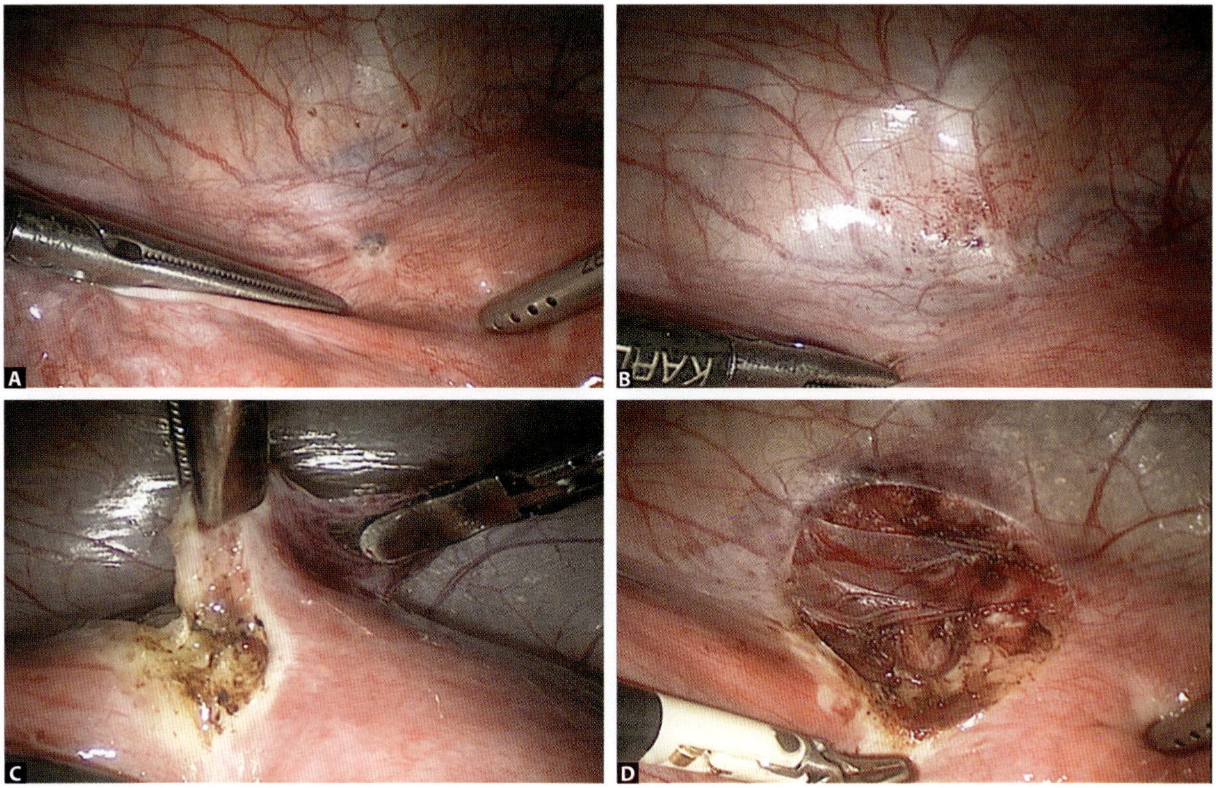

Figs. 24.32A to D: Excision of the endometriotic nodule in the lower anterior uterine wall; (B) Even the adjacent bladder peritoneum appears to be superficially affected because it is hypervascularized and fragile.

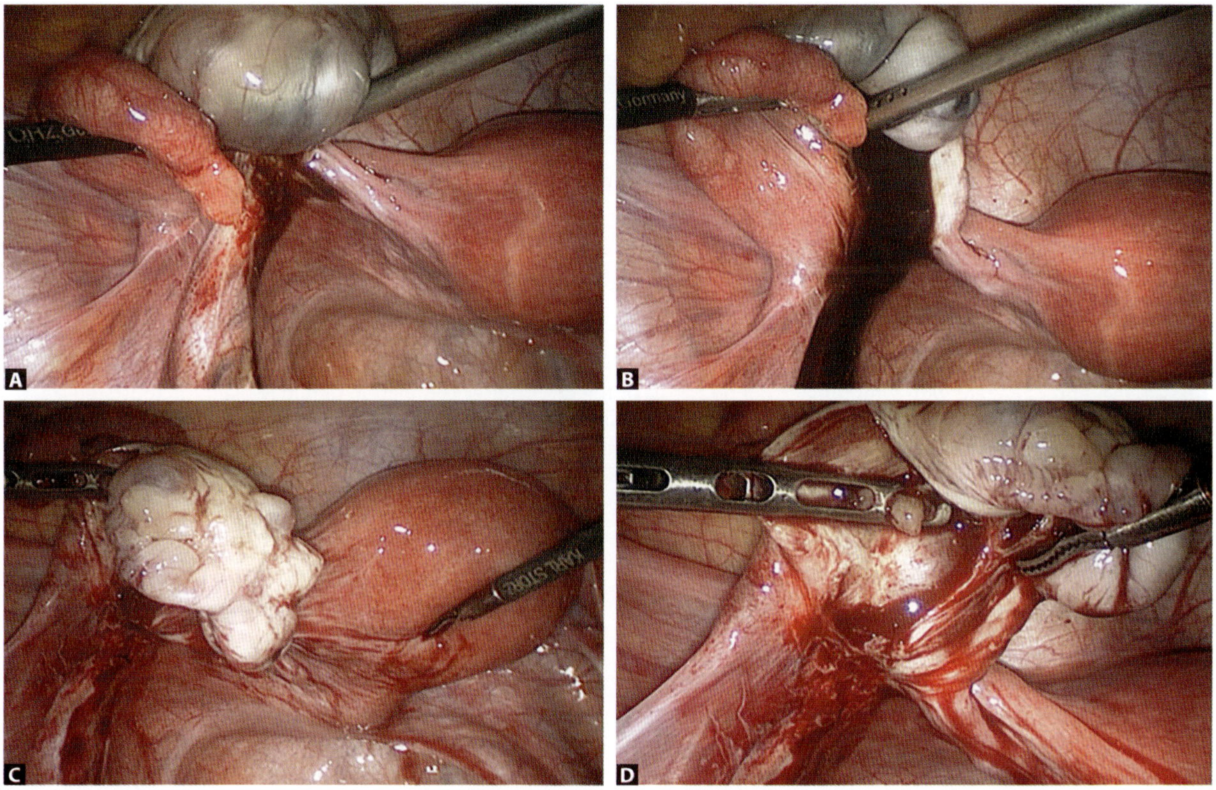

Figs. 24.33A to D: (A and B) Lifting the ovary out of the ovarian fossa and releasing it from its peritoneal adhesion causes the endometrioma to be opened; (C and D) The deep portion of the ovarian fossa is affected and the peritoneal nodule can be demarcated. In most cases, the nodules are connected to the cardinal ligament or the sacrouterine ligament.

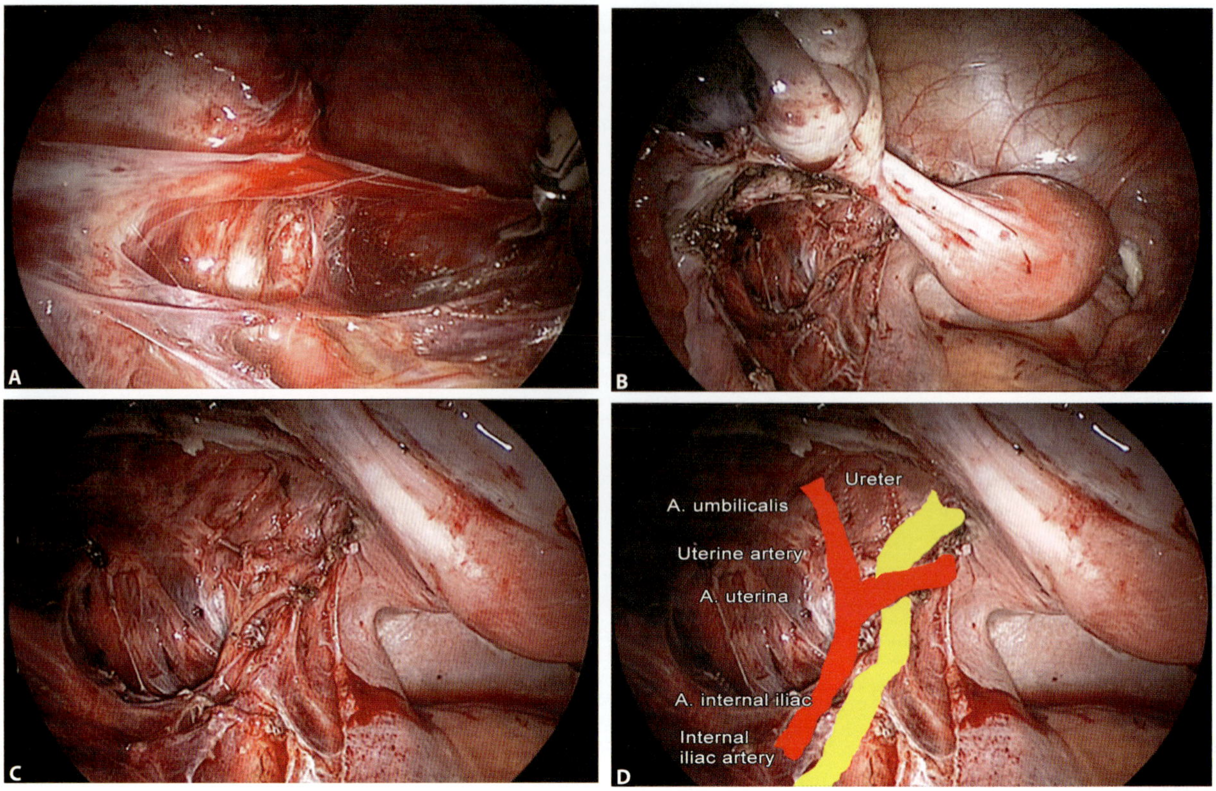

Figs. 24.34A to D: Opening of the peritoneal wall for resection of the symptomatic endometriotic nodule. The ureter and the vessels of the pelvic wall can be separated bluntly from the affected peritoneum and the endometriotic nodule. The ureter or the vessels themselves are very rarely involved and need special surgical treatment when this is the case.

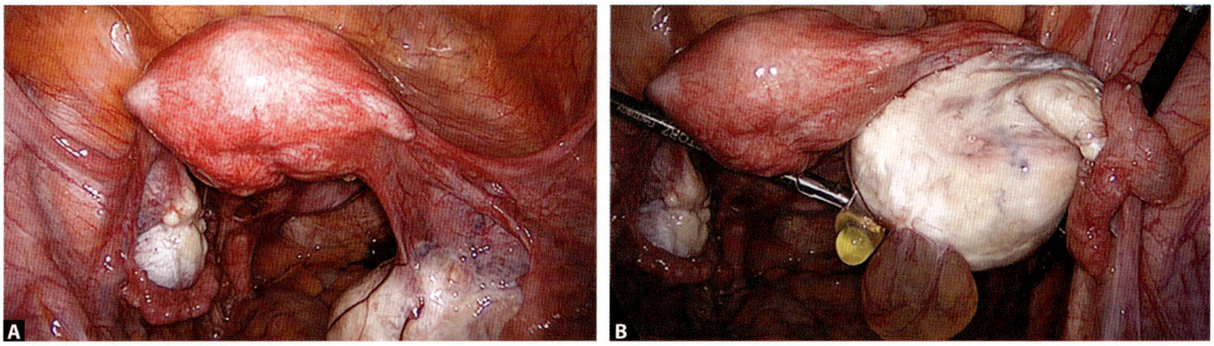

Figs. 24.35A and B: Patient with symptomatic adenomyosis of the uterus after completion of family planning (poststerilization). Lesions of fresh endometriosis are seen on the back wall of the uterus and the right ovary. The symptoms worsened after sterilization because the patient stopped hormonal contraceptive treatment. LTH is now performed.

2–3 cm to clearly visualize the rim of the cervical cap. In cases of postcesarean section, a careful, gentle and nearly blunt dissection should be performed (Figs. 24.47 and 24.48).

3.9 When lateralizing the ureter by pushing the manipulator upward, the uterine artery and vein with its collaterals are fully coagulated near the cervix and dissected.

The key steps of pushing the bladder down from the anterior vaginal fornix prior to incision and distancing the ureters from the uterine vessels at the cervical/vaginal level can be safely performed by stretching the manipulator firmly cranially, to the contralateral side of the exposure (Figs. 24.49A to D).

Step 4: Resection of the vagina from the cervix with the monopolar hook by stretching the manipulator firmly cranially. Intrafascial dissection is performed, leaving the sacrouterine ligaments almost entirely in place (Figs. 24.50 and 24.51).

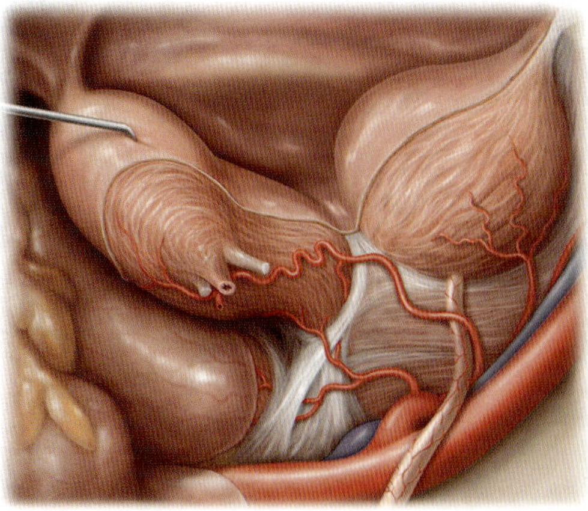

Fig. 24.36: Anatomical illustration showing the relation of the uterine vessel to the ureter in the pelvic wall, as compared to its location close to the uterus. The helical course of the ascending branch of the uterine artery can be easily reproduced. The uterus, bladder and rectum are embedded in a ligament-based pelvic floor.

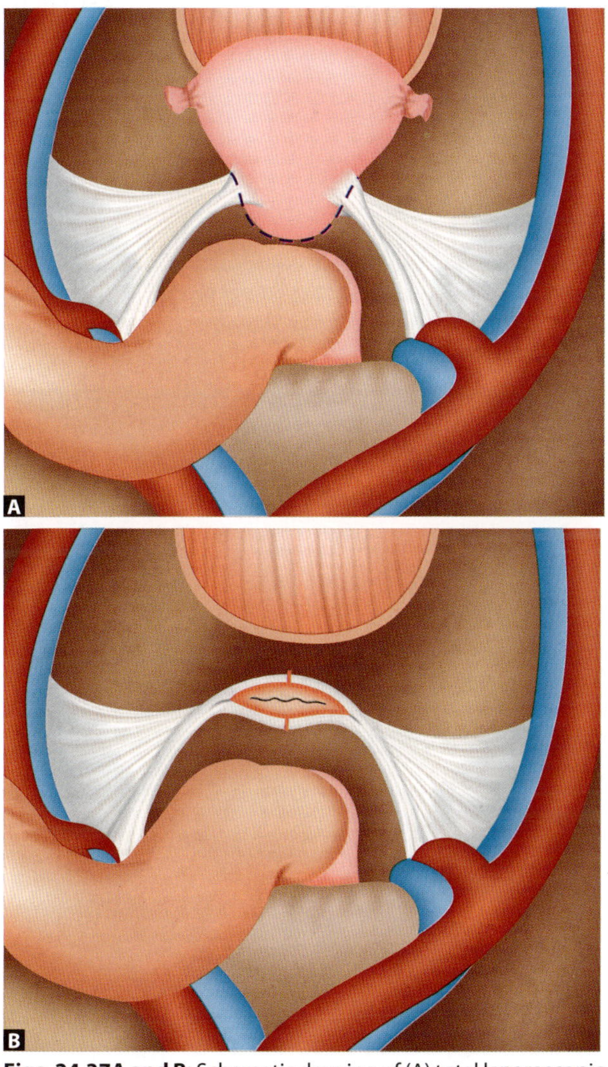

Figs. 24.37A and B: Schematic drawing of (A) total laparoscopic hysterectomy; (B) With the remaining vaginal stump.

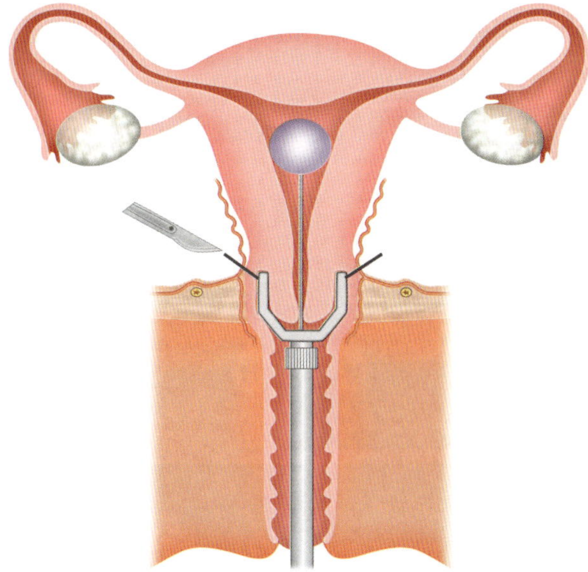

Fig. 24.38: Schematic drawing of the resection line in total laparoscopic hysterectomy. Only the ascending branch of the uterine artery needs to be coagulated and cut with the uterine manipulator. When the surgical technique is performed carefully, the ureter is at a safe distance from the coagulation zone (about 2 cm).

The uterus is then extracted through the vagina or positioned in the vagina to prevent loss of intra-abdominal pressure while still fixed to the manipulator. A large uterus must be morcellated either intraabdominally or transvaginally. In the case of a large benign uterus, visible myomas can be enucleated or the large uterus cut into several smaller pieces that are then extracted through the vagina. As a result, the incision in the lower abdomen need not exceed 5 mm and postoperative pain or the risk of hernia is minimized. Alternatively, a 10- to 12-mm electromorcellator is used to dissect the material, which is then extracted through the abdominal wall. The cutting edge of the morcellator must always be visible during morcellation. Evidence of the absence of any malignancy must be obtained earlier by appropriate preoperative diagnostic investigation. The patient must be informed in advance about the fact that the uterus, depending on its volume, may need to be morcellated.

Step 5: *(Closure technique emphasizing prolapse prevention): A technique for stable fixation of the vaginal or cervical stump*—Vaginal closure with the Te Linde suturing technique modified by Schollmeyer: Hysterectomy is known to be associated with a high risk of pelvic organ pro-

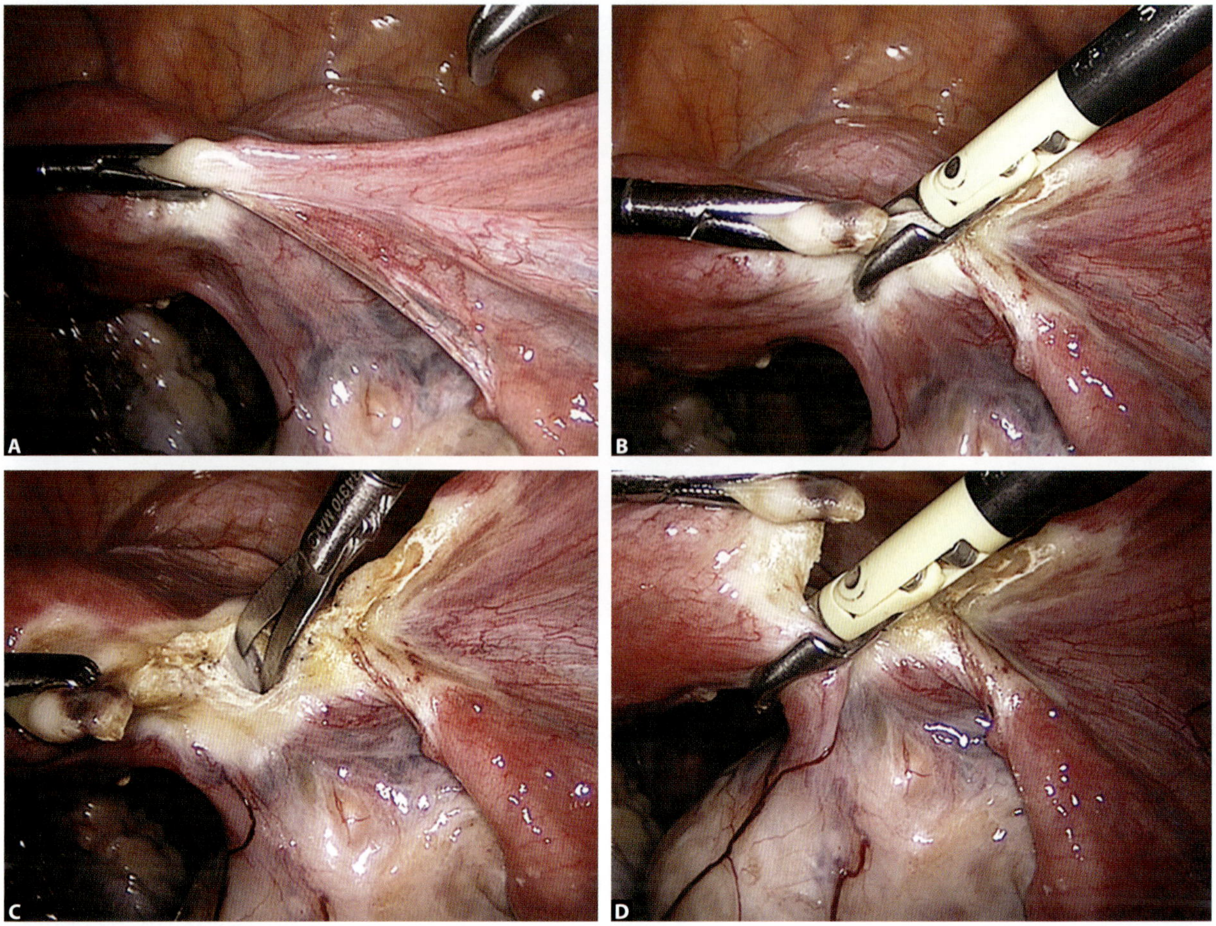

Figs. 24.39A to D: Stepwise coagulation and dissection of the right round ligament (A to C) and the proper ovarian ligament (D).

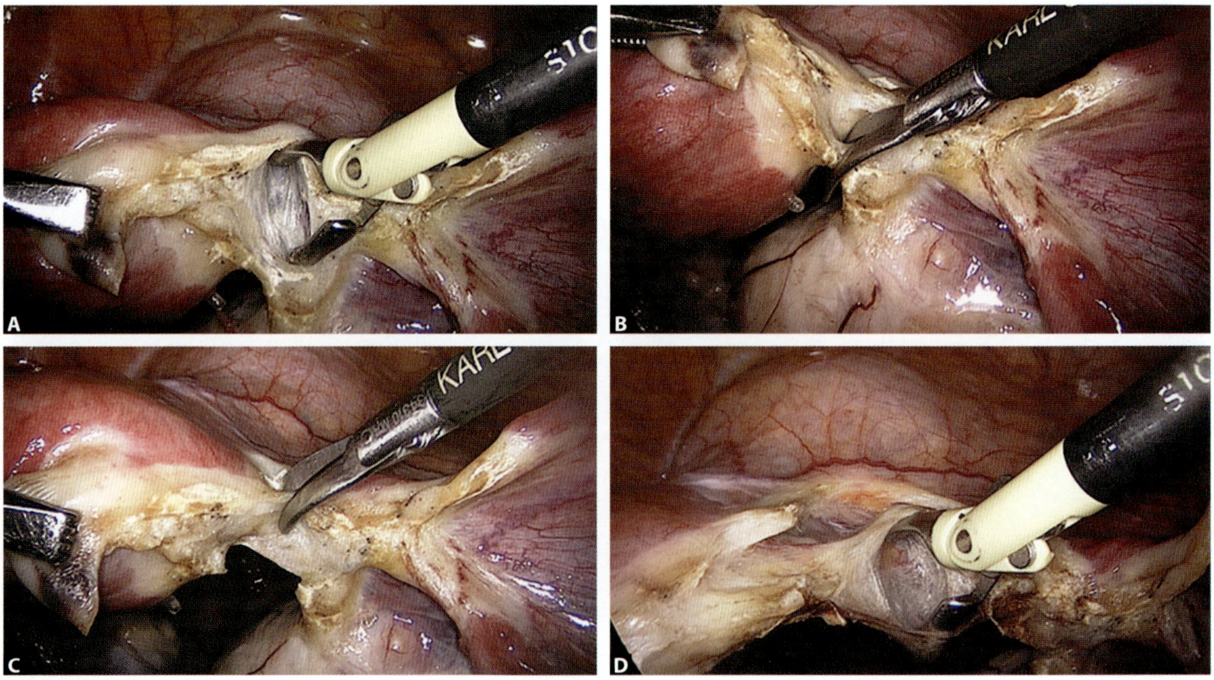

Figs. 24.40A to D: (A and B) The anterior and posterior leaves of the broad ligament are opened; (C) By pulling the uterus upward; (D) The surgical line down to the bladder fat can be opened bluntly.

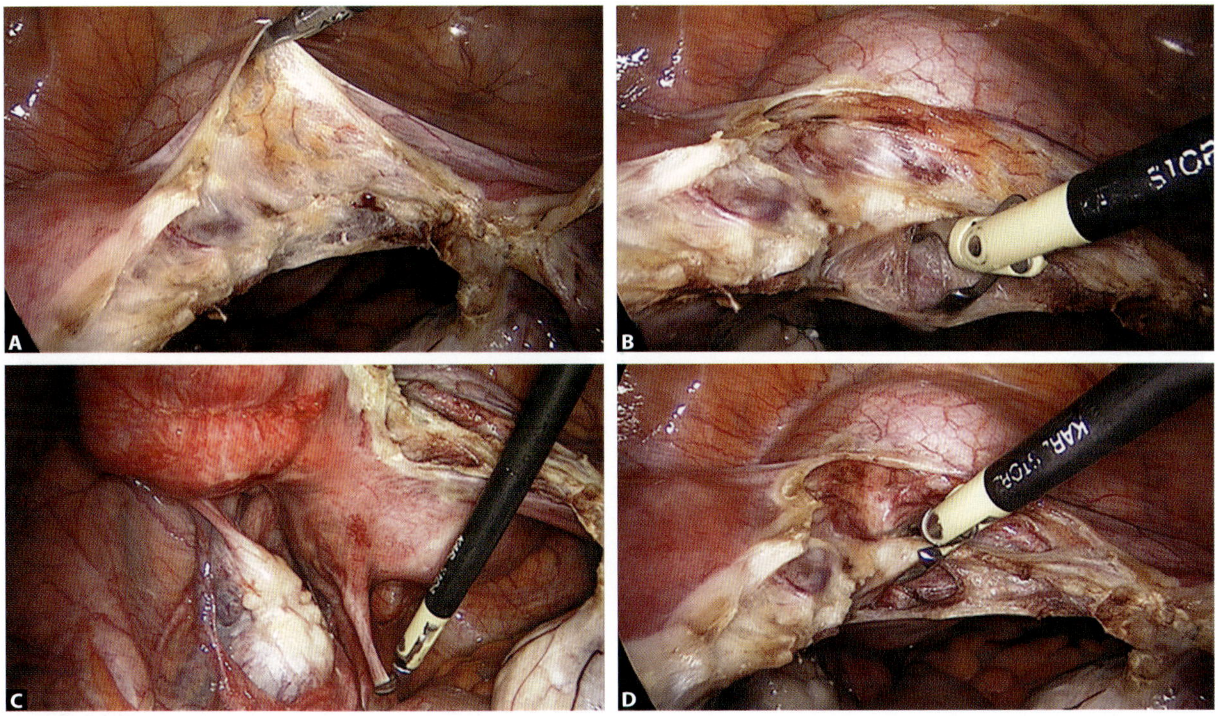

Figs. 24.41A to D: (A) Opening of the bladder peritoneum. The bladder itself is at a safe distance; only the bladder fat and parts of the bladder pillar are seen; (B to D) The ascending branch of the uterine artery can be identified and selectively coagulated. Pulling the uterus upward simultaneously, and pushing it upward with a uterine manipulator are important steps; (C) In benign cases, the cutting line should be above the cardinal ligament. Hysterectomy is then performed by the intrafascial route.

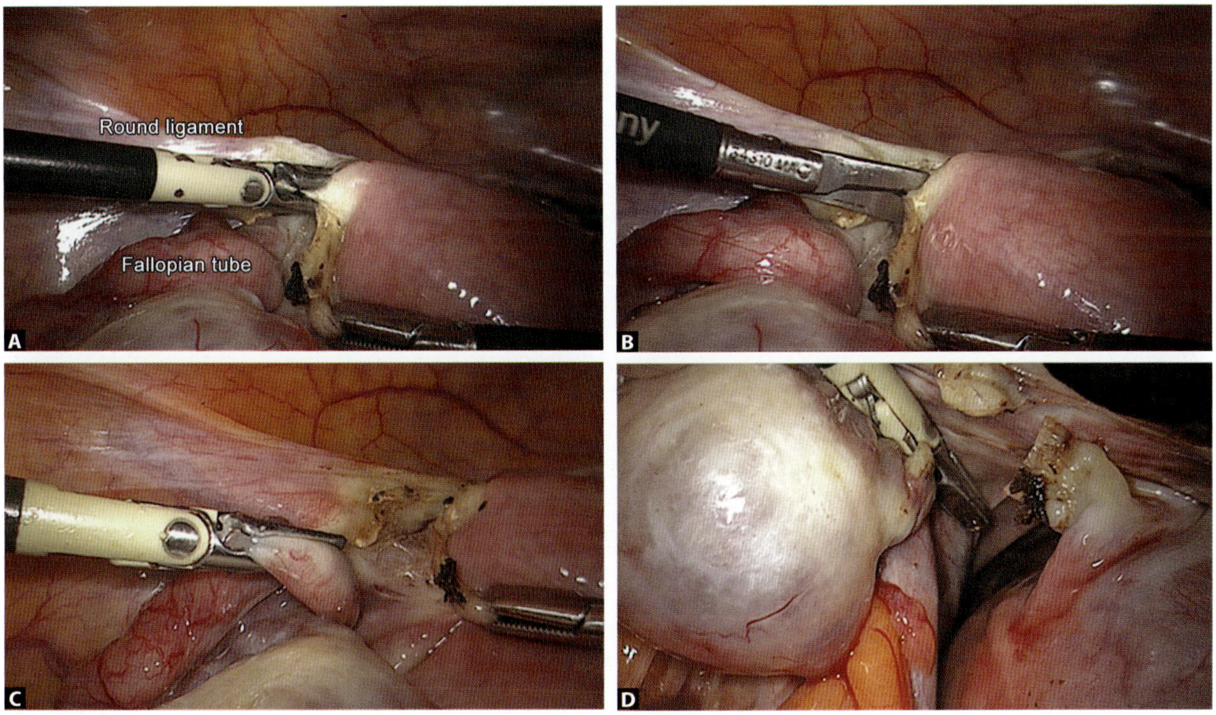

Figs. 24.42A to D: Stepwise coagulation and dissection of the left round ligament and tube (A to C) and the ovarian ligament (D). (A and B) The curved scissors are held with the tip away from the uterine wall; (C and D) After dissecting the fallopian tube, the vessels running underneath must be coagulated before further cutting; (D) In cases of myomas in the lateral aspect, the course of the sacrouterine ligament and the uterus can be visualized by blunt manipulation. The coagulation line should omit this part.

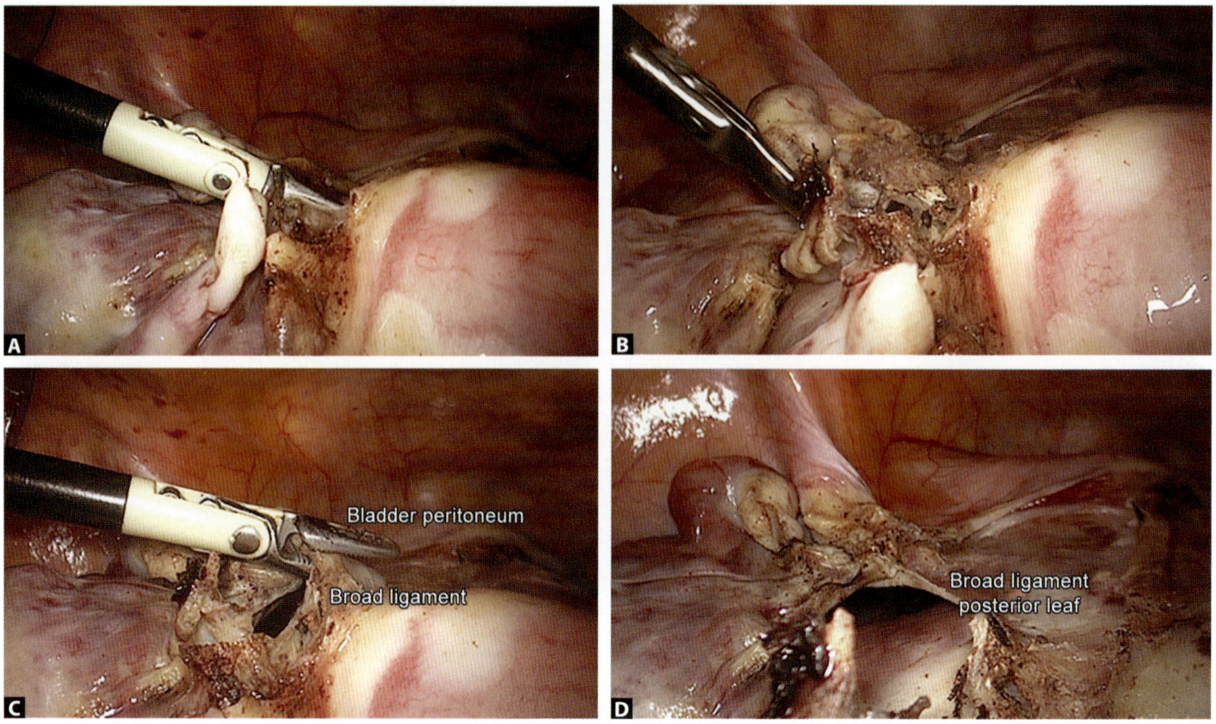

Figs. 24.43A to D: Dissection of the bladder peritoneum as well as the anterior and posterior leaf of the broad ligament on the left side; (D) The bladder peritoneum has already been opened from the right side; the posterior leaf of the broad ligament serves as an anatomic landmark for the uterine vessels.

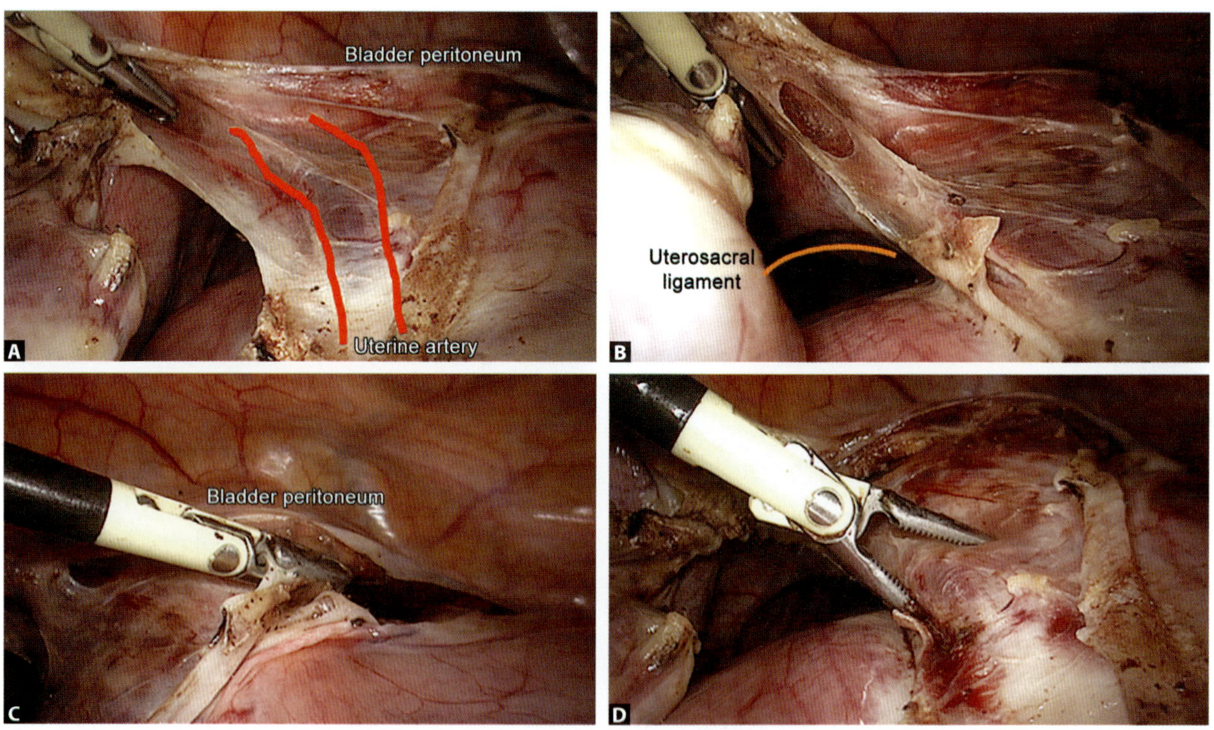

Figs. 24.44A to D: Further opening of the bladder peritoneum and the broad ligament (A to C) and commencement of coagulation of the left uterine vessels (D); The uterine artery functions as an anatomic landmark, leading downward (A). A glance to the back of the uterus shows the cutting edge to be above the conjunction of the sacrouterine ligaments.

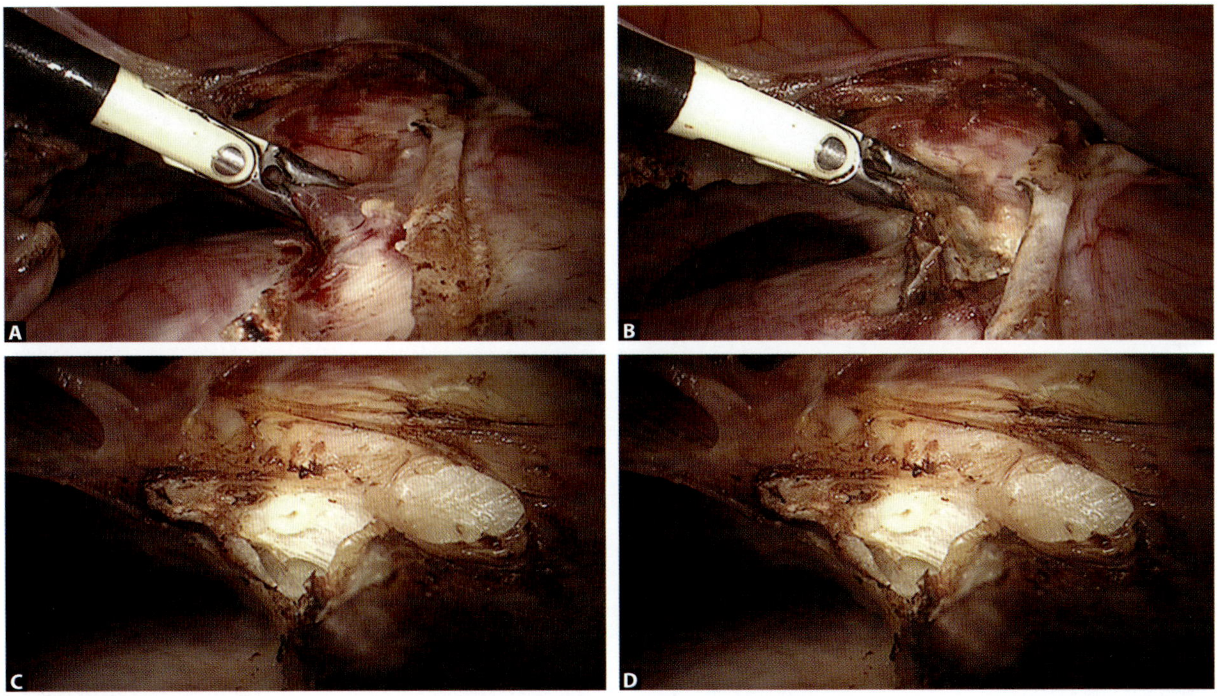

Figs. 24.45A to D: (A) Bipolar coagulation and separation of the uterine vessels on the left side. The area of coagulation should include the upper parts of the artery to avoid any retrograde bleeding after dissection of the vessel; (B) The color of the uterus changes to whitish gray; (C and D) A deep cut can be avoided by using the hook scissors; the uterine artery is dissected in two steps. This permits further coagulation of the tissue lying just behind the artery; venous bleeding can also be avoided.

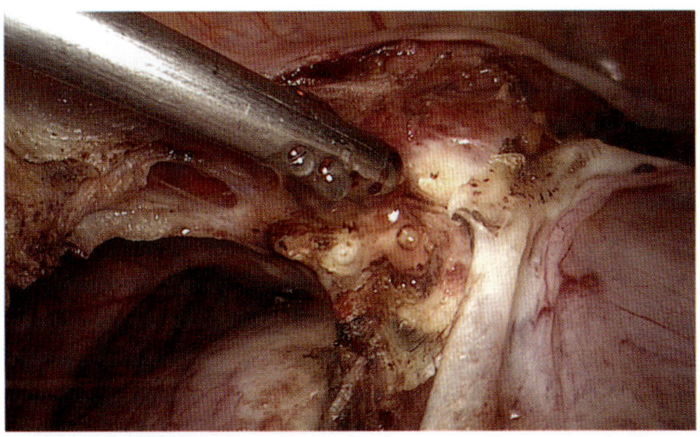

Fig. 24.46: Visualization of the separated left uterine pedicles. A few drops of physiological saline help to achieve more effective bipolar coagulation through the flow of electrolytes, especially when the field of operation is very dry.

lapse; the risk is especially high among multiparous women. This may necessitate pelvic organ prolapse surgery. Given the current high life expectancy of women, organ prolapse may pose a problem in later life and also difficulties in surgical repair (thrombosis, embolism, and infection).[65]

The suturing technique of Te Linde, known from abdominal hysterectomy for closure of the vagina, was modified for laparoscopic use by Bruno van Herendael and further modified by Thoralf Schollmeyer.[66,67]

5.1. Cautious coagulation of the vaginal edge[68] is followed by suturing of the vagina. Coagulation should be performed very carefully to avoid postoperative necrosis of the vaginal stump. Slight residual bleeding is addressed by sutures incorporating the complete vaginal wall. The uterus is either still in the vagina or a glove filled with swabs is placed in the vagina to avoid loss of the pneumoperitoneum. Usually a curved needle and PDS 1-0 is used for single knot suturing, with extracorporeal knots and intracorporeal safety knots. Alternatively, sled needles or even straight needles can be used for easy handling in and out of the 5-mm trocars.

PDS 1-0 extracorporeal knots are used for the following reasons:

- The monofilament thread slides easily through the tissue and does not cause additional damage.
- The monofilament PDS material minimizes the risk of vaginal stump infection.
- The long half-life of the suture material minimizes the risk of vaginal stump dehiscence.[68]
- Extracorporeal knots provide additional strength.

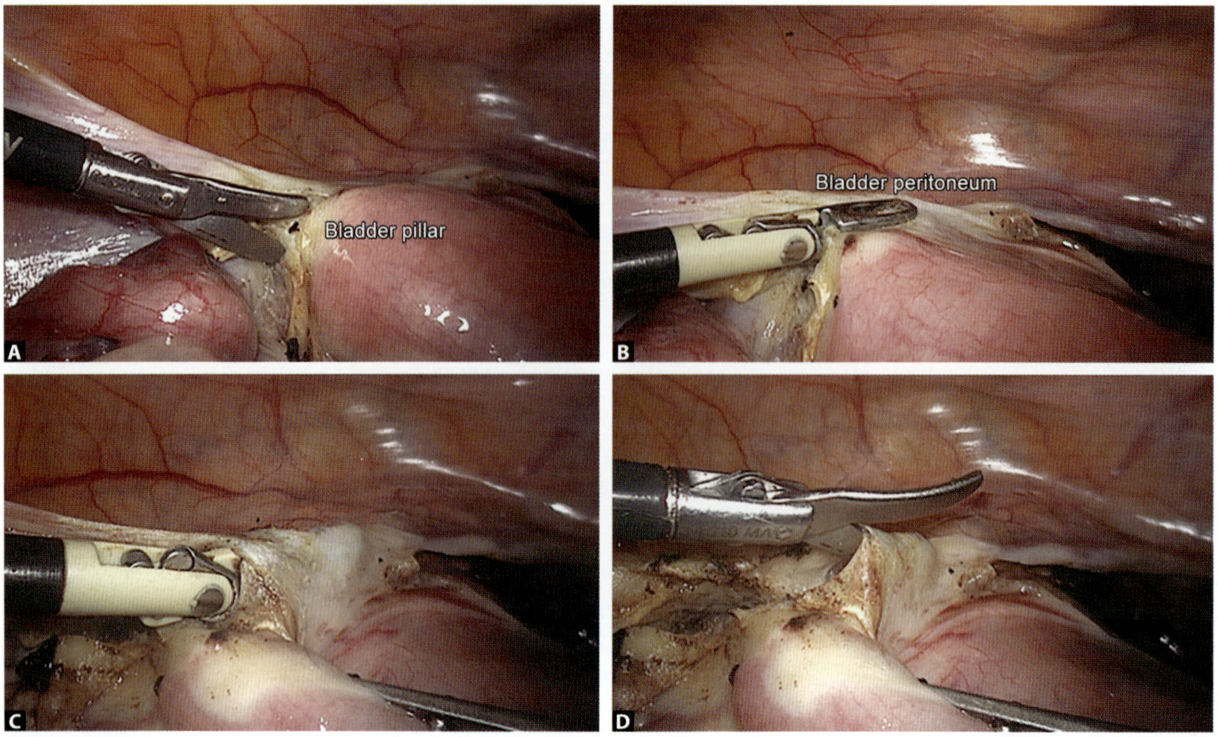

Figs. 24.47A to D: Final dissection of the bladder pillar and the bladder peritoneum from left to right, allowing the CO_2 distension medium to show the way. The bladder is pushed safely downward out of the field of operation and the peritoneal line of the vesicouterine fold is easily identified.

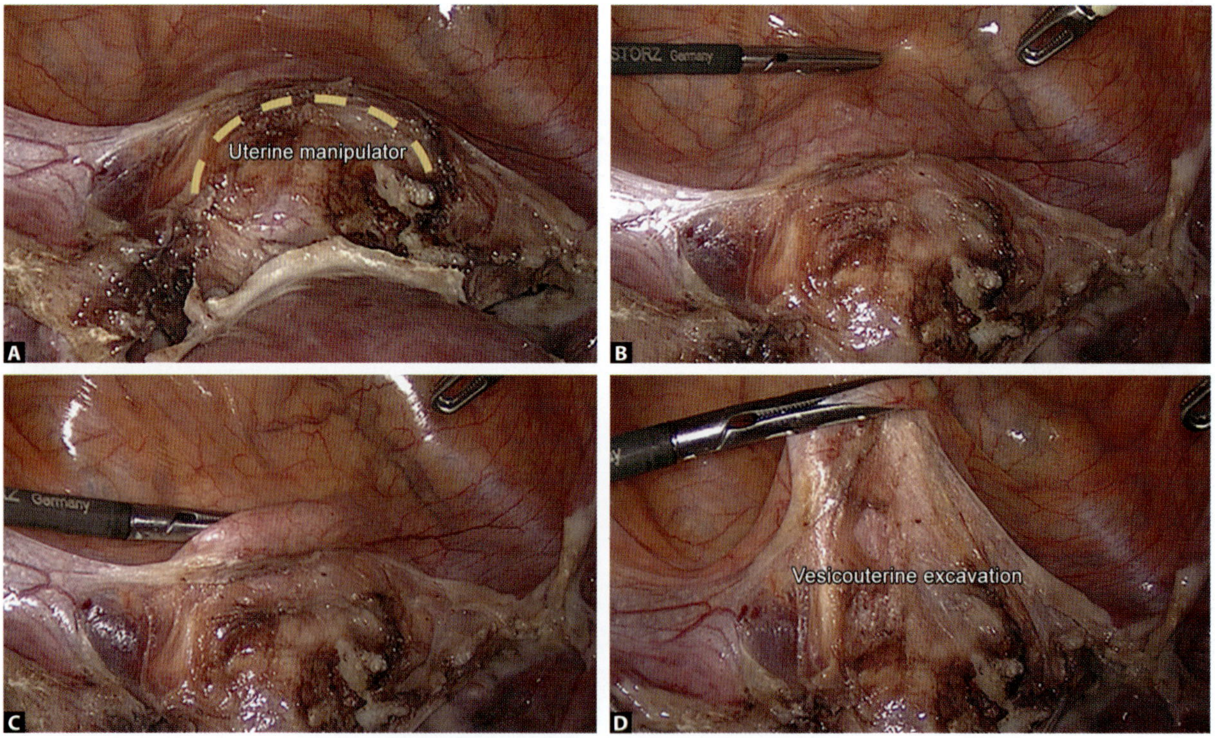

Figs. 24.48A to D: Visualization of the intrauterine manipulator, if inserted (A); (B and C) The bladder cannot always be identified immediately and avoided safely. Exact localization of the bladder is achieved by using a blunt instrument to push the suspected bladder toward the cervix from the balloon of the Foley catheter. The bladder is seen to be elevated and the vesicouterine excavation can be opened to push the bladder further down (D).

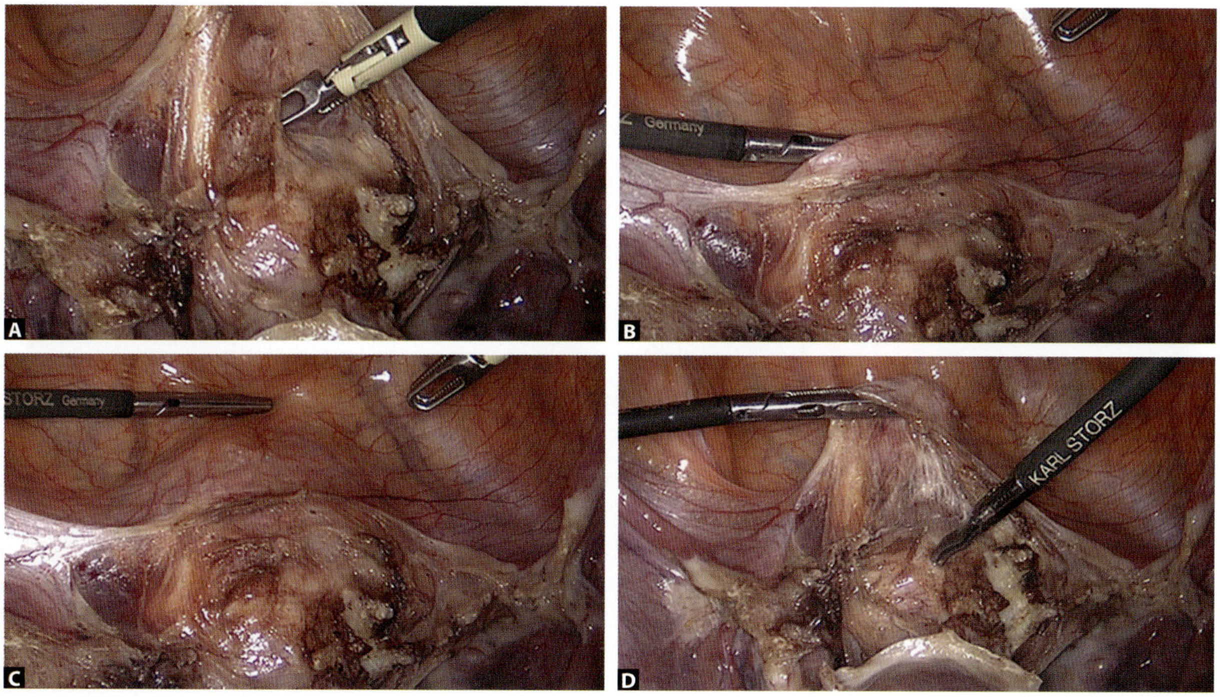

Figs. 24.49A to D: Minimal dissection of the bladder peritoneum—about 1 cm for LSH and 2–3 cm for LTH by opening the vesicouterine excavation. This is easier when a manipulator is inside the vagina and the cervix is pushed upward, but can also be done by traction alone. Once the vesicouterine space has been opened, exposure is achieved easily with a blunt instrument and with no bleeding.

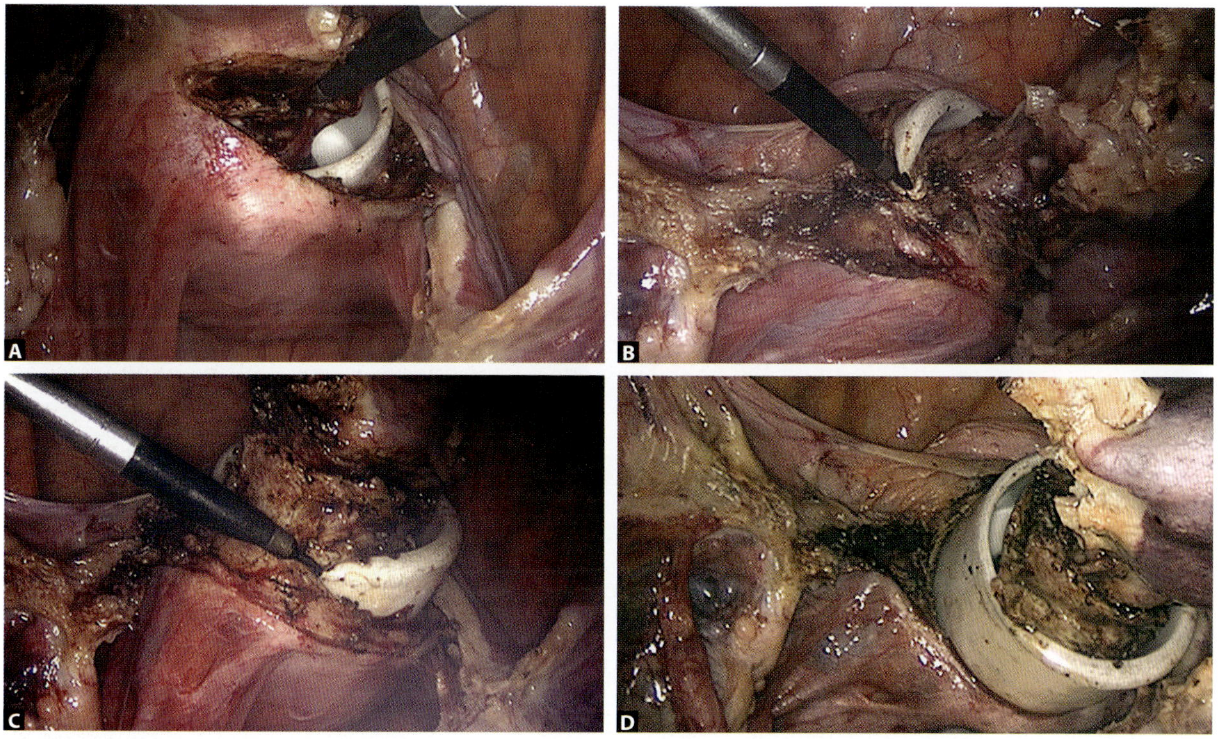

Figs. 24.50A to D: Completion of the dissection of the vagina from the cervix (A to D) and commencement of the transvaginal retraction of the uterine cervix, still grasped by the manipulator forceps. As the monopolar current causes fogging of the lens and the monopolar hook is very sharp, precise exposure under complete sight is essential. This can be achieved under simultaneous retraction/manipulation, using the 30 degrees optical device. The surgeon's vision may worsen immediately when CO_2 gas leaks through the colpotomy. Vision is hindered significantly when this happens and the use of monopolar energy becomes dangerous.

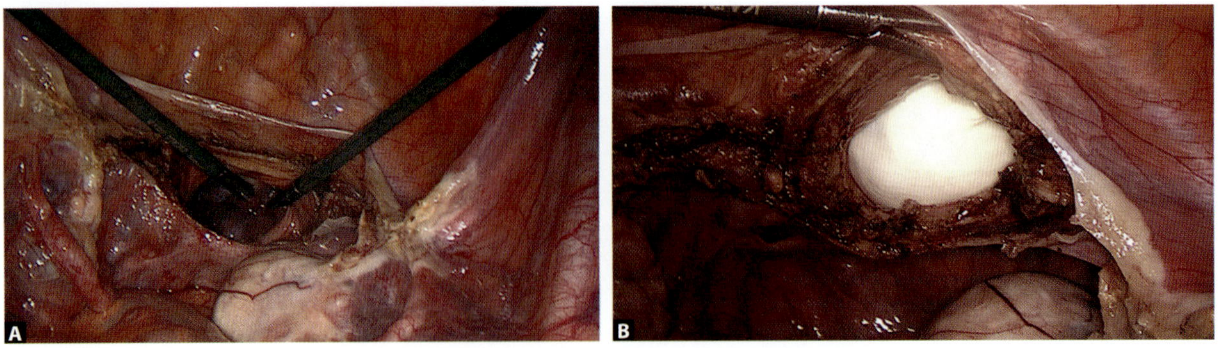

Figs. 24.51A and B: Retraction of uterus through the vagina (A); Introduction of a cotton swab-filled glove transvaginally to hinder the breakdown of the CO_2 pneumoperitoneum (B).

Optionally, both sacrouterine ligaments may be attached to the posterior vaginal wall to prevent vaginal prolapse (McCall culdoplasty).

5.2. *Corner sutures:* The peri-cervical ring is pierced by performing a suture in the right vaginal corner, followed by the corresponding vaginal epithelium. The sutures are made at a distance from the urinary bladder to minimize the risk of bladder laceration.

5.3. In the second step, the needle is passed through the medial aspect of the cardinal ligament in front of the uterine vessels. The second step involves the structures supporting vaginal wall suspension. Extracorporeal knotting with the placement of a deep and strong monofilament suture allows the surgeon to grasp a large quantity of tissue and smoothly glide through the tissue without causing damage.

5.4. Subsequent back-stitching of the vagina is followed by passing the needle through the vaginal epithelium and then, in the third step, through the sacrouterine ligament. The last step may be omitted when the ligament is stitched again once or twice to shorten it. In cases of preexisting descent, this step is absolutely essential.

The needle can now be withdrawn and the suture is completed with an extracorporeal Roeder knot, secured by two to three intracorporeal knots (Figs. 24.52 to 24.58). This procedure is repeated on the contralateral side and ensures that all parts of the endopelvic fascia (vesicouterine, cardinal and sacrouterine ligaments) are connected (Figs. 24.59 to 24.61).

Step 6

6.1. *Vaginal closure:* The remaining vaginal opening in the middle can now be closed with two U- or Z-sutures. These ensure both vertical and horizontal compression of the tissue, and minimize the risk of a vaginal stump hematoma. Neither peritonealization nor drainage is necessary (Figs. 24.62 to 24.64). Physiological reperitonealization occurs during the first two weeks postsurgery. Any additional peritoneal suturing might cause encapsulation of seroma or hematoma and increase the likelihood of postoperative infection as well as pain. If still inside, the uterus or the swab-filled glove is now taken out of the vagina. Figures 24.65A to D provides an overview of the surgical outcome of supracervical and total hysterectomy.

Laparoscopic Subtotal Hysterectomy

In laparoscopic supracervical hysterectomy, resection of the uterine corpus is performed at this stage of surgery. The preceding steps are very similar except for the fact that a manipulator is not needed because the uterus is elevated by traction. The corpus of the uterus is cut with a monopolar loop and the cervical channel is coagulated to prevent spotting. The cervical channel should be closed because of the high risk of ascending infection. Simultaneously, the cervix can be suspended with a strong monofilament suture and extracorporeal knotting. The remaining uterine corpus needs to be morcellated intra-abdominally (Figs. 24.66 to 24.72).

Special Situations

The traditional technique of laparoscopic hysterectomy must be modified in cases of severe adhesions or concomitant deep infiltrating endometriosis. The surgical steps are quite similar to those for oncologic surgery; radical pelvic exposure is essen-

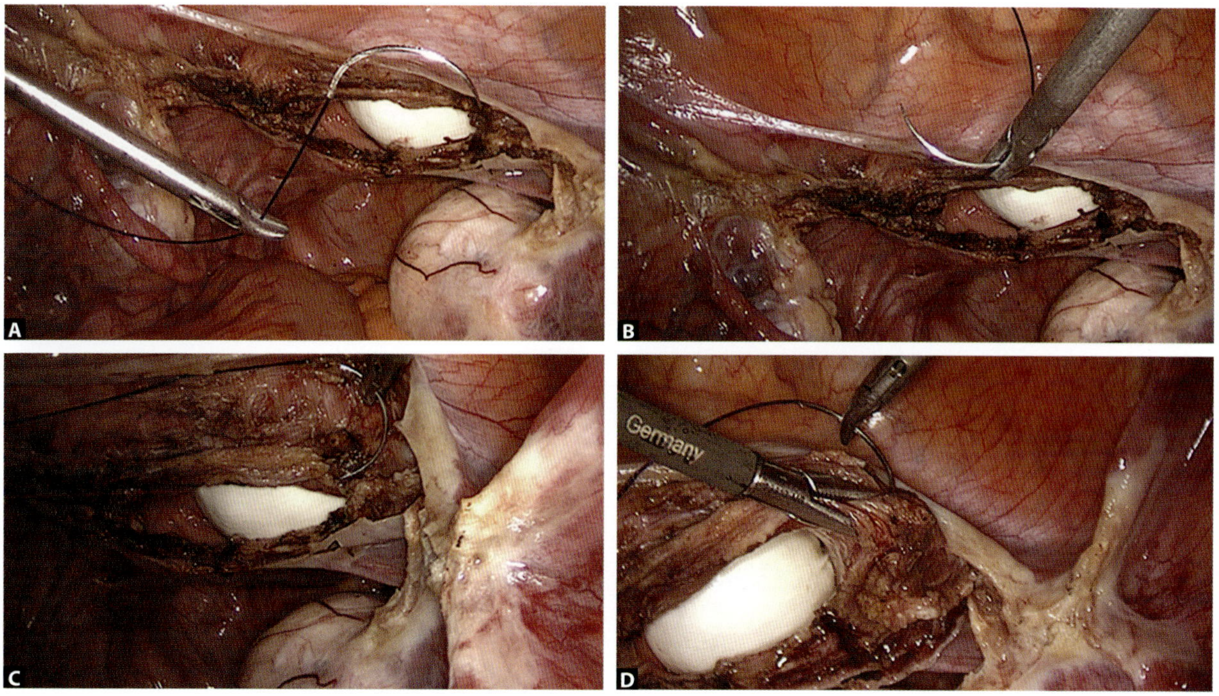

Figs. 24.52A to D: LTH: Right corner suture uniting the anterior and posterior vaginal wall, the posterior peritoneum and the right sacrouterine ligament. The bladder can be omitted under sight. The forceps must be sharp in order to securely grab the vaginal epithelium. When the suture includes the vaginal wall but omits the epithelium, there is a high likelihood of postoperative granulomas.

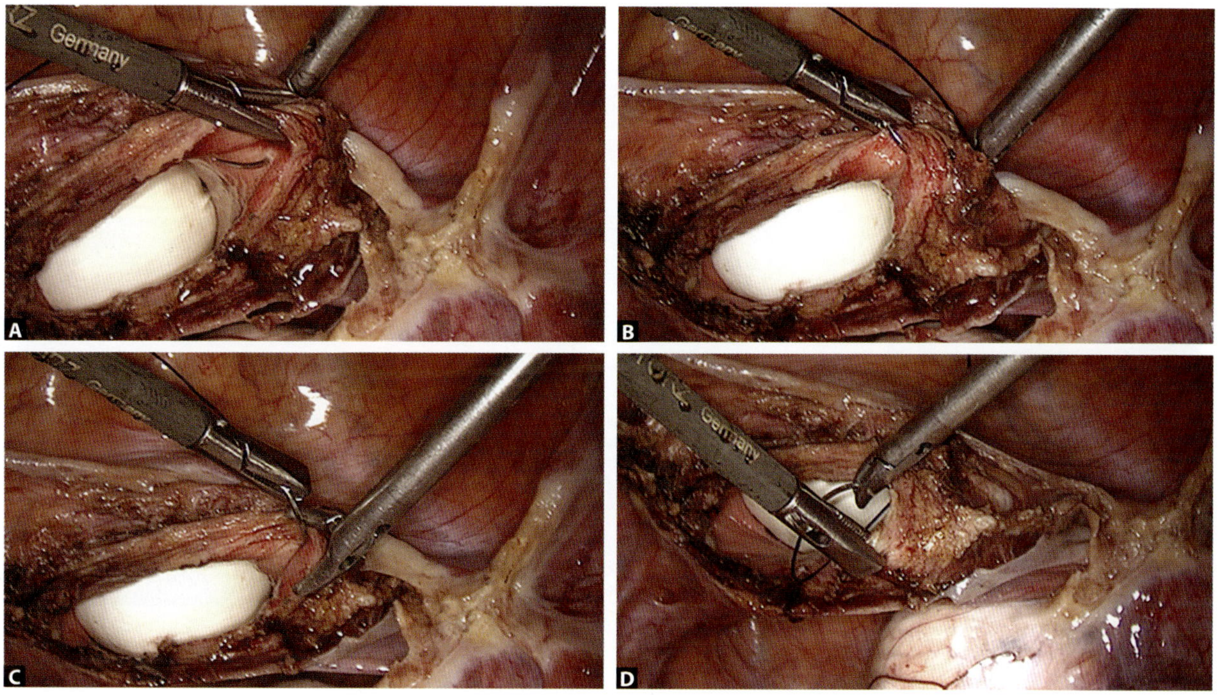

Figs. 24.53A to D: LTH: Continuation of the right corner suture. The 30° optical device permits viewing from below and above into the vagina. The strong paravaginal tissue is grasped in large portions.

tial (Figs. 24.6, 24.33, 24.34 and 24.36). After adhesiolysis, which may be very extensive in severe endometriosis or adenomyosis, the retroperitoneum is opened (Figs. 24.73 to 24.75). The ureter and major vessels are localized, and the crossover of the uterine artery is visualized and exposed (Figs. 24.76A to D). In some cases, clipping the uterine artery just behind its point of departure from the internal iliac artery (Figs. 24.77 to 24.79) is useful for the following reasons:

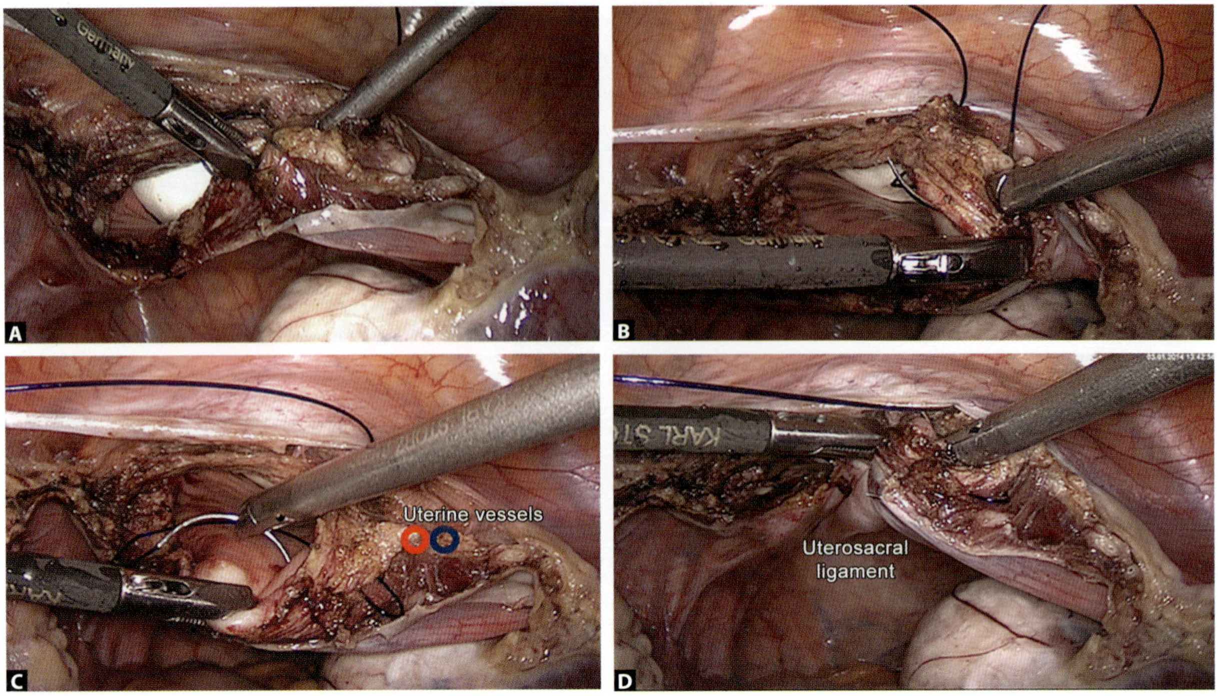

Figs. 24.54A to D: LTH: Continuation of the right corner suture and grasping the right sacrouterine ligament. The vessel stumps are omitted and lateralized. Vessels are compressed mechanically when this type of suture is used.

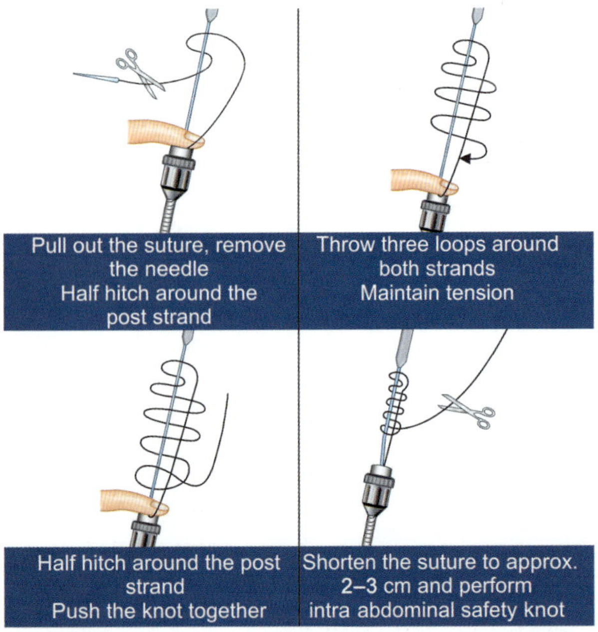

Fig. 24.55: LSH: Finalizing the extracorporeal knot of the PDS suture either with the Roeder knot.

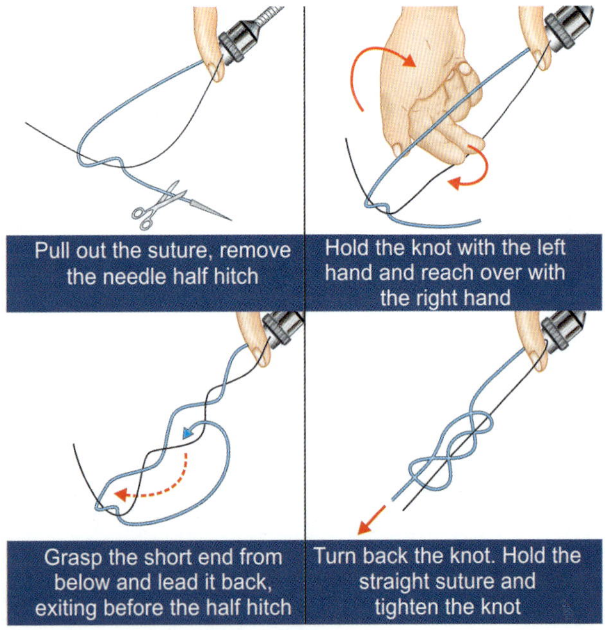

Fig. 24.56: The Von Leffern knot.

- More distal preparation and skeletonization of the uterine artery may be difficult or even impossible.
- Endometriotic scars and nodules are liable to modify the anatomy of the region. This may lead to unexpected bleeding, especially in cases of a large uterus. Clipping of the initial portion of the uterine artery will minimize intraoperative bleeding.
- The proximity of the uterine artery to the ureter and the thermal spread of bipolar instruments may cause secondary coagulation defects of the ureter, which can be avoided by using vessel clips.

At the end of the procedure the abdominal cavity is irrigated with physiological saline solu-

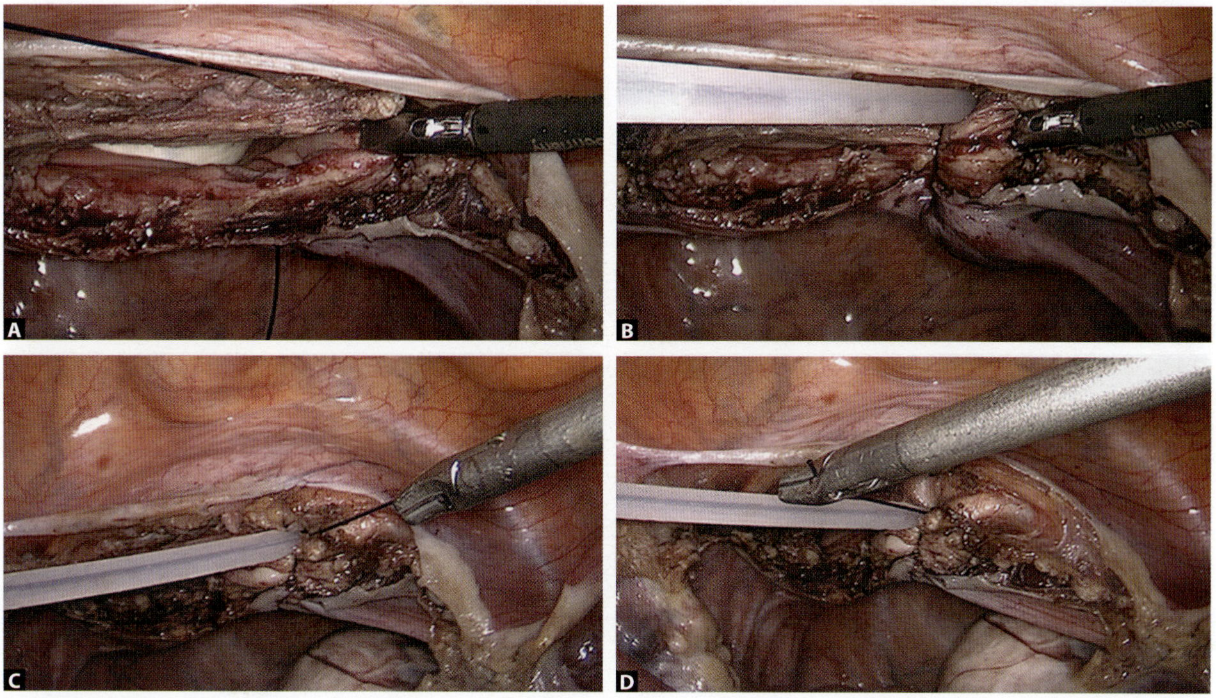

Figs. 24.57A to D: LTH: Completion of the extracorporeal Roeder or von Leffern knot by pushing it down with a plastic push rod. The edge is pulled into the abdomen to preserve intravaginal sensitivity.

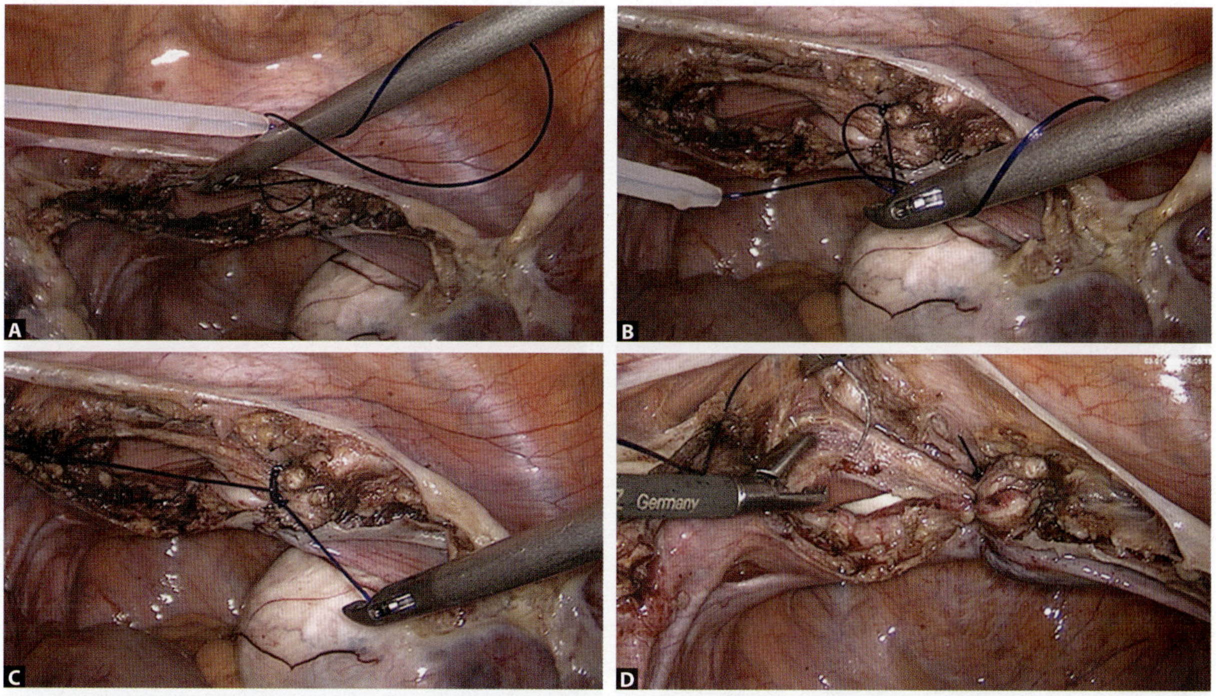

Figs. 24.58A to D: LTH: Placing an intracorporeal knot on the right corner stitch and cutting the thread.

tion and drained. Usually no drains are left in situ (Fig. 24.65).

We established this suture technique because it provides stable fixation of the vaginal end in addition to other safety advantages:

- As the suture is applied parallel to the urethra, kinking of the ureters is avoided. The thread is led through the medial part of the cardinal ligament, along the anterior-posterior access.

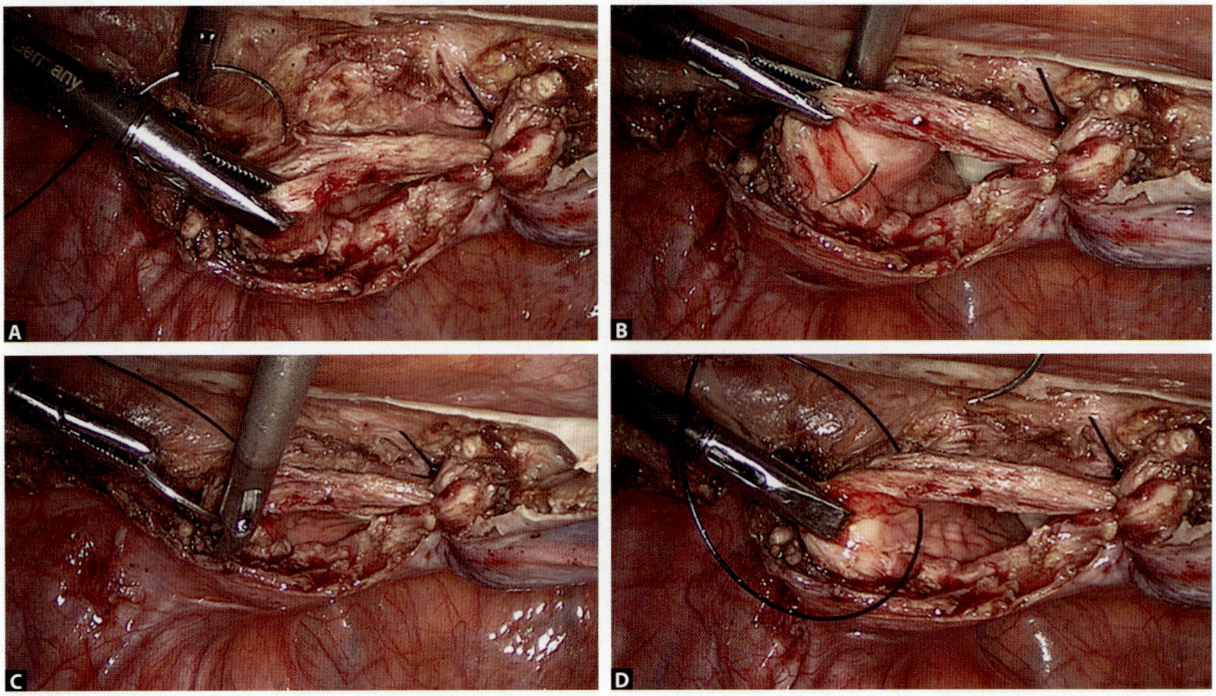

Figs. 24.59A to D: LTH: Left corner suture uniting the anterior and posterior vaginal wall, the posterior peritoneum and the left sacrouterine ligament. The bladder can be avoided under sight. The forceps must be sharp in order to securely grab the vaginal epithelium. When the suture includes the vaginal wall but omits the epithelium, there is a high likelihood of postoperative granulomas.

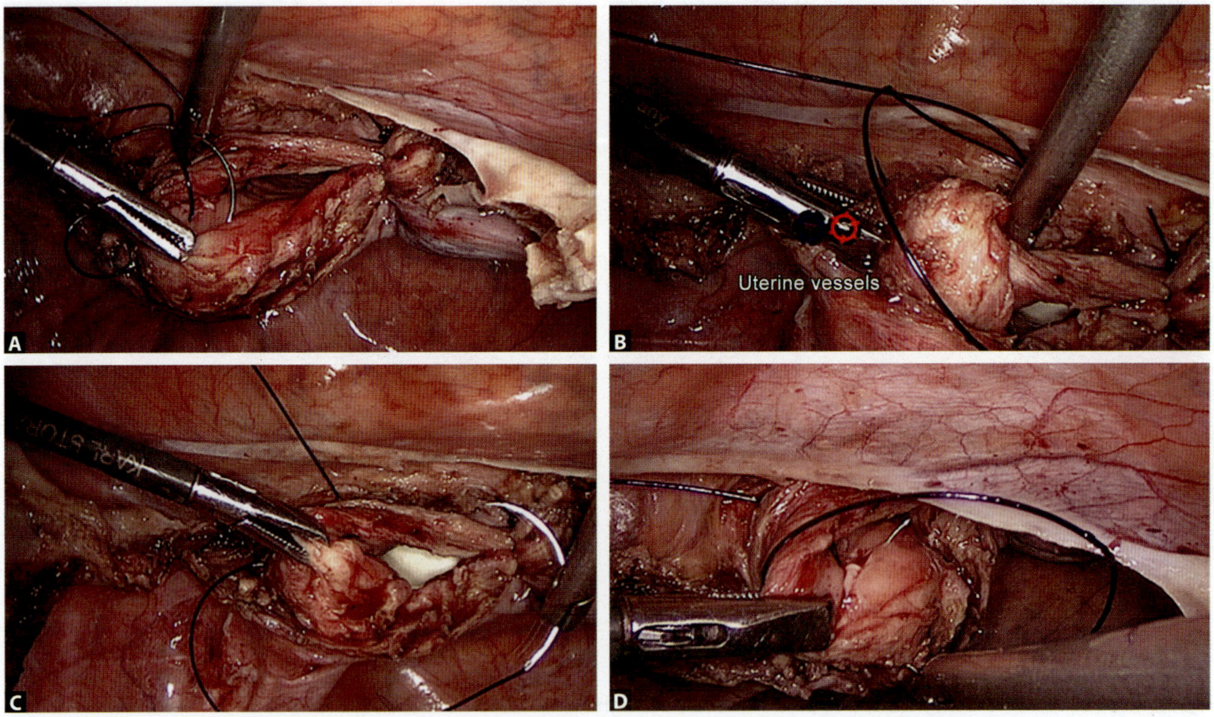

Figs. 24.60A to D: LTH: Continuation of the left corner suture. Vessels are compressed mechanically when this type of suture is used. Approximately 1 cm of the vaginal wall should be included in the suture.

- Compression of small vessels between the vaginal wall and uterine artery within the cardinal ligament minimizes the risk of bleeding.
- Despite good suspension there is no relevant displacement of the vaginal access dorsally, which might increase the risk of a cystocele.

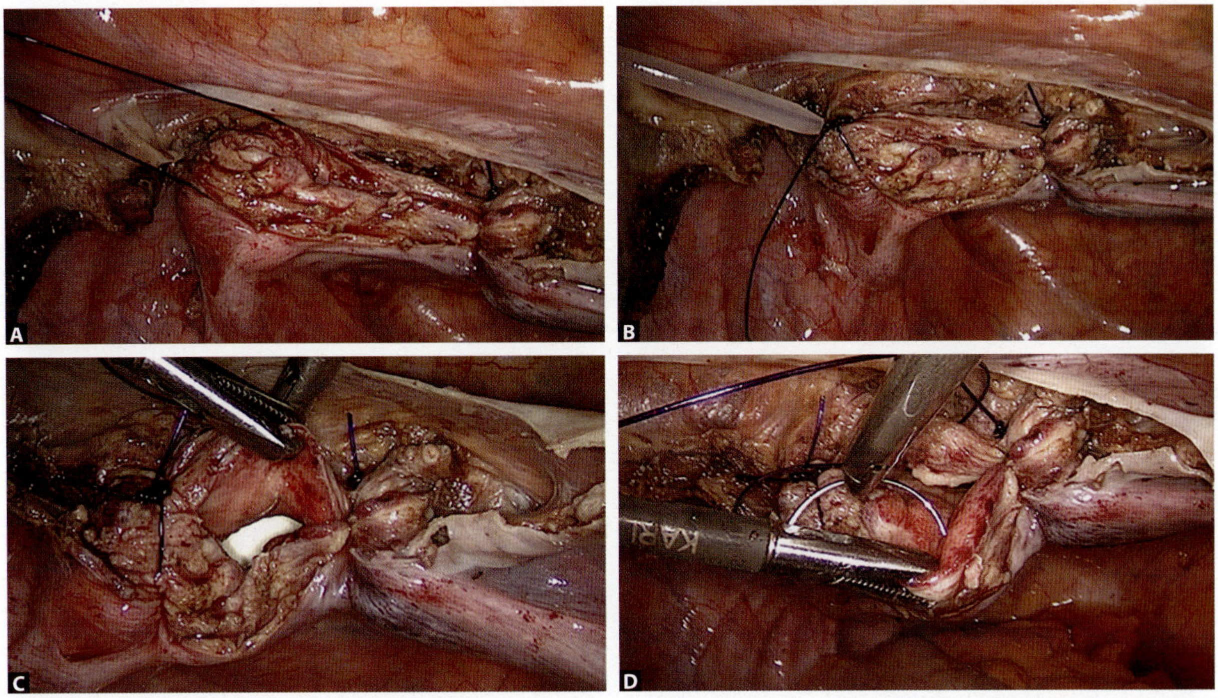

Figs. 24.61A to D: LTH: Completion of the left corner suture. The extracorporeal knot is pushed down with the push rod (A to C). Commencement of a U-stitch or a Z-stitch in the middle (D). It is easier to close the edges when the vaginal cuff is not completely dry. Bleeding ceases largely on its own and further coagulation can be avoided. Severe coagulation on the vaginal wall might increase the risk of vaginal stump infection or dehiscence.

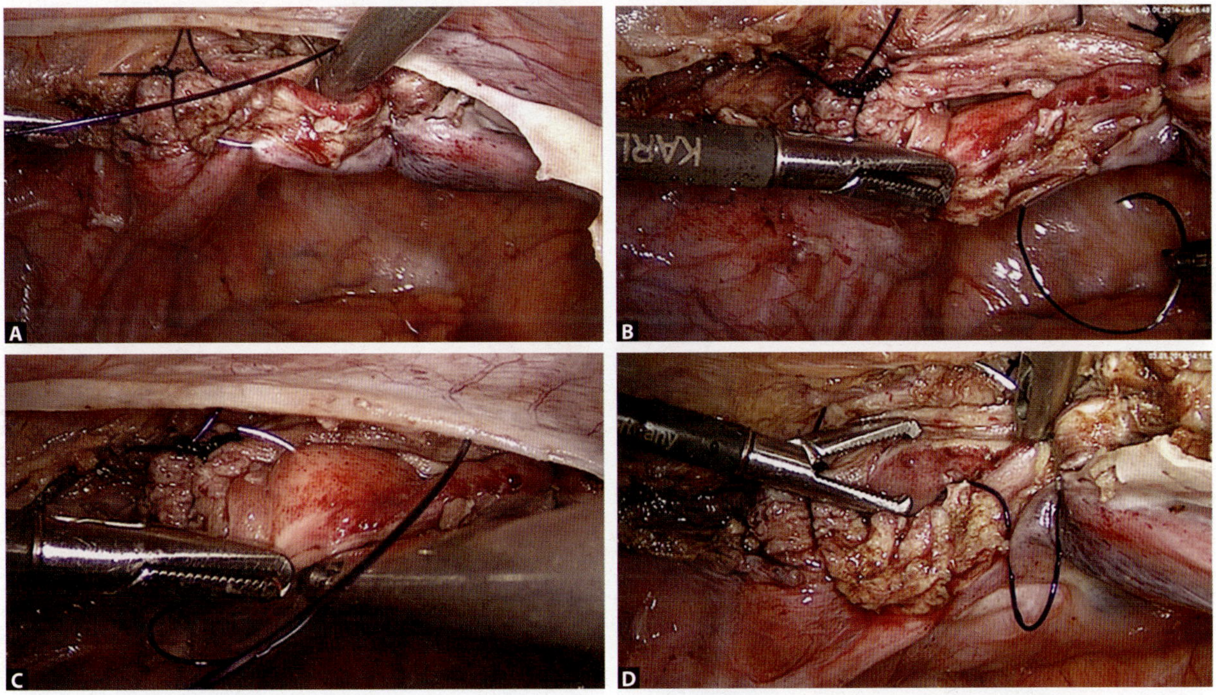

Figs. 24.62A to D: LTH: Final closure of the remaining vaginal opening with a U- or a Z-suture. When performing a U-suture, the suture end should reach the bladder in order to prevent bowel damage.

Posthysterectomy Inspection

The pedicles, bladder, ureters and bowel must be inspected under continuous irrigation with Ringer's lactate or Adept (Baxter). Ureter movement is no proof of integrity. In cases of suspected damage to the ureter or kinking of the ureter while closing the

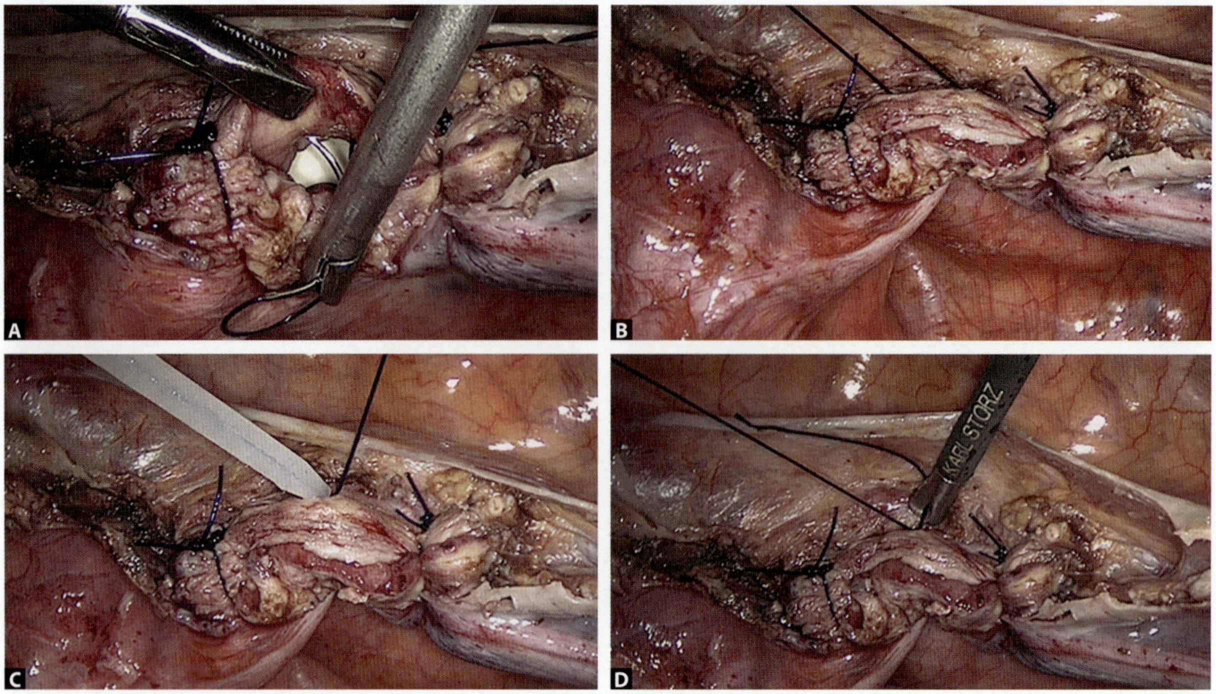

Figs. 24.63A to D: LTH: Completion of the central suture with a U-stitch or a Z-stitch. Extracorporeal suturing is not necessary because the suture is well placed and the tissue mass is adequate.

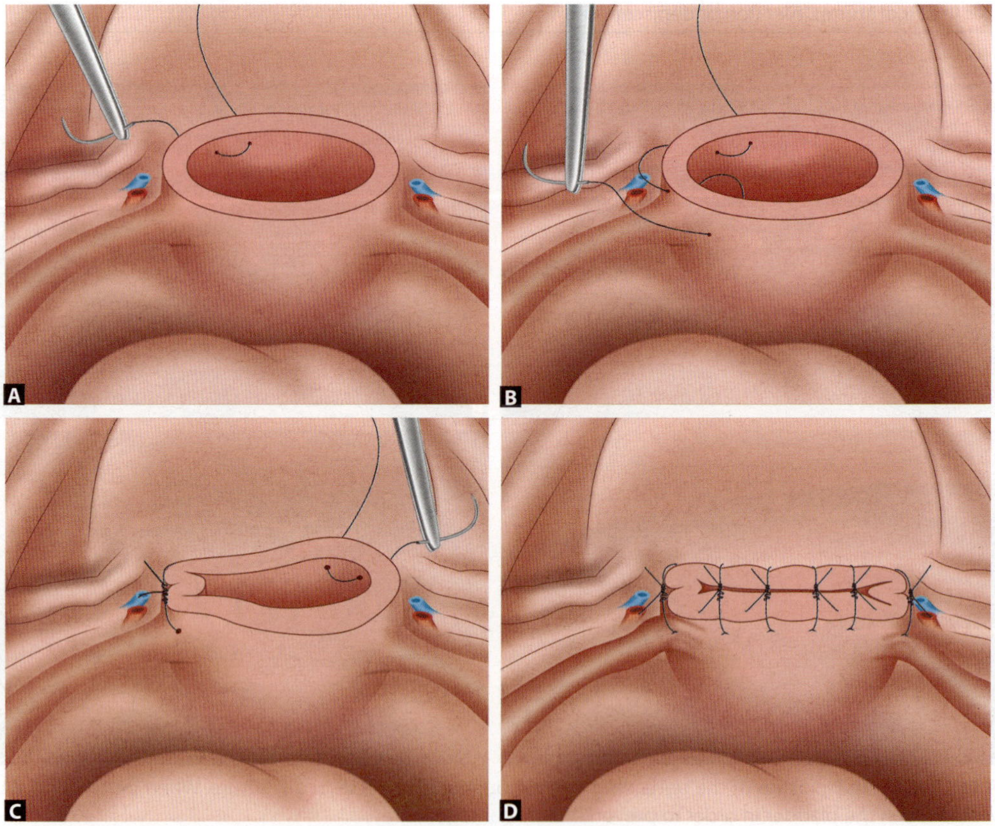

Figs. 24.64A to D: Schematic drawing of vaginal closure after LTH, modified by Schollmeyer. A suture is passed through the endopelvic fascia, 1 cm below the cephalad edge of the vaginal epithelium. The needle is pushed from the vaginal lumen through the vaginal wall, passed between the uterine vessels (median part of the broad ligament), and brought back through the vaginal lumen. The sacrouterine ligament is identified before the suture is passed through. The needle is pushed from the vaginal lumen through the vaginal wall and rectovaginal septum, piercing the sacrouterine ligament. Closure of the vaginal vault with single stiches, U-stiches or Z-stitches. The stitch is drawn through the endopelvic fascia and the vaginal wall, and then out of the vaginal wall and the endopelvic fascia.

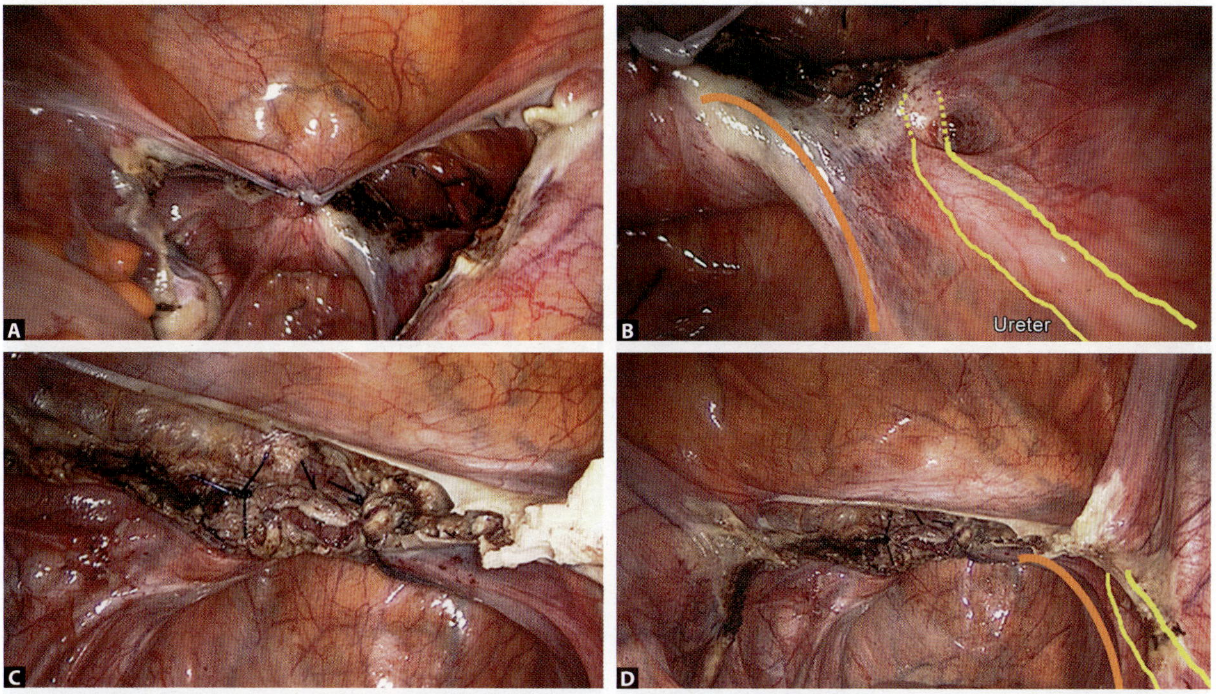

Figs. 24.65A to D: (A and B) Final situs after LASH. The cervical channel is covered with the peritoneum and both sacrouterine ligaments are under slight tension, thus fixing the middle compartment and the cervical ring; (C and D) Final situs after LTH. The vaginal stump has been closed and the sacrouterine ligaments elevated with two corner sutures. The peritoneum closes the cervical channel and draining can be effected from both sides. Both sacrouterine ligaments are under slight tension, thus maintaining the colposuspension. Reperitonealization will occur approximately 2 weeks after the operation. The PDS suture allows safe closure and healing of the vaginal cuff because absorption occurs only after about 6 months. The sacrouterine ligaments and the ureter can be clearly identified. Since the anatomy of the ureter has not been affected, retroperitoneum need not be opened or visualized.

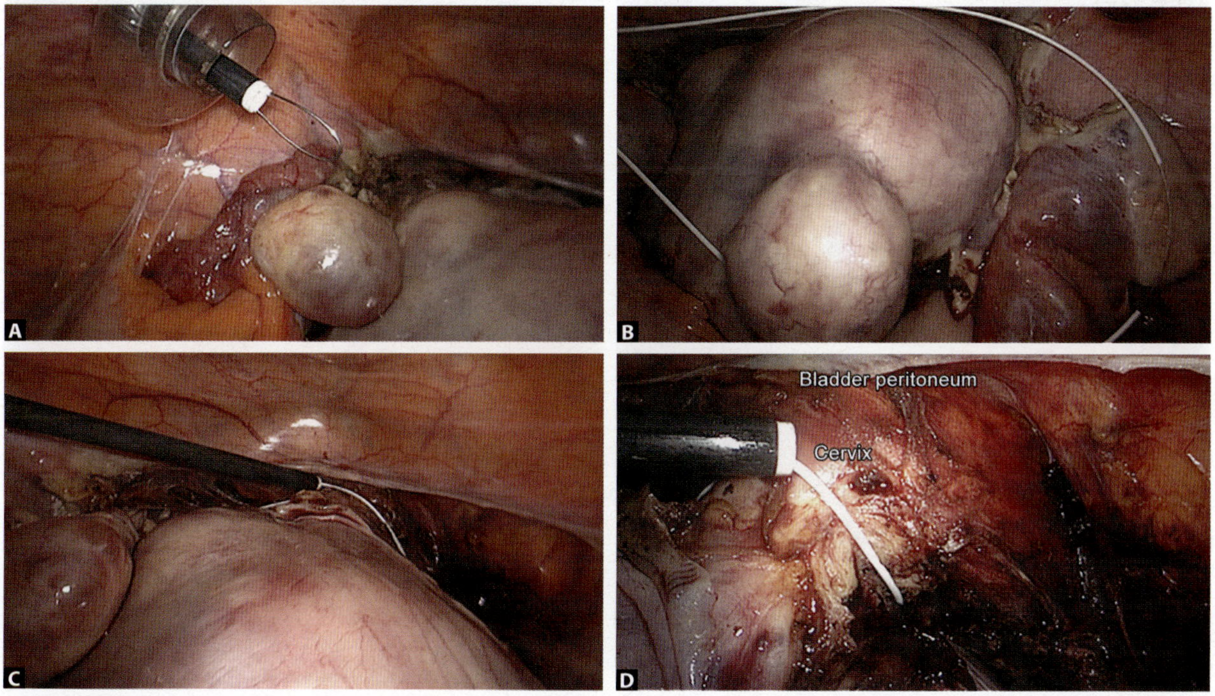

Figs. 24.66A to D: Introduction of a monopolar cutting loop for the cervix and exact placement prior to activation. The whitish uterus is lifted over the loop and the loop is tightened gently. Correct placement between the stumps of the uterine artery and above the conjunction of the sacrouterine ligaments is checked.

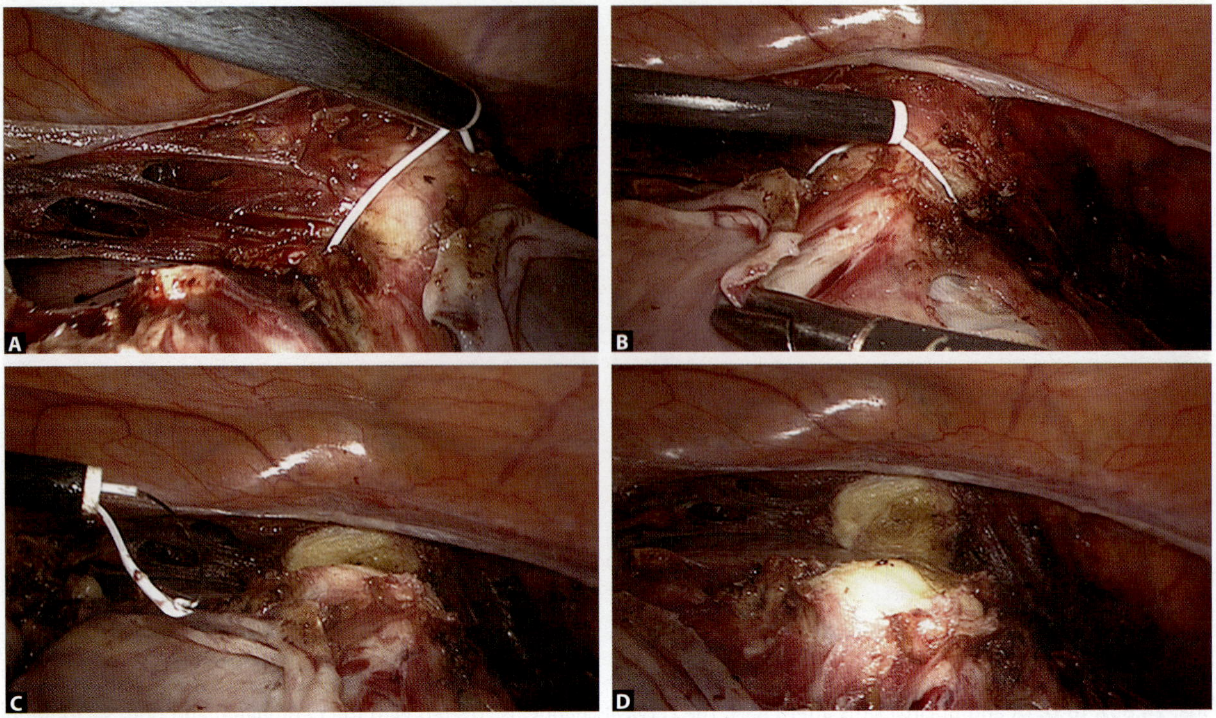

Figs. 24.67A to D: Resection of the uterine corpus from the cervix after placing the cutting loop with the cutting point on the posterior cervix (A and B). Correct placement between the stumps of the uterine artery and above the conjunction of the sacrouterine ligaments is monitored. Dissection of the cervix and uterus is performed (C and D), in this case, LSH by monopolar current only in the non-isolated field. While cutting, the uterine corpus is pulled upward in order to achieve a retrograde conus (B and D).

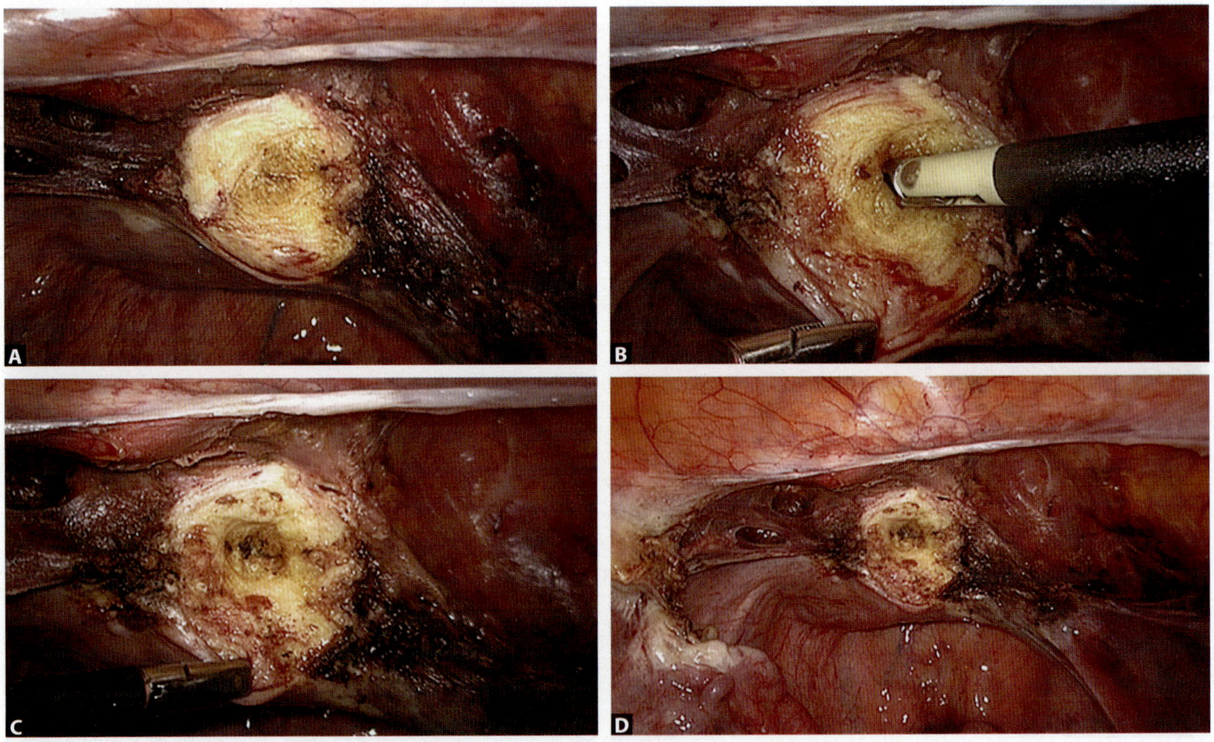

Figs. 24.68A to D: The remaining cervical stump. Extended coagulation should be performed especially in cases of bleeding disorders, adenomyosis of the uterus or endometriosis (A to C); By pulling the uterus upward when cutting the cervix, the resection is performed as an inverse cone (D).

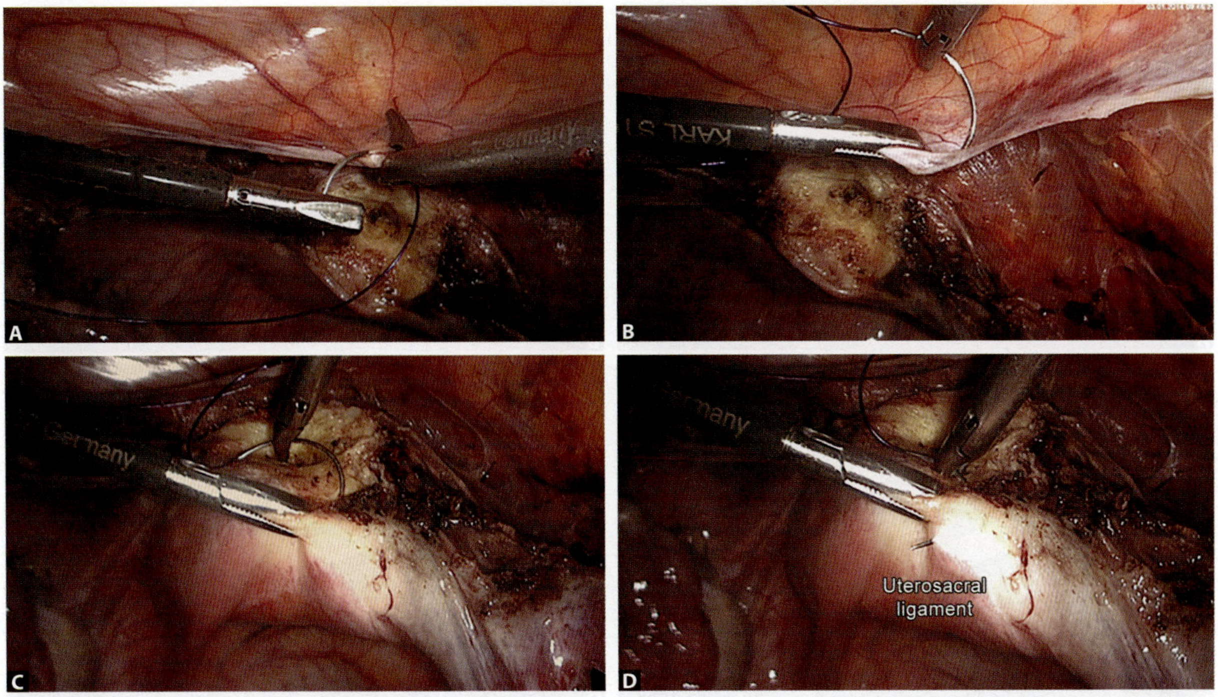

Figs. 24.69A to D: LSH: The conjunction of the sacrouterine ligaments has been omitted; the two ligaments are grasped and included in the suture in order to achieve cervical suspension (A). Connection of the bladder peritoneum to the posterior peritoneum by means of a purse-string suture.

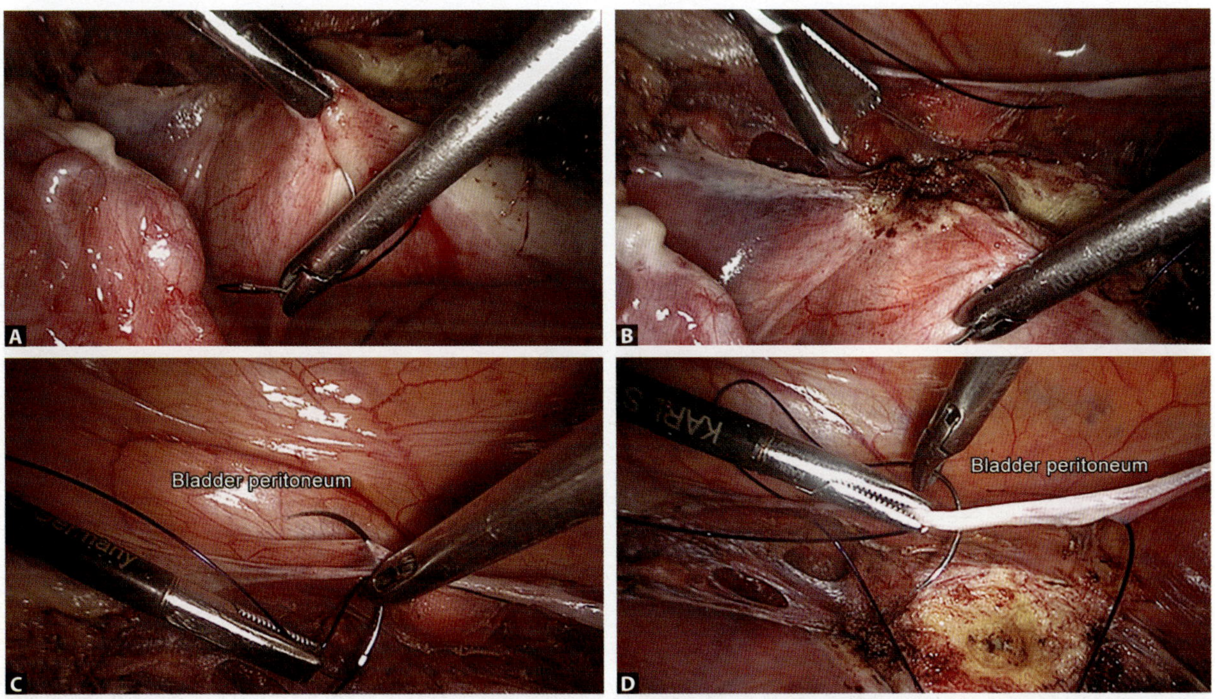

Figs. 24.70A to D: (A and B) The sacrouterine ligaments can be identified and included in the closure of the cervical stump; (C and D) As the bladder has been slightly exposed during the procedure, there is now enough tissue to functionally close the cervical channel.

vagina, the ureter must be visualized by opening the retroperitoneum and ureterolysis performed until the ureter enters the parametria (Figs. 24.79A and B). Alternatively, methylene blue can be injected. If no dye is seen intra-abdominally, severe damage is unlikely. In critical cases the integrity of the ureter

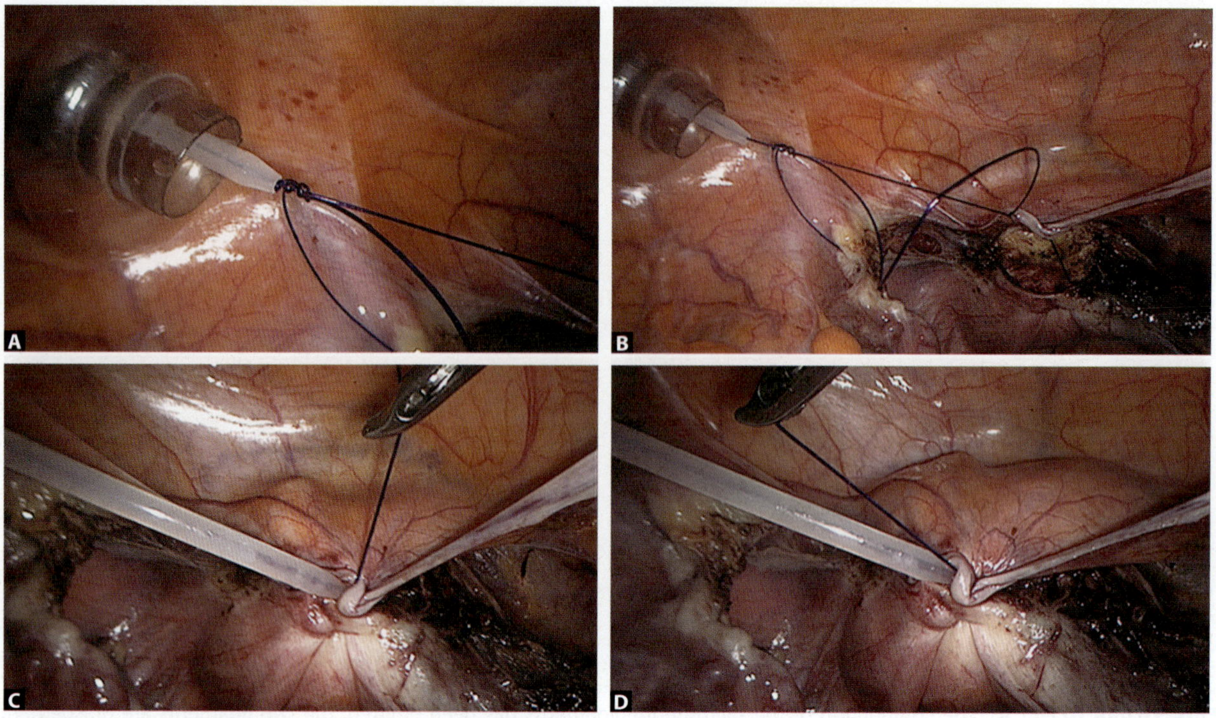

Figs. 24.71A to D: With the extracorporeal knot the peritoneum closes the cervical channel functionally, thus causing cervical suspension. Nevertheless, the sides that have been left out permit draining, if necessary.

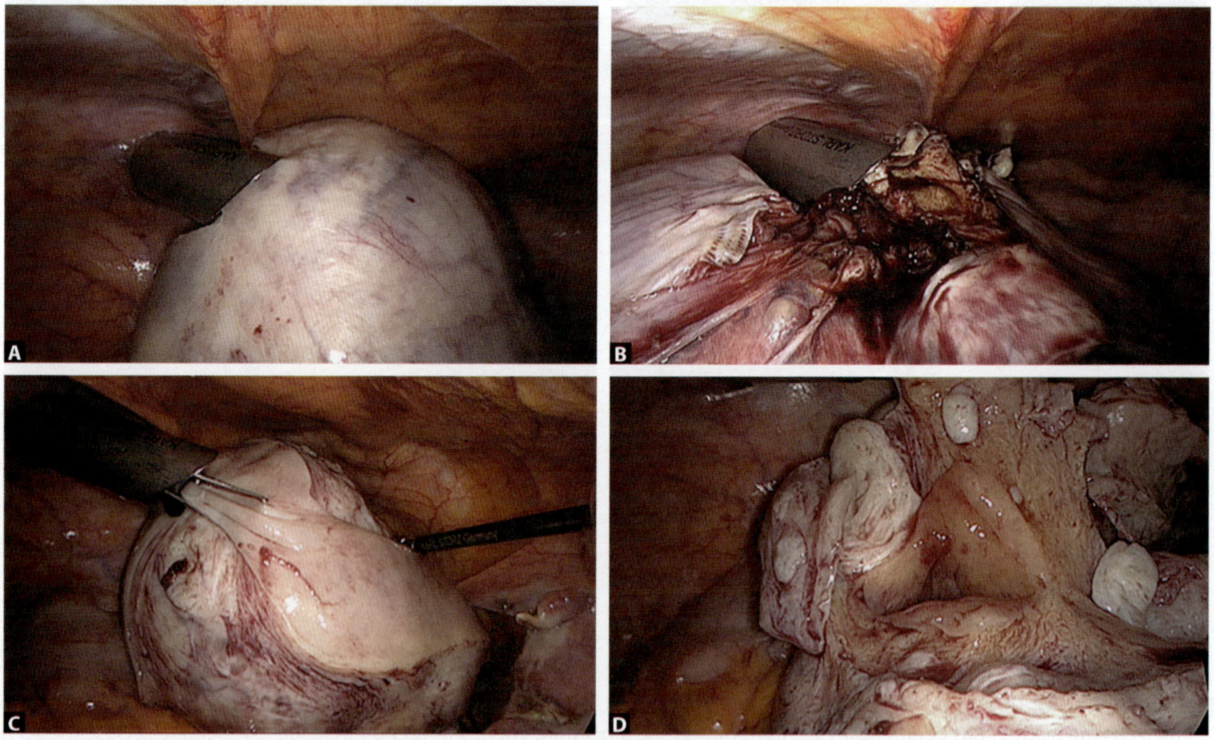

Figs. 24.72A to D: LSH: Morcellation of the myomatous uterus (850 g) under continuous observation of the rotating cutting edge and the protective shield of the morcellator. The protective shield is directed upward towards the abdominal wall in order to avoid severance of the abdominal wall vessels. However, the lower part, especially the small bowel, must be exposed and kept out of the operating area. The surgeon must be patient and avoid cutting into the bowel; the latter is one of the major complications of the LSH procedure.

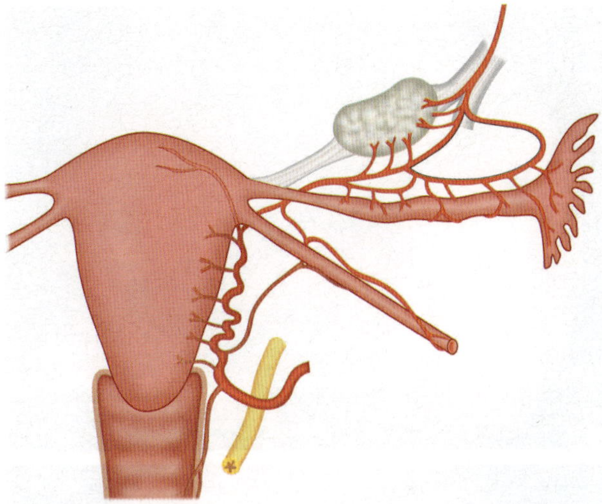

Fig. 24.73: Schematic overview of the typical course of the uterine artery. The safest area to coagulate the uterine artery is the ascending branch close to the uterus. The distance to the ureter is then about 2 cm.

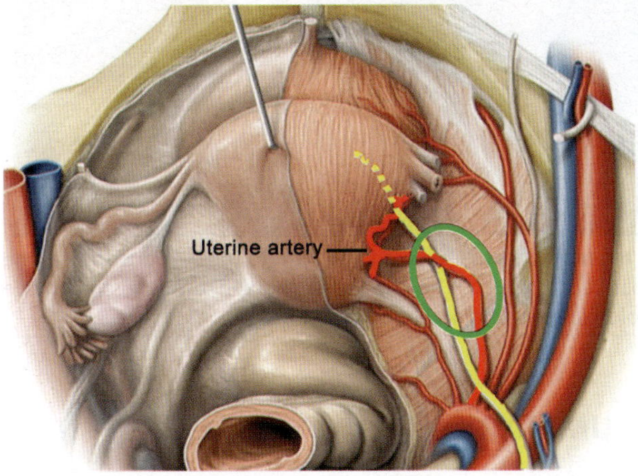

Fig. 24.74: Any uterine pathology will hinder exposure of the lateral uterine wall and the ascending branch of the uterine artery. Furthermore, a radical hysterectomy must include the parametrium and involves a distal resection margin. This might necessitate exposure of the retroperitoneum and localization of the departure of the uterine artery from the internal iliac artery.

can be proven by performing an intravenous pyelogram 2 to 3 days after the operation.

POSTOPERATIVE MANAGEMENT

The urinary catheter is removed; it remains in place only in specific cases. A postoperative cystoscopy is performed in cases of severe endometriosis or adhesions in the upper part of the bladder. Early ambulation a few hours after surgery is good practice. Clear fluids can be ingested 6 h postsurgery, followed by a light diet. Thromboprophylaxis (mechanical and medical) must be used in appropri-

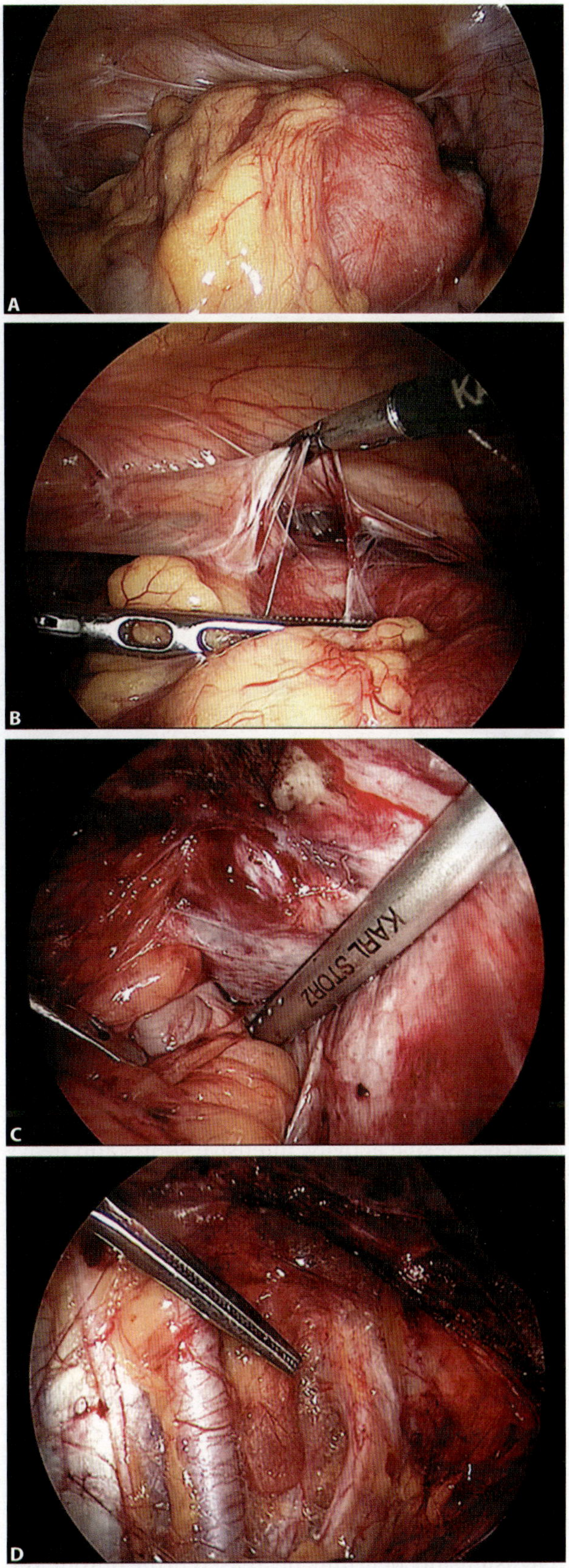

Figs. 24.75A to D: A case of severe adenomyosis of the uterus with adhesions of the bowel (A) and the bladder (B) peritoneum. Access to the lateral aspect of the uterus is blocked (C); A retroperitoneal access is needed (D).

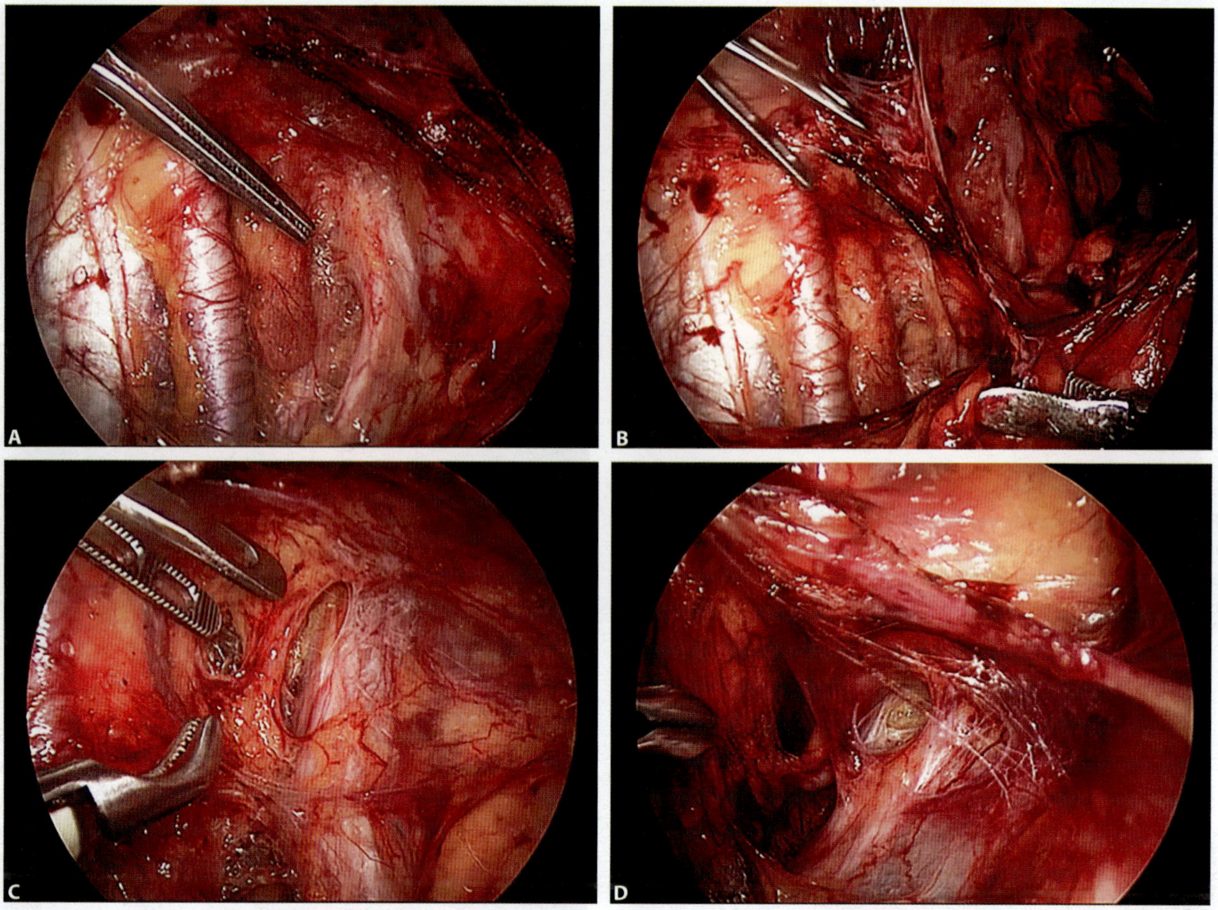

Figs. 24.76A to D: (A) After localization of the external iliac artery, the ureter is usually found adherent to the peritoneum. A large lymph node is found in the intervening area; (B) Opening of the pararectal; and (C) The paravesical fossa; (D) The crossing of the uterine artery is demarcated, the ureter is left in its adventitia to avoid skeletonizing and denudation.

ate cases. The patient can be discharged after 8–12 h. A postoperative ultrasound scan of the renal pelvis should be performed. Ordinary light activities are permitted and the patient may return to work after 4–5 days. Sexual activity, intensive sports and heavy work should be avoided for 6–8 weeks.

The adjuvant medical treatment depends on the patient's intraoperative condition and level of suffering.

ANTICIPATED PROBLEMS

Vital symptoms, pain and temperature must be carefully monitored during the first 8 h. A patient who is discharged early must be given a phone number she may call in case of distress or pain. The insertion of a drain is not necessary. Fever, early pain, abdominal distension, delirium, decreased urine output, the shock index and hypotension must be recognized and attended to immediately, as these may be signs of complications.

SUMMARY

In addition to well-known laparoscopic techniques for endometriosis surgery and hysteroscopic techniques for bleeding disorders, laparoscopic subtotal and total hysterectomy are surgical options for the definitive treatment of adenomyosis of the uterus. The surgical procedure is decided upon jointly by the patient and the doctor. The individual steps described in this chapter help the gynecological surgeon to perform satisfactory surgery for reliable alleviation of the clinical symptoms of adenomyosis in patients who have completed planning their families.

CONCLUSION

- Adenomyosis is a disorder in which endometrial glands and stroma are present within the uterine myometrium. The endometrial glands induce hyperplasia and hypertrophy of the surround-

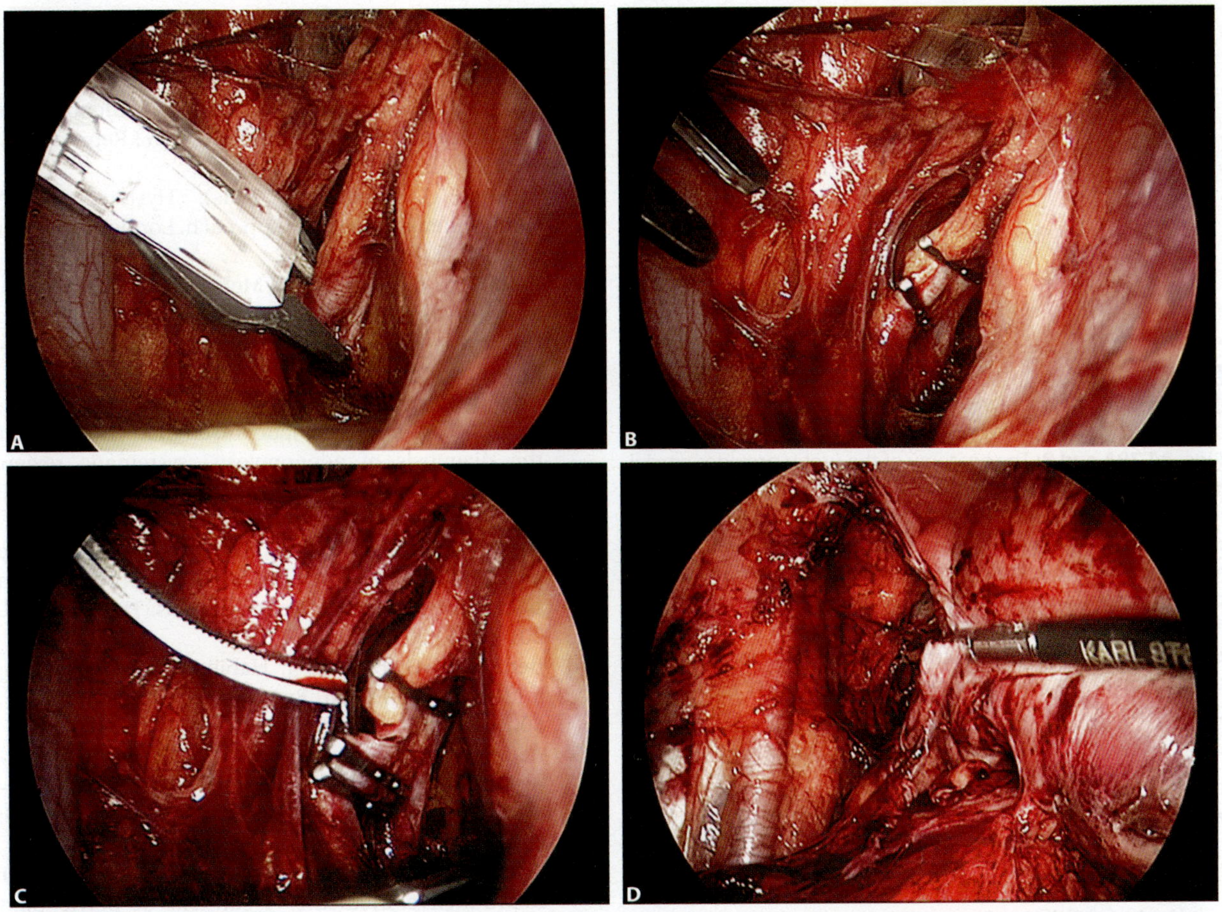

Figs. 24.77A to D: (A and B) Clips can be inserted and the artery can be closed and cut (C); (C) The uterine vein (deep) is just beneath the cut artery; (D) Overview of the exposed region. The uncolored uterus is seen on the right, after closure of both arteries.

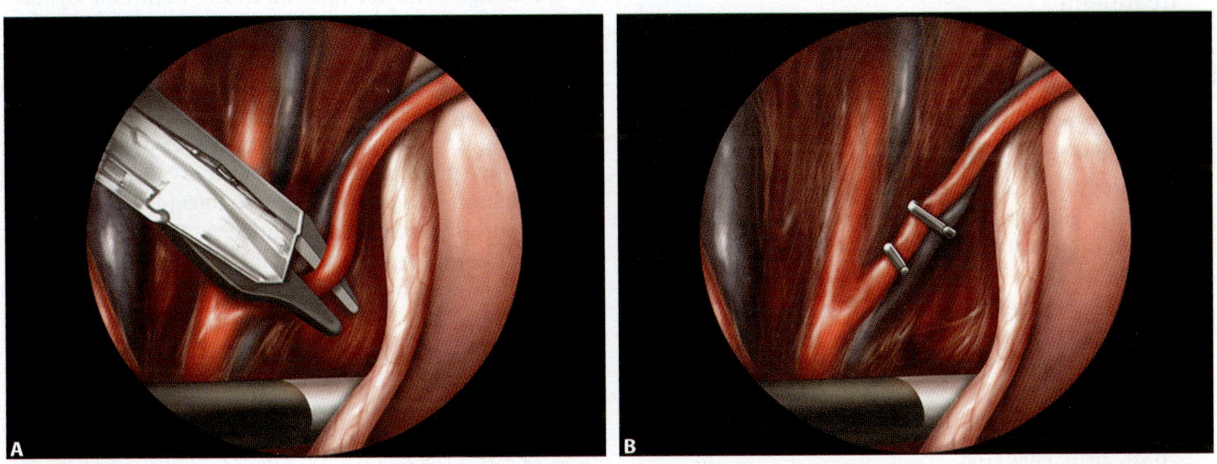

Figs. 24.78A and B: Schematic drawing of the retroperitoneal area where the ureter is undercrossing the uterine artery. The uterine vain is divided into a superficial part and a deep part. Clips can be set after medializing the ureter.

ing myometrium, leading to an enlarged and soft uterus.

- Adenomyosis is marked by menorrhagia and dysmenorrhea; endometriosis is also frequently present.
- The sensitivity and specificity of MRI is high. Nevertheless, vaginal ultrasound is the diagnostic tool of choice. The final diagnosis is established by histological examination of the uterus specimen.

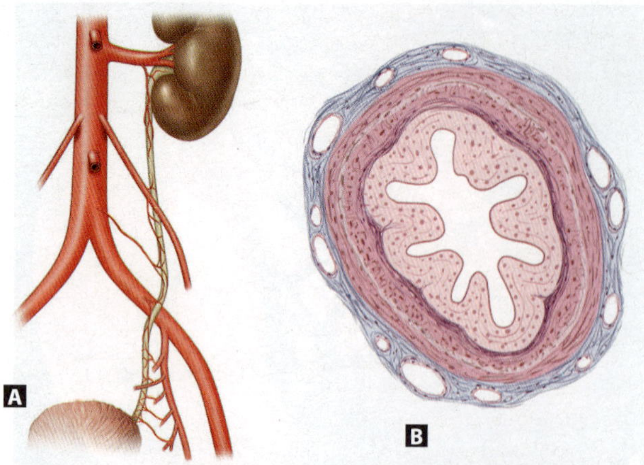

Figs. 24.79A and B: The anatomy of the ureter provides crucial information. (A) Vascular supply is derived from the upper part, including the renal artery, the ovarian artery, and the aorta. In the lower part the ureter is vascularized by the lateral portion, including the iliac vessels and the uterine artery. Blunt dissection causes mild bleeding at the respective location; (B) The histological cross-section shows that the vessels are located in the adventitia. Therefore, electricity or manipulation involving destruction of the adventitia may cause secondary fistula and/or leakage.

- Hysterectomy remains the treatment of choice for women with significant symptoms who have completed planning their families. For those who desire children, the treatment of adenomyosis is similar to that of general endometriosis, which may consist of medical, surgical, or combined treatment.

REFERENCES

1. Olive DL, Schwartz LB. Endometriosis. N Engl J Med. 1993;328(24):1759-69.
2. Kennedy S, Bergquist A, Chapron C, et al. ESHRE guideline for the diagnosis and treatment of endometriosis. Hum Reprod. 2005;20(10):2698-704.
3. Sinaii N, Plumb K, Cotton L, et al. Differences in characteristics among 1,000 women with endometriosis based on extent of disease. Fertil Steril. 2008;89(3):538-45.
4. Engemise S, Gordon C, Konje JC. Endometriosis. BMJ. 2010;340:c2168.
5. Hughes E, Brown J, Collins JJ, et al. Ovulation suppression for endometriosis. Cochrane Database Syst Rev. 2007;18(3):CD000155.
6. Mahmood TA, Templeton A. The impact of treatment on the natural history of endometriosis. Hum Reprod. 1990;5(8):965-70.
7. Templeman C. et al. Adenomyosis and endometriosis in the California Teachers Study. Fertil Steril. 2008;90(2):415-24.
8. Taran FA, Weaver AL, Coddington CC, et al. Understanding adenomyosis: a case control study. Fertil Steril. 2010;94(4):1223-8.
9. Garavaglia E, Audrey S, Annalisa I, et al. Adenomyosis and its impact on women fertility. Iran J Reprod Med. 2015;13(6):327-36.
10. Alkatout I, Mettler L (Eds). Hysterectomy—A Comprehensive Surgical Approach. London; Springer Science; 2016.
11. Reinhold, C, Tafazoli F, Mehio A, et al. Uterine adenomyosis: endovaginal US and MR imaging features with histopathologic correlation. Radiographics. 1999;19(Suppl 1 Special issue):S147-60.
12. Champaneria R, Abedin P, Daniels J, et al. Ultrasound scan and magnetic resonance imaging for the diagnosis of adenomyosis: systematic review comparing test accuracy. Acta Obstet Gynecol Scand. 2010;89(11):1374-84.
13. Vercellini P, Consonni D, Dridi D, et al. Uterine adenomyosis and in vitro fertilization outcome: a systematic review and meta-analysis. Hum Reprod. 2014;29(5):964-77.
14. Benagiano G, Brosens I, Habiba M. Adenomyosis: a life-cycle approach. Reprod Biomed Online. 2015;30(3):220-32.
15. Alkatout I, Egberts JH, Mettler L, et al. [Interdisciplinary diagnosis and treatment of deep infiltrating endometriosis.]. Zentralbl Chir. 2015;141(6);630-8.
16. Practice Committee of American Society for Reproductive Medicine. Treatment of pelvic pain associated with endometriosis. Fertil Steril. 2008;90(5 Suppl):S260-9.
17. Schindler AE. Kombiniertes chirurgisch-hormonelles Management der Endometriose. Zentralbl Gynakol. 1999;121(7):325-9.
18. Zupi E, Marconi D, Sbracia M, et al. Add-back therapy in the treatment of endometriosis-associated pain. Fertil Steril. 2004;82(5):1303-8.
19. Wong CL, Farquar C, Roberts H, et al. Oral contraceptive pill as treatment for primary dysmenorrhoea. Cochrane Database Syst Rev. 2009;(4):CD002120.
20. Moore J, Kennedy S, Prentice A. Modern combined oral contraceptives for pain associated with endometriosis. Cochrane Database Syst Rev. 2000;(2):CD001019.
21. Sheng J, Zhang WY, Zhang JP, et al. The LNG-IUS study on adenomyosis: a 3-year follow-up study on the efficacy and side effects of the use of levonorgestrel intrauterine system for the treatment of dysmenorrhea associated with adenomyosis. Contraception. 2009;79(3):189-93.
22. Mousa NA, Bedaiwy MA, Casper RF. Aromatase inhibitors in the treatment of severe endometriosis. Obstet Gynecol. 2007;109(6):1421-3.
23. Ferrero S, Camerini G, Seracchioli R, et al. Letrozole combined with norethisterone acetate compared with norethisterone acetate alone in the treatment of pain symptoms caused by endometriosis. Hum Reprod. 2009;24(12):3033-41.

24. Alkatout I, et al. Die Rolle der Angiogenese und seiner Inhibitoren in der Gynäkologie. Der Gynäkologe. 2012.
25. Clement PB. The pathology of endometriosis: a survey of the many faces of a common disease emphasizing diagnostic pitfalls and unusual and newly appreciated aspects. Adv Anat Pathol. 2007;14(4):241-60.
26. Stegmann BJ, Sinali N, Liu S, et al. Using location, color, size, and depth to characterize and identify endometriosis lesions in a cohort of 133 women. Fertil Steril. 2008;89(6):1632-6.
27. Wykes CB, Clark TJ, Khan KS. Accuracy of laparoscopy in the diagnosis of endometriosis: a systematic quantitative review. BJOG. 2004;111(11):1204-12.
28. Buchweitz O, Poel T, Dierich K, et al. The diagnostic dilemma of minimal and mild endometriosis under routine conditions. J Am Assoc Gynecol Laparosc. 2003;10(1):85-9.
29. Christensen B, Freie HM, Schindler AE. [Endometriosis—diagnosis and therapy. Results of a current survey of 6,700 gynecologists]. Geburtshilfe Frauenheilkd. 1995;55(12):674-9.
30. Mettler L, Schollmeyer T, Alkatout I. Adhesions during and after surgical procedures, their prevention and impact on women's health. Womens Health (Lond Engl). 2012;8(5):495-8.
31. Alkatout I, Schollmeyer T, Hawaldar NA, et al. Principles and safety measures of electrosurgery in laparoscopy. JSLS. 2012;16(1):130-9.
32. Abbott J, Hawe J, Hunter D, et al. Laparoscopic excision of endometriosis: a randomized, placebo-controlled trial. Fertil Steril. 2004;82(4):878-84.
33. Healey M, Ang WC, Cheng C. Surgical treatment of endometriosis: a prospective randomized double-blind trial comparing excision and ablation. Fertil Steril. 2010;94(7):2536-40.
34. Jacobson TZ, Barlow DH, Garry R, et al. Laparoscopic surgery for pelvic pain associated with endometriosis. Cochrane Database Syst Rev. 2001;(4):CD001300.
35. Crosignani PG, Vercellini P, Biffignandi F, et al. Laparoscopy versus laparotomy in conservative surgical treatment for severe endometriosis. Fertil Steril. 1996;66(5):706-11.
36. Taylor E. Williams C. Surgical treatment of endometriosis: location and patterns of disease at reoperation. Fertil Steril. 2010;93(1):57-61.
37. Yeung PP, Jr, Shwayder J, Pasic RP. Laparoscopic management of endometriosis: comprehensive review of best evidence. J Minim Invasive Gynecol. 2009;16(3):269-81.
38. Alkatout I, Mettler L, Beteta C, et al. Combined surgical and hormone therapy for endometriosis is the most effective treatment: prospective, randomized, controlled trial. J Minim Invasive Gynecol. 2013; 20(4):473-81.
39. Osada H, Silber S, Kakinuma T, et al. Surgical procedure to conserve the uterus for future pregnancy in patients suffering from massive adenomyosis. Reprod Biomed Online. 2011;22(1):94-9.
40. Tsui KH, Lee FK, Seow KM, et al. Conservative surgical treatment of adenomyosis to improve fertility: controversial values, indications, complications, and pregnancy outcomes. Taiwan J Obstet Gynecol. 2015;54(6):635-40.
41. Kovac SR. Route of hysterectomy: an evidence-based approach. Clin Obstet Gynecol. 2014;57(1): 58-71.
42. Schollmeyer T, Elessawy M, Chastamouratidhs B, et al. Hysterectomy trends over a 9-year period in an endoscopic teaching center. Int J Gynaecol Obstet. 2014;126(1):45-9.
43. Lefebvre G, Allaire C, Jeffery J, et al. SOGC clinical guidelines. Hysterectomy. J Obstet Gynaecol Can. 2002;24(1):37-61; quiz 74-6.
44. Stang A, Merrill RM, Kuss O. Hysterectomy in Germany: a DRG-based nationwide analysis, 2005-2006. Dtsch Arztebl Int. 2011;108(30):508-14.
45. Brummer TH, Seppala TT, Harkki PS. National learning curve for laparoscopic hysterectomy and trends in hysterectomy in Finland 2000-2005. Hum Reprod. 2008;23(4):840-5.
46. Prevention, C.f.D.C.a., Women's Reproductive health: Hysterectomy Fact Sheet, D.o.R. Health, Editor. 2009: 1600 Clifton Rd. Atlanta, GA 30333, USA.
47. Hanstede MM, Burger MJ, Timmermans A, et al. Regional and temporal variation in hysterectomy rates and surgical routes for benign diseases in the Netherlands. Acta Obstet Gynecol Scand. 2012;91(2): 220-5.
48. Alkatout I, Bojahr B, Dittmann L, et al. Precarious preoperative diagnostics and hints for the laparoscopic excision of uterine adenomatoid tumors: two exemplary cases and literature review. Fertil Steril. 2011;95(3):119.e5-8.
49. Nieboer TE, Johnson N, Lethaby A, et al. Surgical approach to hysterectomy for benign gynaecological disease. Cochrane Database Syst Rev. 2009; (3):CD003677.
50. Lethaby A, Ivanova V, Johnson NP. Total versus subtotal hysterectomy for benign gynaecological conditions. Cochrane Database Syst Rev. 2006;(2):CD004993.
51. Thakar R, Ayers S, Clarkson P, et al. Outcomes after total versus subtotal abdominal hysterectomy. N Engl J Med. 2002;347(17):1318-25.
52. Gorlero F, Lijoi D, Biamonti M, et al. Hysterectomy and women satisfaction: total versus subtotal technique. Arch Gynecol Obstet. 2008;278(5):405-10.
53. Roovers JP, van der Bom JG, van der Vaart CH, et al. Hysterectomy and sexual wellbeing: prospective observational study of vaginal hysterectomy, subtotal abdominal hysterectomy, and total abdominal hysterectomy. BMJ. 2003;327(7418):774-8.
54. Gimbel H. Total or subtotal hysterectomy for benign uterine diseases? A meta-analysis. Acta Obstet Gynecol Scand. 2007;86(2):133-44.
55. Ascher-Walsh CJ, Tu JL, Du Y, et al. Location of adenomyosis in total hysterectomy specimens. J Am Assoc Gynecol Laparosc. 2003;10(3):360-2.

56. Sarmini OR, Lefholz K, Froeschke HP. A comparison of laparoscopic supracervical hysterectomy and total abdominal hysterectomy outcomes. J Minim Invasive Gynecol. 2005;12(2):121-4.
57. Alkatout I. [Communicative and ethical aspects of physician-patient relationship in extreme situations]. Wien Med Wochenschr. 2015;165(23-24):491-8.
58. Reich H. Laparoscopic oophorectomy and salpingo-oophorectomy in the treatment of benign tubo-ovarian disease. Int J Fertil. 1987;32(3):233-6.
59. Mettler L, Semm K, Lehmann-Willenbrock L, et al. Comparative evaluation of classical intrafascial-supracervical hysterectomy (CISH) with transuterine mucosal resection as performed by pelviscopy and laparotomy—our first 200 cases. Surg Endosc. 1995; 9(4):418-24.
60. Semm K. Hysterectomy via laparotomy or pelviscopy. A new CASH method without colpotomy. Geburtshilfe Frauenheilkd. 1991;51(12):996-1003.
61. Hohl MK, Hauser N. Safe total intrafascial laparoscopic (TAIL) hysterectomy: a prospective cohort study. Gynecol Surg. 2010;7(3):231-9.
62. Schüssler B, Scheidel P, Hohl MK. Hysterektomie Update. Frauenheilkunde aktuell, 2008;3:4-12.
63. Veress J. Neues Instrument zur Ausführung von Brust- und Bauchpunktionen und Pneumothoraxbehandlung. Deutsche medizinische Wochenschrift, 1938;64:1480-1.
64. Alkatout I, Mettler L, Maass N, et al. Abdominal anatomy in the context of port placement and trocars. J Turk Ger Gynecol Assoc. 2015;16(4): 241-51.
65. Altman D, Falconer C, Cnattinguis S, et al. Pelvic organ prolapse surgery following hysterectomy on benign indications. Am J Obstet Gynecol. 2008;198(5): 572.e1-6.
66. Thompson JD, Warshaw J. Hysterectomy. In: Rock JA, Thompson, JD (Eds). Te Linde's Operative Gynecology. Philadelphia, PA: Lippincott Raven; 1996. p. 771-854.
67. van Herendael B. Strategies to prevent vaginal vault descent during hysterectomy. In: Mettler L (Ed). Manual of New Hysterectomy Techniques. New Delhi: Jaypee Brothers Medical Publishers; 2007. p. 82-5.
68. Hur HC, Guido RS, Mansuria SM, et al. Incidence and patient characteristics of vaginal cuff dehiscence after different modes of hysterectomies. J Minim Invasive Gynecol. 2007;14(3):311-7.

Surgical Aspects and Therapeutic Modalities of Deep Infiltrating Diagnosis

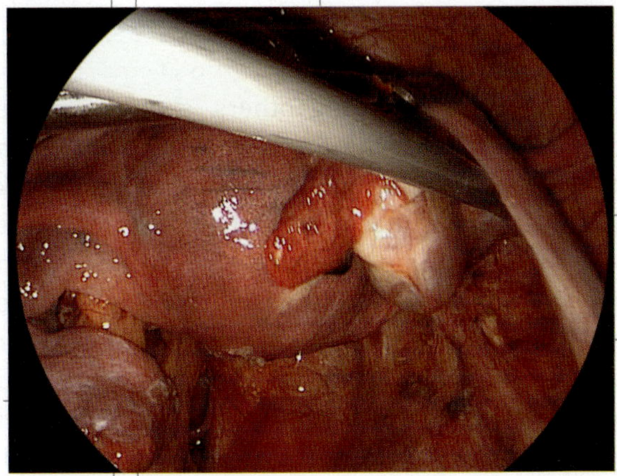

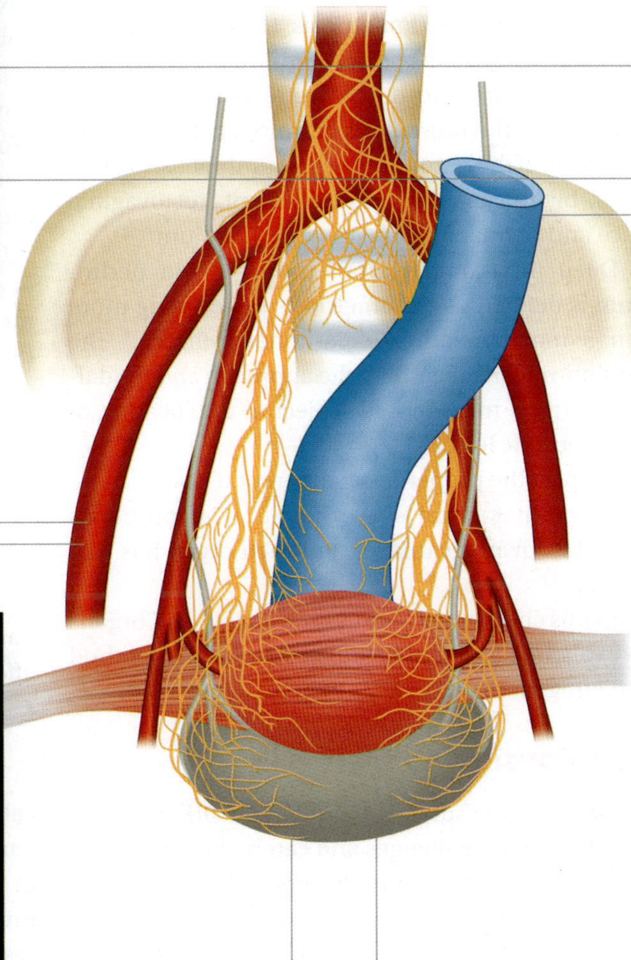

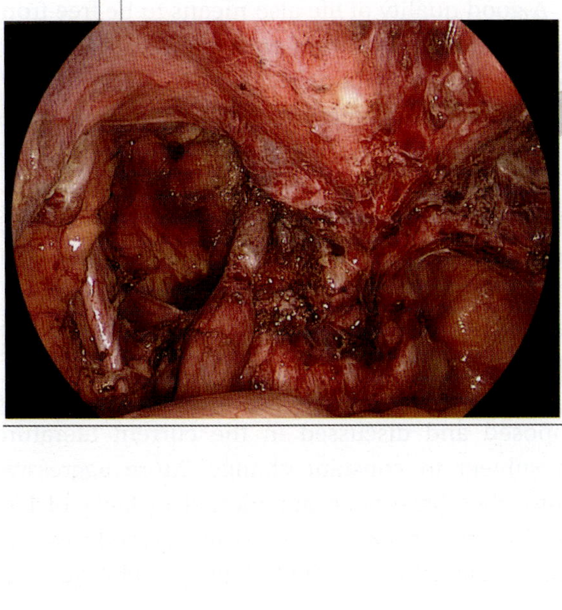

Chapter 25

Surgical Aspects and Therapeutic Modalities of Deep Infiltrating Diagnosis

Ingo von Leffern

INTRODUCTION

Deep infiltrating endometriosis (DIE) means that more than one tissue has been infiltrated by disease, e.g., peritoneum and deeper retroperitoneal structures such as the muscularis or mucosa of the bowel, fatty tissue of the retroperitoneum, umbilicus, nerves, ureter, bladder, sacrouterine ligament, rectovaginal space and vagina, diaphragm or pericardium.

Deep infiltrating endometriosis of the peritoneum is defined as endometriosis penetrating more than 5 mm beneath the peritoneal surface.[1] The decision-making regarding the approach and modality of surgical treatment is subject to the location of endometriotic lesions.

- Respect the properties of different tissues!
- Every anatomical space has its own problems and its own advantages and each organ has that too!

In this chapter, various tissues, spaces and organs are explained and illustrated along with the method of treating them.

Basic Considerations

Considering that surgical treatment of DIE can pose some technical challenges and can be fraught with a multitude of potential complications,[2,3] the first question to be addressed is:

- Why do we opt for a surgical approach and what is the goal to be achieved?

The criteria to be applied when defining the major therapeutic objective are based on quality of life, severity, duration and frequency of symptoms, the patient's individual needs and the anticipated risk of severe complications.

Quality of life, among others, should include sexual function and its level of satisfaction. In a comparative study conducted by U. van den Broeck et al.[3] it was shown, that at 6 months after surgery, the bowel resection group versus the no-bowel-resection group was found to have lower mean levels of the Beck Depression Inventory (BDI) (*P*, 0.05), a lower incidence of "pain during sexual intercourse" and "orgasm problems" (*P*, 0.05) and a lower proportion of patients with severe orgasm problems (*P*, 0.05), measured with the Short Sexual Functioning Scale (SSFS).

These data have demonstrated that radical but fertility-sparing surgery for the treatment of endometriosis—with or without bowel resection—results in comparable and good psychological outcomes concerning depression levels, relationship, satisfaction and sexual function.

A good quality of life also means to be free from pain. Radical resection of endometriosis can be an effective treatment for pelvic pain.[4]

- Nevertheless, sometimes less is more, or in other words, less is even better!

There are two options available for the surgical treatment of bowel or bladder endometriosis: a conservative approach (nodule excision with bowel or bladder shaving and preservation of the organ(s) involved) and a radical approach (segmental bowel resection or partial cystectomy).[5]

It is well known that surgical treatment options proposed and discussed in the current literature are subject to constant change. More aggressive approaches have been abandoned in favor of less invasive tissue-sparing surgical procedures. In recent years, the so-called shaving technique has increasingly gained in acceptance and is now frequently used in those cases where resection was proposed as first-line option for treating endometriosis involving the bowel and/or bladder. It has now become more common for surgeons to even consider medical treatment as an alternative option suited to achieve an effective resolution of the symptoms associated with the disease.[5]

Endometriosis, especially in its more severe form, needs to be treated by highly skilled surgeons capable of coping with the challenges of difficult procedures in an accurate manner. Surgery must be performed by surgeons who are dedicated to endometriosis. It is mandatory that complete treatment be achieved while respecting anatomical integrity and reducing the risk of iatrogenic fertility impairment.

Unlike most other operative procedures, the surgical treatment of DIE should be based on a collaborative multidisciplinary approach. In this way, patients are offered the optimal treatment that should be provided by a team of highly skilled experts.

In patients who wish to have children, a well-adapted treatment strategy should be chosen. In order to preserve integrity of the reproductive organs, in these cases, surgery has to be accomplished in a more conservative and extremely cautious way, that is based on a staged approach in order to prevent postoperative adhesion formation.

In these special cases, we perform a second-look laparoscopy 6 to 8 weeks after primary surgery and carry out adhesiolysis, chromopertubation and prophylaxis for prevention of recurrent adhesions.

Figures 25.1A and B shows the operative situs after primary and secondary surgery in a woman who became pregnant within about 6 months after second-look surgery.

It must be kept in mind that DIE is a benign disease. There is no scientific evidence that 100% surgical removal of disease should be considered the major goal to be achieved in any case.

- Is there a need for complete resection?

Moreover, it is virtually impossible to identify and remove every single endometriosis cell. In a large number of cases lymph nodes are found to harbor endometriotic lesions.[6] To the best of my knowledge these lesions do not cause any disorders or pain, which is why the author advises against attempting a systematic removal.

It is still unclear whether nodules of deep infiltrating endometriosis that do not cause pain should in fact be excised. Another clinical question yet to be answered is whether remnants of endometriosis are a possible cause of relapse.

Conversely, however, it is indisputable that almost complete removal should be attempted to the extent feasible if the patient presents with symptomatic endometriosis. Infertility can be one of these symptoms.

Lacking clear data, the author recommends eradication of visible endometriotic lesions; however, care should be taken in the area of the intestine. The rate of severe complications has led us to exercise due restraint at this site during radical surgery. Occasionally, the need may arise that endometriosis lesions are shaved off the bowel leaving behind a layer of fibrosis that encloses the nodules.

Taking into account that evidence of recurrent disease is most frequently found in the posterior fornix of the vagina[7] and considering that the vaginal cuff commonly heals well, it is important to ensure a complete resection in this region.

SURGICAL APPROACHES AND INSTRUMENTS

- A minimally invasive, laparoscopic approach should be selected, whenever possible

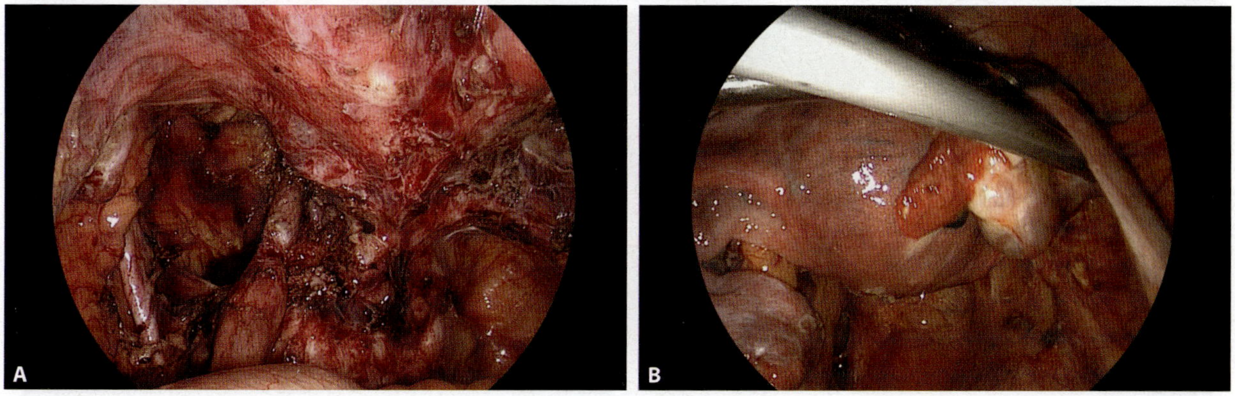

Figs. 25.1A and B: (A) Situs after primary surgery; (B) Situs at second-look surgery.

In the hands of experts, use of the laparoscopic route is less invasive and enables a targeted and accurate surgical treatment of deep infiltrating endometriosis.

Do not hesitate to use an open access, if laparoscopy is not feasible or if the intraoperative situation suggests that conversion to laparotomy seems to be a better option.

Ovariopexy and Hysteropexy

To facilitate laparoscopic access to rectum, pouch of Douglas or to the rectovaginal space, a uterine manipulator (e.g., Valtchev adapter) can be of great help.

From the author's perspective, the use of a temporary ventral uteropexy[8] with a thick, monofilament suture has also proven helpful. The thread is passed through the abdominal wall with a long, straight needle, then guided through the uterine fundus and again withdrawn through the abdominal wall, where the threads are held with a Kocher clamp.

The temporary uteropexy allows a very effective elevation of the uterus without the need for fixing cervix or vagina. This option offers the advantage that no further assistance is needed as is the case with a uterine manipulator.

The same method can also be used for temporary suspension of ovaries for keeping them out of the surgical site. This measure is used by some surgeons for adhesion prevention and involves that the stitches are left in situ for 48–72 h after surgery. So far, there is no authoritative evidence supporting the efficiency of this method in preventing the formation of adhesions. Derived from anecdotal experience of a few surgeons only nonrepresentative samples of cases have been reported so far. Figures 25.2A to H show the technique of ventrolateral ovariopexy.

Instruments

The vast number of different laparoscopic instruments for the surgical treatment of deep infiltrating endometriosis makes it impossible to mention all of them in this chapter.

In the following, the author focuses on the monopolar hook/monopolar needle electrode (Fig. 25.3), an instrument that has always been the subject of controversy among physicians. It is loved by some surgeons and totally rejected by others.

The advantage of this instrument lies in the fact that it allows the surgeon to concurrently cut and

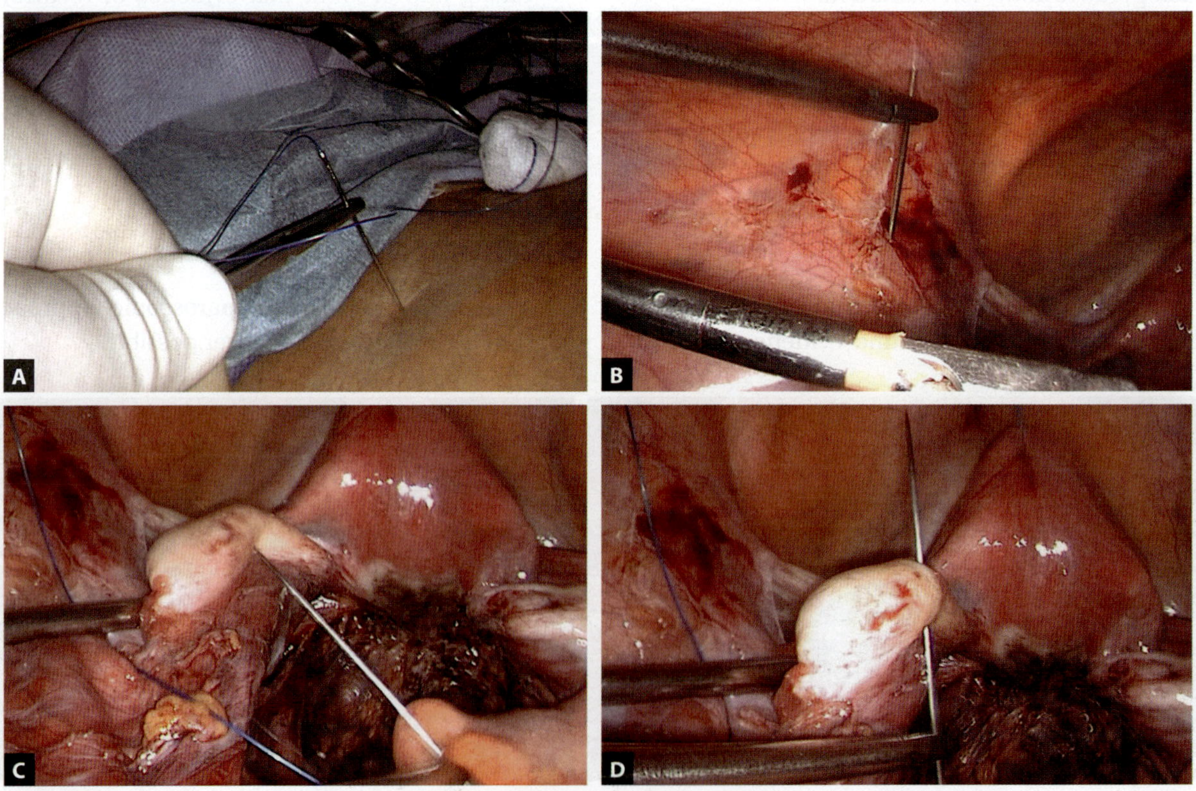

Figs. 25.2A to D

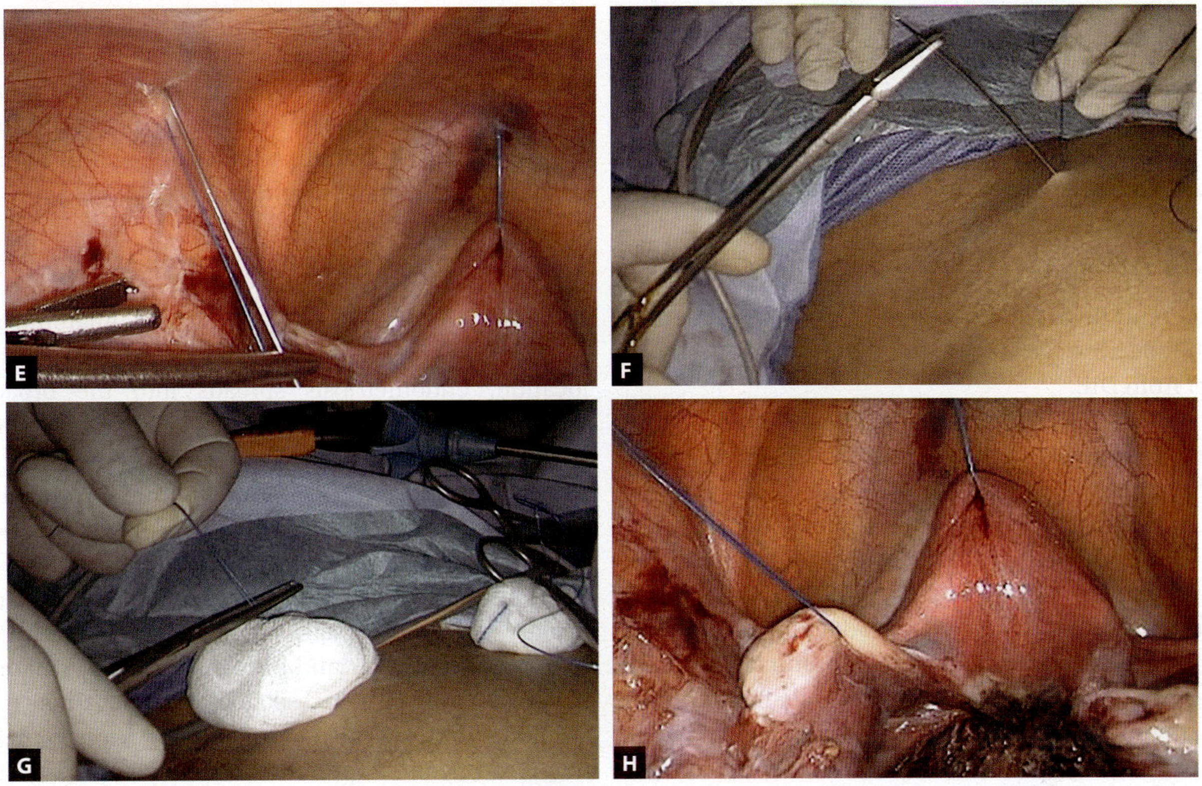

Figs. 25.2E to H

Figs. 25.2A to H: (A) The needle is passed through the abdominal wall; (B) The needle is grasped from inside the abdomen; (C) The needle is placed at the ovary; (D) The needle is passed through the ovary; (E) The needle is passed through the abdomen from inside; (F) Pulling out the thread; (G) Both ends of the suture are held by a Kocher clamp; (H) Final aspect following completion of suspension of the uterus and left ovary.

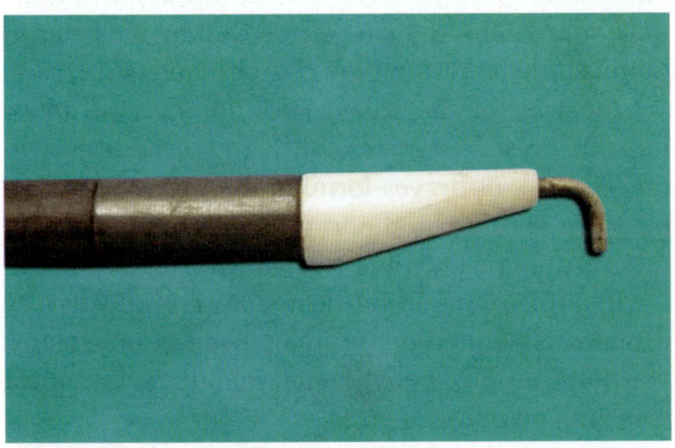

Fig. 25.3: Monopolar hook with a ceramic tip.

coagulate, to cut without coagulation—provided the energy device is adjusted to pure cutting mode, and to cut and coagulate very precisely and millimeter by millimeter—provided an interrupted cutting current is used with very short intervals.

In high-frequency electrosurgery, a cutting current is used to cut through tissue almost without necrosis and without inducing collateral coagulation, offering similar features as those made advantage of in laser surgery.

Another advantage of the monopolar hook/needle is that you can cut without exerting pressure on the tissue. To cut and coagulate, the electrode only has to be in near contact with the target tissue. When using "spray coagulation mode," no contact between the instrument tip and the tissue to be treated is needed at all.

The mass of the electrode is so minimal that it cools immediately in fractions of a second. Iatrogenic burns to adjacent tissue, upon inadvertent contact after shutdown of the current, do not occur.

However, a few disadvantages of monopolar electrodes should also be mentioned. First, monopolar current may spread well beyond the target site into tissue. The direction, in which it spreads, cannot be controlled by the surgeon and is subject to the varying electric conductivity of different tissues.

The use of monopolar current also carries the risk of stimulating distant nerves, which may result in spontaneous muscle jerks or twitches of the body. This is particularly risky while operating close to large blood vessels.

- *Caveat*: Monopolar current must not be used near any nerves since this can result in iatrogenic damage!

Provided these rules are adhered to, the instrument is ideally suited for an atraumatic, quick and in-layer operation. Furthermore, it is very inexpensive.

DIE AND FERTILITY

Endometriosis affects about 10–15% of women of childbearing age and 20% of these patients even suffer from DIE.

Subfertility is a well-known and common problem in patients with endometriosis. Unfortunately, the underlying etiopathological mechanisms of the disease are not yet completely understood.

In endometriosis patients, the management of infertility encompasses surgery, medical treatment and the use of assisted reproduction techniques. In terms of infertility, the use of minimally invasive techniques has been shown to provide better results than those yielded by open surgery approaches.

Based on the current literature, the use of laparoscopic resection techniques has demonstrated a benefit in the treatment of both minimal and moderate endometriosis. In cases of severe endometriosis, data currently available are inadequate. Considering that an extensive surgical intervention is fraught with significant risks, it would not be reasonable to undertake this option in cases where the major objective of treatment is geared toward improving the patient's fertility status.[9]

On the other hand, a literature review by Cohen et al.[10] demonstrated that surgery alone offers a highly spontaneous pregnancy rate in cases of DIE without bowel involvement.

For those women with bowel involvement, the low spontaneous and relatively high overall pregnancy rate suggests that a benefit can be achieved by a combination of surgery and medically assisted reproduction (MAR).

Stepniewska et al.[11] observed three groups of patients for about 4 years after surgery and analyzed the monthly fecundity rate (MFR) of each group. Those patients who underwent surgery for endometriosis with colorectal segmental resection showed a MFR of 2.3%. In those patients with evidence of bowel endometriosis subjected to endometriosis removal, but without bowel resection, a MFR of only 0.84% was revealed. Finally, in the group of patients with DIE, but without any bowel involvement, the MFR was 3.95%. The differences were significant.

Concordant with the results and conclusions of Cohen et al.,[10] it was established that to improve fertility, the affected bowel should better be removed. In a nutshell, DIE of the bowel seems to be associated with a decrease in fertility, which can be partly compensated by adequate surgical treatment.

DIE OF SACROUTERINE LIGAMENT

Sacrouterine ligament is among the anatomical regions most frequently involved by DIE. From this location, endometriosis spreads into the broad ligament, to rectovaginal space, to the pararectal space and to the area surrounding the ureter.

Radical resection of the sacrouterine ligament is complicated by proximity of the ureter, bowel and the nerves of the pelvic plexus. Integrity of these nerves must be preserved. Iatrogenic injury may result in urinary dysfunction and cannot be repaired.[12,13] Atony of the bladder and problems with defecation may result from radical resection of both ligaments.

Refractory neurogenic bladder atony may entail the need for permanent self-catheterization. This serious complication can severely impair the patient's quality of life to a degree exceeding that of endometriosis itself.

Bladder dysfunction and neurogenic atony may occur even years after primary surgery.[14] In the immediate postoperative phase, these symptoms may sometimes remain occult leading to delayed notification of the doctor in charge of follow-up care.

Integrity of the tissue surrounding the ureter must be preserved meticulously to prevent injury to the network of nerves forming the pelvic plexus! If possible, leave behind part of the sacrouterine ligament and some fatty tissue beside the rectum.

If both sacrouterine ligaments are affected by disease, it is sometimes prudent to leave some endometriotic lesions behind and refrain from radical resection on one side.[15]

The vesical plexus is part of the sacral plexus and composed of very delicate nerves that can be difficult to locate. Sometimes, it may be necessary to first trace the larger portions of the pelvic plexus, the sacral roots (Figs. 25.4 and 25.5A) and then follow them caudally to spot the thin branches of the vesical plexus. To identify the sacral roots, dissection is initiated medial to the ureter and lateral to the sacrouterine ligament (Fig. 25.5B).

In the broad ligament, it should be possible to visualize small nerve fibers (Fig. 25.5C) in the pars nervosa inferior to the pars vascularis, which is superior

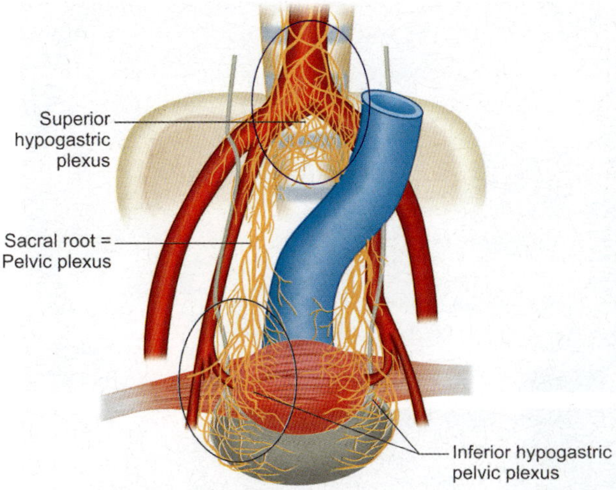

Fig. 25.4: Schematic representation of the pelvic plexus and hypogastric plexus.

to the deep uterine vein. Accordingly, the deep uterine vein constitutes the boundary between pars vascularis and pars nervosa of the broad uterine ligament.

DIE INVOLVING NERVES

Occasionally, nerves are affected by endometriosis, which may lead to muscular dysfunction if motor nerves are involved. Given the involvement of sensory nerves, pain symptoms or sensory discomfort may result from irritation of those nerves.

Cyclical sciatica from intraneural endometriosis of sciatic nerve has been reported[16] as well as cases of DIE affecting a multitude of various other nerves. The literature provides some anecdotal evidence of perineural spread of endometriosis to the lumbosacral plexus along the autonomic nerves and then distally to the sciatic nerve and proximally to the spinal nerves.

Endometriosis may also affect femoral nerves[17] as well as the nerves of the pelvic side wall such as the obturator nerve (Fig. 25.6). Shown in this Figure 25.6 is the obturator nerve after dissection of DIE reaching from the peritoneum to the iliac bone. Intrinsic endometriosis of the ureter was noticeable as well as infiltration of the periosteal layer of the iliac bone, but without affecting the nerve.

As shown in Figure 25.6, endometriosis-associated compression of the obturator nerve was treated by neurolysis carried out in layers.

Deep retroperitoneal nerves can be involved without any prominent signs of DIE visible on the peritoneum. As shown in Figure 25.7A, there is only a small fibrous retraction noticeable on the peritoneum

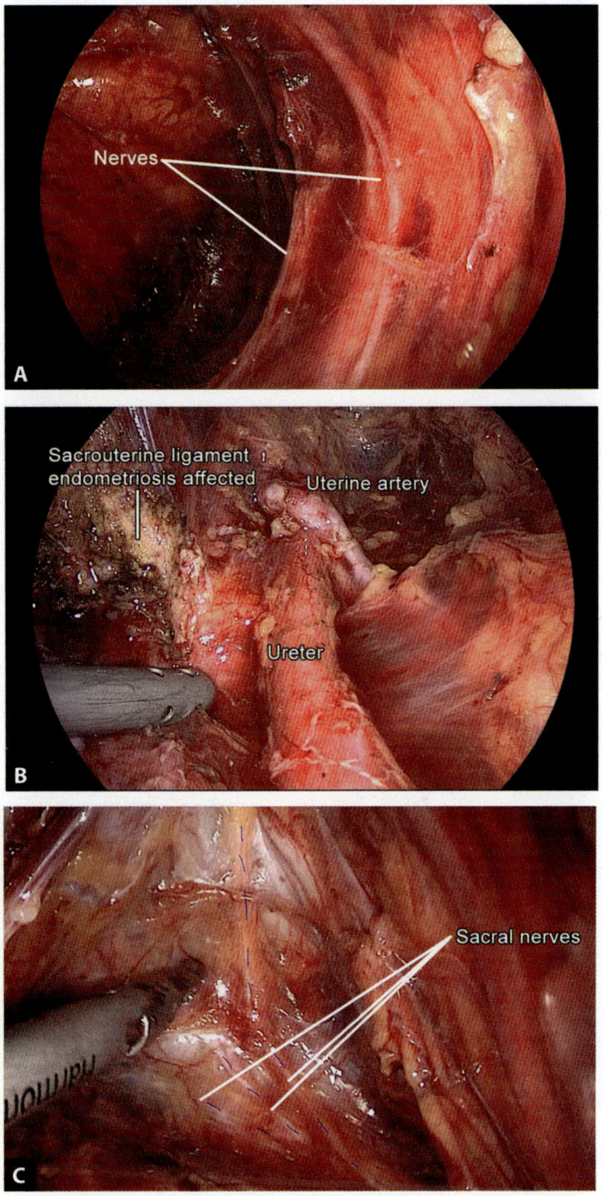

Figs. 25.5A to C: (A) Sacral roots; (B) Anatomical landmarks; (C) Sacral nerves of inferior hypogastric plexus.

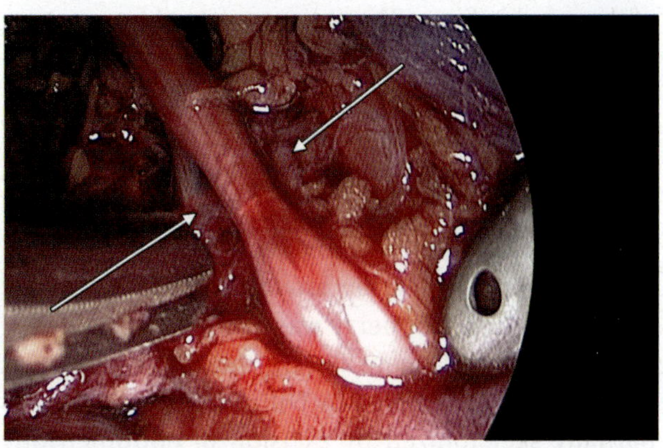

Fig. 25.6: Right obturator nerve with signs of compression.

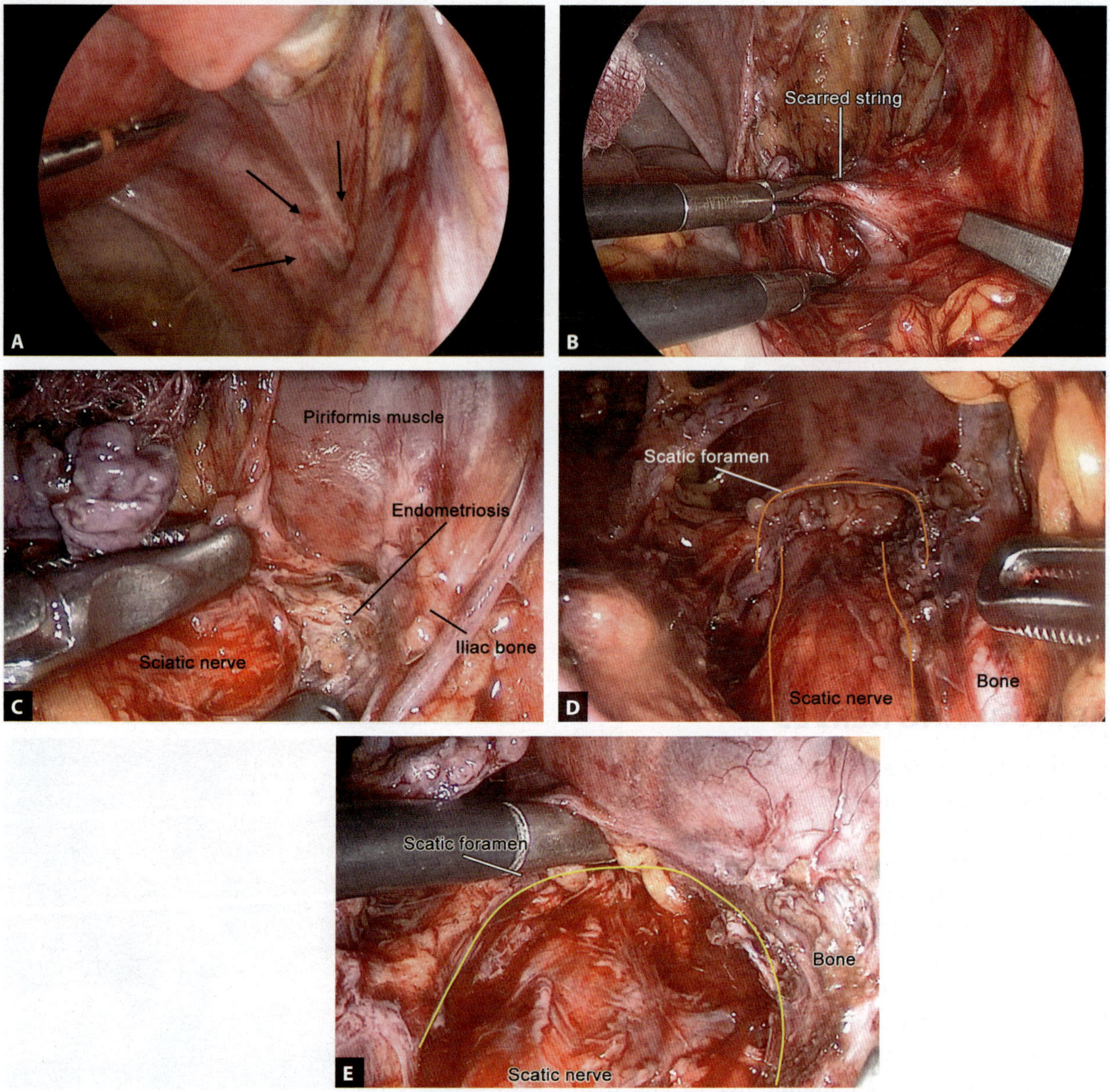

Figs. 25.7A to E: (A) At the site of endometriotic lesions (pointers), the peritoneal wall exhibits signs of retraction; (B) Note the presence of a scarred, string-shaped endometriotic lesion; (C) Endometriosis compressing the sciatic nerve; (D) Sciatic foramen completely infiltrated by endometriosis; (E) View of the sciatic foramen freed from disease.

of the ovarian fossa. The patient suffered from severe cyclic ischialgia. Based on magnetic resonance imaging (MRI) scans, endometriotic involvement was demonstrated in the area surrounding the superior gluteal nerve and the sciatic nerve. Once the peritoneum was opened, a scarred string-shaped lesion (Fig. 25.7B) was revealed to adhere to the obturator foramen and the iliac bone, especially around the greater sciatic notch. The obturator nerve was not involved.

Shown in this Figure 25.7C is the sciatic nerve was encased and constricted by DIE. Once the nerve was partially skeletonized by excision of endometriotic lesions (Fig. 25.7D), marked entrapment of the sciatic nerve became apparent. Upon removal of endometriotic lesions with cold scissors, sciatic foramen was wide open and decompression of the nerve was confirmed (Fig. 25.7E). At follow-up, the patient reported to be free of cyclic sciatica symptoms.

While performing neurolysis, never use electrosurgery (neither monopolar nor bipolar) or any kind of heat-emitting modality (e.g., ultrasound scissors). Dissection should either be performed bluntly or with cold scissors. Occasionally, the use of aqua-jet dissection is feasible.

DIE OF THE URETER

Endometriotic involvement of the ureter is often associated with DIE of the peritoneum. The peritoneal portion in front of the ureter is a predilection area for endometriosis of the pelvic sidewall.

- Anecdotal evidence suggests a predilection of endometriosis to develop on the ureter!

Endometriosis of the ureter may simply be superficial, but may also be more invasive in nature and totally enclose the ureter. As disease progresses, endometriosis can invade deeply into the ureter. This condition is described as "intrinsic ureteral endometriosis."

Secondary to an "entrapped" ureter or if the latter is affected by intrinsic disease, this may result in hydronephrosis, a sequela that constitutes an absolute indication for immediate surgery.

The aim of surgery is to free the ureter from constrictive tissue and to excise endometriosis radically to prevent recurrence of disease, especially in this region.

Utmost care must be taken during ureterolysis, particularly when coming close to the ureter's blood supply. Whenever possible, integrity of the adventitial layer of the ureter should be preserved, while making sure to keep adequate distance from concomitant nerves.

Shown in this Figures 25.8A and B is a ureter affected by intrinsic endometriosis and exhibiting an abrupt change in caliber. Most noticeable is a pronounced dilatation proximally to a segment with severe stenosis. The affected ureter even appears to be deflected even though a stent had been implanted prior to the operation. The stenotic segment and the part of intrinsic endometriosis had to be removed completely.

Stenting with a double-J-stent is imperative in cases of hydronephrosis or stenosis of the ureter. Some surgeons opt for stenting in all cases where ureterolysis is anticipated. The author does not choose this option.

Mostly, the ureter is identified and dissected with ease while obviating the need for stent placement. The use of a stent is often associated with pain and bleeding. Hence, this may result in a dead-end situation in which it remains unclear where pain and bleeding have arisen from.

Partial Resection of the Ureter

In a first step, about 3 to 4 cm of the ureter are excised and then ureteroureterostomy[18] with an end-to-end anastomosis is performed. It is important that the anastomosis is free of tension. To achieve good results, the removed segment should not be too close to the bladder, since blood supply in this region is insufficient.

If end-to-end anastomosis is not feasible because of problems related to the length of the removed part or due to immobility of the ureter, it is recommended to switch to reimplantation of the ureter to the bladder, e.g., by ways of psoas hitch.

Given the lack of experience in urogynecology, it is highly recommended in these cases to call in the assistance of a urologist. In the event of segmental resection, the surgical maneuver is initiated by transection of the ureter at distal (Fig. 25.8C) and proximal sites (Fig. 25.8D) using cold scissors to prevent the risk of necrosis.

Next, the middle part, that needs to be resected is removed (Fig. 25.8E). Make sure that both ends of the ureter are free of scarred tissue, without any signs of endometriosis and with good vascular supply.

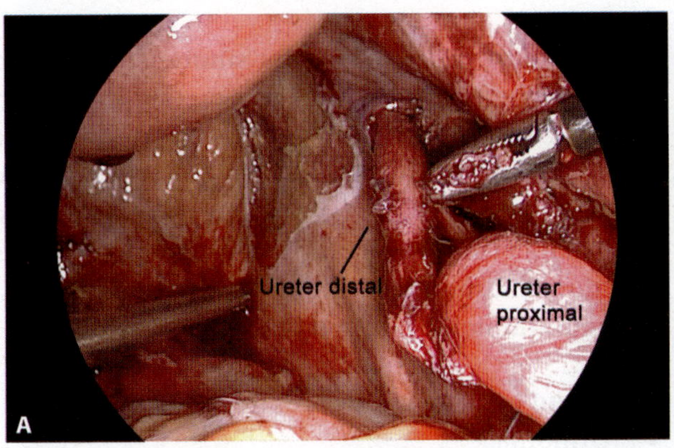

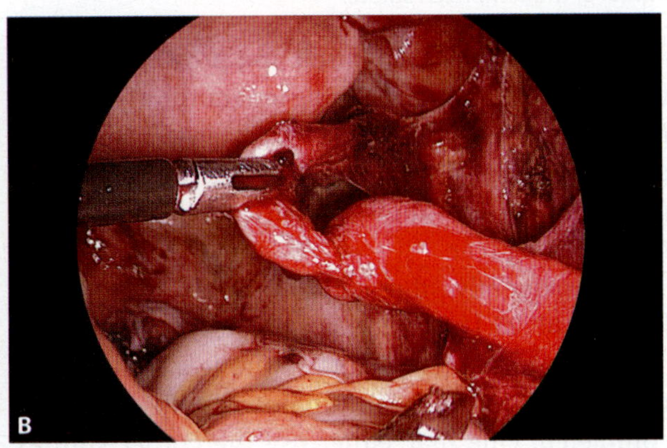

Figs. 25.8A and B

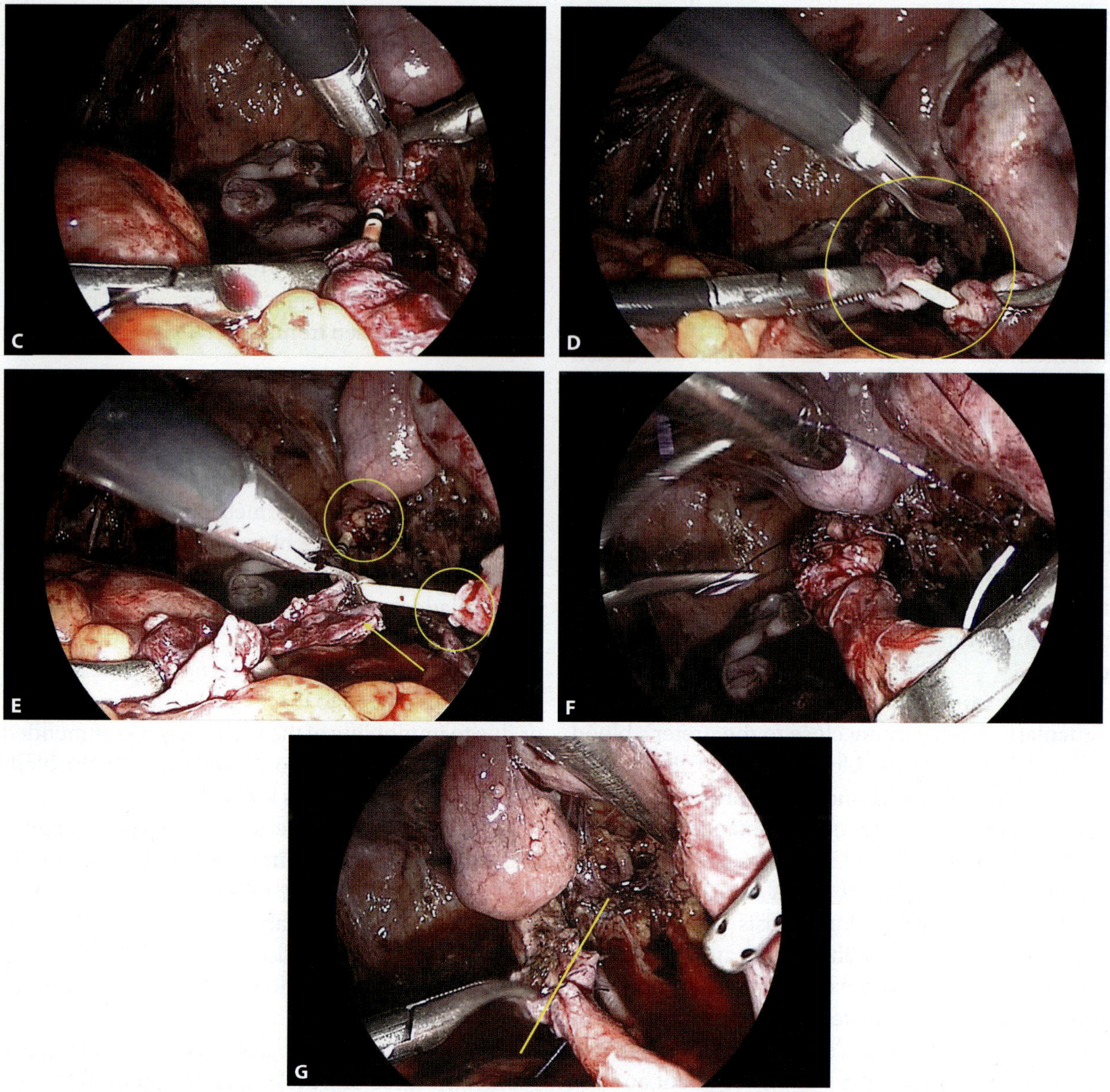

Figs. 25.8C to G

Figs. 25.8A to G: (A) Right ureter with an abrupt change in caliber; (B) Ureter with intrinsic endometriosis; (C) The stenosis is cut free; (D) Proximal transection of the ureter; (E) Removal of the ureteral segment on the indwelling stent; (F) Single knot suture; (G) Final aspect of the completed suture.

In the next step, the distal and proximal ends of the ureter are spatulated using longitudinal incisions that should measure about 7–10 mm in length and be offset by 180° (Fig. 25.9). Spatulating is necessary to prevent the risk of ureter constriction as a result of the shrinking scar.

Subsequently, the corner sutures are placed (Figs. 25.8F, 25.10 and 25.11).

Use of a thin resorbable suture (e.g. USP 5-0) is recommended. Next, anastomosis of the ureter is completed. One may either use the corner sutures to perform a running suture or make a single knot suture (Figs. 25.8G and 25.12).

The short tail of the corner suture is grasped to mobilize the ureter in any direction needed, which affords a good view of the entire circumference of the ureter. A soft drain may be inserted in case of urine leakage and should be left in place for 1 to 2 days. The bladder catheter should be left in place for 3 days and the stent should be removed in about 2–4 weeks. A single antibiotic injection is recommended.

Risks and complications

- Urinoma.
- Urinary infection.
- Recurrence of ureteral stricture.

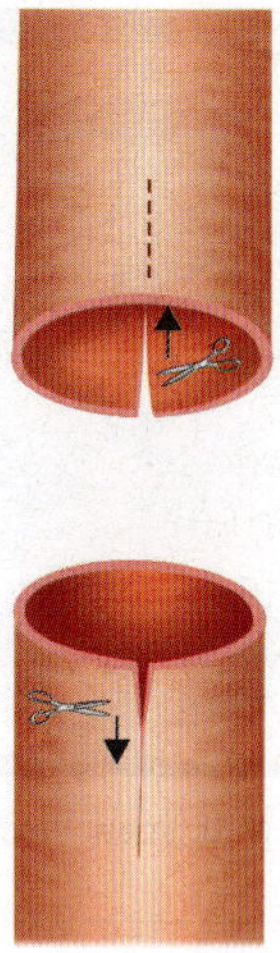

Fig. 25.9: Both ends of the ureter are spatulated.

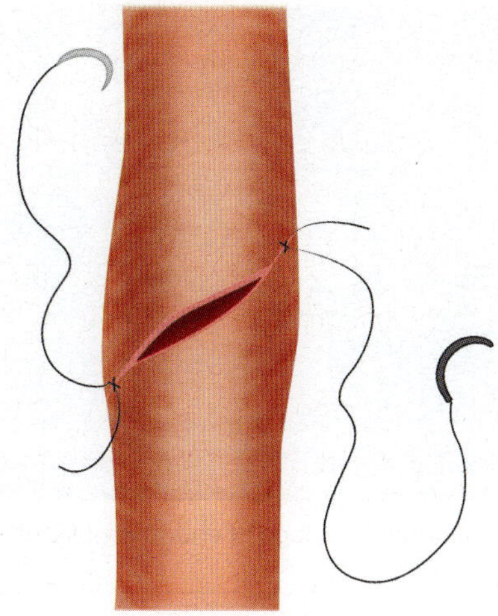

Fig. 25.11: ... completed by knot tying.

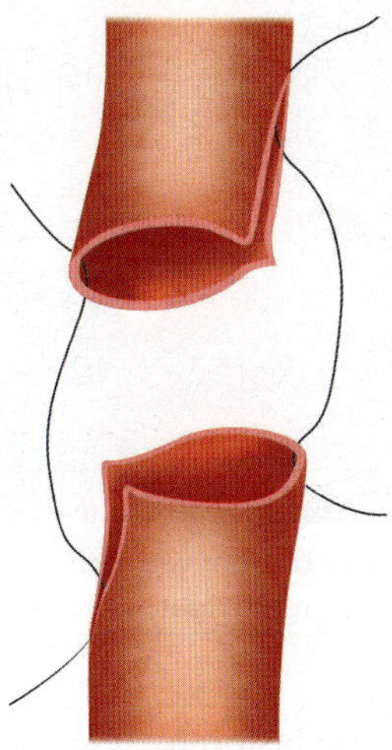

Fig. 25.10: The corner sutures are placed and ....

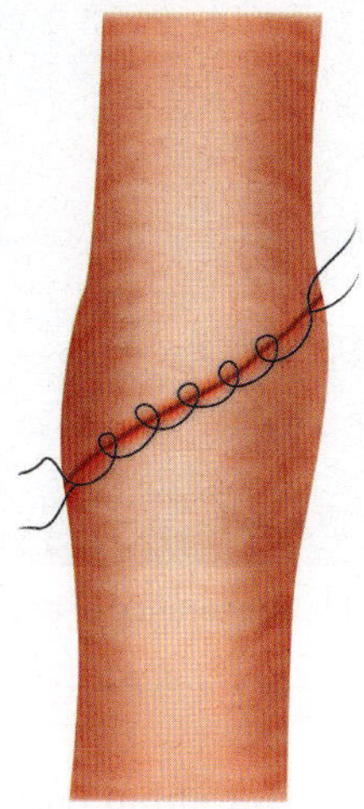

Fig. 25.12: Running suture.

DIE OF THE BLADDER

Most commonly, endometriosis of the urinary bladder may well be identified by ultrasound imaging (Fig. 25.13). In view of its inherent dynamic properties, the vaginal ultrasound probe can be used to move the bladder wall, the uterus or even the endometriotic nodule to differentiate smooth and mobile layers from dense and adherent tissue.Sometimes, an additional MRI exam has shown to be useful to yield additional information (Fig. 25.14). This can be particularly helpful in cases where sonographic density of endometriosis lesions, bladder wall and uterus is similar.

Deep infiltration of the bladder commonly results in bladder pain synchronous with the menstrual cycle and sometimes presenting with micro or macro hematuria. Occasionally, the presence of DIE is recognized during a cystoscopy, but not in all cases.

Often, deep infiltrating endometriotic implants are located at the peritoneal fold between uterus and bladder (Fig. 25.15). Therefore, in most cases, the lesions may encroach on the ventral and cranial wall of the bladder. Depending on the extent of endometriotic growth, the immediate vicinity of the ureteral orifices or the ureters themselves can be involved.

To maintain integrity of the ureter and their ostia, both ureters should be stented before surgery facilitating identification of the ostia. It is vital to make sure that adequate information be obtained on possible abnormalities of the urinary tract.

The prevalence of these abnormalities is about 1:150. Cystoscopy and stenting of ureters can uncover the presence of unknown ureteral duplication. Shown in this Figure 25.16 is an opened bladder with a urethral catheter, and one stent on the right and two stents on the left.

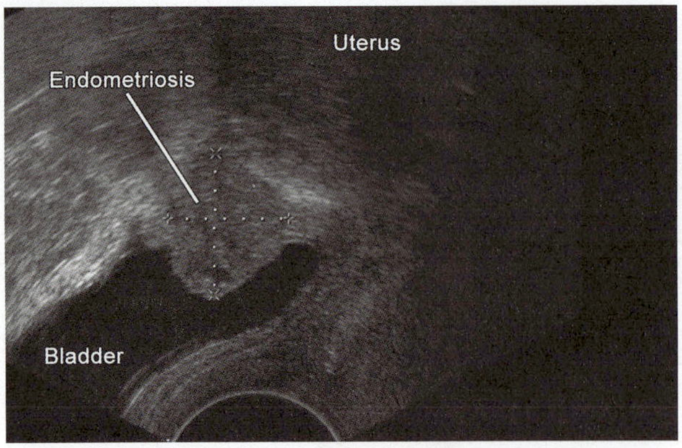

Fig. 25.13: Sonographic image of endometriosis of the bladder wall.

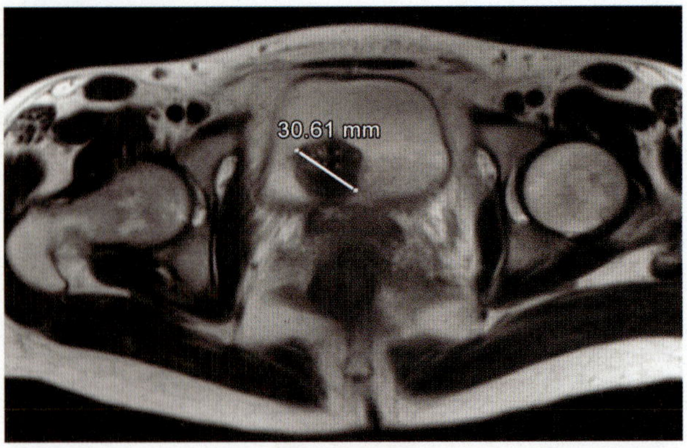

Fig. 25.15: Transverse MRI scan showing an endometriosis nodule.

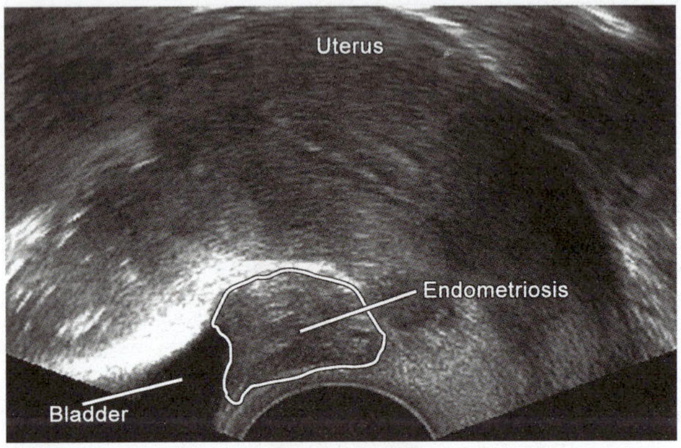

Fig. 25.14: Sonographic appearance of endometriosis between uterus and bladder.

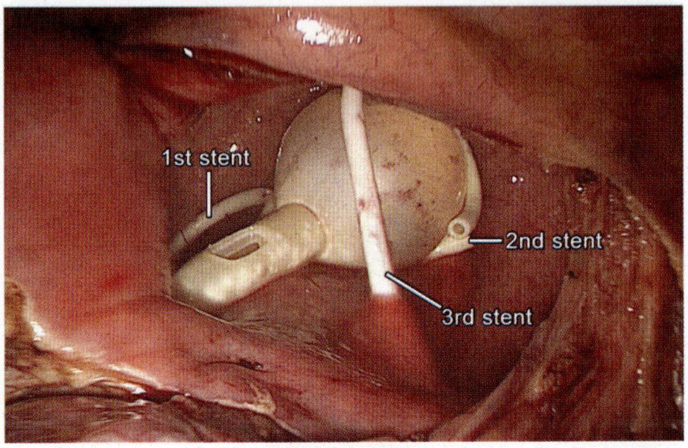

Fig. 25.16: View into a bladder with three stented ureters. One is on the left side, two on the right.

The third stent, and along with it, the proximal right ureter was very close to the removed lesion. The stent helped to identify the intramural part of the ureter. Parts of the bladder wall may easily be resected laparoscopically.

Prior to initiating resection, it has proven helpful to fill the bladder with 200–300 mL of water, which allows for enhanced visualization of margins between the endometriotic lesion and the healthy bladder wall. One may either incise the bladder with a monopolar hook/needle or ultrasound scissors. Do not use undue coagulation and beware of producing wide zones of necrosis. Minor bleedings from the detrusor muscle are acceptable.

Wounds from bladder repair commonly heal very well provided the operating surgeon adheres to the principles of atraumatic dissection, tension-free approximation of wound margins and proper suture techniques.

Occasionally, the lesion can be difficult to identify when obscured by a healthy peritoneum (Fig. 25.17A). In this case, it has proven helpful to trace the site of the lesion by referring to ultrasound or MRI images taken in advance.

After opening the peritoneum, the margins of the lesion need to be circumscribed to prevent excessive removal of healthy bladder tissue (Fig. 25.17B). The lesion should be completely removed, but meticulous care is required at the trigone and ureteric orifices. For this purpose, a full-thickness fenestration is made in the bladder wall at a secure position (Fig. 25.17C), followed by aspiration of saline and insertion of the laparoscope into the bladder (Fig. 25.17D).

While resecting along the circumference of the lesion, constant care must be paid not to transgress the predefined margins. Undue removal of healthy tissue must be avoided to prevent build-up of tension to the suture line placed later in the procedure and potentially resulting in a decrease of bladder capacity.

After resection, the cystostomy is closed with a USP 3-0 resorbable, braided suture. To spare the first knot, it can be helpful to tie a small marker knot at the end of the thread (Fig. 25.17E).

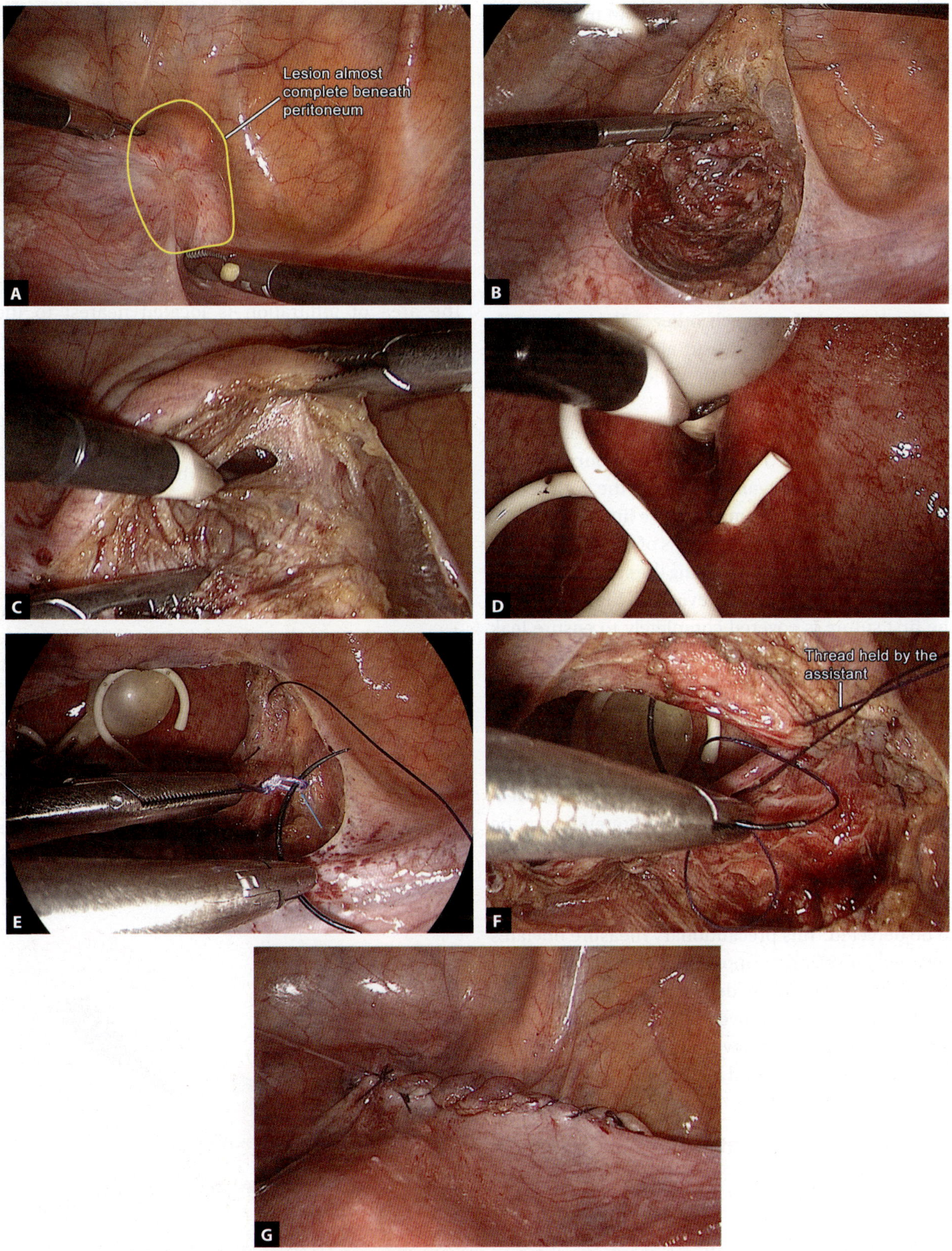

Figs. 25.17A to G: (A) DIE, barely noticeable; (B) Dissection of the endometriotic nodule; (C) The opening is made at a secure position; (D) Localizing the trigone; (E) The needle tip is passed through the loop of the marker knot; (F) Running suture passed through mucosa and detrusor muscle; (G) Suture of peritoneum.

It can also sometimes be helpful to mobilize the bladder prior to the suture of the cystostomy to have a tension-free tissue. This can be performed by widely opening the peritoneum at the ventral fold and by liberating the bladder from the pubic bone.

The continuous suture is initiated from the right side of the cystostomy once the position of the trigone has been confirmed. A two-layer suture is applied for cystostomy closure. At first, the mucosa is closed. Care should be taken to include nearly equal portions of tissue in each bite, which are spaced at similar intervals from each other.[19] The assistant is instructed to align the thread and keep the suture line under moderate tension while placing the running stitches (Fig. 25.17F).

The second-layer suture—of the same material as the first one—is used to reinforce and bury the first suture. Suturing is again started at the right edge, slightly lateral to the primary suture line forming the first layer. Grasp the full thickness of the muscle layer of the detrusor and avoid passing the stitches through the stitch channels made previously. Make sure that the first suture is covered completely to ensure leak tightness of wound closure.

Patency of the suture line is assessed by filling the bladder with 200–300 mL of saline. The use of Methylene Blue is not needed for this purpose.

The peritoneum can be left open allowing blood and coagula to drain off. If the wound does not reveal any signs of hemorrhage, the peritoneum can be closed with a running suture (Fig. 25.17G).

A Foley catheter is inserted and left in place for 4–7 days allowing any signs of secondary bleeding to be detected. This precautionary measure obviates the need for vesical tamponade and helps to prevent the occurrence of suture dehiscence.

The stents are removed 3–4 weeks later in the same session of the follow-up cystoscopy scheduled for monitoring the wound healing process.

Risks and Complications

- Urinary tract infection
- Bleeding
- Wound infection
- Urinoma
- Vesical tamponade
- Voiding dysfunction

DIE OF THE RECTO-VAGINAL SPACE AND VAGINA

Recto-vaginal endometriosis may extend from top of the posterior vaginal wall to the anterior rectal wall and laterally to the uterosacral ligaments. Surgical treatment of DIE of the rectovaginal space is among the most challenging gynecologic operative procedures. This form of endometriosis has been found to become firmly adherent to the nerves that control function of bladder, bowel and sexuality. The area of infiltration is located nearest to the bowel, commonly involves the vagina and may even encroach on the uterine cervix. If the cervix is affected by invasive endometriosis, a complete surgical 100% removal is not feasible without removing the cervix or uterus. Particularly regarding to fertility potential and sexual function, this seems to be a conflict of mutually incompatible goals.

Laparoscopic resection is the treatment of choice for DIE involving the rectovaginal septum, and several authors have reported good clinical outcomes with improvements in symptoms of dysmenorrhea, dyspareunia, and chronic pelvic pain.[13,20-22]

- Nevertheless, damage to pelvic nerves can have a detrimental effect on the patient's quality of life.

To achieve clear resection margins, a combined access should be adopted given involvement of the vaginal wall. Small nodules are sometimes palpable or visible more readily via transvaginal access. Accordingly, it can be helpful to mark the nodules preoperatively with knots (Fig. 25.18), placed during

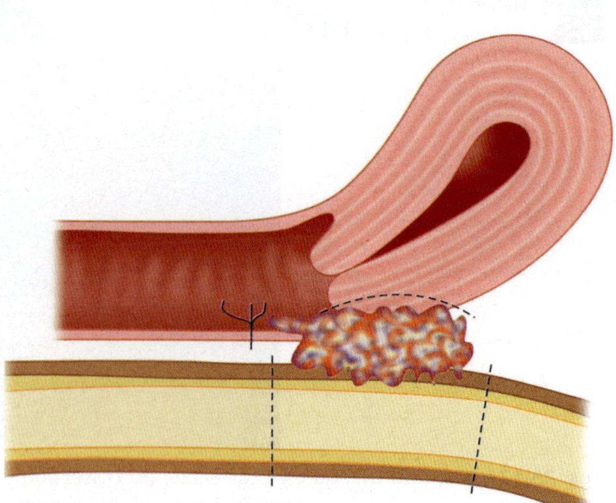

Fig. 25.18: DIE of the rectovaginal space.

laparoscopic inspection at the beginning of the procedure.

Shown in this Figure 25.18 are the resection lines, which are defined to delineate the boundaries for complete surgical removal of DIE.

In cases where the vagina has been opened, the author recommends that wound closure be accomplished by placing a continuous suture with a monofilament absorbable thread (USP 0), which has proven to result in the lowest rate of suture line insufficiency.

There are no specific data available about suture line insufficiency, suture technique and postoperative management. Based on the author's experience, sufficient wound healing can pose a problem, which is why all patients subjected to this type of operative procedure at the author's clinical center are counselled to abstain from sexual intercourse for 8 weeks after surgery. Apart from that, this precaution is aimed at preventing rupture of bowel or vagina, and therefore, women who become pregnant soon after surgery are advised to preauthorize consent to caesarian delivery.

Complications such as anastomotic leakage or rectovaginal fistula can occur after bowel resection and anastomosis. There are reports in the literature on bowel resection and full-thickness discoid excision,[23] with incidence rates for anastomotic leakage, abscess formation and rectovaginal fistula of 0.7%, 0.3% and 0.7%, respectively.

From this, the author draws the conclusion that bowel resection can yield good operative outcomes with an acceptable major complication rate.

DIE OF THE DIAPHRAGM OR PERICARDIUM

The presence of extra-pelvic endometrial deposits (diaphragm, umbilicus) is a rare finding. While most implants are superficial and cause no discomfort, others can be deeply infiltrating. Deep infiltrating endometriosis of the diaphragm can be associated with chest pain, upper quadrant pain and chronic shoulder tip pain.[24]

DIE may be found on and in the diaphragm. The main contributors to the phrenic nerve are the cervical nerves C3, C4 and C5. Considering the common innervation of C5, the presence of shoulder tip pain in young women without clinical findings is an important differential diagnosis.

However, there are also two peripheral innervating sources. The intercostal nerves (T5–T11) and the subcostal nerve which is located at T12. This makes us understand the most common symptoms of diaphragmatic endometriosis, which can manifest as dyspnea, epigastric pain, pain in the chest (pleuritic), shoulder pain and right or left upper abdomen pain. All the symptoms may or may not be cyclic.

Diaphragmatic involvement sometimes causes recurrent catamenial pneumothorax as well. There are some case reports about chronic right shoulder tip pain arising from diaphragmatic DIE.[25,26] The diagnosis of extra pelvic endometriosis is often missed, due to lack of knowledge about the mere existence of this disorder.

Malignant transformation of endometriosis is a rare event. There are very few case reports about transformation of endometriosis of the abdominal wall to either a clear cell carcinoma[27,28] or a papillary serous carcinoma.[29] Because of its rare occurrence, malignant transformation of abdominal wall endometriosis has not been elucidated.

Surgical Therapy

Redwine[30] reports about a small study of eight patients with DIE of the right posterior diaphragm, which is not always visible from the umbilical port site. In all cases, laparoscopic detection of endometriotic lesions was feasible when using a port situated beneath the right costal margin.

In view of the posterior site of infiltration, obscured by the liver, and the presence of full-thickness invasion, laparoscopic treatment was not feasible in all eight patients. Full-thickness resection of the diaphragm resulted in complete eradication of symptoms in seven of eight patients, and good symptomatic amelioration in one patient.

The good news about diaphragmatic endometriosis is that after sound surgical treatment, studies have shown that the condition is far less likely to recur than other forms of DIE.[26]

It seems to make no difference which technique of removal is used. Irrespective of whether vaporization, ablation, hydro dissection, cold scissors excision or ultrasound scissors was used, all these modalities have proven to be similarly efficient.

Based on the experience that has been gained at the author's clinical center, a monopolar hook can be used without problems at the pars membranacea of the diaphragm (nonmuscular part). Using monopolar current at the muscular part triggers jerky movements of the diaphragm, which can lead to pleural rupture.

The occurrence of pleural rupture during laparoscopy is not a critical event because CO_2 gas will be resorbed rapidly because it is readily soluble in blood. A small defect can be closed by placing an absorbable running suture.

Pericardium (Video "Pericardium 17 min" at disc)

Unlike capnopleura, the occurrence of a capnopericardium may result in severe complications. Case reports are extremely rare. One of them was published by Banks-Venegoni et al.[31] reporting on a cardiac arrest arising from a tension capnopericardium that occurred during perorally endoscopic full-thickness myotomy.

In the following, a case report is presented on the occurrence of a capnopericardium encountered at the author's clinical center. Finally, a smart approach will be described explaining how to manage such a special complication successfully during laparoscopy.

A young patient about 30 years of age, presented one year after spontaneous delivery with severe pain in the right shoulder. A review of the patient's history revealed various orthopedic diagnoses as well as a multitude of different unsuccessful attempts of treatment including arthroscopy. Unfortunately, her gynecologist was not alerted to the presence of a clue, namely the finding that pain symptoms were synchronous with the patient's menstrual cycle.

A laparoscopic examination was scheduled to look for any findings suggestive of endometriosis.

At laparoscopy, a few superficial endometriotic lesions were detected in the pelvis, along with multiple nodules seen on both sides of the diaphragm. On the left side, two of them appeared to be of deeply infiltrating type and invaded the posterior diaphragm, next to the liver and adjacent to the falciform ligament (Fig. 25.19A).

Behind the diaphragm, the pulsating movements of the heart could be seen. Endometriosis was found to infiltrate the diaphragm in the area of the pars membranacea. The first nodule was resected by using ultrasonic scissors and intermittent application of a monopolar hook (Fig. 25.19B). During removal of the nodule, some small endometriotic cysts were opened (Fig. 25.19C). An all but full-thickness resection was accomplished and the serous layer of the pericardium was locally exposed (Fig. 25.19D). To stabilize the thin pericardial membrane, the defect was closed with a U-stitch suture (Fig. 25.19E) and a sliding knot tied extra-corporeally.

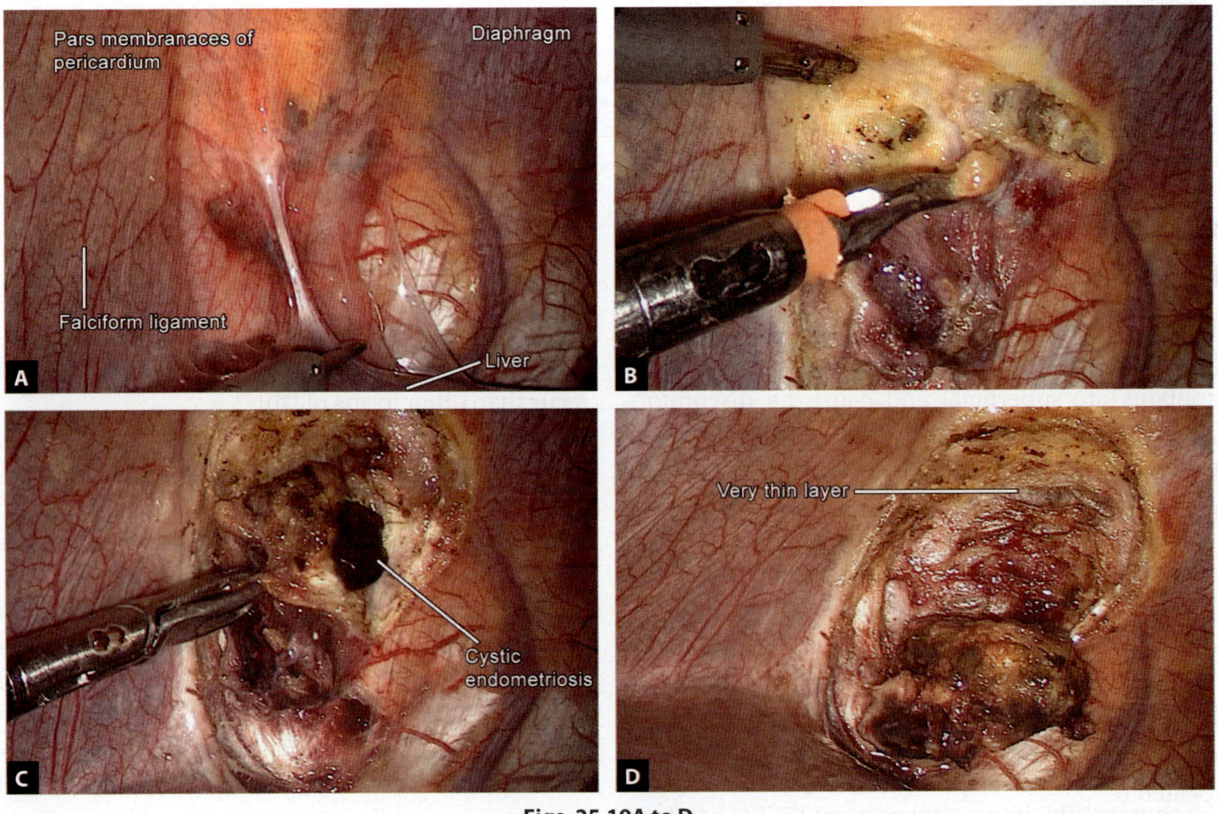

Figs. 25.19A to D

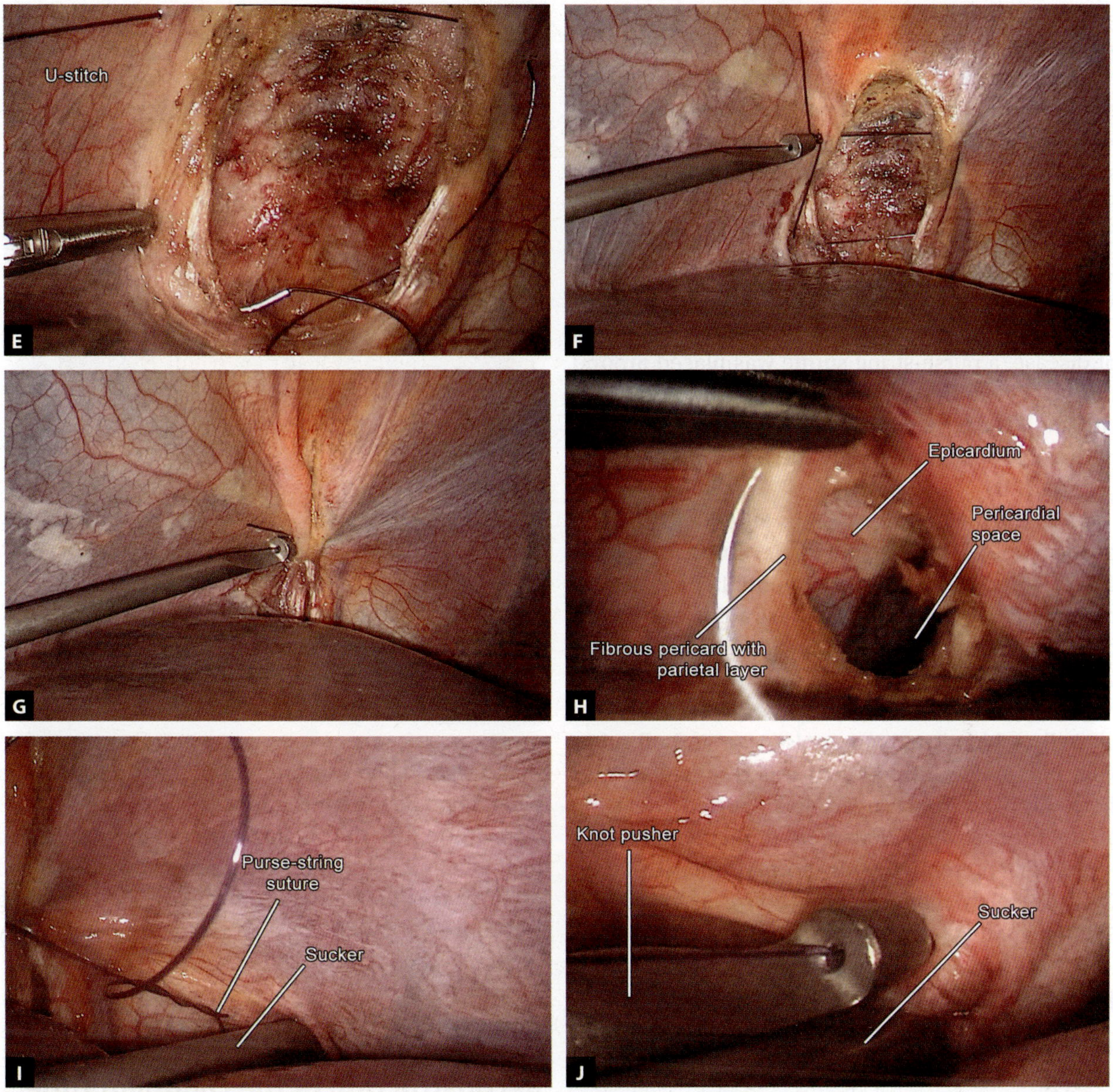

Figs. 25.19E to J

Figs. 25.19A to J: (A) Endometriosis of the diaphragm; (B) Dissection of endometriotic nodule; (C) Opening of a cystic nodule; (D) The pulsating movements of the heart are noticeable; (E) Placing a U-stitch suture; (F) The slipknot is tied down with a knot pusher; (G) Closure of the lesion; (H) Pericardial defect and view into the pericardial space; (I) The suction tube is inserted into the pericardial space after completion of extra-corporeal knot tying; (J) The defect is closed while aspirating the remaining CO_2 gas from the pericardial space.

For extra-corporeal knotting, the author commonly uses a self-locking slip knot named "von Leffern Knot." A monofilament absorbable suture material is applied without undue tensile force allowing the thread to be passed through smoothly and without sawing into the tissue. The knot is tied down with a closed knot-pusher (Figs. 25.19F and G).

Once the first defect had been repaired and closed, the second lesion was excised, again with the aid of an ultrasonic scissors. The nodule was also located in the membranous part of the pericardium. In this case, endometriosis had infiltrated all tissue layers including the parietal serous pericardium, which prompted us to create an opening giving access to the pericardial space.

It was just then when a capno-pericardium occurred and the anesthesiologist was alerted to the presence of a significant decrease in blood pressure and a tachycardia accompanied by a low QRS complex voltage.

To give the anesthesiologist enough time to stabilize the patient, intra-abdominal CO_2 pressure was instantly decreased. All instruments as well as the laparoscope were removed, while making sure that all trocar valves were in an opened state. The patient was stable within a few minutes.

Subsequently, laparoscopy was continued and the lesion was removed completely by resecting all layers of the visceral pericardium. The defect had a size of approximately 1.5 cm in diameter (Fig. 25.19H). From the site of the defect the pulsating movements of the heart could be seen. The epicardium, forming the visceral serous layer of the pericardium, was inspected closely.

To provide for a sustained, long-lasting remission of disease, a purse-string suture was placed around the defect and tied down with an extra-corporeal slip knot. Next, a suction tube was inserted into the pericardial space to aspirate the remaining CO_2 gas (Fig. 25.19I).

While retracting the suction tube, the knot was pushed down while at the same time closing the defect (Fig. 25.19J). Again, monofilament suture material (USP 0) was used for extra-corporeal knot tying. For this purpose, the thread must measure at least 90 cm in length.

The patient's ECG instantly recovered to normal as well as blood pressure, pulse rate and all other vital parameters. The patient was discharged from hospital on day 3 postsurgery and reported to feel fine all the time. At the follow-up examination 10 weeks later, she presented with normal menstruation, remission of dysmenorrhea and above all, absence of shoulder pain.

How to Deal with DIE of Diaphragm

At first, it needs to be established whether the lesion belongs to the pleural or pericardial diaphragm. The latter can be identified by the pulsating movements of the heart. Apart from that, one should be cognizant of where to find the pericardium. Shown in this Figure 25.20 is the pericardium (area between the red interrupted lines) that is situated near the falciform ligament and, in the posterior half of the diaphragm, next to the liver. A small pericardial portion is located above the level of the right liver close to the falciform ligament.

Provided you are clear about the position of the lesion, do not try to open the pericardial space, if there is lack of evidence that this is truly necessary. A lot of endometriotic nodules can be removed by sparing the serous layer.

Considering that you can never be sure about what happens next, it is mandatory to keep in close communication with the anesthesiologist and to make clear what you are planning to do next and what might be the consequences.

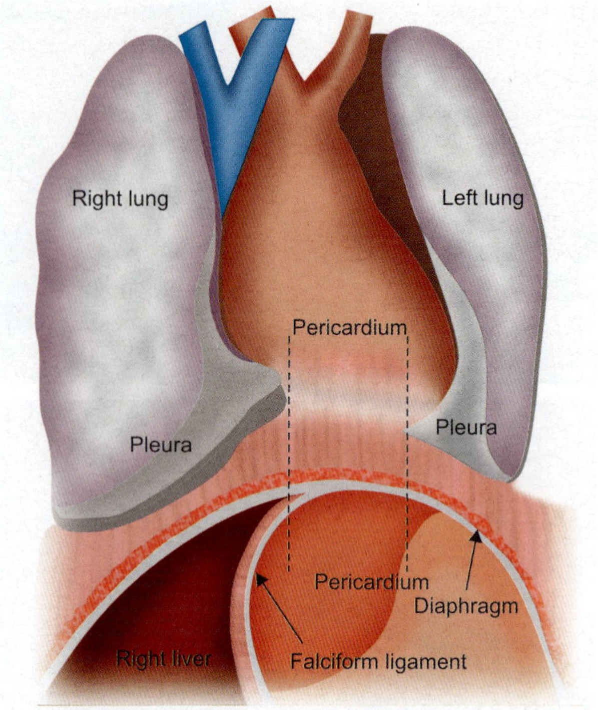

Fig. 25.20: Frontal section demonstrating the topographic relations of the pericardium to neighboring organs.

Suturing in the angle between liver, falciform ligament and diaphragm is not an easy matter. If you do not have adequate skills in laparoscopic suturing techniques, it is safer to convert to an open surgery access.[30]

DIE OF THE FALLOPIAN TUBE

Reconstruction of the Fallopian Tube Using a Forgarty Catheter

In some cases of severe deep infiltrating endometriosis at fallopian tubes, especially with intrinsic endometriosis in the tubes, it is necessary to reconstruct the tubes.

There is no scientific evidence in any kind of splinting the tube but it is helpful and logical. You can use a forgarty catheter (e.g. No. 5) to splint a completely severed tube for better reconstruction and exact suturing. Usually these catheters are used for embolectomy in vascular surgery. The catheters are 80 cm long, so there is enough length to reach from outer abdomen through the tube into the uterine cavity.

They can be inserted through the abdominal wall using a big bore plastic cannula without occupying a trocar. Then it is possible to thread the tube on the catheter beginning with the funnel shaped end of the fallopian tube.

After inserting the catheter into the distal part of the tube, get the tip of the catheter out of the gap between the two ends of the tube (Fig. 25.21A). Then insert the catheter into the proximal end of the tube. (Fig. 25.21B) up to the uterine cavity.

Then you bloc the tip of the catheter in the uterine cavity with 1 or 2 mL saline water. Now it is easy to adapt the lumen of both sides with a few stitches by using 4/0 or 5/0 sutures (Figs. 25.21C and D).

To support a better healing in a correct position and to protect the lumen against stenosis, the catheter can be left in position for a few days. Then it is easy to remove the catheter through the abdominal wall after unblocking the tip.

Take this as one of possible techniques to splint the fallopian tube according to the technique of suturing the ureter.

SUMMARY

Deep infiltrating endometrioses does not respect the borders of tissue layers. Therefore, the principles of good surgical practice are similar to those applied in cancer surgery; however, surgery for DIE can be even more difficult.

Unlike many other diseases, where there is a clear indication for radical surgery, surgeons who opt for surgical treatment of DIE are faced with the need for drawing into account all aspects that are linked to the patient's quality of life.

Radical surgery for deep infiltrating endometriosis has the potential of increasing quality of life and pregnancy rates, but the procedure can also be associated with a multitude of adverse side effects. In the light of this, it is paramount to speak openly to the patient prior to obtaining an informed consent.

All surgeons are required to have an adequate level of experience and skills not only regarding to operative techniques but also in terms of anatomic and functional knowledge. Surgical treatment of DIE often is an interdisciplinary project.

As mentioned before, every layer, every space, each tissue and each organ has its own specific problems and characteristics.

Surgeons should know this and respect the varying properties of tissues when affected by deep infiltrating endometriosis at various anatomical locations.

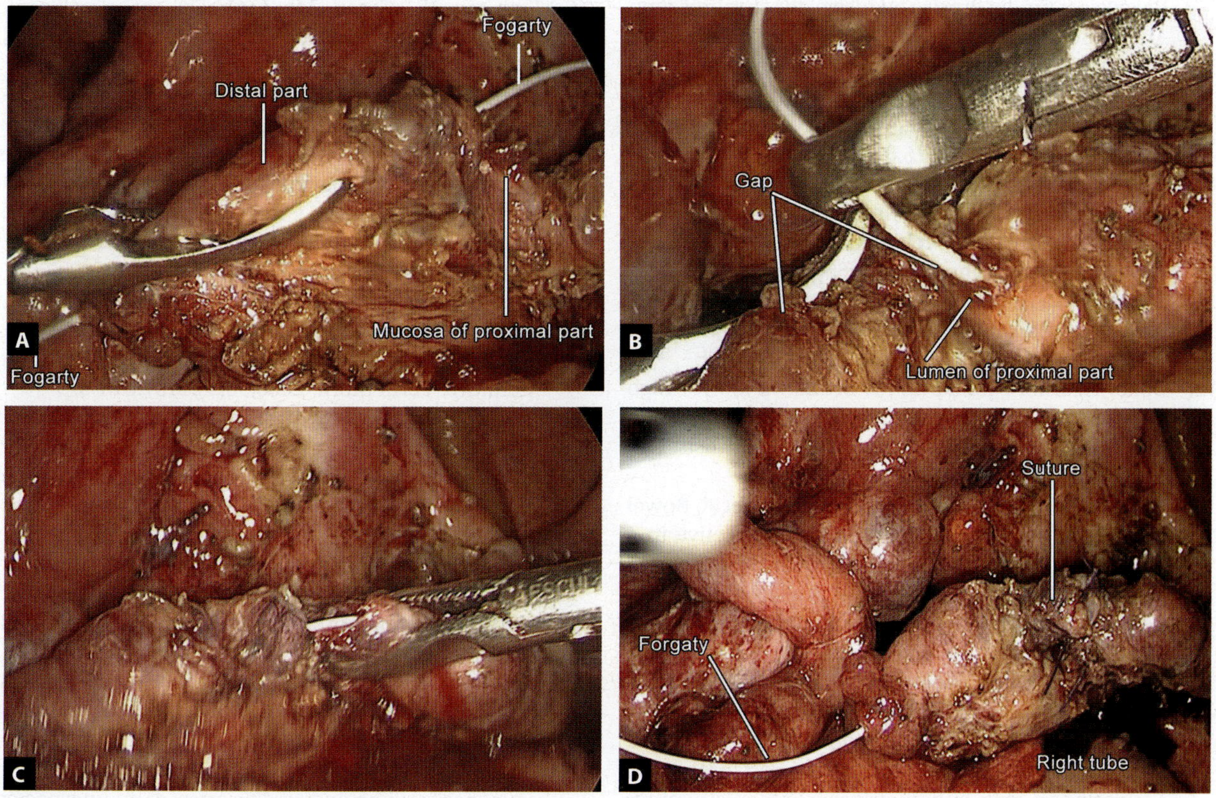

Figs. 25.21A to D: (A) Insertion of catheter in distal part; (B) Insertion of catheter into proximal part; (C) Catheter bridging the gap; (D) Suture is done, catheter still in position.

I thank my beloved wife Barbara von Leffern for preparing the anatomical drawings according to my ideas!

REFERENCES

1. Koninckx PR, Martin D. Treatment of deeply infiltrating endometriosis. Curr Opin Obstet Gynecol. 1994;6(3):231-41.
2. Kondo W, Bourdel N, Tamburro S, et al. Complications after surgery for deeply infiltrating pelvic endometriosis. BJOG. 2011;118(3):292-8.
3. van den Broeck U, Meuleman C, Tomassetti C, et al. Effect of laporoscopic surgery for moderate and severe endometriosis on depression, relationship satisfaction and sexual functioning: comparison of patients with and without bowel resection. Hum Reprod. 2013;28(9):2389-97.
4. Duffy JM, Arambage K, Correa FJ, et al. Laparoscopic surgery for endometriosis. Cochrane Database Syst Rev. 2014;(4):CD011031.
5. Zupi E, Lazzeri L, Centini G. Deep endometriosis: Less is better. J Endometr Pelvic Pain Disord. 2015;7(1):1-2.
6. Mechsner S. Lymphatische Ausbreitungswege der Endometriose. Gyn. 2013;18(6):444–8.
7. Koninckx PR, Ussia A, Adamyan L, Wattiez A, Donnez J. Deep endometriosis: definition, diagnosis, and treatment. Fertil Steril. 2012;98(3):564-71.
8. Ebert AD. Gynäkologische Laparoskopie: Ein Wegweiser für die Praxis ; inklusive der chirurgischen Anatomie des weiblichen Beckens, 2nd edn. Berlin: De Gruyter; 2014.
9. Angioni S, Cela V, Sedda F, et al. Focusing on surgery results in infertile patients with deep endometriosis. Gynecol Endocrinol. 2015;31(8):595-8.
10. Cohen J, Thomin A, Mathieu dE, et al. Fertility before and after surgery for deep infiltrating endometriosis with and without bowel involvement: a literature review. Minerva Ginecol. 2014;66(6):575-87.
11. Stepniewska A, Pomini P, Bruni F, et al. Laparoscopic treatment of bowel endometriosis in infertile women. Hum Reprod. 2009;24(7):1619-25.
12. Bokor A, Csibi N, Lukovich P, Brubel R, Joo JG, Rigo J. Importance of nerve-sparing surgical technique in the treatment of deep infiltrating endometriosis. Orv Hetil. 2015;156(48):1960-5.
13. Wolthuis AM, Meuleman C, Tomassetti C, et al. Bowel endometriosis: colorectal surgeon's perspective in a multidisciplinary surgical team. World J Gastroenterol 2014;20(42):15616-23.
14. Possover M. Pathophysiologic explanation for bladder retention in patients after laparoscopic surgery for deeply infiltrating rectovaginal and/or parametric endometriosis. Fertil Steril. 2014;101(3):754-8.
15. Renner S, Burghaus S, Wimberger P, et al. Veranstaltungsbericht. Operative Verfahren bei Patientinnen mit Endometriose—Ergebnisse eines Expertenworkshops. Geburtshilfe Frauenheilkd. 2015;75(05):417-8.
16. Capek S, Amrami KK, Howe BM, et al. Sequential imaging of intraneural sciatic nerve endometriosis provides insight into symptoms of cyclical sciatica. Acta Neurochir (Wien). 2016;158(3):507-12.
17. Andrade C, Barata S, Antonio F, et al. Laparascopic Neurolysis of deep endometriosis infiltrating left femoral nerve: case report. Surg Technol Int. 2015;27:163-8.
18. Manski D. Ureteroureterostomy: end-to-end anastomosis of the ureter. 2015. Available at: http://www.urology-textbook.com/ureteroureterostomy.html. Accessed January 24, 2016.
19. Jain N. State of the Art Atlas and Textbook of Laparoscopic Suturing. New Delhi: Jaypee Brothers Medical Publishers; 2006.
20. Meuleman C, Tomassetti C, D'Hooghe TM. Clinical outcome after laparoscopic radical excision of endometriosis and laparoscopic segmental bowel resection. Curr Opin Obstet Gynecol. 2012;24(4):245-52.
21. Meuleman C, Tomassetti C, D'Hoore A, et al. Surgical treatment of deeply infiltrating endometriosis with colorectal involvement. Hum Reprod Update. 2011; 17(3):311-26.
22. Meuleman C, Tomassetti C, Wolthuis A, et al. Clinical outcome after radical excision of moderate-severe endometriosis with or without bowel resection and reanastomosis: a prospective cohort study. Ann Surg. 2014;259(3):522-31.
23. Koh CE, Juszczyk K, Cooper MJ, et al. Management of deeply infiltrating endometriosis involving the rectum. Dis Colon Rectum. 2012;55(9):925-31.
24. Freeston JE, Green MJ, King DG, et al. Chronic shoulder pain and diaphragmatic endometriosis. Rheumatology (Oxford). 2006;45(12):1533.
25. Cooper MJ, Russell P, Gallagher PJ. Diaphragmatic endometriosis. Med J Aust. 1999;171(3):142-3.
26. Nezhat C, Nezhat F. Protocols and best practices for treating diaphragmatic endometriosis. Available from: Available at: http://www.nezhat.org/file/Diaphragmatic_Endometriosis_Article.pdf. Accessed January 24, 2016.
27. Bats AS, Zafrani Y, Pautier P, et al. Malignant transformation of abdominal wall endometriosis to clear cell carcinoma: case report and review of the literature. Fertil Steril. 2008;90(4):1197.e13-6.
28. Banks-Venegoni AL, Desilets DJ, et al. Tension capnopericardium and cardiac arrest as an unexpected adverse event of peroral endoscopic myotomy (with video). Gastrointest Endosc. 2015;82(6):1137-9.
29. Omranipour R, Najafi M. Papillary serous carcinoma arising in abdominal wall endometriosis treated with neoadjuvant chemotherapy and surgery. Fertil Steril. 2010;93(4):1347.e17-8.
30. Redwine DB. Diaphragmatic endometriosis: diagnosis, surgical management, and long-term results of treatment. Fertil Steril. 2002;77(2):288-96.
31. Banks-Venegoni AL, Desilets DJ, et al. Tension capnopericardium and cardiac arrest as an unexpected adverse event of peroral endoscopic myotomy (with video). Gastrointest Endosc. 2015;82(6):1137-9.

Adenomyoma Resection in Infertility

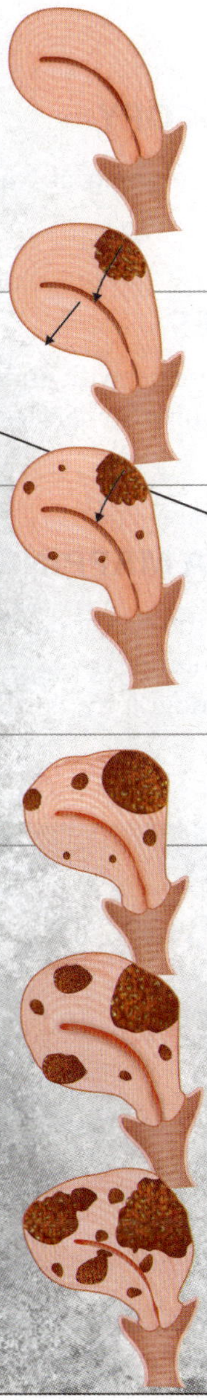

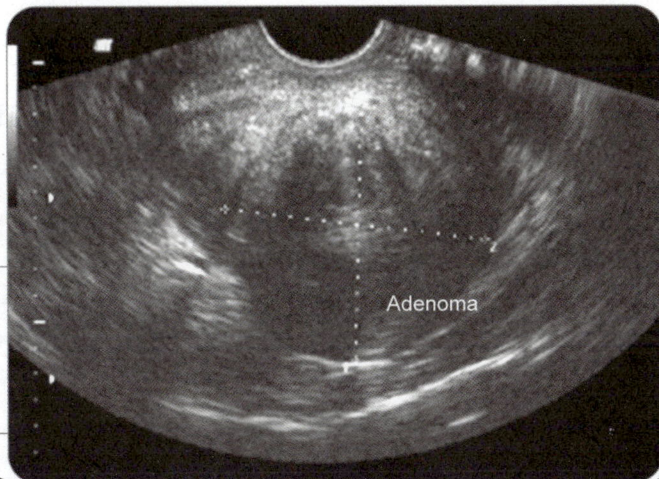

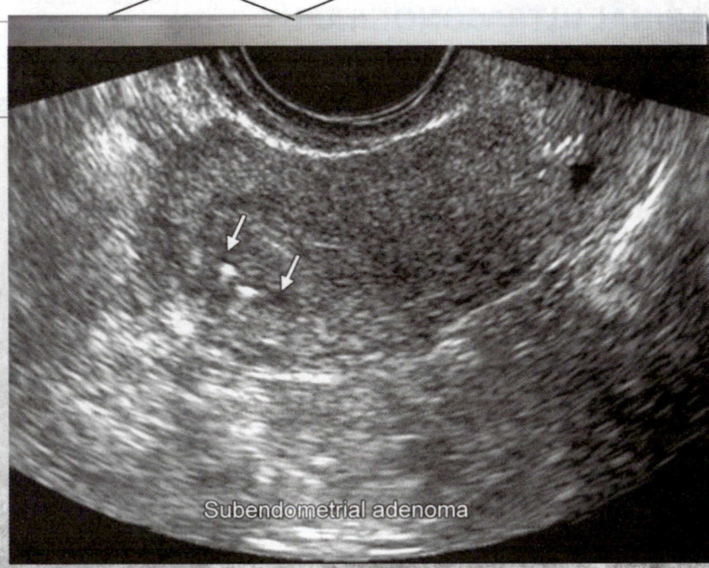

Chapter 26

Adenomyoma Resection in Infertility

Sanjay Patel

DEFINITION

The heterotypic presence of the functioning endometrium glands and stroma within the myometrium at least 2.5 mm deeper to the basal layer is termed as adenomyosis. Common in patients with previous history of MTP, dilatation and curettage or any previous surgery on the uterus.

CLASSIFICATION

As per its morphological occurrence, adenomyoma is classified as: (1) Localised adenomyoma; and (2) Diffuse adenomyosis.

TRANSVAGINAL ULTRASONOGRAPHY

- Adenoma is usually diagnosed on ultrasound. It appears uncapsulated, heterogeneous, and as anechoic areas. All these changes will be more pronounced if the ultrasound is performed during menstruation.
- On color Doppler it may appear as diffuse, increased overall vascularity (PI > 1.18 cm/s)

ADENOMA ON LAPAROSCOPY

Adenoma may be misdiagnosed as a fibroid on ultrasound. If one finds it difficult to find the plane of cleavage during surgery, then it is more likely to be adenoma (Figs. 26.1 to 26.3).

There may be chocolate colored fluid collection in the myometrium (intramyometrial cyst).

ADENOMA ON HYSTEROSCOPY

Hysteroscopy shows increased endometrial vascularity.

COEXISTING PATHOLOGIES

Adenomyosis and adenoma may co-exist with endometriosis, fibroid, endometrial polyp/hyperplasia and uterine adhesions.

PREOPERATIVE ADENOMA MAPPING

We routinely draw a map depicting the size and location of adenoma before starting the surgery.

Intraoperative transvaginal sonography is also done when needed.

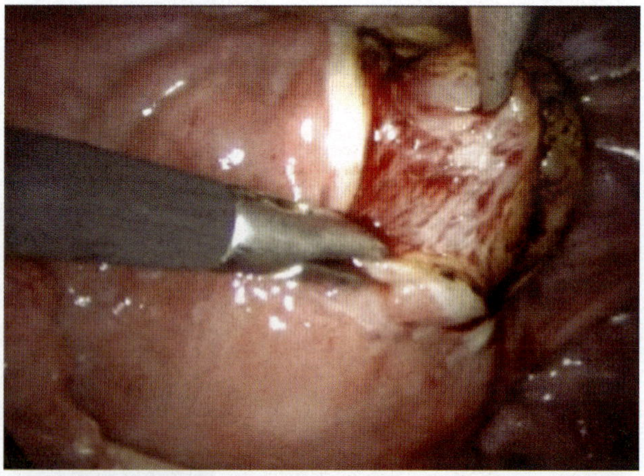

Fig. 26.1: Unclear plane and no capsule visible at myoma enucleation.

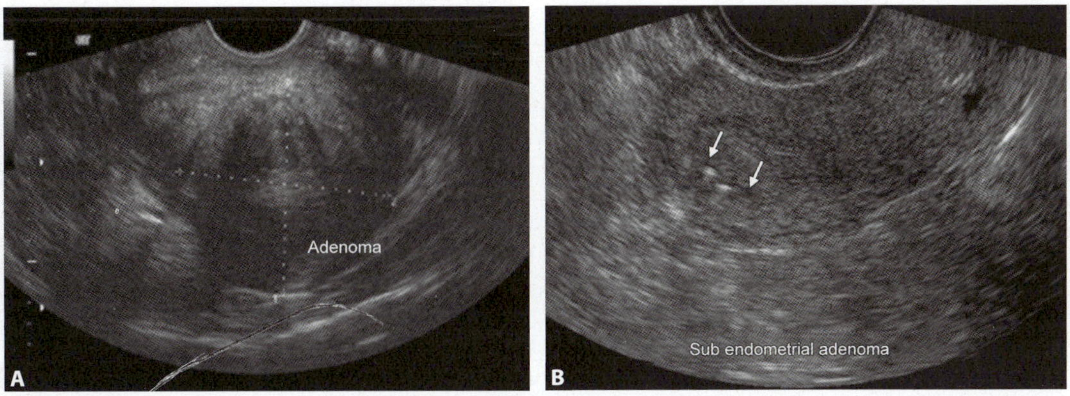

Figs. 26.2A and B: (A) Adenoma with unclear margins in vaginal ultrasonography; (B) Subendometrial adenoma in vaginal ultrasonography.

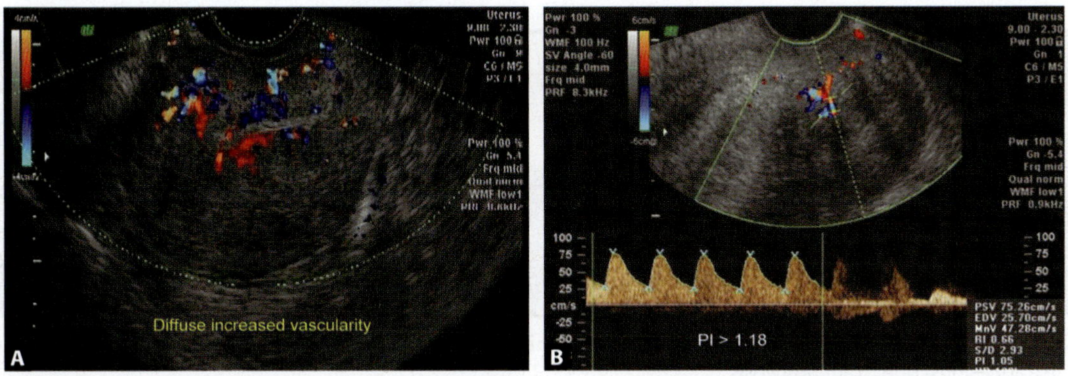

Figs. 26.3A and B: (A) Diffused increased vascularity in vaginal ultrasonography; (B) Increased echogenic area.

AIM OF ADENOMA RESECTION

Resection helps in improving the symptoms by reducing the uterine vascularity, thus improving pain, menorrhagia and fertility. As adenoma/adenomyotic tissue is tough, it is better to use monopolar pure cutting current than scissors. Too much smoke generated during use of monopolar current should be evacuated periodically.

TECHNIQUE OF ADENOMYOMA RESECTION

Three techniques of adenoma resection:

1. Elliptical strip excision technique for Grade I adenoma

Elliptical strip excision would be better for adenoma resection rather than attempting enucleation as in fibroid.

It may be difficult to locate adenoma intraoperatively, for which intraoperative transvaginal sonography is useful.

Adenoma bleeds only minimally. So if the surgeon encounters more bleeding while resecting, then he may have entered the healthy myometrium. The aim of resection is to reduce tension in myometrium (similar to debulking surgery of benign SOL of brain without injuring vital areas of brain), which can be achieved by debulking the affected myometrium, which is sometimes up to 50% leading to hemi-hysterectomy (Figs. 26.2 to 26.14).

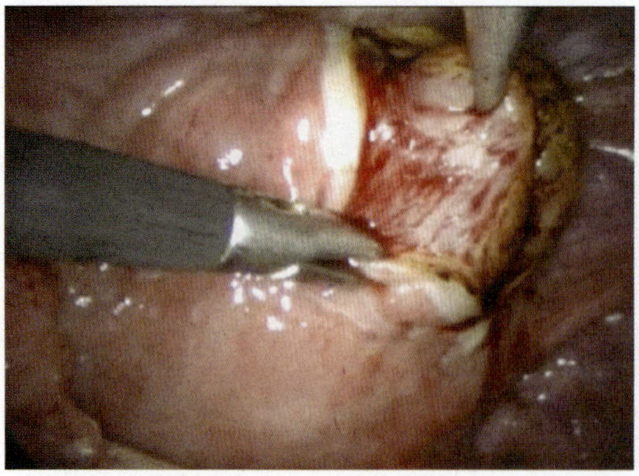

Fig. 26.4: Further enucleation of the adenonmyoma without planes.

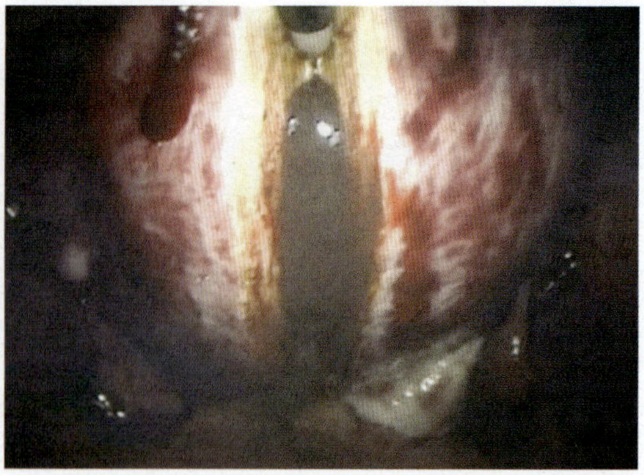

Fig. 26.5: Opening of the fibroid and recognition of chocolate fluid.

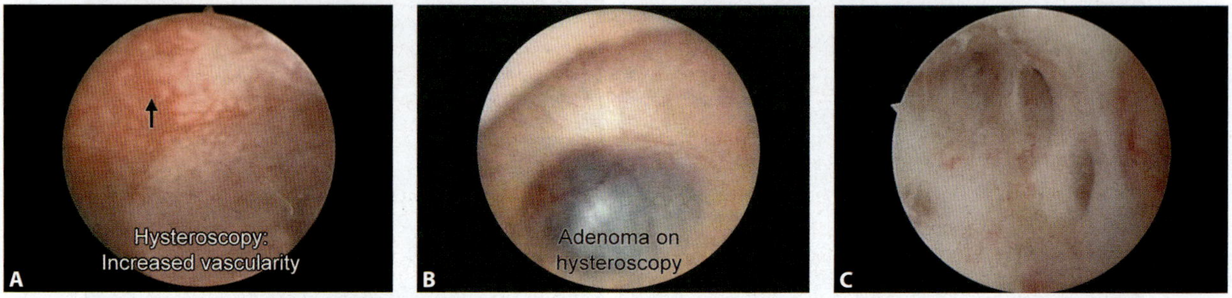

Figs. 26.6A to C: (A) Hysteroscopic sight of adenoma; (B) Subendometrial adenoma on hysteroscopy; (C) Endometrial puckering (looking like adhesions) due to adenomyosis.

2. Hood technique for Grade II without involvement of serosal layer of uterus by disease
3. Slice technique for Grade II with involvement of serosal layer of uterus by disease.

TECHNIQUE OF ENDOSUTURING: INTRACORPOREAL SLIP-KNOT TECHNIQUE

Proper approximation should be done after resection. It can be achieved by intracorporeal slip-knot technique.

First, we take full thickness bite on right edge and then on left edge. Then we place first half hitch and over we place a second half hitch. This makes it a square surgical knot. This loose knot is then slipped as far as down as it goes. This knot is not tightened and is not complete and secured as yet. It is left halfway through. The first stitch acts as an assistant holding the edges together for us.

Then we go for second stitch 1 cm lower down in same manner as the first stitch.

Then we go back to first stitch, which is further tightened completely to secure it further approximating the myometrium.

This is how entire length of myometrium is approximated without leaving any residual dead space.

NEW ADVANCEMENT

With availability of barbed suture, suturing after adenoma resection is less time-consuming and easy.

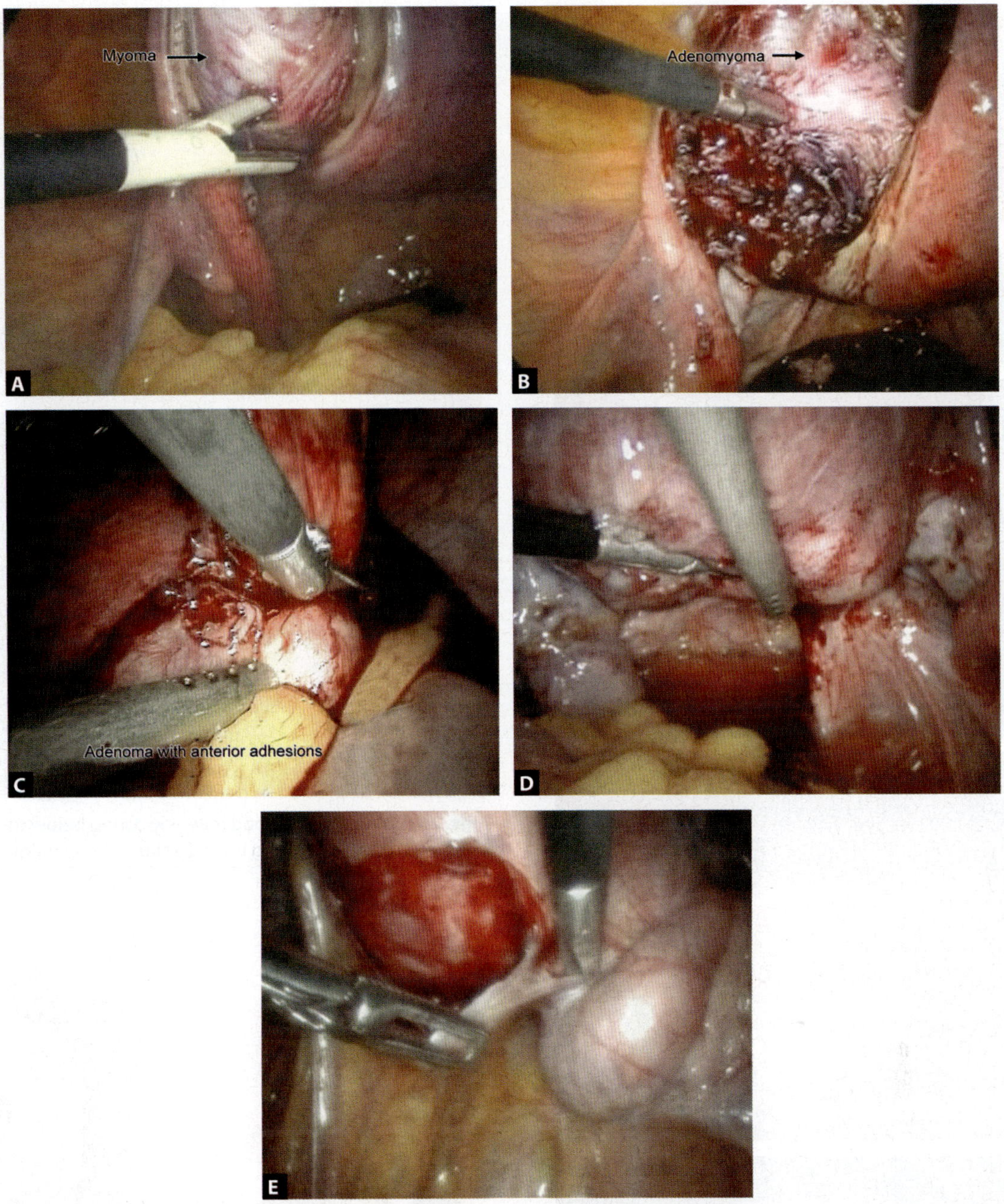

Figs. 26.7A to E: Adenoma with posterior adhesions.

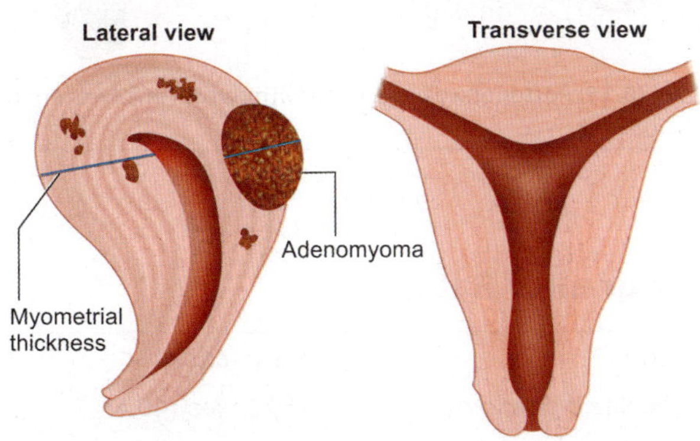

Fig. 26.8: Lateral and transverse view of adenomyotic lesion in ultrasound.

OUR EXPERIENCE

Our series	*1996–2013*
Localized adenoma	285 cases
Diffuse disease	63 cases
Total	348 cases

Symptomatic Improvements

Dysmenorrhea	92%	320 cases
Menstrual loss	84%	292 cases
Recurrence rate after 3 years	38%	132 cases

Note: Recurrence rate is higher in Grade II and Grade III.

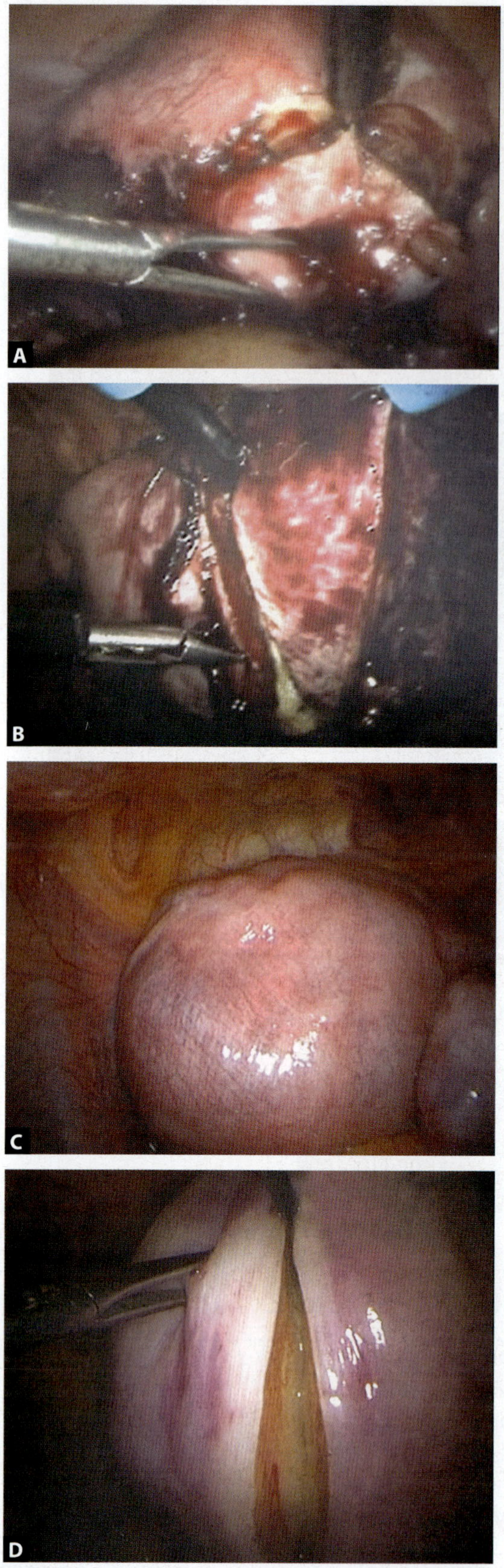

Figs. 26.9A to D: (A and B) Posterior wall fibroid with initial incisions; (C) Posterior wall adenoma with normal serosa; (D) Incision made using monopolar needle.

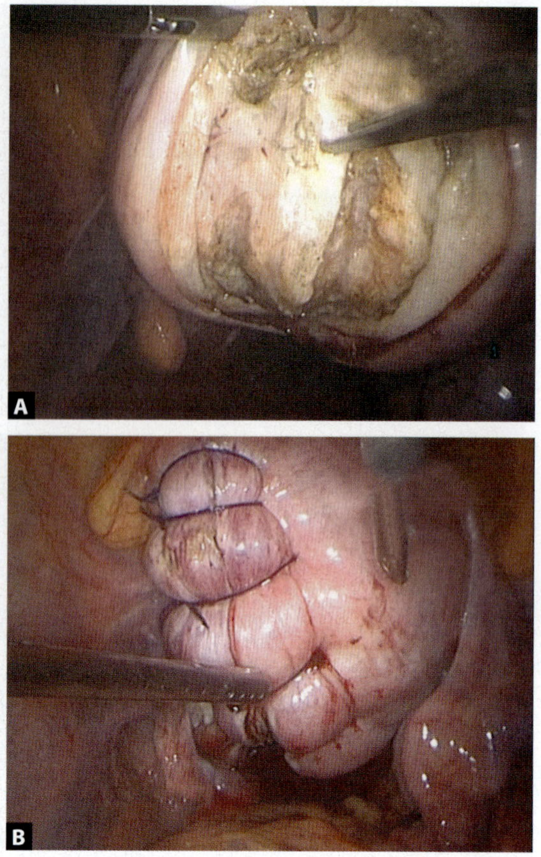

Figs. 26.10A and B: (A) Hood made by coring below the normal uterine serosa; (B) Suturing done by slip-knot technique.

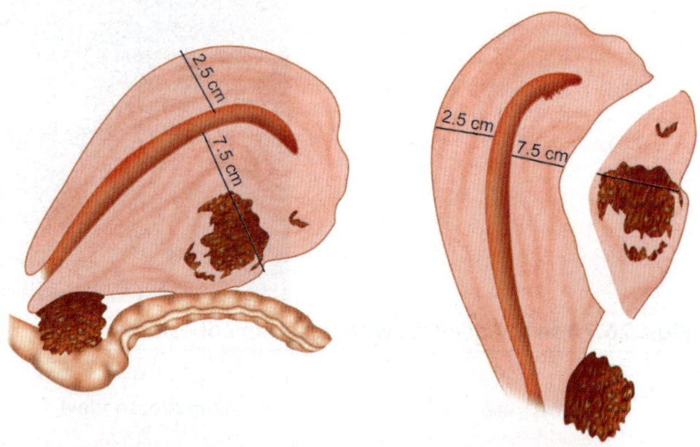

Fig. 26.11: Posterior wall adenoma with serosal involvement by the disease.

Pregnancy Rates

Group	*No. of cases*
Localized adenoma	115 cases (40.4%)
Diffuse adenomyosis	12 cases (19.04%)

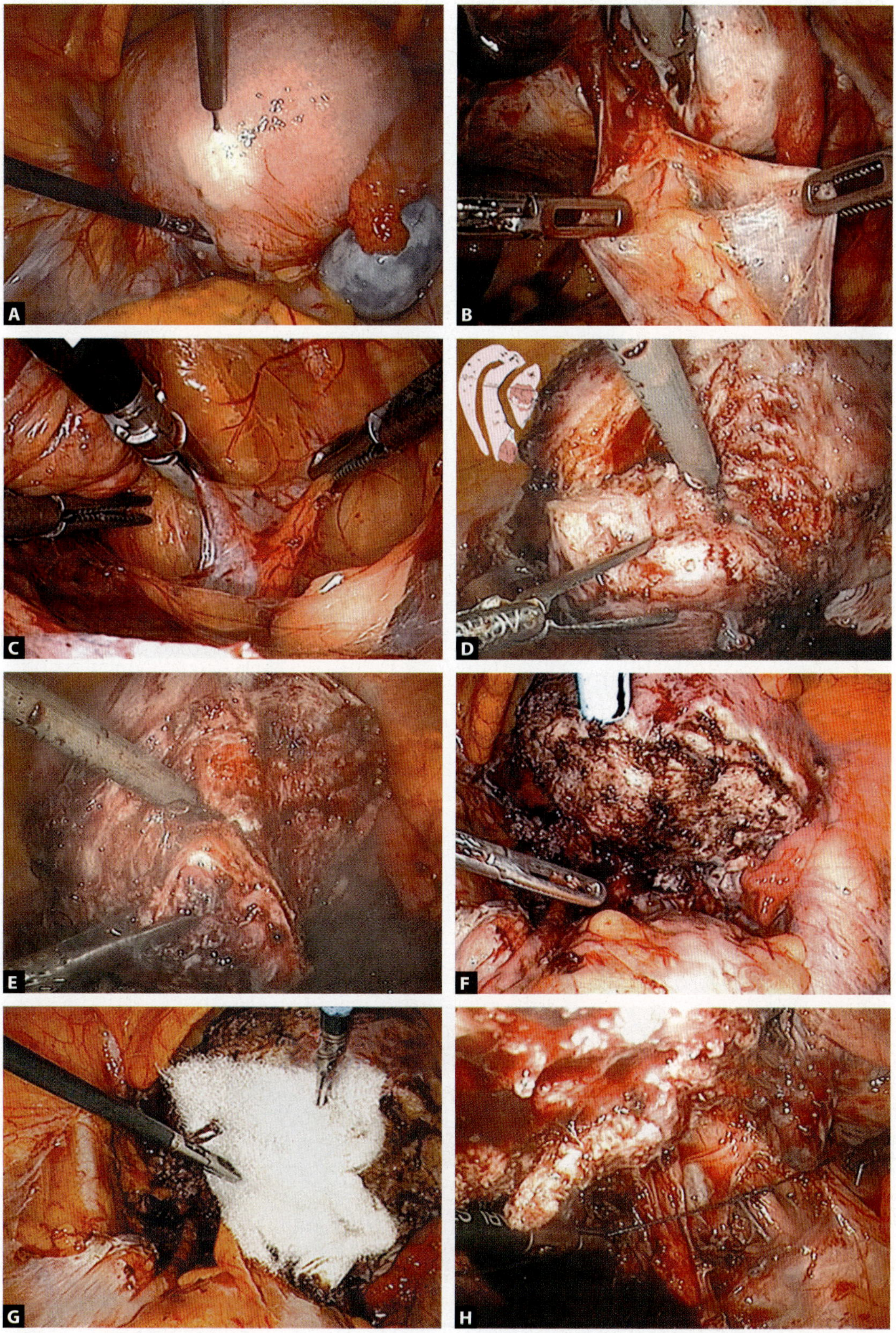

Figs. 26.12A to H: (A) Inj. pitressin (1:200 mL dilution) injected in adenoma; (B) Lateral mobilization of the ureter; (C) Uterine artery ligated at the origin; (D) Slice of adenoma excised; (E) Further enucleation of the adenoma; (F) Half of the adenomyotic posterior wall removed; (G) Surgicel (J&J) placed over the raw area for hemostasis; (H) Internal iliac artery ligated for hemostasis.

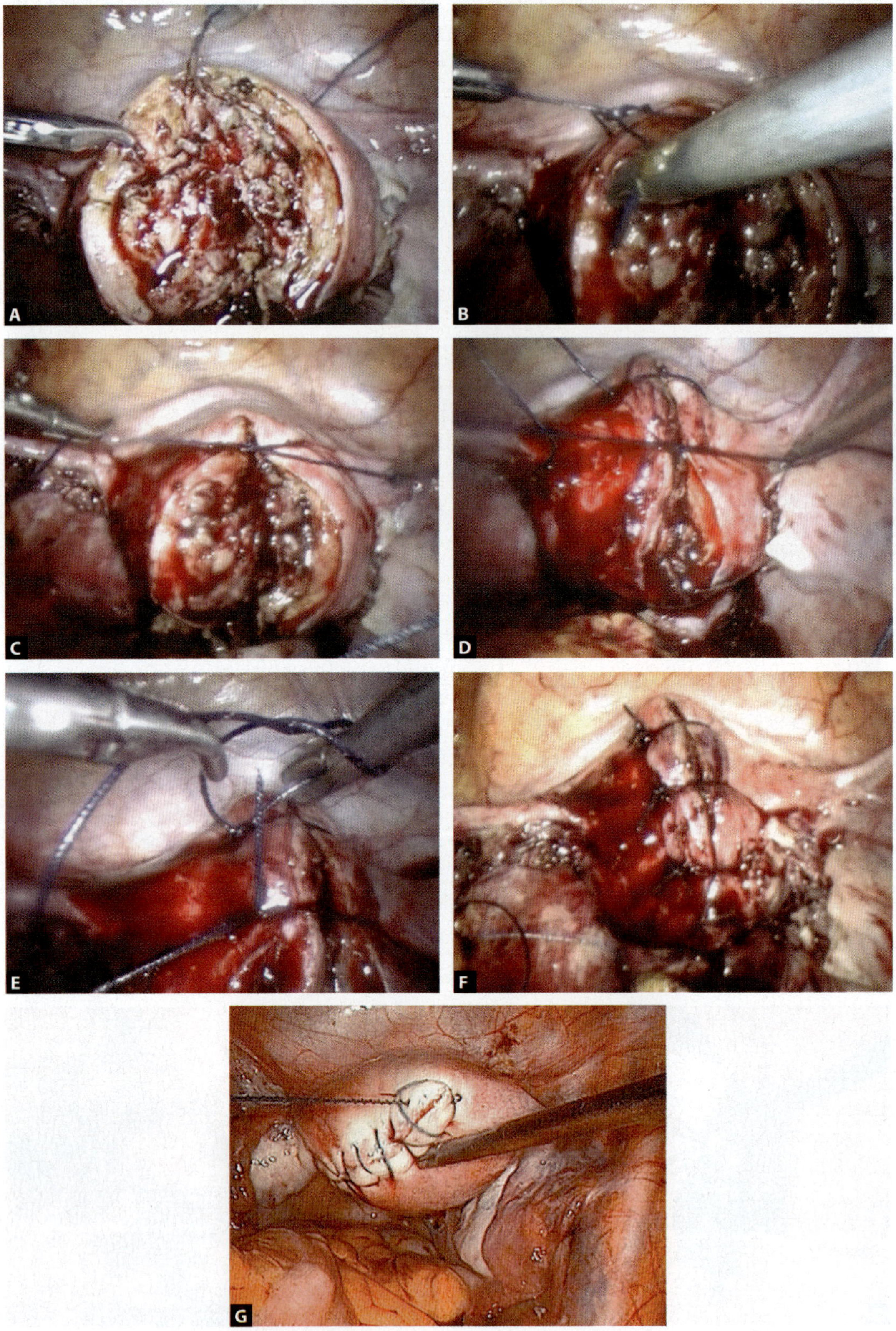

Figs. 26.13A to G: Adenomyomectomy in 7 steps (A-G)

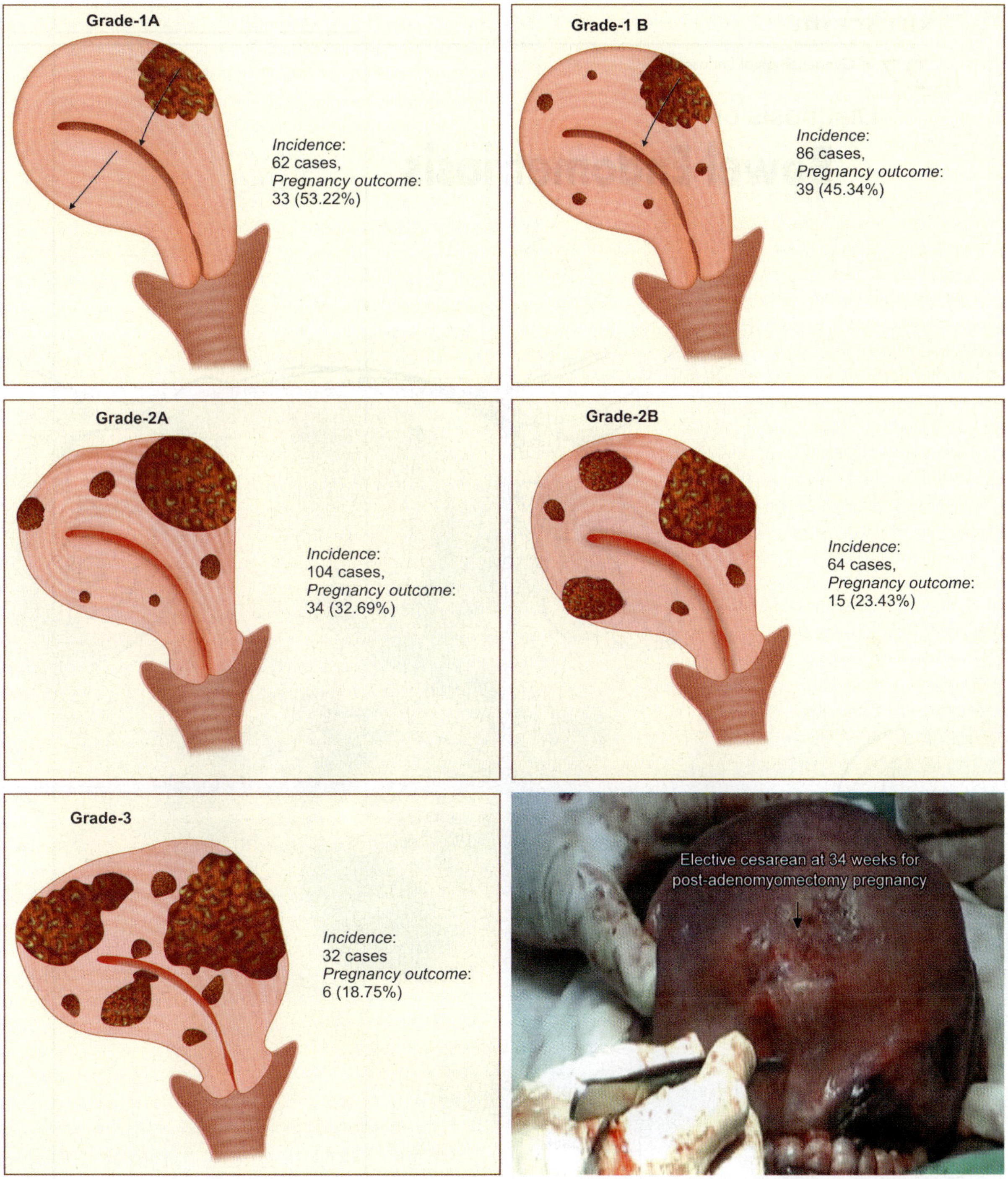

Fig. 26.14: Localizations of intrauterine adnomyosis with elective cesarean section at 34 weeks for post-adenomyotic pregnancy.

CONCLUSION

Adenoma resection is technically more difficult but quite a rewarding surgery in early stage of the disease in terms of fertility and improvement in symptomatology in the patients for whom hysterectomy cannot be advised.

KIEL SCHOOL

27 of Gynaecological Endoscopy

Diagnosis of Bowel Endometriosis

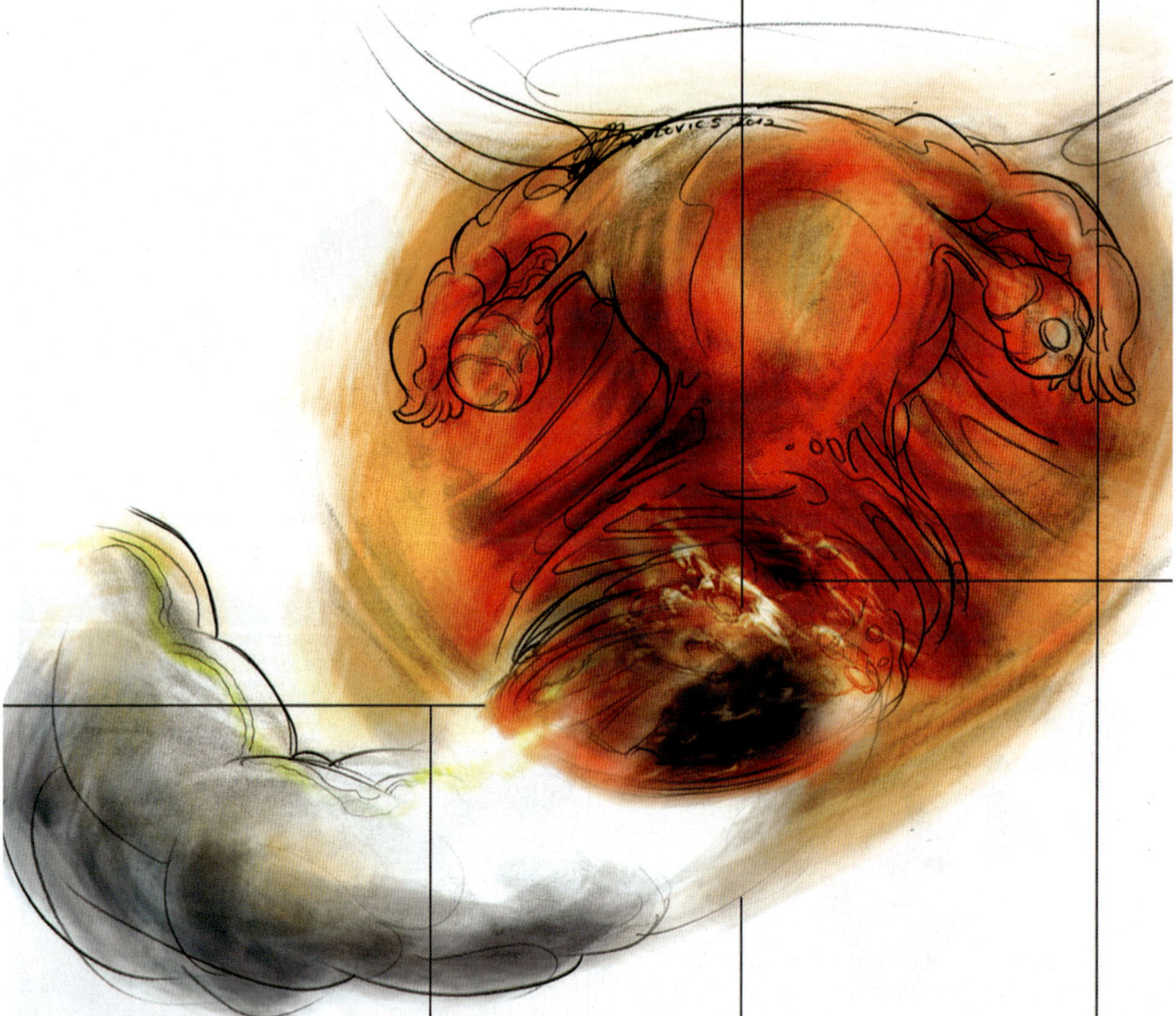

Chapter 27

Diagnosis of Bowel Endometriosis

J Marek Doniec, Mathias SS Löhnert

INTRODUCTION

Endometriosis, one of the most common diseases in gynecology, is often associated with therapeutic setbacks or failures that can be very frustrating for patients and their doctors. Almost 10% of all menstruating females suffer from endometriosis. Although it is a benign disease, pain and discomfort can significantly compromise a patient's quality of life in the long term. The incidence of endometriosis in infertile patients rises to 15–20%.[1]

The staging of endometriosis is usually based on the four-part classification of the American Society for Reproductive Medicine (ASRM).[2] Patients with stage IV disease often suffer from dysmenorrhea, infertility, and diffuse abdominal, pelvic, anal and lower back pain. Symptoms occur predominantly during the menstrual or perimenstrual phase and may take a chronic course.[3,4] If the gastrointestinal tract is involved, endometriosis most commonly affects the rectum and is often associated with anal bleeding and related pain,[5] even though transanal bleeding cannot be singled out as being pathognomonic for bowel endometriosis. To date, the recommended treatment option for rectal endometriosis is still laparotomy with bowel resection, whereas a laparoscopic approach is the preferred method for other cases of deep infiltrating endometriosis.[3,4,6] This underscores the importance of accurate preoperative staging, including the precise localization of extragenital endometriotic foci and possible involvement of the rectal wall.

IS ENDOSCOPIC SCREENING SUFFICIENT?

Rectal endometriosis should be suspected in any woman presenting with pelvic pain associated with defecation or rectal filling and/or transanal bleeding, the latter sometimes occurring synchronously with menstruation. Rectoscopy or colonoscopy can detect intramucosal endometriosis, sometimes accompanied by submucosal involvement, appearing as protrusions of the mucosa caused by the presence of cystic areas. Intramucosal or submucosal endometriosis accounts for 20% of all bowel involvement by endometriosis, because most rectal endometriotic foci are located in the muscularis propria or directly adjacent to the bowel wall. Thus, approximately 80% of all bowel endometriosis is not accessible to digital palpation or endoscopy, and pelvic imaging techniques are necessary for further investigation in patients with suspected rectal endometriosis.

Magnetic resonance (MR) and computed tomographic (CT) imaging of the pelvis is known to have an accuracy of approximately 70% in the diagnosis of rectal endometriotic infiltration.[7] Endorectal ultrasound (ERUS) offers high-resolution images of the rectal wall and perirectal structures and can accurately depict each layer of the rectal wall. Accordingly, ERUS is already a widely accepted modality for the pretherapeutic staging of rectal and anal cancer, with an accuracy greater than 85% for the staging of local intra- and extramural extension of malignant tumors.[8] Detection of a discontinuity in the layered structure of the bowel wall correlates strongly with involvement of the affected layers. In cancer surgery, the greatest disadvantage of ERUS is its inability to differentiate between direct cancer invasion and perirectal inflammatory changes that mimic the malignant invasion of deeper layers. Thus, approximately 10% accuracy is lost in detecting infiltration of the submucosa and muscularis propria. In cancer treatment, of course, staging a lesion as T1 versus T2 has a direct impact on the surgical procedure of choice, i.e., limited excision or radical surgery.

But in the case of endometriosis, poor discrimination between inflammatory changes and endometriotic tissue has no impact on surgical treatment as there is no need for the resection of perirectal lymph nodes. Thus, ERUS can clearly identify affected bowel wall layers to determine whether excision is feasible without opening the bowel, or it would be better to proceed with a segmental resection.

Gastroenterologists prefer endoluminal ultrasound with a flexible probe mounted on the tip of a flexible fiberscope, as commonly used in upper gastrointestinal (GI) endosonography. The use of flexible ultrasound probes extends the access range to the colon and has become a widely accepted modality in gastroenterology units. Colorectal surgeons favor ERUS using a rigid probe that can be introduced directly or through a preplaced rectoscope. Rigid ERUS probes are cheaper, do not require a videoendoscopy unit, provide accurate lesion detection and allow the surgeon to measure the distance to the anal verge and sphincter muscles for planning a sphincter-sparing procedure. In addition, 3D data acquisitions with rigid probe units are simplifying the preoperative visualization of endometriotic foci and their relation to the rectal wall.

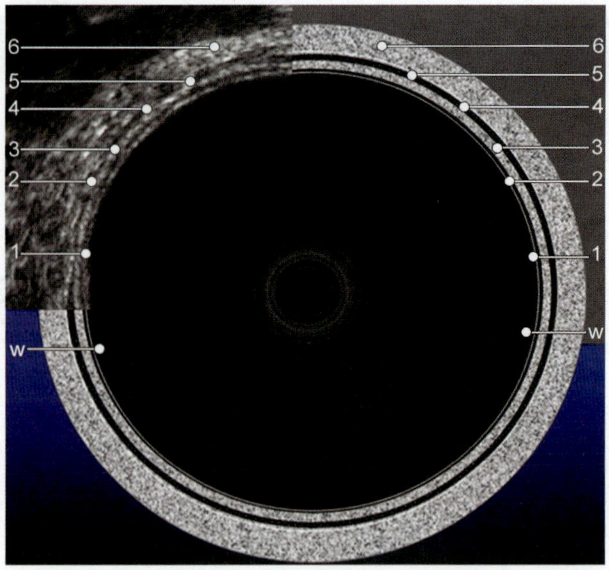

Fig. 27.1: Normal endorectal sonogram: (W) Water; (1) Hyperechoic interface between water-filled balloon and mucosa; (2) Hypoechoic mucosa; (3) Hyperechoic submucosa and interface between submucosa and muscularis propria; (4) Hypoechoic muscularis propria; (5) Hyperechoic margin between muscularis propria and perirectal region or serosa; (6) fatty tissue.

ENDORECTAL ULTRASOUND: ANATOMIC STRUCTURES AND FINDINGS IN ENDOMETRIOSIS PATIENTS

The rigid ultrasound probe is introduced via a rectoscope positioned at the rectosigmoid junction. When a 7.5, 10.0 or 20.0 MHz probe is used, the sonogram displays the bowel wall with three anatomic layers and two artificial layers. Starting from the innermost (luminal) aspect, the first layer is a hyperechoic artificial ring formed by the interface between the water-filled balloon covering the ERUS probe and the mucosa. Next comes a hypoechoic ring (second layer) representing the mucosa of the bowel wall. The second hyperechoic ring (third layer of the wall) consists of the submucosa and a second interface between the submucosa and muscularis propria. The second hypoechoic ring (fourth layer of the wall) corresponds to the muscularis propria and is surrounded by the outer (third) artificial hyperechoic ring (fifth layer), which is formed by the interface between the muscularis propria and perirectal fat or serosa (Fig. 27.1 and Table 27.1).

The imaging appearance of (para)rectal endometriosis depends on the activity of the lesion. Active endometriotic lesions are hypoechoic and include cystic changes, while inactive lesions show heterogeneous echogenicity due to fibrosis. It is very common to find coexisting active and inactive lesions in one patient, so ERUS findings are normally irregular with a mixed hypoechoic and hyperechoic pattern. An asymmetric appearance of perirectal structures with mixed echogenicity in premenopausal women is always suspicious for perirectal endometriosis. This diagnosis can be established by correlating ultrasound findings with the clinical presentation.

The staging of ERUS findings in endometriosis is outlined below.

Stage 1: No relation to the rectal wall, pararectal endometriosis without rectal involvement. ERUS shows asymmetric mixed echogenicity in the perirectal fat. No direct contact with bowel wall structures is observed. The outer hyperechoic (fifth) layer of the bowel wall is not disrupted, and there is no evidence of intramural infiltration.

*Stage 2***:** Endometriotic tissue is in direct contact with the bowel wall. ERUS shows no disruption of the outer hyperechoic layer, which excludes involvement of the rectal wall (Fig. 27.2).

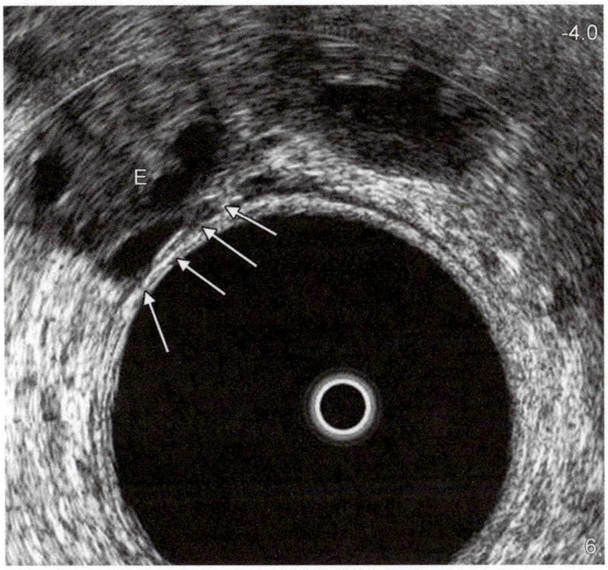

Fig. 27.2: ERUS image of an endometriotic mass (E) (approximately 2 cm) in the cul-de-sac adjacent to the rectal wall. The third hyperechoic layer between the muscularis propria and perirectal region (⇨) is intact and not thickened. This finding excludes involvement of the rectal wall.

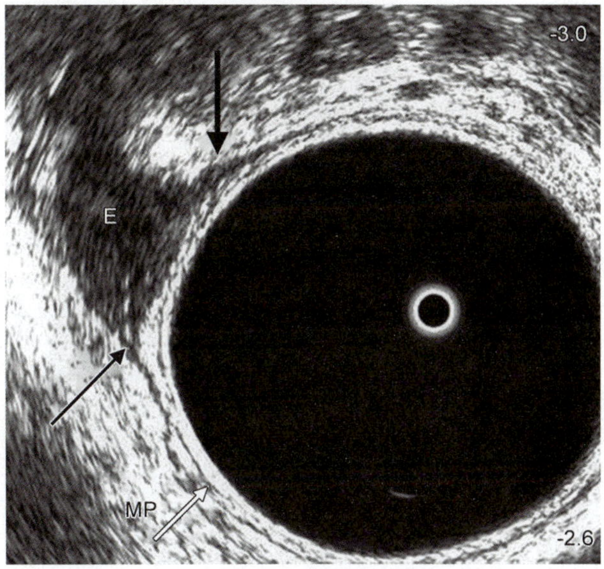

Fig. 27.3: ERUS image of an endometriotic mass (E) (approximately 1.5 cm) infiltrating the rectal wall (between ➔). The third hyperechoic layer, the muscularis propria (MP, ⇨), is thickened, indicating involvement, and cannot be differentiated from the mass. This finding indicates rectal wall involvement with infiltration of the muscularis propria. Normal muscularis propria (MP, second hypoechoic layer).

Stage 3: Infiltration of the bowel wall is detectable by ERUS. The depth of infiltration should be noted:

- Infiltration into the muscularis propria is characterized by disruption of the hyperechoic fifth layer and thickening of the hypoechoic fourth layer (muscularis propria). The hyperechoic third layer (interface) remains intact and is not interrupted (Fig. 27.3).
- Infiltration of the submucosa: The suspected endometriotic tissue is in the third hyperechoic layer or has spread directly through the outer

Table 27.1: Diagnostic imaging modalities used in the preoperative assessment of pelvic endometriosis.

Diagnostic modality	*Advantages*	*Disadvantages*
Endoscopy	Reveals intraluminal findings with high accuracy.	Peri- or intramural masses are detectable only by their visible mass effect. No differentiation from adjacent and infiltrating tumors.
X-ray	Reveals intraluminal findings with high accuracy.	Peri- or intramural masses are detectable only by their visible mass effect.
CT	Reveals intra- and extraluminal findings.	Poor accuracy in differentiating between adjacent invading perimural tumors.
MRI	Accurate depiction of tumor site and involved mural layers. Both intra- and perimural masses are detectable.	Very high cost. Only intrarectal MRI probe provides accuracy comparable to endosonography.
Flexible ERUS	Accurate depiction of tumor site and involved mural layers. Both intra- and perimural masses are detectable. Permits lesion detection into the colon.	High cost, measurement of distance to anal canal is not accurate. Accuracy is examiner-dependent.
Rigid ERUS	Accurate depiction of tumor site and involved mural layers. Both intra- and perimural masses are detectable. Low cost. Accurate measurement of distance to anal canal.	Accuracy is examiner-dependent. Scanning is limited to the rectum and rectosigmoid.

CT, computed tomography; MRI, magnetic resonance imaging; ERUS, endorectal ultrasound.

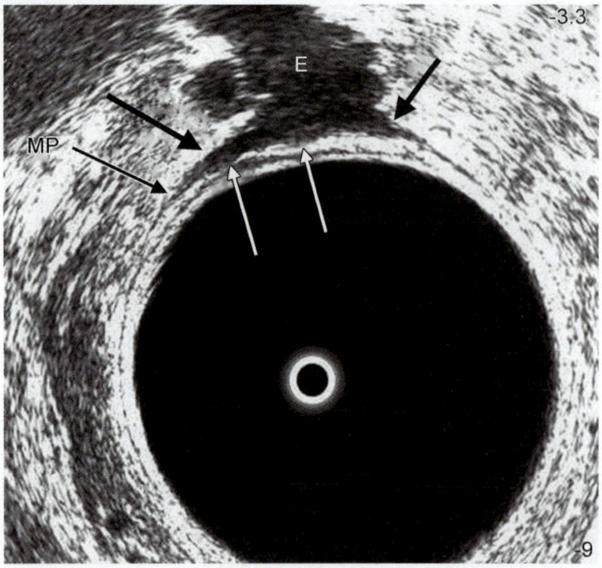

Fig. 27.4: ERUS image of an endometriotic mass (E) (approximately 2.5 cm) infiltrating the rectal wall (between ➡). The third hyperechoic layer, the muscularis propria (MP, ⟶), is thickened, indicating involvement, and cannot be differentiated from the mass. The second hyperechoic layer is irregular (⇨). These findings indicate rectal wall involvement with infiltration of the muscularis propria and submucosa. Normal muscularis propria (MP, third hypoechoic layer).

layers into the third layer. In this case, the submucosa, represented by the third layer, shows an irregular shape with hypoechoic areas in the hyperechoic layer (Fig. 27.4).

- Infiltration of the mucosa: Endometriosis directly involves the mucosa (second hypoechoic layer) or the mucosa and submucosa (disruption of the hyperechoic second layer by a hypoechoic or heterogeneous structure). Full-thickness infiltration through all the outer layers into the hypoechoic second layer indicates involvement of the whole bowel wall.

In our own series, the sensitivity of ERUS imaging for defining the depth of rectal wall infiltration was 76% percent (20/26). Sensitivity for the muscularis propria was 97% (26/27). Overall sensitivity for rectal wall infiltration was 97% (26/27).[8]

MANAGEMENT OF RECTAL ENDOMETRIOSIS

Every patient with transrectal bleeding should have a complete colonoscopy to exclude cancer, polyps and inflammatory disease. If the history suggests external endometriosis as a possible cause of symptoms (menstruation-associated rectal bleeding, anal/pelvic pain, or suspicious pararectal findings by bimanual examination and/or endovaginal ultrasound), ERUS should be performed to detect or exclude endometriosis in the pararectal region. ERUS results are correlated with examiner experience, so the procedure requires an experienced colorectal surgeon who is used to performing ERUS routinely.

If ERUS demonstrates stage 1 or 2 endometriosis (unrelated to the bowel wall or abutting the wall without disrupting the outer hyperechoic layer), the treatment of first choice is primary laparoscopy performed by a gynecologic surgeon without colorectal assistance (Table 27.2).

If ERUS is suspicious for rectal infiltration (stage 3), laparoscopic resection of a rectal wall segment should be performed with the simultaneous help of a colorectal surgeon. In some cases, if the endometriotic mass is less than 10 mm in diameter, the resection can be performed with a linear stapler to cut off a limited portion of the bowel wall and reapproximate the wall in one step.

With an endometriotic mass larger than 10 mm, the infiltration depth does not interfere with the type of resection. In most cases, an anterior rectal resection is necessary for the complete removal of all affected tissue. Experienced colorectal surgeons can perform

Table 27.2: Results of ERUS in 85 patients with suspected rectal involvement by endometriosis and correlation with treatment (conventional laparotomy, laparoscopy or no surgery). The overall sensitivity of ERUS for rectal wall involvement was 97%.

ERUS finding	*Total*	*Laparotomy*	*Laparoscopy*	*Conservative treatment*
No abnormalities	13	2	4	7
Pelvic mass not in contact with the rectal wall	21	6	10	5
Mass abutting the rectal wall	12	4	7	1
Rectal wall infiltration	39	25	7	7
Muscularis propria	32	20	6	6
Submucosa	7	5	1	1

a low anterior rectal resection laparoscopically, so the preferred approach will depend largely on the skills of the surgeon. Conventional resection can be considered in all advanced cases with extensive involvement of the lower third of the rectum in order to preserve the sphincter.

If ERUS confirms the presence of well-circumscribed endometrial lesions that are confined to the mucosa and/or submucosa without affecting the muscularis propria, an endoscopic approach may be considered. A mucosal lesion less than 3 cm in diameter can be treated by endoscopic mucosal resection, similar to a polypectomy. If submucosal spread is found, the authors recommend an endoscopic submucosal dissection as the treatment of choice.

CONCLUSION

ERUS is a useful, noninvasive diagnostic tool in endometriosis, especially in patients with proven or suspected endometriosis involving the bowel wall.

ERUS can safely stratify cases that are appropriate for an endoscopic approach, laparoscopy without bowel resection, a laparoscopic segmental bowel resection, or conventional rectal resection. ERUS provides high sensitivity and specificity for rectal involvement by endometriosis and is recommended in every patient with suspected extragenital pelvic endometriosis.

REFERENCES

1. Farinon AM, Stroppa I, Chiarelli C. Therapy of colorectal endometriosis. Colo Proctol. 1992;14:230-4.
2. The American Fertility Society. Revised American Fertility Society classification of endometriosis: 1985. Fertil Steril. 1985;43(3):351-2.
3. Chapron C, Dubuisson JB. Management of deep endometriosis. Ann N Y Acad Sci. 2001;943:276-80.
4. Koninckx PR, Martin DC. Surgical treatment of deeply infiltrating. In: Shaw RW, editor. Endometriosis. Current Understanding and Management. Oxford: Blackwell Scientific; 1995. p. 264-81.
5. Zwas FR, Lyon DT. Endometriosis. An important condition in clinical gastroenterology. Dig Dis Sci. 1991;36(3):353-64.
6. Schroder J, Lohnert M, Doniec JM, et al. Endoluminal ultrasound diagnosis and operative management of rectal endometriosis. Dis Colon Rectum. 1997;40(5):614-7.
7. Roseau G, Dumontier I, Palazzo L, et al. Rectosigmoid endometriosis: endoscopic ultrasound features and clinical implications. Endoscopy. 2000;32(7):525-30.
8. Doniec JM, Kahlke V, Peetz F, et al. Rectal endometriosis: high sensitivity and specificity of endorectal ultrasound with an impact for the operative management. Dis Colon Rectum. 2003;46(12):1667-73.

KIEL SCHOOL

28 of Gynaecological Endoscopy

Sentinel Lymph Node Detection

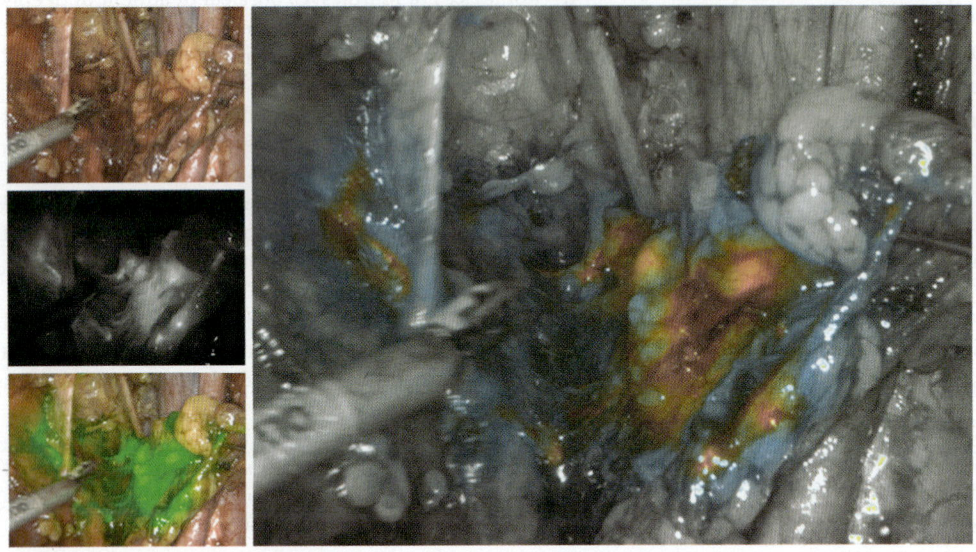

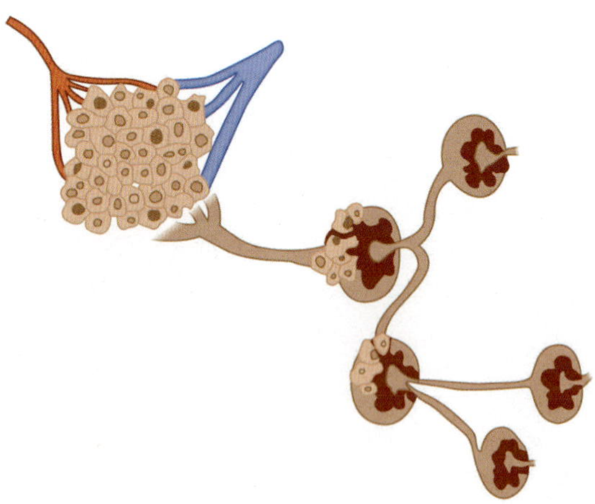

Chapter 28

Sentinel Lymph Node Detection

Andreas Hackethal, Hans-Rudolf Tinneberg

BACKGROUND

Sentinel lymph node biopsy describes a procedure where only one or a couple of specific lymph nodes are detected and removed. They are regarded as responsible for reflecting the extent of lymphogenic metastasis of a tumor. This was first described by Goulds in 1960 when he found that in parotid carcinoma a normal-appearing lymph node between the junction of the anterior and posterior fascial vein contained metastatic disease on frozen section.[1] He studied 28 cases of parotid tumors with investigating the "sentinel node" and did not perform a radical neck dissection in case of negative node. Because of his findings he proposed to abandon the lymphadenectomy in case of negative "sentinel node" on frozen section. The sentinel lymph node describes the first lymph node being drained by the tumor environment (Fig. 28.1). Sentinel means watchman.

The concept of sentinel lymph node states that the sentinel is the first node in the lymphatic basin receiving lymphatic flow from the tumor. Consequently, if the sentinel does not contain metastases, the remainder of the basin will be negative for metastatic disease and a lymphadenectomy will not add to the diagnostic workup or therapeutic benefit. On the contrary, reducing surgical trauma is the main advantage of sentinel node biopsy, therefore reducing the impact to the lymphatic system draining the tumor area with reducing the risk of lymphedema.

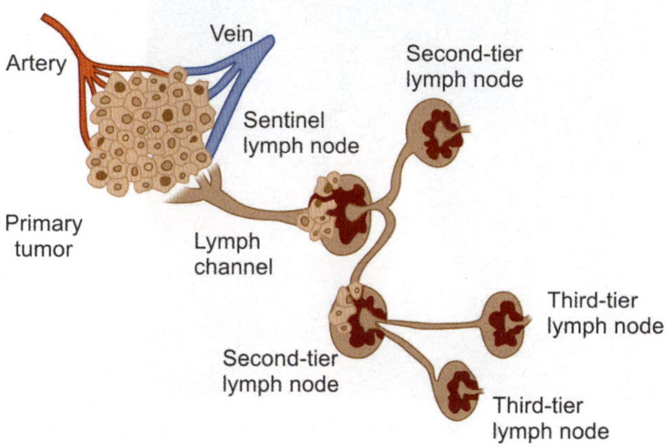

Fig. 28.1: Concept of the sentinel node.

SENTINEL NODE BIOPSY IN CLINICAL USE

Sentinel lymph node biopsy is standard of care in breast cancer and melanoma treatment. Also in vulval cancer, the sentinel concept is recognized and widely used, following the publication of the GOG- 173 and GROINSS V-1 studies.[2,3] Further areas of sentinel node biopsy comprise cervical, endometrial and vulval cancer, colorectal cancer, head and neck cancers, non-small cell lung cancer, thyroid cancer, gastric and esophageal cancers and penile cancer (Table 28.1).

Table 28.1: Overview of first published sentinel node biopsy papers for different entities.

References	*Entity*
4	Penile carcinoma
5	Melanoma
6	Breast cancer
7	Vulvar cancer
8	Thyroid malignancies
9	Nonsmall cell lung cancer
10	Colorectal cancer
11	Gastric cancer
12	Cervical cancer
13	Endometrial cancer

CONVENTIONAL SENTINEL NODE MARKER

In order to detect the sentinel node, traceable material is injected in the environment of the primary cancer. Imaging techniques are used to display the tracer within the lymphatics and lymph nodes. A recent review by Xiong et al. describes the different techniques for lymphatic imaging (Fig. 28.2).

In today's medical surgical routine a filtered sulfur colloid combined with Technetium 99 m with or without blue dye is the most widely used sentinel marker. Preoperative a lymphatic imaging technique is used and intraoperative a gamma probe or Geiger meter is used to identify the sentinel node. During the last years, Indocyanine green has become an excessively investigated marker for sentinel node biopsy.

Techniques of lymphatic imaging

Direct techniques
- Lymphangiography

Indirect techniques
- Lymphography
- Lymphoscintigraphy and single-photon emission computed tomography (SPECT)
- Fluorodeoxyglucose-positron emission tomography FDG-PET/CT and FDG-PET/MRI)
- Magnetic resonance lymphography (MRL)
- Ultrasound and contrast-enhanced ultrasound (CEUS)
- Near-infrared (NIR) fluorescence-guided imaging techniques

Xiong,L.et al, EJSO (2014) 40, 270-276

Fig. 28.2: Direct and indirect techniques of lymphatic imaging.[14]

Indocyanine Green

Indocyanine green (ICG) has been studied in medicine since the 1950s. ICG, a tricarbocyanine dye, is a fluorescent marker, which characteristically lights up in near-infrared light from 806 nm. ICG is highly soluble and binds to albumin, therefore being transported within the lymphatics. The use of ICG as sentinel marker was facilitated with the use of video-laparoscopic surgery and first described for gastric cancer in 2004.[15] Within the last years, studies reporting the use of ICG as sentinel marker in gynecology have been numerous, most of them reporting improved Sentinel detection rates compared to Technetium-99m and blue dye marker (Table 28.2 shows some representative studies).

In short, ICG is diluted and 2.5 mg are injected into the cervix at 3:00 and 9:00 superficially (1 mm) and deep (4 mm). After 5 min, sentinel lymph nodes can be detected laparoscopically with a near-infrared light source and camera. Most helpful is the pinpoint system (Novadaq), which works with an overlay picture of the normal laparoscopic picture and the near-infrared picture at the same time (Fig. 28.3).

Table 28.2: Representative studies evaluating Indocyanine green use as sentinel lymph node marker for gynecological malignancies.

References	*Site/Cancer*	*Detection rate % (n/n)*
16	Cervix	100 (68/68)
17	Endometrium	100
18	Vulva	100% (21/21)

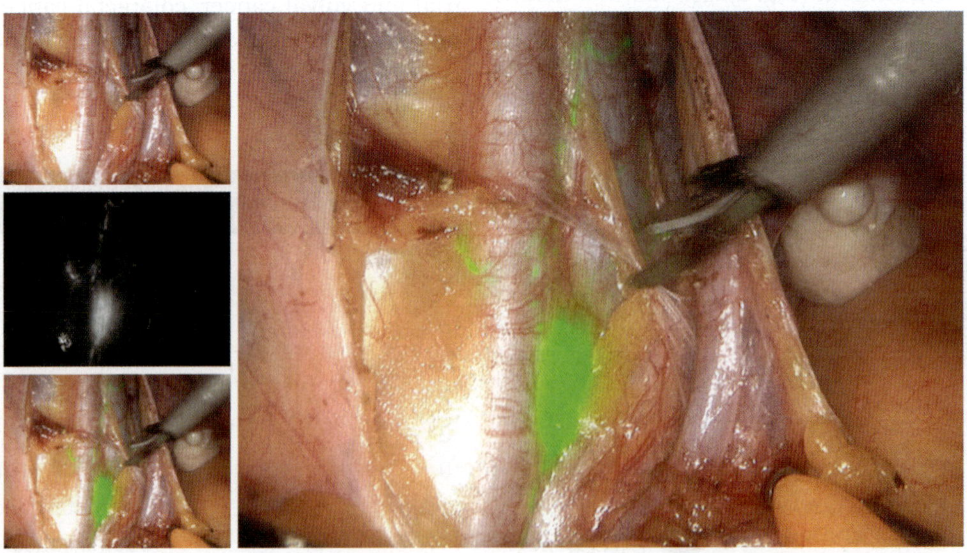

Fig. 28.3: Laparoscopic view during left pelvic sentinel lymphadenectomy with near-infrared overlaid picture. *Left top:* The conventional laparoscopic view, the middle picture showing the near-infrared picture of ICG-positive tissue, the picture at the bottom showing the normal laparoscopic view with ICG fluorescence overlay, also seen large on the right side (Novadaq).

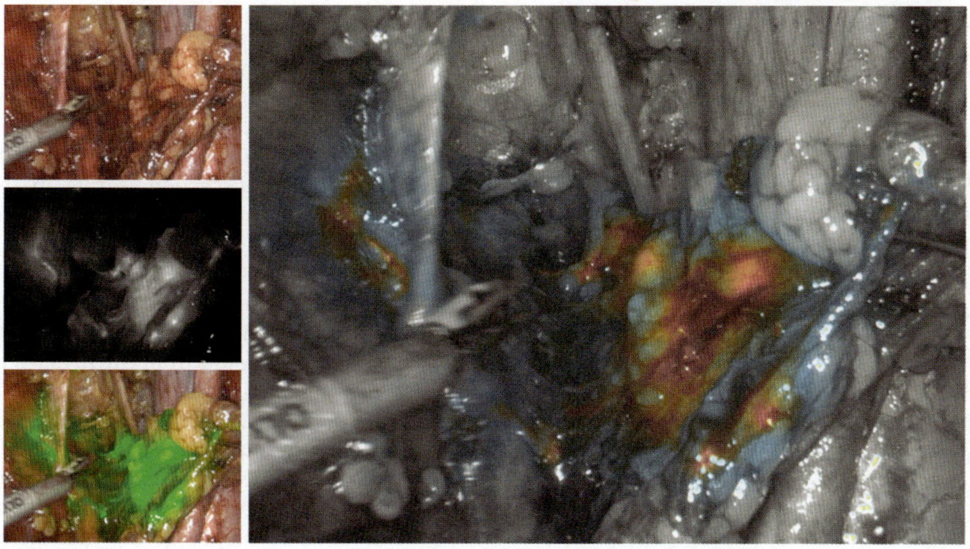

Fig. 28.4: Laparoscopic view during right pelvic sentinel lymphadenectomy with near-infrared overlaid picture. *Left top:* The conventional laparoscopic view, the middle picture showing the near-infrared picture of ICG-positive tissue, the picture at the bottom showing the normal laparoscopic view with ICG fluorescence overlay. On the right side is the ICG color concentration mode shown, reflecting lymph nodes in the red area (Novadaq).

The pin-point system additionally allows an ICG concentration mode on a color basis. With this mode, lymph nodes can be detected more easily (Fig. 28.4).

GYNECOLOGICAL CANCERS

Endometrial Cancer

Endometrial cancer is one of the most common cancers in females. Depending on the infiltration depth and tumor grading hysterectomy and bilateral salpingoopherectomy should be combined with a comprehensive pelvic and paraaortic lymphadenectomy.[19,20] The group of endometrial cancer patients often comprises elderly and obese women with comorbidities. Therefore, a genuine interest is to minimize surgical trauma, if similar oncological outcomes can be achieved. Even though, sentinel lymph node biopsy in endometrial cancer has been investigated since 2001,[13] its regular use is still controversial. A recent meta-analysis published by Lin et al. analyzed 44 studies with 2236 patients.[21] Their pooled overall detection rate was 83%, and the pooled sensitivity 91%. Using ICG increased the overall detection rate to 93%. Lin et al. conclude that there is strong evidence for sentinel node biopsy being an accurate and feasible method for assessment of lymph node involvement in endometrial cancer.[21] This conclusion was also drawn by Bodurtha et al.[22] who published a systematic review and meta-analysis with results from 55 studies and 4915 patient data.[22]

Cervical Cancer

Cervical cancer treatment follows a highly individualized protocol. Since surgery and radiation achieve similar results, it is of outmost importance to assess and evaluate individual tumor parameter and therefore minimize the risk of double treatment, meaning surgery and radiation. Pelvic lymphadenectomy can be considered as one of the keys in cervical cancer treatment. Negative nodes on frozen section may allow for radical hysterectomy, if a complete tumor excision can be achieved. Positive pelvic nodes indicate the necessity for pelvic radiation; therefore no hysterectomy but a paraaortic lymphadenectomy is recommended to define the radiation field.

Sentinel biopsy of pelvic lymph nodes in cervical cancer has been studied extensively and best detection rates and mapping results have been found with tumors less than 2 cm[23,24] Guidelines state to consider the sentinel lymph node biopsy in tumors less than 2 cm (NCCC Guideline, AWMF). However, if no sentinel is detected, a comprehensive lymphadenectomy is recommended (NCCC, AWMF). A recent meta-analysis found the detection rate with use of ICG to be similar to the standard of care, Technetium 99-m with or without blue dye.[25]

Apart from a surgical benefit of minimizing the trauma, the frozen section on a sentinel lymph node is faster than comprehensive lymphadenectomy and may also reduce operating room time and costs.

Vulvar Cancer

The relevance of Sentinel node biopsy in vulvar cancer has been proposed in 1994[7] Up to date, the sentinel concept in vulvar cancer is considered to be an alternative to comprehensive lymphadenectomy and has been adopted within most international guidelines.[20,25-27] Published evidence suggests that unifocal tumors of less than 4 cm maximum dimension might safely be managed by excision of the sentinel lymph nodes identified in either groin (BGCS). However, the patient should be consented preoperatively, if no sentinel node is identified, a comprehensive inguinofemoral lymphadenectomy should be considered. The German AWMF guideline as well as the BGCS state that requirement for Sentinel node biopsy in vulvar cancer should be:

- Cancers measuring less than 4 cm in maximum dimension
- Macroscopic unifocal cancers
- No clinical or on imaging evidence to suspect lymph node metastasis
- No known safety issues for the use of Patent Blue dye and/or technetium-99
- Adequate experience in use of sentinel node biopsy
- Informed patient consent and acceptance of close follow-up

Only recently a new hybrid tracer using indocyanine green with 99m Tc-nanocolloid (ICG 99m Tc-nanocolloid) improved the intraoperative visualization of Sentinel lymph nodes.[28]

PERSPECTIVES

Modern surgical strategies focus on trauma reduction with equal or even improved surgical outcome. Former radical surgery as correlate for consequent and effective cancer treatment is more and more focus of today's discussions. In current medicine, the benefit of a comprehensive lymphadenectomy in certain cancers is questioned or even abandoned and therefore techniques aiming at reducing tissue removal and preservation of nonaffected lymphatics are highly appreciated. Sentinel biopsy in gynecological cancers plays an important role. It was partly adopted to the standard of care. The sentinel node biopsy most likely with use of ICG will become a breakthrough for our daily clinical routine because of its effectiveness, its ease in usage, the availability and the reduction of costs for the health system.

REFERENCES

1. Gould EA, Winship T, Philbin PH, et al. Observations on a "sentinel node" in cancer of the parotid. Cancer. 1960;13:77-8.
2. Van der Zee AG, Oonk MH, De Hullu JA, et al. Sentinel node dissection is safe in the treatment of early-stage vulvar cancer. J Clin Oncol. 2008;26: 884-9.
3. Oonk MH, van Hemel BM, Hollema H, et al. Size of sentinel-node metastasis and chances of non-sentinel node involvement and survival in early stage vulvar cancer: results from GROINSS-V, a multicentre observational study. Lancet Oncol. 2010;11:646-52.
4. Cabanas RM. An approach for the treatment of penile carcinoma. Cancer. 1977;39:456-66.
5. Ross MI, Reintgen D, Balch CM. Selective lymphadenectomy: emerging role for lymphatic mapping and sentinel node biopsy in the management of early stage melanoma. Semin Surg Oncol. 1993;9:219-23.
6. Krag DN, Weaver DL, Alex JC, et al. Surgical resection and radiolocalization of the sentinel lymph node in breast cancer using a gamma probe. Surg Oncol. 1993;2:335-9.
7. Levenback C, Burke TW, Gershenson DM, et al. Intraoperative lymphatic mapping for vulvar cancer. Obstet Gynecol. 1994;84:163-7.
8. Kelemen PR, Van Herle AJ, Giuliano AE. Sentinel lymphadenectomy in thyroid malignant neoplasms. Arch Surg. 1998;133(3):288-92.
9. Little AG, DeHoyos A, Kirgan DM, et al. Intraoperative lymphatic mapping for non-small cell lung cancer: the sentinel node technique. J Thorac Cardiovasc Surg. 1999;117:220-4.
10. Joosten JJ, Strobbe LJ, Wauters CA, et al. Intraoperative lymphatic mapping and the sentinel node concept in colorectal carcinoma. Br J Surg. 1999;86:482-6.
11. Maruyama K, Sasako M, Kinoshita T, et al. Can sentinel node biopsy indicate rational extent of lymphadenectomy in gastric cancer surgery? Fundamental and new information on lymph-node dissection. Langenbecks Arch Surg. 1999;384(2): 149-57.
12. Medl M, Peters-Engl C, Schütz P, et al. First report of lymphatic mapping with isosulfan blue dye and sentinel node biopsy in cervical cancer. Anticancer Res. 2000;20:1133-4.
13. Holub Z, Kliment L, Lukác J, et al. Laparoscopically-assisted intraoperative lymphatic mapping in endometrial cancer: preliminary results. Eur J Gynaecol Oncol. 2001;22:118-21.
14. Xiong L, Engel H, Gazyakan E, et al. Current techniques for lymphatic imaging: State of the art and future perspectives. Eur J Surg Oncol. 2014;40:270-6.
15. Nimura H, Narimiya N, Mitsumori N, et al. Infrared ray electronic endoscopy combined with indocyanine green injection for detection of sentinel nodes of patients with gastric cancer. Br J Surg. 2004;91: 575-9.

16. Buda A, Papadia A, Zapardiel I et al. From conventional radiotracer Tc-99(m) with blue dye to indocyaninee green fluorescence: a comparison of methods towards optimization of sentinel lymph node mapping in early stage cervical cancer for a laparoscopic approach. Ann Surg Oncol. 2016;23: 2959-65.
17. Laios A, Volpi D, Tullis ID. A prospective pilot study of detection of sentinel lymph nodes in gynaecological cancers using a novel near infrared fluorescence imaging system. BMC Res Notes. 2015;8:608.
18. Verbeek FP, Tummers QR, Rietbergen DD, et al. Sentinel lymph node biopsy in vulvar cancer using combined radioactive and fluorescence guidance. Int J Gynecol Cancer. 2015;25:1086-93.
19. Colombo, N., Preti, E., Landoni, F. et al. Endometrial cancer: ESMO Clinical Practice Guidelines for diagnosis, treatment and follow-up. Ann Oncol. 2013;24:vi33-vi38.
20. BGCS Guidelines. https://bgcs.org.uk/BGCS%20Endometrial%20Guidelines%202017.pdf, access 23.4.2017.
21. Lin H, Ding Z, Kota VG, Zhang X, et al. Sentinel lymph node mapping in endometrial cancer: a systematic review and meta-analysis. Oncotarget. 2017 Mar 29. doi: 10.18632/oncotarget. 16662. [Epub ahead of print] Review.
22. Bodurtha Smith AJ, Fader AN, Tanner EJ. Sentinel lymph node assessment in endometrial cancer: a systematic review and meta-analysis. Am J Obstet Gynecol. 2016 Nov 18. pii: S0002-9378(16)32057-9.
23. Cibula D, Abu-Rustum NR, Dusek L, et al. Prognostic significance of low volume sentinel lymph node disease in early-stage cervical cancer. Gynecol Oncol. 2012;124:496-501.
24. Cormier B, Diaz JP, Shih K, et al. Establishing a sentinel lymph node mapping algorithm for the treatment of early cervical cancer. Gynecol Oncol. 2011;122:275-80.
25. Ruscito I, Gasparri ML, Braicu EI, et al. Sentinel node mapping in cervical and endometrial cancer: indocyanine green versus other conventional dyes—a meta-analysis. Ann Surg Oncol. 2016;23:3749-56.
26. Cibula D, Oonk MH, Abu-Rustum NR. Sentinel lymph node biopsy in the management of gynecologic cancer. Curr Opin Obstet Gynecol. 2015;27:66-72.
27. AWMF, German cervical cancer guidelines. http://www.awmf.org/uploads/tx_szleitlinien/032-033OLl_S3_Zervixkarzinom_2014-10.pdf. Accessed March 23, 2017.
28. AWMF, German vulvar cancer guideline. http://www.awmf.org/uploads/tx_szleitlinien/015-059k_S2k_Vulvakarzinom_und_Vorstufen_Diagnostik_Therapie_2016-11.pdf. Accessed April 24, 2017.

KIEL SCH•O L

29 of Gynaecological Endoscopy

Laparoscopic Myomectomy

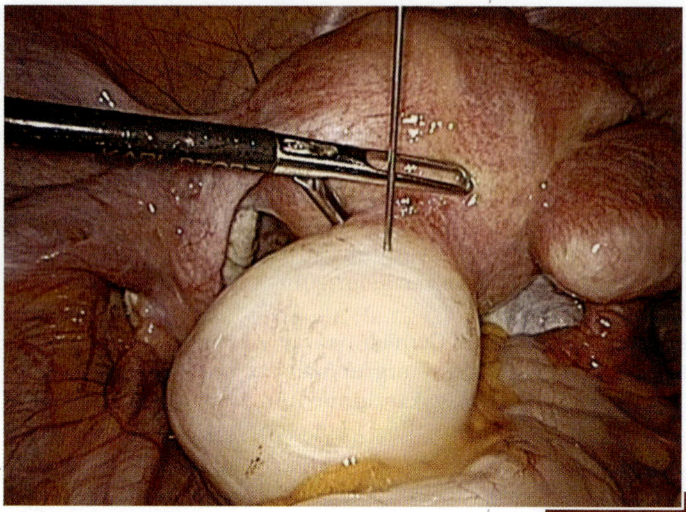

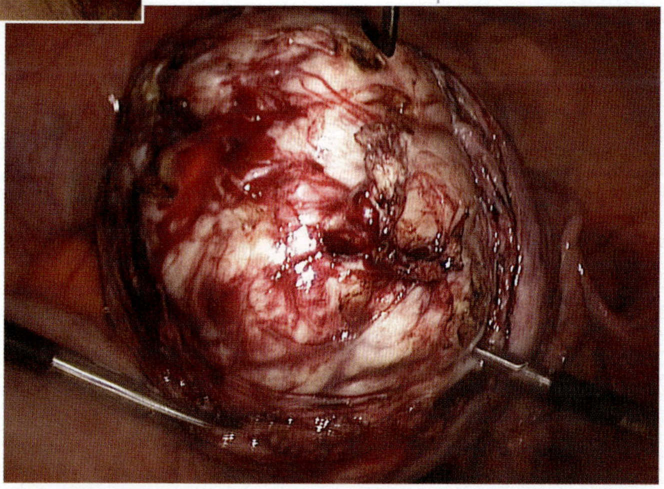

Chapter 29

Laparoscopic Myomectomy

Alfonso Rossetti, Alessandro Loddo

INTRODUCTION

Myomas represent a problem of public health worldwide. The cumulative risk of diagnosis for myomas between the ages of 25 and 44 is approximately 30%.

A myoma is a solid tumor made of fibrous tissue. Hence it is often called a 'fibroid' tumor. Also the designation 'fibroid' is the least accurate. Leiomyoma best describes this neoplasm and refers to any benign tumor of smooth-muscle origin.

The term "leiomyoma" captures the predominant components of these tumors as well as the cell of origin. It is unknown whether a leiomyoma actually transforms into a malignant phenotype termed "leiomyosarcoma." However, the incidence of leiomyosarcoma is extremely low in premenopausal patients when compared to older postmenopausal women, wherein they account for <1% of uterine malignancies. Apart from their tumorigenic potential, they are morphologically similar at the cellular level to normal myometrial smooth muscle cells. Leiomyomas may have single or multiple mutated smooth muscle tumor nodules of varying size attached and/or within the myometrium that are encircled by varying amounts of extracellular fibrous connective tissue.

They are well circumscribed, pseudoencapsulated, solid and pearly white or lightly tanned round masses that may grow as a single nodule or in clusters and may range in size from 1 mm to more than 30 cm in diameter.

The cause of myomas has not actually been determined, but most myomas develop in women during their reproductive years. Myomas do not develop before the body begins producing estrogen. Myomas tend to grow very quickly during pregnancy when the body is producing extra estrogen. Once menopause has begun, myomas generally stop growing and can begin to shrink due to the loss of estrogen.[1]

Luckily, they are most often slow-growing and usually cause no symptoms. Myomas that do not produce symptoms do not need to be treated. Approximately 25% of myomas will cause symptoms and need medical or surgical treatment.

Myomas may cause significant morbidity, including prolonged or heavy menstrual bleeding, anemia, bulk symptoms (low back and pelvic pressure or pain, urinary frequency and constipation), dyspareunia (pain during or after sexual intercourse) and, in rare cases, reproductive dysfunction. Both the economic cost and the effect of fibroids on quality of life are substantial.

Surgery is the mainstay of treatment of fibroids. They represent the most common reason for a woman to have a hysterectomy. In addition to hysterectomy and abdominal myomectomy, various minimally invasive procedures have been developed to treat fibroids.[2-4]

Laparoscopic myomectomy is now a well standardized procedure. Kurt Semm reported the first laparoscopic myomectomy in 1979. Nevertheless, it is still a controversial one, especially in regard to the volume and number of the myomas to be removed and the supposed higher risks during following pregnancies. Moreover, laparoscopic myomectomy is still considered a technique for surgeons mastering advanced laparoscopy. The concept could be true only regarding the ability of endoscopic suturing, which is indispensable in this kind of surgery. For this reason a thorough training in suturing is necessary before confronting ourselves with the laparoscopic myomectomy. Besides, the past experience of more than 20 years is allowing us to easily deal with myomas otherwise considered challenging and risky.

Furthermore, laparoscopic myomectomy presents all the recognized advantages of minimally invasive surgery as lower hemoglobin drop (2.17 vs. 1.33%, $p < 0.001$), lower postoperative pain ($p < 0.05$) , lower febrile morbidity (26.2 vs 12.1%, $p < 0.05$) and faster recovery ($p < 0.05$) in comparison with traditional laparotomic procedure.[5]

No significant differences were found between laparoscopic and laparotomic myomectomy with regard to pregnancy rate and abortion rate.[6] Recent findings demonstrate improved fertility rates in women undergoing laparoscopic myomectomy: in fact, laparoscopic myomectomy could reduce the risk of postoperative adhesions compared with laparotomy (32.9% vs 80%).

OPERATIVE INDICATIONS

Traditionally, symptomatic fibroids have been treated with myomectomy or hysterectomy performed by laparotomy. Hysterectomy is the most common major gynecological intervention in the world and is commonly used to treat fibroids.

For women who desire future pregnancies or retain their uterus for other reasons, myomectomy is still the operation of choice. In an effort to reduce the cost, morbidity and lifestyle impact of major surgery, various less invasive surgical procedures, including minilaparotomy and operative endoscopy (laparoscopy or hysteroscopy), have been introduced over the years. Medical treatments may be useful in some cases and for the short term, but does not lead to a cure.

Medical management includes oral contraceptives, menopausal hormone therapy, GnRH (gonadotropin-releasing hormone) agonist therapy, antiprogestins, progesterone-containing intrauterine devices (IUDs) and nonsteroidal anti-inflammatory drugs (NSAIDs).

The standard medical treatments for menorrhagia can be used also if they are less effective in the presence of fibroids. Prostaglandin synthetase inhibitors work well in a certain percentage of women and GnRH agonists or danazol can be useful in some instances.

For example, GnRH agonists are often used as preoperative adjunctive therapy to surgery. They cause downregulation of estrogen receptors, which decreases fibroid growth. GnRH agonist therapy also helps to optimize hematocrit levels that may have declined secondary to menorrhagia from fibroids.

Mifepristone is a synthetic steroid that competitively binds to intracellular progesterone receptor, thereby blocking the effects of progesterone and causing significant shrinkage in fibroids. Raloxifene is a selective estrogen receptor modulator (SERM) that has been reported to cause a significant reduction in fibroid size.

Indications to myomectomy are infertility, recent and significant enlargement and symptoms (pelvic pain or abnormal uterine bleeding). Inclusion criteria are the presence of at least one symptomatic myoma >4 cm and the absence of submucous myomas, which can be removed by hysteroscopy. No upper limit to myoma size is posed, as long as the myoma can be mobilized. Usually a number of myomas for patients equal or inferior to eight are the indication to myomectomy but in some case the number of myomas could be higher.[7-12]

While some authors suggest that no more than three or four myomas with diameter <7–8 cm are to be removed, others believe in the individual choice based on pathologic findings and surgical skill. In practice, the choice of surgical approach is largely dependent on surgical expertise.

Our results show that the upper limit that should be proposed mostly depends on other characteristics (i.e., location, depth of penetration, mobilization capability) of the myoma rather than the mere number or size. Nevertheless, it has to be recognized that our previous studies have demonstrated that the recurrence rate and especially the complication rate are higher in case of multiple myomas.[13-15]

In select cases, mostly when hysterectomy is advocated for a number of myomas, the patient could be given the option of alternative microinvasive approaches as the cryoablation or the myolysis, uterine artery embolization (UAE) or magnetic resonance imaging (MRI)-guided focused ultrasound (MRgFUS).

All these procedures have as rationale the elimination of major blood supply, which leads to a myoma shrinkage between 40% and 80%. The procedures are intended to remove the symptoms although not the myomas. A combined procedure, as a classic laparoscopic myomectomy following the less invasive approaches as the UAE, has the advantages of an easier removal of the fibroids, reduced blood loss, lower recurrence and complications rate.

Uterine artery embolization is a percutaneous, image-guided procedure performed by interventional radiologist. It is an option available to women who wish to avoid surgery, are poor surgical candidates or wish to retain their uterus, and also if given the relatively new nature of this procedure, very little information is available in order to make estimations of recurrence, persistence, incidence of premature menopause, outcome of pregnancy, quality of life and need for subsequent therapy.[16]

It consists in the placement of an angiographic catheter into the uterine arteries via a common femoral artery approach and injection of embolic agents (in most cases, polyvinyl alcohol particles or tris-acryl gelatin microspheres) into both uterine arteries until the flow becomes slow.

The proposed mechanism of uterine artery embolization is that occluding or markedly reducing uterine blood flow at the arteriolar level will produce an irreversible ischemic injury to the fibroids, causing them to undergo necrosis and shrink, while the normal myometrium is able to recover. For reasons not fully understood, the normal myometrium receives a new blood supply from the vaginal and ovarian vasculature, whereas the fibroids become avascular.

In MRI-guided focused ultrasound, the clinician uses MRI to guide ultrasound energy (i.e., sound waves from ultrasound) directly to the fibroid. The highly focused ultrasound beam (very different from ultrasound used for imaging studies) causes the temperature in the target tissue to rise (55–90°C), enough to induce coagulative necrosis within a few seconds.

The clinician can monitor the thermal destruction of the fibroid during the procedure with the MRI and avoid damage to nearby tissue or structures.

Thermal destruction is monitored in real time using MRI estimates of the tissue temperatures achieved. Each fibroid is treated separately, and total treatment times are generally longer than an hour for most women.

In case of very large myomas, a combined treatment (UAE followed by laparoscopic myomectomy) could be advised. Myomectomy will be easier, quicker and with a minor risk of hemorrhage.

PREOPERATIVE EVALUATION, TESTING AND PREPARATION

Routine preoperative workout includes ultrasound and hysteroscopy. Hysteroscopy will give information about the degree of submucosal involvement or whether an hysteroscopic approach could be indicated. Ultrasound examination should give the surgeon information about the number and localization of the myomas. Particular attention has to be paid for intramural myomas regarding their distance from the serosa and from the endometrium. Ultrasound should be able to rule out an adenomyoma and/or a sarcoma, or at least, in doubtful cases, to address the necessity of a MRI. Common signs of adenomyosis are uterine enlargement in the absence of myomas, asymmetric enlargement of the posterior or anterior abdominal wall, anechoic lacunae or cysts of various size, lack of contour abnormality or mass effect, hyperechoic islands or nodules, finger-like projections or linear striations and increased echotexture of the endometrium.[17]

While in case of a myoma vasculature typically circumscribes the mass, in patients with diffuse or focal adenomyosis—the vascular architecture appears unremarkable, with the vessels following their normal course perpendicular to the endometrial interface even if the vessels are slightly more dilated than radial artery of a normal uterus.

Uncertainty in defining the site and more particularly the extent of adenomyosis make it difficult to determine the feasibility and accuracy of complete excision when conserving the uterus. Unless the adenomyosis is well defined, as in an adenomyoma, it is not possible to be certain of cure after excision. Typically an adenomyoma (focally involved uterus) has poorly defined margins because they merge with the surrounding normal myometrium. In contrast, myomas compress the surrounding myometrium and have clear-cut, well-circumscribed margins. The latter can be enucleated, whereas the former cannot. In fact, fibroids grow inside normal myometrium, which they displace as in benign tumor. When fibroids are removed, a capsule demarcates them from normal myometrium. The cavity is then repaired leaving the uterus similar to what is was prior to growth of myoma, except for the presence of a scar. Adenomyosis infiltrates normal myometrium so that excision of the diseased area subtracts myometrial mass from the total uterine volume. This can cause a reduction in myometrial capacity during pregnancy and the production of scars with reduced tensile strength.

Particular attention has to be paid in ruling out sarcomas. In case of rapidly growing or degenerated myomas—especially when not responsive to GNRh analogs therapy, MRI evaluation, total LDH and LDH isozyme type 3 assay are recommended.[18]

Although all these newly developed techniques are by now easily available, an effort should be made to focus on how they are applicable. In fact, it is impractical to use MRI of the uterine lesion as a method of investigation in all cases. Therefore, a preoperative algorithm should be proposed in order to avoid the occurrence of unexpected leiomyosarcoma (LMS) diagnosis on the pathological postoperative report.

Preoperative evaluation should start from clinical and ultrasonographic findings suspect of LMS. Only in the highly suspected cases a pelvic MRI examination should be performed.

Table 29.1 shows the clinical risk criteria according to the ACOG report.[19] Patients should be examined by transvaginal and/or trans-abdominal sonography with Gray-scale imaging, color and directional power Doppler imaging, using a convex trans-abdominal 2.5–5.5-MHz transducer and a 5.5–8.5-MHz vaginal probe. The number of every single uterine mass has to be reported and the longitudinal, transverse and anterior-posterior diameters are measured. Volume (V) of the mass is estimated using the following formula: $V = \text{length} \times \text{width} \times \text{diameter} \times 0.52$.

Table 29.1: Clinical risk criteria according to ACOG statement.

Clinical risk criteria:
• *Age:* > 35 years (women younger than age 35 years seem to have the lowest incidence. The mean age of the patients with LMS was significantly higher than that of patients with LM. The highest incidence of uterine sarcoma is in women over age 65). • Postmenopausal status • Uterine size • Rapid uterine growth • Certain treatment (tamoxifen® or pelvic radiation) • Hereditary conditions (Lynch syndrome or hereditary leiomyomatosis and renal cell cancer).
Symptoms:
• Hyperpolymenorrhea • Abnormal genital bleeding • Dysmenorrhea • Palpable abdominal mass • Lower abdominal pain • Lumbago • Pressure symptoms (Urinary frequency, dysuria, bowel symptoms).

Grayscale imaging is also used to evaluate absence or presence of calcifications, presence of cystic necrosis or hemorrhage and to describe the echo pattern of the lesion (homogeneous or inhomogeneous).

A subjective, semiquantitative assessment of the amount of blood flow within the examined lesion is made with power Doppler images (color score), describing the vascularity of the central and peripheral region of the lesion as marked, moderate, mild, or not appreciable (Table 29.2).

It is also recommended that all patients undergo: LDH and isoenzyme 3 assay, Pap smear and hysteroscopy with biopsy in any case of uterine bleeding plus Ca 125 assay.

Patients clinically evaluated, with blood test assays and ultrasound examination, and considered "low risk" can undergo surgery without further investigations.

It is recommended to send the other patients for MRI evaluation. MRI provides a better image to delineate the exact location and characteristics of the LMs but should be considered only for women in

Table 29.2: Ultrasound criteria to evaluate the risk score. A score > 19 with associated clinical risk is considered to be the indication to MRI.

Color score	
1	No blood flow is found
2	Only minimal flow is detected
3	Only mild flow is detected
4	Numerous vessels are present
The scores for both central and peripheral regions are combined with a maximum vascular score of 8 [21].	
II levels ultrasound criteria	
Echo pattern	Homogeneous or inhomogeneous with mixed echogenic and poor echogenic parts
Necrotic, cystic, hemorrhagic changes	
Single lesion	
Presence or absence of central vascularization	
Distribution of tumoral vascularization: A high vascularity score	
Size	Diameter > 8 cm
Presence or absence of calcifications	

whom the nature of the pelvic mass is uncertain after clinical assessment followed by pelvic ultrasound. In fact, MRI is far more expensive and less accessible than ultrasound, and it is therefore impractical to use as a method of investigation in all cases.

All MRI examinations are performed on 1.5–3 T units. T1-, T2-weighted and diffusion-weighted imaging images are acquired; apparent diffusion coefficient maps are derived from diffusion-weighted images. Conventional MRI images are reviewed for the following items: size of the tumor (the greatest diameter), signal intensity of the tumor on T1- and T2-weighted images, tumor margin, endometrial involvement, intratumoral hemorrhage and unenhanced areas in the tumor. Tumor–myometrium contrast ratio is also evaluated.

Signal intensity (SI) on diffusion-weighted imaging images is judged as high when it shows equal or higher signal than that of the endometrium and on the basis of this finding, patients are included in two groups the diffusion-weighted imaging intermediate- or high-intensity group or in the diffusion-weighed imaging low-intensity group; diffusion-weighted imaging intensity is compared to the corresponding apparent diffusion coefficient values.

Correlation between conventional MRI findings (T1- and T2-weighted images), diffusion-weighted imaging intensity and corresponding apparent diffusion coefficient (ADC) values is evaluated in order to exclude or suspect the presence of an LMS.

Only the patients who are considered "low risk" after MRI imaging will undergo minimal invasive surgery (MIS) involving an intra-abdominal morcellation, unless the morcellation can be carried out in a contained bag.

Proper informed consent has to be given to the patient explaining the potential risk of sarcoma morcellation and upstaging and the difficulties we are encountering to give an actual risk (given the heterogeneity of papers that leads to inadequate or confounding data). A risk-sharing process has to be undertaken. According to the AAGL Statement, these risks should be weighed against the benefits of minimal invasive surgery. The risks of laparotomy should be noted, including wound infections, blood transfusions, longer recovery and the potential for life-threatening complications such as venous thrombotic disease.[20]

Considering the fact that no one is challenging the benefits of minimal invasive surgery for the patients and that the recent audit of the Food and Drug Administration (FDA) on July 11, 2014, has stated that the data in the literature are at best "very weak," it is obvious that new prospective trials will have to be designed to obtain more reliable answers. At the same time there are no significant data suggesting that surgeons should stop offering young infertile patient access to laparoscopic myomectomy.

On the other hand it could be recommended to perform total laparoscopic hysterectomies instead of supracervical hysterectomies, with morcellation of the specimen through the vagina, possibly in a bag.

There are no evidence-based medicine data showing that supracervical hysterectomy is better for the patient on the long run compared to total laparoscopic hysterectomy.[21] All the patients must have Pap-smear evaluation, at least second-level US examination, LDH assessment and hysteroscopy with endometrial biopsy in case of Abnormal Uterine Bleeding (AUB).

Preference to SCH can be justified only in case of Pelvic Organ Prolapse (POP) repair after evaluation of the endometrium of the patient and LDH assessment, second level US and of course Pap smear. Techniques for single or multiport laparoscopic morcellation in newly designed sturdy bags have already been described but the safety of this technique will have to be studied.

From the data we have at our disposal, it appears that the risk of unexpected sarcomas found after a laparoscopic intra-abdominal morcellation is probably over estimated by some articles cited by the FDA, but it is generally agreed that the odds of a woman with uterine fibroids having an unsuspected cancer are likely higher than had been assumed in the past. Thus, we need to have more data that show how safe and reliable the diagnostic presurgical tools are, so as to differentiate between low- and high-risk patients.

GnRH agonists are prescribed for 3 months only in patients with very large myoma; otherwise it is very difficult to mobilize or in case of severe anemia due to persistent menometrorrhagia to improve hemoglobin concentration before surgery. At least a week before the procedure, an autologous transfusion is collected. A standard bowel preparation and short-term antibiotics prophylaxis (as cefoxitin 2 g) are given to the patients.

PATIENT POSITIONING IN THE OPERATING SUITE

Under general endotracheal anesthesia, the patient is positioned in lithotomic position (Fig. 29.1) with arms tucked at the sides to allow free movements for the surgeons and to avoid brachial plexus injury. The legs are abducted at 90°. A Foley catheter is placed in

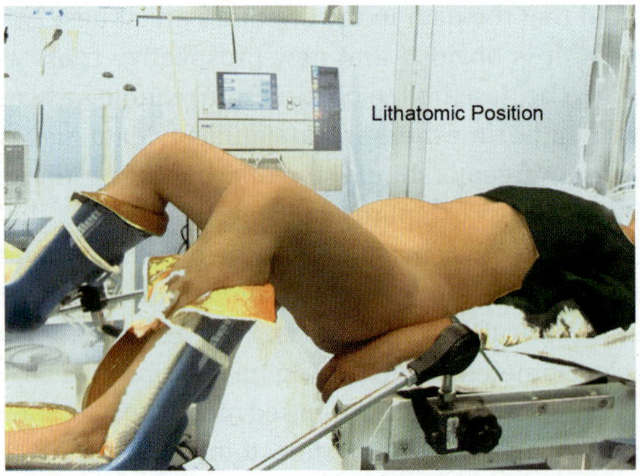

Fig. 29.1: Correct patient positioning for laparoscopic myomectomy.

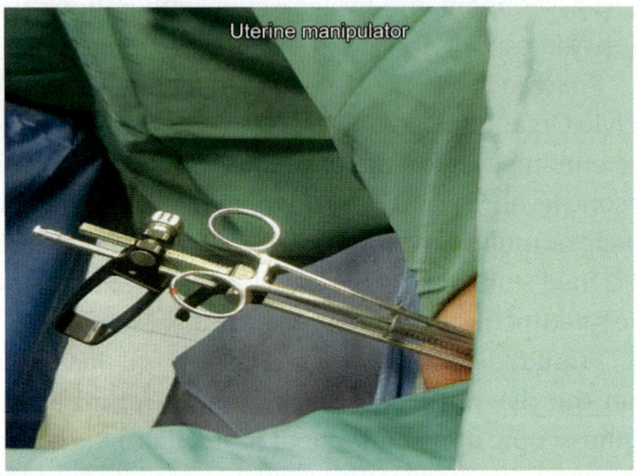

Fig. 29.2: Valtchev™ uterine manipulator inserted into the cervix.

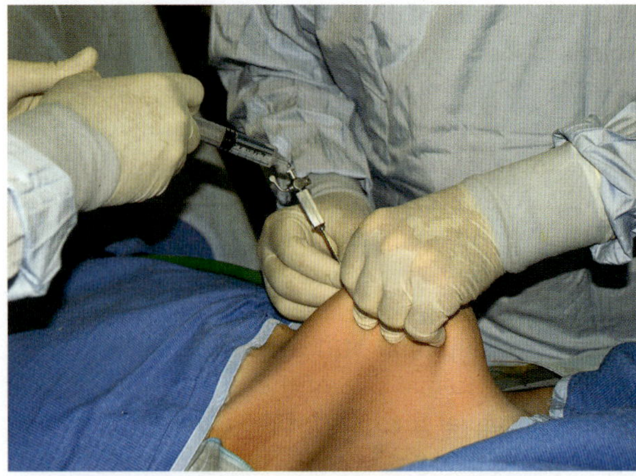

Fig. 29.3: Veress needle insertion inside the umbilicus.

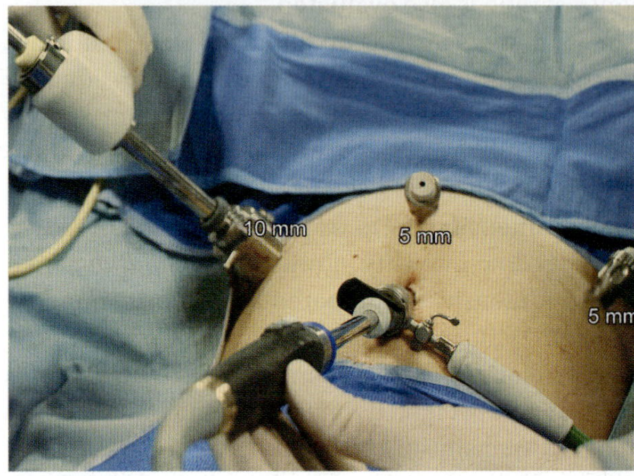

Fig. 29.4: Standard trocars disposition.

Box 29.1: Operative set-up.
❖ Lithotomy, abducted legs, general anesthesia
❖ 2 TV monitors at the feet of the patient
❖ Surgeon left, 1st assistant right, 2nd assistant between the patient's legs
❖ 1 optical trocar, 2 suprapubic 5 mm trocars, 1 suprapubic 10 mm trocar
❖ Foley catheter
❖ Uterine manipulator

the bladder. The cervix is grasped with a tenaculum, dilated with Hegar cones and a uterine manipulator (Valtchev™, Conkin Surgical Instruments, Toronto, Canada or MUR 18™, Sofar, Trezzano Rosa, Italy) (Fig. 29.2) is inserted to allow a correct exposure of the myomas and strong countertractions during enucleation and suturing. (Box 29.1).

The abdomen is insufflated with CO_2 at a preset first trocar entry pressure of 18 mm Hg through Veress needle inserted at the umbilicus (Fig. 29.3).

Positioning and Placement of Trocars

In most cases, video laparoscopy is performed with a 10-mm laparoscope in standard umbilical position. Myomectomies are performed with standard technique (with three ancillary suprapubic ports) (Figs. 29.4 and 29.5). Two suprapubic access routes (5 and 10 mm) are inserted lateral to the deep inferior epigastric arteries and slightly higher than usual: in fact, the accessory trocars should be inserted sufficiently high to provide an easy approach to the myomas for the laparoscopic instruments. A third trocar (5 mm) is inserted in the midline, level or higher than the other two.

In case of very large myoma, trocar insertion sites should be changed. The option of open abdominal entry should be considered to minimize the risk of lacerating the uterus, if it reaches or exceeds the midline. Using the Palmer point to insert the Veress needle could be another option, especially if adhesions are suspected (Fig. 29.6). Obviously there is a

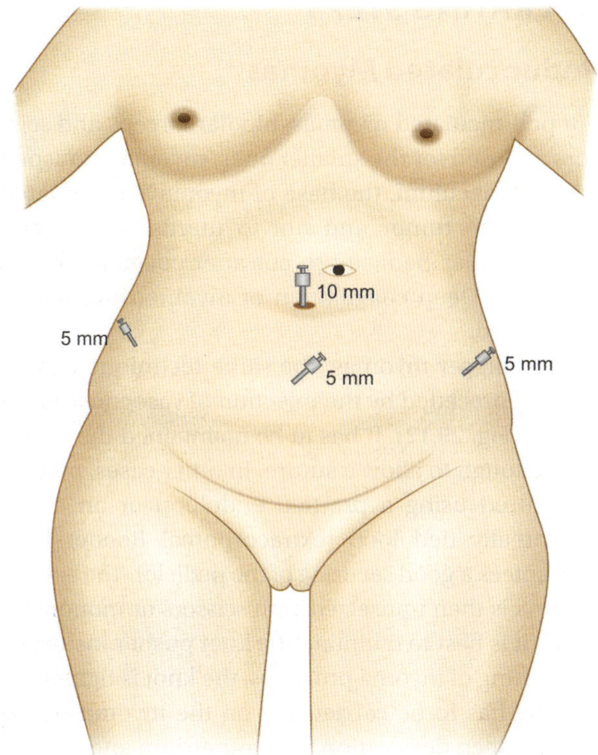

Fig. 29.5: Drawing of standard disposition.

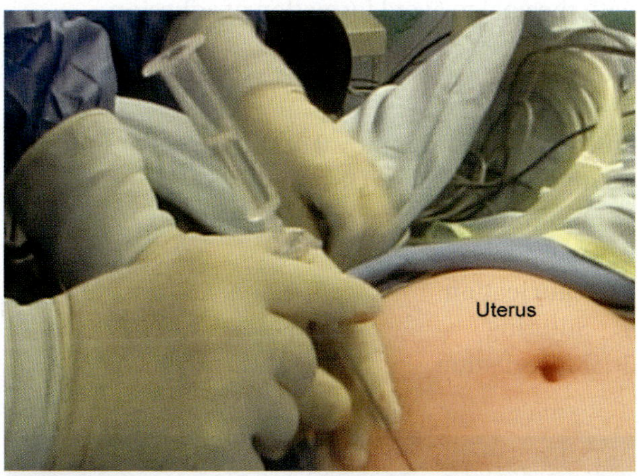

Fig. 29.6: Palmer point Veress needle insertion.

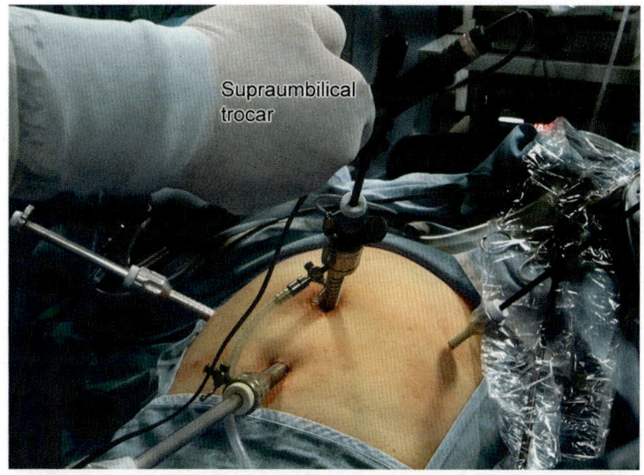

Fig. 29.7: Optic trocar placed in supraumbilical position.

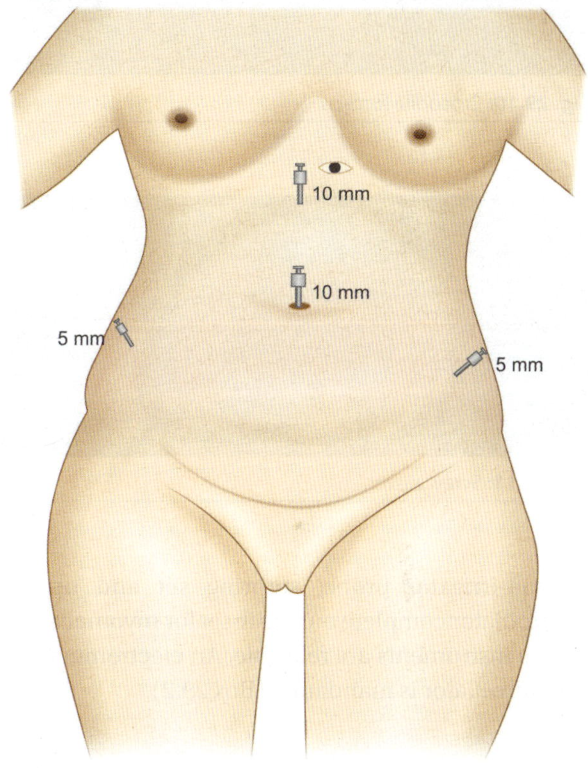

Fig. 29.8: Middle trocar placed through the umbilicus.

physical limit to the space of maneuver of our instruments and to the angle of vision represented by the space between the distended abdominal wall and the uterus. The goals are better exposure and handling of the instruments without the hindrance of uterus.

In this case, optic trocar should be placed up to 10 cm above the umbilicus (supraumbilical trocar) (Figs. 29.7 and 29.8). The middle trocar should be placed through the umbilicus or even higher. The other two lateral trocars should be placed according to uterine size and location of myomas. The higher the uterus the higher the ancillary trocars should be inserted, at umbilical line or even some centimeters further up.

OPERATIVE TECHNIQUE

Bipolar coagulation forceps, monopolar hook, hook scissors, grasping forceps, tenaculum (Fig. 29.9), crocodile forceps (Fig. 29.10) and screw driver (Fig. 29.11),

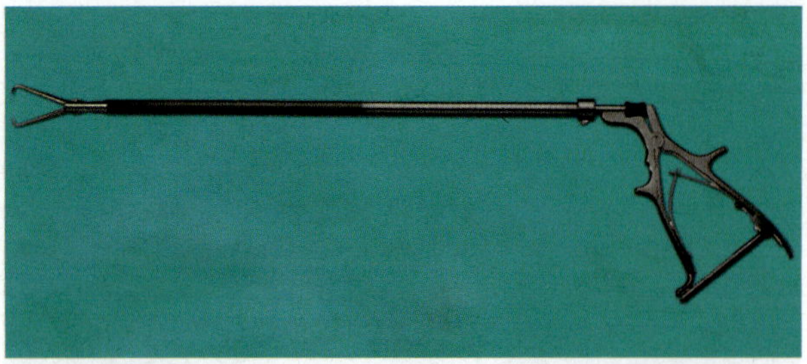

Fig. 29.9: Tenaculum.

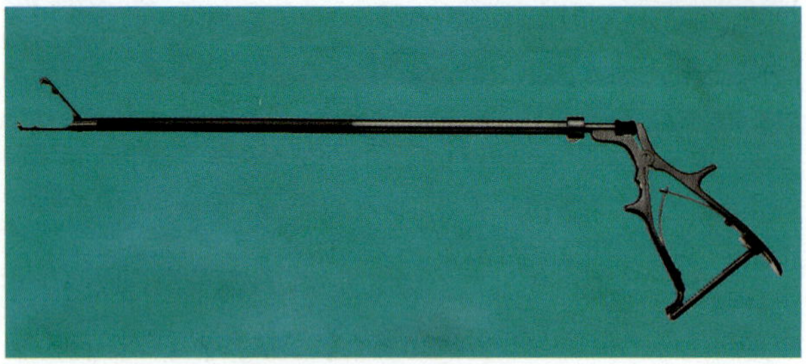

Fig. 29.10: Crocodile forceps.

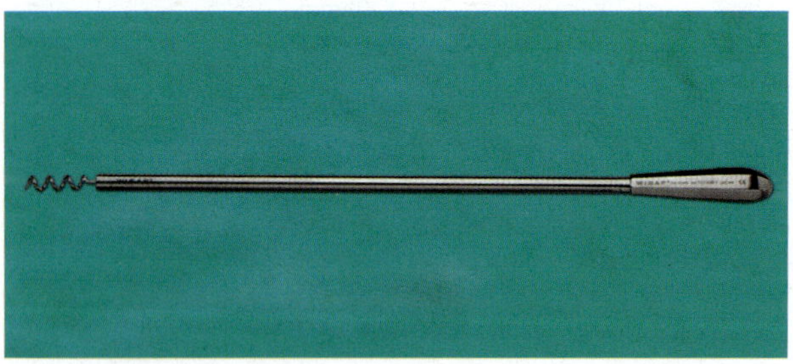

Fig. 29.11: Screw driver.

suction-irrigator probe, suturing set and uterine manipulator complete our basic set for myomectomy. All the instruments are reusable. An electromechanical morcellator is mandatory (Box 29.2).

Box 29.2: Basic set for myomectomy.
• 1 Hooked scissors
• 2 Grasping forceps
• 1 Monopolar hook
• 1 Tenaculum 10 mm or myoma screw
• 1 Washing-suction device
• 2 Needle holders
• 1 Counter needle holder
• 1 Knot pusher
• 1 Uterine manipulator
• Electromechanical morcellator

OPERATING STEPS

Pedunculated Myomas

For pedunculated myomas, bipolar forceps and scissors are used for the smaller ones; myoma is grasped with a tenaculum, the base of myoma is coagulated next to the tumor and not to uterus. Serosa and then vascular pedicle are cut after coagulation has occurred. Deep coagulation of myometrium has to be avoided.

For bigger myomas, the same technique can be utilized preceded by the injection of vasoconstrictive agents (Fig. 29.12). It has to be maintained the serosa long enough to allow a suture. In other cases, pedicle is secured using a pre-tied endoloop or an extracorporeally tied loop (extracorporeal Roeder knot guarantees a good securing of the pedicle). The stalk of myoma is then transected with scissors or monopolar hook. It is best to maintain the knot pusher inside. As the cutting of myoma proceeds, the knot is tightened. Cutting has to be carried out on the myoma site to avoid a deep desiccation of myometrium and to have enough uterine serosa to allow to apply a suture on the transected myoma pedicle. Suture is performed not only to achieve an optimal hemostasis but also with the goal to avoid formation of adhesion.

Subserosal and Intramural Myomas

The technique for removal of subserosal or intramural myomas consists of five steps:

1. Infiltration of vasoconstrictive agents
2. Incision
3. Enucleation
4. Suturing
5. Morcellation

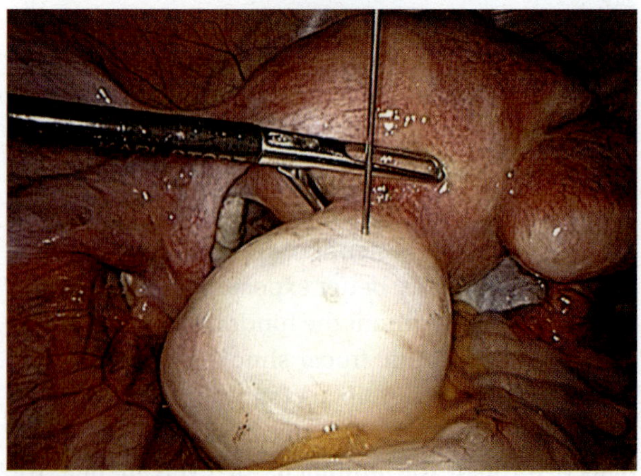

Fig. 29.12: Vasoconstrictive agents injection.

Infiltration of Vasoconstrictive Agents

To reduce vascularization and blood loss, we inject diluted ornitin vasopressin or diluted (20 IU: 500 mL) argipressin.[22] Vasoconstrictive agent is injected laparoscopically with a laparoscopic needle (lacking the laparoscopic needle, a common needle for epidural anesthesia is used transabdominally) (Fig. 29.13). The substance is injected between myometrium and myoma capsule, looking for the cleavage plane, all around the myoma circumference, until blanching occurs. It is useless to directly inject the vasopressin inside the myoma. The use of diluted vasoconstrictive agents has allowed a minor use of electrosurgery to achieve hemostasis and dissection in favor of sharp dissection.

Incision

For subserosal and intramural myomas, both for anterior and posterior myomas, a vertical incision (hysterotomy) is made on serosa overlying the myoma down and through the myoma pseudocapsule with a unipolar hook or scissors and high cutting current (Fig. 29.14). This is the crucial point of the myomectomy procedure: incision is continued until the cleavage plane is found and most of the myoma surface is freed from the surrounding myometrium. Instead of a monopolar hook, it is possible to use ultrasonic energy both reusable (SonoSurg™, Olympus, Japan) and disposable (Ace™, J&J, Cincinnati, OH) (Figs. 29.15 and 29.16). Vertical incision is advantageous when the surgeon sutures through the midline port. If the surgeon sutures through lateral port or in the vertical zone, a transversal incision is recommended.

Enucleation

After exposure of myoma, grasping forceps is positioned to apply tractions on the myoma and expose

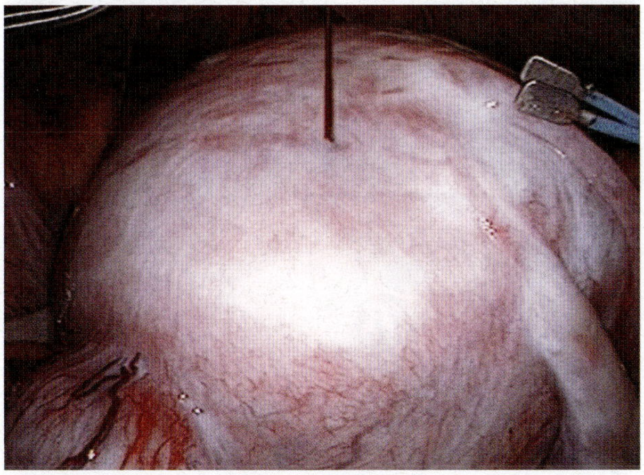

Fig. 29.13: Injection performed with laparoscopic needle.

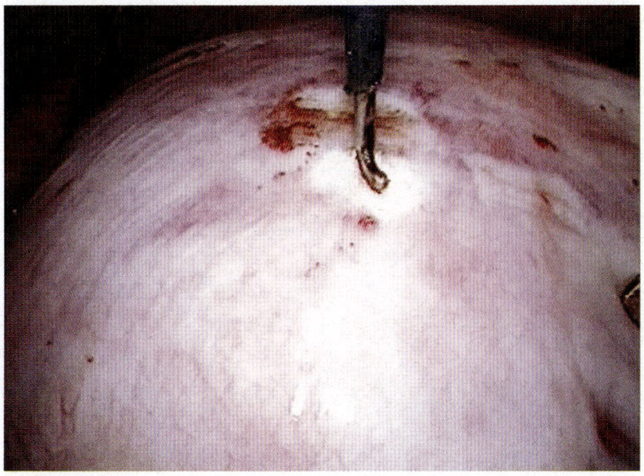

Fig. 29.14: Vertical incision made with unipolar hook.

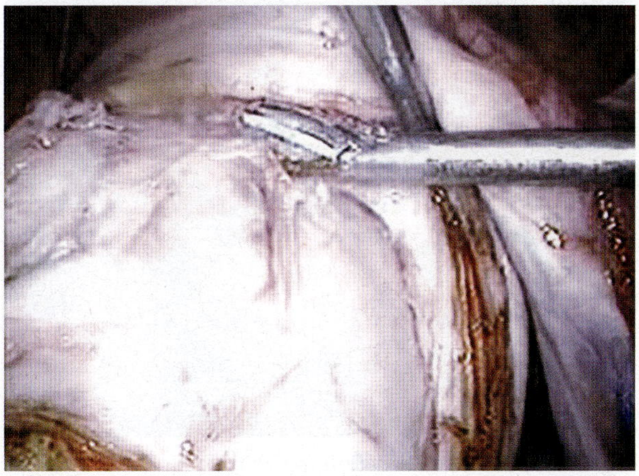

Fig. 29.15: Incision and enucleation performed with ultrasonic energy.

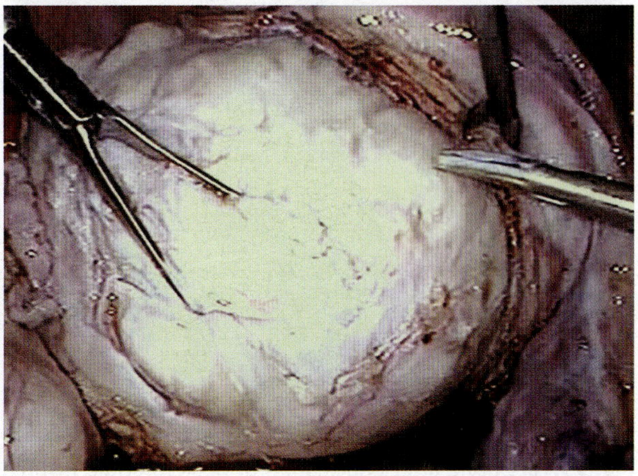

Fig. 29.16: Traction on the myoma with a tenaculum.

the cleavage plane. Tractions on myoma applied with tenaculum or a myoma screw with a countertraction on the uterus facilitate the dissection. Actions exercised by the grasping forceps consist not only of simple pulling out, but also of the use of torsional force and luxation of the myoma (Fig. 29.17). Countertraction is achieved with any forceps used as lever between myoma and myometrium and is also applied by the second assistant through the uterine manipulator. Mechanical enucleation is carried out whenever is possible. Division of some residual connective fibers surrounding myoma is obtained with unipolar hook or with ultrasonic energy, the latter having the advantage of less tissue charring.

The only exception to this technique is in case of unsuspected adenomyosis. In this situation the cleavage plane does not exist and excision can only be carried out with monopolar hook, sharp cutting or ultrasonic energy device.

Suturing

For subserosal or intramural myomas, suturing is usually done along one or two layers depending on the depth of incision. It consists of bringing the entire thickness of the edges of myomectomy site together to prevent the formation of hematomas. Large, curved needles (CT 1, 30 to 40 mm) swaged to polyglactin suture (1 or 0 Vycril®, Johnson & Johnson, Somerville, KY, USA) are used. For one-layer sutures, we use interrupted, simple or more frequently cross-stitches, tied intracorporeally. In a majority of cases it is necessary to make a suture in two layers. In this case, suturing is usually carried out along different planes: one larger stitch reaching the deep layers and one more superficial suture to introflect the serosa (Figs. 29.18 to 29.20). In fact, after deeper layers have been approximated, to avoid a too tight compression on the tissues with consequent risk of necrosis while

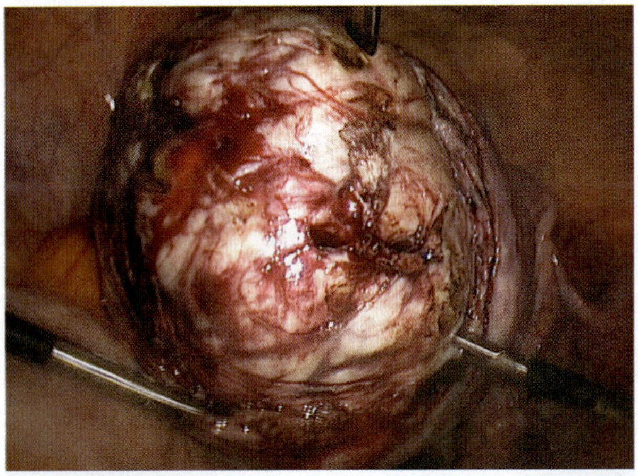

Fig. 29.17: Enucleation performed with traction and countertraction maneuvers.

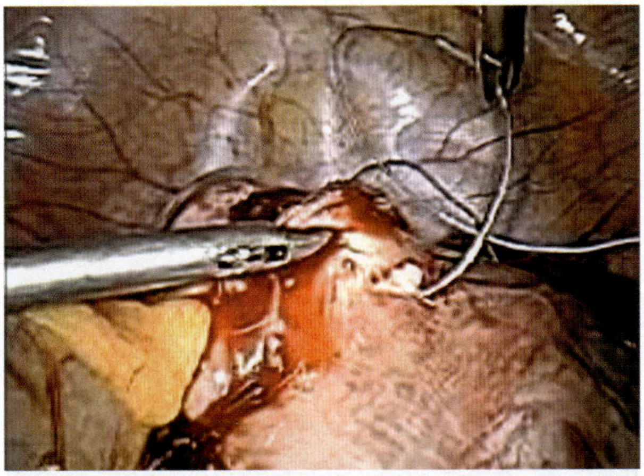

Fig. 29.19: Suture in case of anterior myoma.

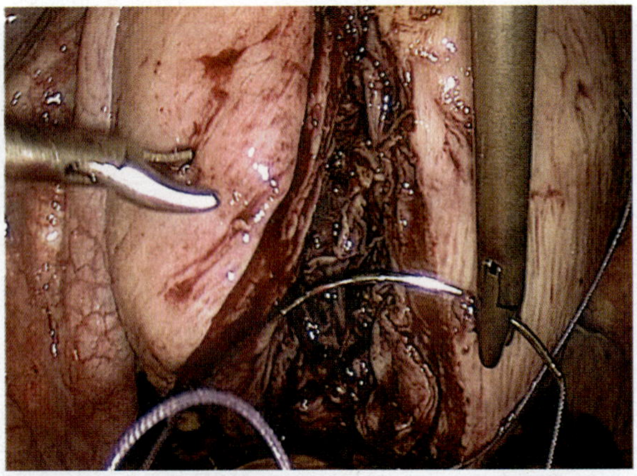

Fig. 29.18: Suture after enucleation of posterofundic myoma with large curved needles.

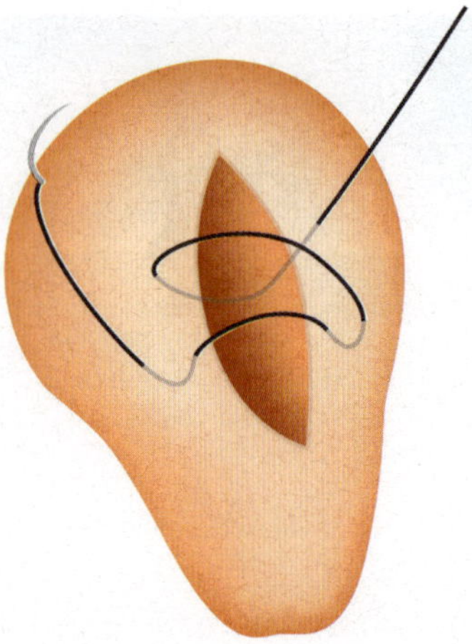

Fig. 29.20: Our suturing technique.

at the same time securing the hemostasis, it is recommended to apply introflecting sutures. In and out closer to the margin on one side and in next to the margin and out again on the other side (Fig. 29.21). Suturing technique differs according to myoma location. In case of posterior myoma, when suturing through the midline trocar, the needle is positioned on the needle holder with its convexity directed toward the uterus. In this case the curvature of the needle is directed upward toward sacrum. In case of anterior myoma, the needle is also again positioned on the needle holder with the convexity turned toward the uterus, slightly oblique on the instruments axis, but the curvature is positioned upward directed toward the abdominal wall.

Whenever is possible, to facilitate suturing, the second assistant should try to keep the uterus in an upright position or better, to transform anterior myoma into a posterior one by retroverting uterus.

As for double-layer closures, a running suture can also be used: it is applied first in the deeper plane starting from the apex of the myomectomy scar to the base, continuing along the more superficial plane from the base to the apex. The suture is in the end tied intracorporeally with the tail of running suture. In any case it is imperative to avoid leaving dead spaces, which could cause hematomas, which, in turn, could bring to fistulas or indentation formation.

In the last years, some products have been proposed to facilitate closure of the hysterotomy site in laparoscopic myomectomy. One of the latest and more successful proposal is the uni- or bidirectional knotless barbed suture, a suture whose barbs penetrate inside the tissue and lock them in place, eliminating the need for knots to tie the suture.

Although further studies are needed, it seems they can facilitate the closure of uterine wall during laparoscopic myomectomy, reducing the time required to suture the uterine wall defect, the total duration of surgery and the intraoperative blood loss.

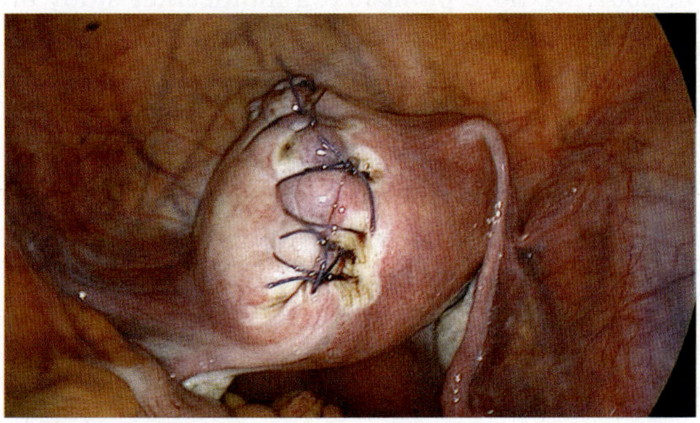

Fig. 29.21: Uterus after suture completion.

Morcellation

The morcellator knife is a classic lancet with an interchangeable blade, transformed into an endoscopic instrument that can be inserted easily through a 10-mm-diameter trocar. The blade can have an automatic retraction system, which, if is set in the standby position, ensures security. The mass to be cut is held between two grasping forceps for easy cutting with the blade, under permanent visual control. After morcellation, extraction of the masses is performed through a posterior culdotomy or through an enlarged port. The system, even though inexpensive, is obviously time-consuming and a more invasive extraction is necessary.

Since 1993, with the development of Steiner morcellator, several systems of electromechanical morcellation have been available. In each system, a cylinder with a coring knife or cutter at its intra-abdominal end is placed inside the trocar sleeve and it is rotated by an electrical microengine attached to trocar. Cylindrical tissue blocks are cut step by step out of the main specimen and removed from the peritoneal cavity through the cannula with a pulling of the grasping forceps.

Of course, the removed tissue has to be suitable for histological examination. These systems are useful for myoma removal or for removal of entire uterus after supracervical hysterectomy. It has to be pointed out that the task of morcellator is to transform an ellipsoid form such as a myoma into a cylindrical one in order to be removed from the abdominal cavity through a trocar sleeve. In practice, this process is influenced by several conditions.

Factors Influencing Myoma Morcellation

- Tissue resistance
- Myoma volume
- Cannula diameter
- Torsional stress

The first variable factor is due to consistency and tissue resistance of each myoma. This resistance depends on the proportion between the connective component of myoma and myometrial component and on the presence of calcifications. The resistance to cutting strength varies inside the myoma itself and mostly from myoma. It is obvious that another important factor is the myoma diameter.

Considering myoma as a spheroid, its volume will exponentially increase while increasing its diameter

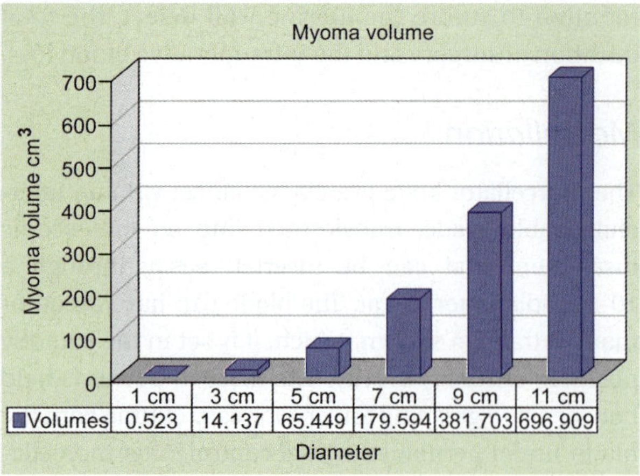

Fig. 29.22: Myoma volume increases exponentially with diameter growth.

(Fig. 29.22). Another factor influencing the speed of tissue removal is the diameter of cutting cannula. In fact, volume of the cylinders of the removed tissue varies with diameter of the blade, the length being constant.

Moreover, it has to be stressed that increasing the cannula diameter the length of the skin incision (and especially of the fascial incision) will increase. Furthermore, the skin incision will be about 20% wider than the cannula diameter, resulting in greater postoperative discomfort. Obviously, cutting strength is strictly connected to rotating speed of the blade. On the other hand, an increasing of the torsional stress applied to the specimen together with a not constant tissue resistance can lead to the tearing of cylinder inside the cannula, thus increasing the time of myoma removal.

The key point of myoma morcellation is to be able to "peel" the external aspect of the myoma rotating on its surface while cutting the myoma in stripes.

A new morcellator on the market is the PKS™ PlasmaSORD™ (Olympus, Japan) bipolar morcellator, which is the first completely bladeless solid organ removal device (SORD) based on the use of the PK® Technology that delivers a proprietary pulsed RF energy waveform. The myoma is vaporized inside the cannula.

Nevertheless, and despite improvements in morcellating systems, myoma morcellation is still the most time-consuming part of the entire procedure. Operative time is significantly positively correlated with the dominant myoma diameter and the number of myomas.

Closure of the fascia at the port site where the morcellator is used is recommended.

Intraligamentous Myomas

As regards intraligamentous myomas, they usually are to be considered as pedunculated or subserosal myomas arising into the broad ligament. They can develop into anterior or posterior or both leaves of the ligament. Depending on their position and proximity to dangerous structures, their removal can become challenging. Peritoneum surrounding myoma is incised with cold scissors and bipolar forceps. Myoma is gently enucleated by the surrounding areolar tissue through the use of scissors, bipolar forceps and graspers. Ultrasonic energy is handy for dissection and hemostasis of smaller vessels avoiding the necessity to continuously changing instruments. In other cases hemostasis can be achieved with bipolar coagulation of the major vessels reaching the myoma paying attention to dangerous structures such as the ureter or uterine vessels. When the base of myoma has been reached, coagulation of blood supply is obtained with bipolar forceps. If necessary, especially when the myoma has a subserosal-intramural component, a suture is applied.

If hemostasis is optimal, there is no need to close the peritoneum.

Postoperative Care

Postoperative course is typical of minimally invasive surgery. The Foley catheter is removed on day 1. The bowel function resumes mostly after 24 h. Antibiotics are administered to the patient given the high risk of postoperative fever. The patient is usually discharged on day 1 or 2 and returns to work in 2 weeks.

Management of Procedure-specific Complications

In 2007, we have published a multicenter study on complications of laparoscopic myomectomy. Out of 2,050 myomectomies, total complication rate was 11.1% (225/2,050 cases).

Box 29.3 shows a detailed description of minor and major complications occurring during and after laparotomic myomectomy. Minor complications occurred in 187 cases (9.1%) and major complications in 38 cases (2.02%). Particularly, 70 patients (3.4%) contracted a urinary tract infection, 105 patients (5.1%) had unexplained transient pyrexia, which resolved quite promptly, and 12 reported manipulator

Box 29.3: Complications (total procedures: *N* = 2050).

Major complications	*N*	*%*
Hematomas**	10	0.48
Hemorrhages	14	0.68
Sarcomas	2	0.09
Redo surgeries	2	0.09
Postoperative renal failure	1	0.04
Bowel injury	1	0.04
Uterine rupture*	1	0.26§
Procedure failings	7	0.34
Total	**38**	**2.02**
Minor complications		
Cystitis	70	3.41
Fever > 38	105	5.11
Manipulator lesions	12	0.58
Total	**187**	**9.11**
Total complications	**225**	**11.1**

* Adenomyosis; ** Two cases with double complication.
§ Data on uterine rupture are reported using the number of pregnancies (386 cases) as the denominator.

lesions (0.6%). With regard to major complications, intraoperative bleedings occurred in 14 cases (0.7%), one of these requiring transfusion. Transvaginal US in the postoperative period revealed the presence of 10 (0.5%) hematomas at the site of myomectomy scar. There were two cases of serious secondary hemorrhages, which were also responsible for the other two blood transfusions (for a total of 0.14%) and readmission to surgery (0.09%): one of these had a laparoscopic hysterectomy because of a severe hemorrhage from the left uterine artery and the other underwent a drainage of a hematoma in the broad ligament under ultrasound vision. Failure to complete planned surgery occurred in seven cases (0.34%): in one case, we converted to laparoscopic hysterectomy because of a large intraligamentous myoma occupying most of the lateral part of uterus, after uterine vessels were skeletonized. We converted to laparotomy in three cases because of anesthesiology problems: in two cases for lack of space and possibility of mobilization of very large myomas and in one case because of a suspect sarcoma. Bowel injury occurred in one patient (0.04%) who had a previous laparoscopic myomectomy 10 years before and was presenting a leiomyomatosis peritonealis disseminata with multiple myomas arising from the right round ligament, the right uterosacral ligament and the peritoneum of the pouch of Douglas. The myomas were all removed. The patient had a late bowel perforation on postoperative day 13, which was treated with thorough peritoneal washing, laparoscopic suturing and drainage, without colostomy. Leiomyomatosis peritonealis disseminata (LPD) is a rare disease.

We have found three cases of LPD in patients who had previous laparoscopic myomectomy in the early 1990s while manual morcellation was still in use, making myoma removal a very tiring and frustrating part of the procedure. This frequency leads to wonder whether the incomplete removal of pieces of myoma missed at morcellation can cause the intraperitoneal regrow of these myoma particles.

We had two cases (0.09%) of unexpected sarcoma. In one case, malignancy was immediately recognized and the procedure converted to laparotomy. In the second case the frozen section failed in making a correct diagnosis. Although distressing, this incidence is very low considering that the incidence of leiomyosarcoma in uterine myomas is estimated to be between 0.13 and 0.29% and that after hysterectomy in patients with presumed benign disease, histological diagnosis of leiomyosarcoma was made in 0.49% of the patients. Probably the incidence is low partly because of a thorough diagnostic workout before scheduling a laparoscopic myomectomy (US, RMN, LDH isoenzyme 3 assay) and partly because of the younger age of the patients: in fact presence of sarcomas increases steadily from the fourth to seventh decades of age. It is obvious that morcellation of sarcoma due to frozen section failure is a serious problem. Nevertheless, this event has been reported also during vaginal or laparoscopic hysterectomy with morcellation. Considering patients inadvertently operated on for leiomyosarcomas the rate of pelvic recurrence at 3 months was increased in patients who mistakenly underwent uterine morcellation for sarcoma but this difference was not statistically significant. Overall and disease-free survival was similar in all patients with sarcomas.

During follow-up after surgery 386 (22.9%) patients conceived after laparoscopic myomectomy with a pregnancy rate in patients wishing pregnancy of 69.8%.

We had one (0.26%) spontaneous uterine rupture at 33 weeks gestation in a patient who had had 8-cm adenomyoma. In this case mechanical enucleation of myoma was impossible because of the characteristics of adenomyosis whose fibers merge with surrounding myometrium, making impossible the delineation of a cleavage plane and subtracting substance to uterus. In fact, adenomyosis infiltrates normal myometrium so that excision of the diseased area subtracts myometrial mass from the total uterine volume. This can cause a reduction in myometrial capacity during pregnancy and production of scars with reduced tensile strength. Nineteen reports of uterine rupture after laparoscopic myomectomy have been reported so far, although the precise frequency is difficult to evaluate. All are case reports never related to the real number of myomectomies performed and reflecting isolated cases in early experience with laparoscopic myomectomy. In only one study of a series of over 100 births after laparoscopic myomectomy, uterine rupture rate was 1%. Authors cite application of excessive tissue coagulation and use of unsuitable suture size (3-0 and 4-0) with following risk of intramural hematomas, indentations and uterine fistulas as possible contributing factors. In one case of 4-cm subserosal myoma suture was not performed because hemostasis was already achieved with bipolar forceps. In another case in which the uterine wall suture was not used, uterine rupture occurred after a spontaneous vaginal delivery. Uterine ruptures occurred in two cases of pedunculated myomas removed after transecting the stalk with bipolar forceps without suture. The problem gave rise to doubts about how solid is the uterine wall after laparoscopic myomectomy for patients desiring pregnancy. Laparoscopic-assisted myomectomy (LAM) has been recently advocated to be less technically demanding and less time-consuming thus being a more effective technique to prevent defective healing because with this method it would be possible to perform a better suturing, but a case of spontaneous uterine rupture after LAM has been reported as well as complications related to laparotomy.

It should be stressed that the risk, even if low, does also exist when a laparotomy is made and results to be 1 out of 40–60 uterine ruptures, event that occurs in 1 out 1,500 pregnancies. In a retrospective review of pregnancy, which comprehended 14 years of activity in a university teaching hospital, the incidence of ruptured uterus was 0.24% in patients with previous myomectomy scars and 4.1% in those with previous primary cesarean sections. Even uterine ruptures of the unscarred uterus or after hysteroscopic resection have been reported. Nevertheless, attention that has been focused on the problems caused when first laparoscopic myomectomies have been immediately reported, which has not always applied to old standardized procedures such as laparotomic myomectomy. In our experience, we always made uterine suture meticulous as possible, using 1 or 0 sutures and applying if needed "Figure of eight" sutures in two different planes. The use of diluted POR8 or pitressin has allowed a minor use of electrosurgery to achieve hemostasis and dissection in favor of sharp dissection. In this way we tried to avoid defective scarring secondary to tissue necrosis. The risk of 0.26% for uterine rupture is quite acceptable and even favorable in comparison with laparotomy. Moreover, the use of vasoconstrictive agents appears to favorably decrease the risk of hemorrhages during myomectomy, as previously reported.

Results based on statistical logistic regression analysis showed that the probability of complications significantly rises with an increase in the number, dimension of myomas (OR: 2,11, $p < .01$) and with the intraligamentous location of myomas (OR: 2.19, $p < .05$) (Fig. 29.4) (Tables 29.3 and 29.4).

Table 29.3: Probability of developing complications computed on the basis of a logistic regression analysis after applying the forward stepwise procedure (underscored).

Number of cases: 1827; Complications 225			
Variables	*Final model*		
	Odds ratio	*95% CI*	*p value*
Myoma size			
1–5 cm	1		—
>5 cm	1.48	0.88–2.46	.13
N° of myomas removed per patient			
1	1		—
2–3	<u>1.73</u>	1.07–2.82	.02
>3	<u>4.46</u>	2.59–7.66	.001
Depth of infiltration			
Pedunculated	1		—
Subserosal	0.72	0.36–1.43	.29
Intramural	<u>1.48</u>	1.05–2.20	.05
Intraligamentous	<u>2.36</u>	1.22–4.59	.01
Vasoconstrictive agents during surgery			
No	1		—
Yes	0.94	0.56–1.59	.82
Age	0.98	0.94–1.01	.29
Hemoglobin before surgery	1.29	0.87–1.92	.38
Hemoglobin after surgery	1.63	1.06–2.51	.02
Operative time	0.99	0.99–1.00	.88

Table 29.4: Probability of developing major complications computed on the basis of a logistic regression analysis after applying the forward stepwise procedure (underscored).

Number of cases: Total 2050; Major complications: 38			
Variables	*Final model*		
	Odds ratio	*95% CI*	*p value*
Myoma size			
1–5 cm	1		–
>5 cm	6.88	3.40–13.79	.001
N° of myomas removed per patient			
1	1		–
2–3	1.01	0.70–2.12	.39
>3	1.31	1.09–2.66	.01
Depth of infiltration			
Pedunculated	1		–
Subserosal	0.78	0.56–1.62	.45
Intramural	1.20	0.66–21.09	.14
Intraligamentous	6.44	3.20–10.82	.03
Vasoconstrictive agents during surgery			
No	1		–
Yes	0.20	0.06–0.62	.005
Age	0.98	0.93–1.05	.93
Hemoglobin before surgery	0.50	0.35–0.71	.001
Hemoglobin after surgery	2.71	0.77–9.45	.12
Operative time	1.03	1.01–1.04	.001

RESULTS AND OUTCOME

Although common, the incidence of febrile morbidity after laparoscopy is anyway much lower than those associated with the conventional approach.

The use of laparoscopic route has been proved to reduce hemorrhagic risk associated with myomectomy. This result is confirmed by our series: important blood loss was reported in only 0.68% of the cases, with requirement for transfusion in 0.14%.

Three hundred and eighty-six (22.9%) patients conceived after laparoscopic myomectomy with a pregnancy rate in 69.8% of patients wishing pregnancy. Miscarriage was 20% resulting in a normal rate. Eighty-one percent of women delivered at term by elective cesarean section; in the other cases there was a normal vaginal delivery. These data are in accordance with many other favorable results of pregnancy outcome, which demonstrate improved fertility rates reported after laparoscopic myomectomy.

We studied vascularization of uterine wound after laparoscopy by means of transvaginal color Doppler ultrasonography in comparison with vascularity of the contralateral intact myometrium. In this way it was also possible to check for defective healing (hematomas, indentations) along the uterine scar in the immediate postoperative period. Transvaginal color flow Doppler was used to study myometrial and fibroid arterial supply. The equipment used was Esaote Biomedica color Doppler AU4 IDEA with a transvaginal multifrequency (5-6.5-7.5 MHz) probe for imaging and a pulsed Doppler system (3.5-4.7MHz) for blood flow analysis. Wall filters (100 Hz) were used to eliminate low-frequency signals. Blood flow impedance expressed as resistance index (RI), pulsatility index (PI) and blood velocity were preoperatively calculated from the 5th to the 8th day of menstrual cycle to study blood flow in the main arteries supplying identifiable fibroid and in the arteries of the contralateral myometrium. Thirty patients were randomized for laparoscopic or laparotomic myomectomy. Examinations were performed before, between 7 and 15, and between 30 and 45 days after the surgery. Blood flows were measured in the arteries supplying myomectomy wound and in the arteries of the contralateral myometrium. Serial sonographic examinations were performed so as to determine the morphology and volume of "scars."

Sonographic evaluations performed 7–15 days after the intervention showed a remarkable accentuation of the vascularity at the level of the myomectomy scar along with a further slight reduction in Pulsatility Index (PI) and Resistance Index (RI). The following US examinations demonstrated a progressive reduction in hypervascularity that 45 days after surgery was absolutely undistinguishable from vascularity of the surrounding myometrium. PI and RI gradually increased to be the same as the indexes in the intact myometrium. The myomectomy wound showed as only one ultrasonic pattern in a highly echogenic area with an ill-defined, heterogeneous myometrial texture. A progressive reduction in scar's size was also reported. Moreover, US postoperative examinations showed the absence of hematomas in the site of the myomectomy wound. US findings after laparoscopic or laparotomic myomectomy were comparable ($p = 0.2$). The healing process after laparoscopic myomectomy seems to be as safe and uneventful as after laparotomic myomectomy: the size of uterine wound decreased steadily from the day after the procedures to day 30–40 when it was possible to assess the healing process. Vascularization at the site of myomectomy scar was also comparable after lapa-

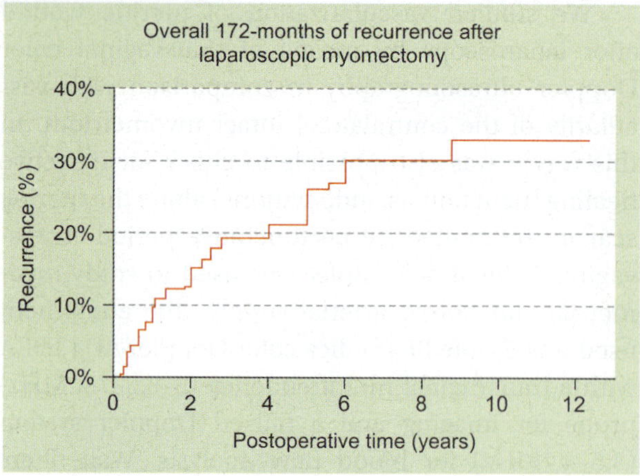

Fig. 29.23: Recurrence rate.

roscopic and laparotomic procedures. Results of this study make us believe that the risk of uterine rupture is more related to incorrect technique for tissue approximation rather than to endoscopic suturing itself.

We have prospectively followed up patients over a 14-year period and we have seen a 21.3% of recurrence rate (Fig. 29.23).

Most recurrence was seen at US with a mean of 29 months (±29 SD) after surgery (range 2–105). Quantitative estimates of the risk of recurrence according to the various considered prognostic factors showed, according to other authors' results, that both the number of myomas removed and the depth of penetration were positively associated with the risk of recurrence. As the number of enucleated fibroids increased, the risk of residual fibroids and recurrence tended to increase.

Another independent risk factor was the use of GnRH analogs prior of the intervention. The use of the Intra Operative Ultrasound Guidance helps to detect and remove the smaller myomas (Fig. 29.24).

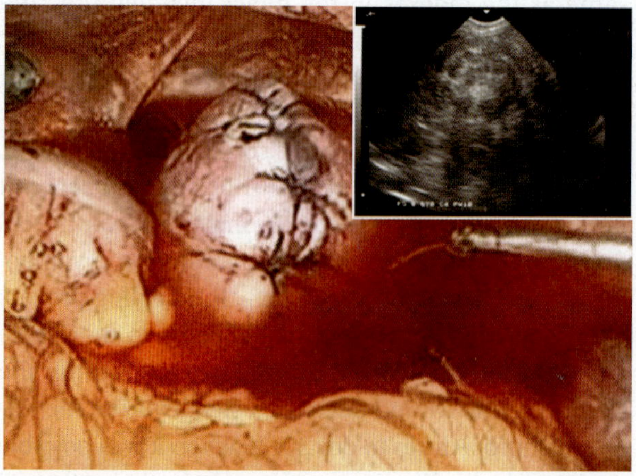

Fig. 29.24: Intraoperative ultrasound guidance.

In fact the frequency of patients with residual fibroids calculated in relation to the number of enucleated fibroids showed that the frequency tended to increase as the number of fibroids increased and that almost all the patients with 10 or more fibroids had residual ones.

CONCLUSION

Laparoscopic myomectomy can be considered a safe technique with a low failure rate (0.34%) and good results in term of pregnancy outcome (pregnancy rate in patients wishing childbearing of 65%) and recurrence rate.

Complication rates (10.5%) appear to be more than acceptable in comparison with the complication rates reported after laparotomic myomectomies (12–39%). It would be invalid to claim that laparoscopic myomectomy is safer than laparotomic myomectomy because the comparison is unmatched, but it would appear that laparoscopic surgery can at least compete with traditional surgery with regard to safety.

Considering the high recurrence rate also with laparotomy and the consequent risk of repeated surgery, we think that patients should be offered the least invasive surgical approach available.

REFERENCES

1. Blake RE. Leiomyomata uteri: hormonal and molecular determinants of growth. J Natl Med Assoc. 2007;99(10):1170-84.
2. Viswanathan M, Hartmann K, McKoy N, et al. Management of uterine fibroids: an update of the evidence. Evid Rep Technol Assess. 2007;154:1-122.
3. Lumsden MA. Embolization versus myomectomy versus hysterectomy. Which is best, when? Hum Reprod. 2002;17(2):253-9.
4. Tropeano G, Amoroso S, Scambia G. Non-surgical management of uterine fibroids. Hum Reprod Update. 2008;14(3):259-74.
5. Mais V, Ajossa S, Guerriero S, et al. Laparoscopic versus abdominal myomectomy: a prospective, randomized trial to evaluate benefits in early outcome. Am J Obstet Gynecol. 1996;174(2):654-8.
6. Seracchioli R, Rossi S, Govoni F, et al. Fertility and obstetric outcome after laparoscopic myomectomy of large myomata: a randomized comparison with abdominal myomectomy. Hum Reprod. 2000;15(12):2663-8.
7. Dubuisson JB, Chapron C. Laparoscopic myomectomy today. A good technique when correctly indicated. Hum Reprod. 1996;11(5):934-5.
8. Dubuisson JB, Chapron C, Verspyck E, et al. Laparoscopic myomectomy. 102 cases. Contracept Fertil Sex. 1993;21(12):920-2.

9. Miller CE, Johnston M, Rundell M. Laparoscopic myomectomy in the infertile woman. J Am Assoc Gynecol Laparosc. 1996;3(4):525-32.
10. Dubuisson JB, Chapron C, Fauconnier A, et al. Laparoscopic myomectomy fertility results. Ann N Y Acad Sci. 2001;943:269-75.
11. Takeuchi H, Kuwatsuru R. The indications, surgical techniques, and limitations of laparoscopic myomectomy. JSLS. 2003;7(2):89-95.
12. Dubuisson JB, Chapron C, Fauconnier A. Laparoscopic myomectomy. Operative technique and results. Ann N Y Acad Sci. 1997;828:326-31.
13. Malzoni M, Sizzi O, Rossetti A, Imperato F. Laparoscopic myomectomy: a report of 982 procedures. Surg Technol Int. 2006;15:123-9.
14. Sizzi O, Rossetti A, Malzoni M, et al. Italian multicenter study on complications of laparoscopic myomectomy. J Minim Invasive Gynecol. 2007;14(4):453-62.
15. Rossetti A, Sizzi O, Chiarotti F, et al. Developments in techniques for laparoscopic myomectomy. JSLS. 2007;11(1):34-40.
16. Donnez J, Dolmans MM. Uterine fibroid management: from the present to the future. Hum Reprod Update. 2016;22(6):665-86.
17. Dartmouth K. A systematic review with meta-analysis: the common sonographic characteristics of adenomyosis. Ultrasound. 2014;22(3):148-57.
18. Goto A, Takeuchi S, Sugimura K, et al. Usefulness of Gd-DTPA contrast-enhanced dynamic MRI and serum determination of LDH and its isozymes in the differential diagnosis of leiomyosarcoma from degenerated leiomyoma of the uterus. Int J Gynecol Cancer. 2002;12(4):354-61.
19. Bogani G, Cliby WA, Aletti GD. Impact of morcellation on survival outcomes of patients with unexpected uterine leiomyosarcoma: a systematic review and meta-analysis. Gynecol Oncol. 2015; 137(1):167-72.
20. Brown J. AAGL advancing minimally invasive gynecology worldwide: statement to the FDA on power morcellation. J Minim Invasive Gynecol. 2014;21(6):970-1.
21. Kives S, Lefebvre G, Wolfman W, et al. Supracervical hysterectomy. J Obstet Gynaecol Can. 2010;32(1): 62-8.
22. Rossetti A, Paccosi M, Sizzi O, et al. Dilute ornitin vasopressin and a myoma drill for laparoscopic myomectomy. J Am Assoc Gynecol Laparosc. 1999;6(2):189-93.

30 Specific Features of Myomectomy

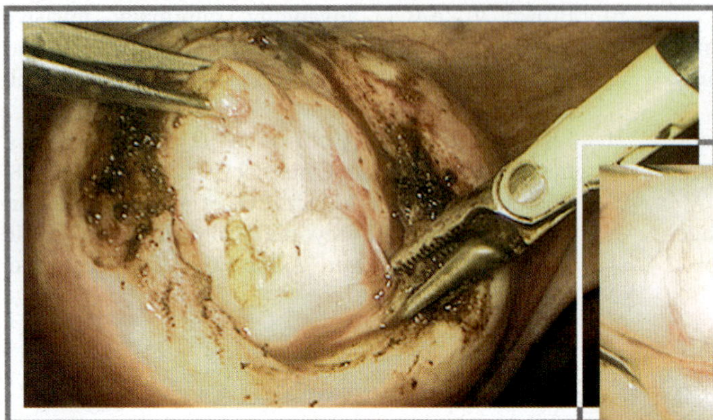

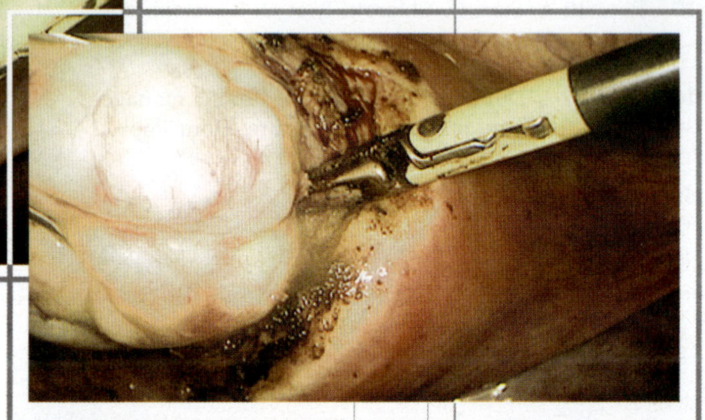

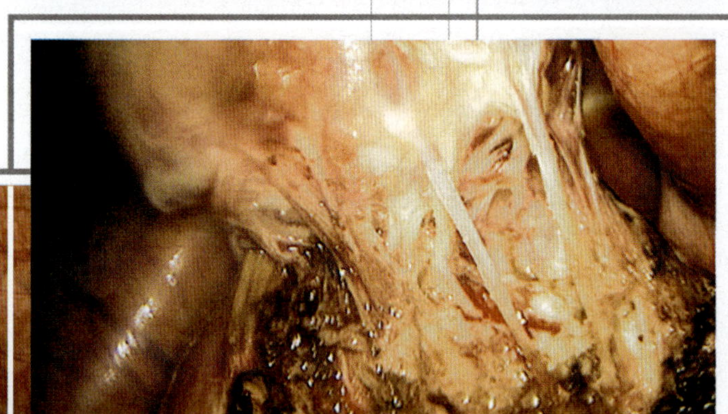

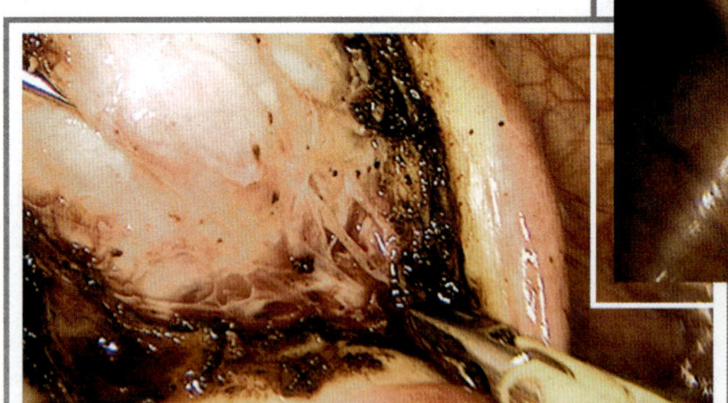

Chapter 30

Specific Features of Myomectomy

Ibrahim Alkatout, Liselotte Mettler

GENERAL

Uterine fibroids are the most frequent benign tumors of the female genital tract. Fibroids are associated with a variety of clinical problems, e.g., pain and pressure symptoms, bleeding disorders, bulk-related symptoms or infertility. For women wishing to preserve their uterus, fibroids can be surgically removed by hysteroscopy, laparoscopy or laparotomy. While hysterectomy remains the only definitive solution, many alternative treatment possibilities for uterine preservation are available today. The indication for a specific treatment has to be taken carefully after considering alternative treatment methods, such as expectant management, medical treatment or interventional radiologic methods, and after obtaining informed consent from the patient. The optimal method of treatment takes into account the patient's interests and wishes and the practical feasibility in the clinical setup. Surgical skills and experience play an important role as surgical procedures on the uterus are not without risk and can lead to severe complications. The decision to operate anticipates an improvement of the initial situation and, therefore, the ideal surgical approach is of utmost importance. Today, a sequence of laparoscopic and hysteroscopic surgical steps with adequate instrumentation and knowledge of suturing guarantees a satisfying surgical outcome of myomectomy if hysterectomy is not desired.

INTRODUCTION

One of the multiple treatment possibilities for myomas considering all laparoscopic surgical, medical or interventional techniques is total laparoscopic hysterectomy (TLH) or subtotal laparoscopic hysterectomy (SLH). As SLH is a much less invasive procedure, a good number of patients with myomas can consider a subtotal approach. However, only a total laparoscopic hysterectomy (TLH) can offer 100% protection from new fibroid formation, later sarcoma formation, uncontrolled bleedings, cervical and endometrial cancer or any other problems arising from the uterus.

In spite of numerous theories, the etiology of fibroid formation remains unclear. While a genetic disposition must be given, as Africans have a much higher frequency of multiple myomas than Caucasians certain up- and down-regulations in the genes of patients with and without myomas have been described. However, as yet no clear guidelines for the prevention of fibroids are available. Hereditary leioyomatosis and renal cell carcinoma syndrome are a rare syndrome involving fibroids. Individuals with the gene that leads to both fibroids and skin leiomyomas have an increased risk of developing a rare case of kidney cell cancer (papillary renal cell carcinoma).

Understanding which genes are involved in fibroids does not automatically tell us why fibroids develop or how to control them. From our understanding of fibroid behavior, we would guess that genes involved in estrogen or progesterone production, metabolism or action are involved. Unfortunately, science is seldom that straightforward. Most guesses regarding these "candidate genes" turn out to be wrong and much research is still required to find out how these genes lead to disease. There are also small variations, called polymorphisms, in genes that may play a role in influencing the risk of fibroids. Both polymorphisms and mutations are changes in the sequence of genes, but the difference is in the degree of change. A mutation makes a major change in the gene that leads to a change in the protein the gene is coding for. For example, it can change amino acid from alanine to glycine or cause that protein to be prematurely cut off.

GENETICS OF FIBROIDS, GENOTYPE AND PHENOTYPE

The discovery of the structure of DNA by Watson and Crick revolutionized biology and medicine. They discovered that DNA carries the code for life in a ladder-like structure. Today, it is known that the genes from a single person take up the space of 400,000 times the distance from the earth to the moon or 1,000 times the distance from the earth to the sun, which works out to 150 billion kilometers.[1,2]

Before going further, it is important to define the terms genotype and phenotype. Genotype is the pattern of genes that you inherit. For example, with eye color, brown is a dominant color and is represented by a "B." Blue is a recessive trait and represented by a "b." Therefore, a person can have "BB," "bb" or "Bb" as genotypes for eye color. Each person gets two copies of the gene, one originally from his or her mother and the other from his or her father. The dominant gene will always dominate; it has the power to trump a recessive trait. Phenotype is physical manifestation, or end result, of the genotype. Although there are three different genotypes (BB, bb, or Bb), there are only two phenotypes: brown eyes and blue eyes. People with "BB" or "Bb" genotype have brown eyes because brown is the dominant trait; only people with "bb" genotype have blue eyes.

We believe that fibroids are a common phenotype that represents many different underlying genotypes. In other words, in our view, fibroids can arise through multiple pathways. In this case, "Bb" might represent two different genes that code for the estrogen receptor beta, which influences the action of estrogen on a fibroid tissue. A "B" gene may make the fibroid more sensitive to this hormone and therefore more likely to grow. In addition, probably multiple genes influence fibroids so that in addition to "Bb" we may also have "Pp" for progesterone receptors, "Ff" for fibrotic factors and so on. This information would be most helpful in advancing treatment as women who carry a high risk of recurrent fibroids and have completed their family planning might choose to have a hysterectomy because of the higher chance of their having an additional surgery. We currently have some clinical information (based on physicians' clinical experience with many patients) to predict prognosis for recurrence after myomectomy, but our clinical information for alternative forms of treatment options is limited.

Evidence for the Role of Genes in Fibroid Development and Growth

Studies of women with fibroids suggest several reasons to suspect that genes play a role in fibroid formation. The first is that both women in a pair of identical twins are twice as likely to have had a fibroid-related hysterectomy as both women in a pair of fraternal (nonidentical) twins. Identical twins share 100% of their genes, while fraternal twins share only 50% of their genes. This suggests that genes that identical twins share make them more likely to form fibroids, since both are identical and nonidentical twins have equal exposure to environmental factors. This difference between identical and fraternal twins has been observed in a general population of women undergoing hysterectomy and a population of women with fibroids leading to hysterectomy.[3,4]

There is also evidence that women who have close relatives, such as mother or sister, with fibroids are much more likely to have fibroids themselves.[5,6] This propensity is called familial aggregation. Just as with breast cancer, if you have many relatives affected by fibroids, your risk of disease is likely to be increased.

Molecular Genetics and Genome-wide Scan for Fibroid Genes

Finally, in the age of molecular genetics, we can scan markers across the complete sets of DNA, or genomes, of many people to find genetic variations associated with a particular disease. This process is called a genome-wide scan. This is a common approach to finding genes in complex diseases, such as diabetes, asthma and heart disease. With a genome-wide scan, women who are sisters and both have fibroids (an affected sibling pair) are recruited to participate in the study. Their DNA is studied for common genes. If hundreds of women are studied, each region of every chromosome can be examined, and it can be determined which genes are shared by sisters who share the fibroid phenotype but are different in many other respects. This approach often produces novel genes that were not previously thought to be involved in the disease process.[7-10]

MICROSCOPIC FACTS AND FIBROID VIABILITY

Fibroids are composed primarily of smooth muscle cells. The uterus, stomach and bladder are all organs made of smooth muscle. Smooth muscles cells are arranged so that the organ can stretch, instead of being arranged in rigid units like the cells in skeletal muscle in arms and legs that are designed to "pull" in a particular direction. In women with fibroids, tissue from the endometrium typically looks normal under the microscope. Sometimes, however, in submucosal fibroids there is an unusual type of uterine lining that does not have the normal glandular structure. The presence of this abnormality, called aglandular functionalis (functional endometrium with no glands), in women having bleeding disorders is sometimes a clinical clue for their doctors to look more closely for a submucosal fibroid.[11] A second pattern of endometrium, termed chronic endometritis, can also suggest that there may be a submucosal fibroid, although this pattern can also be associated with other problems, such as retained products of conception and various infections of the uterus. Hysterectomy is not the only solution for treating fibroids; distinctions in size, position and appearance have to be taken into account when deciding upon the best treatment option. If we understand these issues, we may be able to tell why some women have severe bleeding and other women with a similarly sized fibroid have no problem.

COSTS OF FIBROIDS

In fact, accurately capturing all the costs attributable to uterine fibroids will help us move toward more, and more effective, innovative therapies. When deciding whether or not to launch a new concept, companies typically look at the amount currently spent for other treatments. The economics of fibroids has chiefly been discussed in terms of the health care costs of hysterectomy. This in itself is a huge amount of money. According to a recent estimate, in the United States, more than $2 billion is spent every year on hospitalization costs due to uterine fibroids alone.[12] Additionally, one study estimates that the health care costs due to uterine fibroids are more than $4,600 per woman per year.[13]

When you incorporate all the costs of fibroids, however, the way of treatment becomes even more significant. Let us consider what costs arise:

- The costs of myomectomy, uterine artery embolization (UAE) and other minimally invasive therapies
- The costs of birth control pills and other hormonal treatments to control bleeding
- The costs of tampons, pads and the adult diapers many women require to contain bleeding
- The costs of alternative and complementary therapies
- The cost of doing nothing (for many women this means missing work or working less productively during their period).

WHY HYSTERECTOMIES IN FIBROID PATIENTS?

Why should a patient have hysterectomy today when so many alterative treatment possibilities are available? First, up to a certain size of the enlarged uterus, laparoscopic subtotal hysterectomy completely solves the problem and if women want to eliminate every risk of recurrent fibroids, hysterectomy is their only choice. Hysterectomy also solves coexisting problems, such as adenomyosis, endometriosis and endometrial polyps or cervical dysplasia, and there is no danger of ever leaving a sarcoma or carcinoma behind.

REVIEW OF ALL UTERINE-PRESERVING TREATMENT POSSIBILITIES FOR FIBROIDS

The surgical treatment of fibroids can be differentiated between less invasive and more invasive surgical techniques. Time and type of treatment have to be chosen individually and are dependent on the patient and the treating gynecologist (Tables 30.1 and 30.2).

Expectant Management

Wait and see is a possibility if patients are asymptomatic, decline medical or surgical treatment or have contraindications to any kind of treatment. However, existing data describe the possibility that fibroids can shrink substantially either by optimizing endocrinological disorders, such as hypothyroidism, or during the postpartum period.[14,15]

To pursue the idea of expectant management, the pelvic mass must definitely be classified as a fibroid

Table 30.1: Uterine fibroids or myomatous uterus.

Asymptomatic	*Symptomatic*
Conservative treatment	Operative treatment
No acute need for action	Acute need for action
Medical therapy	Primary operative treatment
Expectant management	Delayed operative treatment with medical pretreatment

Table 30.2: Treatment options for uterine fibroids.

Treatment options for uterine fibroids							
Alternative				*Surgical*			
Uterine artery embolization		*Myomectomy*				*Hysterectomy*	
High intensity focused ultrasound	Hysteroscopic	Laparoscopic	Abdominal	Robotic assisted	Vaginal	Laparoscopic	Abdominal
Miscellaneous methods (myoma coagulation, myolysis)						- supracervical - total	

and differentiated from an ovarian mass. Complete blood count (CBC) should be normal, especially in patients with severe symptoms, such as menorrhagia or hypermenorrhea. Women must also be informed that the risk of miscarriage, premature labor and delivery, abnormal fetal position and placental abruption is increased during pregnancies with uterine fibroids.[16]

Medical Therapy

The benefit of medical treatment in the management of women with symptomatic fibroids is still difficult to prove. Medical therapy can provide adequate symptom relief, especially in cases where hypermenorrhea is the leading problem. The benefit of symptom improvement decreases in long-term treatment periods so that more than 50% undergo surgery within two years.[17]

Nevertheless, there has been a shift in traditional thinking that medical treatment of fibroids is solely based on the manipulation of steroid hormones. A deeper analysis and understanding of specific genes or pathways associated with leiomyomatosis may open new possibilities for prevention and medical treatment.[18]

Primarily as a preoperative treatment to decrease heavy bleedings in patients with fibroids, hormonal treatment with selective progesterone modulators, such as ulipristal acetate 5–10 mg daily, have become widely used over the last 2 years.[19-21]

Alternative Treatment Methods

If the patient does not want to undergo surgery or there are contraindications to surgery, there are alternative procedures:

Uterine Artery Embolization (*UAE*): This minimally invasive therapeutic option allows an occlusion of the specific arteries supplying blood to the fibroids. A catheter is introduced via the femoral artery under local anesthesia and particles are injected to block the blood flow to the fibroid. This can be an effective treatment option if the uterus should not be removed, surgery is contraindicated and family planning is completed. It results in myoma shrinkage of up to 46%. Nevertheless, there is still a significant rate of postinterventional complications.[22,23]

Magnetic Resonance-guided focused Ultrasound (*MgRf-US*): This is a more recent treatment method for uterine fibroids in premenopausal women. For this procedure, patients should have completed their family planning. In this noninvasive thermoablative technique multiple waves of ultrasound energy are converged on a small volume of tissue, resulting in maximal thermal destruction. The limiting factors are size, vascularity and access.[24,25]

Uterine-preserving Surgical Treatment of Fibroids

Indications

Surgical removal of fibroids is still the main pillar in the treatment of leiomyomas. Hysterectomy is the only definitive solution and can be performed as supracervical or total hysterectomy. Myomectomy performed by hysteroscopy, conventional laparoscopy or laparoscopy with robotic assistance and by the open or vaginal approach are alternative surgical methods.

Indications for surgical therapy of uterine fibroids are the following:

- Abnormal uterine bleeding disorders (hypermenorrhea, dysmenorrhea, menorrhagia and metrorrhagia)
- Bulk-related symptoms
- Primary or secondary infertility and recurrent pregnancy loss.

COUNSELING AND INFORMED CONSENT

Patients undergoing an operative procedure have to be informed of the risks and potential complications as well as alternative operating methods. Counseling before surgery should include discussion of the entry technique and the associated risks: injury of the bowel, urinary tract, blood vessels, omentum and other surrounding organs and, at a later date, wound infection, adhesion-associated pain and hernia formation.

Counseling needs to integrate the individual risk dependent on the body mass index (BMI) of the patient. Depending on medical history, it is important to consider anatomical malformations, number of vaginal births, midline abdominal incisions, history of peritonitis or inflammatory bowel disease.[26]

MYOMECTOMY

Myomectomy is a surgical treatment option for women who have not completed their family planning or who wish to retain their uterus for any other reason. The enucleation of fibroids by any method is an effective therapy for bleeding disorders or displacement pressure in the pelvis. Nevertheless, the risk of recurrence remains after myomectomy. Furthermore, if any other pathologies might be causative or only co-causative for the symptoms (such as adenomyosis uteri), these problems will persist.[27] Complications arising at myoma enucleations and pregnancy-related complications have been investigated extensively. All operating possibilities, especially laparoscopic versus laparotomic, but recently also laparoscopic versus robotic-assisted myomectomy have been evaluated. Uterine rupture or uterine dehiscence is rare and occurs in less than 1% of laparoscopic cases and even less seldom in robotic-assisted and laparotomic cases. Careful patient selection and preparation, as well as suture techniques, appear to be the most important variables for myomectomy in women of reproductive age.[28,29] Uteri with multiple fibroids have an increased number of uterine arterioles and venules. Therefore, myomectomy can lead to a significant blood loss and corresponding arrangements should be made.[30]

Hysteroscopic Myomectomy

Submucosal fibroids have their origin in myometrial cells underneath the endometrium and represent about 15–20% of all fibroids. Before the establishment of hysteroscopy as a minimally invasive and effective treatment method, these myomas were removed by hysterotomy or even hysterectomy. Increased surgical training, improvement of technology and the widespread use of hysteroscopic myomectomy have made it a safe, fast, effective and cheap method of fibroid resection while preserving the uterus.[31]

Patient selection concentrates on intracavitary submucous and some intramural fibroids. More than 50% of the fibroid circumference needs to be protruding into the uterine cavity. Deep myometrial leiomyomas require advanced operative skills and have an increased risk for perioperative complications and incomplete resection. The depth of myometrial penetration correlates with the volume of distension fluid absorbed.[32,33] Few data are available on the size of myoma that prevents the use of the hysteroscopic approach. The European Society of Hysteroscopy suggests to limit the myoma size to 4 cm but the few existing data report a significant increase of complications in fibroids that are >3 cm. Surgical skills determine the size and number of myomas that can be resected.[34]

Prior to hysteroscopy, knowledge of the patient's medical history is important e.g., history of cesarean section or any other reason to expect an anatomical disorder. A vaginal ultrasound scan must be performed to precisely determine the uterus location, size and all cervical and uterine pathologies.[35] If available and feasible, fluid hystero-sonography should be performed to better differentiate the relationship of leiomyoma to the endometrial cavity and the myometrium. No prophylactic antibiotic is required to prevent surgical site infection.

The first step is the dilation of the cervical channel with Hegar dilators up to Hegar 9. The most commonly used instrument for fibroid resection is monopolar or bipolar wire loop. Using a monopolar device the fluid medium must be nonelectrolytic, using a bipolar device the fluid medium is isotonic.[36] A continuous flow allows the clearance of blood out of the uterine cavity to improve visualization. Furthermore, the resected pieces can be retracted. Nevertheless, the surface of myoma and time needed for resection increase the risk of excessive fluid absorption.[37]

The resectoscope is inserted through the cervix into the uterine cavity and after distension with fluid the uterine cavity is carefully inspected. The monopolar resectoscope requires a cutting current of 60–120 W. Bipolar resectoscopes offer the possibility of simultaneous cut and coagulation. The wire loop passes easily through the tissue. The incision starts at the highest point of the myoma. Only in pedunculated fibroids might the incision cut the peduncle first. The loop is then moved toward the surgeon using the spring mechanism and simultaneously the entire resectoscope is gently pulled backward. The wire loop must be in view of the surgeon during the whole procedure. This motion is repeated until the whole myoma has been resected and the surrounding myometrium (depth) and endometrium (side) can be differentiated. All resected specimen is sent to the pathologist. In cases of heavy bleeding and reduced vision endometrium and the cutting surface have to be reinspected. These areas can be desiccated with the coagulating current.

The resected area will be recovered by surrounding endometrium during the following weeks. The complication rate is low (0.8–2.6%).[37,38] Complications that can occur, especially after extensive resection, are uterine perforation or excessive fluid absorption. Absorption of distension fluid might result in hyponatremia or volume overload.[39] The recurrence rate is about 20% in a follow-up period of more than 3 years.[34]

Laparoscopic Myomectomy

With the improvement of laparoscopic techniques and skills myomectomy can be performed laparoscopically in most women. The laparoscopic approach is usually used for intramural or subserosal fibroids. The main advantage compared to abdominal myomectomy is decreased morbidity and a shorter recovery period. Nevertheless, laparoscopic myomectomy is limited by surgical expertise and especially laparoscopic suturing skills.[40,41] Selection criteria for laparoscopic myomectomy are location, size and number of fibroids. Nevertheless, these characteristics are variable in relation to the surgical expertise. Preoperative imaging is performed by vaginal ultrasound to assess the precise features of the leiomyomas.[30,35,42,43]

Laparoscopic myomectomy starts with the usual placement of ports and trocars. After placement of the initial port in the umbilicus or higher up in the midline, depending on the size of fibroids, two or three ancillary trocars are placed in the lower abdomen about 2 cm medial of each iliac crest and possibly in the midline.[30,44,45] Myomectomy can lead to severe bleeding that will complicate the procedure due to reduced vision. Vessel bleeding is controlled by bipolar electrosurgical power tools. Intraoperative bleeding can be reduced using vasopressin or other vasoconstrictors. Vasopressin is diluted (e.g., 20 units in 100 mL of saline) and injected into the planned uterine incision site. Vasopressin constricts the smooth muscle in the walls of capillaries, small arterioles and venules. Nevertheless, due to side effects the surgeon should pull back the plunger of the syringe before insertion to check that the needle is not inserted intravascularly.[46-48] Alternatively, misoprostol can be administered vaginally about one hour before surgery to reduce blood loss.[49]

Uterine incision is preferably made vertically as this allows a more ergonomic suturing of the defect. The incision is performed with a monopolar hook directly over the fibroid and carried through deeply until the entire myoma tissue has been reached (Figs. 30.1 to 30.6).

After exposure of the myoma, it is grasped with a tenaculum or sharp forceps and traction and countertraction are applied. The removal of the myoma can easily be performed with blunt and sharp dissecting devices. Capsular vessels should be coagulated before complete removal of the myoma as coagulation becomes more difficult if traction is unsuccessful and bipolar coagulation occurs in the remaining myometrium wall. Subsequent to removal, myoma is morcellated with an electromechanical device under direct vision and at a safe distance to all structures, such as the small bowel, to avoid inadvertent injury. The myoma tissue is removed and sent for pathologic evaluation. Uterine defect is closed with delayed absorbable sutures in one or two layers, depending upon the depth of the myometrial defect. It is important that the suture starts at the deepest point to avoid any cavity that might lead to a weak uterine wall. Furthermore, we tie the knot extracorporeally so that the knot can be pushed into the deep layers with full strength (Figs. 30.7 A to D).

Alternatively, barbed sutures, such as V-lock, can be used to tighten the tissue or a third ancillary trocar can be inserted to hold the suture tight. The security of the uterine closure has bearing on the risk of uterine rupture in subsequent pregnancy. Different kinds of adhesion prevention barriers can be applied (Figs. 30.8 A to E).[50-52] Women should wait at least 4 to 6 months before attempting to conceive.[53]

Abdominal Myomectomy

Abdominal or open myomectomy has its origin in the early 1900s as a uterus-preserving procedure.

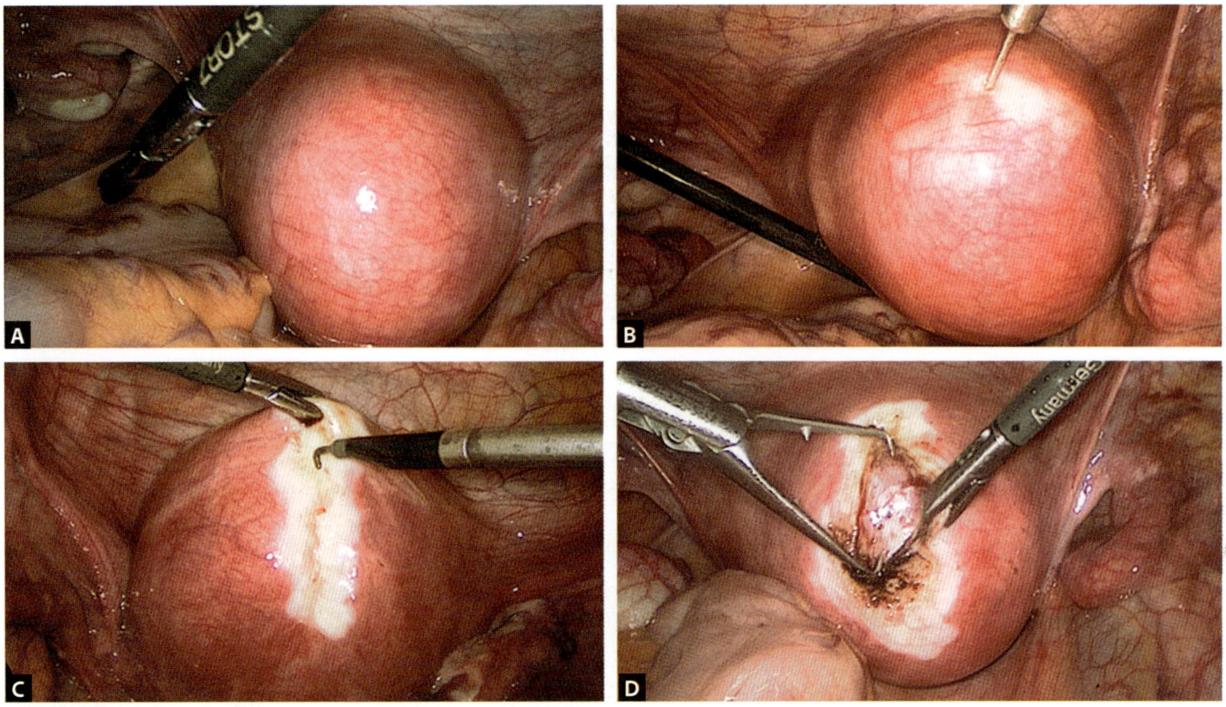

Figs. 30.1A to D: Laparoscopic myoma enucleation. (A) Situs of a fundal/anterior wall fibroid; (B) Prophylactic hemostasis with 1:100 diluted vasopressin solution (Gylcilpressin) in separate wells. The injection intends to separate the pseudocapsule from the fibroid and reduces bleedings; (C) Bipolar superficial coagulation of the longitudinal incision strip and opening of the uterine wall with the monopolar hook or needle up to the fibroid surface; (D) Grasping of the fibroid and beginning of the enucleation. The pseudocapsule remains within the uterine wall and is pushed off bluntly.

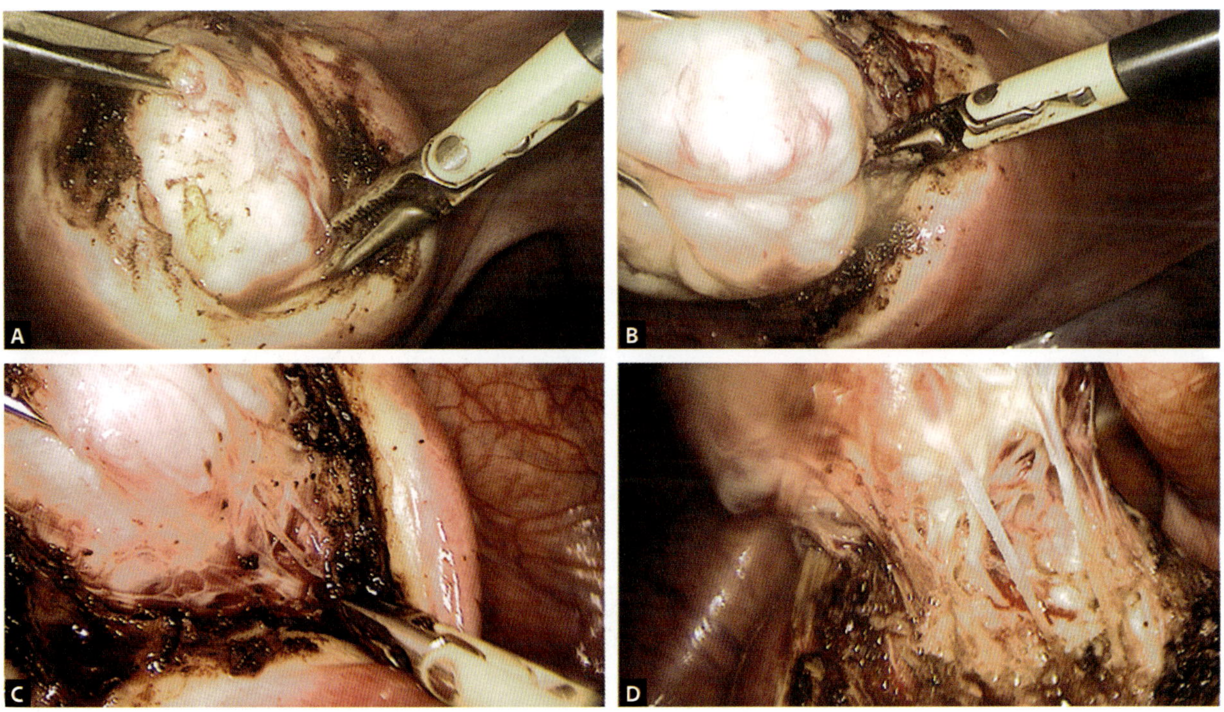

Figs. 30.2A to D: Laparoscopic myoma enucleation. (A) Traction of the fibroid with a tenaculum and blunt delineation from the capsule; (B) Focal bipolar coagulation of basic vessels; (C) Continuous enucleation of the fibroid under traction and specific coagulation of capsule fibers containing vessels; (D) Magnification of remaining capsule fibers to be coagulated and cut.

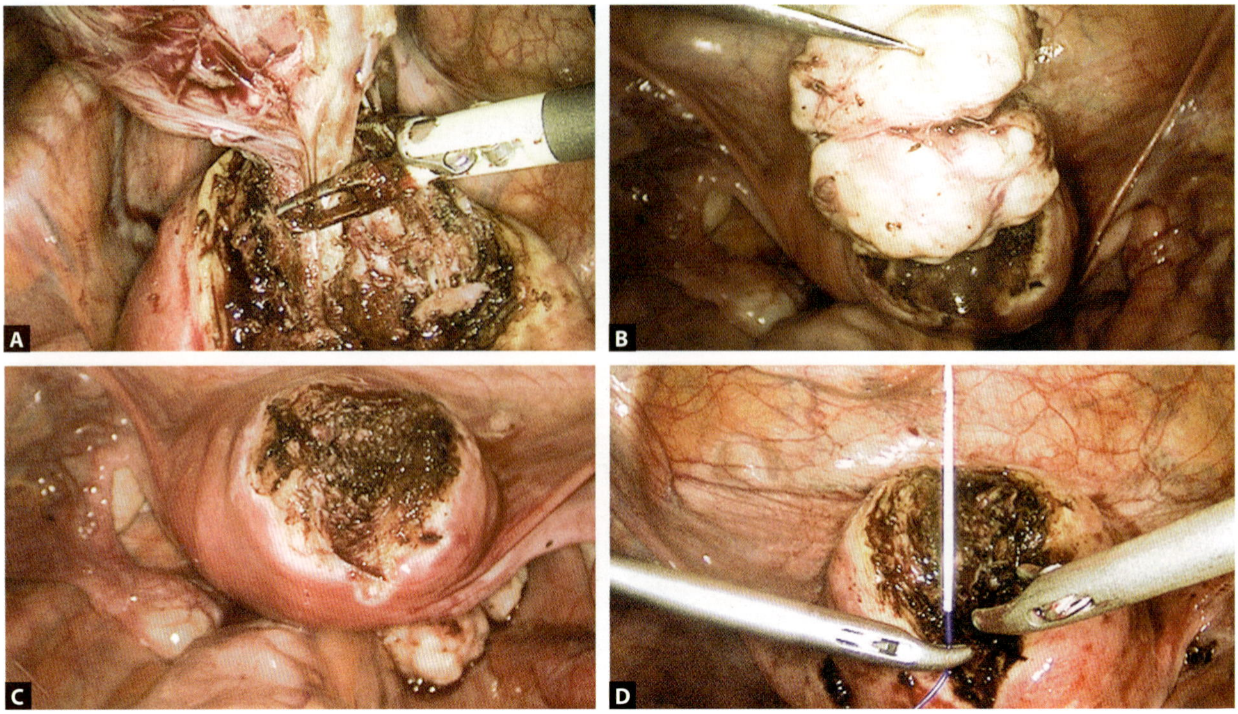

Figs. 30.3A to D: Laparoscopic myoma enucleation. (A) Final coagulation of the capsule vessels; (B) Double belly fibroid after complete enucleation; (C) Minimal coagulation of bleeding vessels under suction and irrigation; (D) Approximation of wound edges with either straight or round sharp needle and a monofilar late-absorbable suture.

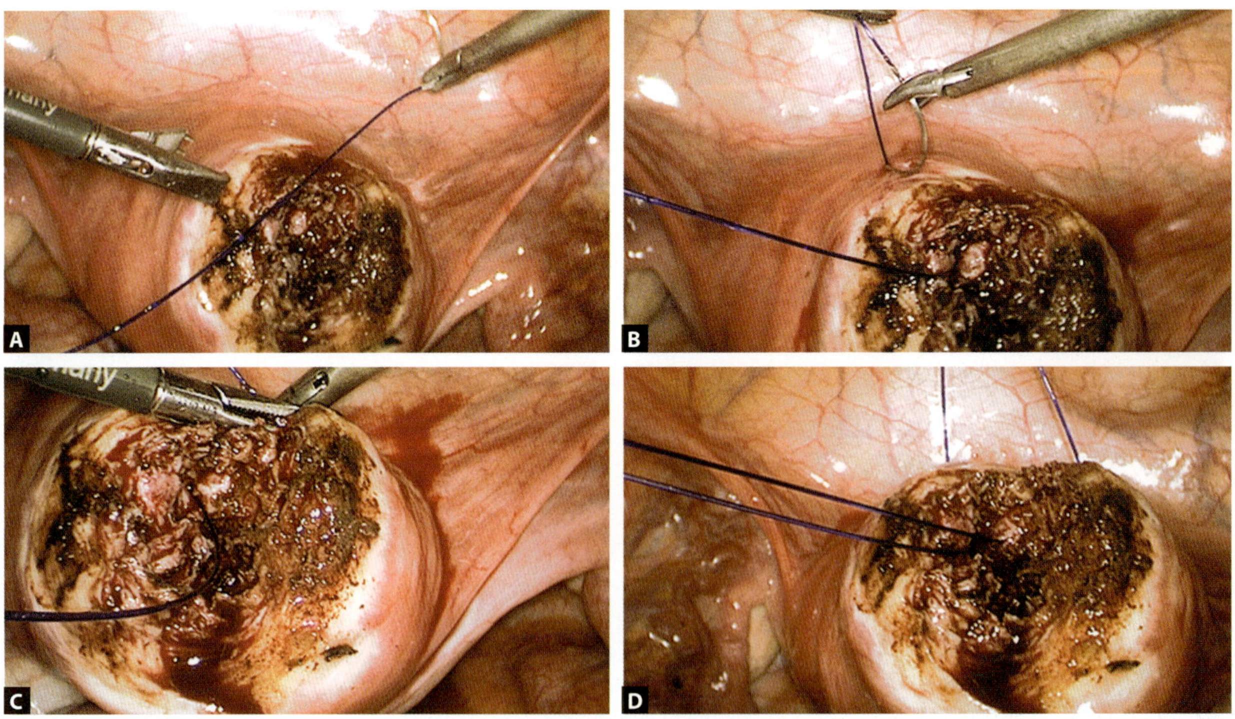

Figs. 30.4A to D: Laparoscopic myoma enucleation. (A) Advantage of round needle stitch. The wound angle is elevated safely and completely by elevation with Manhes forceps. Deeper layers of the myometrium can be grasped more easily using a round needle; (B) Needle exit and simplified regrasping with the right needle holder; (C) Final stitch to invert the knot; (D) Extirpation of the needle and completion of the extracorporeal knot and preparation to push down the extracorporeal knot.

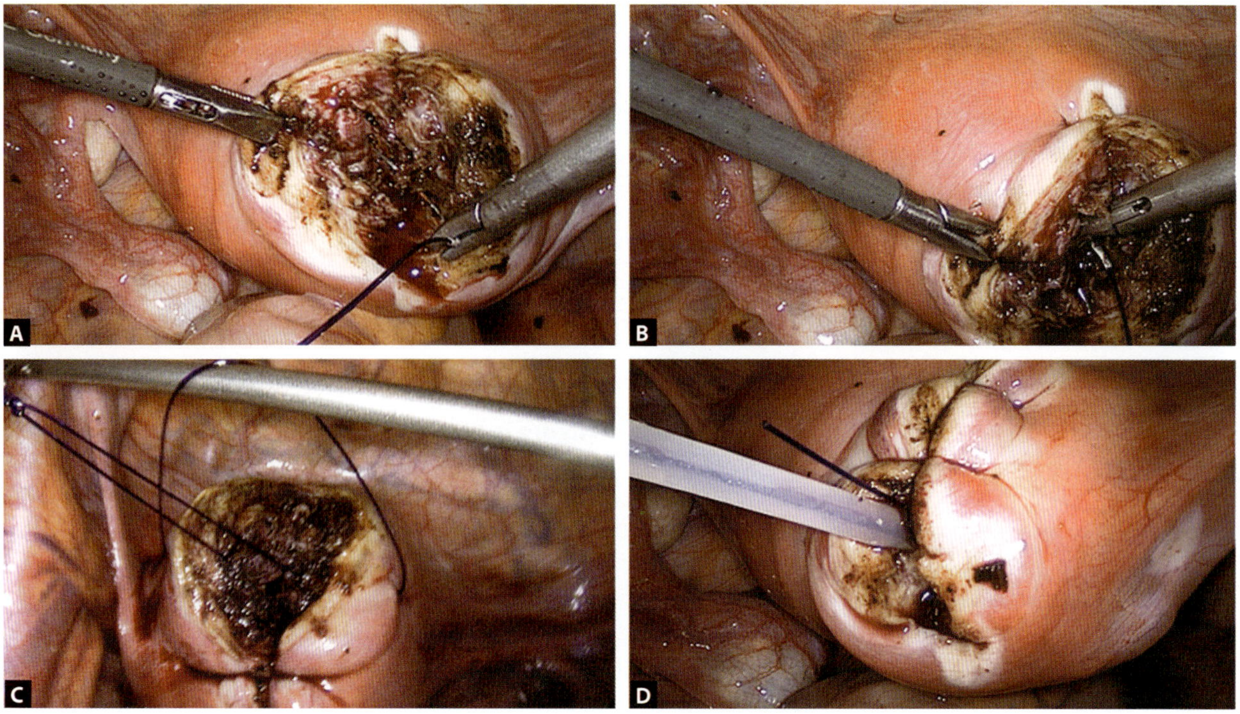

Figs. 30.5A to D: Performance of the extracorporeal "von Leffern" knot. (A) Pulling out the suture, removing the needle, half hitch; (B) Holding the knot with the left hand and reaching over with the right hand; (C) Grasping the short end from below and leading it back, exiting before the half hitch; (D) Turning back the knot. Holding the straight suture and tightening the knot.

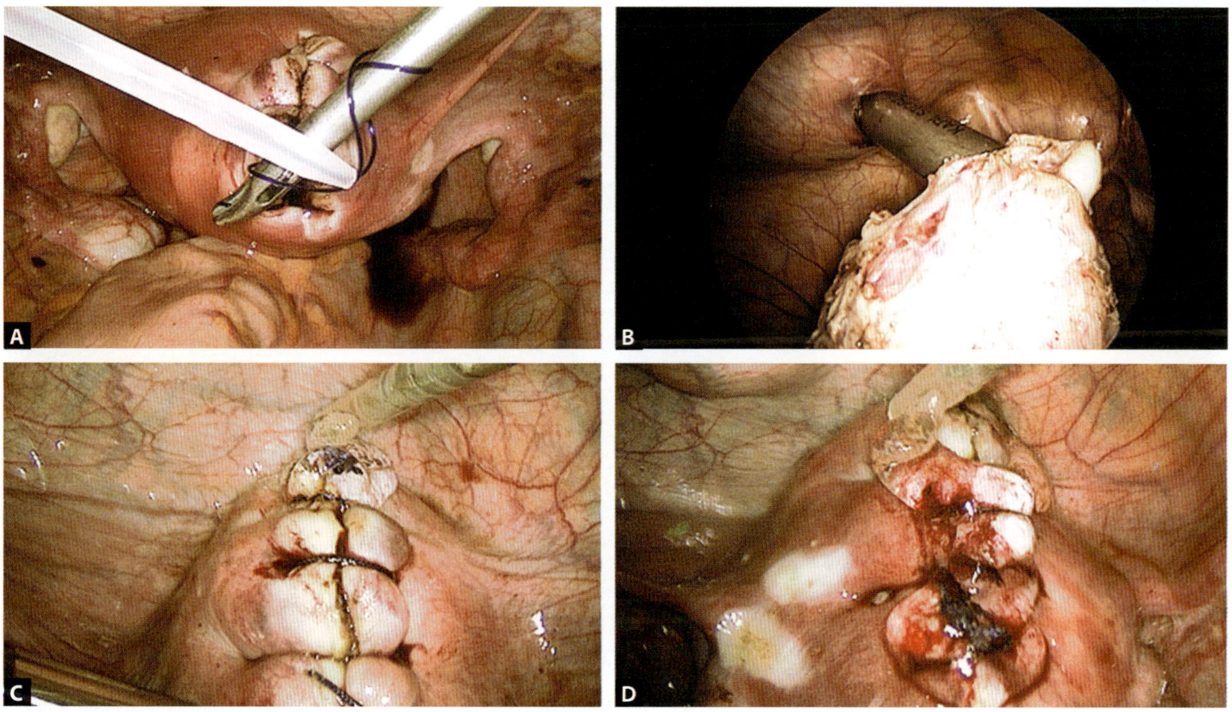

Figs. 30.6A to D: Laparoscopic myoma enucleation. (A) Second single stitch starting as deep as possible in the uterine wound; (B) Exit of the needle on the left wound margin (just next to the Manhes forceps); (C) Completion of the stitch and preparation of the extracorporeal von Leffern knot. The needle holder elevates the thread to avoid tearing of the uterine wall while pulling through the monofilar thread (PDS); (D) The extracorporeal knot is pushed down with a plastic push-rod and deposited deep in the wound minimizing the external suture part.

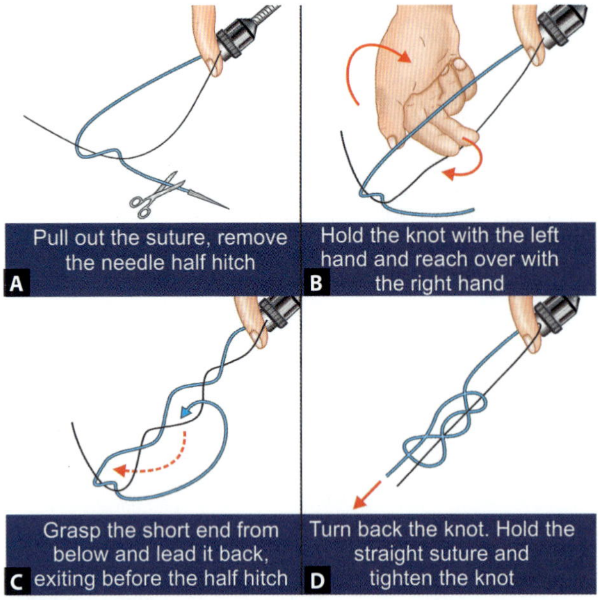

Figs. 30.7A to D: Laparoscopic myoma enucleation. (A) Intracorporeal safety knot performed extracorporeally; (B) Morcellation of the fibroid with the Rotocut morcellator (Storz) in an apple-peeling manner; (C) Final situs showing the extracorporeal sutures to adapt the uterine wound edges; (D) Application of Hyalo Barrier (Nordic Pharma) for adhesion prevention.

Today, it is mostly performed for women with intramural or subserosal myomas and less frequently for submucosal localization. Since the introduction of endoscopic procedures, the indication for abdominal myomectomy has become rare. It becomes an option if hysteroscopic or laparoscopic myomectomy is not feasible or if a laparotomy is required for any other reason. The indication to exclude uterine sarcomas has to be taken very strictly; however, uterine sarcoma is a very rare malignancy and the rate of sarcoma after clinical diagnosis of myoma is very low. The risk of severe complications in association with open surgery is higher than with hysteroscopic or laparoscopic moymectomy. Prophylactic antibiotics should be given for any abdominal fibroid operation.[54,55] After the Pfannenstiel incision either a vertical or transverse uterine incision is performed.[56] Myoma enucleation is performed by traction on the myometrial edges, e.g., with Allis clamps. After exposure of the fibroid it can be extirpated. Pseudocapsule is typically dissected bluntly. Uterine defects are closed with sutures in several layers to reapproximate the tissue and achieve hemostasis without excessive bipolar coagulation.

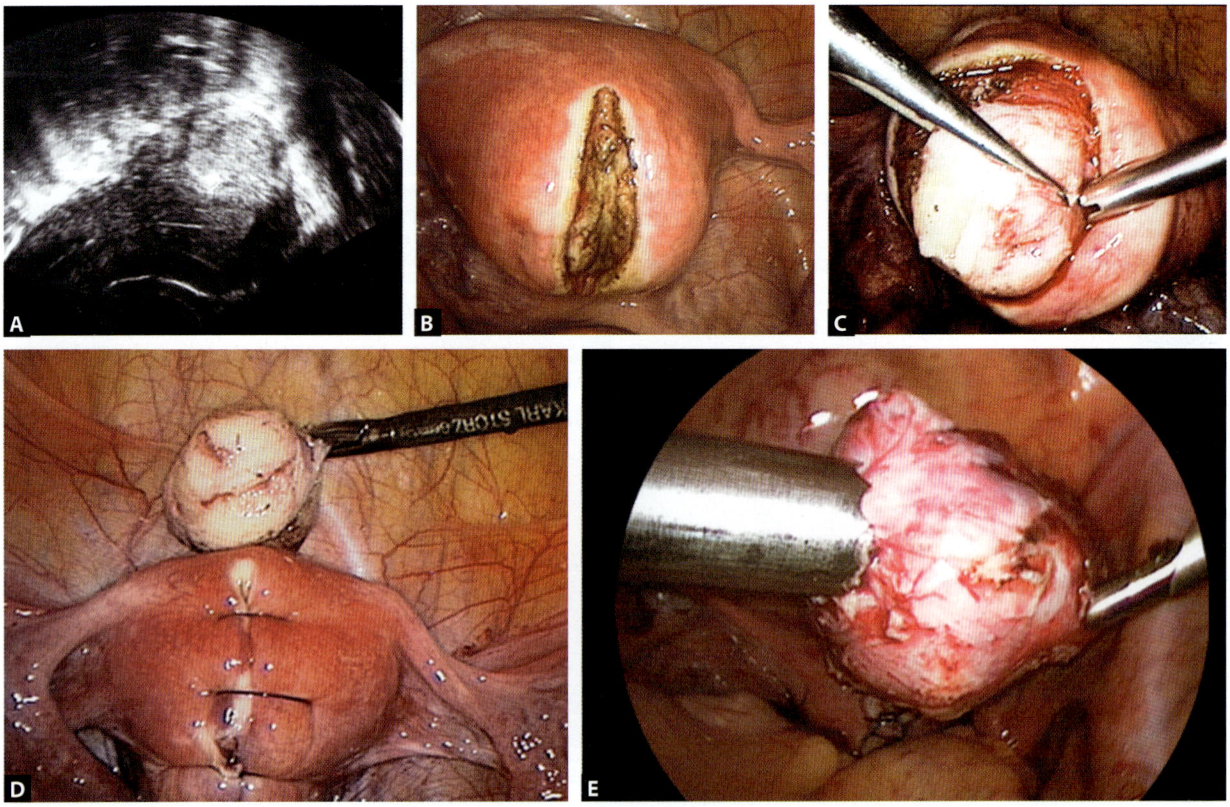

Figs. 30.8A to E: (A) Transvaginal ultrasound shows a 3.5-cm intramural myoma in the back wall of the uterus; (B) Intraoperative uterotomy just above the myoma after injection of vasopressin. The uterotomy includes the myometrium and the myoma capsule and is done with a monopolar needle. All different tissue layers can be differentiated; (C) Intraoperative sight of the myoma and its surrounding vascularized capsule; (D) Reconstruction of the uterine wall after excision of the tumor; (E) Removal of the myoma by morcellation.

Robotic Myomectomy

Robot-assisted laparoscopic myomectomy is a relatively new approach. The advantages of robotic surgery are three-dimensional imaging, mechanical improvement, including seven degrees of freedom for each instrument, stabilization of the instruments within the surgical field and improved ergonomics for the surgeon. Technical difficulties are decreased as suturing is easier than during conventional laparoscopy; however, there are few data comparing robot-assisted with conventional laparoscopic myomectomy.[57-59] The advantages compared to abdominal myomectomy are decreased blood loss and shorter recovery time. Nevertheless, operation duration and operating costs are much higher than for conventional procedures. Furthermore, robotic devices are large and bulky. Robotic surgery is limited by the lack of tactile feedback and additional team training is necessary to minimize the risk of mechanical failure.[60] To date, no advantage compared to conventional laparoscopy could be demonstrated regarding blood loss or operative duration. A more secure myometrial closure has not yet been proven. In obese patients robot-assisted surgery might be beneficial.[61]

HYSTERECTOMY AS TREATMENT FOR MYOMAS

As fibroids are also the most common indication for hysterectomy (30% of hysterectomies in white and 50% of hysterectomies in black women), specific focus is given to hysterectomies within this chapter. The decision for a hysterectomy in a multifibroid uterus depends on the wish of the patient, her health status, whether childbearing has been completed and on the combined decision with the doctor. Only if the patient suffers from metrorrhagia does the disorder need to be examined preoperatively in more detail as this may be a sign of endometrial cancer or sarcoma. Nevertheless, the combined evaluation of MRI and tumor makers preoperatively leads to a more specific diagnosis of rapidly growing uterine masses or adnexas in the case of a leiomyomatous uterus or adnexal tumors. Only in cases where malignancy is not suspected is a simple TLH or SLH recommended, otherwise an oncological approach has to be selected. Hysterectomy as TLH or SLH is recommended for the following indications:

- Acute hemorrhage with nonresponse to other therapies
- Completion of family planning and current or increased future risk of other diseases, such as cervical intraepithelial neoplasia, endometrial hyperplasia or an increased risk of uterine or ovarian cancer. Precondition for the indication for hysterectomy is that these risks can be eliminated or decreased by hysterectomy.
- Failure of previous treatment
- Completion of family planning and significant symptoms (e.g., multiple fibroids or adenomyosis) and the desire for a definitive solution.

The main advantage of hysterectomy over all other therapeutic possibilities is the definitive solution in eliminating all existing symptoms and the risk of recurrence. Nevertheless, the advantage of a definitive solution that allows freedom from future problems can be an obstacle if family planning has not been completed or the patient has a personal inhibition against the removal of the central genital female organ.[62] These issues must be discussed in advance with the patient before the decision for a hysterectomy is taken. Furthermore, for a solitary submucous, subserous, pedunculated or intramural myoma, the complication rate of a hysterectomy has to be compared with the complication rate of myomectomy. The operational risks have to be compared to the operational risks of hysteroscopy, laparoscopic fibroid enucleation or conservative management. With the advances in cervical cancer screening the prevention of future cervical or uterine pathologies is no longer a relevant indication for hysterectomy. The decision must be tailored to meet the needs of each individual patient.

Laparoscopic hysterectomy was first introduced in 1989 with the aim of reducing morbidity and mortality of abdominal hysterectomy to the level reached with vaginal hysterectomy. Laparoscopic assistance for vaginal hysterectomy can be of advantage if there is a need for adhesiolysis, a need to treat endometriosis simultaneously, a need to treat large leiomyomas and to ensure an easier and safer adnexectomy. If feasible, vaginal hysterectomy allows a more rapid and less painful recovery than open or laparoscopic surgery and is much cheaper.[63]

Should Ovaries and/or Fallopian Tubes be Removed or Left in Place at Hysterectomy?

Ovaries

Generally, ovaries are not removed when a hysterectomy is performed for uterine fibroids. Removing uterus alone will cure bleeding and size-related symptoms caused by fibroids. When treating fibroids it is not necessary to remove ovaries or fallopian tubes as is sometimes the case when treating other diseases, such as endometriosis or gynecologic cancers.

Many physicians were taught that at a set age (which varies between 35 and 50) women should be told that removal of the ovaries is recommended as part of the surgery, with the speculation of "while we are there, we may as well." The general teaching has been that ovaries do not have any function after menopause and the risk of ovarian cancer increases with increasing age, so removing the ovaries near the time of menopause was a no-lose proposition. This was especially true if hormone replacement therapy could be used to help younger women transition to the time when they would naturally go through menopause.

However, more recent research suggests that although after menopause the ovaries produce little estradiol (the major estrogen in premenopausal women), they produce a tremendous amount of androgens (usually thought of as male hormones).[64] It is thought that these androgens may be important in maintaining mood and sex drive.[65-67] In addition, risks of hormone replacement have become clearer, and many women choose to use hormones following menopause.[68,69] Most women are aware of the research from the Women's Health Initiative demonstrating significant complications with postmenopausal hormone replacement therapy. However, it is not widely known that the risks are lower for women without a uterus, who are able to take estrogen alone.[69] Recently the association of premature loss of ovarian function and the increasing risk of heart disease has also been investigated.[70]

Considering all these factors, there are good reasons to retain the ovaries if possible. The major reason to remove them at the time of fibroid surgery is if the woman has a high risk of ovarian cancer.

Fallopian Tubes

According to new research presented at the Annual Clinical Meeting of the American College of Obstetricians and Gynecologists in 2013, bilateral salpingectomy at hysterectomy, with preservation of the ovaries, is considered a safe way of potentially reducing the development of ovarian serous carcinoma, the most common type of ovarian cancer. Increasing evidence points toward the fallopian tubes as the origin of this type of cancer. Removing fallopian tubes does not cause the onset of menopause, as does the removal of ovaries.

Prophylactic removal of fallopian tubes during hysterectomy or sterilization would rule out any subsequent tubal pathology, such as hydrosalpinx, which is observed in up to 30% of women after hysterectomy. Moreover, this intervention is likely to offer considerable protection against later tumor development, even if the ovaries are retained. Thus, we recommend that any hysterectomy should be combined with salpingectomy. Women undergoing hysterectomy with retained fallopian tubes or sterilization have at least a doubled risk of subsequent salpingectomy. Removal of fallopian tubes at hysterectomy should therefore be recommended.[71,72]

For this reason, once reproductive function is completed the tubes of a female of reproductive age should be removed while ovaries should remain to support the female well-being. Beyond the reproductive age, tubes should always be removed with uterus while ovaries, as previously discussed, are routinely removed only above the age of 65 years.

Abdominal Hysterectomy

As the indication for abdominal hysterectomy in benign diseases has become very rare, it is not discussed in this chapter.[73]

Vaginal Hysterectomy

Before beginning vaginal hysterectomy, a bimanual pelvic examination is performed to assess uterine mobility and descent and to exclude unsuspected pathology of the adnexa. Only then can a final decision be made whether to proceed with a vaginal or abdominal approach. The operation starts with entry into the cul de sac or the vesicovaginal fold. Here we describe the posterior peritoneal opening. The uterosacral ligaments are identified and clamped, including the lower portion of the cardinal ligaments. In the next step the vesicovaginal space is opened and after identification of the peritoneal fold it is cut and the cardinal ligaments are ligated, including the uterine vessels. Most adnexa can be removed by grasping the ovary and clamping the infundibulopelvic ligament. The uterus can then be enucleated stepwise from the remaining peritoneal fold at a safe distance from the bladder. The peritoneum can either be closed or left open and the vaginal epithelium is reapproximated in either a vertical or a horizontal manner.

A myomatous uterus has to be morcellated in a circular manner. Sometimes it is necessary to enucleate large solitary myomas or perform intramyometrial coring, especially in cases of diffusely enlarged uteri.[74,75]

Subtotal Laparoscopic Hysterectomy (SLH)

Supracervical (subtotal) hysterectomy was first described by Semm in 1990 and in another technique by Lyons. The operative technique is similar to total laparoscopic hysterectomy. Only after occluding the ascending branch of uterine artery is uterine corpus resected as a reverse conus down to the endocervical canal.[76] For SLH and TLH the trocar placements are the same as for laparoscopic myomectomy and depend on the size of the uterus (see above). There is no need to perform ureterolysis at the beginning of the operation as the ureter is at a safe distance if the suturing line is kept strictly at the uterine wall. The infundibulopelvic ligament and the round ligament are divided from the pelvic side wall and, if the adnexa are to remain in situ, division of the adnexa from the uterus is performed. The broad ligament is then opened, dissected and each leaf separately coagulated. The bladder is separated from the uterus by opening the vesicouterine ligament and pushing the bladder downwards for about 1–2 cm. This is followed by presentation of the ramus ascendens of the uterine artery and division of the uterine pedicles with the same stepwise dissection of the left adnexa. A thorough inspection of the cervix then takes place. Cervix is separated from uterus with the help of electric cutting loop or any other cutting instrument. This is followed by coagulation of the cervical canal and closure of the peritoneum over the remaining cervical stump for infection and adhesion prevention. However, the peritoneum can also be left open, according to surgeon preference. Afterwards, morcellation of the uterine body is performed and, if the adnexa are also resected, they should be put into an endo bag for extraction.

As morcellation techniques are described in detail in other chapters of the book, the importance of this technique is not dealt with here.

Total Laparoscopic Hysterectomy (TLH)

Subtotal laparoscopic hysterectomy (SLH) should be avoided if adenomyosis uterus is suspected because part of the endometrial glands remain in the cervical and paracervical channel. These can cause an early recurrence or persistence of the symptoms although the few existing data offer no direct confirmation of this view.[77,78]

Surgical steps are identical to LSH, the only difference being that a uterine manipulator is placed in the vagina before the operation. After separation of the bladder from uterus, the bladder is pushed and dissected down 2–3 cm to clearly visualize rim of the cervical cup. In cases of postcesarean section, a gentle, blunt and intermediate sharp dissection has to be carried out. After uterus has been lateralized by pushing up the manipulator, uterine artery and vein with collateral vessels are completely coagulated near cervix and dissected. Vagina is resected from cervix with monopolar hook by firmly stretching the manipulator cranially and carefully performing an intrafascial dissection leaving the sacrouterine ligaments almost completely in place. This is in accordance with the CISH technique introduced by Kurt Semm.[79] The uterus is then retracted through vagina while still fixed to manipulator. If the uterus is too large, it has to be morcellated either intra-abdominally or transvaginally. Vagina is closed with two corner sutures and one or two sutures in between corner sutures. Sacrouterine ligaments and the middle portion of vagina are stitched and elevated by the corner sutures to prevent vaginal prolapse or enterocele formation at a later time. Peritonealization and drainage are not required.

With the improvement of endoscopic surgery and above all the improvement in endoscopic suturing laparoscopic-assisted vaginal hysterectomy has become obsolete, especially as this technique does not include a suspension of the cardinal and sacrouterine ligaments.

CONCLUSION

Treatment options for uterine leiomyomas vary. The choice of treatment should be made on an individual basis taking into account the following factors: the patient's level of suffering due to bleeding disorders or displacement-caused pain, the status of family planning and the patient's preferences regarding the different treatment options.

In *asymptomatic women* expectant management is suggested except for hydronephrosis caused by displacement or hysteroscopically resectable submucous fibroids in women who pursue pregnancy.

In *postmenopausal women* without hormonal therapy fibroids usually shrink and become asymptomatic. Therefore, expectant management is the method of choice. However, sarcoma should be excluded if a new or an enlarging pelvic mass occurs in a postmenopausal woman. Surgical treatment is the option if leiomyomas are symptomatic. If there are contraindications to operative procedures or hysterectomy is declined by the patient for personal reasons, any of the alternative treatment options can be considered (medical, embolization or guided ultrasound).

In *premenopausal women* appropriate submucosal leiomyomas should be resected hysteroscopically if women wish to preserve their childbearing potential and/or they are symptomatic (e.g., bleeding, miscarriage). Intramural and subserosal leiomyomas in women who wish to preserve their fertility can be removed laparoscopically. Nevertheless, an appropriate surgical technique and advanced laparoscopic skills are necessary. If this cannot be guaranteed, abdominal myomectomy has to be recommended or referral to a laparoscopic center to maximize the possibility and safety of pregnancy after uterine reconstruction. The risk of uterine rupture in pregnancy following myomectomy needs to be discussed with the patient.

Robotic assistance makes laparoscopic suturing easier and offers surgery with three-dimensional vision; however, costs are still high. Further developments in robotic assistance, including force feedback, will catch more of our attention in the future.

For *women who have completed their family planning,* hysterectomy is the definitive procedure for relief of symptoms and prevention of recurrence of fibroid-related problems. With increasing experience in laparoscopic hysterectomies, the risk of side effects has become manageable. In relation to compliance and individuality of the patient, a suitable solution can be either laparoscopic supracervical or total laparoscopic hysterectomy.

REFERENCES

1. Watson JD, Crick FH. Molecular structure of nucleic acids; a structure for deoxyribose nucleic acid. Nature. 1953;171(4356):737-8.
2. Watson JD Crick FH. Genetical implications of the structure of deoxyribonucleic acid. Nature. 1953;171(4361):964-7.
3. Treloar SA, et al. Pathways to hysterectomy: insights from longitudinal twin research. Am J Obstet Gynecol. 1992;167(1):82-8.
4. Snieder H, MacGregor AJ, Spector TD. Genes control the cessation of a woman's reproductive life: a twin study of hysterectomy and age at menopause. J Clin Endocrinol Metab. 1998;83(6):1875-80.
5. Vikhlyaeva EM, Khodzhaeva ZS, Fantschenko ND. Familial predisposition to uterine leiomyomas. Int J Gynaecol Obstet. 1995;51(2):127-31.
6. Van Voorhis BJ, Romitti PA, Jones MP. Family history as a risk factor for development of uterine leiomyomas. Results of a pilot study. J Reprod Med. 2002;47(8):663-9.
7. Al-Hendy A, Salama SA. Catechol-O-methyltransferase polymorphism is associated with increased uterine leiomyoma risk in different ethnic groups. J Soc Gynecol Investig. 2006;13(2):136-44.
8. Tsibris JC, Segars J, Coppola D, et al. Insights from gene arrays on the development and growth regulation of uterine leiomyomata. Fertil Steril. 2002;78(1):114-21.
9. Wang H, Mahadevappa M, Yamamoto K, et al. Distinctive proliferative phase differences in gene expression in human myometrium and leiomyomata. Fertil Steril. 2003;80(2):266-76.
10. Gross K, Morton C, Stewart E. Finding genes for uterine fibroids. Obstet Gynecol. 2000;95 (4 Suppl 1):60.
11. Patterson-Keels LM, Selvaggi SM, Haefner HK, et al. Morphologic assessment of endometrium overlying submucosal leiomyomas. J Reprod Med. 1994;39(8):579-84.
12. Flynn M., Jamison M, Datta S, et al. Health care resource use for uterine fibroid tumors in the United States. Am J Obstet Gynecol. 2006;195(4):955-64.
13. Hartmann KE, Birnbaum H, Ben-Hamadi R, et al. Annual costs associated with diagnosis of uterine leiomyomata. Obstet Gynecol. 2006;108(4):930-7.
14. Peddada SD, Laughlin SK, Miner K, et al. Growth of uterine leiomyomata among premenopausal black and white women. Proc Natl Acad Sci USA. 2008;105(50):19887-92.
15. Laughlin SK, Hartmann KE, Baird DD. Postpartum factors and natural fibroid regression. Am J Obstet Gynecol. 2011;204(6):496 e1-6.
16. Zaima A, Ash A. Fibroid in pregnancy: characteristics, complications, and management. Postgrad Med J. 2011;87(1034):819-28.
17. Marjoribanks J, Lethaby A, Farquhar C. Surgery versus medical therapy for heavy menstrual bleeding. Cochrane Database Syst Rev. 2006;(2):CD003855.
18. Al-Hendy A, Lee EJ, Wang HQ, et al. Gene therapy of uterine leiomyomas: adenovirus-mediated expression of dominant negative estrogen receptor inhibits tumor growth in nude mice. Am J Obstet Gynecol. 2004;191(5):1621-31.
19. Donnez J, Tatarchuk TF, Bouchard P, et al. Ulipristal acetate versus placebo for fibroid treatment before surgery. N Engl J Med. 2012;366(5):409-20.
20. Donnez J, Vazquez F, Tomaszweski J, et al. Long-term treatment of uterine fibroids with ulipristal acetate. Fertil Steril. 2014;101(6):1565-73 e1-18.
21. Donnez J, Hudecek R, Donnez O, et al. Efficacy and safety of repeated use of ulipristal acetate in uterine fibroids. Fertil Steril. 2015;103(2):519-27.e3.
22. Edwards RD, Moss RG, Lumsden MA, et al. Uterine-artery embolization versus surgery for symptomatic uterine fibroids. N Engl J Med. 2007;356(4):360-70.

23. van der Kooij SM, Bipat S, Hehenkamp WJ, et al. Uterine artery embolization versus surgery in the treatment of symptomatic fibroids: a systematic review and metaanalysis. Am J Obstet Gynecol. 2011;205(4):317.e1-18.
24. Kim HS, Baik JH, Pham LD, et al. MR-guided high-intensity focused ultrasound treatment for symptomatic uterine leiomyomata: long-term outcomes. Acad Radiol. 2011;18(8):970-6.
25. Funaki K, Fukunishi H, Sawada K. Clinical outcomes of magnetic resonance-guided focused ultrasound surgery for uterine myomas: 24-month follow-up. Ultrasound Obstet Gynecol. 2009;34(5):584-9.
26. Royal College of Obstetricians and Gynecologists. Preventing entry-related gynaecological laparoscopic injuries. RCOG Green-top Guideline. 2008;49:1-10.
27. Wallach EE, Vlahos NF. Uterine myomas: an overview of development, clinical features, and management. Obstet Gynecol. 2004;104(2):393-406.
28. Kim MS, Uhm YK, Kim JYm et al. Obstetric outcomes after uterine myomectomy: laparoscopic versus laparotomic approach. Obstet Gynecol Sci. 2013;56(6):375-81.
29. Lonnerfors C, Persson J. Pregnancy following robot-assisted laparoscopic myomectomy in women with deep intramural myomas. Acta Obstet Gynecol Scand. 2011;90(9):972-7.
30. Mettler L, Schollmeyer T, Tinelli A, et al. Complications of uterine fibroids and their management, surgical management of fibroids, laparoscopy and hysteroscopy versus hysterectomy, haemorrhage, adhesions, and complications. Obstet Gynecol Int. 2012:2012;791248.
31. Di Spiezio Sardo A, Mazzon I, Bramante S, et al. Hysteroscopic myomectomy: a comprehensive review of surgical techniques. Hum Reprod Update. 2008;14(2):101-9.
32. Emanuel MH, Hart A, Wamsteker K, et al. An analysis of fluid loss during transcervical resection of submucous myomas. Fertil Steril. 1997;68(5):881-6.
33. Wamsteker K, Emanuel MH, de Kruif JH. Transcervical hysteroscopic resection of submucous fibroids for abnormal uterine bleeding: results regarding the degree of intramural extension. Obstet Gynecol. 1993;82(5):736-40.
34. Hart R, Molnar BG, Magos A. Long term follow up of hysteroscopic myomectomy assessed by survival analysis. Br J Obstet Gynaecol. 1999;106(7):700-5.
35. Mettler L, Sammur W, Alkatout I, et al. Imaging in gynecologic surgery. Womens Health (Lond Engl). 2011;7(2):239-48; quiz 249-50.
36. Varma R, Soneja H, Clark TJ, et al. Hysteroscopic myomectomy for menorrhagia using Versascope bipolar system: efficacy and prognostic factors at a minimum of one year follow up. Eur J Obstet Gynecol Reprod Biol. 2009;142(2):154-9.
37. Loffer FD, Bradley LD, Brill AI, et al. Hysteroscopic fluid monitoring guidelines. The ad hoc committee on hysteroscopic training guidelines of the American Association of Gynecologic Laparoscopists. J Am Assoc Gynecol Laparosc. 2000;7(1):167-8.
38. Jansen FW, Vredevooqd CB, van Ulzen K, et al. Complications of hysteroscopy: a prospective, multicenter study. Obstet Gynecol. 2000;96(2):266-70.
39. Propst AM, Liberman RF, Harlow BL, et al. Complications of hysteroscopic surgery: predicting patients at risk. Obstet Gynecol. 2000;96(4):517-20.
40. Parker WH, Rodi IA. Patient selection for laparoscopic myomectomy. J Am Assoc Gynecol Laparosc. 1994;2(1):23-6.
41. Lefebvre G, Vilos G, Allaire C, et al. The management of uterine leiomyomas. J Obstet Gynaecol Can. 2003;25(5):396-418; quiz 419-22.
42. Alkatout I, Bojahr B, Dittmann L, et al. Precarious preoperative diagnostics and hints for the laparoscopic excision of uterine adenomatoid tumors: two exemplary cases and literature review. Fertil Steril. 2011;95(3):1119 e5-8.
43. Dueholm M, Lundorf E, Hansen ES, et al. Accuracy of magnetic resonance imaging and transvaginal ultrasonography in the diagnosis, mapping, and measurement of uterine myomas. Am J Obstet Gynecol. 2002;186(3):409-15.
44. Alkatout I, Schollmeyer T, Hawaldar NA, et al. Principles and safety measures of electrosurgery in laparoscopy. JSLS. 2012;16(1):130-9.
45. Alkatout I, Stuhlmann-Laeisz C, et al. Organ-preserving management of ovarian pregnancies by laparoscopic approach. Fertil Steril. 2011;95(8): 2467-70.e1-2.
46. Kongnyuy EJ, Wiysonge CS. Interventions to reduce haemorrhage during myomectomy for fibroids. Cochrane Database Syst Rev. 2011;(11):CD005355.
47. Zhao F, Jiao Y, Guo Z, et al. Evaluation of loop ligation of larger myoma pseudocapsule combined with vasopressin on laparoscopic myomectomy. Fertil Steril. 2010;95(2):762-6.
48. Tinelli A, Mettler L, Malvasi A, et al. Impact of surgical approach on blood loss during intracapsular myomectomy. Minim Invasive Ther Allied Technol. 2013;23(2);87-95.
49. Celik H, Sapmaz E. Use of a single preoperative dose of misoprostol is efficacious for patients who undergo abdominal myomectomy. Fertil Steril. 2003;79(5):1207-10.
50. Mettler L, Sammur W, Schollmeyer T, et al. Cross-linked sodium hyaluronate, an anti-adhesion barrier gel in gynaecological endoscopic surgery. Minim Invasive Ther Allied Technol. 2013;22(5):260-5.
51. Mettler L, Schollmeyer T, Alkatout I. Adhesions during and after surgical procedures, their prevention and impact on women's health. Womens Health (Lond Engl). 2012;8(5):495-8.
52. Tulandi T, Murray C, Guralnick M. Adhesion formation and reproductive outcome after myomectomy and second-look laparoscopy. Obstet Gynecol. 1993;82(2):213-5.
53. Tsuji S, Takahashi K, Sugimura K, et al. MRI evaluation of the uterine structure after myomectomy. Gynecol Obstet Invest. 2006;61(2):106-10.
54. D'Angelo E, Prat J. Uterine sarcomas: a review. Gynecol Oncol. 2009;116(1):131-9.

55. Mukhopadhaya N, De Silva C, Manyonda IT. Conventional myomectomy. Best Pract Res Clin Obstet Gynaecol. 2008;22(4):677-705.
56. Discepola F, Valenti DA, Reinhold C, et al. Analysis of arterial blood vessels surrounding the myoma: relevance to myomectomy. Obstet Gynecol. 2007;110(6):1301-3.
57. Pundir J, Pundir V, Walavalkar R, et al. Robotic-assisted laparoscopic vs abdominal and laparoscopic myomectomy: systematic review and meta-analysis. J Minim Invasive Gynecol. 2013;20(3):335-45.
58. Barakat EE, Bedaiwy MA, Zimberg S, et al. Robotic-assisted, laparoscopic, and abdominal myomectomy: a comparison of surgical outcomes. Obstet Gynecol. 2011;117(2 Pt 1):256-65.
59. Mettler L, Clevin L, Ternamian A, et al. The past, present and future of minimally invasive endoscopy in gynecology: a review and speculative outlook. Minim Invasive Ther Allied Technol. 2013;22(4):210-26.
60. Schollmeyer T, Mettler L, Jonat W, et al. Roboterchirurgie in der Gynäkologie. Der Gynäkologe. 2011;44(3):196-201.
61. George A, Eisenstein D, Wegienka G. Analysis of the impact of body mass index on the surgical outcomes after robot-assisted laparoscopic myomectomy. J Minim Invasive Gynecol. 2009;16(6):730-3.
62. Falcone T, Parker WH. Surgical management of leiomyomas for fertility or uterine preservation. Obstet Gynecol. 2013;121(4):856-68.
63. Garry R, Fountain J, Brown J, et al. EVALUATE hysterectomy trial: a multicentre randomised trial comparing abdominal, vaginal and laparoscopic methods of hysterectomy. Health Technol Assess. 2004;8(26):1-154.
64. Adashi EY. The climacteric ovary as a functional gonadotropin-driven androgen-producing gland. Fertil Steril. 1994;62(1):20-7.
65. Shifren JL. The role of androgens in female sexual dysfunction. Mayo Clin Proc. 2004;79(4 Suppl):S19-24.
66. Buster JE, Kingsberg SA, Aquirre O, et al. Testosterone patch for low sexual desire in surgically menopausal women: a randomized trial. Obstet Gynecol. 2005;105(5 Pt 1):944-52.
67. Nyunt A, Stephen G, Gibbin J, et al. Androgen status in healthy premenopausal women with loss of libido. J Sex Marital Ther. 2005;31(1):73-80.
68. Manson JE, Hsia J, Johnson KC, et al. Estrogen plus progestin and the risk of coronary heart disease. N Engl J Med. 2003;349(6):523-34.
69. Anderson GL, Limacher M, Assaf AR, et al. Effects of conjugated equine estrogen in postmenopausal women with hysterectomy: the Women's Health Initiative randomized controlled trial. JAMA. 2004;291(14):1701-12.
70. Parker WH, Broder MS, Liuz Z, et al. Ovarian conservation at the time of hysterectomy for benign disease. Obstet Gynecol. 2005;106(2):219-26.
71. Dietl J, Wischhusen J, Hausler SF. The post-reproductive Fallopian tube: better removed? Hum Reprod. 2011;26(11):2918-24.
72. Guldberg R, Wehberg S, Skovlund CW, et al. Salpingectomy as standard at hysterectomy? A Danish cohort study, 1977-2010. BMJ Open. 2013;3(6):pii e002845.
73. AAMIG, W. AAGL position statement: Robotic-assisted laparoscopic surgery in benign gynecology. J Minim Invasive Gynecol. 2013;20(1):2-9.
74. Meeks GR, Harris RL. Surgical approach to hysterectomy: abdominal, laparoscopy-assisted, or vaginal. Clin Obstet Gynecol. 1997;40(4):886-94.
75. Mazdisnian F, Kurzel RB, Coe S, et al. Vaginal hysterectomy by uterine morcellation: an efficient, non-morbid procedure. Obstet Gynecol. 1995;86(1):60-4.
76. Jenkins TR. Laparoscopic supracervical hysterectomy. Am J Obstet Gynecol. 2004;191(6):1875-84.
77. Berner E, Ovigstad E, Myrvold AK, et al. Pelvic Pain and patient satisfaction after laparoscopic supracervical hysterectomy: prospective trial. J Minim Invasive Gynecol. 2014;21(3):406-11.
78. Alkatout I, Mettler L, Betata C, et al. Combined surgical and hormone therapy for endometriosis is the most effective treatment: prospective, randomized, controlled trial. J Minim Invasive Gynecol. 2013;20(4):473-81.
79. Semm K. Hysterectomy via laparotomy or pelviscopy. A new CASH method without colpotomy. Geburtshilfe Frauenheilkd. 1991;51(12):996-1003.

KIEL SCHOOL

31 of Gynaecological Endoscopy

Laparoscopic Myoma Therapy

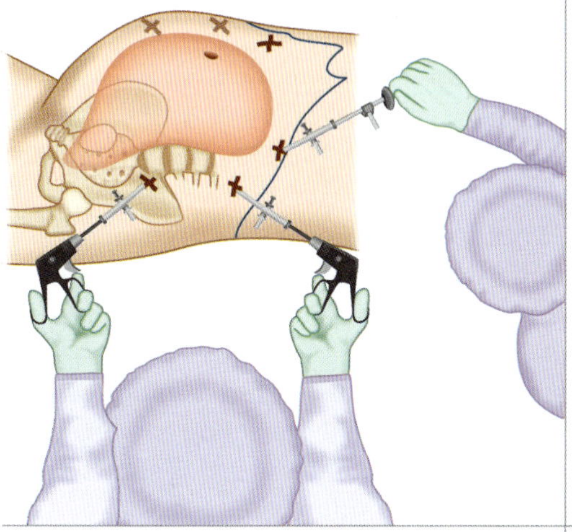

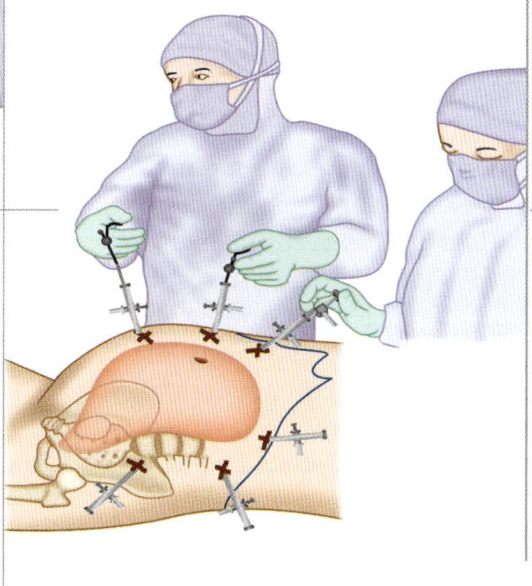

Chapter 31

Laparoscopic Myoma Therapy

Garri Tchartchian, Bernd Bojahr, Khulkar Abdusattarova, De Wilde RL

PLASTIC UTERUS RECONSTRUCTION AFTER LAPAROSCOPIC MYOMECTOMY

Plastic uterus reconstruction (PUR) after myomectomy is a specific and technically complex surgical procedure. PUR restores the uterus after myomectomy of multiple, large and deep intramural myomas. Plastic uterus reconstruction has its importance in patients with existing or potential wish for pregnancy.[1] Furthermore, PUR can be applied in patients who have completed family planning and who wish to preserve their uterus. The goal is to completely restore the anatomy and function of the uterus. As such, one has to make use of a variety of surgical and organ-sparing techniques.

The PUR procedure can be accomplished both by laparoscopic means as by laparotomy, yet, the route of access does not influence the PUR procedure.[2] Nevertheless, open myomectomy is associated with a higher risk for the formation of adhesions.[3] That is why laparoscopic myomectomy is preferred when one can choose a method, which can guarantee a similar efficiency.[4,5] Indeed, the suture technique is identical to ensure efficient successful sutures, the microsurgical treatment of the uterus and the double-layer sutures with the laparoscopic approach have to be performed as during an open microsurgical treatment.

Basic Rules of the PUR Technique

- To avoid postoperative complications, the uterine tissue has to be protected. As such, instruments should be used atraumatically to touch and manipulate the tissue.[6,7] This avoids defects, which could lead to formation of adhesions, pain, infections, and, in some cases, insufficient sutures.
- Bipolar surgical techniques should not be used automatically in the vicinity of the serosa.[8] In areas where such techniques are used, necrosis is a potential complication, which, in turn, can lead to the formation of adhesions and abovementioned complications.
- Myometrium should be spared as much as possible to ensure maximal protection and preservation of the native myometrial layers allows better wound healing and suture sufficiency.[9]
- After uterotomy, uterus should only be touched atraumatically from the inside of the myometrial area. Precautions should be taken to ensure maximum protection of the tunica serosa of the uterus.
- Careful punctual hemostasis should be achieved while minimizing thermal damage to the myometrium.
- Drying out of the tissue should be avoided; the wound surface should be continuously rinsed with Ringer's lactate solution, similar to a microsurgical operation procedure by laparotomy.[10]
- The closure should be performed in double layers using microsurgical procedures.[11] As such, the tunica muscular is closed with interrupted or continuous stitches using thickness 0–1. The closure of the tunica serosa is done subserosally with continuous stitches using threads with thickness 2/0–4/0.
- When necessary, adhesion prophylactic agents can be used in the area of uterorrhaphy.
- Diligent hemostasis should be performed and the abdominal cavity flushed to remove any blood remnants. Bleeding in the area of uterorrhaphy should have stopped completely.
- A Douglas drainage can be placed for 24 h; this monitors postoperative bleeding.

PUR Surgical Procedure

- *Trocar placement (Fig. 31.1):* For myomas up to a size of 7 cm, umbilicus is used as an access for the optical trocar. For larger and multiple myomas, an epigastric placement can be selected to provide a better overview and more manipulation space. The PUR technique requires three trocars: one trocar in both the left and right lower abdomen and one trocar in the middle. The size of the myomas determines the position of the trocars: the larger the fibroids, the more cranially the trocars are inserted.
- *Distribution of instruments:* Usually, the myoma drilling device is introduced via the left trocar. The forceps are inserted via the right trocar. The bipolar forceps to control blood supply and introduce preparation instruments (e.g., jet grasper, which aquadissects myomas) is inserted through the middle trocar.

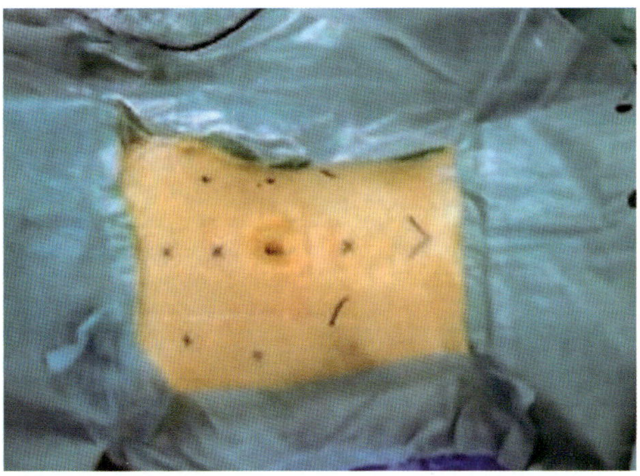

Fig. 31.1: Trocar placement. Plastic uterus reconstruction technique makes use of three trocars: the optical trocar is inserted though the umbilicus or epigastric area and two working trocars are introduced in the left and right lower abdomen.

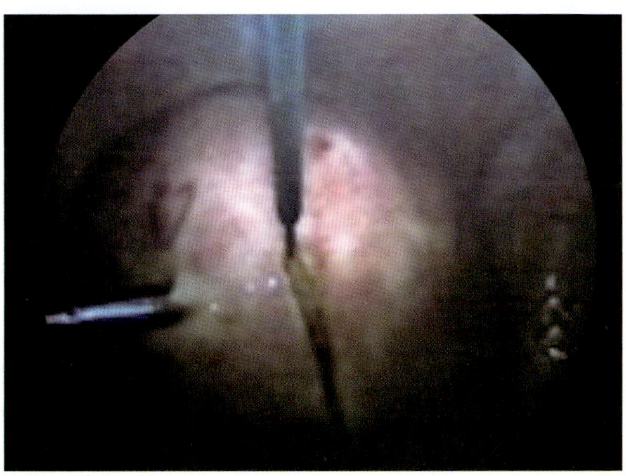

Fig. 31.2: Uterotomy with monopolar needle.

- *Hemostasis:* To minimize the chance of bleeding, Vasopressin is diluted with saline (10 units of Vasopressin (20 IU), diluted in 100 mL of saline) or an adrenaline solution is used.
- Uterotomy (Fig. 31.2)
- *Exposure of the uterine wall:* The myoma is fixed using the myoma drill (Figs. 31.3A to C).

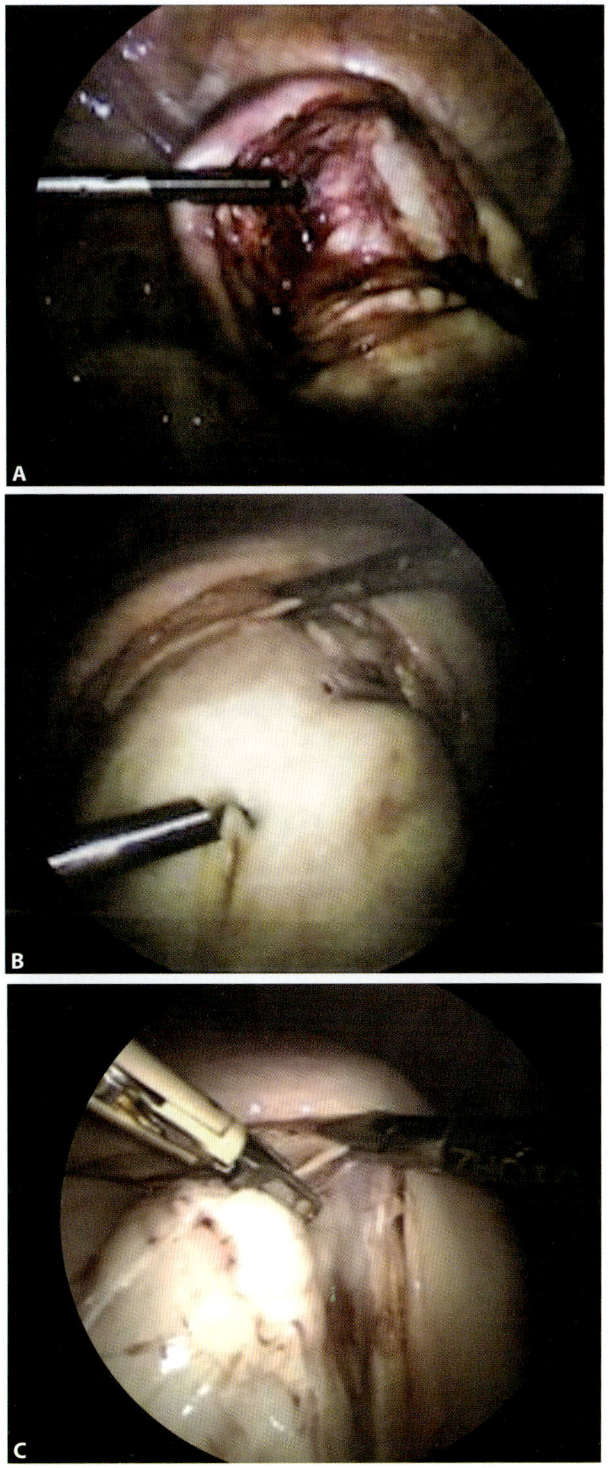

Figs. 31.3A to C: Myoma fixation with myoma drill.

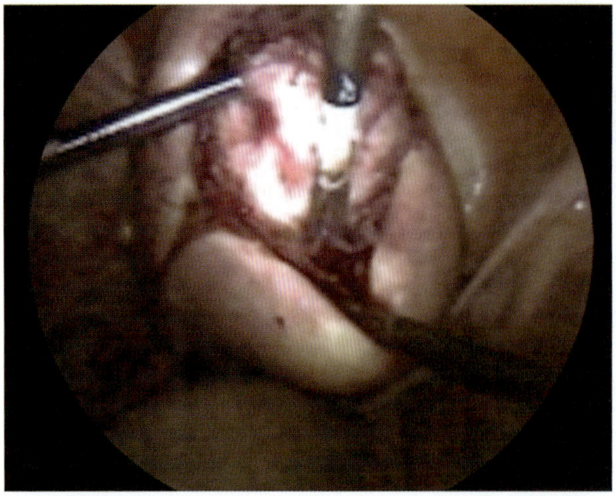

Fig. 31.4: Exposure of uterine wall.

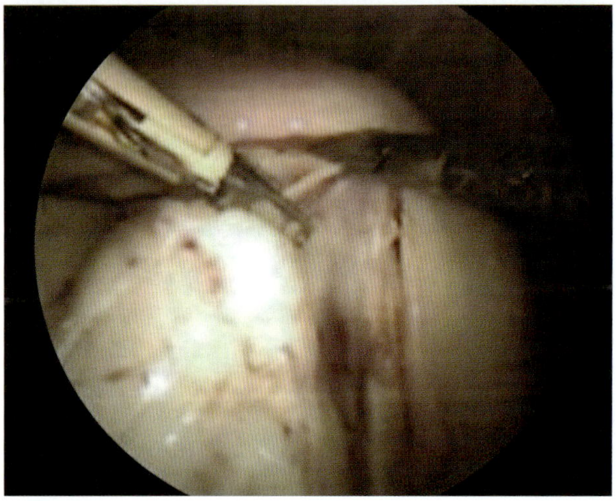

Fig. 31.5: Bipolar forceps for punctual homeostasis and control of bleeding.

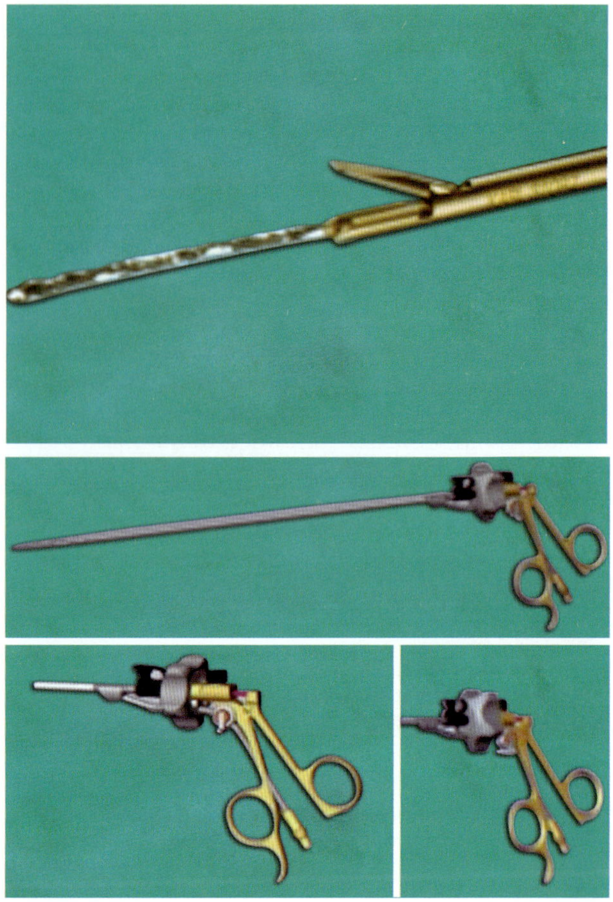

Fig. 31.6: Jet grasper.

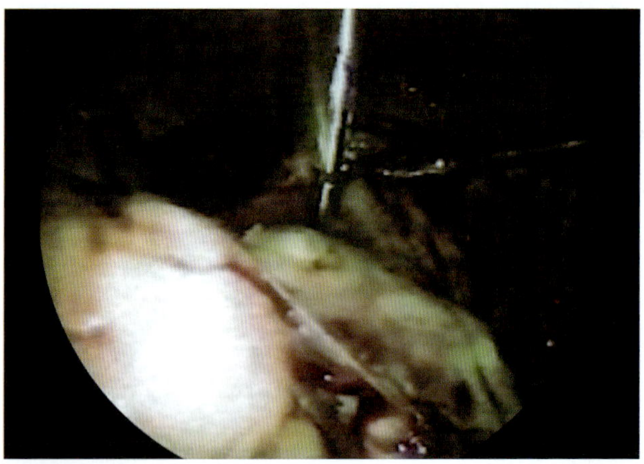

Fig. 31.7: Myomectomy using jet grasper.

The uterine wall is grasped and exposed from the inside of the myometrium using the forceps which is introduced via the right trocar (Fig. 31.4).

The bipolar forceps for punctual hemostasis (Fig. 31.5) and eventually the jet grasper, are inserted alternately through the middle trocar.

The jet grasper was developed specifically to dissect the plane between myoma and myometrium by means of aquadissection. It allows exposure by using the mechanical forceps of the jet grasper with simultaneous aquadissection. As such, myometrium and uterine cavity are maximally protected (Fig. 31.6).

- *Exposure of the contralateral uterine wall:* After complete exposure of the whole uterine wall, the instruments in left and right trocars are interchanged, and when necessary the left uterine wall is operated in a mirror-like manner.

  The bipolar coagulation and aquadissection remain in the middle trocar.
- *Myomectomy:* Subsequently, the myomectomy is performed while protecting the myometrium and the cavum uteri, using jet grasper when necessary (Fig. 31.7).

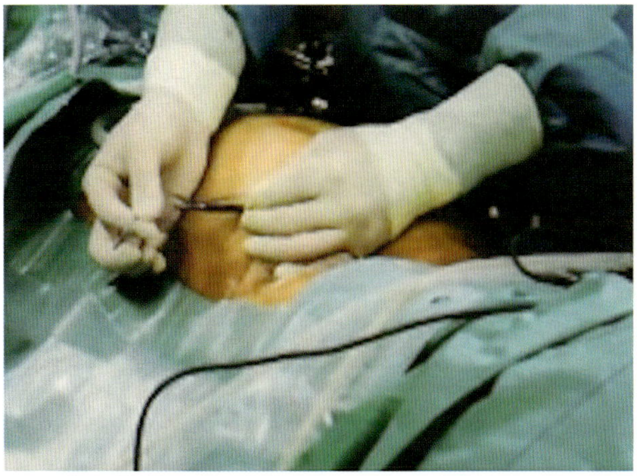

Fig. 31.8: Pointed forceps is introduced thought the right working trocar.

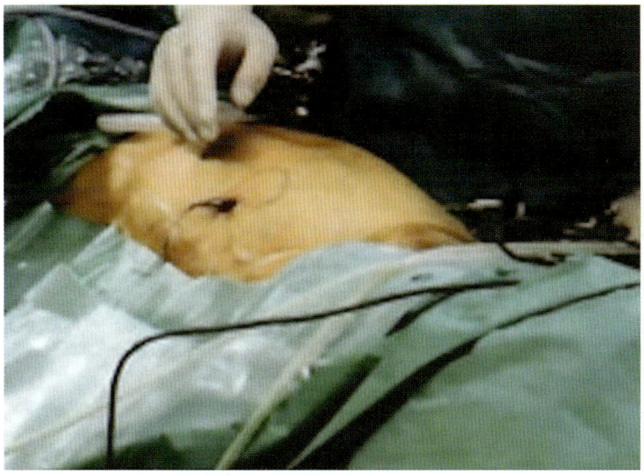

Fig. 31.9: Insertion of the needle and thread.

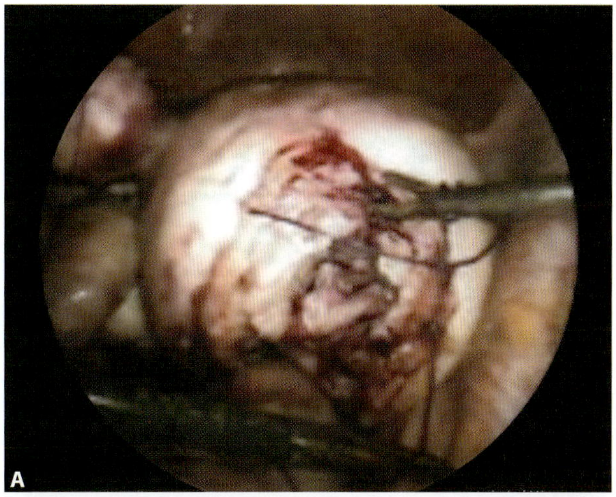

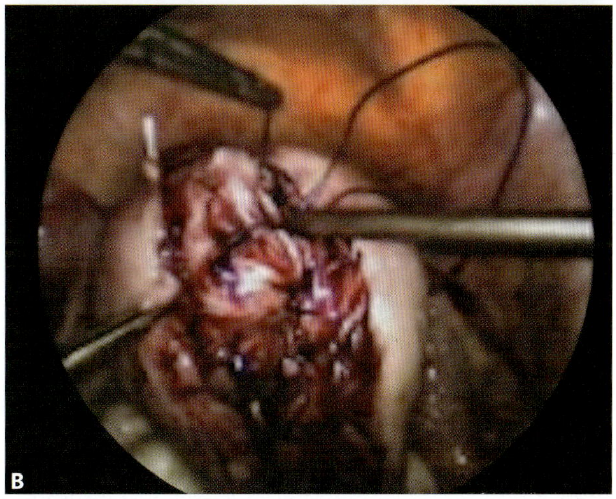

Figs. 31.10A and B: Closure of the first layer of the myometrium with simple interrupted stiches avoiding the serosa.

- *Inserting suture equipment:* First, the pointed forceps is guided through the right trocar into the abdominal cavity (Fig. 31.8).

  Then a thread with thickness 0-1 and length of 20–25 cm is grasped in the middle and pulled into the abdominal cavity with one single movement without the left trocar tube. The needle follows the thread and because of the round shape of the needle, it is efficiently and safely inserted into the abdominal cavity (Fig. 31.9).
- *Double-layered sutures:* The first layer of myometrium is closed with simple interrupted or continuous stitches without piercing the uterine cavity. The needle is avoiding the serosal layer (Figs. 31.10A and B).

  The serosal suture is performed continuously with a thread strength of 2/0 (Figs. 31.11A to D).
- *Lavage:* Next, an extensive lavage of the abdomen is performed as an additional measure to avoid adhesion formation in the area of uterotomy.
- *Douglas drainage:* A Douglas drainage is placed during 24 h to monitor postoperative bleeding.

Postoperative Management

Patients who underwent a laparoscopic myomectomy using PUR technique should be observed postoperatively for at least 24–48 h. Circulatory and inflammatory parameters as well as postsurgical bleeding signs are checked to early detect potential complications such as formation of hematoma, inflammation or postoperative bleeding. An insufficiency in suturing the myometrium leads to a risk of uterine rupture during pregnancy and childbirth.[12] On the first and second or third postoperative day, checkup and control of laboratory parameters seem obligatory. After an open myomectomy using PUR technique, patients are discharged later.

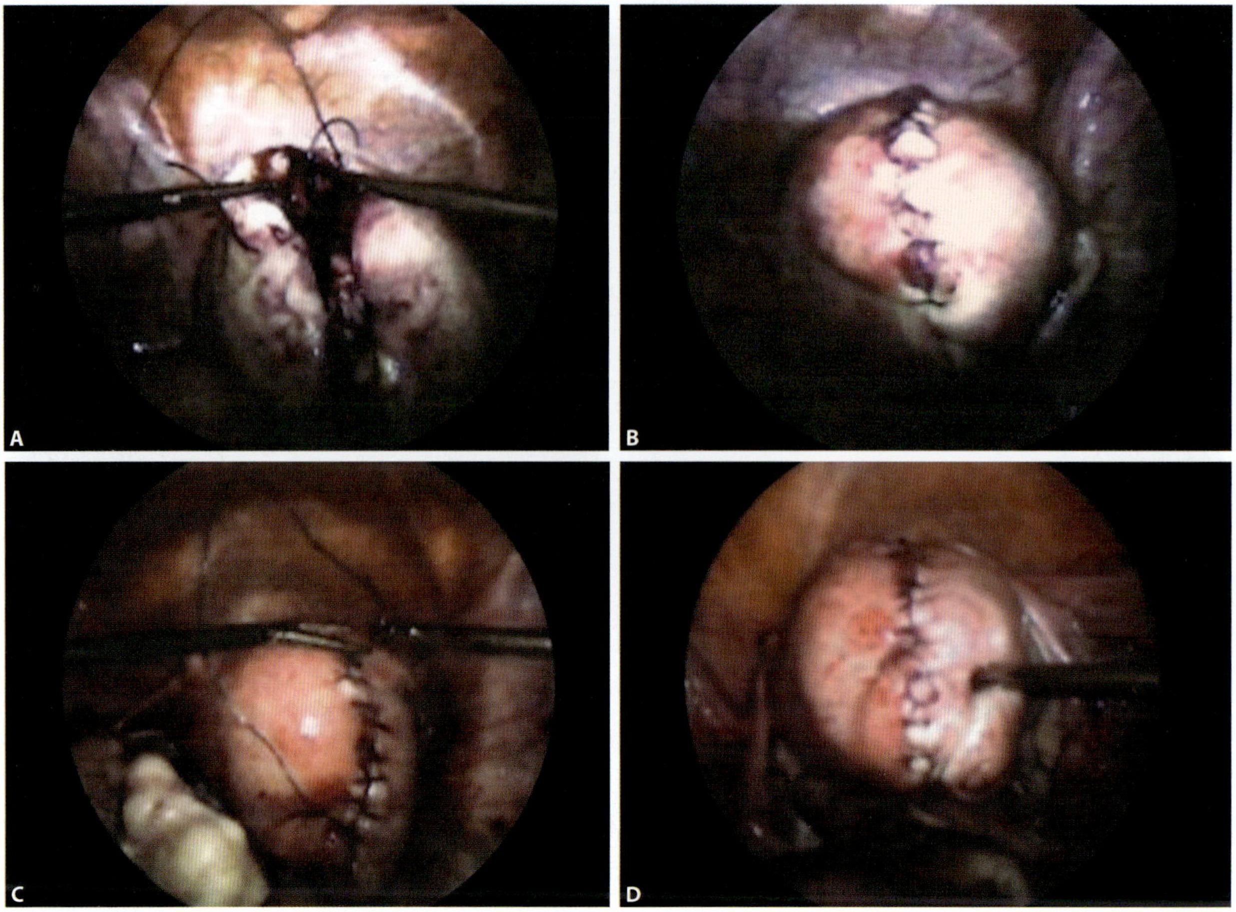

Figs. 31.11A to D: Closure of serosal mucosa with continuous suturing.

The patient should be informed about the side effects and consequences of surgery preoperatively and again postoperatively. An explanation should be given about the prevalence of uterine rupture during pregnancy as well as intrapartially. Depending on the number, size and position of the myomas, a planned caesarean section might be recommended as birth modus.

LAPAROSCOPY-ASSISTED COMBINED HYSTERECTOMY (LACH) FOR LARGE UTERI WITH CHANGEOVER TECHNIQUE

In the last decades, there is an apparent shift in favor of laparoscopic hysterectomy techniques because of advantages such as shorter convalescence, minor trauma and less pain. When a complete hysterectomy is indicated in difficult cases such as in case of a very large uterus and/or nulliparity per vaginam, an abdominal hysterectomy (AH) usually is applied.[13] Indeed, the preconditions for laparoscopy-assisted vaginal hysterectomy (LAVH) are sufficient space for vaginal manipulation and an ideal uterus size with an estimated weight of up to 400 g.[14] Furthermore, a total laparoscopic hysterectomy (TLH) should be avoided as well, since it could have higher complication rate.[15] To solve this, we developed a special surgical technique for the laparoscopic removal of a very large uterus: the laparoscopic combined hysterectomy (LACH) with "changeover-technique." For laparoscopic abscission and morcellation of uterine corpus, the LACH method uses the "changeover-technique," which means that the position of team changes from the left side of the patient to the right side. Once the laparoscopic phase of the surgery is completed, the uterine cervix is removed per vaginam, which adds an additional time of up to 10 min the surgery. This technique allows to combine the advantages of both the vaginal hysterectomy (VH) and the laparoscopic supracervical hysterectomy (LASH) in terms of their complication rate.[16] The "changeover-technique" can also be used in LASH given a difficult-case-uterus (*see* next chapter).

The LACH Surgical Procedure

After urinary bladder catheterism and vaginal disinfection, the patient is placed in the Trendelenburg position. The surgeon and assistant start the operation on the left side of the uterus. A Veress needle is used to ensure an intra-abdominal pressure of 15 mm Hg in the peritoneum. In LACH with "changeover technique," it is preferred to introduce the optical trocar through the Palmer's point. Two 5 mm working trocars are placed on the left axillary line of the abdomen 8–10 cm from each other with the lower trocar at about the height of the uterotubal junction (Figs. 31.12A to D). The placement of three trocars on the left side of the patient allows for a better visualization of the area of the left parametria, left adnexa and left round ligament. In this type of procedure, we mainly use these four instruments: seizing forceps, bipolar coagulator, Metzenbaum scissors and a palpation probe. The seizing forceps enters through the upper working trocar and is used to control the position of the uterus, manipulate the sealing and abscising of the adnexa and mobilize the uterus (by fixating the round ligament at its proximal end). The round ligament, fallopian tube and ovary ligament are coagulated with bipolar current and then transected.

Next, the left half of the plica vesicouterina is lanced and the urinary bladder is prepared toward caudally. To avoid injuries to ureter and urinary bladder, it is recommended to visualize the ureter before parametrization. After parameterization, the uterine vessels are coagulated with bipolar current on the left side and then dissected using the scissors. Using bipolar, as opposed to monopolar current and scissors for abscission, allows for better control and thus higher safety. When the left side is finished, a second optical trocar is placed symmetrically to the Palmer's point under the right costal arch with laparoscopic observation. Then, the surgical team changes position to the right of the patient for the second phase of the "changeover technique." Again, two working trocars are placed, this time along the

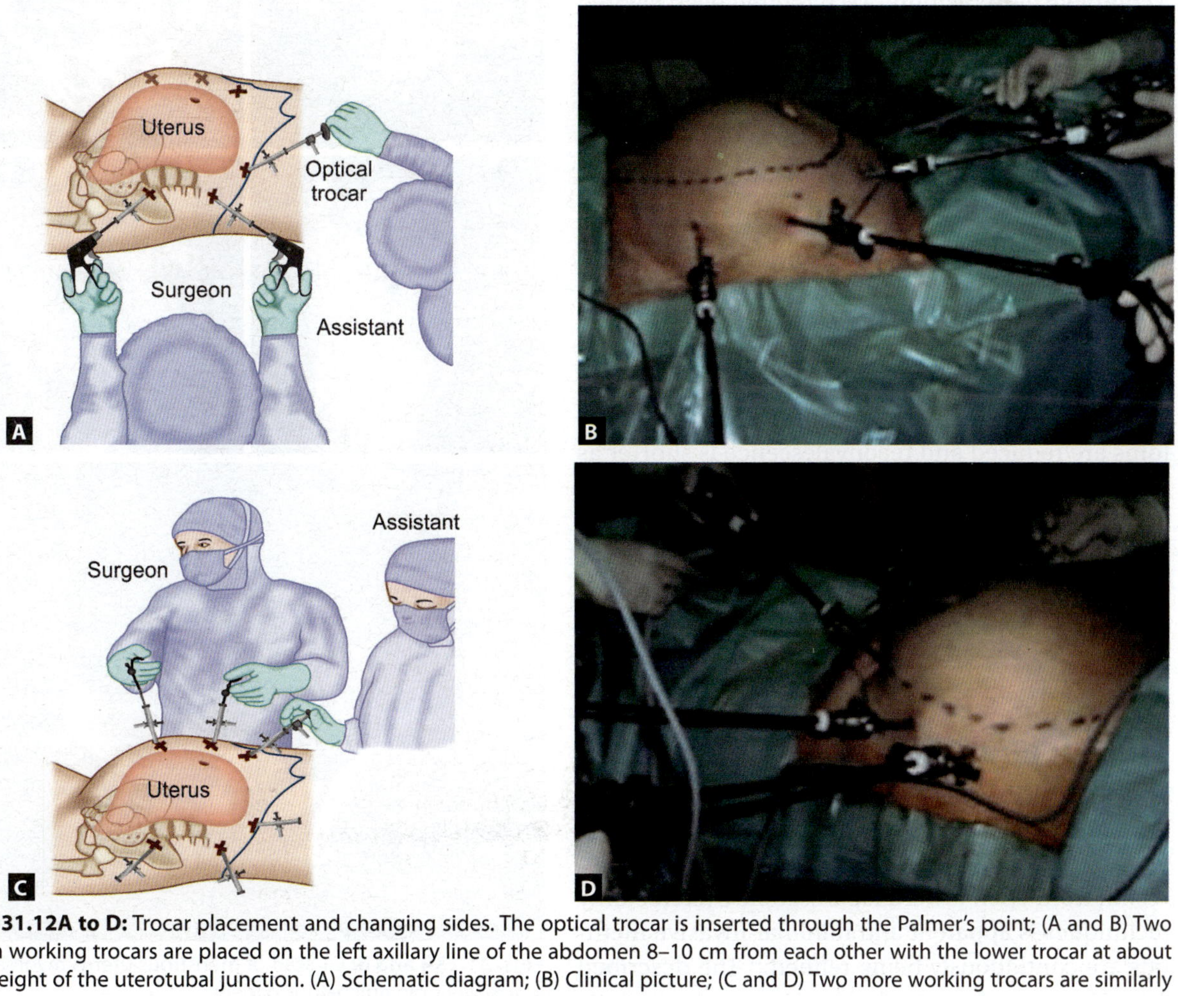

Figs. 31.12A to D: Trocar placement and changing sides. The optical trocar is inserted through the Palmer's point; (A and B) Two 5 mm working trocars are placed on the left axillary line of the abdomen 8–10 cm from each other with the lower trocar at about the height of the uterotubal junction. (A) Schematic diagram; (B) Clinical picture; (C and D) Two more working trocars are similarly placed on the right axillary line. (C) Schematic diagram; (D) Clinical picture.

right axillary (Figs. 31.12A to D), and the same surgical steps are now performed on the right side. During LASH, the endocervical canal is coagulated and the uterine cervix can be peritonealized after abscission of the uterine corpus. In LACH however, we remove the uterine cervix per vaginam later. Afterward, the left incision is prolonged to 15 mm and the uterine corpus is morcellated and removed from the abdominal cavity. Next, the patient is repositioned for the vaginal phase of surgery. The uterine cervix is trimmed circularly. The urinary bladder is pushed cranially and the rectouterine excavation is lanced. After abscission of the sacrouterine ligaments, parametria and uterine vessels. The clamps are replaced by ligatures and a circular peritonealization under extraperitonealization of the adnexal stumps is performed. Finally, the vaginal stump is closed through simple interrupted stitches.

Conclusion

When patients with large uteri or nulliparity require a complete hysterectomy, AH has often been favored as an alternative to LAVH since TLH is known for urological higher complication risks.[17] Yet, abdominal hysterectomy still has a higher complication rate than VH or LSH.[18] The combination of VH and LASH, the two safest surgical techniques regarding complication rates, presents a safe and low-risk alternative to TLH and AH. Indeed, in our prospective study comparing LACH with LAVH in 101 cases, we noted a very low complication rate (in less than 0.4% of subjects). With no conversion to laparotomy, no blood transfusion nor reoperations. Furthermore, because of minimal-invasive approach, pain symptoms are reduced and reconvalescence is shorter as compared to AH.

We can conclude that LACH using the "changeover technique" is a safe and low-risk surgical technique performing a total hysterectomy in large uterine myomata.[19]

LAPAROSCOPY-ASSISTED SUPRACERVICAL HYSTERECTOMY (LASH) WITH CHANGEOVER TECHNIQUE

A shift from open toward laparoscopic hysterectomy techniques is apparent and minimal-invasive methods are continuously being refined.[11] The described "changeover-technique" is an operation technique, which is applicable in all cases where large clusters of growth are found. Here, we present an exemplary case where the "changeover technique" is used for the LASH treatment of a uterus, which reached beyond the umbilicum and up to the costal arch.

Case Presentation

A 47-year-old nulliparous patient with a monstrous uterus myomatosus. Anamnesis revealed that its existence was known for 12 years and kept growing since. Because of fearing laparotomy, the patient had declined surgical therapy. We suggested LASH, informed about the risks, side effects and alternatives and after the patient's consent, we planned the surgery. Before surgery, we performed imaging diagnostics by means of computed tomography (CT) of the abdomen (Figs. 31.13A and B).

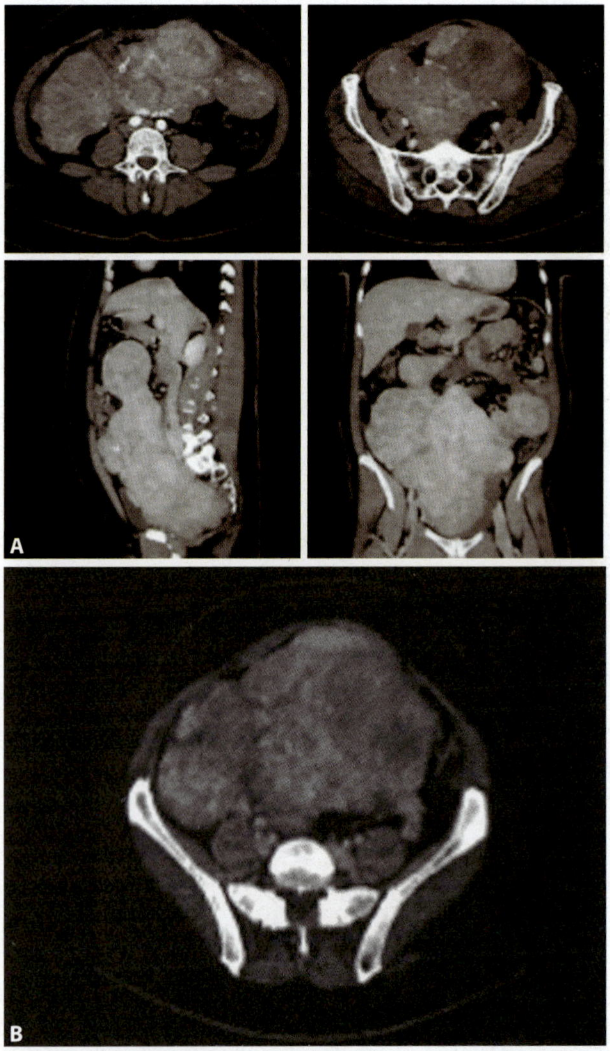

Figs. 31.13A and B: CT scan of monstrous uterus myomatosus of a 47-year-old nulliparous patient.

Surgical Procedure of LASH with "Changeover Technique"

Based on the estimation of an operating time of approximately 3 h, the patient was placed in a flat supine position. Furthermore, prophylactic measures to avoid a compartment syndrome were carried out intraoperatively. Furthermore, prophylactic measures to avoid a compartment syndrome were carried out intraoperatively; flat positioning of legs, periodic leg movements, regular change of position and mechanical activation of circulation.

Following the "changeover technique," we inserted six trocars. On the left side, those included one trocar in left lower abdomen, one in middle abdomen and one in upper abdominal (Fig. 31.14).

The three trocars on the right were placed in a mirror-like fashion. The trocar in the left upper abdominal, in the area of the costal arch, was used for the introduction of camera (Fig. 31.15).

Parameterization was started on the left side. After abscission of adnexa and parametria, plica vesicouterina was exposed. After uterine bladder was pushed caudally, the surgeon and his team switched their position from the left to the right side of the patient. Two working trocars were already placed on the right side previously (lower and middle right abdomen) while the optical trocar was introduced via the right upper abdomen. The surgery proceeded analogically as on the left side. Indeed, as was seen on the CT scan (Figs. 31.13A and B), there were multinodal, intraligamentary and parametric myoma on the right side of the patient. Accordingly, further exposure and protection of the ureter was performed by visualization and preparation as well as abscission of the right adnexa, parametria and blood vessels (Figs. 31.16A to C).

Next, the corpus uteri was abscised and the cervix peritonealized with a purse-string suture (Figs. 31.17A and B).

After morcellation, corpus uteri was removed from the abdominal cavity by power morcellation (Fig. 31.18).

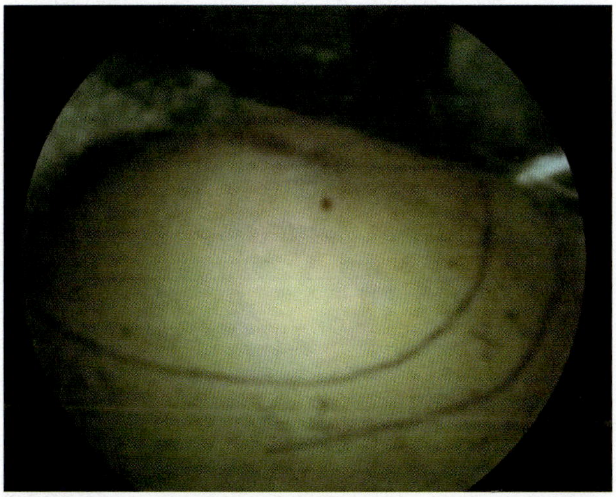

Fig. 31.14: Positions of the three trocars on the left side of the patient.

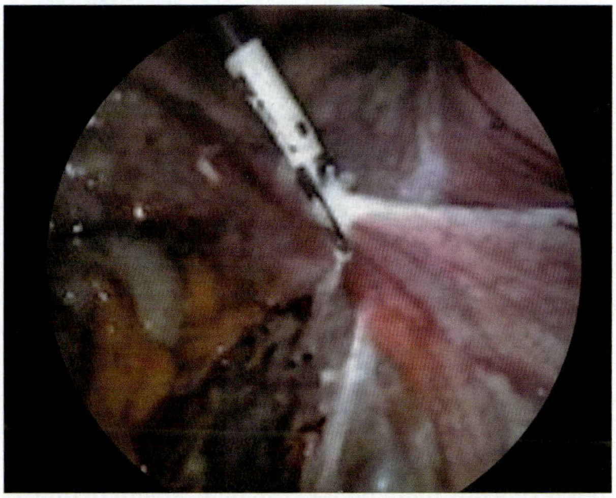

Fig. 31.15: The trocar in the upper abdomen was used to introduce the camera.

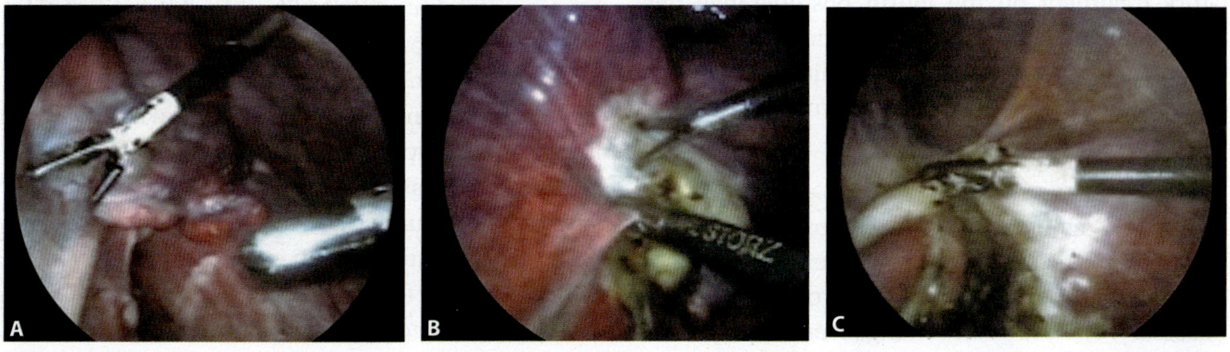

Figs. 31.16A to C: From the right side of the patient, exposure of the uterus was performed as well as abscission of the right adnexa and blood vessels.

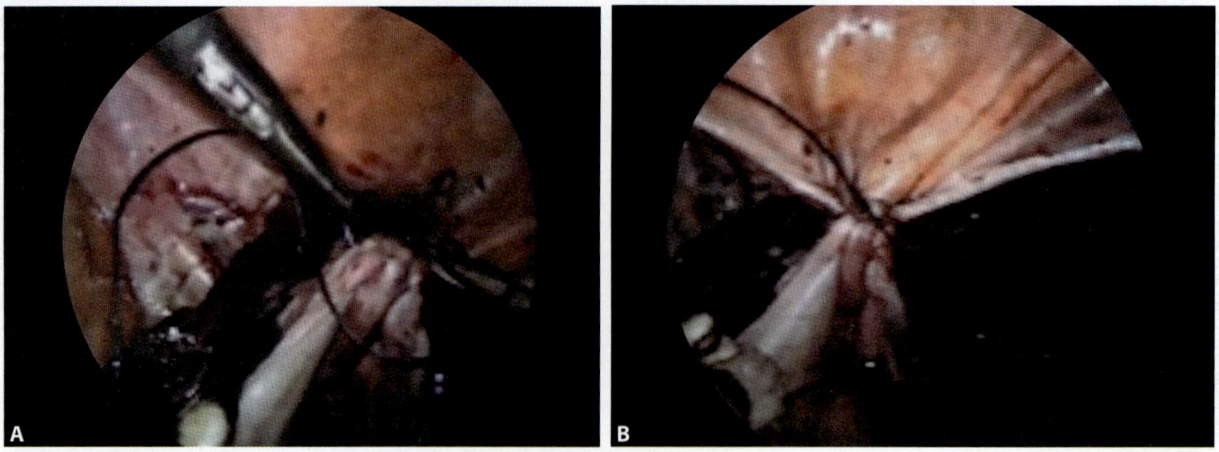

Figs. 31.17A and B: Peritonealization of the cervix with a purse-string suture.

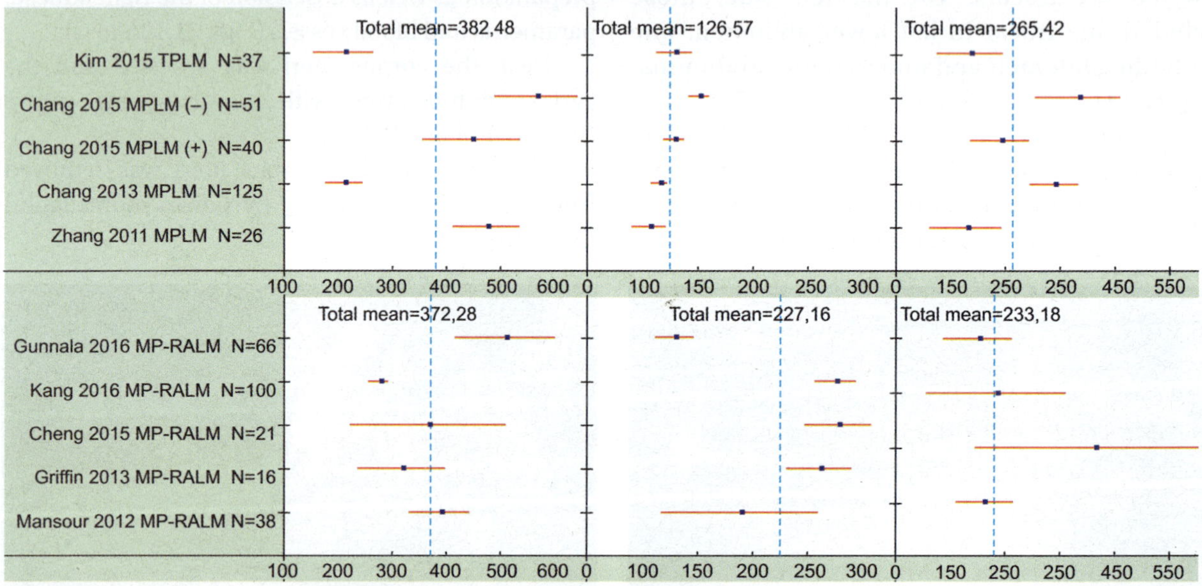

Fig. 31.18: Laparoscopic and robotic myomectomies for large uterine myoma (mean and 95% CI) by different studies.

Postoperative Considerations

Histological analysis of the removed specimen did not reveal any malignancy. The total weight of uterus was 4065 g. No postoperative complications arose and the patient was able to be released into ambulatory treatment on the fourth postoperative day. Postoperative imaging diagnostics did not reveal any conspicuous intra-abdominal findings. Moreover, urinary tract and bladder were shown to be intact.

Conclusion

At our MIC clinic in Berlin, we regularly apply the "changeover technique" for the removal of large uteri. So far, no conversion to laparotomy has been necessary. The use of the "changeover technique" for total or subtotal hysterectomy is useful and advisable when a high uterine weight is expected.

DISCUSSION

Laparoscopic Myomectomy along with Advanced Technologies

The issue of preservation of reproductive function in women with uterine fibroids deserves special attention, due to an increase in the number of middle-aged women who are still planning first or subsequent pregnancies, the topic is growing in social importance. Laparoscopic myomectomy (LM) is acknowledged as gold standard uterus-preserving surgical procedure and has provided an efficacious outcome for patients with regard to the low morbidity and short-hospital stay.[11] However, the use of a laparoscopic approach to treat large intramural myomas is technically demanding and time-consuming procedures, which is required highly qualified surgical skills. Problematic aspects of LM to treat large intramural myomas include the difficulties of cleavage, performing a strong and layered closure for the uterine incision and the tissue extraction. Furthermore, the evaluation of perioperative risk factors of LM revealed that the combination of enlarged uterine volume of ≥750 cm³, dominant myoma diameter of ≥12 cm and also a duration of the surgery can be independent predictors of complications.[20,21] In recent years, robotic assisted laparoscopic myomectomy (RALM) has gained to treat the large intramural myomas; however, perioperative and long-term results of this mode remain under debate.[22]

Our review focused on the comparison of LM with RALM in cases of the large intramural myomas with a mean diameter of more than 7.5 cm.[22-30] The total number of myomectomies was 520, out of which 279 cases were performed by conventional laparoscopic approach and 241 cases by laparoscopically assisted robotic technique (Fig. 31.18). The total mean weight of the retrieved myomas in the LM was 382.48 ± 267.17 g, compared to 372.28 ± 368.86 g in the RALM group. The mean operative time was significantly longer with RALM; 227.16 ± 103.80 min, compared to LM with mean operative time of 126.57 ± 42.36 min. Moreover, the total mean estimated blood loss was slightly lower in the RALM in comparison with LM, 233.18 ± 276.28 mL and 265.42 ± 244.16 mL, respectively. The intraoperative complication rate in conventional LM and RALM was approximately the same at 6.4% and 6.3%, respectively. In addition, the conversion rate in the RALM was slightly higher than in LM (0.82% and 0.71%). The postoperative operative complication rate in LM was 2.8% and RALM was 2.9%. Thus, the review of 520 cases reveal that conventional LM and RALM are feasible and safe to treat the large intramural myomas; perioperative and postoperative complication rates were approximately similar, but the conversion rate was slightly higher in RALM. Nevertheless, there is concern regarding the significantly prolonged duration of surgery in RALM procedures. There were no cases of undiagnosed uterine malignancies.

In addition, adhesions are common sequels of myomectomy, which can be reason of long-term complications such as abdominal or pelvic pain, subfertility and intestinal obstruction and it can lead to technical difficulties during the assisted-reproduction procedures.[31] To date, several modifications in surgical techniques and various pharmacological and nonpharmacological modalities have been introduced to prevent adhesions formation. A new dissection tool, the "jet grasper" (KARL STORZ®) was utilized in our experience to reduce surgical trauma during tissue dissection, as well as preserving vascular integrity by decreasing the use of electrocoagulation during laparoscopic procedures. The hydrodissection of tissues can reduce the risk of perioperative bleeding and long-term postoperative adhesion formation. Furthermore, we conducted a randomized clinical study to test a new developed bioabsorbable anti-adhesion agent Actamax™. The results of this study reveal that the hydrogel was effective in reducing adhesions, particularly following myomectomy.[32]

In conclusion, laparoscopic myomectomy with plastic uterus reconstruction is a safe and reliable procedure even in the presence of large intramural myomas. Moreover, the introduction of new advanced technologies, such as jet grasper and training and acquiring surgical skills may decrease complications associated with laparoscopic myomectomy. In addition, antiadhesion agents can decrease the risk of postoperative adhesion formation following myomectomy. Also, the RALM could be considered as alternative to LM, yet with longer duration of operation time.

Minimal-invasive Hysterectomy for Large and Extremely Large Uterine Myoma[1]

Hysterectomy remains the definitive treatment mode of uterine myomas due to complete elimination of symptom recurrence. When hysterectomy procedures performed using minimal-invasive laparoscopic approaches are compared to laparotomy procedures, the patient's risk of morbidity and mortality is decreased.[33] To date, there are various types of laparoscopic hysterectomy techniques to treat the large uterus myomatosus. However, the technical challenges exist in each of those methods, which can be explained by limited access to uterine vessels, risk of complications due to poor exposure, difficulty in extracting the uterus and the duration of the procedure.

In this review, the total number of women who underwent minimally invasive hysterectomies for large uterine myomata was 1,600; majority of patients (1,303 or 81.43%) had a mean uterus weight between 500 and 1,000 g, while 279 patients (17.43%) had a mean uterus weight between 1,000 and 5,500 g.[34-48] Of those 1,303 cases, 568 were laparoscopic subtotal

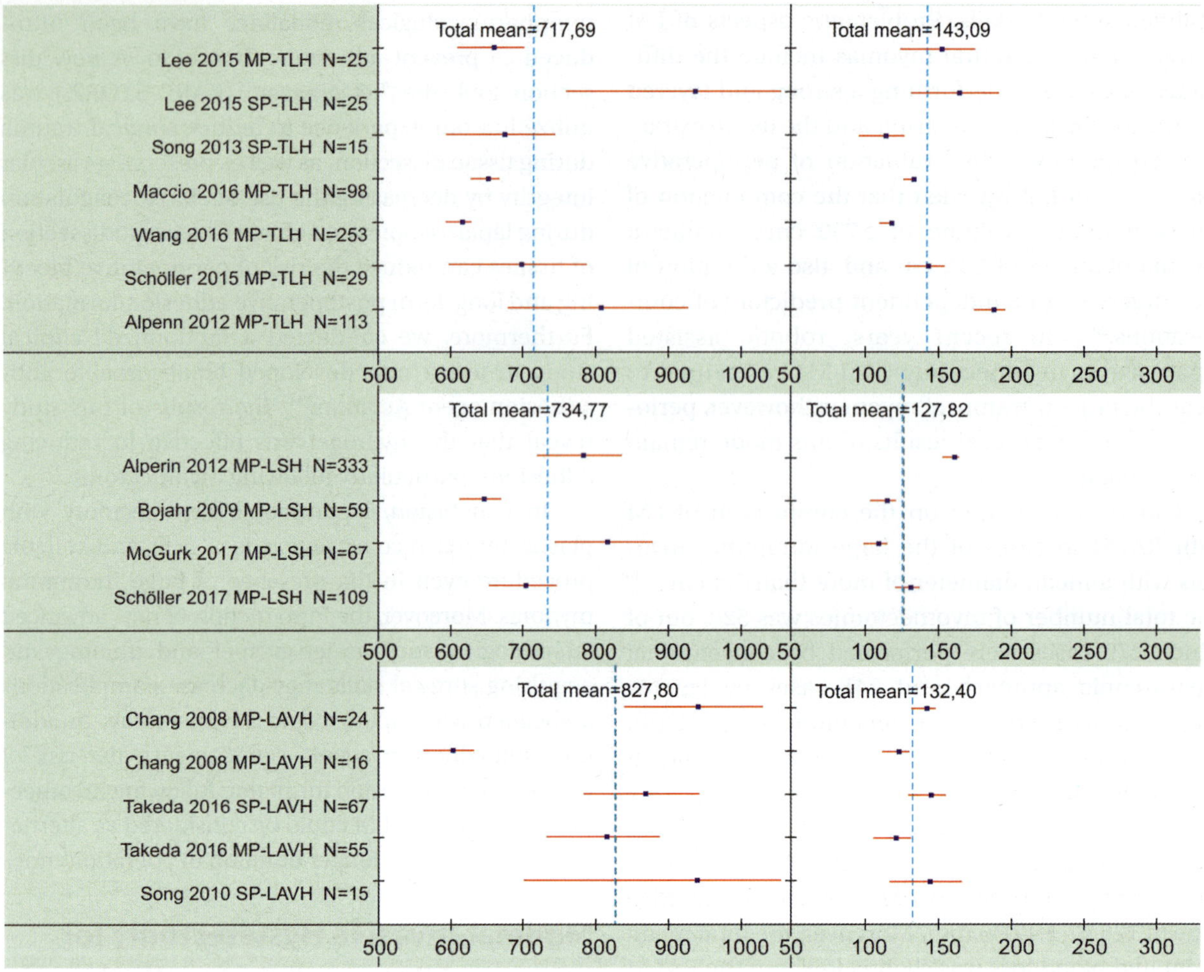

Fig. 31.19: Duration of surgeries and weights of large uterine myomata (mean and 95% CI) in laparoscopic hysterectomies by different studies.

hysterectomies (LSH), 558 were laparoscopic total hysterectomies (TLH) and 177 were laparoscopy-assisted vaginal hysterectomies (LAVH) (Fig. 31.19). The total average uterine weight for LAVH technique was higher (827.00 ± 269.72 g) as compared to cases treated with TLH and LSH (717.69 ± 345.93 g and 734.77 ± 443.75 g, respectively). The operation time was shortest in LSH (127.82 ± 52.53 min) while longer operation times were needed with TLH (143.09 ± 58.27 min) and LAVH (132.40 ± 53.80 min). The rate of conversion to laparotomy due to the high uterine weight and technical challenges was significantly lower in the LAVH group (2.3%) as compared to TLH (5.7%) and LSH (4.5%). Also, Schöller et al. (2017) recently reported a high rate of intraoperative conversion to laparotomy in both LSH (16.5%) and TLH (41.4%) procedures.

The total complication rate in LSH was 4.6%, while it was 6.1% in TLH. More specifically, the intraoperative complication rate in TLH was 2.9%, of which 1.4% required blood transfusion due to bleeding, 0.35% were intestinal contusion, 0.17% bladder injury, 0.35% vascular injuries and 0.53% subcutaneous emphysema. The postoperative complication rate in TLH was 3.2%, 1.25% vaginal stump infections, 0.34% urine retention, 0.53% ileus, 0.17 % umbilical hernia, 0.17% pelvic hematoma, 0.17% vaginal cuff dehiscence, 0.34% pelvic infection, 0.17% pulmonary edema and 0.17% lower limb venous thrombosis. Of 4.6% complications with LSH, 2.4% were intraoperative; 1.8% hemorrhage requiring blood transfusion and 0.42% visceral injuries. The postoperative complication rate in LSH was 2.2%, of which 0.89% were uterine retention, 0.18% incarcerated hernia, 0.18% ileus and 0.89% wound infection. Even though the overall complication rate in LAVH was 7.7%, which is higher than in TLH and LSH groups; it can be accounted for the low number of patients in this group. In the LAVH group, intraoperative complications occurred in 1.3% of cases; 0.74% were associated

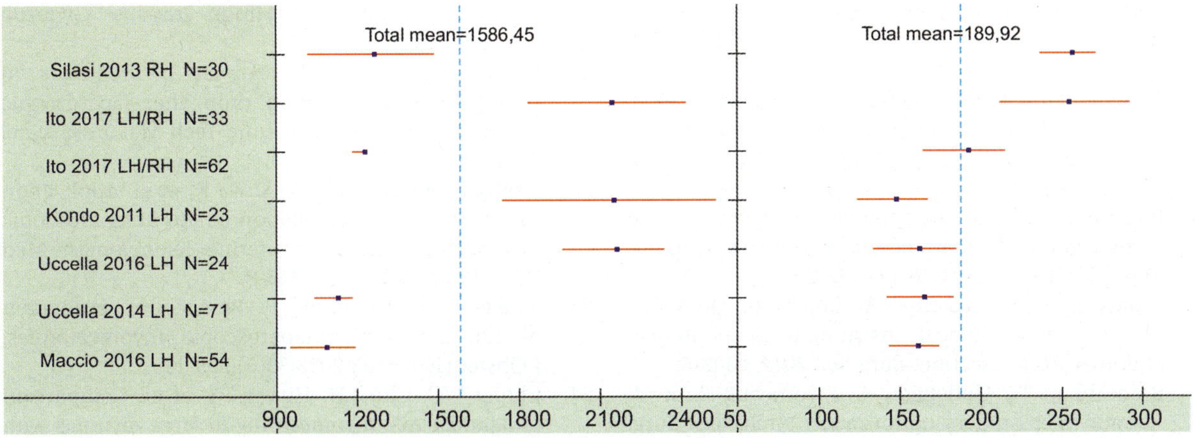

Fig. 31.20: Duration of the surgeries and weights of extremely large uterine myomata (mean and 95% CI) in laparoscopic and robotic-assisted hysterectomies by different studies.

with hemorrhage and 0.56% with bladder injury. The postoperative complication rate observed in LAVH was 6.4%, 2.46% vaginal bleeding, 2.25% ileus and 1.69% pelvic abscess. Furthermore, minimally invasive approaches were applied for the hysterectomy of an extremely large uterus in 279 patients (Fig. 31.20). A majority of cases were total hysterectomies, which were performed either by laparoscopic (229 cases) or robotic assistance techniques (42 cases). The mean uterus weight was 1568.45 ± 675.33 g. The mean duration of the surgery was 189.92 ± 83.25 min; however, in robotic hysterectomies the duration of surgery was significantly prolonged. The intraoperative complication rate was 3.74%, of which 2.02% were hemorrhage requiring blood transfusion and 1.72% bowel lesions. The rate of postoperative complications was 6.2%; the majority of cases were blood transfusion (3.53%), followed by lower urinary tract infections (0.67%), vaginal vault hematoma (0.67%), surgical site infection (0.67%), urinary retention (0.33%) and vaginal bleeding (0.33%). The total referred conversion rate to laparatomy was 5.9%. Thus, in laparoscopic hysterectomies for large uteri, the rate of conversion to open surgery is high due to its technically challenges such as limited operative field, restrictive instrument range of motion and limited access to uterine vascular pedicles. To overcome these limitations, laparoscopic hysterectomies of large uteri should be modified.

Therefore, the newly developed laparoscopic combined hysterectomy (LACH) technique is an option. LACH integrates the advantages of two surgical approaches: LSH with low risk of urological and vascular injuries, shorter duration of the surgery and also using the natural orifice of a vaginal route of VH. Comparative analysis of 101 cases of LACH and LAVH with a mean uterus weight of 738.61 g reveals that there were no significant differences in intraoperative and postoperative outcomes, and the duration of the surgery was significantly shorter in LACH. Moreover, no operation was converted to laparotomy and no urinary tract injuries or severe perioperative complications occurred.

CONCLUSION

Our results show that, in experienced hands, LACH can be considered as a safe and feasible procedure to treat large uterus myomata with significant advantages over the AH and TLH, when LAVH is contraindicated. Moreover, LACH can minimize the risk of conversion, perioperative and postoperative complications associated with technical challenges during laparoscopic hysterectomies in cases of large uterine myomata.

REFERENCES

1. Hirschelmann A, De Wilde RL. Plastic and reconstructive uterus operations by minimally invasive surgery? A review on myomectomy. GMS Interdiscip Plast Reconstr Surg DGPW. 2012;1:Doc09.
2. Hackethal A, Westermann A, Tchartchian G, et al. Laparoscopic myomectomy in patients with uterine myomas associated with infertility. Minim Invasive Ther Allied Technol. 2011;20(6):338-45.
3. De Wilde RL, Bakkum EA, Brolmann H, et al. Consensus recommendations on adhesions (version 2014) for the ESGE Adhesions Research Working Group (European Society for Gynecological Endoscopy): an expert opinion. Arch Gynecol Obstet. 2014; 290(3):581-2.
4. Tchartchian G, Hackethal A, Herrmann A, et al. Evaluation of Spray Shield Adhesion Barrier in a single center: randomized controlled study in 15 women

undergoing reconstructive surgery after laparoscopic myomectomy. Arch Gynecol Obstet. 2014;290(4): 697-704.

5. Hirschelmann A, Tchartchian G, Wallwiener M, et al. A review of the problematic adhesion prophylaxis in gynaecological surgery. Arch Gynecol Obstet. 2012;285(4):1089-97.
6. Rakotomahenina H, Rajaonarison J, Wong L, et al. Myomectomy: technique and current indications. Minerva Gynecol. 2017;69(4):357-69.
7. Tchartchian G, Hackethal A, Bojahr B, De Wilde RL. The new surgical instrument in peritoneal endometriosis resection. Surg Sci. 2012;3:403-5.
8. Brahmbhatt JV, Gudeloglu A, Liverneaux P, et al. Robotic microsurgery optimization. Arch Plast Surg. 2014;41(3):225-30.
9. Roeder HA, Cramer SF, Leppert PC. A look at uterine wound healing through a histopathological study of uterine scars. Reprod Sci. 2012;19(5):463-73.
10. Litta P, Pluchino N, Freschi L, et al. Evaluation of adhesions after laparoscopic myomectomy using the Harmonic Ace and the auto-crosslinked hyaluronan gel vs Ringer's lactate solution. Clin Exp Obstet Gynecol. 2013;40(2):210-4.
11. Dubuisson JB, O'Leary T, Feki A, et al. Laparoscopic myomectomy. Minerva Ginecol. 2016;68(3):345-51.
12. Kim HS, Oh SY, Choi SJ, et al. Uterine rupture in pregnancies following myomectomy: a multicenter case series. Obstet Gynecol Sci. 2016;59(6):454-62.
13. Kho RM, Abrao MS. In search for the best minimally invasive hysterectomy approach for the large uterus: a review. Clin Obstet Gynecol. 2017;60(2): 286-95.
14. Mettler L, Ahmed-Ebbiary N, Schollmeyer T. Laparoscopic hysterectomy: challenges and limitations. Minim Invasive Ther Allied Technol. 2005; 14(3):145-59.
15. Harmanli OH, Tunitsky E, Esin S, et al. A comparison of short-term outcomes between laparoscopic supracervical and total hysterectomy. Am J Obstet Gynecol. 2009;201(5):536e1-7.
16. Tchartchian G, Heldmann P, Bojahr B, et al. The laparoscopic-assisted combined hysterectomy: a new surgical concept compared to the classical laparoscopic-assisted vaginal hysterectomy by a prospective study. Gynecol Obstet Invest. 2017; 82(3):223-9.
17. Tan-Kim J, Menefee SA, Reinsch CS, et al. Laparoscopic hysterectomy and urinary tract injury: experience in a health maintenance organization. J Minim Invasive Gynecol. 2015;22(7):1278-86.
18. Tchartchian G, Dietzel J, Bojahr B, et al. No more abdominal hysterectomy for myomata using a new minimally-invasive technique. Int J Surg Case Rep. 2010;1(1):7-8.
19. Cohen SL, Ajao MO, Clark NV, et al. Outpatient hysterectomy volume in the United States. Obstet Gynecol. 2017;130(1):130-7.
20. Vargas MV, Moawad GN, Sievers C, et al. Feasibility, safety, and prediction of complications for minimally invasive myomectomy in women with large and numerous myomata. J Minim Invasive Gynecol. 2017;24(2):315-22.
21. Watrowski R, Jager C, Forster J. Predictors of postoperative hemoglobin drop after laparoscopic myomectomy. Wideochir Inne Tech Maloinwazyjne. 2017;12(1):81-7.
22. Zhang P, Song K, Li L, Yukuwa K, et al. Application of simultaneous morcellation in situ in laparoscopic myomectomy of larger uterine leiomyomas. Med Princ Pract. 2011;20(5):455-8.
23. Sankaran S, Odejinmi F. Prospective evaluation of 125 consecutive laparoscopic myomectomies. J Obstet Gynaecol. 2013;33(6):609-12.
24. Chang WC, Chu LH, Huang PS, et al. Comparison of laparoscopic myomectomy in large myomas with and without leuprolide acetate. J Minim Invasive Gynecol. 2015;22(6):992-6.
25. Kim SM, Baek JM, Park EK, et al. A comparison of single-, two- and three-port laparoscopic myomectomy. JSLS. 2015;19(4):pii: e2015.00084.
26. Kang SY, Jeung IC, Chung YJ, et al. Robot-assisted laparoscopic myomectomy for deep intramural myomas. Int J Med Robot. 2017;13(2): Epub 2016. Mar 16.
27. Mansour FW, Kives S, Urbach DR, et al. Robotically assisted laparoscopic myomectomy: a Canadian experience. J Obstet Gynaecol Can. 2012;34(4):353-8.
28. Cheng HY, Chen YJ, Wang PH, et al. Robotic-assisted laparoscopic complex myomectomy: a single medical center's experience. Taiwan J Obstet Gynecol. 2015;54(1):39-42.
29. Griffin L, Feinglass J, Garrett A, et al. Postoperative outcomes after robotic versus abdominal myomectomy. JSLS. 2013;17(3):407-13.
30. Gunnala V, Setton R, Pereira N, et al. Robot-assisted myomectomy for large uterine myomas: a single center experience. Minim Invasive Surg. 2016;2016:4905292.
31. Bruggmann D, Tchartchian G, Wallwiener M, et al. Intra-abdominal adhesions: definition, origin, significance in surgical practice, and treatment options. Dtsch Arztebl Int. 2010;107(44):769-75.
32. Trew GH, Pistofidis GA, Brucker SY, et al. A first-in-human, randomized, controlled, subject- and reviewer-blinded multicenter study of Actamax Adhesion Barrier. Arch Gynecol Obstet. 2017;295(2): 383-95.
33. Neis KJ, Zubke W, Romer T, Schwerdtfeger K, et al. Indications and Route of hysterectomy for benign diseases. Guideline of the DGGG, OEGGG and SGGG (S3 Level, AWMF Registry No. 015/070, April 2015). Geburtshilfe Frauenheilkd. 2016;76(4):350-64.
34. Lee J, Kim S, Nam EJ, et al. Single-port access versus conventional multi-port access total laparoscopic hysterectomy for very large uterus. Obstet Gynecol Sci. 2015;58(3):239-45.
35. Song T, Lee Y, Kim ML, et al. Single-port access total laparoscopic hysterectomy for large uterus. Gynecol Obstet Invest. 2013;75(1):16-20.
36. Maccio A, Chiappe G, Kotsonis P, et al. Surgical outcome and complications of total laparoscopic

hysterectomy for very large myomatous uteri in relation to uterine weight: a prospective study in a continuous series of 461 procedures. Arch Gynecol Obstet. 2016;294(3):525-31.

37. Wang H, Li P, Li X, et al. Total laparoscopic hysterectomy in patients with large uteri: comparison of uterine removal by transvaginal and uterine morcellation approaches. Biomed Res Int. 2016;2016:8784601.
38. Scholler D, Taran FA, Wallwiener M, et al. Laparoscopic supracervical hysterectomy and laparoscopic total hysterectomy in patients with very large uteri: a retrospective single-center experience at a major university hospital. Geburtshilfe Frauenheilkd. 2017; 77(3):251-6.
39. Alperin M, Kivnick S, Poon KY. Outpatient laparoscopic hysterectomy for large uteri. J Minim Inv Gynecol. 2012;19(6):689-94.
40. Bojahr B, Tchartchian G, Ohlinger R. Laparoscopic supracervical hysterectomy: a retrospective analysis of 1000 cases. JSLS. 2009;13(2):129-34.
41. McGurk L, Oliver R, Odejinmi F. Laparoscopic supracervical hysterectomy for the larger uterus (>500 g): a case series and literature review. Arch Gynecol Obstet. 2017;295(2):397-405.
42. Chang WC, Huang SC, Sheu BC, et al. LAVH for large uteri by various strategies. Acta Obstet Gynecol Scand. 2008;87(5):558-63.
43. Takeda A, Hayashi S, Imoto S, et al. Gasless single-port laparoscopic-assisted vaginal hysterectomy for large uteri weighing 500g or more. Eur J Obstet Gynecol Reprod Biol. 2016;203:239-44.
44. Silasi DA, Gallo T, Silasi M, et al. Robotic versus abdominal hysterectomy for very large uteri. JSLS. 2013;17(3):400-6.
45. Ito TE, Vargas MV, Moawad GN, et al. Minimally invasive hysterectomy for uteri greater than one kilogram. JSLS. 2017;21(1):pii: e2017.00045.
46. Uccella S, Casarin J, Marconi N, et al. Laparoscopic versus open hysterectomy for benign disease in women with giant uteri (>/=1500 g): feasibility and outcomes. J Minim Invasive Gynecol. 2016;23(6):922-7.
47. Uccella S, Cromi A, Serati M, et al. Laparoscopic hysterectomy in case of uteri weighing >/=1 kilogram: a series of 71 cases and review of the literature. J Minim Invasive Gynecol. 2014;21(3):460-5.
48. Kondo W, Bourdel N, Marengo F, et al. Is laparoscopic hysterectomy feasible for uteri larger than 1000 g? Eur J Obstet Gynecol Reprod Biol. 2011;158(1):76-81.

KIEL SCHOOL

32 of Gynaecological Endoscopy

Fertility-enhancing Endoscopic Surgeries

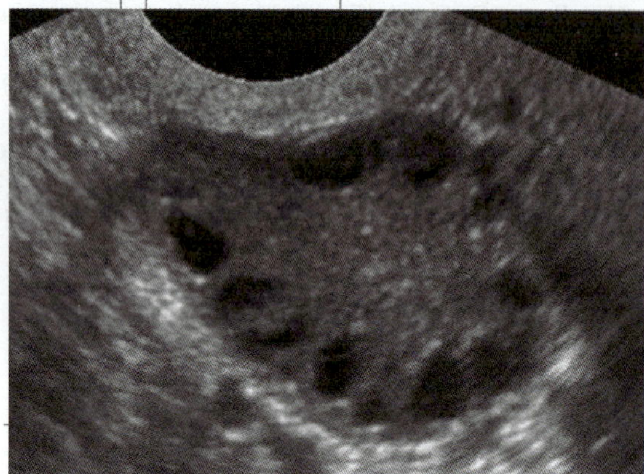

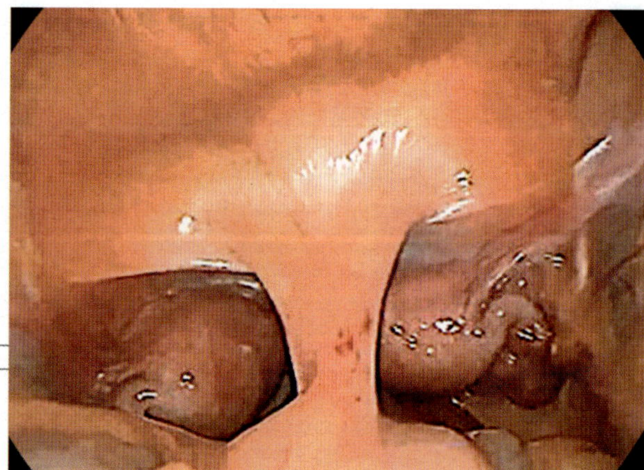

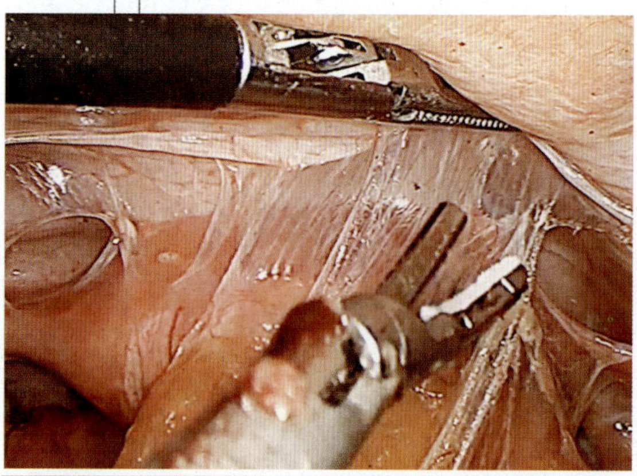

Chapter 32

Fertility-enhancing Endoscopic Surgeries

Meenu Agarwal

"Of all the rights of women, greatest is to be a mother."

—Lin Yutang

INTRODUCTION

Every effort must be made to maximize the chances of success in an assistant reproductive technology (ART) cycle. Failure of an ART cycle is a psychological, physical and financial disaster for the patient as well as a disappointment for the treating clinician. The results of ART can be enhanced in certain cases by a surgical approach.

The role of surgery to improve fertility was recognized and adopted way back in 1970s by Swolin and Gomel.[1] This was replaced by laparoscopic route in 1980s because of its minimally invasive route, better magnification, less postoperative pain and lesser duration of hospital stay. Simultaneously there was the development of ART, which led to further enhancement of reproductive outcomes. The surgery and ART are not interchangeable but work in tandem with each other to give the optimal benefit to the patient.

Fertility-enhancing endoscopic surgeries not only enhance the results of ART but also aid in spontaneous conceptions, slow down the progression of pathologies like fibroid or endometriosis and improve concomitant symptoms such as pain and bleeding. The various indications of endoscopic surgeries will be covered in the following headings.

POLYCYSTIC OVARY SYNDROME

Stein and Leventhal in 1935 reported that several women undergoing wedge resection (which was started as a biopsy from the bilaterally enlarged ovaries) experienced a resumption of ovulation. This was attributed to the reduction of hyperplastic central stroma (Fig. 32.1). As a result, wedge resection was practiced for many years as the surgical treatment for polycystic ovarian disorder for the initiation of ovulation in infertility cases. However, with the advent of clomiphene citrate and gonadotropins wedge resection slowly waned in its popularity. In 1984, it was reported that in women with PCOS, electrocautery of the ovarian capsule during laparoscopy resulted in high rate of ovulation and pregnancy.

Technique

Stabilize the Ovary with a Grasper

Three to four punctures on each side with a monopolar needle perpendicular to the ovarian surface to a depth of 4–10 mm. (The idea is to reduce the stroma and not to puncture the cysts on the ovarian surface) (Fig. 32.2).

Always cool down the ovary with normal saline before releasing it.

Select the patients well. One should employ medical treatment to its fullest before resorting to laparoscopic ovarian drilling (LOD).

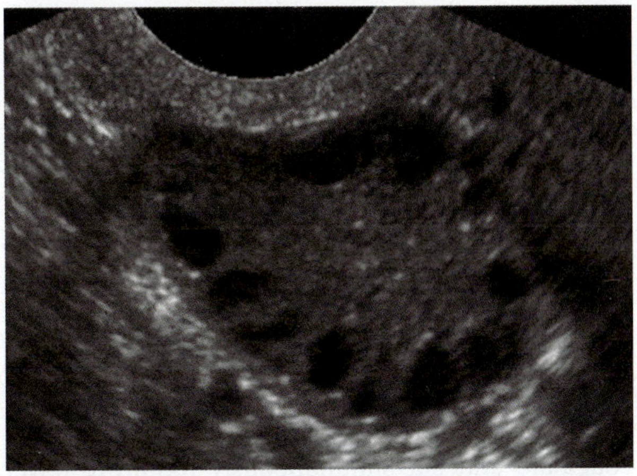

Fig. 32.1: USG appearance of polycystic ovaries.

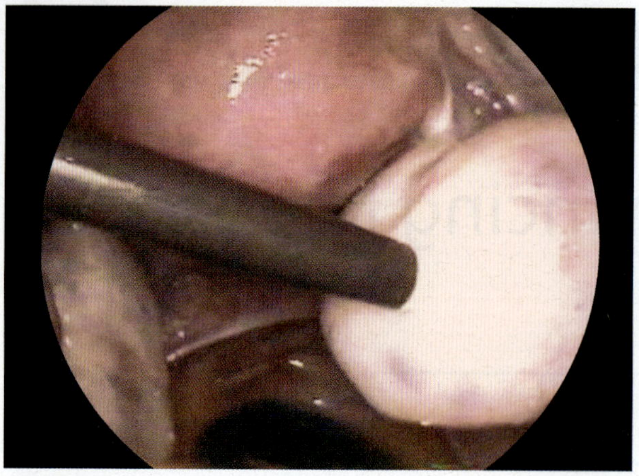

Fig. 32.2: Laparoscopic electrocauterization of ovarian surface.

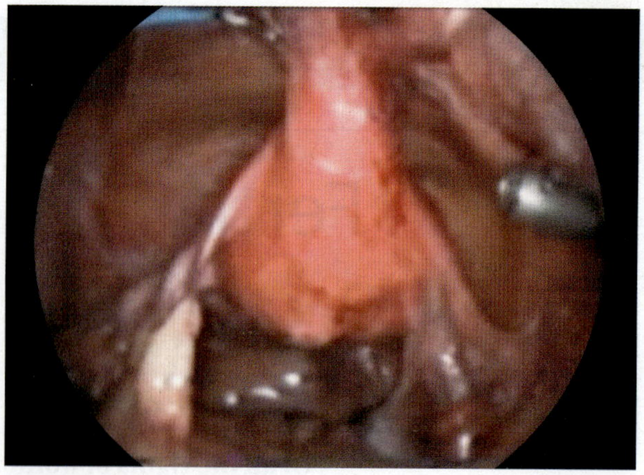

Fig. 32.3: Fundus of the uterus adherent to anterior abdominal wall.

PELVIC ADHESIONS

Adhesions are abnormal connective tissue (band of scar tissues) between tissues and organs in the form of fibrous adhesive bands. Normally internal organs and tissues have slippery surfaces, but the adhesions can cause them to stick together causing a restrictive movement, which may lead to pain and infertility. The pelvic adhesions arise as a result of tissue irritation caused by a spectrum of infection and inflammation or from trauma (e.g., post-surgical) (Figs. 32.3 to 32.5).

Hulka was first to publish a classification of pelvic adhesions based on the extent of ovarian involvement (surface area percentage) and the nature of adhesions.[2] We may find pelvic adhesions to be a cause of infertility and the adhesiolysis may improve the fimbrio-ovarian relationship leading to a spontaneous conception. In many cases, it may facilitate ovum pickup (OPU) and Embryo transfer procedures giving us a better clinical pregnancy rate (CPR) and take home baby rates.

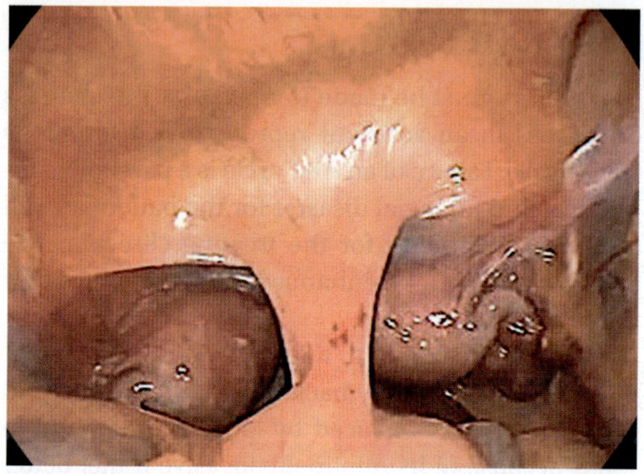

Fig. 32.4: Bicornuate uterus with congenital anteroposterior adhesion band.

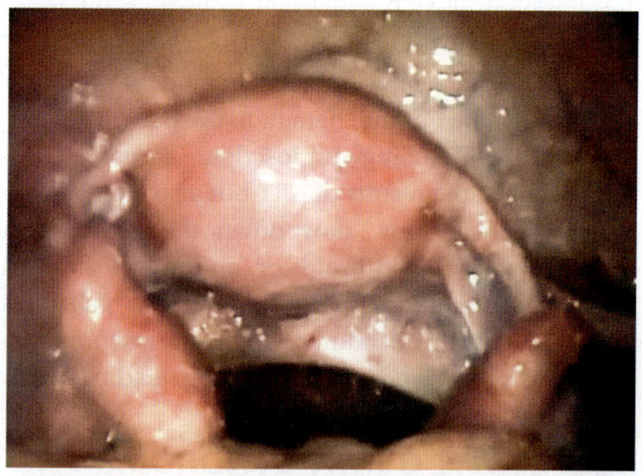

Fig. 32.5: A case of genital Kochs with bilateral tubes adherent.

Technique

Sharp dissection is the primary technique used for adhesiolysis to reduce the risk of reformation of adhesions. Apply tension over the adhesion with forceps and cut with scissors (Fig. 32.6). Blunt or rounded scissors with one stable blade and one movable blade are used to dissect adhesions sharply. Hook scissors are not so useful for the dissection of adhesions.

We may use monopolar current on the scissors and judiciously use blend or cutting. The use of harmonic scalpel has gained popularity as it can grasp, coagulate and cut simultaneously requiring fewer instruments change in and out of port sites.

Start with simple adhesions and then go to the complex ones. Always first bring the anatomy back to normal as far as possible by dissecting the adhesions before starting any surgical procedure. No risk should be taken with thick and small bowel adhesions which do not interfere with fertility.

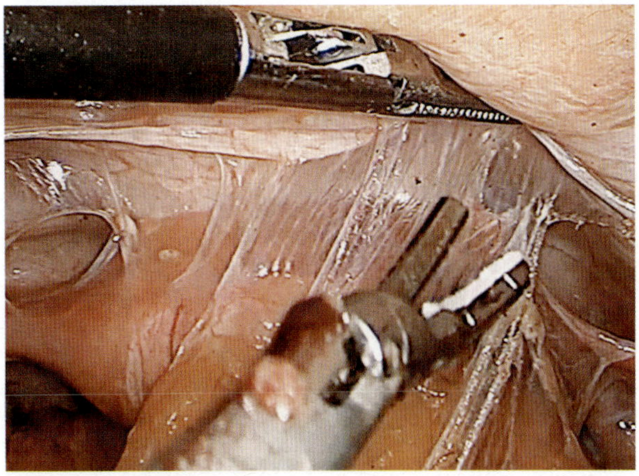

Fig. 32.6: Adhesions between the uterus and bladder.

MYOMECTOMY

Uterine fibroids are the most common benign tumors occurring in women of the reproductive age group (Fig. 32.7). Fibroids are present in approximately 5–10% of the patients presenting with infertility; however, they are found to be the sole identified factor in only 1–2.4% of the infertile patients.[3] According to Somigliana et al. myomas negatively affect the pregnancy rates[4] and submucosal fibroids strongly interfere with the chance of pregnancy. The impact of intramural myomas is less dramatic, even though it is statistically significant. In general, these effects appear to be more relevant when considering the take home baby rate rather than the clinical pregnancy rate. As expected, sub-serosal fibroids do not play a role in fertility.

Many studies have shown that the size of the fibroids is positively related to implantation failure, especially when the diameter of the fibroid is more than 4 cm.[5]

Approximately 50% of the women with infertility and myomas become pregnant after myomectomy.

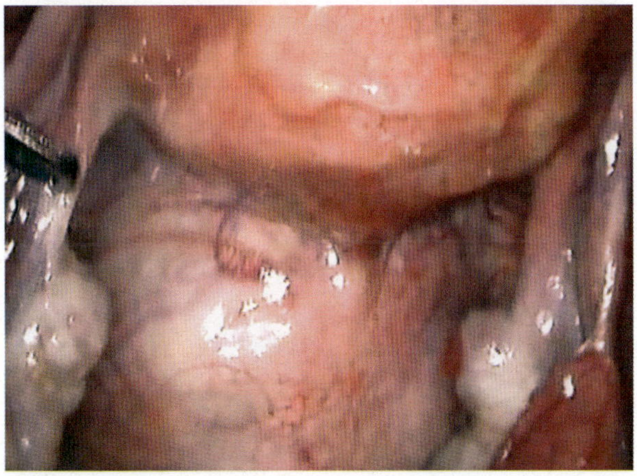

Fig. 32.7: Cervical fibroid.

Mapping of fibroids describing the exact number, size and location of the myomas helps in the planning of the surgery (Figs. 32.8 and 32.9).

Technique

- If using ipsilateral secondary ports, then plan a transverse incision.
- Inject dilute vasopressin (use 6 drops in 100 mL of normal saline).
- Alternatively, in large myomas, we can apply clips on uterine artery and on infundibulopelvic ligament bilaterally, which can be gently removed with a grasper at the end of the surgery. This reduces the blood loss during surgery and has reported a lesser recurrence rate of fibroids.
- Give a linear cut with a monopolar needle or the active blade of harmonic scalpel exposing the fibroid.
- Fibroid tissue is different from the myometrium so it is important to keep incising till the fibroid is seen and then stabilize the fibroid either with a myoma screw or with a tenaculum (we prefer tenaculum) and slowly and gently push the myometrium with bipolar forceps coagulating the tissue as and when required. We can also use harmonic blade here or a combination of bipolar and scissors depending on the surgeon's preference.
- Always check the integrity of endometrium by instilling some amount of dilute methylene blue in the uterine cavity.

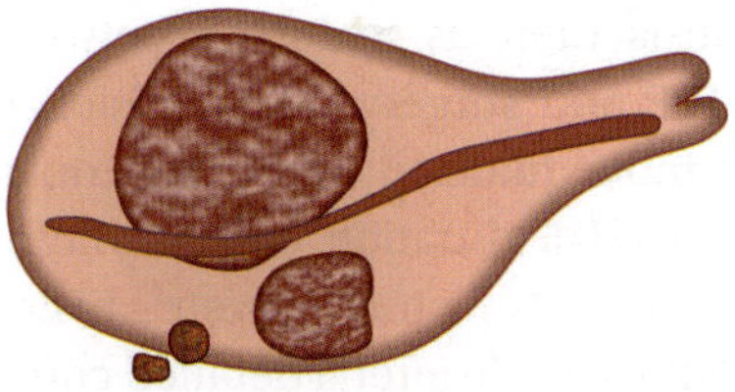

Fig. 32.8: Mapping of intramural myoma.

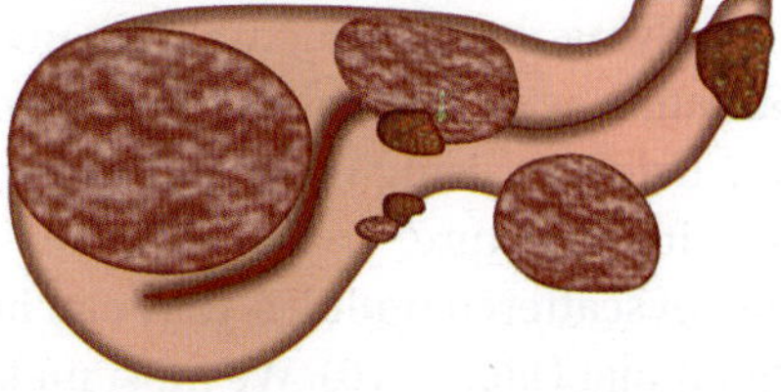

Fig. 32.9: Mapping of large intramural myoma indenting the endometrium.

- It is not drastic if the endometrial cavity is opened but we must make sure not to include endometrium in the sutures as that can cause micro fistulae, leading to increased risk of scar ectopic pregnancy.
- The defect is closed in one or two layers depending on the thickness of the edges to be closed, interrupted, continuous or Figure of 8 interrupted, vicryl 1-0 or barbed, depending on surgeon's preference. When using a barbed suture, it's debatable to cover it with a continuous 1-0 vicryl for the prevention of bowel complications at a later date.

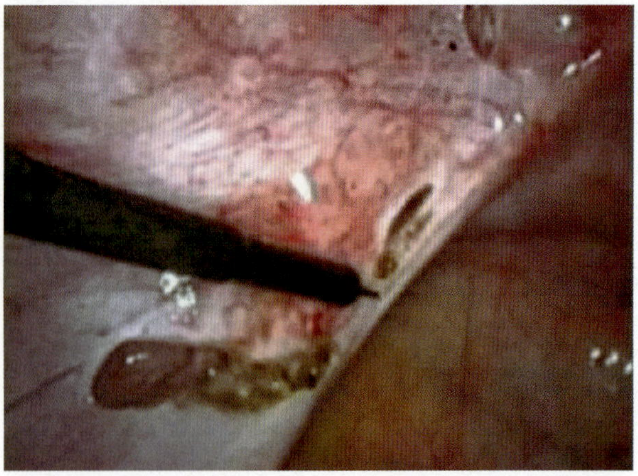

Fig. 32.10: Excision of the scattered nodules.

ENDOMETRIOSIS

Many studies suggest that prevalence of endometriosis among the reproductive age group is 11%. The most common symptoms in women with endometriosis are progressive dysmenorrhea and infertility. Laparoscopy with the histological evidence of ectopic endometrial epithelium is the gold standard to establish a firm diagnosis.

The role of laparoscopic surgery for minimal to mild endometriosis has long been an accepted mode of treatment. There is also evidence that ablation of lesions in minimal to mild endometriosis prior to in vitro fertility (IVF) results in higher live birth rates.

In the management of endometriotic cysts, ovarian cystectomy though preferred over incision and drainage, has been associated with significantly diminished AMH after surgery.

In cases of infertility due to moderate to severe endometriosis there is a debate between directly going for IVF and surgery. The decision to operate should be individualized depending on the age of the patient, AMH, duration of infertility, any other associated infertility factors, obstetric history and the decision of the couple after a detailed counseling.

Technique

In minimal to moderate endometriosis, the lesions can be excised with scissors. In cases where the lesion is overlying a vital structure like ureter, then an in infiltration with normal saline just under the lesion may help in raising it up and protecting the underlying vital structure.

In cases of scattered nodules, they can be cauterized using bipolar (Fig. 32.10). We must make sure to look at the post surface of ovaries and into the pouch of Douglas for the presence of endometriotic nodules and if present, coagulate them. A biopsy must always be taken from these nodules to confirm the histopathological diagnosis of the disease treating it by electrocoagulation at the same time.

In the case of an endometriotic cyst, there is an historical debate between incision and drainage or cystectomy, the former has higher chances of recurrence and the latter reduces the ovarian reserve. An in-between approach, i.e., do a cystectomy till the base and then coagulate the base at this point of time, seems to be the preferred approach by most of the surgeons (Fig. 32.11).

In case of the associated infertility factors like bilateral blocked fallopian tubes or male factor infertility, a judicious approach needs to be taken whether to operate or not to operate in such cases. A laparoscopic surgery in such cases would be indicated only if the cyst might interfere in the OPU, previous implantation failures and a large cyst (more than 4 cm). If possible it's a good approach to first freeze

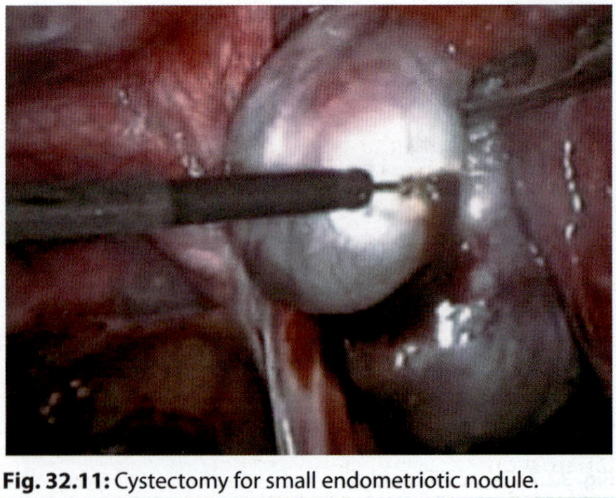

Fig. 32.11: Cystectomy for small endometriotic nodule.

the embryos and then go for the surgery followed by downregulation of the ovary and embryo transfer.

In moderate to severe endometriosis with infertility, the decision to operate or to go for IVF will depend on the clinical history, age and the ovarian reserve of the patient. Currently, in such cases, there are no randomized, controlled trials comparing the outcome of endoscopic infertility surgery before IVF or go for IVF directly. In cases of previous implantation failures with IVF with grade III or IV endometriosis, a surgical intervention in the form laparoscopy is justified. At the time of surgery, a patient approach with the clearance of all adhesions, getting the normal anatomy back is the aim of the surgery. Ovarian reserve tests like AFC count, AMH testing and day 2 serum FSH before and after the surgery must be performed, documented and informed to the patient.

HYDROSALPINGES

Hydrosalpinges are common encounters in infertility patients going for ART. On ultrasonography (USG), they appear as fluid-filled cavities surrounding the ovary with septa inside (waist sign or beads on a string). These lesions look like oval-shaped cysts with fine septae. The USG scan to look for hydrosalpinges is best performed at midcycle as the fluid tends to accumulate during the follicular phase. The presence of fluid in the endometrial cavity in the mid-follicular phase may also lead to the suspicion of subclinical hydrosalpinx.

Hydrosalpinx reduces the pregnancy rates for various reasons and must be treated before IVF. There may be a direct effect on embryos, as well as an alteration in uterine implantation. The proposed mechanism by which embryo toxicity occurs begins with a leakage of the fluid from the hydrosalpinx into the uterine cavity. This fluid may not only be harmful to embryos but may also have an effect on uterine receptivity and implantation mechanisms. In addition to improving overall pregnancy rates by removal of the diseased tubes, it has been suggested that treatment decreases the rate of miscarriage compared with those with untreated hydrosalpinges.[6]

A Cochrane review confirmed that the odds of pregnancy were increased with laparoscopic salpingectomy for hydrosalpinges prior to IVF (OR = 1.75, 95 percent CI 1.07 to 2.86), as were the odds of ongoing pregnancy or live birth (OR = 2.13, 95 percent CI 1.24 to 3.65). All these data demonstrate that laparoscopic salpingectomy for hydrosalpinges is the preferred procedure for improving pregnancy rates.

Technique

The tube can be removed using progressive bipolar coagulation and scissors or harmonic if available. We start at the fimbrial end and go to the proximal isthmic end of the tube (Fig. 32.12).

We should try to take the mesosalpinx close to the tube so as to avoid compromising the blood supply to the ovary. After the fallopian tube has been removed the proximal stump of the tube should be coagulated to prevent an ectopic pregnancy in the stump (Figs. 32.13 and 32.14).

In difficult cases (or sometimes if the patient does not want salpingectomy even after detailed counseling), a clipping (Fig. 32.15) or detachment of the tube with bipolar coagulation and scissors can be done at the isthmic end of the tube.

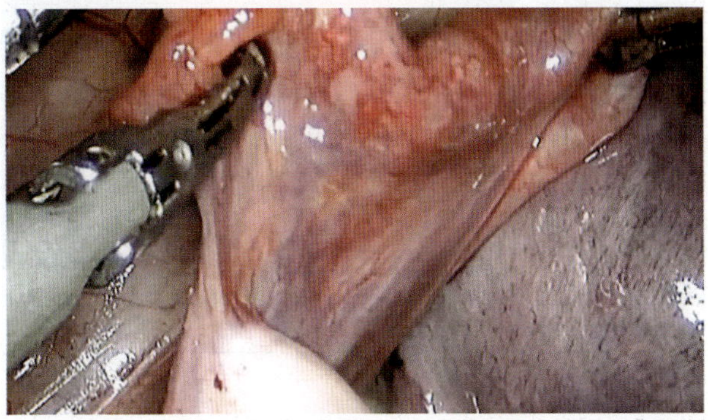

Fig. 32.12: Starting from the fimbrial end of the tube takes the mesosalpinx close to the tube.

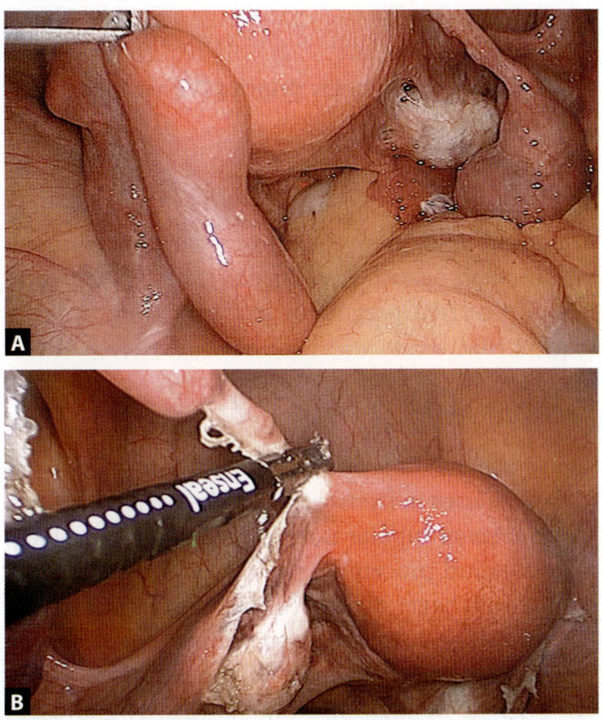

Figs. 32.13A and B: Salpingectomy for hydrosalpinx.

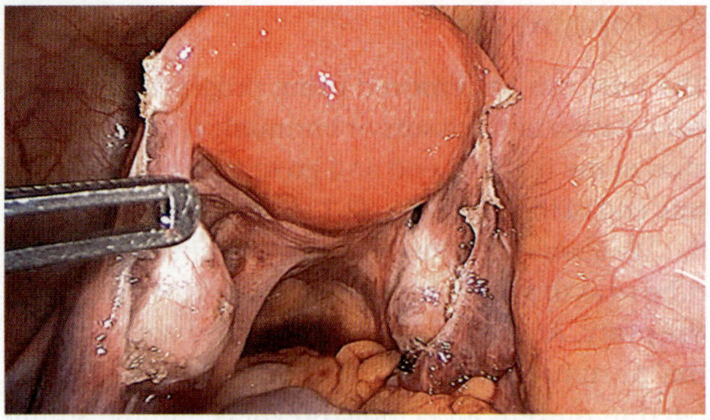

Fig. 32.14: Bilateral salpingectomy.

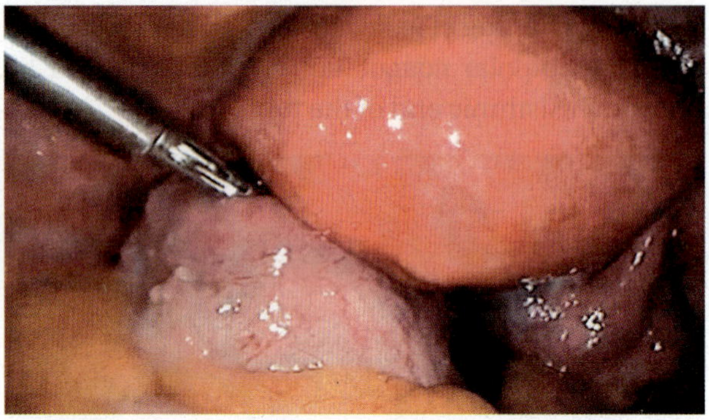

Fig. 32.15: Clipping the distal isthmic end of the tube to delink it from the uterine cavity.

HYSTEROSCOPIC SURGERIES

- Septum resection
- Adhesiolysis
- Myomectomy
- Routine hysteroscopy prior to IVF with endometrial injury

Septum Resection

A uterine septum is the most common congenital anomaly causing reduced reproductive outcome, recurrent pregnancy loss and preterm labor (Fig. 32.16).

Technique

Septum resection is one of the most satisfying surgical procedures in hysteroscopy. We can use scissors, monopolar or bipolar needle or resectoscope loop. In a standard procedure, the cervix is progressively dilated with hegar dilators to insert the resectoscope. A pure cutting current is used. Both the ostia should be visualized before starting the procedure. The uterine septa is divided midway between the anterior and posterior part, starting from the apex and going

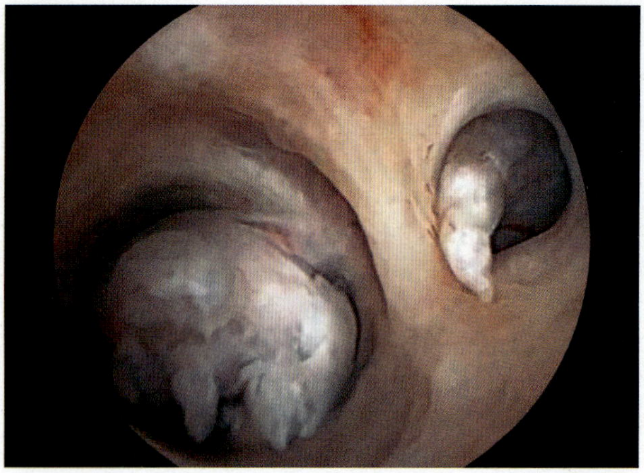

Fig. 32.16: An unusual case of uterine septum with polyp in each cornu.

transversely on either side. The cavity opens out as we progress in the resection until it reaches an endpoint where we would see both the ostia in the same view and at this point we may encounter slight bleeding which means that we have reached the myometrium.

Lateral Metroplasty

In women with hypoplastic and T-shaped uterus lateral metroplasty increases the size of the cavity and improves the clinical pregnancy rates and live birth rates. The procedure should be planned in the postmenstrual phase or anytime in a downregulated cycle and if the patient is on oral contraceptive pills.

Technique

After cervical dilatation, an operative hysteroscope (4 mm) with a side operating channel (to insert a 5 French monopolar hook) is introduced. With glycine as the distension media, an incision on the lateral wall of uterus is performed from fundus to the isthmus, decreasing the depth of the incision as we advance down (Fig. 32.17).

Generally, two or three incisions in the same depth are performed (Fig. 32.18). The procedure is repeated on the other lateral wall of the uterus. By the end of the procedure, we should be able to see both ostia in the same hysteroscopic field. We can also use scissors or a bipolar or monopolar needle to do lateral metroplasty but it requires slightly higher level of skills.

Postoperatively patient is put on oral estrogen tablets for about 2 weeks or until she gets her one cycle. The patient is followed up with a transvaginal 3D ultrasound for the cavity assessment.

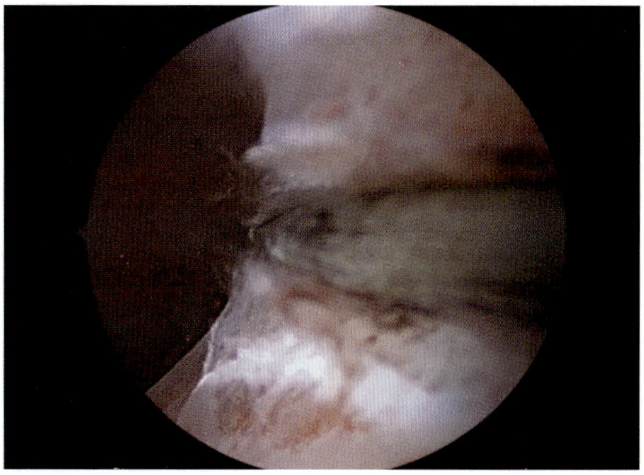

Fig. 32.17: Lateral metroplasty by monopolar hook.

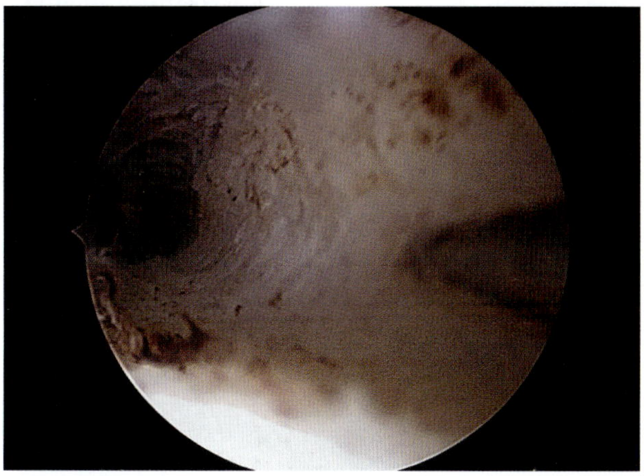

Fig. 32.18: *Lateral metroplasty:* Two to three incisions in the same depth.

Hysteroscopic Myomectomy

For women with submucous myomas presenting with infertility, hysteroscopic myomectomy is the treatment of choice. If the location is accessible like in type 0 and 1 (European Society of Hysteroscopy Classification), these myomas can be resected hysteroscopically with proven fertility outcomes.

It is important to know that the submucous fibroids which are smaller in size, with a smaller base, less penetration into the myometrium and preferably on anterior or posterior wall are low complexity surgeries. Bigger size submucous fibroids (more than 5 cm) with lesser penetration and broader base can be considered for medical treatment or removed by laparoscopic route.

The procedure is classically done using a resectoscope, which could be supported by monopolar or bipolar energy. Gynecologists borrowed this technology from urologists. Neuwirth and Amin[11] reported the first case of using a resectoscope for the treatment of a submucosal myoma in 1976 and the urologists had been using this device for decades before its use in gynecology.

Technique

The procedure should be planned in the postmenstrual phase or anytime in a downregulated cycle and if the patient is on oral contraceptive pills. The endometrial atrophy eases the surgical procedure.

After cervical dilatation the hysteroscope is introduced. The myoma is resected bit by bit with the help of resectocopic loop till we reach the base. At this stage if the procedure is incomplete, the hysteroscope with the loop is removed and the uterus massaged bimanually for a few seconds. Alternatively a Pitocin drip can be started to help the uterus contract so virtually all of the fibroid could be squeezed into the cavity, allowing the surgeon to completely remove it.

Inj. vasopressin diluted in normal saline can be injected into cervical stroma at 12,3,6 and 9 o'clock position helps in reducing the blood loss intraoperatively.

Intrauterine Adhesions

Hysteroscopy is the gold standard for the diagnosis and treatment of intrauterine adhesions (Figs. 32.19 and 32.20).

There are no controlled trials to assess the impact of adhesions and the role of surgical treatment prior to an ART cycle. In some women, we require more than one sitting to get an optimal result. Postoperative hormonal treatment with estrogen can be given to facilitate the growth of endometrium and to decrease the regrowth of adhesions.[7] The estrogen replacement therapy has not been evaluated in properly

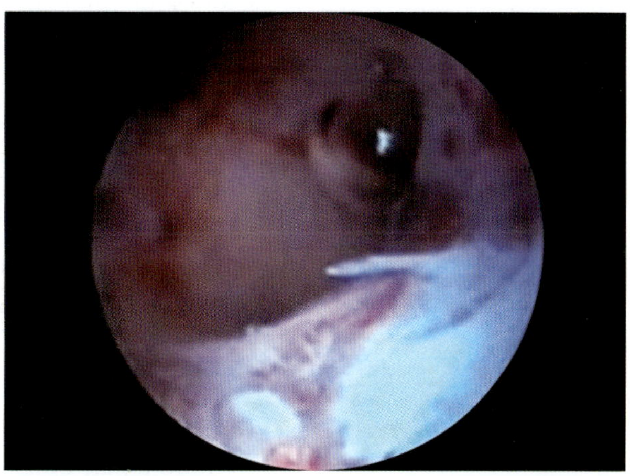

Fig. 32.19: Adhesions on the lateral wall of uterus.

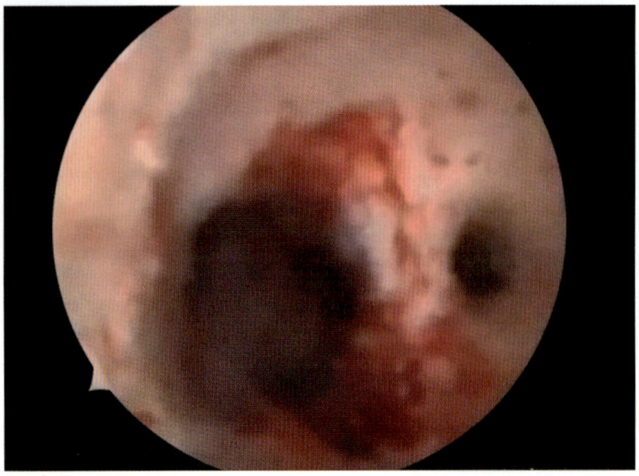

Fig. 32.20: Thick anteroposterior adhesion band.

designed clinical trials and we are still in the infancy stage for the newer anti adhesive adjuvants.

We should look at the surgical result rather than the severity of the disease to get a green signal to go ahead with IVF and the women can be offered surrogacy wherever appropriate.

Technique

These adhesions are usually lysed with scissors and can also be performed as an office procedure.

In some cases we can also use monopolar needle with pure cutting current with glycine distension media. As the incidence of genital tuberculosis is high in India we always send the endometrium for histopathology/PCR DNA/culture for Kochs culture.

Routine Hysteroscopy Prior to IVF with Endometrial Scratching

The relationship between endometrial injury and successful implantation has been found in clinical studies in different IVF populations.[8] This effect probably is due to the local inflammation, which is conducive to the implantation. There is recent evidence that suggests that the local injury doubles the live birth rate of women undergoing IVF.[9]

It was shown in recent Cochrane review based on 591 women that endometrial injury in the previous cycle significantly increases the odds of live birth.[10]

Technique

It is planned in the luteal phase of the cycle prior to the planned IVF cycle. It can be done as an office procedure with an endometrial pipelle biopsy inserted transcervically or in conjunction with the mock embryo transfer with diagnostic hysteroscopy. A 5 French grasper in introduced from the side channel of office hysteroscope and the tip is gently moved touching and scratching the fundus area. A slight movement of the hysteroscope in the horizontal plane allows the free movement of the grasper tip.

TIPS AND TRICKS

- Ovarian drilling should only be considered for patients after exhaustive medical management has failed.
- Only three to four punctures on each to a depth of 4 mm. The idea is to reduce the stroma and not to puncture the cysts.
- Always cool down the ovary with thorough irrigation before leaving it.
- The surgeon's skill level plays a role in adhesion formation. Gentle handling of the tissue, minimal blood loss, use of antiadhesive barriers and minimally invasive surgery decrease the risk of adhesion formation.
- For ovarian endometrioma, excision of the endometrioma capsule, instead of drainage and coagulation will increase the pregnancy rates and reduce the recurrence rates.
- In severe grade III or grade IV endometriosis a judicious decision should be taken to choose between surgery and IVF.
- Myomas should be removed when they distort the cavity or intramural and large.
- Adnexal masses should be removed when they exceed 5 cm and persist for more than 3 months.
- Patients with hydrosalpinx going for IVF should be counseled for salpingectomy or delinking the fallopian tube by clipping will improve the implantation rates.
- During hysteroscopic myomectomy, inj. vosopressin diluted in normal saline injected into cervical stroma at 12, 3, 6 and 9 o'clock positions helps in reducing the blood loss intraoperatively.
- Hysteroscopic adhesiolysis is recommended to all women with intrauterine adhesions prior to ART.
- Routine hysteroscopy with endometrial scratching can be performed as an office procedure in the preceding luteal phase to improve the results of implantation.

REFERENCES

1. Gomel V. Salpingostomy by microsurgery. Fertil Steril. 1978;29(4):380-7.
2. Hulka JF. Adnexal adhesions, a prognostic staging and classification system based on a 5 year survey of fertility surgery. Am J Obstet Gynecol. 1982;144(2): 141-8.
3. Benecke C, Kruger TF, Siebert TI, et al. Effect of fibroids on fertility in patients undergoing assisted reproduction. A structured literature review. Gynecol Obstet Invest. 2005;59(4):225-30.
4. Somigliana E, Vercellini P, Daguati R, et al. Fibroids and female reproduction: A critical analysis of evidence. Hum Reprod. 2007;13(5):465-76.
5. Eldar-Geva T, Meagher S, Healy DL, et al. Effect of intramural, subserosal, and submucosal uterine fibroids on the outcome of assisted reproductive technology treatment. Fertil Steril. 1998;70(4):687-91.
6. Spielvogel K, Shwayder J, Coddington CC. Surgical management of adhesions, endometriosis, and tubal pathology in the woman with infertility. Clin Obstet Gynecol. 2000;43(4):916-28.
7. Kodaman PH, Arici A. Intra-uterine adhesions and fertility outcome: how to optimize success? Curr Opin Obstet Gynecol. 2007;19(3):207-14.
8. El-Toukhy T, Sunkara S, Khalaf Y. Local endometrial injury and IVF outcome: a systematic review and meta-analysis. Reprod Biomed Online. 2012;25(4):345-54.
9. Narvekar SA, Gupta N, Shetty N, et al. Does local endometrial injury in the nontransfer cycle improve the IVF-ET outcome in the subsequent cycle in patients with previous unsuccessful IVF? A randomized controlled pilot study. J Human Reprod Sci. 2010;3(1): 15-9.
10. Nastri CO, Gibreel A, Raine-Fenning N, et al. Endometrial injury in women undergoing assisted reproductive techniques. Cochrane Database Systematic Rev. 2012;7: C0009517.
11. Neuwirth RS, Amin HK. Excision of submucous fibroids with hysteroscopic control. Am J Obstet Gynecol. 1976; 126(1):95-9.

KIEL SCH•OL

33 of Gynaecological Endoscopy

Hysterectomies

Total Laparoscopic Hysterectomy (TLH)

Technique 1

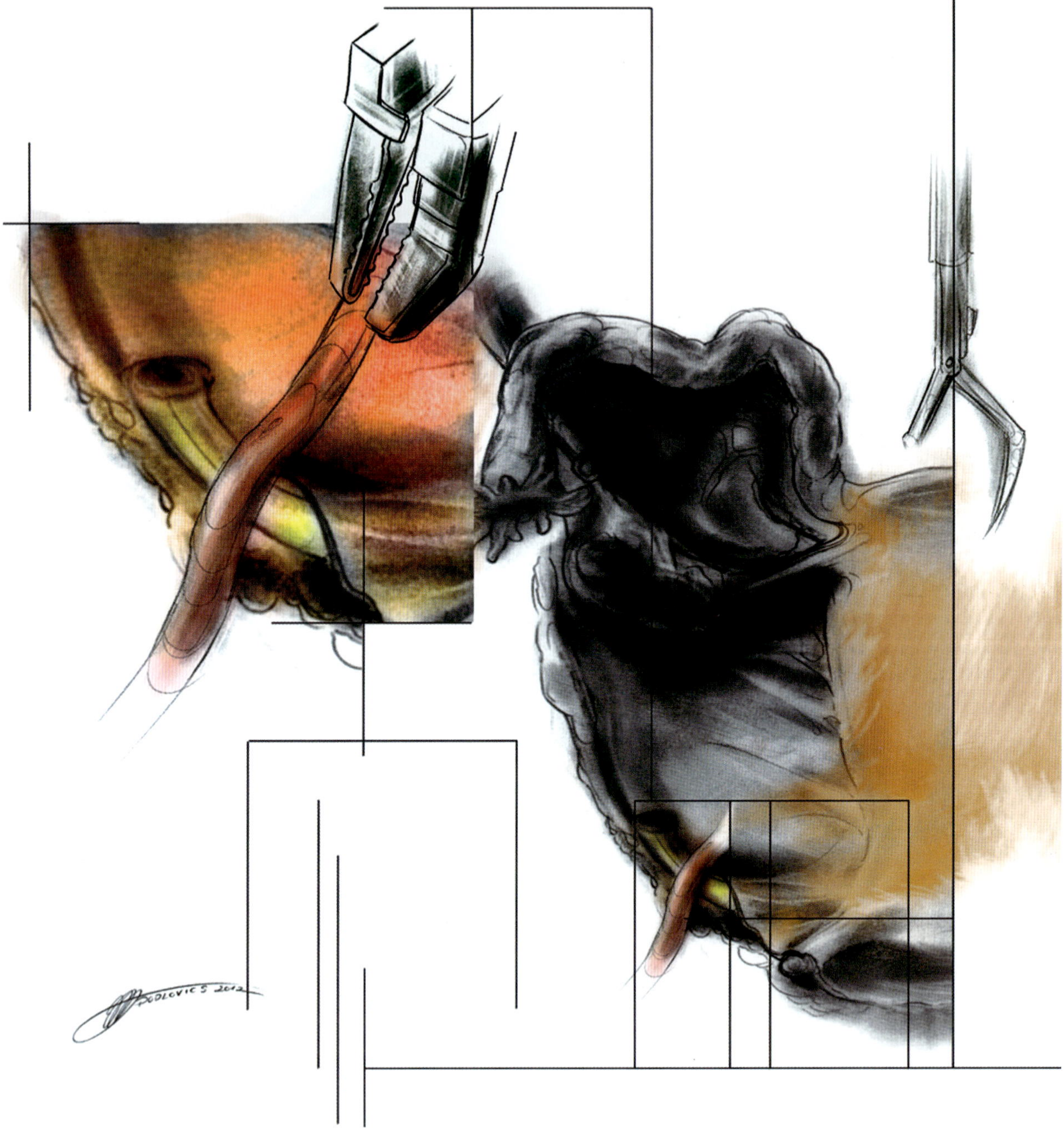

Chapter 33

Technique of Routine Total Laparoscopic Hysterectomy with a Dissection of Uterine Vessels at Internal Iliac Level and Using a Uterine Manipulator

Bernd Holthaus, Susanne Denny

PREPARATION

The patient will be placed in the laparoscopic lithotomy position with both arms positioned alongside the patient. She is then cleaned, draped and the bladder catheterized with a standard Foley's catheter. With a speculum placed in the vagina, a vulsellum is attached to the anterior cervical lip to gently pull down uterus and a sound inserted into the cervical canal to measure the uterine length. According to vaginal width and length of the uterine cavity the Hohl manipulator (Fig. 33.1) is assembled and inserted into vagina and cervical canal and vulsellum removed.[1] The ceramic cup needs to sit snugly over the cervical body and thus stretch the fornix firmly over its rim. To safeguard and maintain correct positioning of the cervical cup the manipulator is pushed in at all times.

One purpose of the manipulator is to move uterus within the abdominal cavity to facilitate optimal exposure to all sides when isolating the organ. Therefore the patient needs to be placed right at the end of the operating table to allow the manipulator to be angled right down for maximum elevation of uterus.[2]

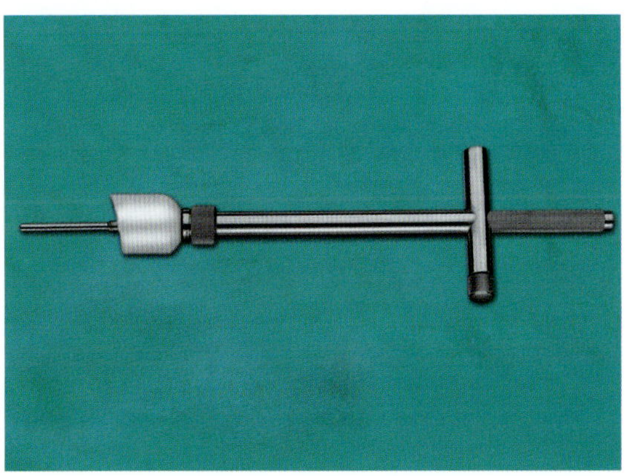

Fig. 33.1: Uterus manipulator by Prof Hohl K Storz, Tuttlingen.

TROCARS, INSTRUMENTS AND THE START

Together with the 10-mm umbilical port, three 5-mm instrument ports are used—one about 2 cm suprapubically, the other two in the right and left iliac fossa. Preferred instruments include reusable graspers, bipolar forceps, Metzenbaum's scissors connected with a unipolar electrode, monopolar hook electrode and two needle holders. The rim of the cup is located in two ways: (1) A gentle "knocking" motion with the tip of a grasper along the cervicovaginal region will reveal the hard surface of the cup under the vaginal tissue. (2) A gentle "step" in the vaginal tissue created by the rim of the cup can normally be visualized after the vesical tissue has been pushed down well below the rim. Laparoscopic hysterectomy is now under way.

OPENING OF PELVIC SIDEWALL

After complete visual exploration of the abdominal cavity (Fig. 33.2) both round ligaments are dissected about 2 cm medially from the pelvic sidewall (Fig. 33.3A). From here the anterior leaf of the broad ligament is opened up in the direction of the uterovesical fold. Bladder peritoneum is now elevated and bladder pushed and dissected down to expose the anterior vaginal wall approximately 1–2 cm below the rim of the cervical cup (Fig. 33.3B).

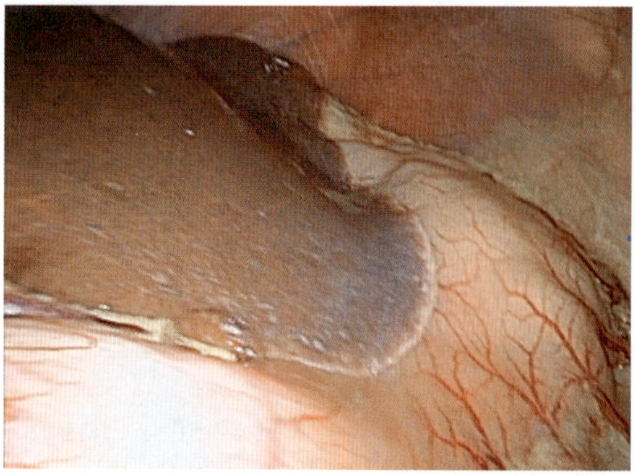

Fig. 33.2: Upper abdomen.

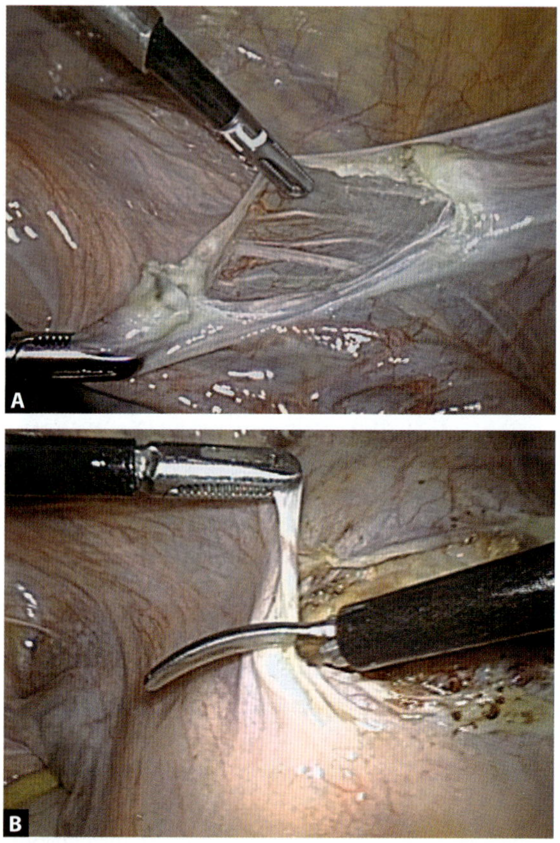

Figs. 33.3A and B: (A) Dissection of round ligament; (B) Dissection of bladder.

IDENTIFICATION AND DISSECTION OF UTERINE VESSELS AT INTERNAL ILIAC LEVEL

Now the opening of the broad ligament is continued in the cranial direction (Fenestration Fig. 33.4A), i.e. from the round ligament to the tubo-ovarian pedicle at the level of its iliac crossing. With proper medialization of the tubo-ovarian pedicle the fine 'spider web'

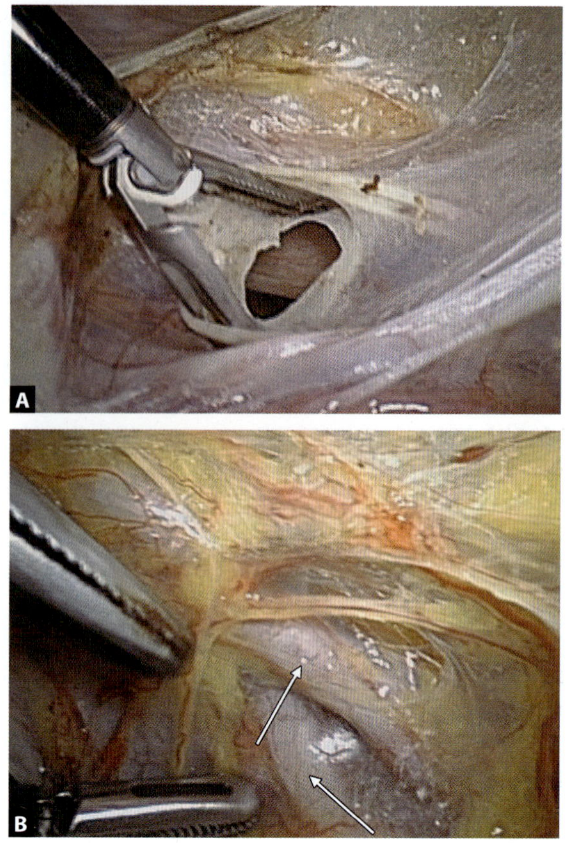

Figs. 33.4A and B: (A) Fenestration of broad ligament; (B) Uterine artery crossing ureter right side.

of retroperitoneal connective tissue is exposed. With gentle and blunt dividing movements of the closed grasping forceps the external and internal iliac vessels and ureter should be identified (Fig. 33.4B). Following the course of the internal iliac artery the bifurcation of the uterine artery is soon exposed.

While ureter is medialized uterine artery is coagulated and dissected just medially to the point of its origin at the internal iliac artery (Fig. 33.5).

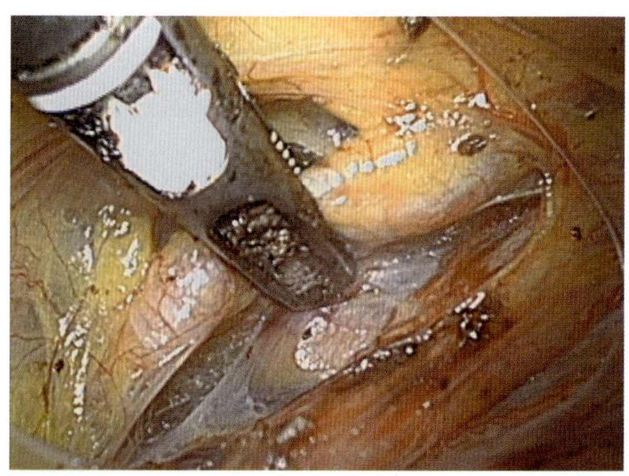

Fig. 33.5: Coagulation of uterine artery left side.

This normally exposes one or two uterine veins, which may then also be coagulated and dissected.

DISSECTION OF PARAMETRIA AND SACROUTERINE LIGAMENTS

For this step — the uterine end of the dissected round ligament is medialized thus exposing the posterior leaf of the broad ligament. This is now fenestrated, which allows easy and safe lateralization of the ureter while the parametria are coagulated and dissected along the uterine wall and cervix. Bladder pillar and uterine vessels are now coagulated and dissected. Elevation of uterus will also expose the sacrouterine ligaments for dissection.

The commonly high risk of inadvertent blood loss from uterine pedicle is minimized by above described coagulation and dissection of uterine vessels at pelvic sidewall level. However, this maneuver may be omitted, which will simplify and shorten the procedure by 5–15 min.

The key elements, pushing the bladder down from the anterior vaginal fornix prior to incision as well distancing ureter from the uterine vessels at cervicovaginal level are only safely facilitated by stretching the manipulator firmly cranially and to the contralateral side of preparation.

WITH OR WITHOUT BILATERAL SALPINGO-OOPHORECTOMY

If adnexa are to remain in situ, the fallopian tube and ovarian ligament are coagulated and dissected close to the uterus and the broad ligament dissected in the direction of the earlier fenestration (Fig. 33.6).

Likewise, if a bilateral salpingo-oophorectomy (BSO) is required the suspensory ovarian ligament is coagulated and dissected close to ovary and meso-ovary dissected in the direction of fenestration. Here again, fenestration is a useful point of orientation to safeguard the ureter.

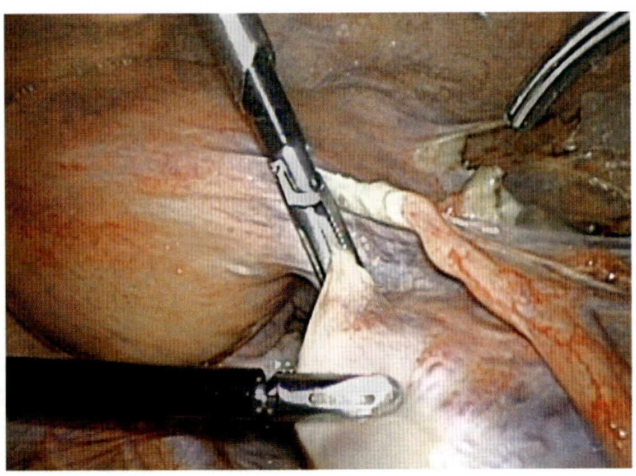

Fig. 33.6: Dissection of adnexa.

REMOVAL OF UTERUS

Vaginal fornix is now incised using a monopolar hook electrode, which is guided along the ceramic rim of the manipulator (Figs. 33.7A and B).

Uterus is then pulled into the vaginal canal for removal. To prevent loss of intra-abdominal inflation pressure uterus may be left in vagina until the cuff is closed with two to four "figure-of-8" stitches using size 0 Vicryl. Alternatively uterus is removed and pneumoperitoneum maintained by occluding vagina with a large, moisturized swab (Figs. 33.8A and B).

Optionally, both sacrouterine ligaments may be attached to posterior vaginal wall to prevent vaginal prolapse (McCall-culdoplasty). Also, pelvic peritoneum may be closed with a 3-0 Vicryl suture in a continuous unlocked fashion.

At the end of the procedure the abdominal cavity is irrigated with normal saline solution and drained. We normally do not leave any drains in situ.

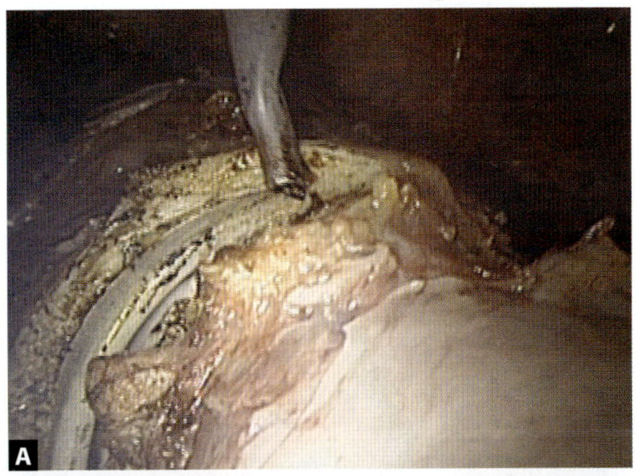

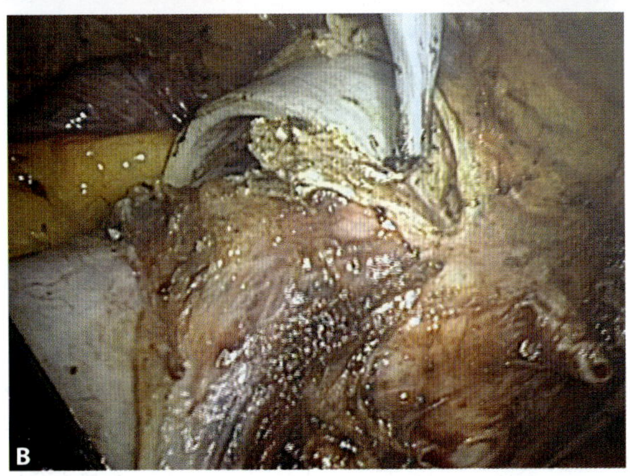

Figs. 33.7A and B: Opening the vagina with a monopolar hook dissection of adnexa.

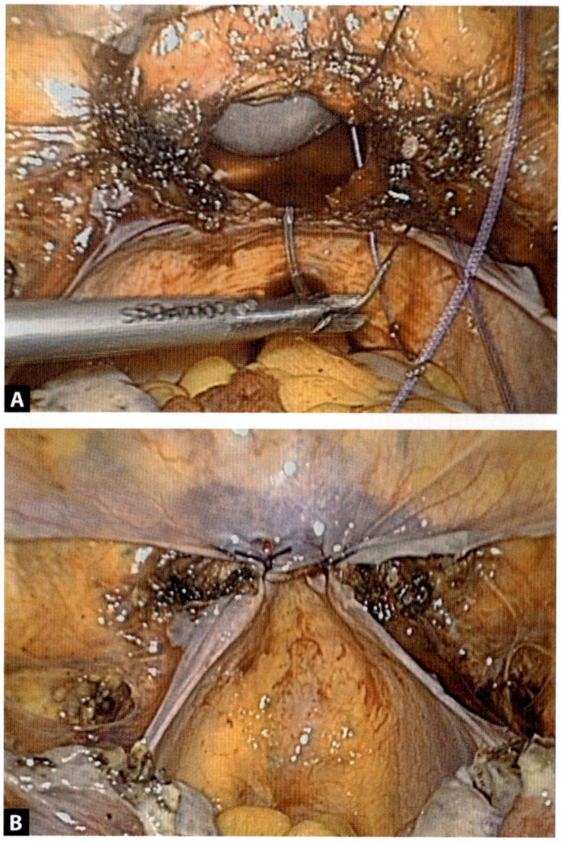

Figs. 33.8A and B: Suturing the vagina.

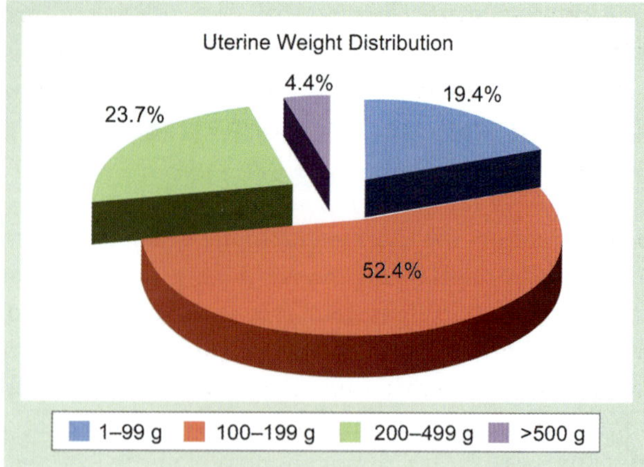

Fig. 33.9: Uterine weight (in grams).

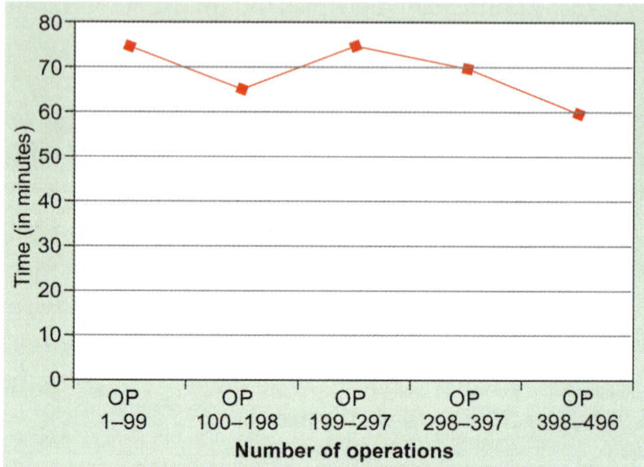

Fig. 33.10: Operating time (in minutes) since introduction.

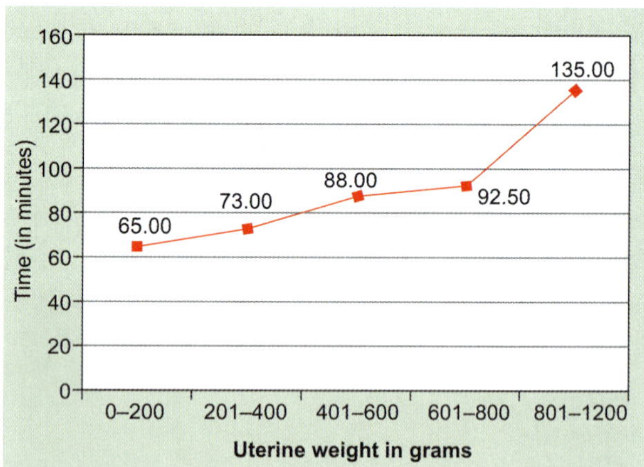

Fig. 33.11: Operating time (in minutes) according to uterine weight.

RESULTS

Since its introduction in 2008 we performed about 2,000 procedures with this technique in our department. The data below have been collected retrospectively.

Mean patient age was 45.03 years, and 15.9% of patients were nulliparous while the mean number of children in the multiparous group was 1.7. The mean body mass index (BMI) was 271.1 ± 4.8. Of the patients 66% had an operation.

The mean uterine weight was 191.46 g with a range of 27–1222 g (Fig. 33.9).

Over time, the mean operating time dropped from 80 min to 55 min with a range from 25 to 285 min (Fig. 33.10).

The operating time seems to depend not only on the surgeons' experience but also on factors such as the number of previous operations, uterine weight and body mass index (BMI) of the patient. We have shown the operating time according to four defined groups of uterine weight: Group 1, 1–99 g; group 2, 100–199 g, group 3, 200–500 g and group 4, over 500 g (Fig. 33.10)). From group 1 to group 4 the mean operating time rose from 65 to 135 min (mean) (Fig. 33.11).

Blood loss was evaluated according to the drop of hemoglobin (Hb). The mean drop in Hb was 1.02 g/dL (range 0.3–4.7 g/dL). No patient required a blood transfusion. The mean hospital stay was 3.7 days (range 1.4–8).

Complications were recorded and defined as minor or severe (Fig. 33.12). Minor complications are hematoma at the level of the vaginal suture, thrombosis, suture dehiscence and infection.

Severe complications include injury to bladder, ureter, bowel and vessels, fistula formation and conversion to laparotomy.

In 92.6% of the procedures we had no complications. In 5.8% of the cases we experienced minor complications: Twelve patients developed a hematoma at the level of vaginal suture. After we changed our suturing technique from continuous to a number of figure-of-8 stitches we experienced no further hematoma. Another 12 patients had some form of infection and 4 patients developed a deep venous thromboembolism. In two cases we observed a vaginal suture dehiscence.

In 1.6% of patients ($n = 8$) we experienced severe complications: Four cases of bladder injury, two ureteric lesions and two patients developed a vesicovaginal fistula. In one case we had to convert to a laparotomy. All these patients had at least one previous operation.

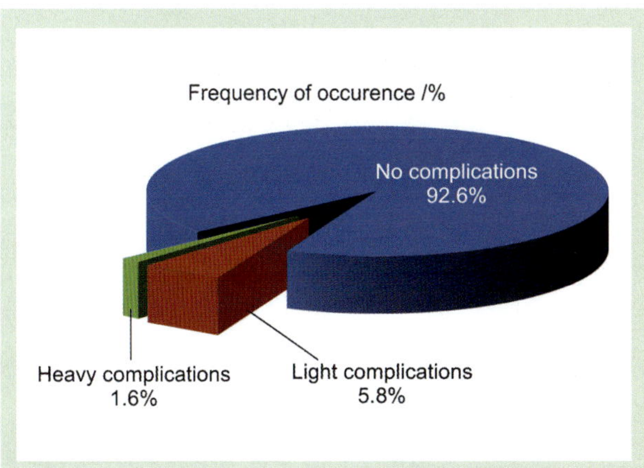

Fig. 33.12: Complication rate.

TIPS AND TRICKS

There is an easy way to insert a large needle into the abdomen for suturing the vagina.[3] Take the suture about 2 cm above the needle with a needle holder (outside the abdomen). You then follow your 5 mm incision with the tip of the needle holder. There is then no problem to get inside the abdomen. The needle will follow the suture. It is very easy to suture the vagina with large needles.

CONCLUSION

We believe the above described technique of total laparoscopic hysterectomy is a safe and valid procedure, which, in experienced hands, may result in a lower overall complication rate compared with the conventional open technique within reasonable operating times and with the additional benefit of a shorter procedure-to-dischargetime. Obviously there is a certain learning curve required for the whole team including theater staff but for the endoscopically experienced surgeon this is an easy-to-learn technique. In our department TLH has become the standard form of hysterectomy leaving very few indications for the conventional open technique (TAH).

REFERENCES

1. Hohl MK. Der Uterus manipulator n. Hohl. Endo World Gyn Nr. 16 D, Tuttlingen, Deutschland; Karl Storz Ltd; 2001.
2. Mueller A, Oppelt P, Ackermann S, et al. The Hohl instrument for optimizing total laparoscopic hysterectomy procedure: J Minim Invasive Gynecol. 2005:12(5);432-5.
3. Alkatout I, Mettler L, editors. Hysterectomy, A Comprehensive Surgical Approach. Berlin: Springer; 2017. 1577 p.

Hysterectomies
Total Laparoscopic Hysterectomy **(TLH)**
Technique 2

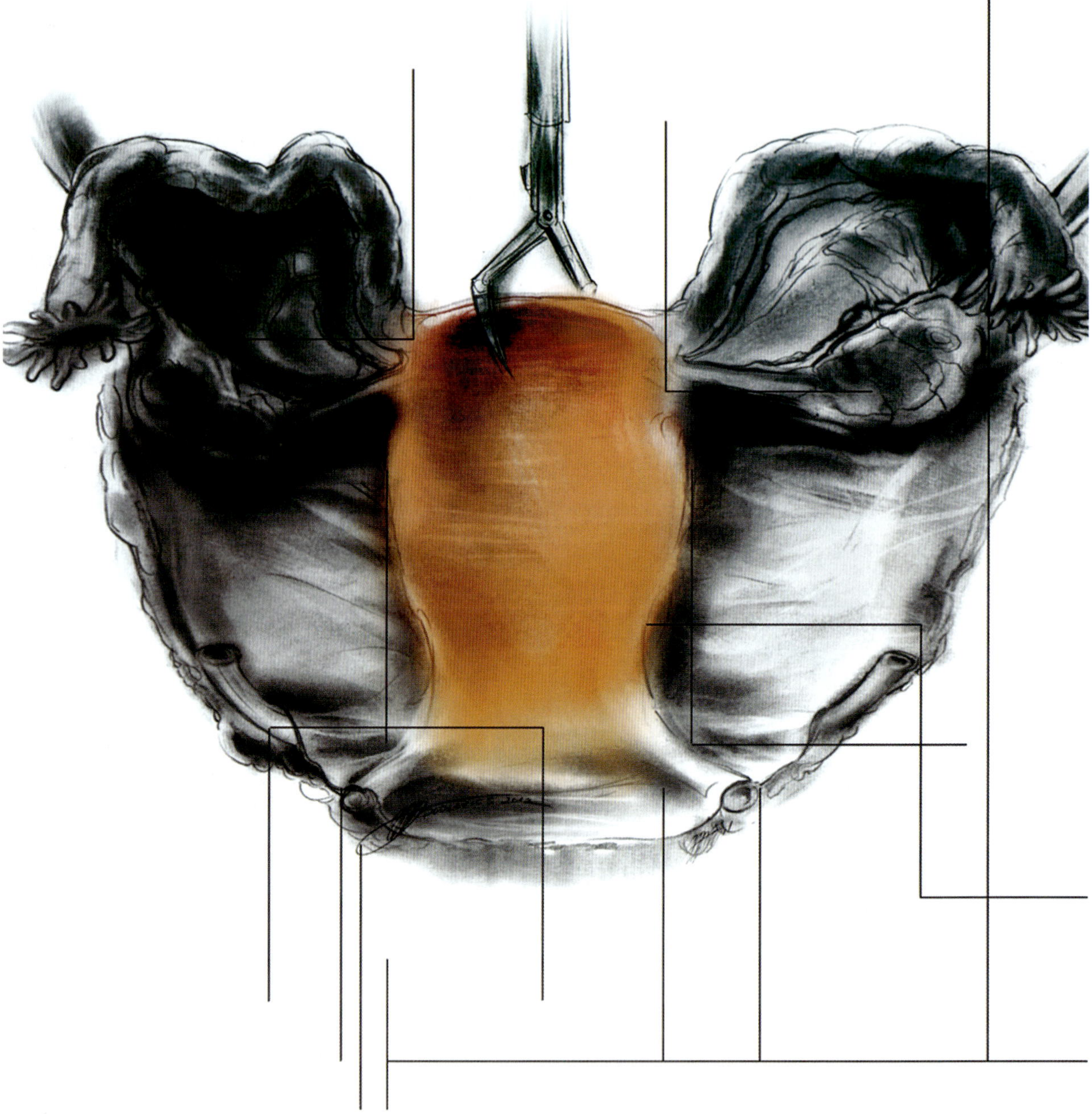

Chapter 34

Total Laparoscopic Hysterectomy

Liselotte Mettler, Ibrahim Alkatout, Mohamed Elessawy

TEACHING YESTERDAY AND TODAY

Hysterectomy is a standard gynecological operation that is taught during training as vaginal and abdominal hysterectomy.

Personal experience and daily teaching, however, have shown that the changeover to laparoscopic hysterectomy is not only difficult, but also complicated. This can only be avoided by making the operation more structured and teaching it as early as possible.[1]

Classical Teaching of Hysterectomy

Most gynecological surgeons start their clinical training with abdominal hysterectomy under professional supervision. The access routes are wide open and even large uteri can be dissected easily without endangering important structures, such as the uterine artery and urinary bladder.

This phase is followed by the vaginal hysterectomy approach, which is more challenging for the surgeon. Anatomy is suddenly twisted upside down and the surgeon depends on a well-trained assistant to have a good anatomical view despite the tiny opening.

A new aspect gains importance in the vaginal and laparoscopic approach: the correct indication to prevent a conversion to laparotomy.

The following preliminary considerations are essential for the surgeon:

- Main indications for the hysterectomy approach?
- Adequate vaginal access?
- Has the patient already given birth? Is the uterus descendible?
- What happens in the case of cesarean section?
- Can the adnexa be reached?
- Is a prolapse therapy essential?
- How to deal with a large uterus?
- How to control the vaginal morcellation?

Vaginal hysterectomy is only possible after mastering the previous considerations.

By the end of clinical training period, surgeons performing both vaginal and abdominal hysterectomies should have acquired sufficient expertise to master most hysterectomy constellations.

Current Teaching Methods

Today, the training that takes place in large clinics runs along completely different lines due to the internal rotation process.

On the one hand, the trainees have little experience of abdominal or vaginal hysterectomy and on the other hand, there is a general lack of experience with extended laparoscopic operations, quite different from the time when most of the authors of this book began their laparoscopic training.

Due to pericervical dissection total laparoscopic hysterectomy (TLH) should be considered a distinct surgical procedure, when compared to laparoscopic supracervical hysterectomy (LSH) and laparoscopic-assisted vaginal hysterectomy (LAVH), and it should be taught by experienced surgeons (Video 34.1).

That is why systematic reviews[2,3] report increased complication rates, especially urinary tract complications, increased risk of bleeding and relatively long operation times, and recommend it only as a subordinate option.

These problems, however, do not occur in experienced centers[4] where TLH complication rates are more or less the same as those of other laparoscopic operations, when performed by experienced surgeons.

Hohl reported that the complication rates of experienced and nonexperienced surgeons performing

TLH are very low (2.7%) and are more or less the same if the surgeons have been taught and have learnt the TLH in structured steps.[1]

Surgeons should therefore concentrate on a streamlined training program for their junior staff that combines all surgeons' experience to achieve a steep learning curve for the trainees.

For this reason, the focus of this chapter lies more in the didactic domain rather than in demonstrating specific features for experienced surgeons.

Concept of Total Laparoscopic Hysterectomy in the Kiel School

The development of the Kiel School's TLH technique is based on the works of Semm and Mettler in Kiel, but has incorporated crucial developments from other centers.[5,6]

This has led to a structured technique, reproducible in all its separate steps.

Intrafascial Hysterectomy and Total Atraumatic Intrafascial Laparoscopic (TAIL™) Hysterectomy

The basic concept of laparoscopic hysterectomy was developed by Kurt Semm.[5,7] Nevertheless, the instruments and techniques (endotherm and loop) used at that time did not keep pace with the concept of classic intrafascial supracervical hysterectomy (CISH), which was the main reason for the technique not duly spreading. Furthermore, most of the gynecologists at that time were not ready to support laparoscopic hysterectomy.

Advancements in instruments and constant training considerably improved the situation.

Thanks are due to Hohl for taking up the concept of the classical intrafascial hysterectomy and developing it further with the introduction of his manipulator. The development began in 1992 and the Hohl manipulator (Karl Storz, Tuttlingen, Germany) has been available on the market since 2002. Hohl called the method "TAIL hysterectomy. The Kiel School very quickly decided to include this procedure in its curriculum.

Descent Prevention

The concept of intrafascial hysterectomy (TAIL™) already includes the first step of descent prevention by preserving ligament structures. It is well known that bladder ptosis plays an important role in patients due to undergo a hysterectomy. This concern is justified as proven by numerous studies, which indicate that often an inadequate prolapse prophylaxis is carried out at vaginal hysterectomy (the preferred approach of all specialist associations).[8,9]

It was therefore Kiel School's main concern to integrate descent prevention into its concept. This has been achieved by adopting the modification by van Herendael to the vaginal closure stitches of Te Linde.[10] For further details refer to chapter "Strategies to Prevent Vault Descent at the Time of Hysterectomy."

Treatment of Vaginal Vault Prolapse

There are well-established methods (Amreich-Richter and sacrocolpo suspension) for the treatment of the central defect in descensus uteri as well as another method, pectopexy by Noé, which is easier and quicker to perform as well as quicker to learn.[11]

Experienced surgeons who excise large uteri know that after removal of a large uterus a relaxation of the middle compartment often occurs as the non-stressed ligaments are hypotrophic and cannot perform their function properly.

In summary, different concepts are available during laparoscopic hysterectomy for the conservation of important ligaments and the fixation and reconstruction of severed structures.

HOW TO LEARN LAPAROSCOPIC HYSTERECTOMY?

The TLH can be approached in many ways. This depends on the surgeon's skills and experience.[12,13] For a comprehensive overview of TLH and all other surgical procedures own for hysterectomy, we recommend you read our new book, *Hysterectomy—A Comprehensive Surgical Approach.*[14] Those who have already performed an LSH will encounter new techniques from step 4 onward.

For this reason, the TLH is described didactically in all its different steps:

1. Preparation for total laparoscopic hysterectomy
2. Placement of the trocars
3. Separation of the adnexa from the uterus or the pelvic wall
4. Dissection of the broad ligament
5. Dissection of the bladder peritoneum
6. Dissection of the uterine artery

7. Excision of the uterus
8. Retrieval of the uterus or morcellation
9. Vaginal closure
10. Conclusion of the operation.

Laparoscopically trained surgeons will already be familiar with some of these steps. According to surgeons' experience, during training insecurity begins at step 4 and ends at step 10. This makes it necessary to discuss each step of the TLH separately.

Step 1: Preparation for Total Laparoscopic Hysterectomy

When preparing for the TLH operation, the surgeon has to think through the indication and the intraoperative findings he expects to encounter. He has to take into consideration the weight of the patient, the presence of infections, endometriosis or adhesions. Focus lies on the variables directly related to hysterectomy.

How Large is the Uterus?

The size of uterus determines the placement and diameter of trocars.

Trocars (including the optic trocar) should be placed more cranially in cases of larger uteri. For further details refer to chapter "Laparoscopic Combined Hysterectomy Using the 'Changeover Technique' for Very Large Uterine Myomata."

The diameter of trocars is also very important. If uterus cannot or should not be removed through vagina, it must be morcellated.

The diameter of morcellator should match the size of the uterus. If the uterus cannot be removed vaginally, you should choose the largest morcellator to work efficiently.

Provided that the morcellator will later be used in the left lower area, a 10 mm instead of a 5 mm trocar can be primarily used. This can, for example, facilitate the insertion of a curved needle for vaginal closure.

These preoperative considerations with regard to trocars should enable a smooth operation with a higher efficiency. Surgeons at the Kiel School use three different trocar settings in their daily routine (Table 34.1). This is very important to give the assistant and nurse a feeling of security and minimize the materials used during the operation.

Assistance

The surgeon's working procedure depends significantly on the intraoperative assistance he receives.

If the assistant is inexperienced and at the beginning of his/her training period (camera holder), the surgeon is obliged to perform all of the operation steps himself. An inexperienced camera holder is fully occupied with holding the picture still, focusing the procedure in the middle of the screen, keeping the optic clean and making use of the advantages of a 30° optic during the operation. If an experienced surgeon is assisting, the operation steps can be divided between two surgeons. An experienced assistant can hold the camera and at the same time use the scissors or a grasper while the first surgeon, in addition to the left trocar, can also use a suprasymphyseal trocar for the right hand. For further details refer to chapter "Technique of Routine Total Laparoscopic

Table 34.1: A possible trocar setting.

Conditions	Optic trocar 30° (mm)	Lower left (mm)	Lower right (mm)	Advantages
Small uterus (work with bipolar coagulation and scissors)	5/10	5	5	Smallest possible trauma by the trocars, uterus transvaginally removed + No fascial stitches, less painful
Middle-sized uterus	5/10	10	5	Morcellator planned in the lower left region + Easy insertion of the curved needle
Large uterus	10	10	10	Morcellator planned, bilateral insertion of the tenaculum is possible + Possible insertion of different combi-instruments (NightKNIFE® 10 mm)

Hysterectomy with a Dissection of Uterine Vessels at Internal Iliac Level and Using a Uterine Manipulator."

Intrauterine Manipulator

The Hohl manipulator is a part of the Kiel School's standard setting (Fig. 34.1).

During the operation the manipulator can be moved either by the assistant or by the surgeon. The critical moment, when uterus is removed through vagina, requires precise interaction between the moving hand (left hand at the manipulator) and the cutting hand (right hand at the monopolar hook) (Fig. 34.2).

It is the surgeon's responsibility to guide the inexperienced assistant in the correct application of the manipulator. The surgeon should control and readjust the movement of manipulator during the procedure. Otherwise the overview and the safety of the operation will be endangered.

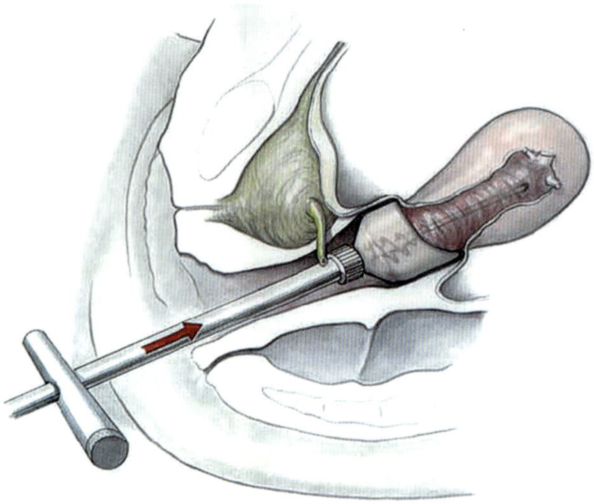

Fig. 34.1: Application of Hohl manipulator. Pushing adjacent structures away creates a secure plane for dissection.
Source: MK Hohl.

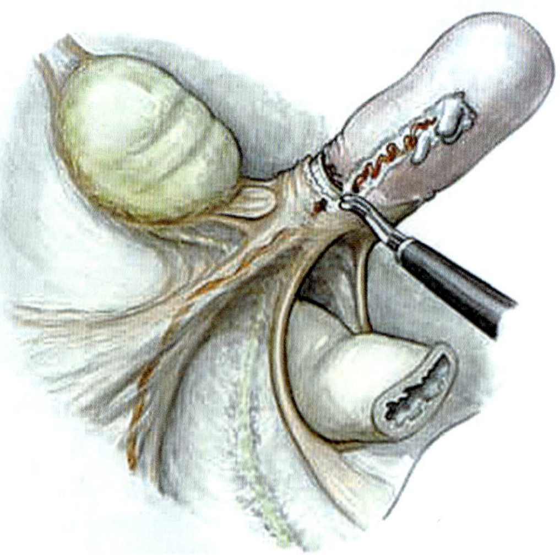

Fig. 34.2: Uterine artery appears separately and can be safely coagulated and ligated. The Hohl manipulator creates a sufficient distance from the urinary bladder.
Source: MK Hohl.

Mangeshikar Uterine Mobilizer

For the last two years we have preferred to use Mangeshikar manipulator, which presents essential advantages.

The Mangeshikar Uterine Mobilizer was developed with the idea of maximizing uterine manipulation in multiple axis or directions to facilitate excellent exposure for surgical dissection during the total laparoscopic hysterectomy and colpotomy (Fig. 34.3).

Is it Necessary to Use a Manipulator?

Every experienced surgeon knows that it is not mandatory to use a manipulator. Nevertheless, in Kiel surgeons have decided to use a manipulator for the following reasons:

- The Hohl manipulator is easy to handle, reusable and durable.
- The uterus can be moved in all directions (Fig. 34.4).
- The ceramic cap creates a flat surface to work on.
- There is very little or virtually no need for bladder dissection due to the manipulator's cap.
- After cesarean section, application of the manipulator for bladder dissection is useful and safe.
- Application of the manipulator imitates the classical movements during abdominal and vaginal hysterectomy so that the ureters are kept out of the operation field.
- The cap allows intrafascial hysterectomy, which preserves the ligaments and avoids vaginal shortening.

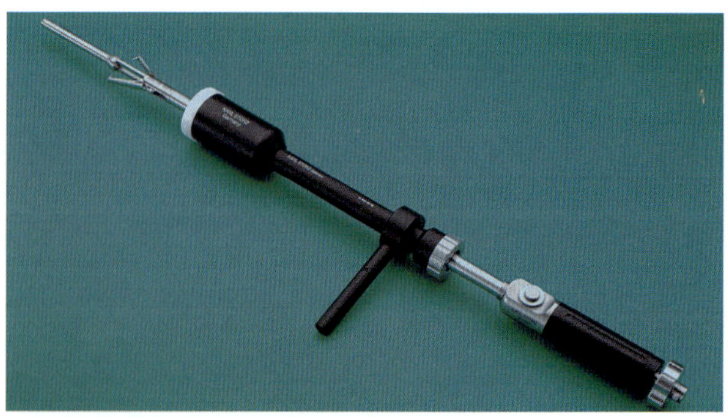

Fig. 34.3: Separation of the round ligament with NightKNIFE (BOWA, Gomaringen, Germany).

- The smooth cutting edge is useful during vaginal occlusion.

Points to be Considered

- Monopolar electricity can be used on the ceramic cap. Ultrasound destroys this apparatus
- Intrafascial hysterectomy causes a marked reduction in the size of the opening to the vagina because of the preservation of the circular ligaments. For this reason, larger-sized uteri have to be morcellated more frequently.

Ultimately, the advantages of application of the uterus manipulator outweigh any disadvantages.

Preparation (Insertion of the Adapter/ Manipulator)

Surgeons begin with an examination of the vaginal wall with speculum (exclusion of a fresh or undiscovered endometriosis).

After the disinfection of vagina, bladder evacuation or Foley catheter insertion, a vaginal examination is performed.

An assessment is made of the size, consistency and mobility of the uterus and the nature of adnexa. A careful examination of sacrouterine ligaments and palpation of the retrocervical area is also carried out.

Examination under anesthesia is a rapid, effective and inexpensive method, which allows further assessment of the patient in addition to the simple gynecological examination.

Next follows the insertion of the manipulator, which is technically easy. Two parameters are important: diameter of the cervix and length of the uterus. Once these measurements have been taken, the manipulator can be individually adapted (Video 34.2).

Step 2: Placement of the Trocars

The localization of trocars has been previously discussed. All trocars are to be placed under vision. Trocar systems are available that can be fixed into the abdominal wall to prevent their slipping and ensure a smooth procedure. These are especially recommended during long operations.

Step 3: Separation of the Adnexa from the Uterus or the Pelvic Sidewall

Following a 360° view of the operative field, the small intestine is elevated from the small pelvis in order to start hysterectomy. A prospective examination of the operation field, including the bladder surface, Douglas pouch and adnexa, should be carried out.

Preservation of the Adnexa: Begin on the right side. Push the uterus to the left to stretch the right adnexa.

Creating a Coagulation Mark: If you work with two 5-mm instruments, it is useful to make a coagulation mark on the right round ligament. The Manhes forceps can then grasp the uterus from the left without bleeding at that site.

Transection of the Round Ligament: The next step is to coagulate the middle of round ligament and separate it. Note that this has to be performed in two steps due to the presence of a small artery (Sampson's artery, a branch of the ovarian artery anastomosing with uterine artery) below the round ligament that also has to be coagulated (Fig. 34.4).

Separation of the Tubes: The fallopian tubes are coagulated and separated with coagulation of the underlying vessels to prevent excessive bleeding [ramus tubarius anastomoses with the rete ovarii under the tubes (Figs. 34.5A to D)].

Prophylactic excision of the fallopian tubes is discussed in a separate chapter.

Use of Sealing Instruments: The rest of the procedure depends on the instruments used. In the case of sealing instruments, it is sufficient to coagulate until you reach the cap of the manipulator. At this site the sealed double-layered peritoneum should

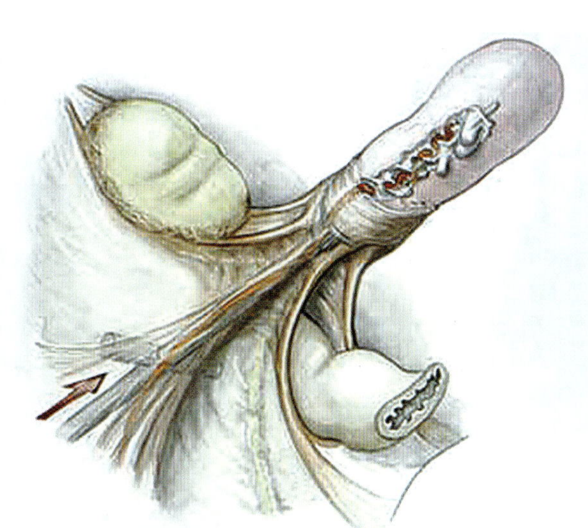

Fig. 34.4: By moving the Hohl manipulator the ligaments are clearly demonstrated and can be preserved during intrafascial hysterectomy.
Source: MK Hohl.

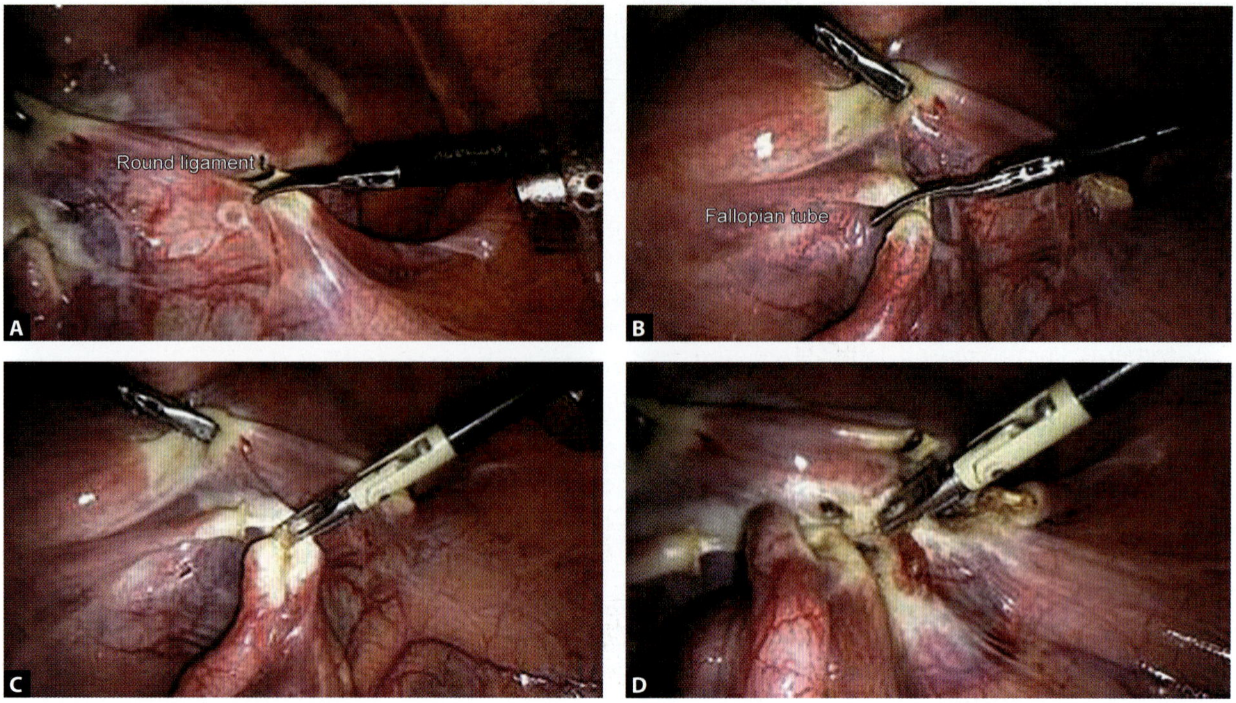

Figs. 34.5A to D: Division of the tube.

be reopened to undermine and separate the bladder peritoneum. You can then search for, coagulate and separate the ascending branch of the uterine artery.

With Adenectomy

Begin on the right side: push the uterus to the left to stretch the right adnexa.

The adnexa on the right side are pushed cranially from the left to stretch the ligamentum infundibulum pelvicum. Direct coagulation under the ovary gives wide and secure distance to the ureters. Further dissection of the ureters is not normally necessary.

If adhesions (resulting from infections or endometriosis) are apparent, the risk of ureter injury is very high and hence their visualization is very important.

Continue stretching the adnexa cranially, coagulating and excising the structures till the point of emergence of adnexa from uterus.

Adenectomy can be performed as a separate step at the beginning of operation to keep a clear view. At the end both adnexa are separately removed through vagina. The advantage lies in a better view of the retrouterine area.

Step 4: Dissection of the Broad Ligament

By using classical instruments, the broad ligament can be dissected and each leaf separately coagulated and excised.

During abdominal hysterectomy the surgeon always applies the clamp on the lower edge of uterus to prevent bleeding from the uterine artery. This is not the case in laparoscopic hysterectomy because the artery is kept safely in view and the surgeon keeps a clear distance away from it. Beginning the operation in the middle of the broad ligament creates a safe distance to the uterine artery.

One of the most important steps is when dissection of the broad ligament ends and identification and transection of the uterine artery begins (Figs. 34.6A to D).

Based on their experience with the LSH operation, surgeons in Kiel cranially coagulate the uterine artery before it divides into its uterine and vaginal branches.

The advantages can be summed up as follows:

- The operational direction is targeted lateral to the uterus. This direction is automatically away from and preserves the ureters and opening of broad ligament (Figs. 34.7A to D).
- Application of the Hohl manipulator distances the uterine artery from the ureters.
- The vessel stump, which is created, enables coagulation and ligation of possible uterine artery bleeding with prevention of thermal damage because of the safe distance to the ureters (Figs. 34.8A to D).
- The large dissection gap allows removal of uterus from vagina and prevents an accidental opening of the vessels already coagulated (Figs. 34.10 and 34.12).

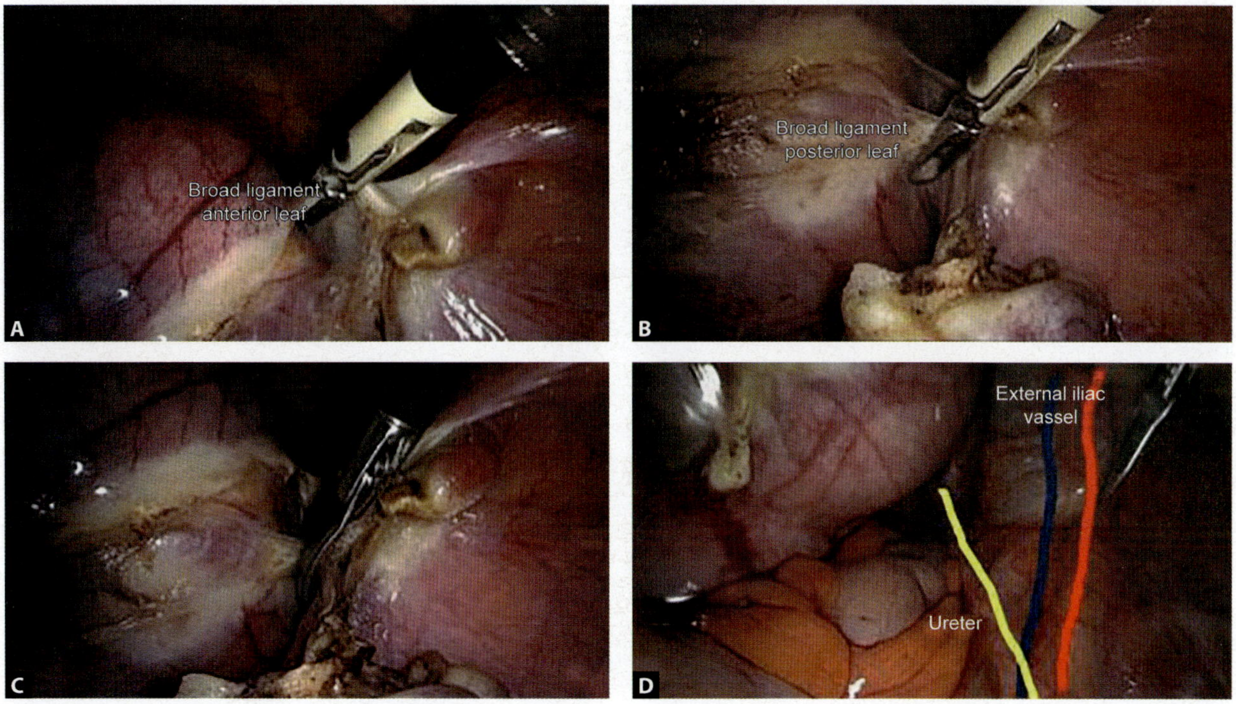

Figs. 34.6A to D: Division of the broad ligament.

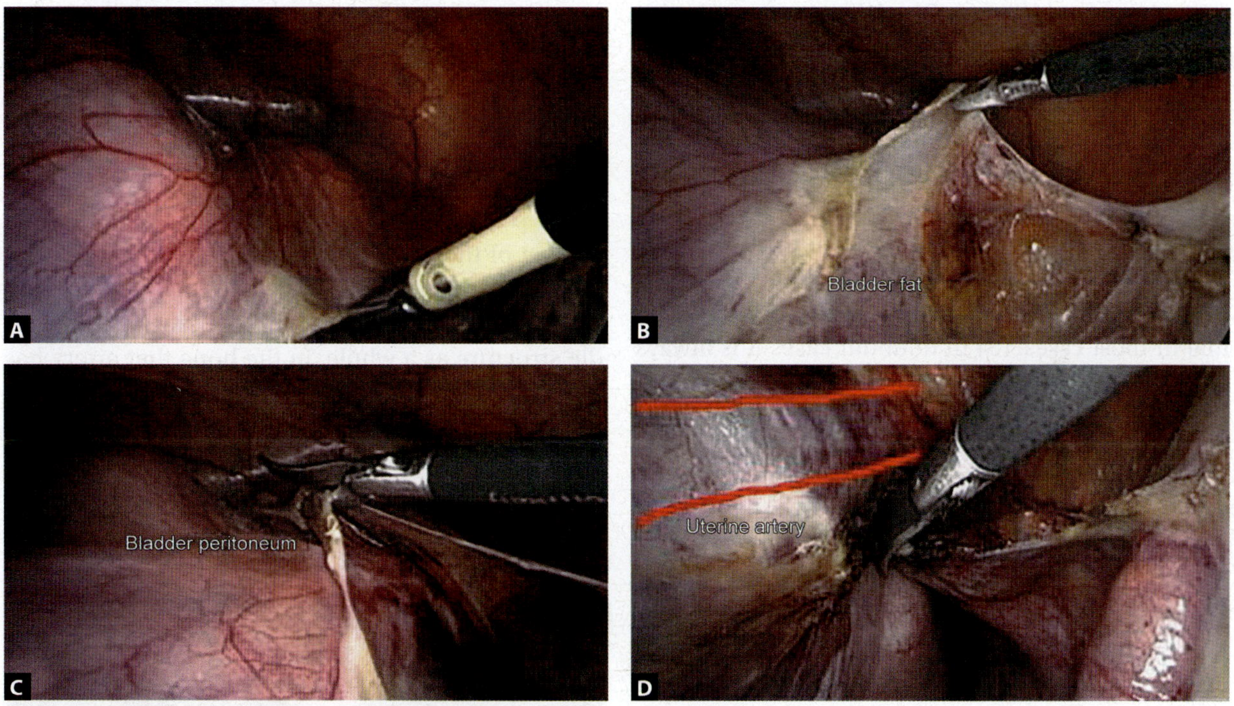

Figs. 34.7A to D: Coagulation of the uterine artery.

Step 5: Dissection of the Bladder Peritoneum

Urinary bladder dissection is not necessary in most TLH cases if the original method of TAIL^{TM}, according to Hohl, is applied. Nevertheless, it should be explained here because it can be necessary in cases after cesarean section and it involves an increased risk of bladder injury if the following points are neglected.

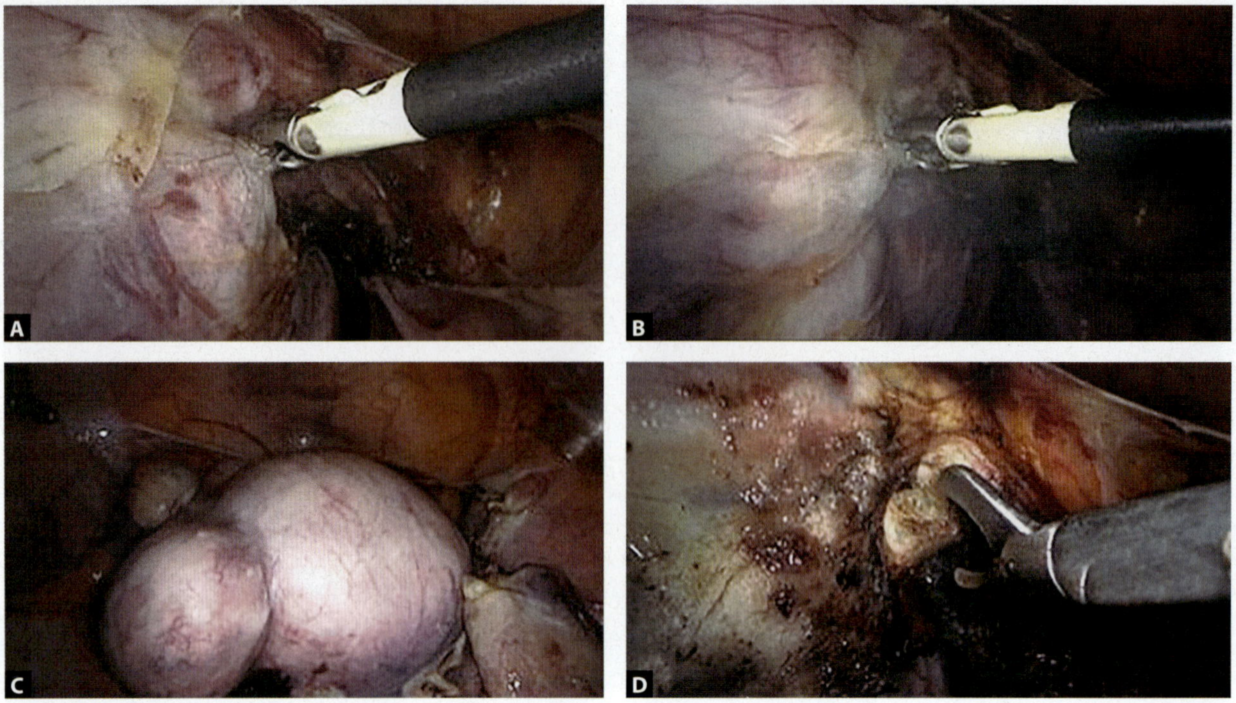

Figs. 34.8A to D: Opening of the bladder peritoneum.

Viewing the Urinary Bladder

Exposing the urinary bladder may be problematic for inexperienced surgeons. The first steps, however, are relatively simple and not dangerous. (1) First, the Hohl manipulator can be retracted slightly backward. The cranial edge of the urinary bladder should then be visible. (2) After restoring the normal anatomy urinary bladder can be moved cranially using a blunt instrument. The upper edge of bladder becomes visible in most cases. (3) In doubtful cases it is always possible to fill the urinary bladder with fluid, preferably methylene blue, to promptly detect and correct bladder defects in cases of massive adhesions.

Urinary Bladder Dissection

Urinary bladder dissection should be done with sharp scissors and not bluntly (Fig. 34.7). Minimize the use of electricity to prevent thermal injury to the bladder wall. Scissor dissection requires an exact mastery of anatomy, but allows a layer-specific dissection. Hold the scissors with the tip facing the vaginal edge, namely from above to below. However, the most important step is bladder elevation, which is performed with a blunt object holding both the bladder and its peritoneum. Only then can you detach the bladder centrally from the anterior vaginal wall. The advantage of this dissection is that there is sufficient tissue for vaginal occlusion at the end of the procedure.

Step 6: Dissection of the Uterine Artery

A key point of the TLH is the coagulation and dissection of the ascending uterine artery. During this procedure the vessel should always be under vision (Fig. 34.9). Total coagulation of tissue-vessel bundle structure as a whole, in the hope that artery has been coagulated, has many disadvantages. It spoils the surgeon's chance to gain a good overview of the anatomy. In cases of thick bundle structures the electrical energy is insufficient to coagulate the vessel tissue bundle at once which sometimes makes

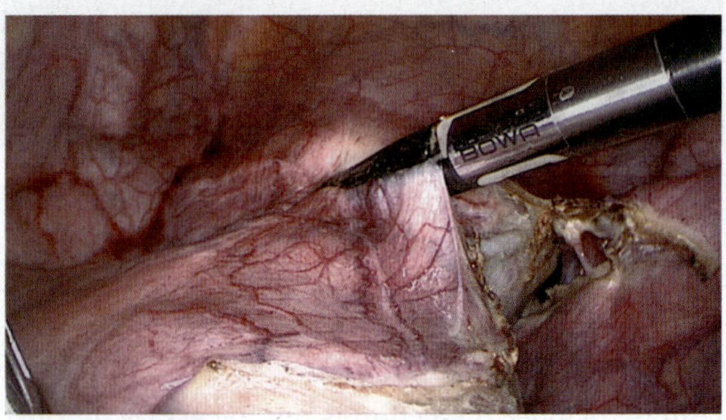

Fig. 34.9: Cutting of the uterine artery.

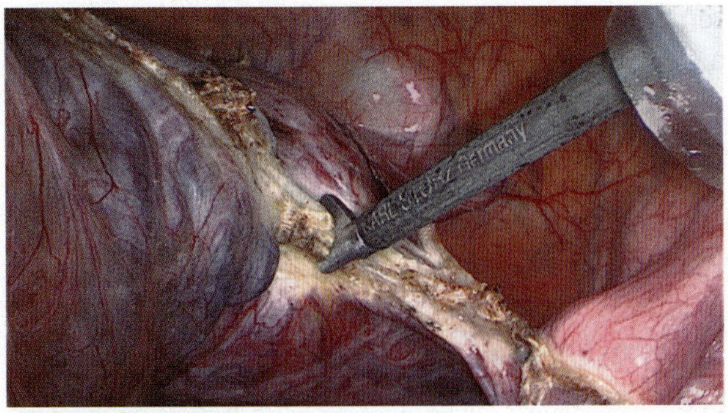

Fig. 34.10: Well-prepared gap and landmark for opening the vagina on the left side.

it necessary to repeatedly coagulate and dissect the bundle structures.

If you have the impression that diathermy is not working effectively during coagulation, it is probably due to dryness and electrolyte depletion in the tissue. A current flow is then no longer possible. The answer is to moisten or cautiously wash with a saline solution. The effect is immediately noticed after further coagulation.

Make sure to additionally coagulate retrograde to prevent excessive bleeding from the uterus.

After sufficient coagulation the artery can be cut-off with one clean stroke (Figs. 34.9 and 34.10). The vessel is always easy to identify later on by its clean, smooth cut surface. Afterward, proceed in the same way to dissect the accompanying vein, usually the venous plexus. Thorough and careful dissection prevents unnecessary bleeding during excision of the uterus.

A complete interruption of the uterine blood supply is recognized by a blue discoloration.

Step 7: Excision of the Uterus

The Hohl manipulator provides several advantages during excision of the uterus out of the vagina. In addition to the previously described aspects with modification of the anatomical structures (forcing back of the ureters), vagina is not shortened as the curved cap adapts to vaginal anatomy. It is also possible to use the monopolar hook and work safely and effectively. Minimal lateral usage of electrical energy prevents further damage of the vaginal epithelium and decreases the risk of delayed wound healing at the vaginal end.

Surgeons begin at 12 o'clock position while observing the urinary bladder (Fig. 34.11). First, dissect to the right. If the surgeon is holding the manipulator, he only has to make minimal movements and can fix the monopolar hook.

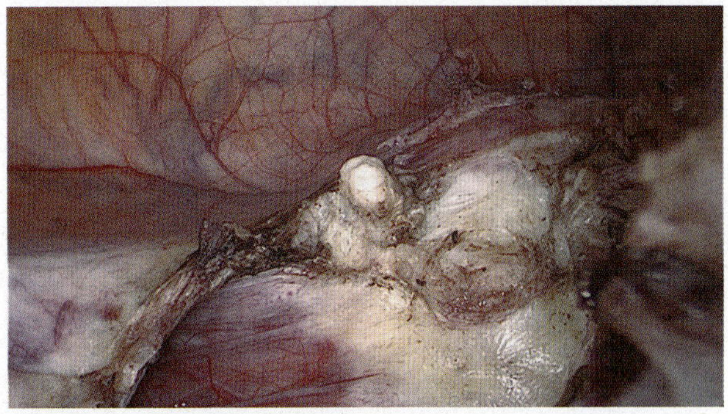

Fig. 34.11: Opening of the vagina with monopolar hook.

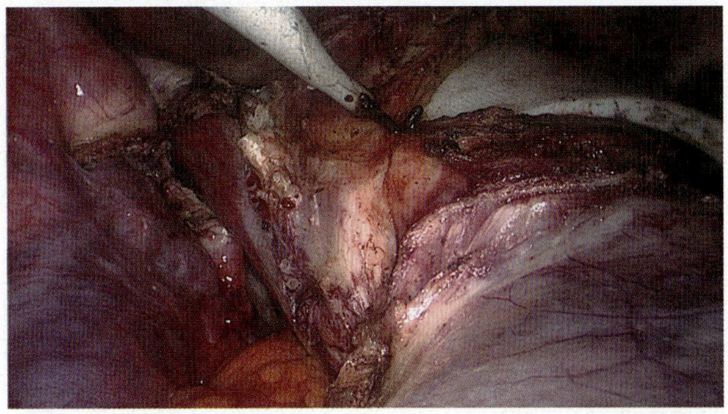

Fig. 34.12: Opening of the vagina using the gap and landmarks.

Continue in cranial direction, exactly in the middle of both stumps of the cut uterine artery branch (Fig. 34.12).

Now, you can slightly rotate the manipulator to keep working at the highest point and hence create the described platform, which enables a clean preparation.

By now you will have reached the insertion site of the sacrouterine ligament on the right side. Here, it is important to continue opening the vagina from its cranial aspect to preserve the ligamentous structure and provide a good suspension of the vaginal end. The ligaments are not separated as is the case with classical hysterectomy.

Further excision is done till the middle. The monopolar hook is then put on the left side and the process of starting at 12 o'clock position is repeated on the left till you reach the point of dissection.

Step 8: Retrieval or Morcellation of the Uterus?

Retrieval of the Uterus

Small and medium-sized uteri are pulled into vaginal canal for removal (Fig. 34.13). Vagina is then closed gas-tight and pneumoperitoneum is maintained.

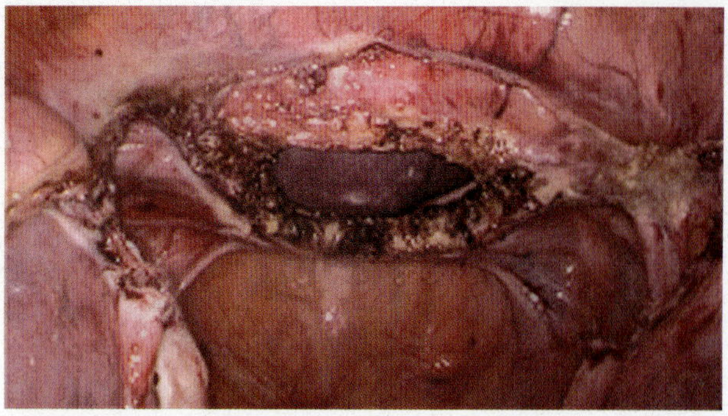

Fig. 34.13: Withdrawal of the uterus and deposition in the vagina.

If uterus is very small and cannot produce a gas-tight seal, it can be removed. A glove filled with two three swabs fulfills this function after being moistened and placed in vagina. In many cases the proportion of vaginal opening and the size of uterus do not allow primary removal of uterus.

You then have to decide, as after a vaginal hysterectomy, how uterus is to be removed. Laparoscopic morcellation is usually the quicker and easier solution.

Forced vaginal removal of uterus is associated with an increased risk of excessive bleeding necessitating repeated uterine vessel or vaginal wall coagulation.

Morcellation of Uterus

In cases of large uteri that cannot be taken out transvaginally intraabdominal piecemeal removal is necessary. A morcellator is then used. In Kiel, surgeons use the Rotocut G1 (Karl Storz, Tuttlingen, Germany).

Pay careful attention during intraabdominal use of an instrument with a rotating knife. The surgeon should always have the tip of the apparatus under vision throughout the whole procedure to avoid accidental bowel injury. This is relatively challenging for the camera holder.

Morcellator can be inserted from the lower left region; sometimes the incision must be widened under visual control. The blunted tip of the mandarin can be applied nontraumatically.

When inserting the Rotocut G1 in the left lower abdomen, it is possible, due to its construction, to place it on the abdominal wall. The design of the sleeve provides a good control of the instrument on the surface of uterine fibroids or the uterus.

A continuous movement of the forceps at a constant speed of the blade allows a maximum profit of removed tissue. Tissue avulsion usually occurs when a change in consistency takes place (from fibroid to myometrium or vice versa).

At the end of the morcellation process it is essential to thoroughly remove even the smallest tissue residues. A thorough stitching of the fascia closes the vaginal incision.

Step 9: Vaginal Closure

Laparoscopic vaginal closure is one of the most difficult steps of the TLH for beginners for the following reasons:

- The awkward blunt angle between the vertical opening of the vagina and the instruments (needle holder)
- The resulting even more awkward angle between the fixed needle and the vertical stitching area
- The relatively wide distance/depth of the operative field
- Lack of skill in suturing and knotting.

After cautious coagulation of the vaginal edge, suturing can begin. Surgeons mainly use a curved needle and polydioxanone (PDS) 2-0 for single-knot suturing with extracorporeal knots and intracorporeal safety knots for the following reasons:

- The monofilament thread easily slides through the tissues and does not cause additional damage.
- The monofilament PDS material minimizes the risk of vaginal infection.
- The long half-life of the thread prevents the risk of early vaginal dehiscence.
- Extracorporeal knots provide extra strength.

Corner Stitch: Surgeons first begin with the right corner stitch piercing the pericervical ring, followed by the corresponding vaginal epithelium. Surgeons pierce away from urinary bladder to minimize the risk of bladder injury during suturing (Fig. 34.14).

During the second step the needle passes through medial aspect of the cardinal ligament in front of the

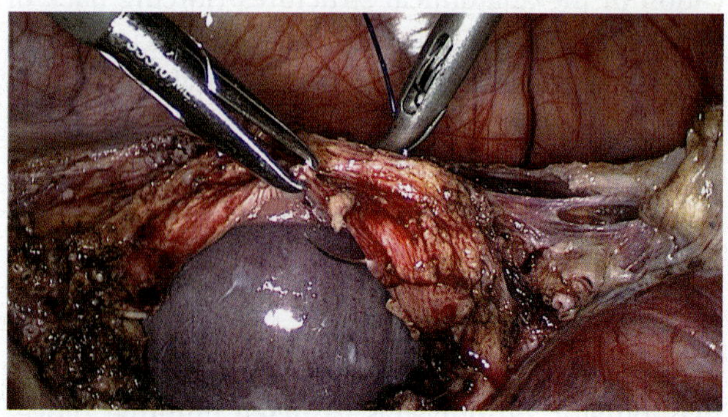

Fig. 34.14: First corner stitch on the right.

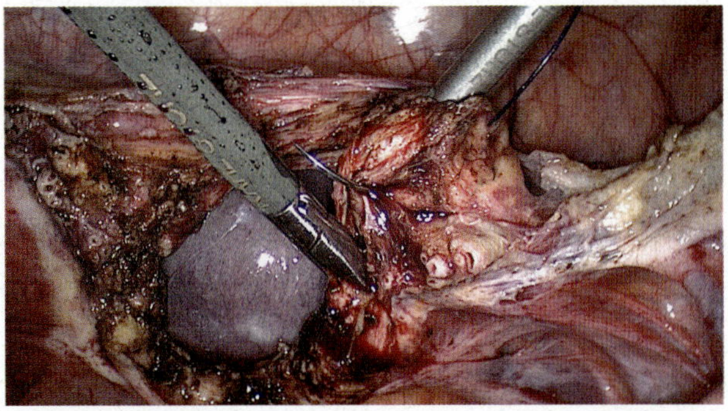

Fig. 34.15: Second corner stitch on the right side through the medial part of the cardinal ligament. Modified suture by van Herendael.

uterine vessels (Fig. 34.15). The second step involves the structures supporting vaginal wall suspension. Subsequent back stitching of the vagina is followed by passing the needle through vaginal epithelium and then in the third step through the sacrouterine ligament. The last step involves piercing the ligament once or twice to shorten it. This is not necessary in cases without prolapse.

The needle can now be withdrawn and the suture is completed with an extracorporeal Roeder knot, secured by two or three intracorporeal knots (Fig. 34.16).

The procedure is repeated on the contralateral side (Fig. 34.17).

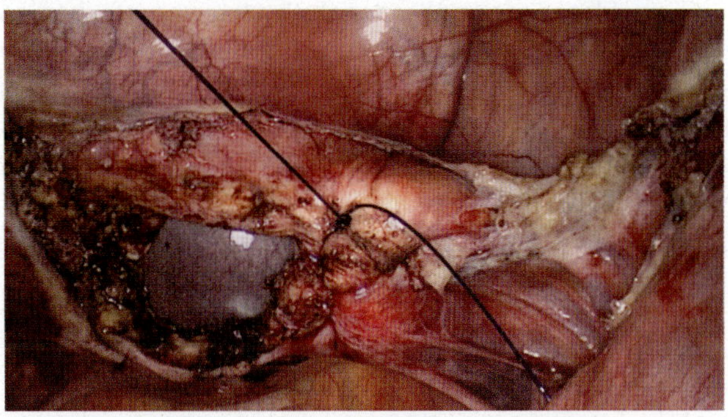

Fig. 34.16: Right corner suture at vaginal cuff closure.

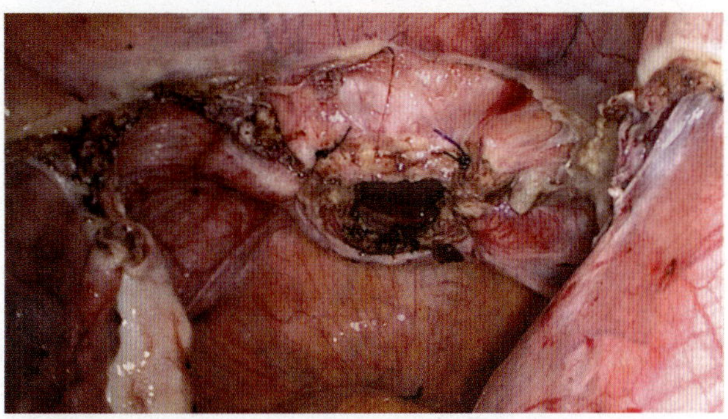

Fig. 34.17: Right and left corner suture of vaginal cuff closure associated.

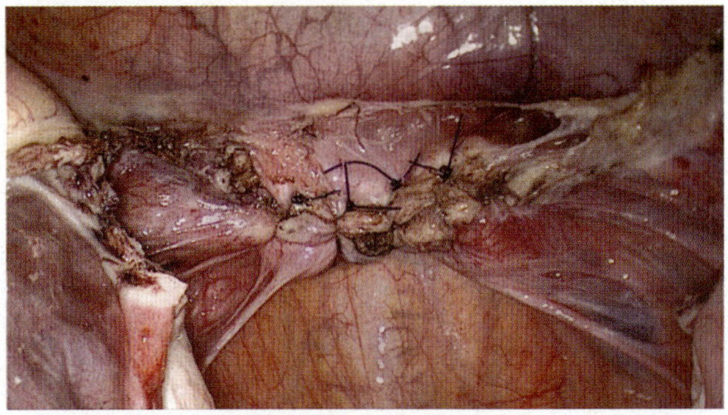

Fig. 34.18: Closed vaginal cuff by extracorporeal knotting technique.

The remaining vaginal opening can be closed with two Z-stitches. These guarantee both vertical and horizontal compression of tissues and minimize the risk of vaginal hematoma formation (Fig. 34.18).

Neither peritonealization nor drainage is required. If still inside, uterus or tampoon glove should be removed from vagina.

Step 10: Conclusion of the Operation

At the end of the operation, a 360° view of the whole operative field is carried out to detect and remove any possibly scattered material after morcellation. The peritoneum can now be irrigated to remove any remaining blood and to assure hemostasis at all sites.

Before removing the instruments, the urine output should be checked for flow and presence of blood.

The instruments can be removed after checking all incisions.

Peritoneum is first closed with the bipolar forceps and then fascia is closed with single-knot Vicryl stitches under visual control, followed by its skin sutures.

CONCLUSION

General

- Preliminary considerations before surgery takes place: indications, personal setting (camera holder, assistant)
- Make use of the opportunity to examine the patient under anesthesia to avoid unpleasant surprises.
- Check the intraoperative instrument setting.
- Minimize the number of instruments.
- Insert a manipulator, instruct the beginner and control the manipulator during the operation.

During the Procedure

- Beginning in the middle part of the round ligament ensures a safe distance to the ascending uterine vessels and markedly reduces the risk of bleeding
- A clean cutting of the uterine artery leaves clearly visible stumps
- Urinary bladder dissection only if necessary and then with sharp scissors
- Use a manipulator. It makes the operation easier, lowers the risk of injury and allows the preservation of ligament structures
- Practice suturing and knotting for vaginal closure on a suitable model before the operation
- Always keep the morcellator in the field of vision to prevent bowel injuries.

REFERENCES

1. Hohl MK, Hauser N. Safe total intrafascial laparoscopic (TAIL) hysterectomy: a prospective cohort study. Gynecol Surg. 2010;7(3):231-9.
2. Donnez O, Donnez J. A series of 400 laparoscopic hysterectomics for benign disease: a single centre, single surgeon prospective study of complications confirming previous retrospective study. BJOG. 2010;117(6): 752-5.
3. Nieboer TE, Johnson N, Lethaby A, et al. Surgical approach to hysterectomy for benign gynecological disease. Cochrane Database Syst Rev. 2009;(3): CD003677.
4. Brummer TH, Seppälä TT, Härkki PS. National learning curve for laparoscopic hysterectomy and trends in hysterec- tomy in Finland 2000-2005. Hum Reprod. 2008;23(4):840-5.
5. Hirst A, Dutton S, Wu O, et al. A multi-center retrospective cohort study comparing the efficacy, safety and cost- effectiveness of hysterectomy and uterine artery embolisation for the treatment of symptomatic uterine fibroids. The HOPEFUL study. Health Technol Assess. 2008;12(5):1-248.
6. Semm K. Hysterectomy via laparotomy or pelviscopy. A new CASH method without colpotomy. Geburtshilfe Frauenheilkd. 1991;51(12):996-1003.
7. Mettler L, Sammur W, Schollmeyer T. Hysterectomy for uterine disease in 2010: from past to future. Clinical Medicine Insights: Reproduc Health. 2010;4: 7-22.
8. Semm K. [CISH (pelviscopic intrafascial hysterectomy–without colpotomy), TUMA (total uterine mucosa ablation) and IVH (intrafascial vaginal hysterectomy)]. Gynakologe. 1993;26(6):378-84.
9. Cruikshank SH, Kovac SR. Randomized comparison of three surgical methods used at the time of vaginal hysterectomy to prevent posterior enterocele. Am J Obstet Gynecol. 1999;180(4):859-65.
10. RCOG. Management of Posthysterectomy Vaginal Vault Prolapse. Green-top Guideline, 2007.
11. van Herendael B. Strategies to prevent vaginal vault descent during hysterectomy. In: Mettler L (Ed). Manual of New Hysterectomy Techniques. New Delhi: Jaypee Brothers Medical Publishers (P) Ltd; 2007. pp. 82-5.
12. Banerjee C, Noé KG. Laparoscopic pectopexy: a new technique of prolapse surgery for obese patients. Arch Gynecol Obstet. 2011;284(3):631-5.
13. Elessawy M, Schollmeyer T, Mettler L, et al. The incidence of complications by hysterectomy for benign disease in correlation to an assumed preoperative score. Gynecol Obstet. 2015;292(1): 127-33.
14. Alkatout L, Mettler L, editors. Hysterectomy: A Comprehensive Surgical Approach. Cham, Switzerland: Springer; 2017.

Stepwise Approach to Total Laparoscopic Hysterectomy

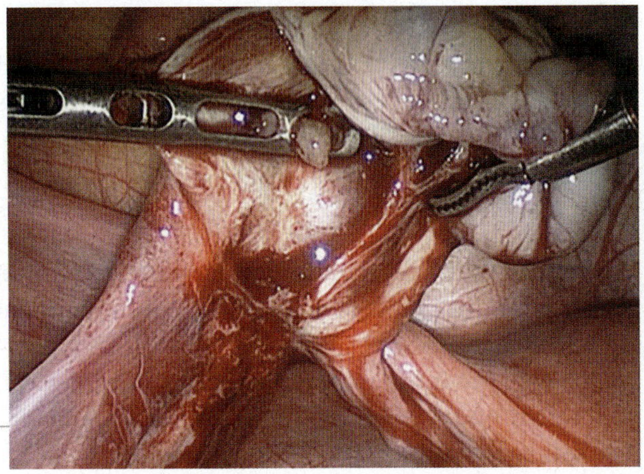

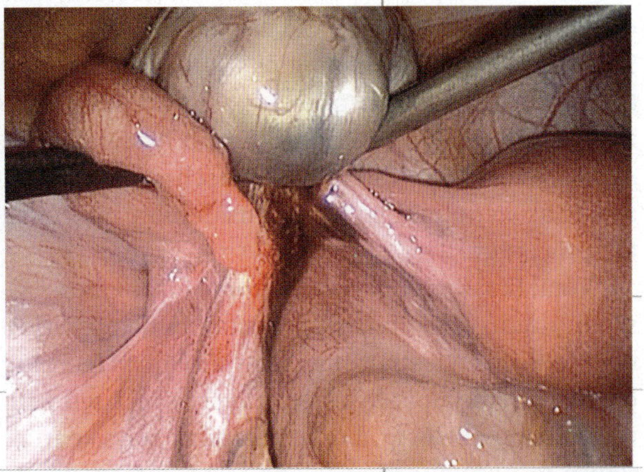

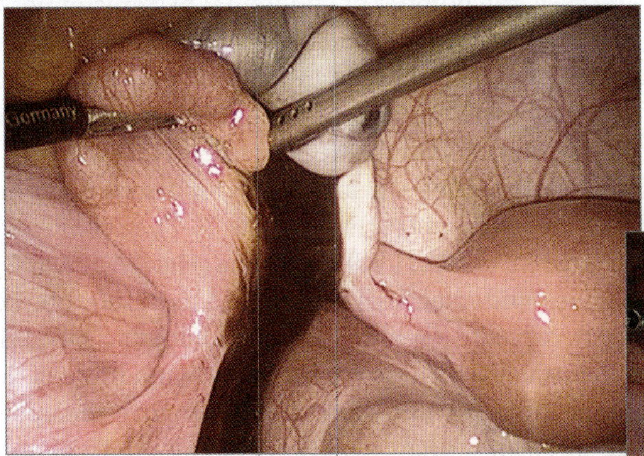

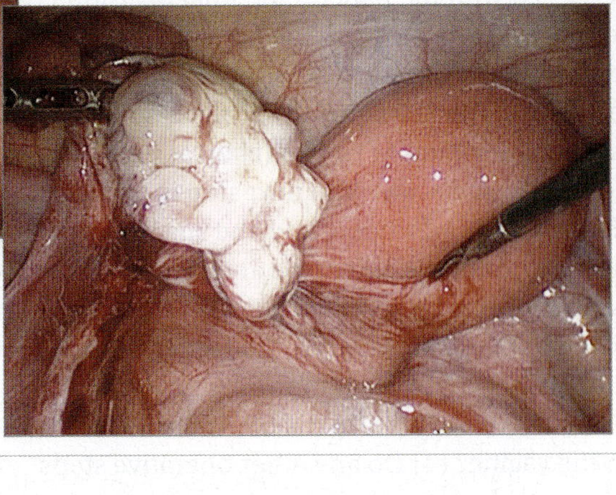

Chapter 35

Stepwise Approach to Total Laparoscopic Hysterectomy

Ibrahim Alkatout, Liselotte Mettler

BACKGROUND

The basic concept of laparoscopic hysterectomy was developed by Kurt Semm and Liselotte Mettler in the 1980s. However, the instruments and techniques used at the time (endotherm and loop) did not keep pace with the development of intrafascial hysterectomy. Advancements in instruments, technical support and consistent training have considerably improved the procedure.

Total laparoscopic hysterectomy for the normal-sized uterus has become a standard operation with low complication rates and a regular learning curve. Laparoscopic hysterectomy is associated with reduced blood loss, shorter hospital stays, earlier return to normal activities and fewer infections. Its major advantage over vaginal hysterectomy is the possibility to simultaneously treat comorbidities, such as endometriosis or adhesions. Laparoscopic supracervical/subtotal hysterectomy is a useful alternative. Its advantages and disadvantages need to be discussed with the patient; the final decision is made jointly by the doctor and the patient.

Antibiotic prophylaxis should be given for all types of hysterectomy. The first step is a correct assessment of the size and location of uterus (clinical examination and ultrasound scan). The next step is to determine the positions of trocars and the manipulator. The following questions have to be answered: (1) Are disposable instruments required? (2) Are more than two ancillary trocars necessary? What trocar diameter should be used and what is the best location? (3) Is morcellation necessary or can the uterus be removed through the vagina? (4) Do any other operative steps have to be considered, such as the treatment of endometriosis, adnexal masses, or adhesions? (5) How is the vaginal cuff to be closed?

Oophorectomy and/or salpingectomy should be considered; their advantages and disadvantages should be included in the patient's counseling.

INTRODUCTION

Hysterectomy is one of the most frequently performed operations in gynecological surgery. International gynecological societies recommend vaginal hysterectomy as the most acceptable technique. However, operative endoscopic methods have gained widespread acceptance in the last two decades, and play a much more important role than the traditional approaches of abdominal and vaginal hysterectomy. With regard to hysterectomies performed for benign disease, the number of abdominal hysterectomies is decreasing, the number of vaginal hysterectomies varies, but laparoscopic and robotic-assisted laparoscopic procedures are on the increase,[1] the trend is visible throughout the world (Fig. 35.1).[2]

The most frequent indications for hysterectomy are uterine leiomyomas (Figs. 35.2 to 35.7), adenomyosis (Figs. 35.8 to 35.11), adenomyoma (Figs. 35.12A to D), diffuse endometriosis (Figs. 35.13 to 35.18), uterine prolapse, and therapy-resistant idiopathic bleeding abnormalities. These constitute 60% and more of the indications for hysterectomy.[3] Alternative therapeutic strategies, such as uterine artery embolization or focused ultrasound therapy have been developed in Germany[4] and other countries[5] over the last ten years. Conservative operative management and the introduction of ulipristal acetate have reduced the number of hysterectomies. Hysterectomy rates depend not only on the indication but also on the age group, family planning and the centers at which the patients are treated. The indications for hysterectomy in general have now been adapted to the patients' wish to

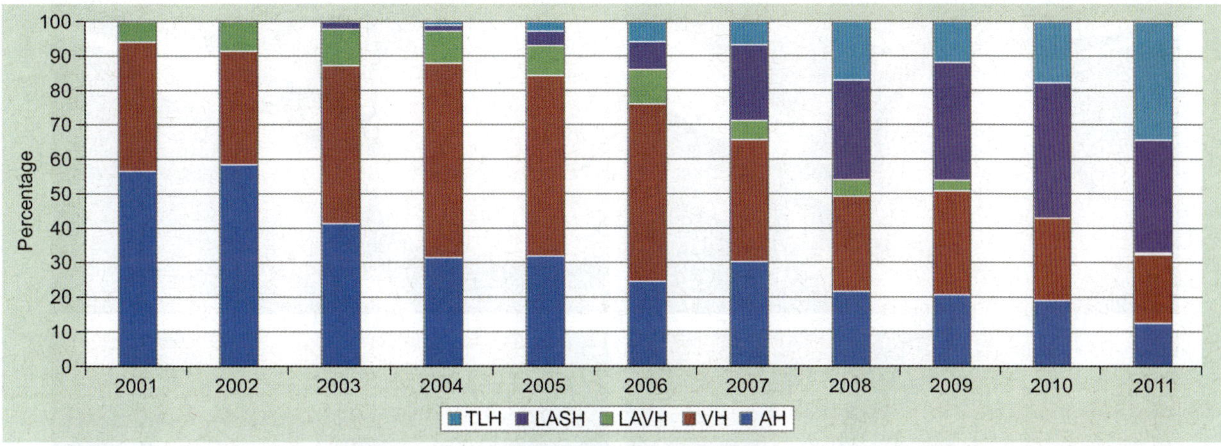

Fig. 35.1: Development of surgical techniques from 2002 to 2010 at the department of obstetrics and gynecology, University of Kiel, Germany.

Abbreviations: AH: Abdominal hysterectomy; LAVH: Laparoscopically assisted vaginal hysterectomy; LSH: Laparoscopic supracervical hysterectomy; TLH: Total laparoscopic hysterectomy; VH: Vaginal hysterectomy.

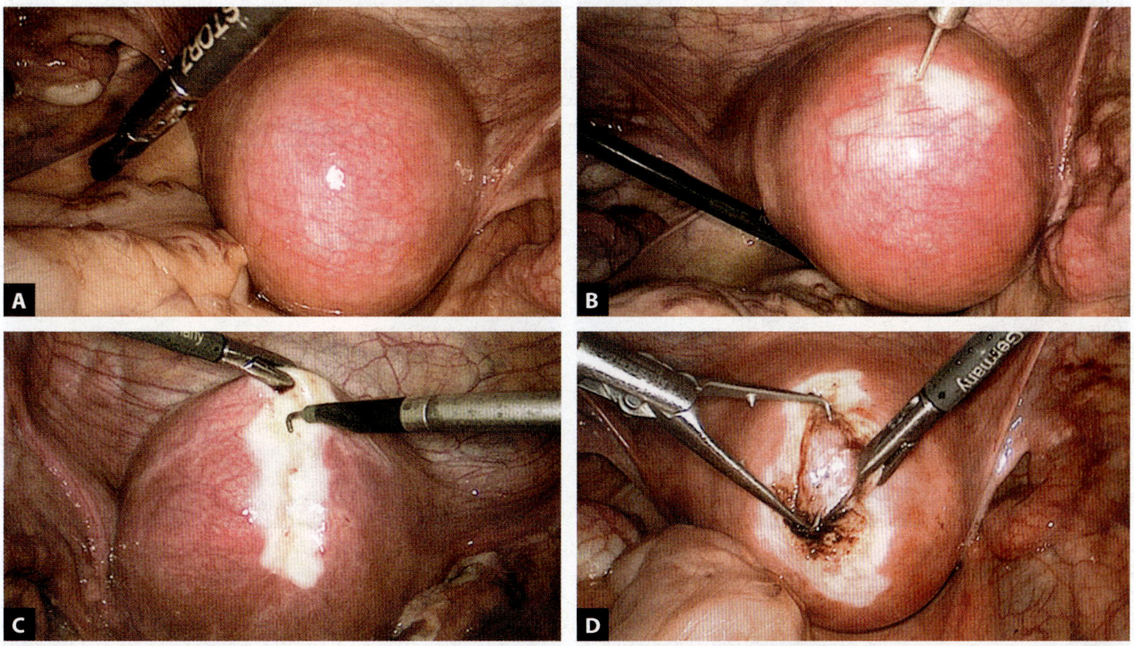

Figs. 35.2A to D: Laparoscopic myoma enucleation. (A) Situs of a fundal/anterior wall fibroid; (B) Prophylactic hemostasis with 1:100 diluted vasopressin solution (Gylcylpressin) in separate wells between the superficial and healthy tissue of the myometrium, and the capsule/fibroid surface. The purpose of the injection is to separate the pseudocapsule from the fibroid and reduce bleeding; (C) Bipolar superficial coagulation of the longitudinal incision strip and opening the uterine wall above the myoma with a monopolar hook or needle until one reaches the myoma; (D) Grasping the fibroid and starting the enucleation. The pseudocapsule remains within the uterine wall and is pushed off bluntly.

retain their uterus.[6,7] Hysterectomy is also performed for malignant diseases of the inner genital organs (endometrium or cervix, ovaries and fallopian tube). Endoscopic surgery is only performed for endometrium and cervical cancer. Table 35.1 summarizes the indications for hysterectomy.

Once the decision to perform hysterectomy has been made, the physician and patient must decide whether the procedure will be performed abdominally, vaginally or with laparoscopic or robotic

Table 35.1: Five major diagnostic categories that constitute indications for hysterectomy.
• Uterine leiomyomas
• Endometriosis and adenomyosis uteri
• Pelvic organ prolapse
• *Pelvic pain or infection (other than endometriosis):* pelvic inflammatory disease, adhesions
• Abnormal uterine bleeding of known and unknown origin
• Malignant and premalignant disease

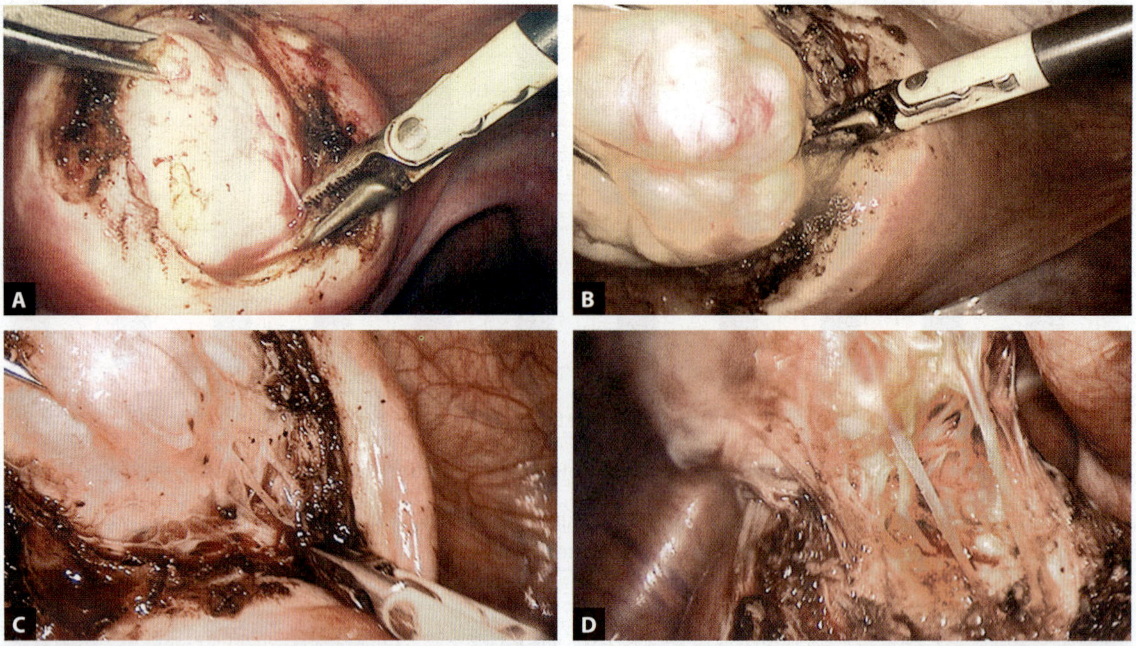

Figs. 35.3A to D: Laparoscopic myoma enucleation. (A) Traction of the fibroid with a tenaculum and blunt demarcation from the capsule; (B) Focal bipolar coagulation of basic vessels; (C) Continuous enucleation of the fibroid under traction and specific coagulation of capsule fibers containing vessels; (D) Magnification of the remaining capsule fibers to be coagulated and cut.

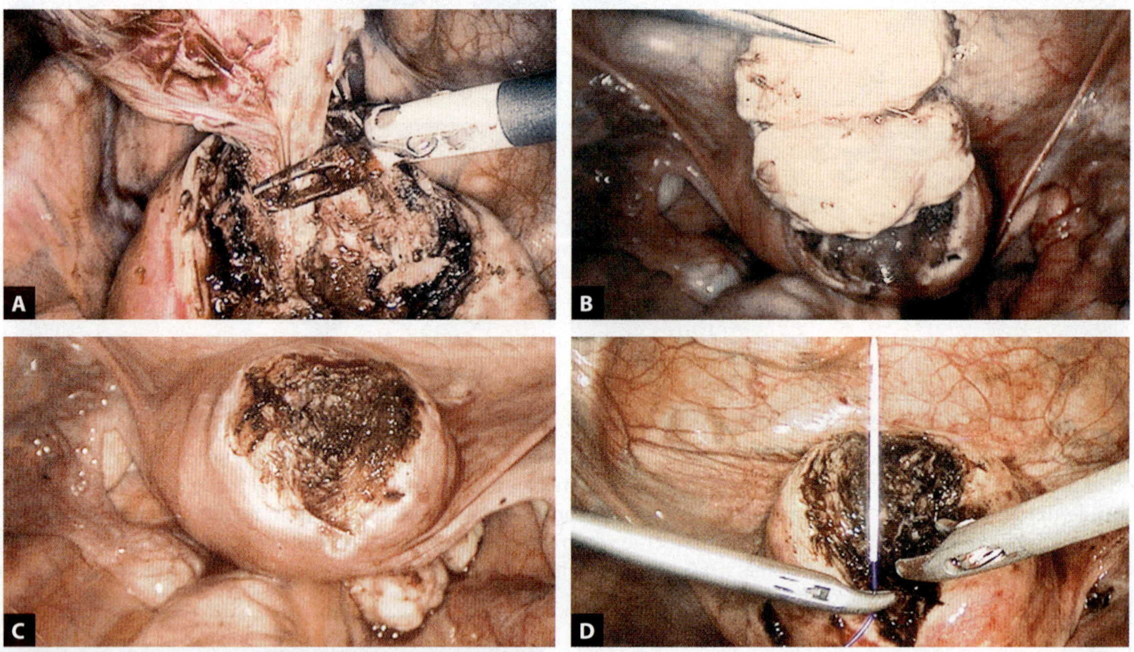

Figs. 35.4A to D: Laparoscopic myoma enucleation. (A) Final coagulation of the capsule vessels; (B) Double belly fibroid after complete enucleation; (C) Minimal coagulation of bleeding vessels under suction and irrigation; (D) Approximation of the wound edges with a straight or round sharp needle and a monofilar late-absorbable suture.

assistance.[8-10] Each of these approaches has its advantages and disadvantages, which must be explained to the patient (Fig. 35.19). The surgeon's familiarity with the technique and the economic resources of the hospital are also important considerations (Table 35.2).

The foremost advantage of endoscopic treatment is the fact that the surgeon is able to address other intraabdominal comorbidities simultaneously, such as endometriosis or severe adenomyosis in the adjacent organs (sacrouterine ligaments, cardinal

Table 35.2: Vaginal versus abdominal versus laparoscopic hysterectomy. Robot-assisted laparoscopic hysterectomy is included in the category of laparoscopic hysterectomies.

Vaginal hysterectomy compared to abdominal hysterectomy	
Advantages	Shorter hospitalization (mean difference 1 day, 95% CI 0.7–1.2)
	More rapid return to normal activities (mean difference 9.5 days, 95% CI 6.4–12.6)
	Fewer infections or fever (OR 0.42, 95% CI 0.21–0.83)
	Possibility of regional anesthesia
Disadvantages	No simultaneous surgery of comorbidities
	More difficulties in simultaneous adnexal surgery
Laparoscopic hysterectomy compared to abdominal hysterectomy	
Advantages	Less blood loss (mean difference 45.3 mL, 95% CI 17.9–72.7)
	Shorter hospital stay (mean difference 2 days, 95% CI 1.9–2.2)
	More rapid return to normal activities (mean difference 13.6 days, 95% CI 11.8–15.4)
	Fewer wound infections or fever (OR 0.32, 95% CI 0.12–0.85)
Disadvantages	Longer operating times (mean difference 10.6 min, 95% CI 7.4–13.8)
	More urinary tract injuries (OR 2.61, 95% CI 1.22–5.60)
Laparoscopic hysterectomy compared to vaginal hysterectomy	
Advantages	Simultaneous surgery for comorbidities
	Almost independent of the preoperative assessment
Disadvantages	Similar outcomes except longer operating times (mean difference 41.5 min, 95% CI 33.7–49.4)
	More expensive

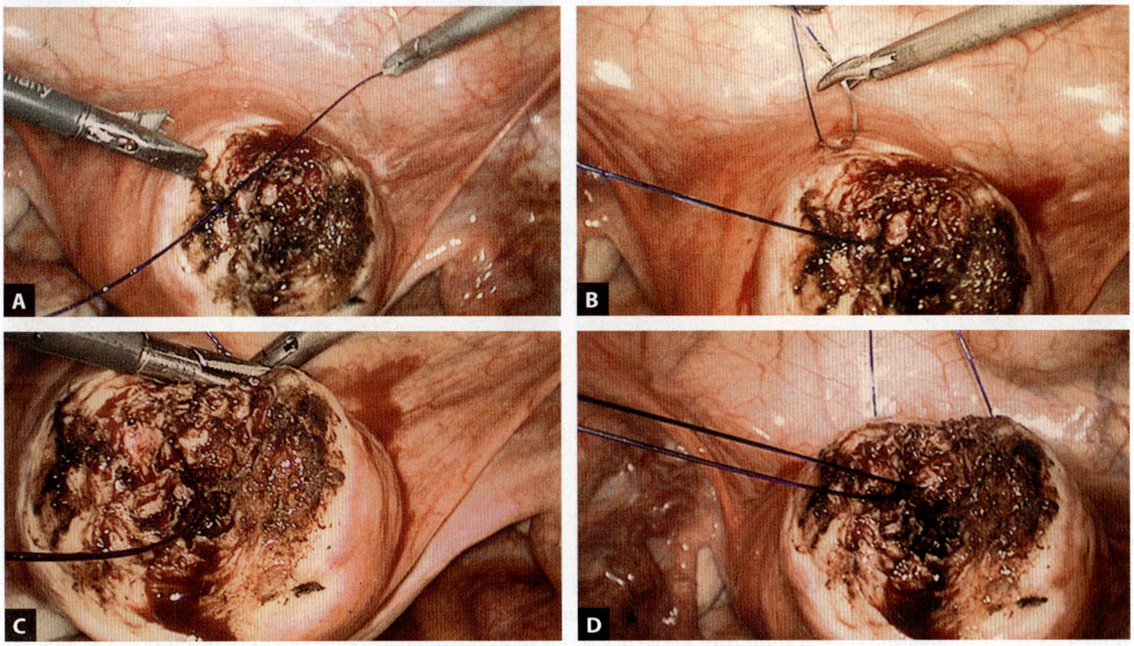

Figs. 35.5A to D: Laparoscopic myoma enucleation. Advantages of a circular needle stitch. (A) The wound angle is elevated safely and completely when raised with a Manhes forceps; (B) Deeper layers of the myometrium can be grasped more easily with a circular needle; (B) Needle exit and simplified re-grasping with the right needle holder; (C) Final stitch to invert the knot; (D) Extirpation of the needle, completing the extracorporeal knot, and preparing to push down the extracorporeal knot.

ligament, bladder and/or bowel), as well as adhesions. Although uterine-preserving operative strategies are still controversially discussed and the results are not consistently promising, the only reliable treatment for adenomyosis is total hysterectomy. Since the disease is confined to uterus, ovaries can be preserved.

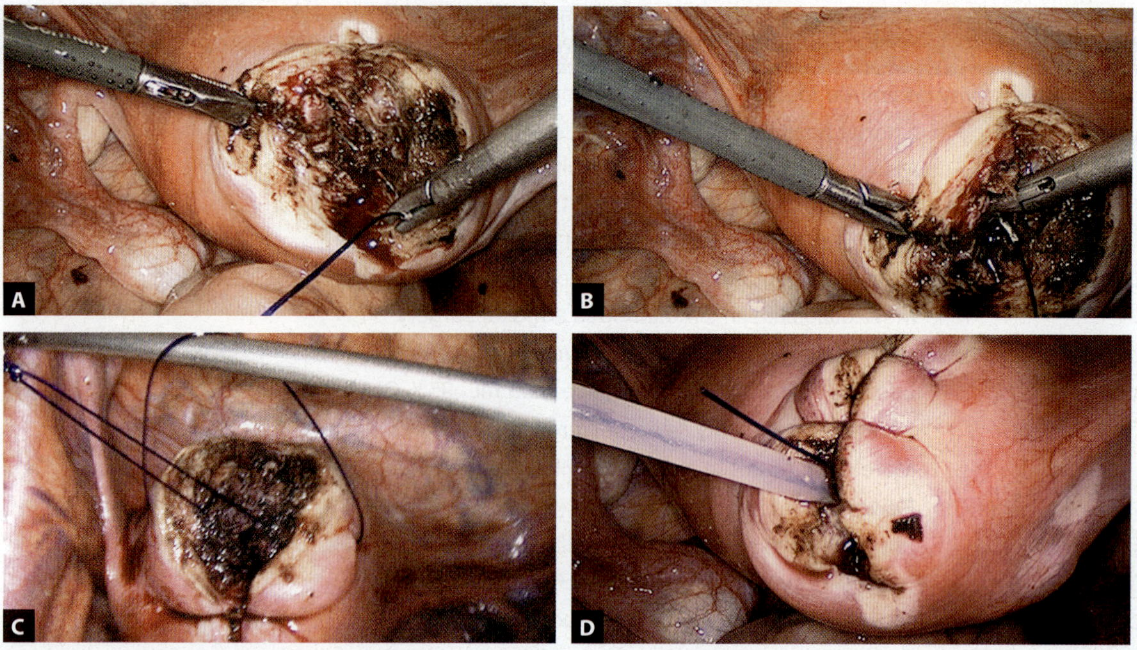

Figs. 35.6A to D: The extracorporeal "von Leffern" knot. (A) Pulling out the suture, removing the needle, half hitch; (B) Holding the knot with the left hand and reaching over with the right hand; (C) Grasping the short end from below and leading it back, exiting before the half hitch; (D) Turning back the knot. Holding the straight suture and tightening the knot.

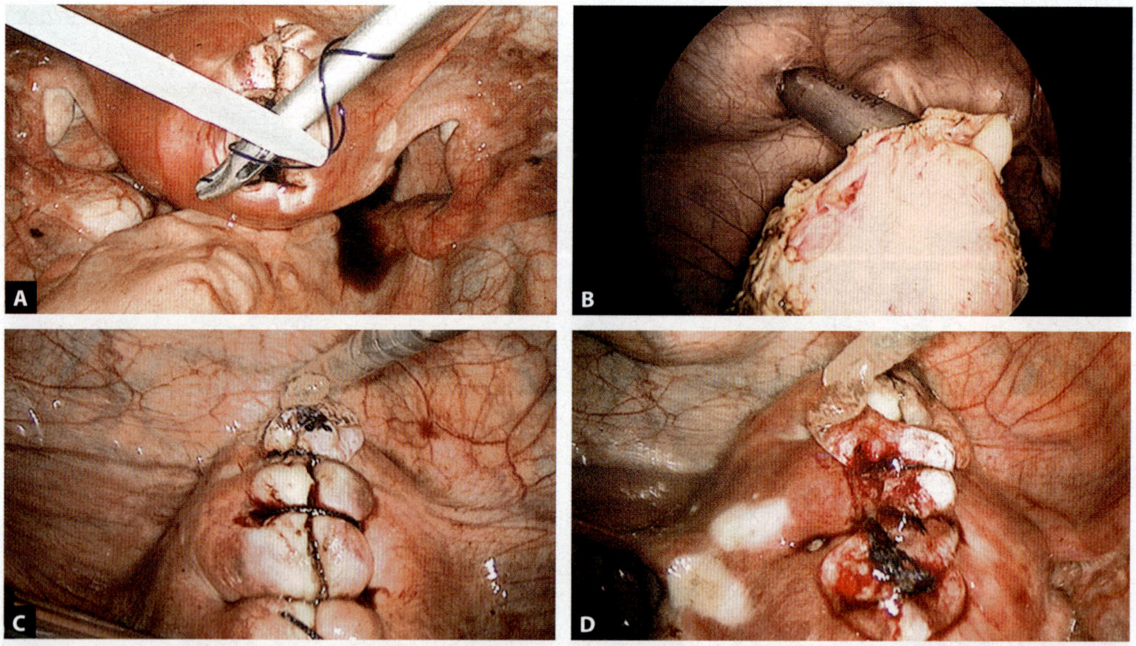

Figs. 35.7A to D: Laparoscopic myoma enucleation. (A) Second single suture starting as deep as possible in the uterine wound; (B) The needle exits on the left wound margin (immediately adjacent to the Manhes forceps); (C) Completing the stitch and preparing the extracorporeal von Leffern knot. The needle holder elevates the thread to avoid tearing the uterine wall when pulling the monofilar thread (PDS); (D) Pushing down the extracorporeal knot with a plastic pushrod into the depth of the wound to dump the knot, thus minimizing the size of the external part of the suture.

In many cases, conservative medical or conservative surgical treatment signifies undertreatment of the patient, who may then need surgery later on. Subtotal hysterectomy is a compromise that meets the requirements of patients, society and doctors. It is the least invasive approach of hysterectomy. However, the patient must provide her informed consent regarding disadvantages of the remaining cervix. Only laparoscopic total hysterectomy (LTH) provides complete protection from renewed fibroids, prevents

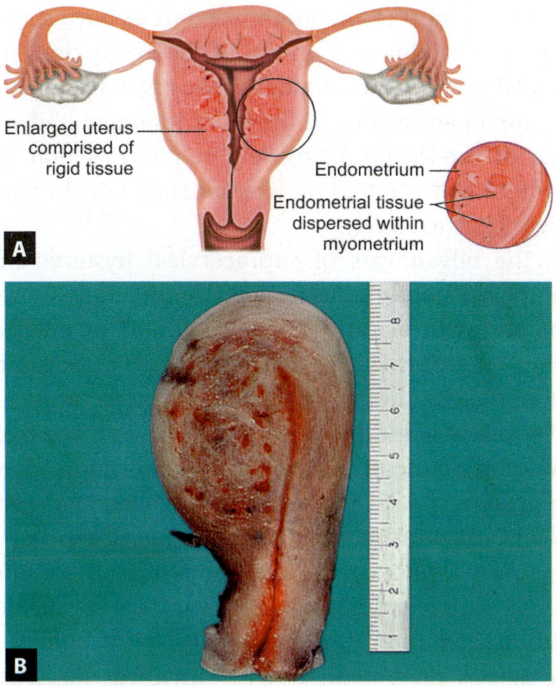

Figs. 35.8A and B: (A) Schematic illustration of an enlarged uterus with adenomyosis. Endometriosis glands are dispersed within the myometrium; (B) Anatomical specimen in a sagittal cut. The posterior wall is much thicker than the anterior wall, with endometriosis glands spread diffusely in the myometrium wall.

subsequent carcinoma of the cervix or sarcoma, cell spilling when cutting the corpus and during morcellation, uncontrolled bleeding and other problems arising from the uterus. The persistence or recurrence of adenomyosis-related symptoms in subtotal hysterectomy continues to be a subject of debate.

TOTAL VERSUS SUBTOTAL (SUPRACERVICAL)

Independent of the surgical technique (subtotal or total hysterectomy), endoscopic surgery is a desirable goal. Some women wish to retain their cervix, believing that it may affect their sexual satisfaction after hysterectomy. Removal of cervix is known to cause excessive neurologic and anatomic disruption, thereby leading to greater surgical and postoperative morbidity, vaginal shortening, subsequent vault prolapse, abnormal cuff granulations and a propensity for fallopian tube prolapse. These issues were addressed in a systematic review of three randomized trials focused on total versus subtotal hysterectomy for benign gynecological conditions. The conclusions were as follows:[11]

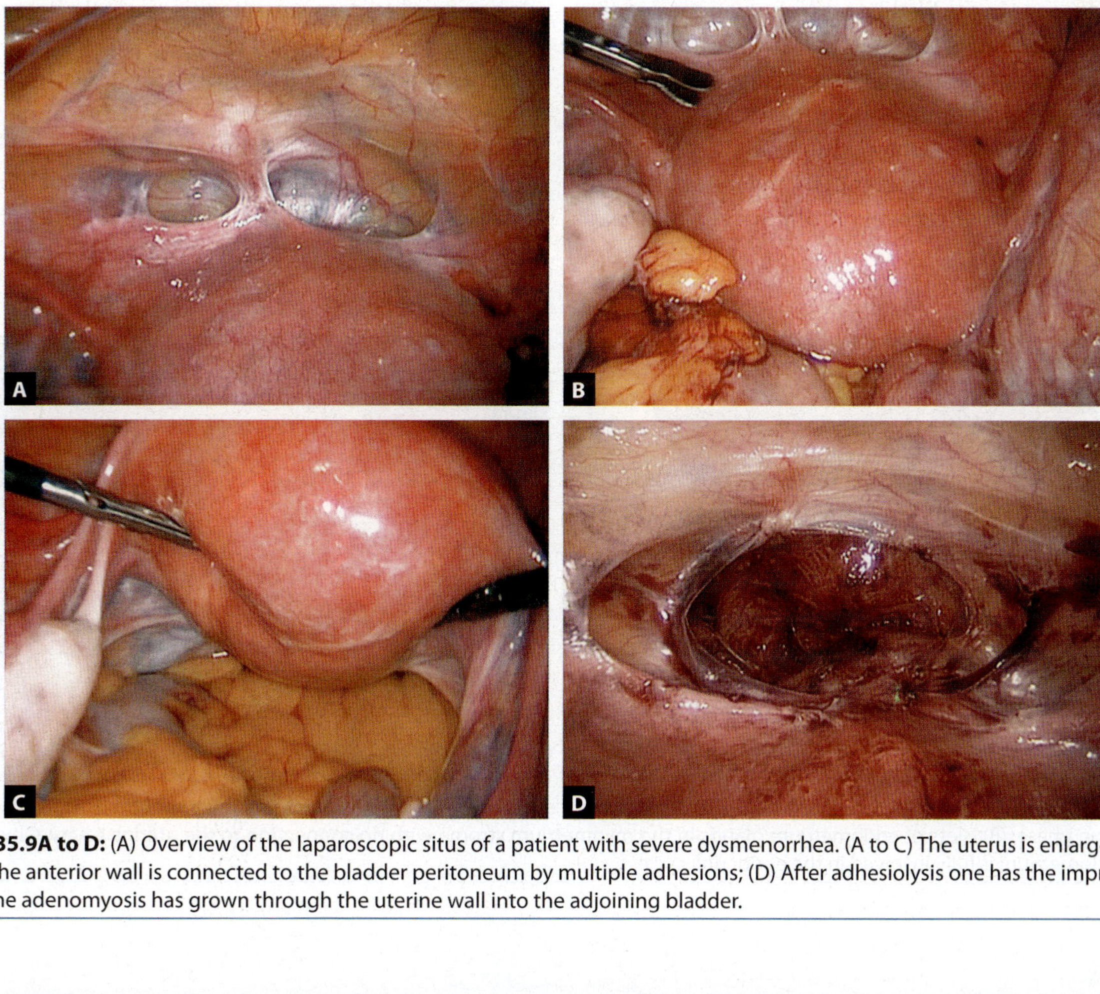

Figs. 35.9A to D: (A) Overview of the laparoscopic situs of a patient with severe dysmenorrhea. (A to C) The uterus is enlarged and soft. The anterior wall is connected to the bladder peritoneum by multiple adhesions; (D) After adhesiolysis one has the impression that the adenomyosis has grown through the uterine wall into the adjoining bladder.

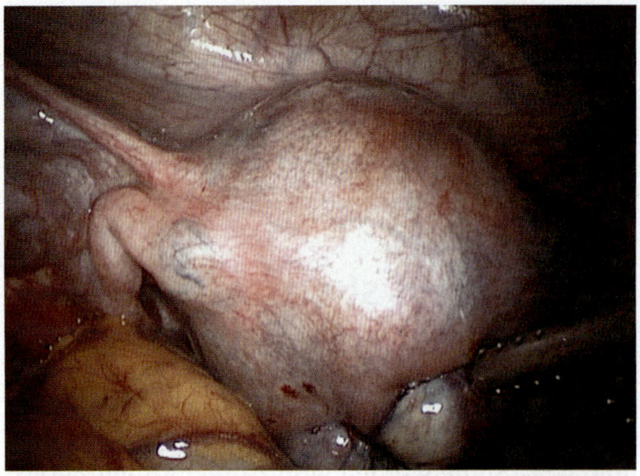

Fig. 35.10: Patient with severe dysmenorrhea and dyspareunia. The injection of blue dye exposes the intramural vessels, which seem to be massively increased. This picture is also typical of adenomyosis of the uterus.

- No difference was noted in rates of incontinence, constipation or measures of sexual function (sexual satisfaction, dyspareunia).
- The duration of surgery and the quantity of blood loss during surgery were significantly less during subtotal hysterectomy compared with total hysterectomy. However, there was no difference in the likelihood of the patient needing a transfusion.
- Febrile morbidity was less likely and ongoing cyclic vaginal bleeding one year after surgery more likely after subtotal hysterectomy.
- No difference was noted in the rates of other complications, recovery from surgery or readmission rates.

In the short term, randomized trials have shown that preservation or removal of the cervix does not affect the rate of subsequent pelvic organ prolapse.

The anatomical and therefore functional advantage of the cervix being left in place is that the cardinal and uterosacral ligaments remain in place (Figs. 35.20 to 35.24).

The advantages of supracervical hysterectomy compared to abdominal hysterectomy include shorter operating times and a shorter length of hospital stay when performed laparoscopically. Furthermore, patients who undergo subtotal hysterectomy are able to withstand loads earlier because there is no risk of vaginal cuff dehiscence.[12] Some studies have reported a shorter recovery period following subtotal hysterectomy, but this finding is not supported by data from randomized trials. In a prospective cohort study, supracervical hysterectomy was associated with greater improvement in short-term quality of life scores than total hysterectomy, but no difference was registered in postoperative pain or return to activities of daily living.[13] There may also be fewer injuries to the urinary tract because dissection is not performed as close to the cervix or as deep into the pelvis as in total hysterectomy. However, clinical trials designed to demonstrate this clinical observation have not been performed yet.

Other differences include posthysterectomy body image and health status. Women who underwent subtotal hysterectomy reported a significantly better body image and health-related quality of life than those who underwent total hysterectomy. Both groups reported an improvement in sexual satisfaction.[14]

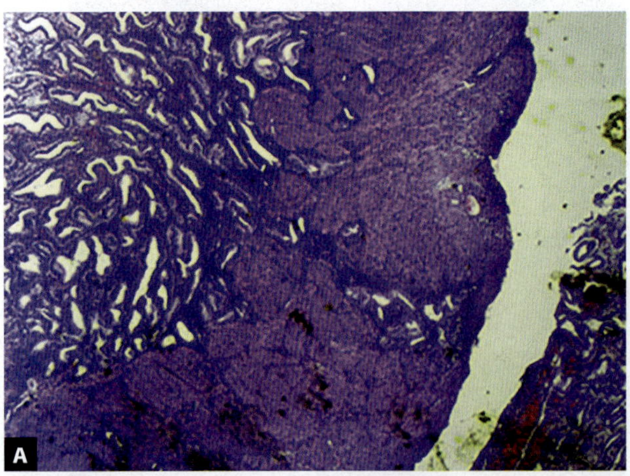

A

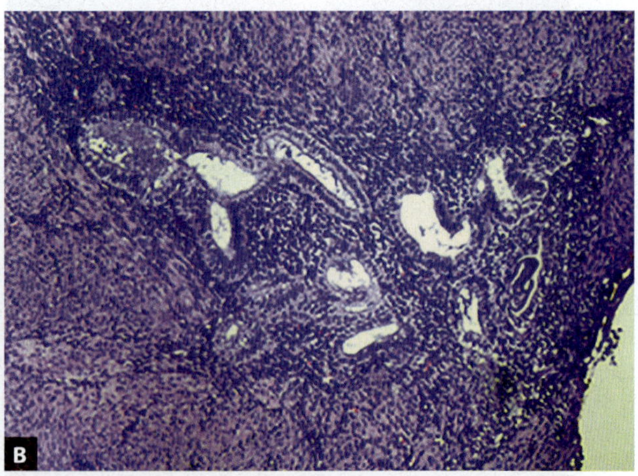

B

Figs. 35.11A and B: (A) Low magnification of a piece of ablated endometrium with the adjoining myometrium tissue in the early secretion phase; (B) Islets of endometrium glands in the myometrium stroma with no connection to the uterine cavity. Obviously, the endometrium is fully involved in the endocrine cycle.

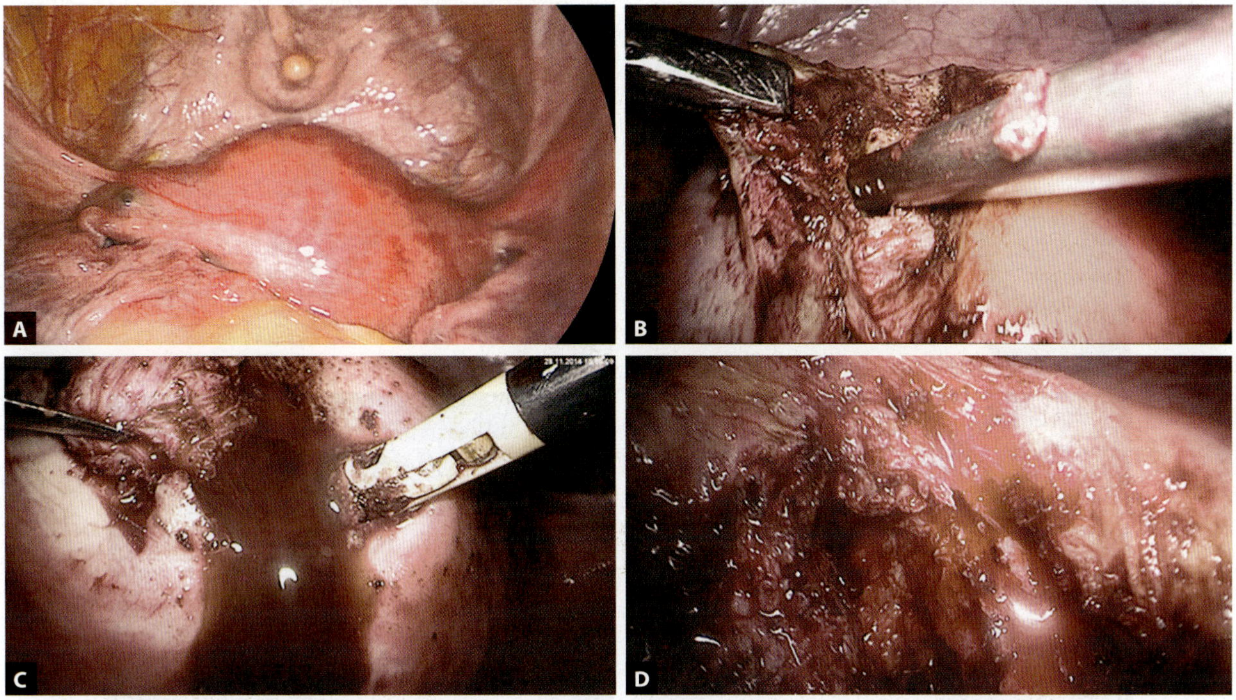

Figs. 35.12A to D: (A) Overview of an asymmetrical uterus; endometriosis is suspected at the left tube and a central space-occupying lesion is seen; (B) Opening the central intramural lesion, which was suspected to be a fibroid; (C) Chocolate-like fluid after entering the adenomyoma; (D) On the magnification even the wall layers, including the mid-endometrium tissue can be seen.

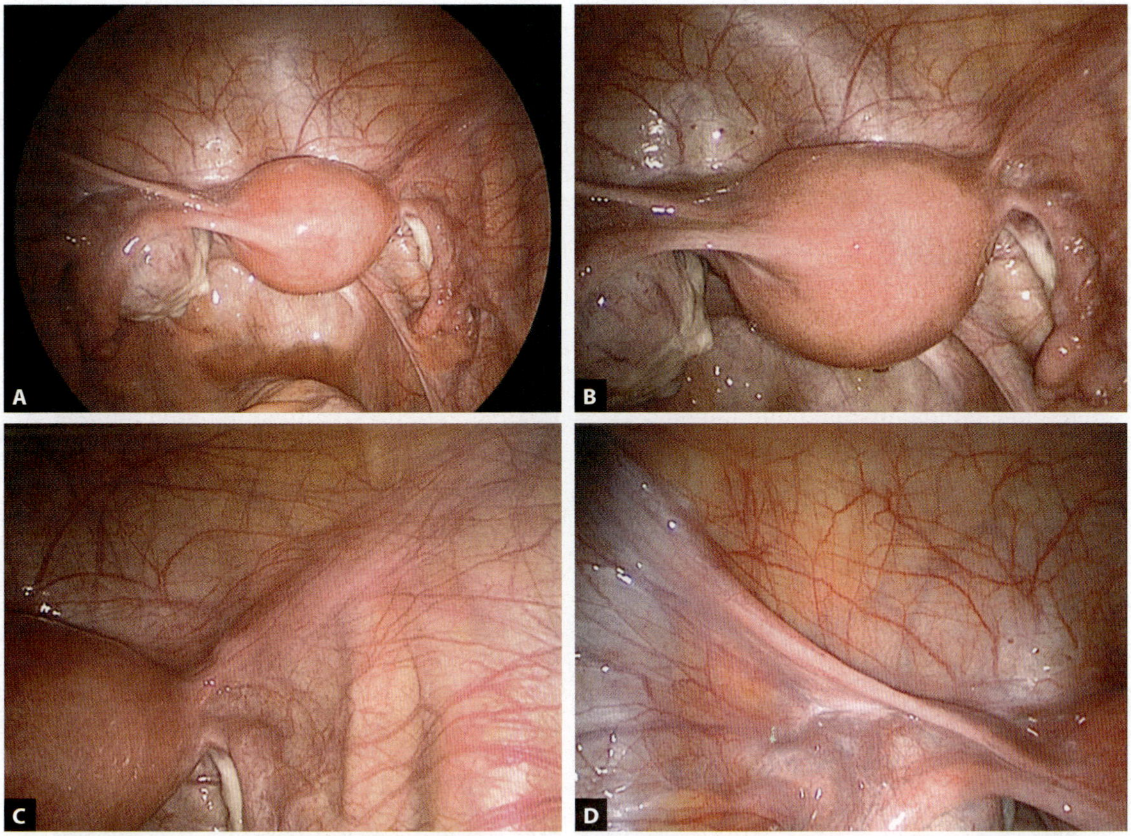

Figs. 35.13A to D: Laparoscopic overview of a patient with dysmenorrhea. (A and B) An enlarged and irregular uterus with hypervascularization of the serosa. The chronic disease has caused an asymmetry of the round ligaments; (C) Right side is much shorter than; (D) Left side.

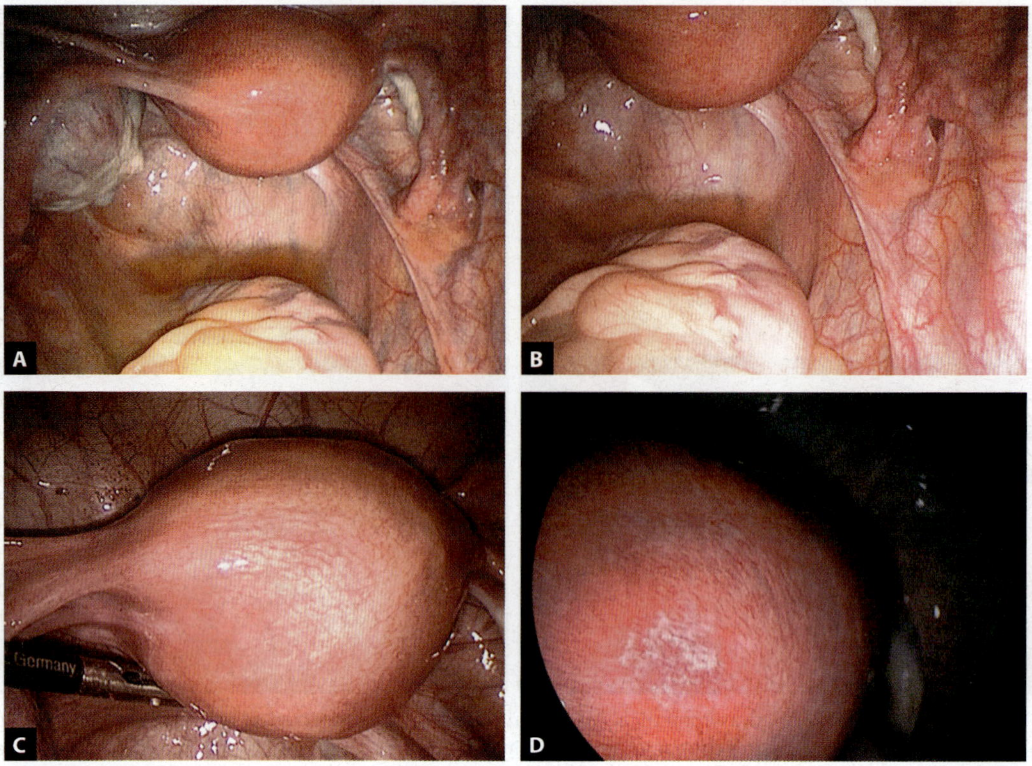

Figs. 35.14A to D: (A and C) The uterus appears to be less mobile but somehow fixed in the pelvis; (B) The peritoneum above the ureter is under tension and can be demarcated from the sacrouterine ligament; (C) The surface of the uterus is hypervascularized; (D) The outflow of the tubes seems to be steep.

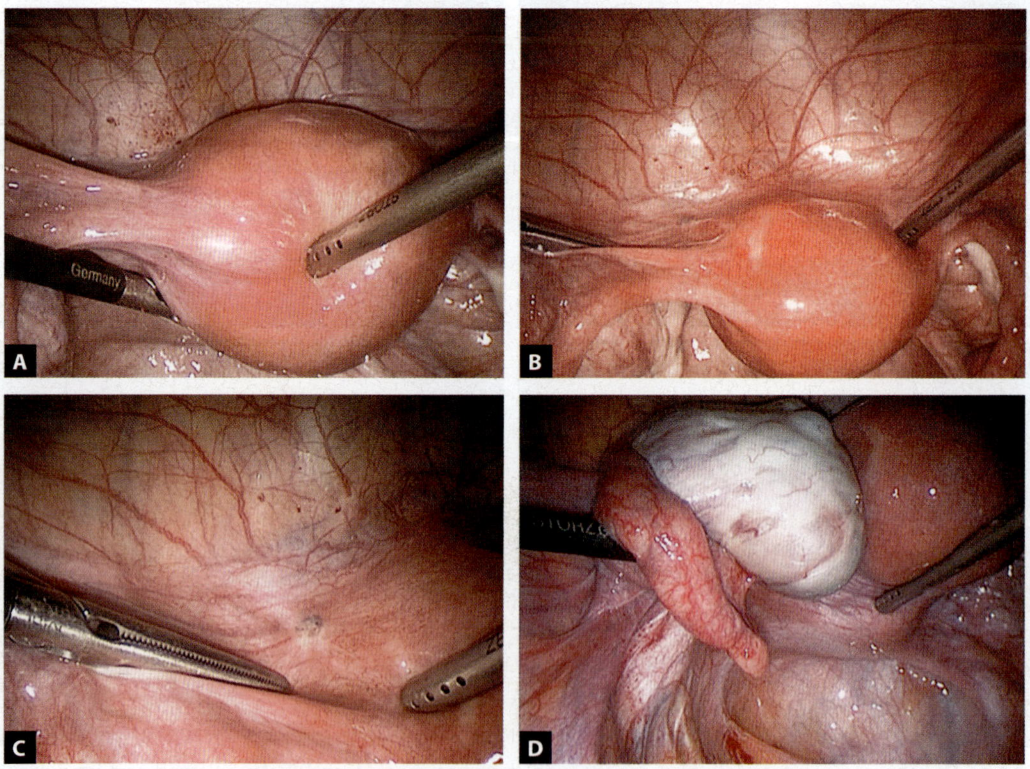

Figs. 35.15A to D: (A) Palpating the uterus with a blunt instrument shows that its consistency is less soft; (B) It is tight but hypervascular; (C) Endometriotic nodule on the lower uterine anterior wall; (D) Fixed and enlarged cystic left ovary in the ovarian fossa. The ureter can be demarcated behind the peritoneum and is lifted to the fixed area.

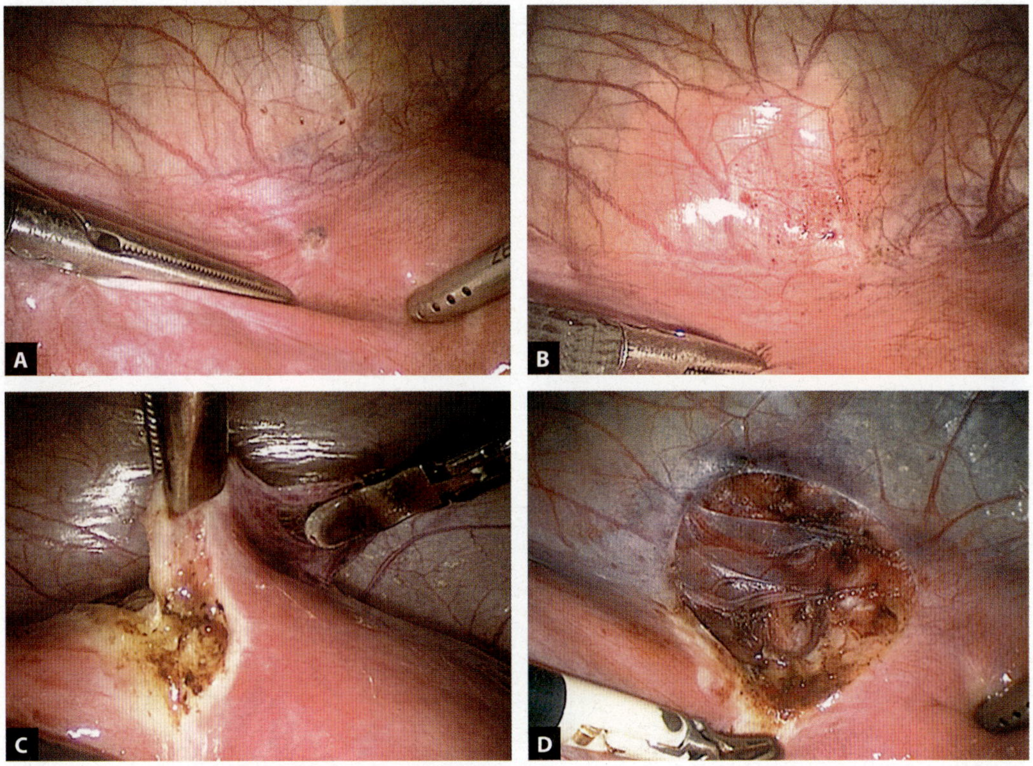

Figs. 35.16A to D: Excision of the endometriotic nodule of the lower anterior uterine wall; (B) Even the adjacent bladder peritoneum appears to be superficially affected because it is hypervascularized and fragile.

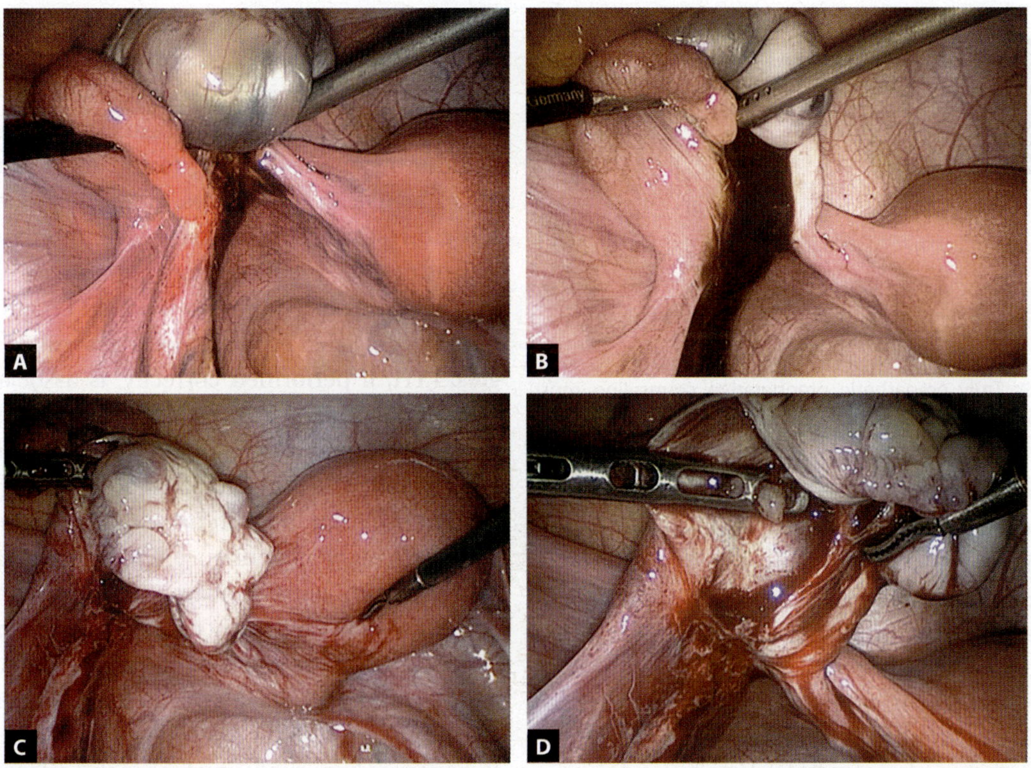

Figs. 35.17A to D: (A and B) Lifting the ovary out of the ovarian fossa and releasing it from its peritoneal adhesion leads to opening of the endometrioma; (C and D) The depths of the ovarian fossa are affected by disease, as proven by the demarcation of the peritoneal nodule. These nodules are usually connected to the cardinal ligament or the sacrouterine ligament.

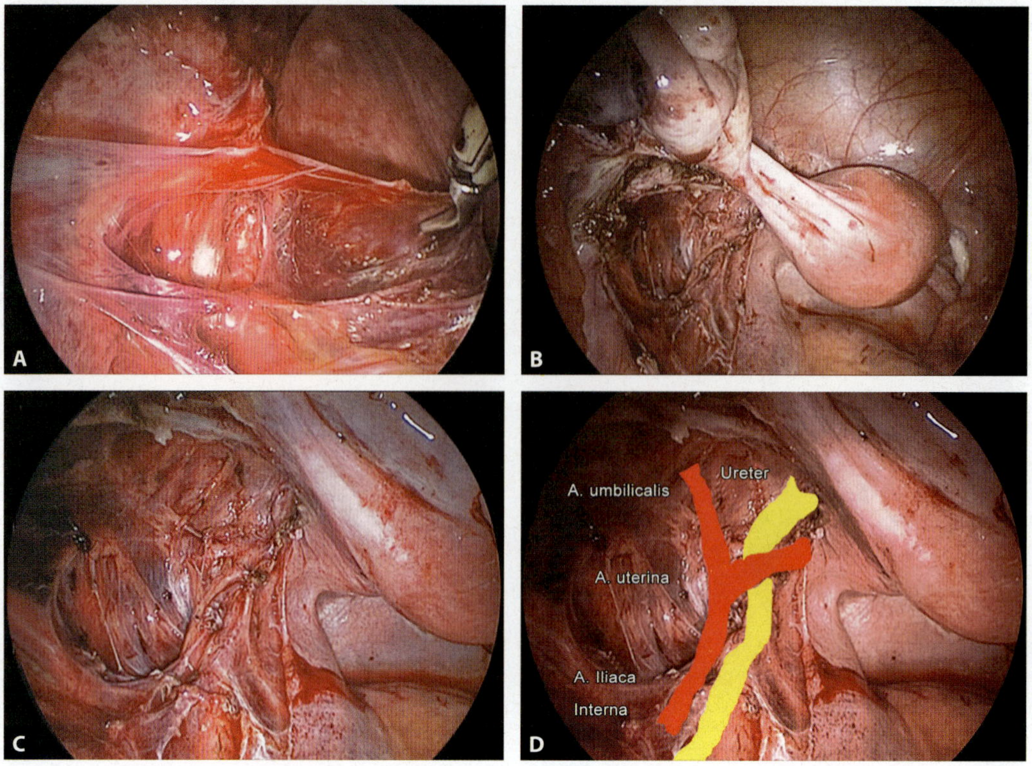

Figs. 35.18A to D: Opening the peritoneal wall for resection of the symptomatic endometriotic nodule. The ureter and vessels of the pelvic wall can be separated bluntly from the peritoneum and the endometriotic nodule. The ureter or the vessels themselves are very rarely affected. If they are, the condition calls for special surgical treatment.

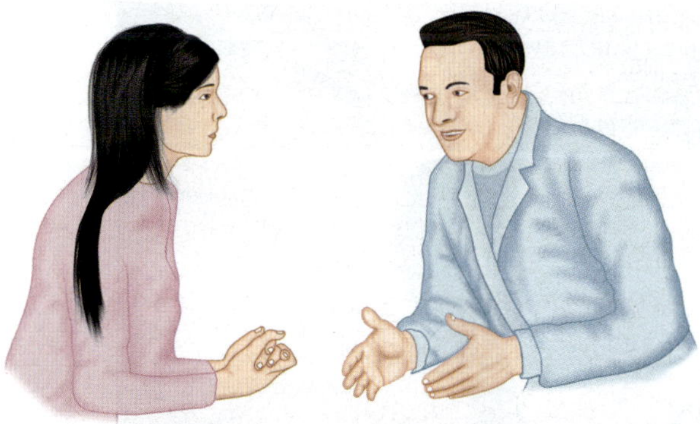

Fig. 35.19: Truly empathetic preoperative counseling must include congruence and respect for the patient.

The only absolute contraindication for subtotal hysterectomy is a malignant or premalignant condition of the uterine corpus or cervix.

Extensive endometriosis is a relative contraindication because these women may experience persistent dyspareunia when the cervix is retained. The significance of adenomyosis has been underestimated so far. The uterus is morcellated in the abdomen. If the morcellated uterus is not collected in a bag, adenomyosis may spread into the abdominal cavity. The patient may experience persistent pain in the central segment of the lower abdomen. In laparoscopic supracervical hysterectomy (LSH), the involvement of the cervix or the retrocervical/precervical space is ignored. Very often the sacrouterine ligaments or the lateral cardinal ligaments leading to the ovarian fossa are also affected. In these cases, either the adenomyosis has grown through the uterine wall into the adjacent organs or there is concomitant endometriosis. To rule out all causes of symptoms, it would be advisable to remove all visible endometriosis-associated pathologies. LTH, if performed correctly, is associated with very few additional risks or side effects. Therefore, in cases of adenomyosis of the uterus we explain the situation to the patient in detail and advise LTH [personal statement]. Arguments in favor of LTH include fewer cases of urinary incontinence, less prolapse and cervical stump problems. However, subtotal hysterectomy is performed faster in most cases and seems to be associated with fewer intraoperative and postoperative complications. We lack convincing data concerning the advantages of simultaneous removal of the cervix; the cervix is very rarely involved in the disease.[15,16]

Elective supracervical hysterectomy should be preceded by cervical cytology confirming the absence

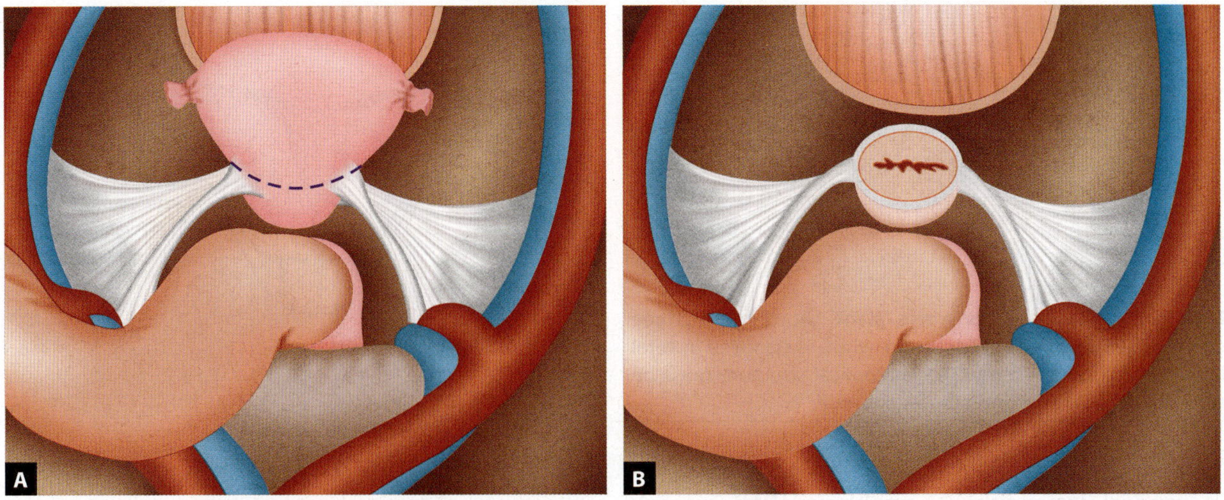

Figs. 35.20A and B: Schematic illustration of subtotal or supracervical hysterectomy with the remaining cervical stump. The sacrouterine ligaments and the cardinal ligament remain untouched. The medial compartment is not opened.

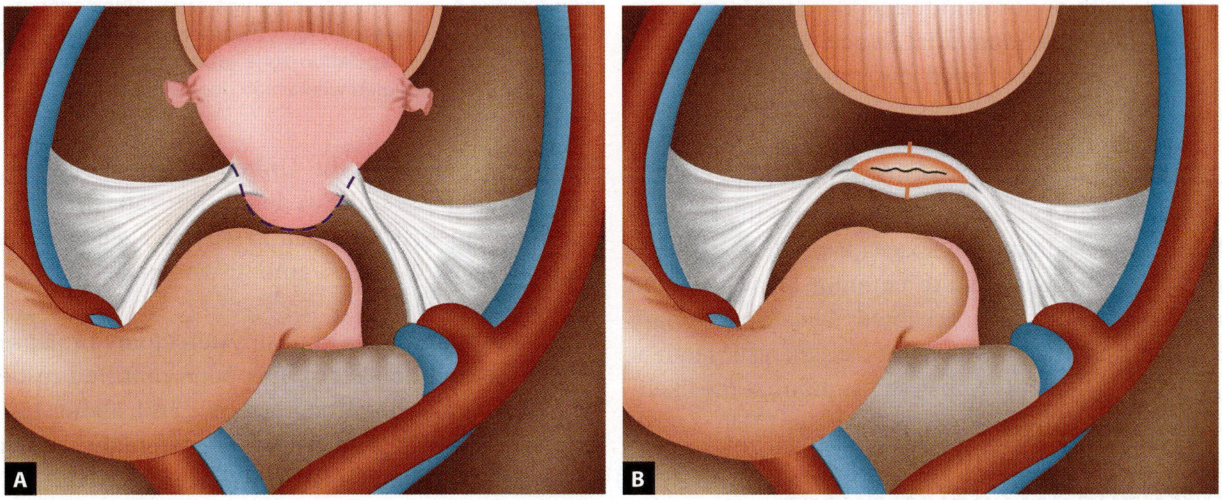

Figs. 35.21A and B: In comparison, in laparoscopic total hysterectomy the middle compartment is opened and the cervix is enucleated out of its bed. In intrafascial hysterectomy, the surrounding ligaments remain intact and the vaginal stump is retained.

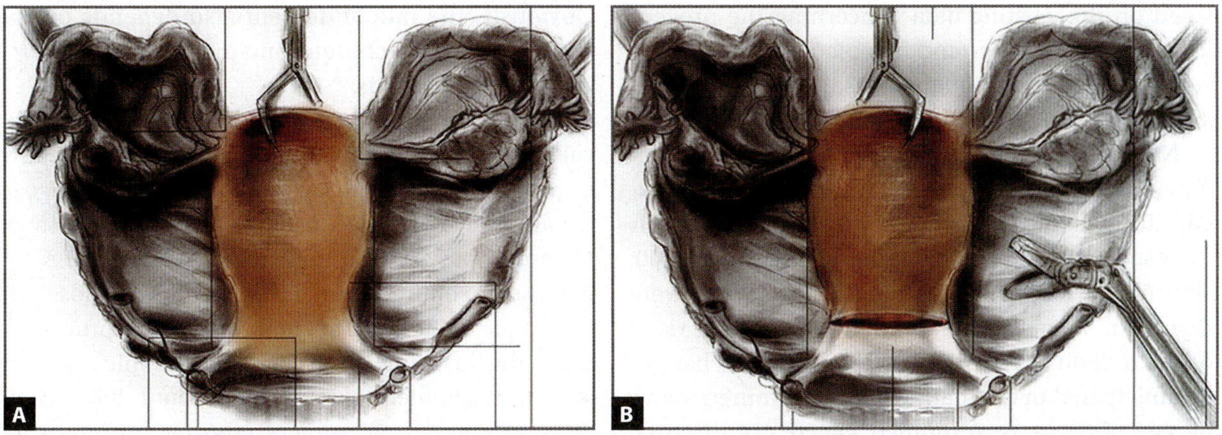

Figs. 35.22A and B: Overview of subtotal and total hysterectomy with reference to the surrounding tissue. The sacrouterine ligaments are omitted in both procedures.

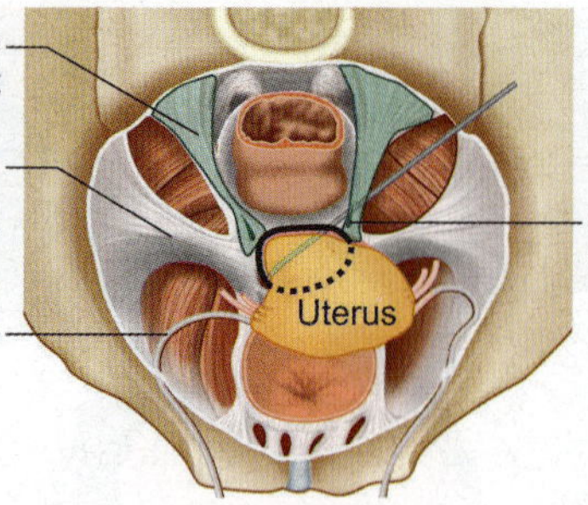

Fig. 35.23: Imaginary transverse plane showing the three compartments and the cervical ring, which is removed in total laparoscopic hysterectomy. The anatomical structure must be reconstructed when closing the vaginal cuff.

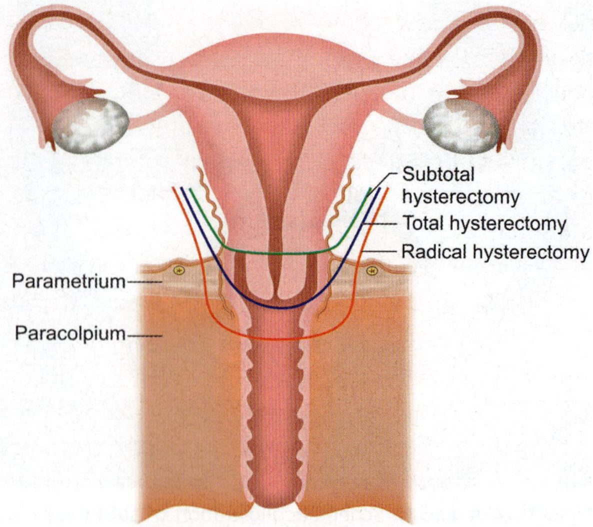

Fig. 35.24: Schematic illustration of the resection line in subtotal, total, and radical laparoscopic hysterectomy. Only the ascending branch of the uterine artery needs to be coagulated and cut with the uterine manipulator in benign cases. When adhering closely to this operative technique, the ureter is located at a safe distance from the coagulation zone (about 2 cm). All radical procedures are associated with a high degree of risk.

of cervical intraepithelial neoplasia (PAP smear). Women who have had a supracervical hysterectomy should be screened for cervical cancer according to standard guidelines for their age and risk status. In patients with abnormal uterine bleeding (especially metrorrhagia), endometrial cancer or any type of sarcoma should be ruled out prior to performing supracervical hysterectomy.

Sometimes the cervix needs to be removed later as a separate procedure. This approach is associated with frequent damage to the bowel and the bladder because the anatomical spaces cannot be exposed clearly and adhesions are common. However, the approach is readily accepted because primary surgery is associated with fewer risks than subsequent procedures. Patients who wish to minimize the likelihood of subsequent surgery may prefer LTH.

WILL THE FALLOPIAN TUBES OR OVARIES BE REMOVED IN HYSTERECTOMY?

Based on the existing data concerning the prevention of ovarian cancer and fallopian tube disorders, we recommend a simultaneous salpingectomy after appropriate counseling.

Notwithstanding the above facts, the number of pelvic floor corrections has increased very markedly throughout the world in recent years. This is a consequence of demographic changes. In 2000, 34.8 million women (12.7%) in the United States were 65 years or older. By 2030 this number will have risen to 70.3 million (20%). Similar demographic changes are anticipated in Germany.[17] In 2011, women above the age of 65 years accounted for 20% of the total population; the percentage will rise to 35% by 2060. This development will be less striking in other European countries, the United Kingdom, France, the Netherlands and Sweden.[17] The rate of pelvic organ prolapse (POP) repair in women aged 65 years and above is 30–50%[18]; among women older than 80 years it is still 11%.[19]

The reported rates of posthysterectomy prolapse vary. The cumulative risk has been reported to be 1% at 3 years after hysterectomy, and about 15% fifteen years later. The risk is 5.5-fold higher when hysterectomy is performed for a descensus. Incidence rates of 46% have been reported elsewhere.[19-22] Apart from the risk of a preexisting descensus, vaginal deliveries and age are discussed as reasons for the risk doubling with each advancing decade of life.[23] Obviously, the rate of descent also depends on the applied surgical technique and measures for the prevention of descensus.[24]

Total laparoscopic hysterectomy involves removal of the uterus and the cervix. The entire procedure is performed laparoscopically. The specimen can usually be removed through the vaginal vault. Laparoscopic-assisted vaginal hysterectomy (LAVH) has been entirely replaced by the endoscopic technique, which has become a standard procedure since the learning curve for laparoscopic suturing is now favorable. Taking into account the advantages of endoscopic surgery (shorter hospital stay, faster recovery, better cosmetic result and fewer infections), the question arises as to whether the risk of posthysterectomy prolapse after LSH can be reduced by preserving the existing structures of the pelvic floor in the middle compartment or reconstructing them. In cases of preexisting defects, LTH provides sufficient fixation of the pelvic floor and thus minimizes the risk of a posthysterectomy prolapse. Mesh implants such as those used for sacrocolpopexy may be employed in both procedures simultaneously.

Our multimodality concept of laparoscopic intrafascial hysterectomy is aimed at the removal of all concomitant pathologies that might also be responsible for the patient's symptomatic condition, and simultaneously reducing the risk of posthysterectomy prolapse:

- Removal of all concomitant pathologies, such as adhesions or endometriosis spots, and demarcating the extent of adenomyosis.
- Intrafascial hysterectomy with preservation of existing ligaments, yet opening the medial compartment when performing total laparoscopic hysterectomy:
- *Technique 1:* Primary uterine artery clipping/ligation
- *Technique 2:* Classic intrafascial hysterectomy
- A technique of stable fixation of the vaginal stump.

DEVELOPMENT OF LAPAROSCOPIC HYSTERECTOMY TECHNIQUES AND INSTRUMENTS

The popularity of laparoscopic hysterectomy rose gradually after Harry Reich's initial publication of the procedure.[25,26] A number of approaches evolved, such as laparoscopically assisted vaginal hysterectomy (LAVH), LSH, LTH and laparoscopic intrafascial hysterectomy. LTH had a steep learning curve and was initially associated with rather high complication rates.[5] The development of new instruments and consistent training improved the situation. The introduction of the intrauterine manipulator helped to develop the classic intrafascial concept, which, today, is the aim of every gynecological surgeon performing TLH. Hohl used Kurt Semm's procedure of classic intrafascial supracervical hysterectomy (CISH)[27] and developed it further with the use of his manipulator.[28] The majority of the available manipulators are well accepted because they are easy to handle, reusable and durable. Uterus can be moved in all directions while the elliptical long tip of the manipulator eases out vaginal and paravaginal tissue intraabdominally. The manipulator can be pushed straight toward the field of operation, especially when cutting the uterus off the vagina with the monopolar hook and targeting the tip of the manipulator.

The large majority of manipulators are provided with a ceramic cap that creates a flat surface to work on. Consequently, dissection of the bladder is usually not necessary. It should be noted that the use of the manipulator for bladder dissection is useful and safe even after a cesarean section. The application of the manipulator imitates the classical movements during abdominal hysterectomy; the ureters are kept out of the field of operation. The cap allows intrafascial hysterectomy, which preserves the ligaments and avoids vaginal shortening. The smooth cutting edge is useful for vaginal occlusion (Figs. 35.25A to I).

Points to be considered:

- Monopolar electricity can be used on the ceramic cap. Bipolar current causes a larger defect, bearing the risk of subsequent wound healing problems and vaginal cuff dehiscence. The fact that ultrasound is liable to destroy this apparatus must be taken into account when using ultrasound for dissection during hysterectomy.
- Intrafascial hysterectomy involves a much smaller opening to the vagina and preserves the circular ligaments. Large uteruses may need to be morcellated. Extended endometriosis or adenomyosis may involve the circular ligaments, which then have to be removed.[28]

The other instruments may be of the disposable or reusable type. Disposable tissue sealing instruments are faster and need not be replaced frequently. However, the instruments are costly and fusion of the layers of tissue results in a less clear overview of the anatomical structures. Bipolar forceps are essential. Extracorporeal sutures (PDS 1.0) are helpful, although intracorporeal sutures (Vicryl) are sufficient for vaginal closure. The monopolar hook facilitates the removal of endometriotic spots and the uterus from the manipulator, but can be replaced by bipolar forceps and scissors. In cases of a large uterus, the tenaculum can be used to lift out the uterus; a morcellator avoids troublesome comminution of the uterus.

PREOPERATIVE CONSIDERATIONS AND PREPARATION

When severe endometriosis (Figs. 35.26A to D) is suspected on vaginal examination (Figs. 35.27A and B) and the ultrasound scan is correlated with the patient's medical history, it will be necessary to perform further diagnostic investigations such as MRI, cystoscopy, rectoscopy, or endosonography (Figs. 35.28 and 35.29). Radical interdisciplinary surgery can then be planned and performed (Figs. 35.30 to 35.32).

Hysterectomy must always be accompanied by antibiotic protection, such as a second-generation cephalosporin. In cases of suspected bowel involvement, a single shot of metronidazole is also essential. The antibiotic should be applied about 30 min before the start of the operation.

The instruments consist of trocars, a uterine manipulator (for LTH only), needle holders and sutures. Additionally one needs an instrument for coagulation, graspers, scissors, window forceps and a suction irrigation unit. If a robotic setup is available, the instruments must be adjusted accordingly. A thermofusion device with an integrated knife is optional.

PREREQUISITES

Obesity or comorbidities, a large uterus or a uterus with multiple myomas is no contraindication for a

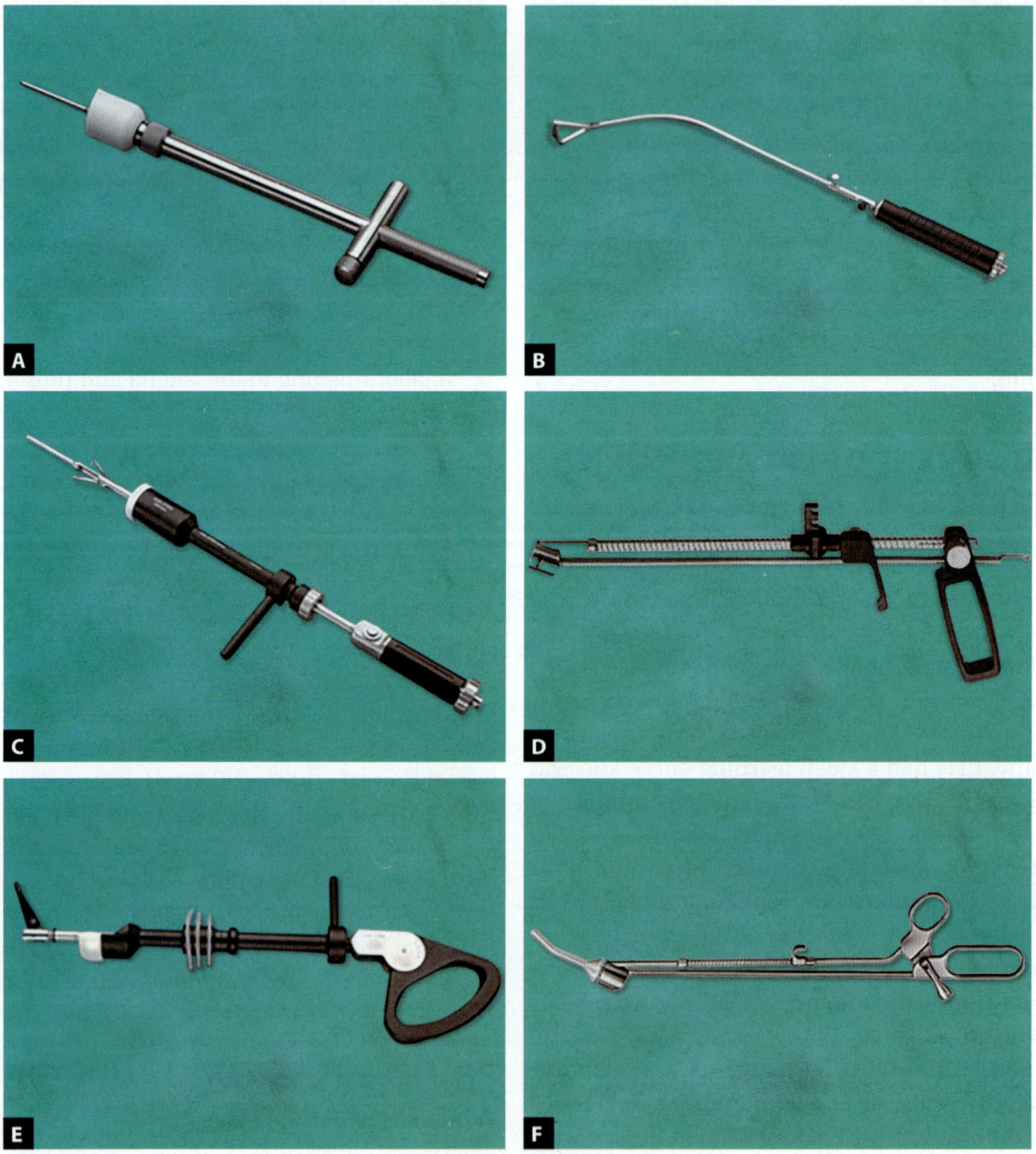

Figs. 35.25A to F

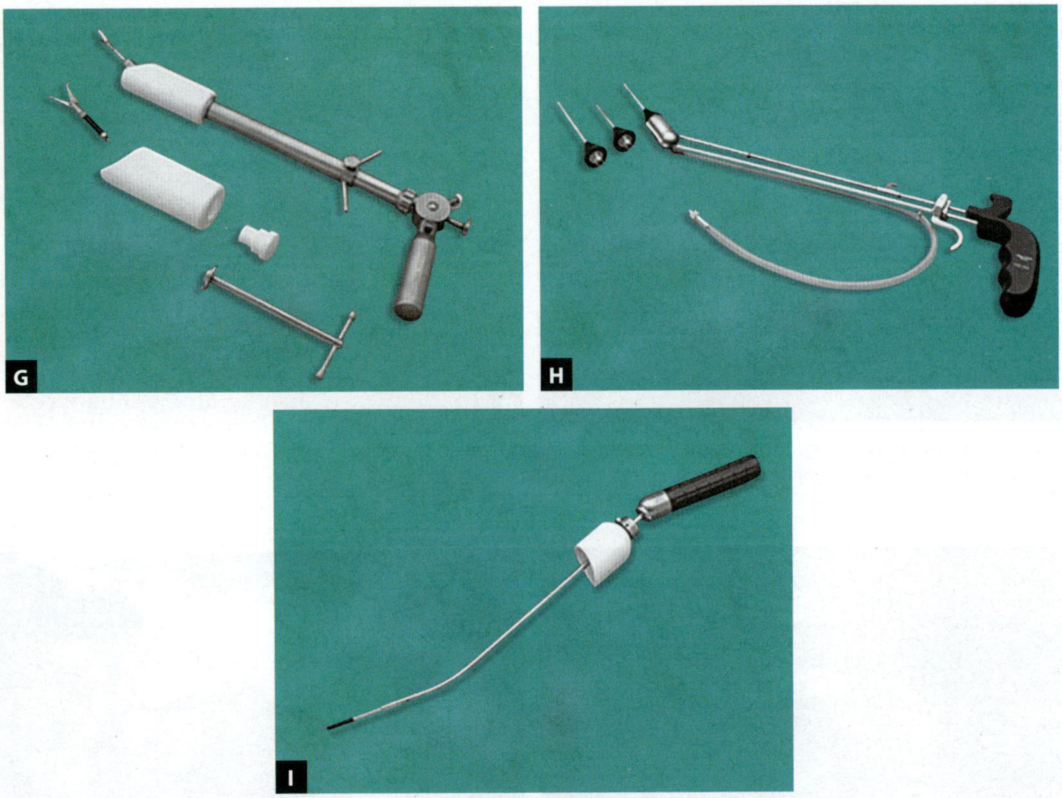

Figs. 35.25G to I

Figs. 35.25A to I: (A) Hohl manipulator (Storz); (B) Dionisi uterine manipulator (Storz); (C) Mangeshikar uterine manipulator (Storz); (D) RfQ uterine manipulator; (E) Clermont-Ferrand uterine manipulator (Storz); (F) Braun uterine manipulator; (G) Koninckx uterine manipulator (Storz); (H) Tintara uterine manipulator (Storz); (I) Donnez uterine manipulator (Storz).

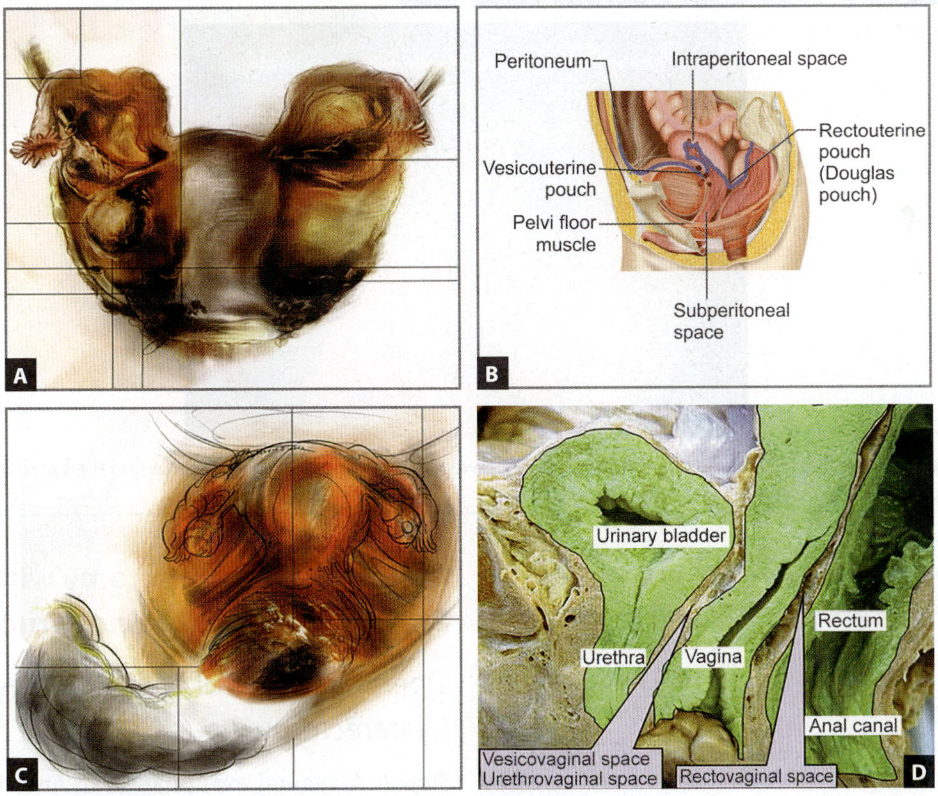

Figs. 35.26A to D: Severe endometriosis in relation to anatomical landmarks.

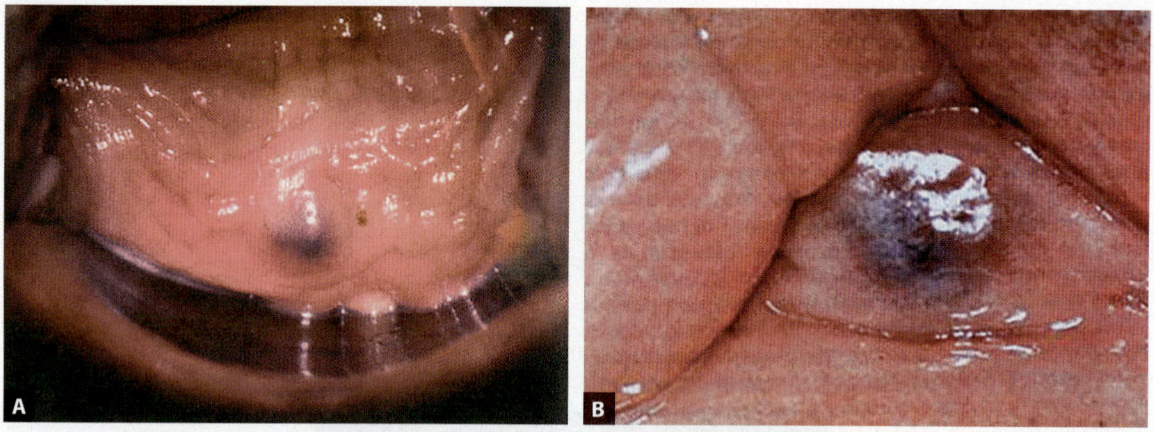

Figs. 35.27A and B: Vaginal photograph of a small endometriotic nodule in the dorsal vaginal wall and another patient with severe deep infiltrating endometriosis involving the vagina.

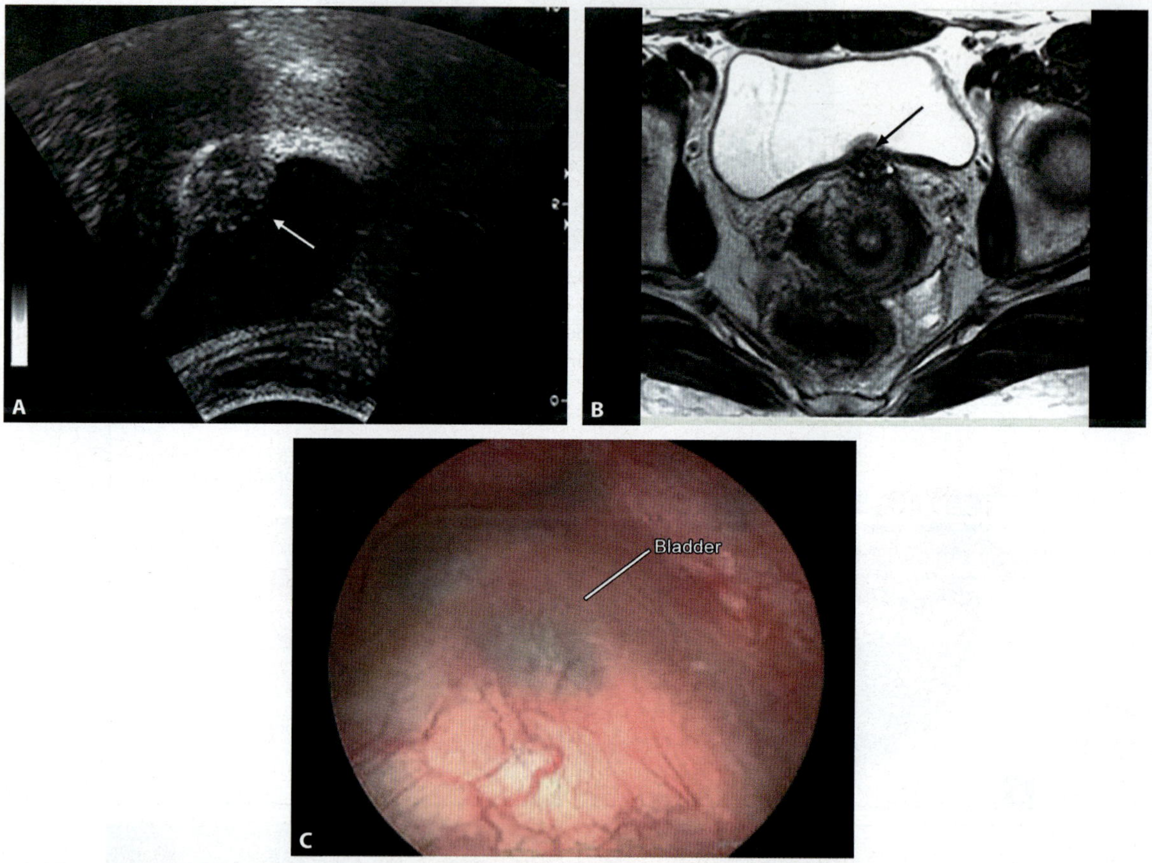

Figs. 35.28A to C: (A) Vaginal ultrasound of a solitary nodule between the anterior wall of the uterus and the bladder (vesicovaginal space); (B) MRI scan; (C) Cystoscopy of the same patient.

laparoscopic procedure. However, in these cases the preoperative assessment and the anesthesia procedure must be discussed with the patient in advance. The trocars may need to be placed higher in the abdominal wall and the surgeon may need more than the usual two ancillary trocars. In cases of a large uterus, the need for morcellation and its risks must be explained to the patient.

Intrafascial Hysterectomy with Preservation of Existing Structures

Operative Steps of Total Laparoscopic Hysterectomy

Step 1: A vaginal examination in anesthesia is performed first using the manipulator. When no further

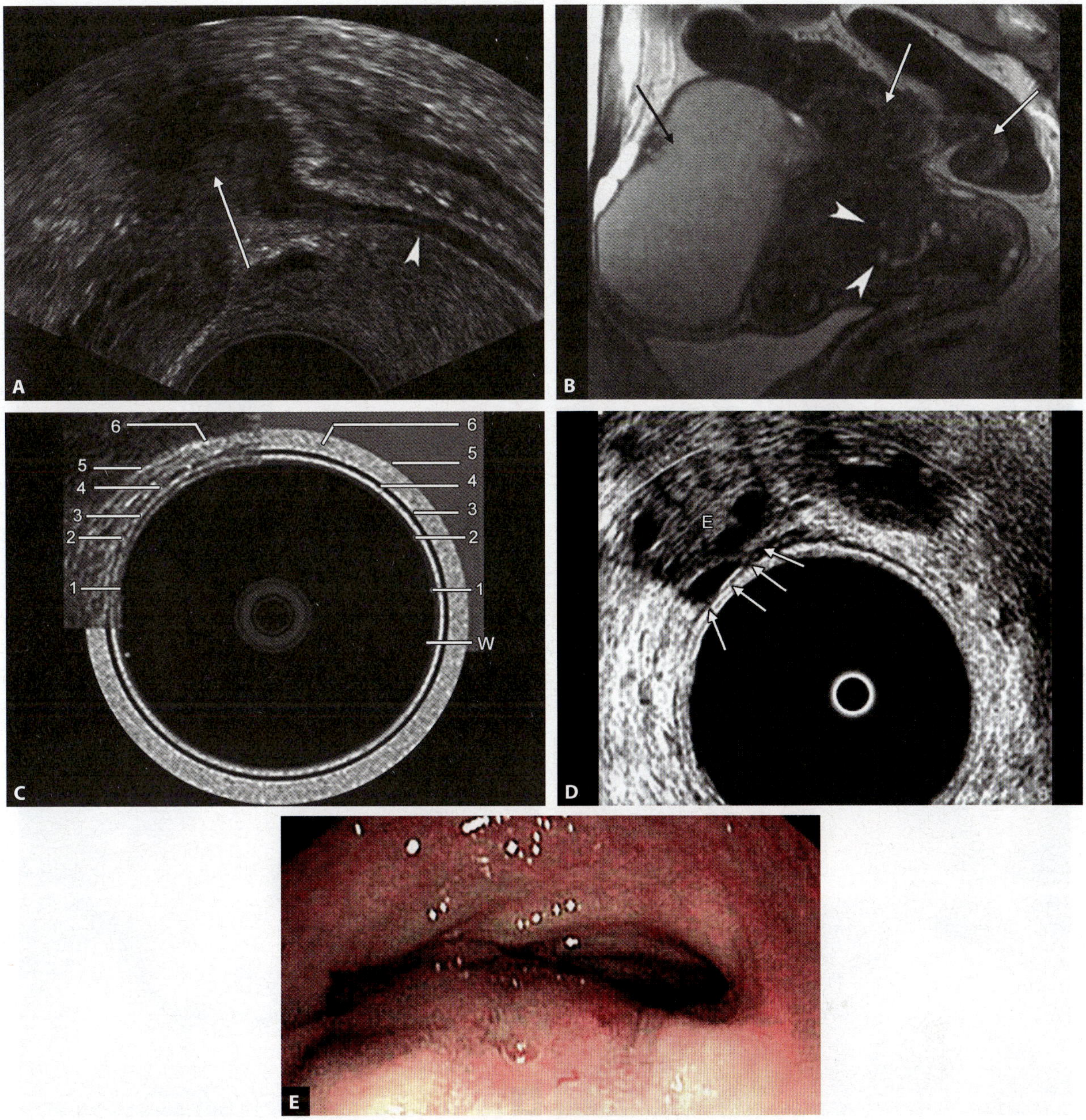

Figs. 35.29A to E: (A) Vaginal ultrasound of a solitary nodule between the lower back wall of the uterus/cervix and the rectum (rectovaginal space); (B) MRI scan; (C and D) Endosonography; (E) Rectoscopy.

vaginal or rectal pathologies are found, the manipulator is inserted.

Step 2: **Port placement—**The first step of the operation is placement of the uterine manipulator (Fig. 35.25).[29] A number of entry techniques are available; direct entry under sight has become very popular in the last few years. Nevertheless, the traditional entry technique described by Kurt Semm and Liselotte Mettler from the University Hospitals Schleswig-Holstein, Kiel, in the 1980s, and still used at the Kiel School of Gynecological Endoscopy is shown here.

Optic Trocar

Veress Needle Technique and CO_2 Gas

To insert Veress needle, the operating table needs to be in horizontal position. Trendelenburg tilt is carried out after creating a pneumoperitoneum. The most common site of entry for Veress needle is the umbilical area. As the wall layers are thinnest at this level, a deep incision will ensure access to the peritoneal cavity. Before incising the skin it would be advisable to palpate the course of the aorta and identify

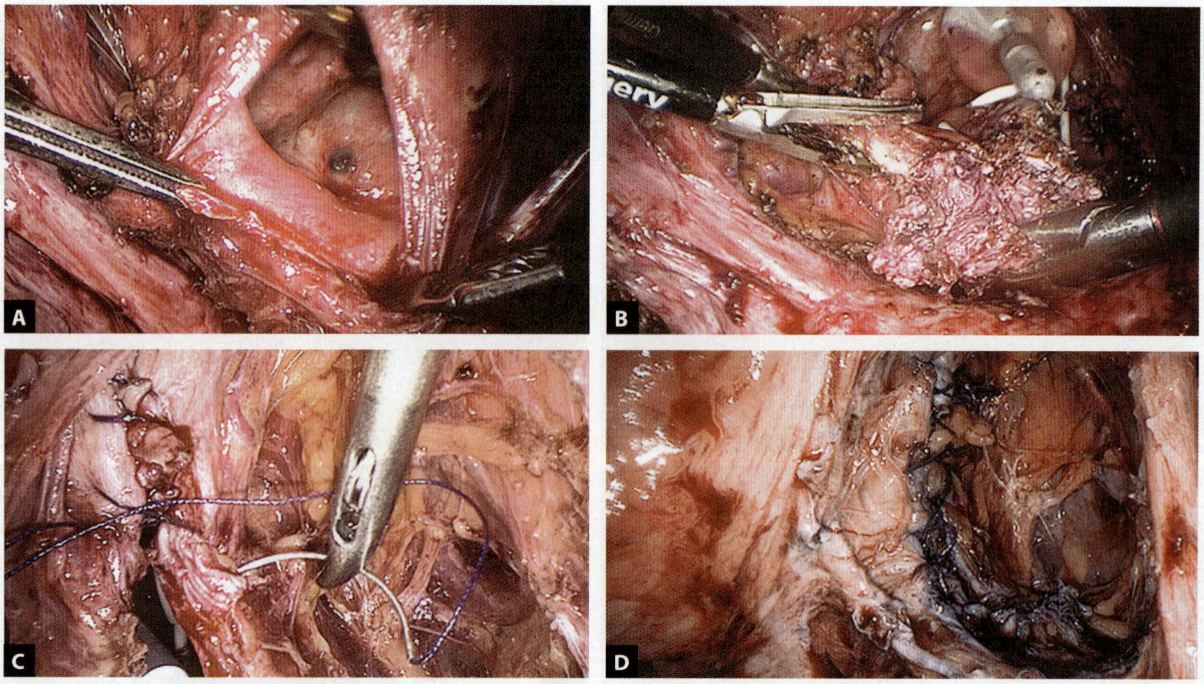

Figs. 35.30A to D: Resection of a solitary nodule in bladder endometriosis. (A) The nodule is seen after opening the bladder. Two double J-catheters are placed in both ureters so that; (B) The nodule can be cut out with an energy device; (C and D) Closure of the bladder in two layers.

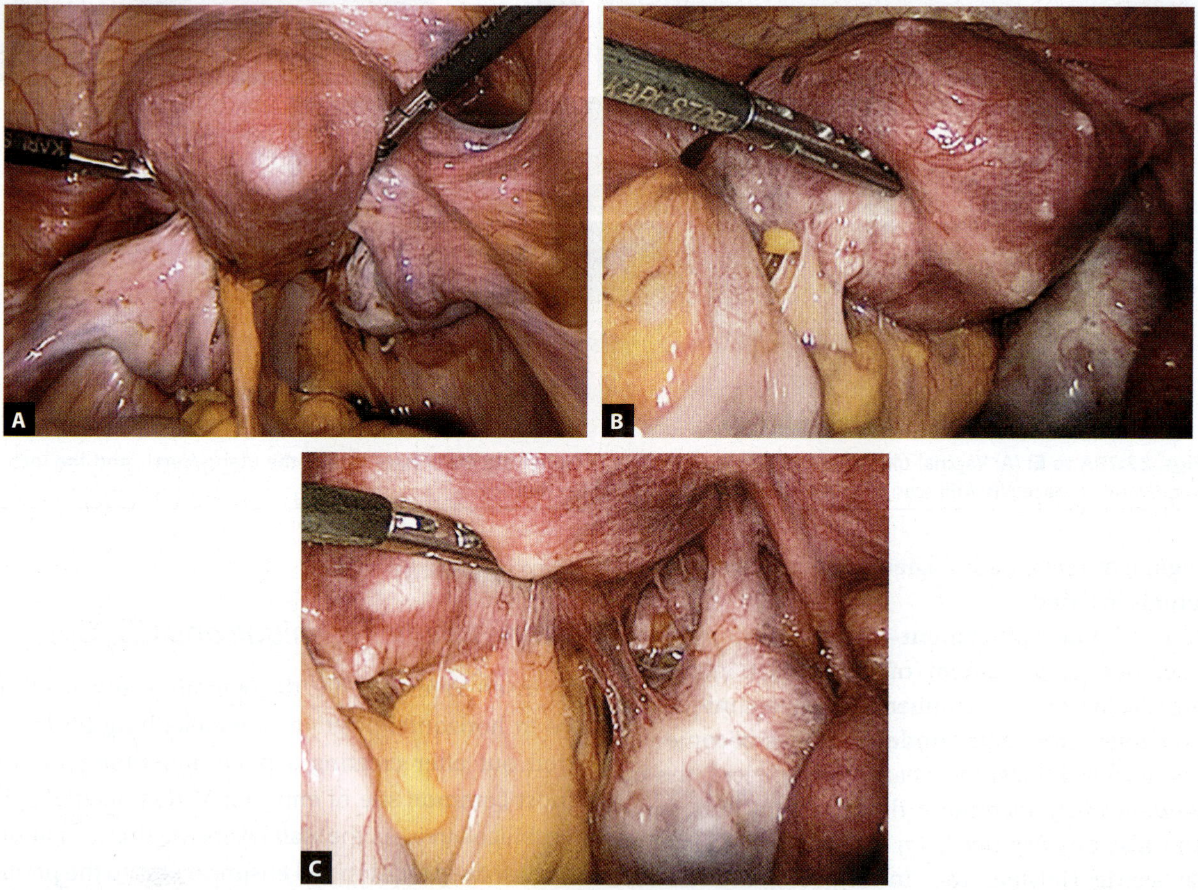

Figs. 35.31A to C: Overview of severe deep infiltrating endometriosis associated with adenomyosis of the uterus, affecting the lower sigmoid colon/rectum.

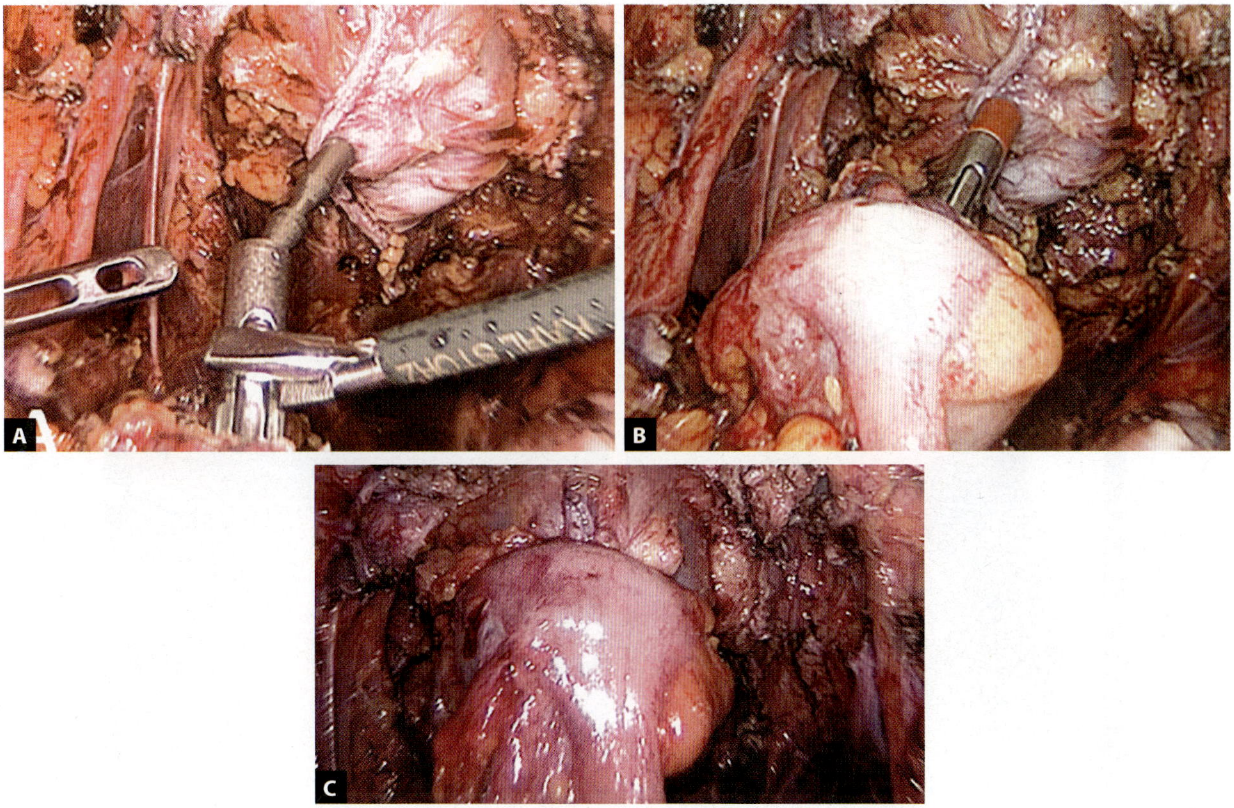

Figs. 35.32A to C: Endoscopic re-anastomosis can be performed after partial bowel resection.

iliac bifurcation. This will permit inspection and palpation of abdomen in order to detect any unusual masses (Figs. 35.33 to 35.35).[30]

The Veress needle must be tested to ensure that the valve springs, and that gas flow is between 6 and 8 mm Hg. In this position the insertion of the primary instrument at a 45° angle toward the uterus involves the least risk of damaging the major vessels coursing downward retroperitoneally. The abdominal wall should be lifted before inserting the instrument. In obese patients the insertion angle is close to 90°, whereas in slim patients the angle is close to 45°. If the first attempt fails, a second attempt is made before selecting an alternative entry site. Before placing Veress needle, a number of safety checks should be performed in order to minimize the risk of complications.

Two clicks: Usually *two clicks* are heard: the first after perforation of the muscle fascia and the second after perforation of the peritoneum. Proper needle placement is ensured by keeping the Veress needle between the thumb and the index finger.

Aspiration test: Injection of 5–10 mL of physiological saline solution results in negative aspiration when Veress needle is correctly placed and yields a blood-tinged aspirate, or one with intestinal contents when the needle is placed in a blood vessel or the intestine.

Hanging drop test and "fluid in flow": With Veress needle placed in the abdominal cavity, lifting the abdominal wall creates negative intraabdominal pressure. A drop of water is then placed on the open end of the Veress needle. If the needle is correctly positioned, water will move down the shaft.

Any movement of the needle after placement must be avoided as this may convert a small needlepoint injury into a complex and threatening tear. After ensuring that the Veress needle has been positioned correctly, the insufflation is started. Once adequate gas flow and pressure have been achieved, the influx can be raised so that 2–3 L of CO_2 gas can be insufflated per minute until 3–6 L have been insufflated, depending on the patient's size and obesity. After an insufflation volume of about 300 mL, percussion of the liver region will confirm the *loss of liver dullness*, which is a reliable sign of proper positioning of Veress needle and creation of pneumoperitoneum. Abdominal pressure should then be increased to 20–25 mm Hg before inserting the primary trocar because this maximizes the distension of the abdominal wall from all underlying structures (Figs. 35.36A to C).[27]

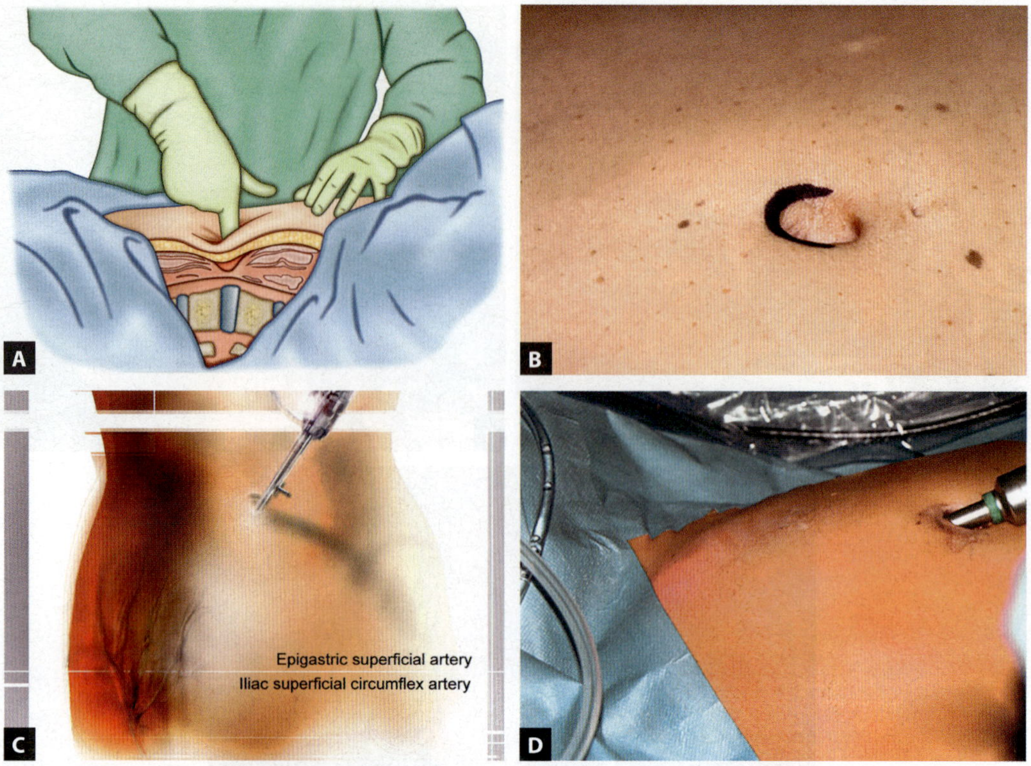

Figs. 35.33A to D: (A) Typical point of palpation in the subumbilical region. The fingertip is pointing to the promontory. (B to D) Subumbilical incision and local palpation reveal the short distance from the skin to the spine. Diaphanoscopy illuminates the region of insertion of the ancillary trocars while demarcating the superficial epigastric artery and the superficial circumflex iliac artery.

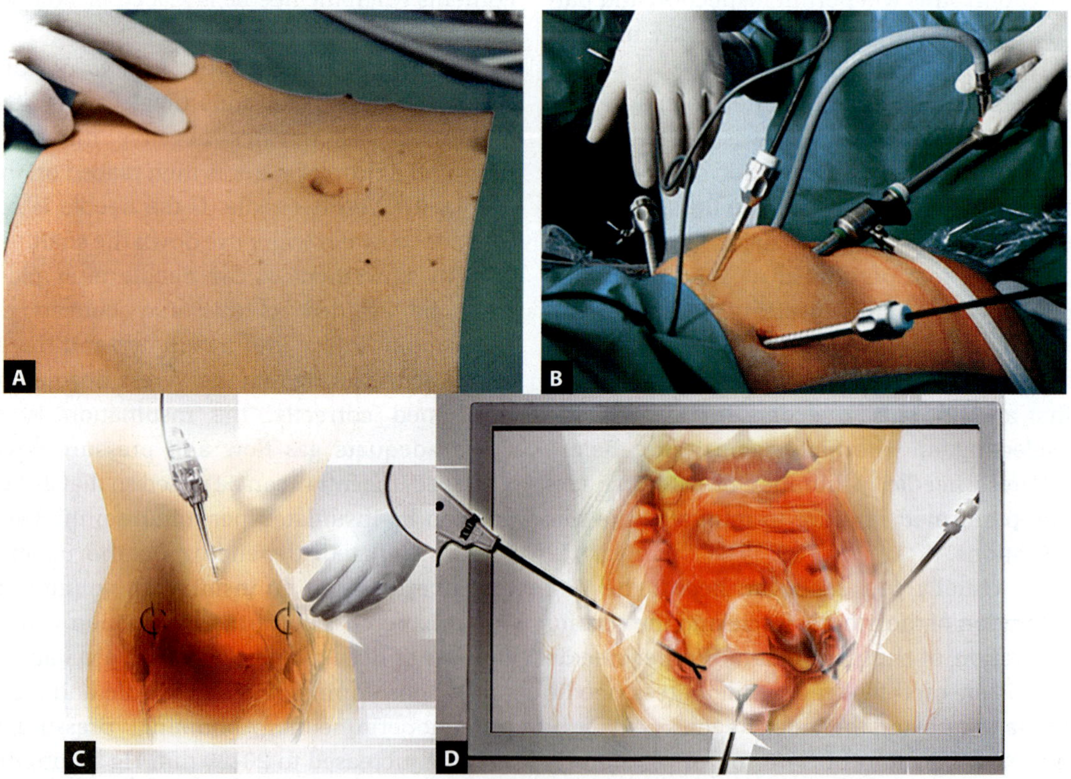

Figs. 35.34A to D: (A and C) Point of insertion from the outside (two thumbs medial to the anterior superior spine), at a 90° angle to the surface, with penetration of all layers of the abdominal wall. Trocar insertion site lateral to the lateral umbilical fold; (B and D) Overview after insertion of the laparoscope and 3 ancillary trocars.

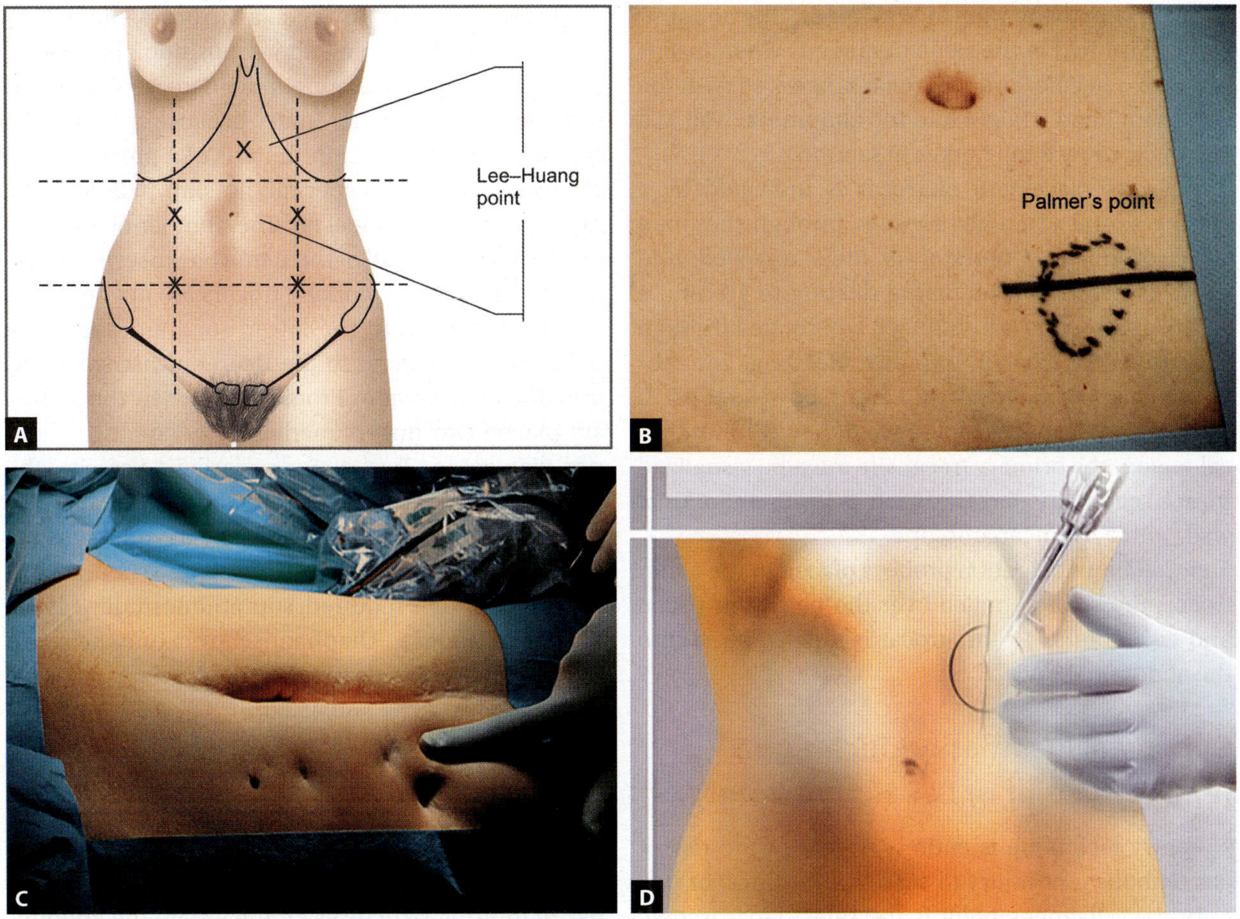

Figs. 35.35A to D: Alternative entry site showing. (A) In cases of a large uterus, especially at or above the level of the umbilicus, the Lee-Huang point. This point is recommended for video-assisted laparoscopy; (C) In cases of anticipated adhesions in the region of Palmer's point; (B to D) Palmer's point is situated in the midclavicular line, about 3 cm below the costal margin.

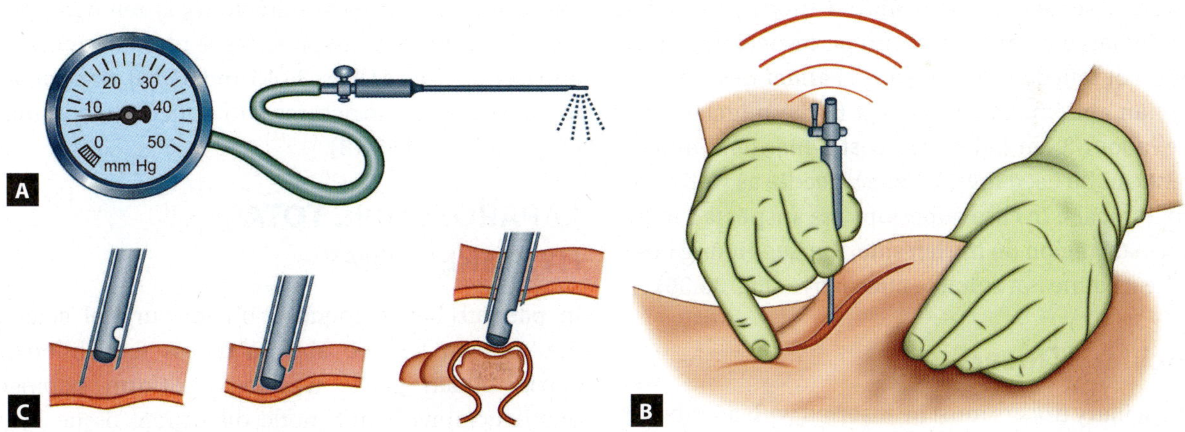

Figs. 35.36A to C: Veress needle and its insertion. The safety mechanism avoids damage or injury to the bowel or vessels.

The optic trocar is inserted in two steps. In the first step, a 5 mm optic trocar and the laparoscope are inserted to confirm pneumoperitoneum and the absence of local adhesions. Dilation to 10 mm is achieved in the second step, either under sight or blindly, thus ensuring optimum visibility during the operation.

Step 1: Entry is performed by a Z technique in the following manner: After proceeding forward with the trocar forward to about 1.5 cm, the tip is moved to about 1.5 cm to the right at a 90° angle. The abdominal wall is lifted in the same manner as when inserting Veress needle, and the trocar is screwed with the dominant hand straight into the abdominal wall at a 90° angle, toward the hollow of sacrum.

Correct placement of trocar is indicated by a hissing sound when gas escapes through the open valve of trocar. Obturator is then removed and trocar is held in place. Before dilating to 10 mm, a 5 mm laparoscope is introduced and rotated through 360° to check visually for any bleeding, intraabdominal abnormality or adherent bowel loops. If the surgeon suspects adherence of bowel in umbilical region, the primary trocar site must be visualized from a secondary port site, such as lower abdominal wall, with a 5 mm laparoscope.

Step 2: A blunt palpation probe is placed in the 5 mm trocar; the shaft is pulled over the palpation probe and taken out. A 10-mm trocar is then screwed into the abdominal cavity.[27]

Subcostal Insufflation Technique (Palmer's Point or Lee Huang Point)

No entry technique is entirely devoid of the risk of gas embolism or injury to vessels, intestines, or urinary tract. Palmer's point is the safest laparoscopic entry point because it is least likely to be affected by adhesions.

For all patients with a significantly higher risk of adhesion, a history of abdominal surgery including cesarean section, a large fibroid uterus, umbilical hernia, large ovarian cysts, preperitoneal gas insufflation or failed umbilical entry, Palmer described in 1974 an abdominal entry point in the midclavicular line, about 3 cm below the costal margin. Palmer's point can be used for the Veress needle as well as for small trocars. In case adhesions are suspected in the subcostal region on the left side, the Lee Huang point in the midline is a suitable alternative (Fig. 35.35).[27]

Ancillary Trocars

All ancillary trocars must be inserted with an intraabdominal pressure of 15–20 mm Hg under direct vision. The inferior epigastric vessels are visualized laparoscopically whereas the superficial vessels can be visualized by diaphanoscopy.

Once the tip of trocar has pierced peritoneum, it should be angulated in the direction of uterine fundus under visual control until the port is placed correctly and the sharp tip can be removed.

Before inserting any ancillary trocars, the patient is moved into Trendelenburg position. Premature Trendelenburg positioning may increase the risk of retroperitoneal vascular injury because the iliac vessels are located exactly in the axis of a preconceived 45° insertion angle, especially in slim patients with minimal retroperitoneal fat. The number of ancillary trocars is variable; all of them must be inserted under direct vision. If two working trocars are needed, they should be placed in the lower quadrant above the pubic hairline lateral to the deep epigastric vessels from the interior view. From exterior view the trocars are placed two fingers medial to the anterior superior iliac spine. Two major superficial vessels—the superficial epigastric artery and the superficial circumflex iliac artery—must be avoided. These vessels can be visualized by diaphanoscopy. When a third ancillary trocar is required, suprapubic midline is the most common site. Diaphanoscopy cannot be relied upon to locate the deep vessels, especially in obese patients (Figs. 35.37 and 35.38).

Finger-tapping from outside can be used to verify correction positioning of the trocar. A small skin incision should be performed before trocar sleeve is inserted. The trocars must be inserted by the shortest route at a 90° angle to the skin surface so that the risk of injuring structures on the way to the abdominal wall is minimized. When inserting a trocar in the midline, the Foley catheter must be identified in order to avoid accidental bladder perforation.[27,31]

Step 3: **Surgical steps—Resection of endometriosis:** The primary sept in hysterectomy is removal of all visible endometriosis spots. These may be superficial and easy to excise (Figs. 35.15 and 35.16), or adherent to more delicate structures and difficult to eliminate (Figs. 35.17 and 35.18).

LAPAROSCOPIC TOTAL HYSTERECTOMY

In patients being operated on for surgical staging, the surgeon will be able to assess the abdomen, pelvis, obtain pelvic washings, perform salpingo-oophorectomy, lymph node dissection, tissue biopsies and omentectomy in addition to laparoscopic hysterectomy.

Technique 1: Primary Uterine Artery Ligation

The next step is to coagulate and separate the round ligament near the pelvic side wall (Fig. 35.39A).

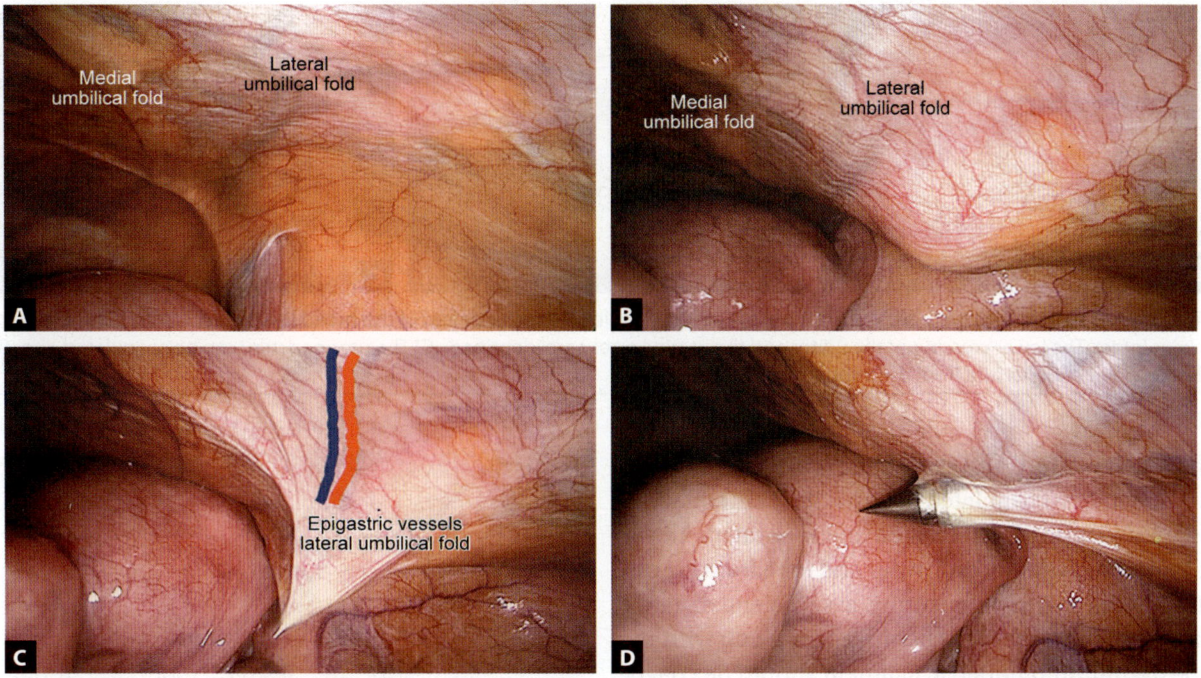

Figs. 35.37A to D: Secondary trocar placement, entry in the right lower abdomen. (A) Three different plicae are visualized; (B) The palpating finger is showing the area lateral to the lateral umbilical fold; (C) Entry of the sharp ancillary trocar lateral to the lateral umbilical fold; (D) Once the peritoneum has been penetrated, the trocar points to the fundus of the uterus in order to avoid injury to the major vessels and the bowel.

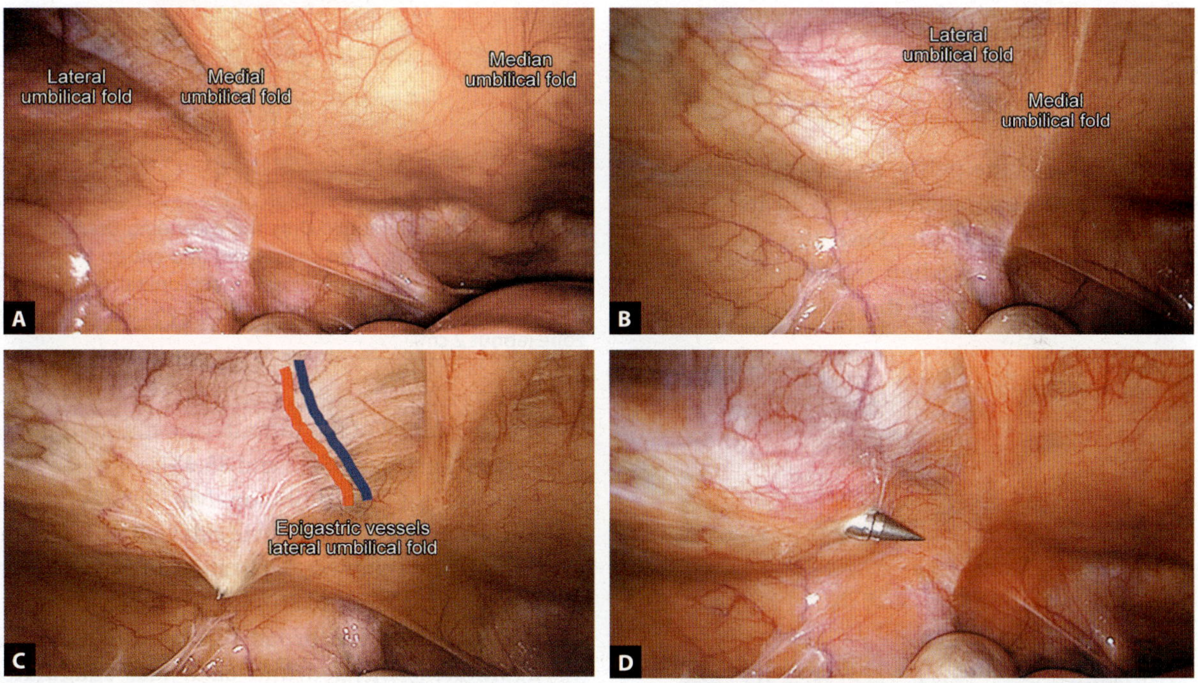

Figs. 35.38A to D: Secondary trocar placement, entry in the left lower abdomen. (A) The three plicae are visualized; (B) The palpating finger is showing the area lateral to the lateral umbilical fold; (C) Entry of the sharp ancillary trocar lateral to the lateral umbilical fold; (D) Once the peritoneum has been penetrated, the trocar points to the fundus of the uterus in order to avoid injury to the major vessels and the bowel.

The peritoneum is then incised further. The anterior leaf of the broad ligament is opened to the bladder fold and bladder is pushed downward. The posterior leaf of the broad ligament is visualized and the ureters are lateralized. The retroperitoneal space is then exposed, the course of the ureters demonstrated and the site of exit of the uterine artery from the iliac artery visualized (Fig. 35.39B). The crossing point of

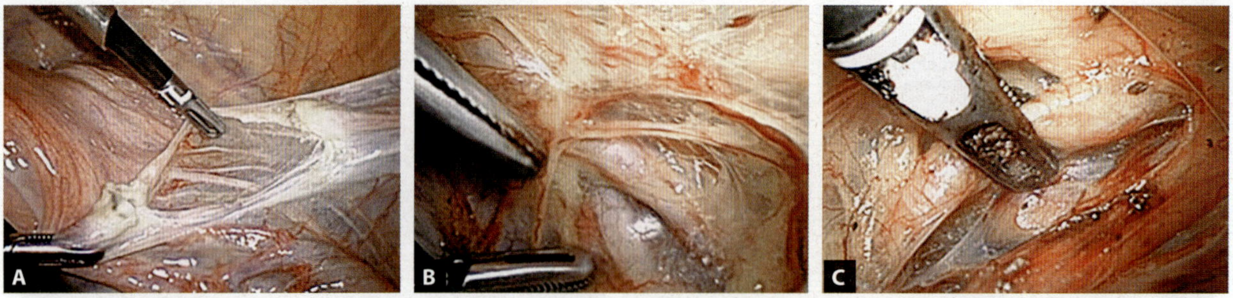

Figs. 35.39A to C: Technique 1: (A) The first step consists of opening the anterior leaf of the broad ligament; (B) The round ligament is kept intact. The lower crossing of the ureter and the uterine artery are identified; (C) The uterine artery can be coagulated directly after its point of departure from the internal iliac artery.

the uterine artery and the ureter is exposed and the uterine artery coagulated (Fig. 35.39C). The bladder pillar is identified, coagulated and separated. This is followed by separation of ovary and tube from uterus. If the adnexa—after ensuring a sufficient distance from the ureters—are to be dissected along with the uterus, infundibulopelvic ligament should be coagulated and mesosalpinx and mesovarium dissected in the direction of fenestration. Fenestration is a useful point of orientation to safeguard the ureter.[32-34]

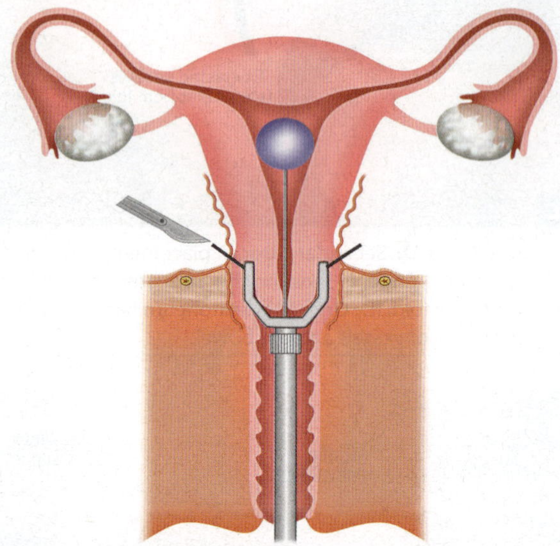

Fig. 35.41: Schematic illustration of the resection line in total laparoscopic hysterectomy. Only the ascending branch of the uterine artery needs to be coagulated and cut on the uterine manipulator. When adhering closely to this operative technique, the ureter is located at a safe distance from the coagulation zone (about 2 cm).

Technique 2: Classic Intrafascial Hysterectomy

Surgical steps:

1. Inspection of the pelvis, tracing the ureters and planning the operation (Figs. 35.40 and 35.41).
2. Start on the right side. Push the uterus in the opposite direction when separating the adnexa or the ligaments from the pelvic sidewall, with the assistance of the intrauterine manipulator or by traction (Figs. 35.42 and 35.43).
3. Division of infundibulopelvic ligament and round ligament from pelvic sidewall or, when the adnexa are retained, separation of adnexa from uterus (Figs. 35.44 to 35.48).
4. Dissection of the broad ligament: The broad ligament is opened and each leaf coagulated separately (Figs. 35.49 to 35.51). This is not possible when a sealing and cutting instrument is used, because the two leaves of the broad ligament are sealed together. The direction of exposure is as close to uterus as possible but as distant as necessary, thus avoiding exposure close to the sidewall and the ureter (Figs. 35.52A to D).

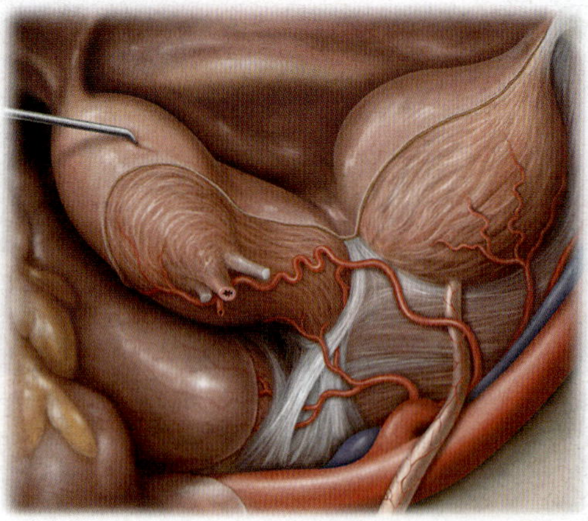

Fig. 35.40: Anatomical illustration showing the relation of the uterine vessel to the ureter in the pelvic wall, compared to its location close to the uterus. The helical course of the ascending branch of the uterine artery can be easily followed. The uterus, bladder and rectum are embedded in a ligament-based pelvic floor.

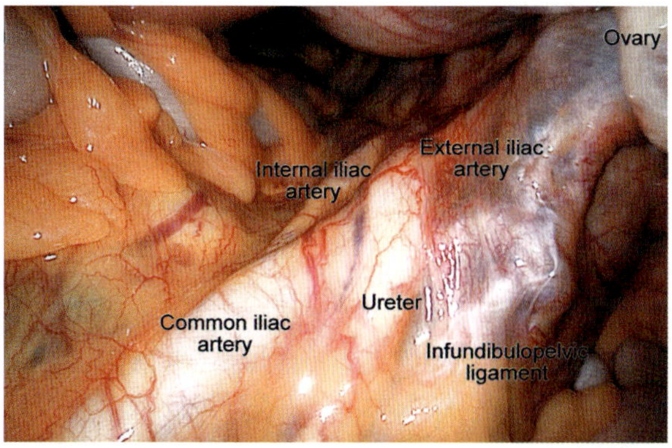

Fig. 35.42: Preliminary inspection of the uterus and the surrounding organs. The lower pelvis as well as the ligaments, vessels and the ureter can be differentiated in relation to the uterus. In slim patients the crossing of the ureter and the common iliac artery can be seen. The infundibulopelvic ligament is identified and held towards the lateral wall in order to obtain a better view of the field of surgery.

5. Separation of the bladder from the uterus by opening the vesicouterine ligament and pushing the bladder downward by about 1–2 cm (Figs. 35.51B and C).
6. Presentation of the ascending branch of uterine artery and separation of uterine pedicles (Figs. 35.53A to D).
7. Identical stepwise dissection of the left adnexa (Figs. 35.54 and 35.55), opening of the bladder peritoneum and broad ligament (Figs. 35.56A to D), and dissection of the uterine vessels (Figs. 35.57 and 35.58) on the left side. A thorough inspection of the cervix is performed.
8. After separation of the bladder from uterus, the bladder is pushed and dissected down by 2–3 cm to clearly visualize the rim of cervical cap. In cases of postcesarean section, a careful, gentle and nearly blunt dissection should be performed (Figs. 35.59 to 35.61).
9. While lateralizing ureter by pushing the manipulator upward, uterine artery and vein with its collaterals are fully coagulated near cervix and dissected.

The key steps of pushing the bladder down from the anterior vaginal fornix prior to incision and distancing ureters from uterine vessels at the cervical/vaginal level can be safely performed by stretching the manipulator firmly cranially, to the contralateral side of the exposure.

Step 4:

1. In laparoscopic supracervical hysterectomy, resection of uterine corpus is performed at this stage of surgery. The steps of exposure are very similar until this point, except for the fact that there is no need for a manipulator and elevation of uterus is achieved by traction. The corpus of the uterus is cut with a monopolar loop and the cervical channel coagulated to prevent spotting. The cervical channel should be closed because of the risk of ascending infection. Simultaneously,

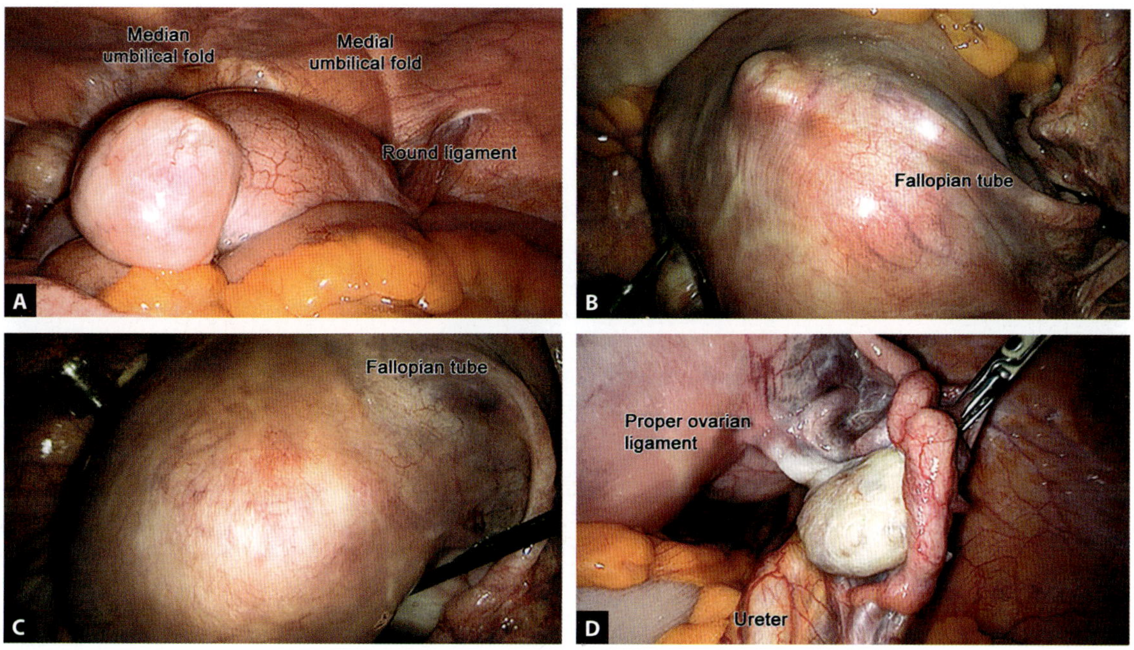

Figs. 35.43A to D: Reconstruction of the anatomy of the right pelvic wall. The bifurcation of the common iliac artery and the crossing of the ureter are clearly visible. The infundibulopelvic ligament and the ovarian vessels are situated lateral to the ureter. The infundibulopelvic ligament might be fixed to the bowel (especially on the left side) and cause difficulties when exposing the adnexa.

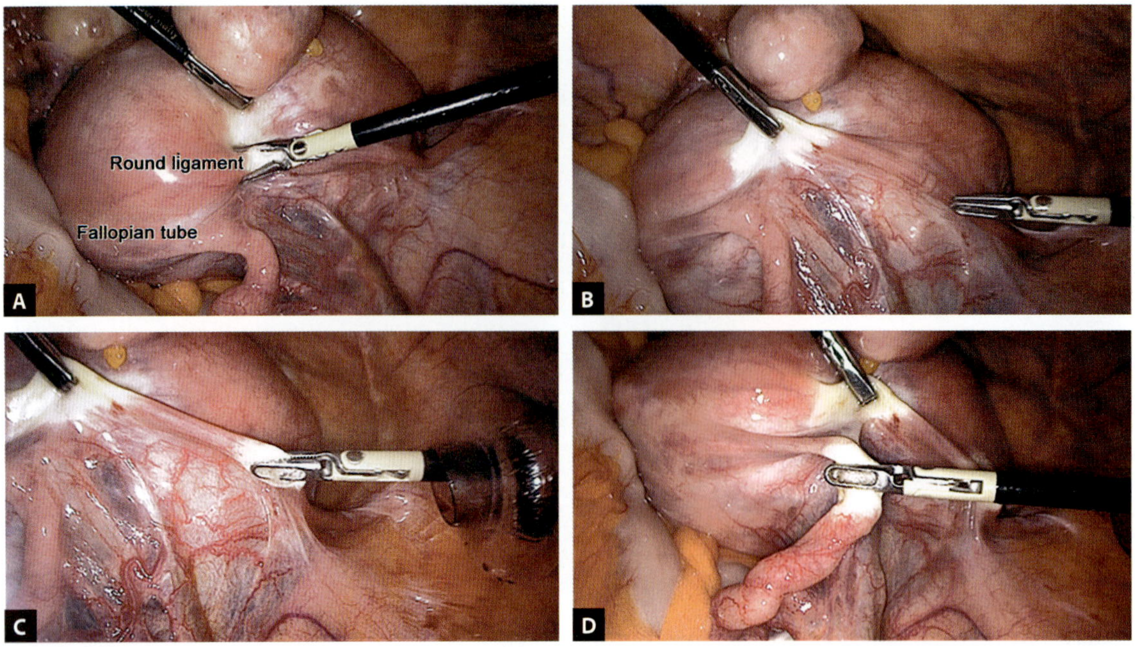

Figs. 35.44A to D: Stepwise bipolar coagulation of the right tube and the right round ligament. (A and B) The round ligament is coagulated so that a sharp instrument can be used to pull the tissue without causing bleeding that might impede vision (C and D).

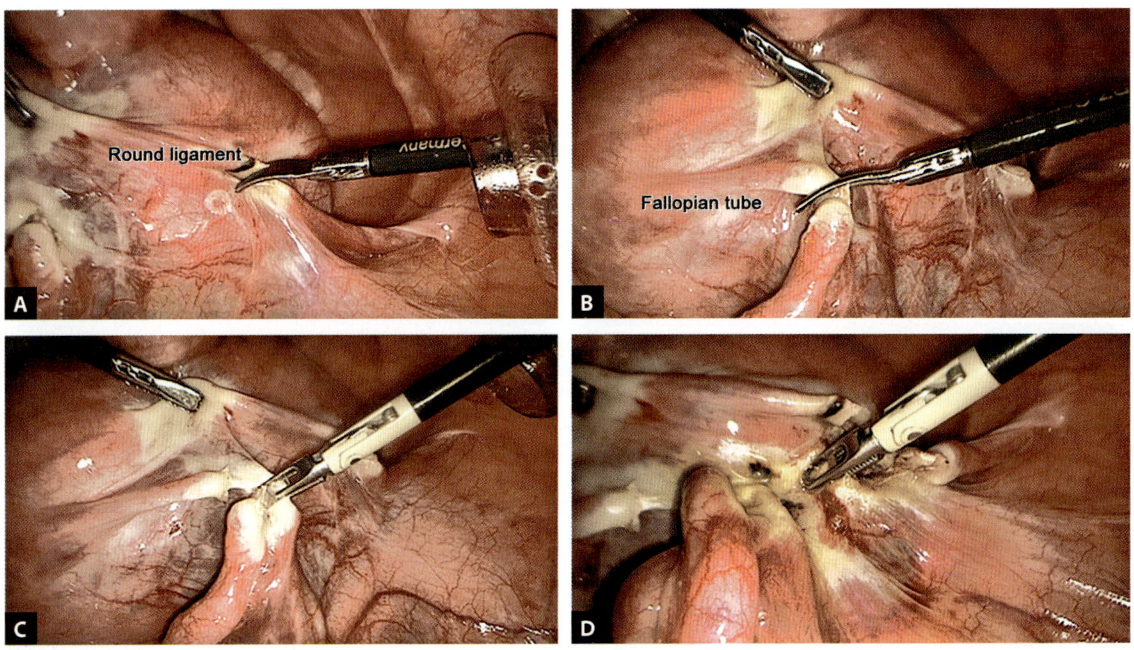

Figs. 35.45A to D: Stepwise dissection of the right tube and the round ligament. (A and B) The curved scissors are held with the tip away from the uterine wall; After dissecting the fallopian tube, the vessels running underneath must be coagulated before further cutting (C and D).

cervix can be suspended using a strong monofilament suture with extracorporeal knotting (Figs. 35.62 and 35.63).

2. Resection of vagina from cervix with the monopolar hook by stretching the manipulator firmly cranially. Intrafascial dissection is performed, leaving the sacrouterine ligaments almost completely in place (Figs. 35.64 to 35.66).

Uterus is then extracted through vagina or positioned in vagina to prevent the loss of intraabdominal pressure while still fixed to the manipulator (Figs. 35.67A and B). A large uterus must be morcellated either intraabdominally or transvaginally. In cases of a large benign uterus, visible myomas can be enucleated or the large uterus cut into several smaller pieces, which are then extracted through vagina.

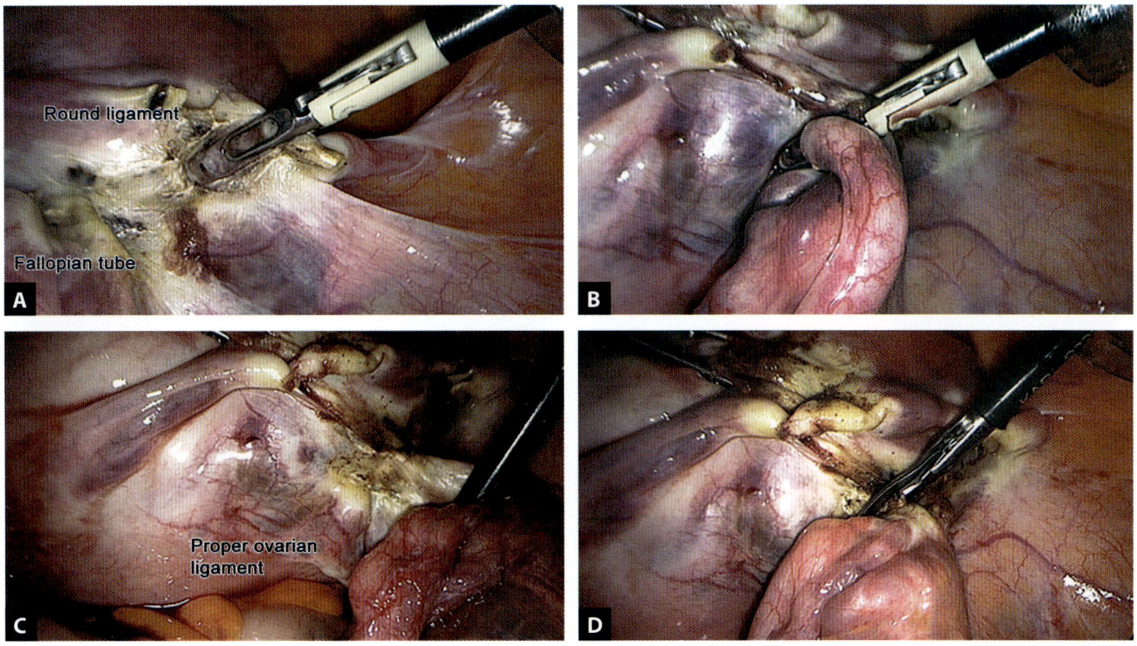

Figs. 35.46A to D: Continuous stepwise dissection and exposure for opening the broad ligament. (A and C) With traction on tissue, the line of exposure can be easily demarcated; (B and D) Coagulation involves the entire tissue, but the cutting line strictly omits the uterine wall. Cutting the tube at this stage provides a better overview for exposure in the following steps. The tube can be removed easily after the hysterectomy.

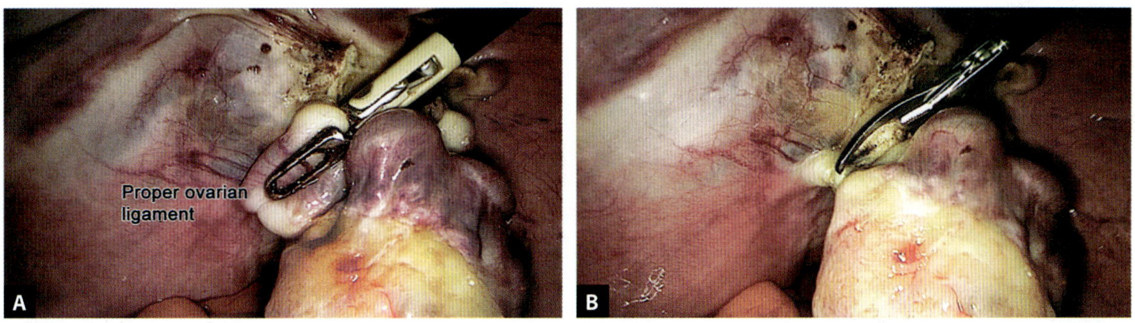

Figs. 35.47A and B: Coagulation of the proper ovarian ligament and dissection without involving the uterine or the ovarian wall.

As a result, incision in the lower abdomen need not exceed 5 mm and postoperative pain or the risk of hernia is minimized. Alternatively, a 10–12 mm electromorcellator is used to dissect the material, which is then extracted through the abdominal wall. The cutting edge of the morcellator must always be visible during morcellation. Evidence of the absence of any malignancy must be obtained earlier by appropriate preoperative diagnostic investigation. The patient must be informed in advance about the fact that the uterus, depending on its volume, may need to be morcellated.

Step 5: **(Classical closure)**—After removing uterus, vaginal cuff and peritoneum are closed with two Vicryl 0 Z-sutures, or with a running suture with or without separate knotting of the lateral edges. Suturing may be performed intraabdominally or extraabdominally. This simple and economical concept can be adapted to almost all techniques of open surgery.

Step 6: **(Alternative closure technique emphasizing prolapse prevention):**

1. *A technique for stable fixation of the vaginal or cervical stump.*
2. *Vaginal closure with Te Linde suturing technique modified by Schollmeyer.*

Hysterectomy is known to be associated with a high risk of pelvic organ prolapse; the risk is especially high among multiparous women. This may necessitate pelvic organ prolapse surgery. Given the current high life expectancy of women, organ prolapse may pose a problem in later life and also

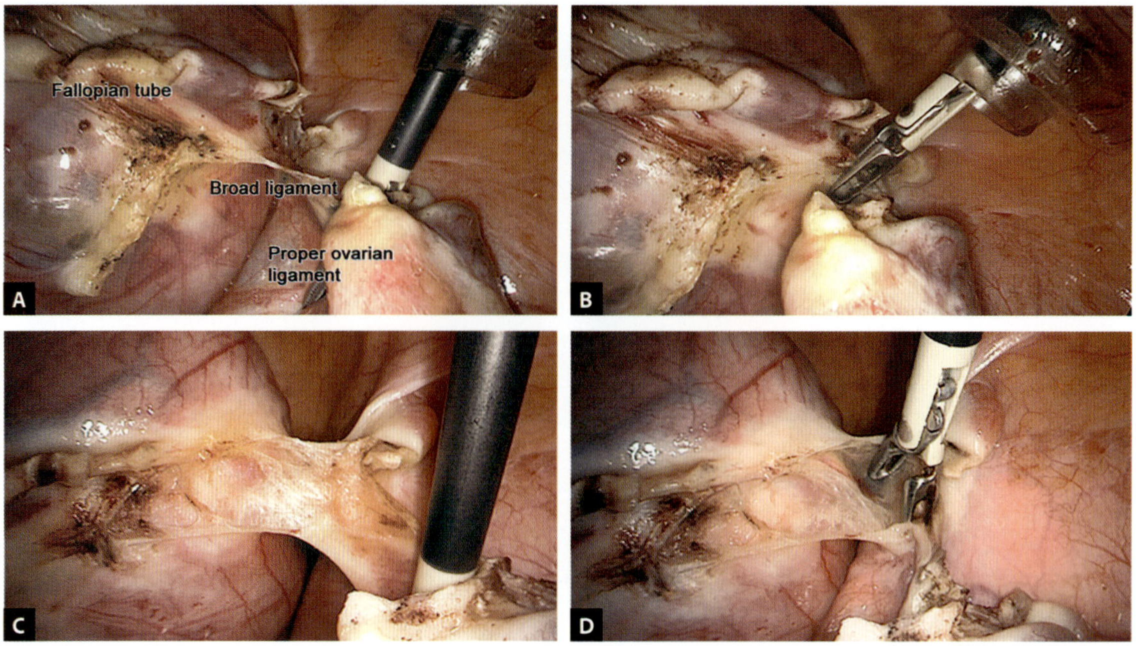

Figs. 35.48A to D: Dissection of the proper ovarian ligament and opening the broad ligament. (A) After the proper ovarian ligament has been dissected, the adnexa falls to the lateral aspect; (B to D) The broad ligament can then be identified and separated into its two leaves.

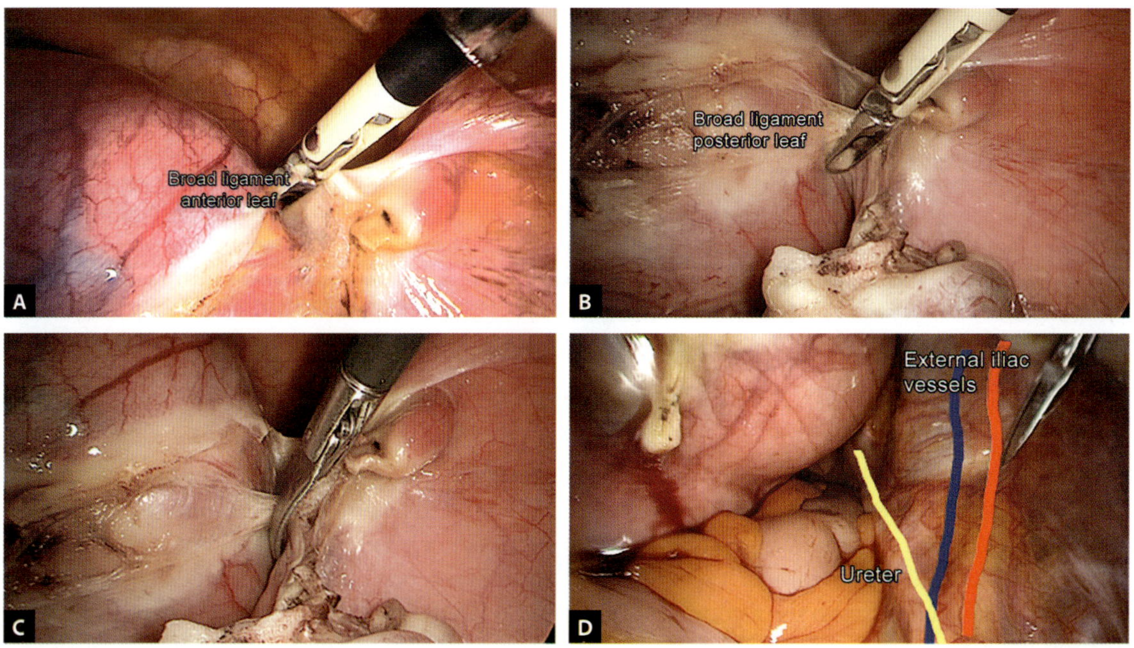

Figs. 35.49A to D: (A to C) Separation of the anterior and posterior leaf of the broad ligament in relation to the; (D) Ureter and the pelvic vessels; (A to C) The broad ligament is coagulated and dissected as close to the uterus as possible without affecting the uterine artery. As the two leaves are separated, the ascending branch of the uterine artery can be visualized easily and omitted. The tip of the scissors is directed strictly away from the uterine wall using the curved blade.

difficulties in surgical repair (thrombosis, embolism, and infection).[35]

The suturing technique of Te Linde, known from abdominal hysterectomy for the closure of vagina, was modified for laparoscopic use by Bruno van Herendael and further modified by Thoralf Schollmeyer.[36,37]

- Cautious coagulation of the vaginal edge[38] is followed by the suturing of vagina. Coagulation should be performed very carefully to avoid postoperative necrosis of the vaginal stump. Slight residual bleeding is addressed by sutures incorporating the complete vaginal wall. The uterus

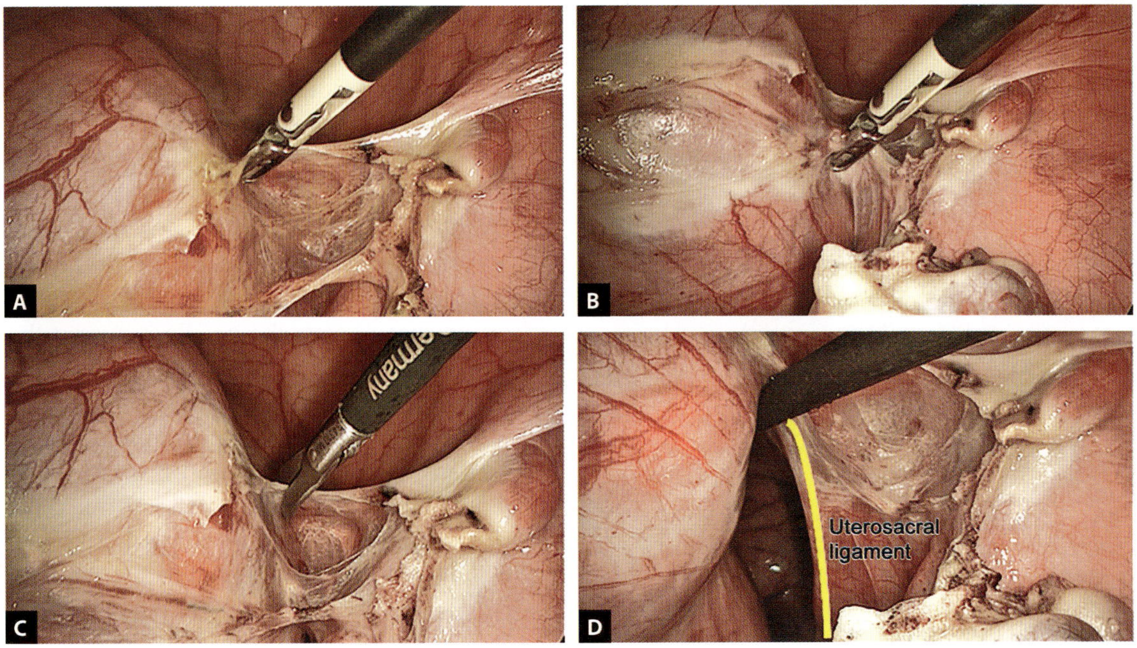

Figs. 35.50A to D: (A to C) Final separation of the leaves of the broad ligament close to the pelvic floor; (D) The sacrouterine ligament. The uterus is pushed to the left side; the bladder peritoneum is close by. (D) By blunt manipulation the course of the sacrouterine ligament can be visualized; the line of coagulation should omit this part.

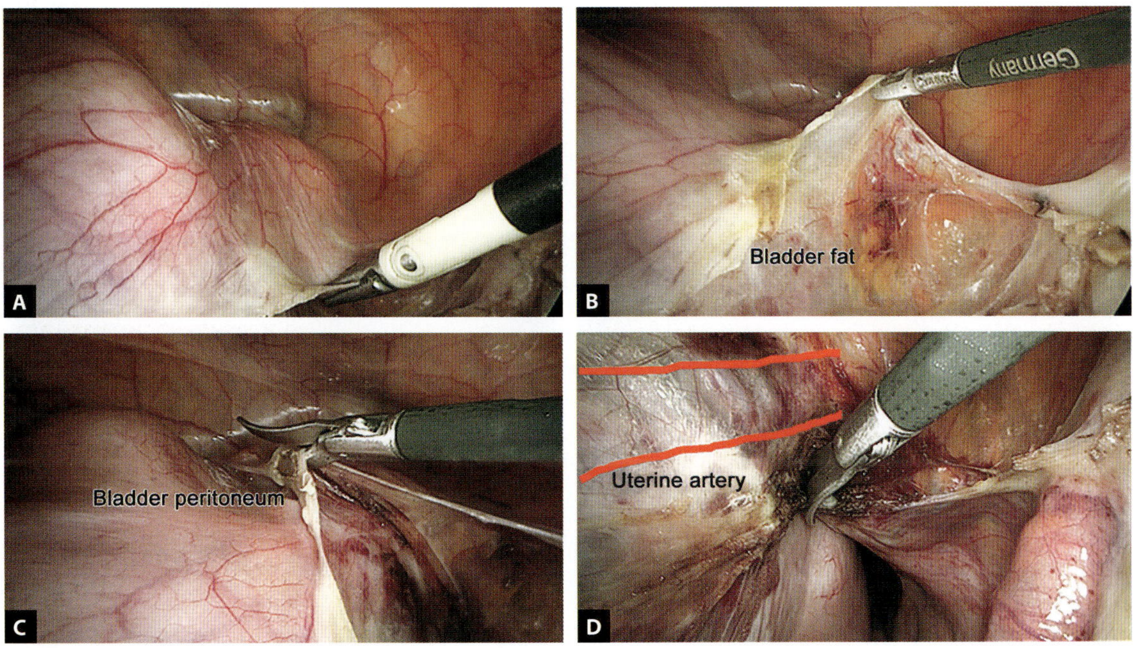

Figs. 35.51A to D: (A to C) Opening the bladder peritoneum from the right side. The beginning of the bladder peritoneum can be easily demarcated; the cutting line should be neither above this zone nor too far into the caudal aspect. Gas enters the created space and shows the beginning of the bladder pillar; (D) The uterine vessel bundle is freed by coagulating and dissecting above and below it. The ureter is at a safe distance lateral to this area of exposure.

is either still in the vagina or a glove filled with swabs is placed in the vagina to avoid loss of the pneumoperitoneum. Usually a curved needle and PDS 1-0 is used for single-knot suturing, with extracorporeal knots and intracorporeal safety knots. Alternatively, sled needles or even straight needles can be used for easy handling in and out of the 5 mm trocars.

PDS 1-0 extracorporeal knots are used for the following reasons:

- The monofilament thread slides easily through the tissue and does not cause additional damage.

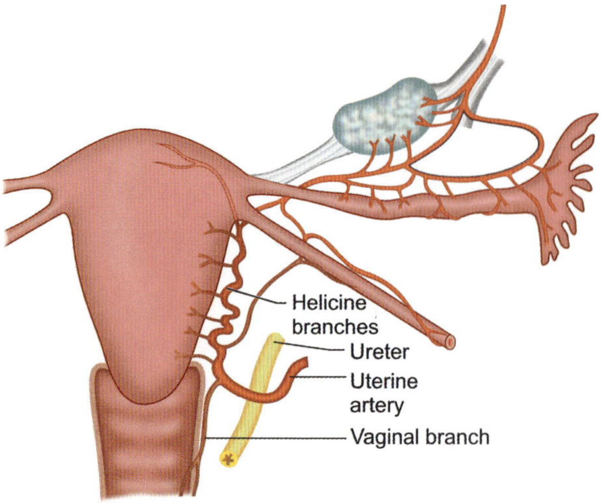

Fig. 35.52: Anatomical schematic illustration showing the spiral structure of the ascending uterine artery. Exposure too close to the uterus may cause arterial bleeding, which can only be stopped after complete coagulation of the uterine artery on the opposite side. The field of surgery would be greatly disturbed by antegrade or retrograde bleeding. The ureter is close to the surgical field only in the lowest part. Pushing the uterus away lateralizes the ureter and moves it to the side.

- The monofilament PDS material minimizes the risk of vaginal stump infection.
- The long half-life of the suture material minimizes the risk of vaginal stump dehiscence.[38]
- Extracorporeal knots provide additional strength.

Optionally, both sacrouterine ligaments may be attached to posterior vaginal wall to prevent vaginal prolapse (McCall culdoplasty).

- *Corner sutures:* The pericervical ring is pierced by performing a suture in the right vaginal corner, followed by the corresponding vaginal epithelium. The sutures are made at a distance from the urinary bladder to minimize the risk of bladder laceration (Figs. 35.68 and 35.69).
- In the second step, the needle is passed through medial aspect of the cardinal ligament in front of uterine vessels (Figs. 35.70A to D). The second step involves the structures supporting vaginal wall suspension. Extracorporeal knotting with the placement of a deep and strong monofilament suture allows the surgeon to grasp a large quantity of tissue and smoothly glide through the tissue without causing damage (Figs. 35.71 to 35.73).
- Subsequent back-stitching of the vagina is followed by passing the needle through vaginal epithelium and then, in the third step, through sacrouterine ligament. The last step may be omitted when ligament is stitched again once or twice to shorten it. In cases of preexisting descent, this is absolutely essential.

The needle can now be withdrawn and the suture is completed with an extracorporeal Roeder knot, secured by two to three intracorporeal knots (Figs. 35.74A to D). This procedure is repeated on

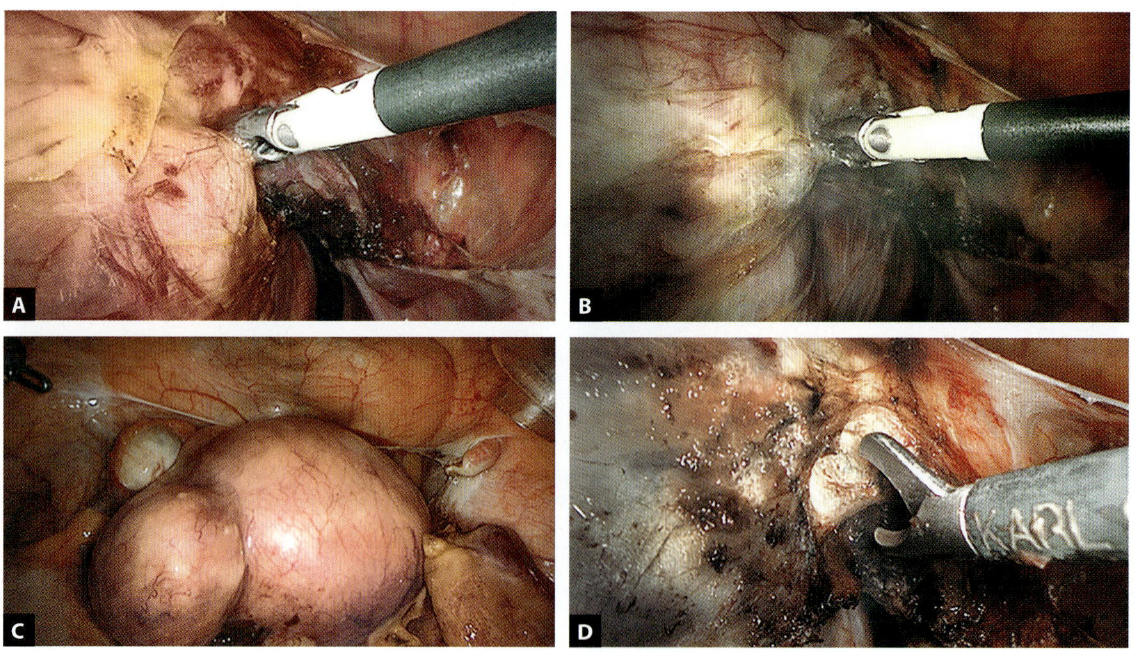

Figs. 35.53A to D: Bipolar coagulation and dissection of the uterine vessels. (A and B) The area of coagulation must include the upper part of the artery to avoid retrograde bleeding after dissecting the vessel; (C) The color of the uterus changes to whitish/grey; (D) A deeper cut can be avoided by using the hook scissors; the uterine artery is dissected in two steps. This allows further coagulation of the tissue lying just behind the artery and avoids cumbersome venous bleeding.

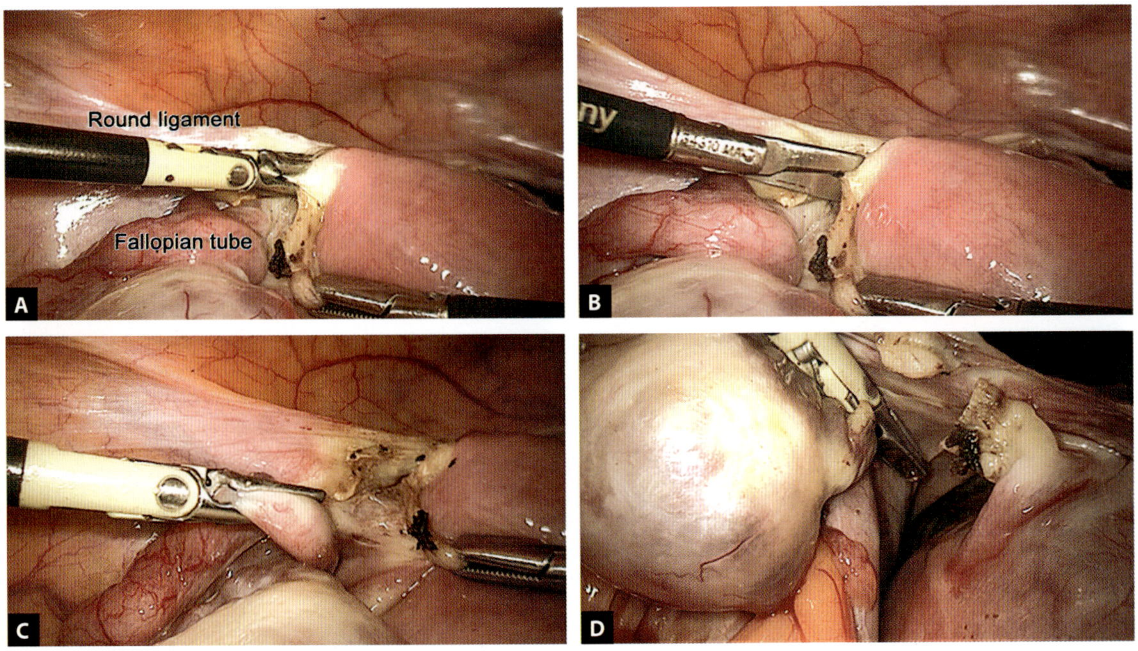

Figs. 35.54A to D: (A to C) Stepwise coagulation and dissection of the left round ligament and tube; (D) The ovarian ligament; (A and B) The curved scissors are held with the tip away from the uterine wall; (C and D) After dissecting the fallopian tube, the vessels coursing below must be coagulated before further cutting; (D) By blunt manipulation, the course of the sacrouterine ligament and the uterus can be visualized in patients with lateral myomas. The line of coagulation should omit this part.

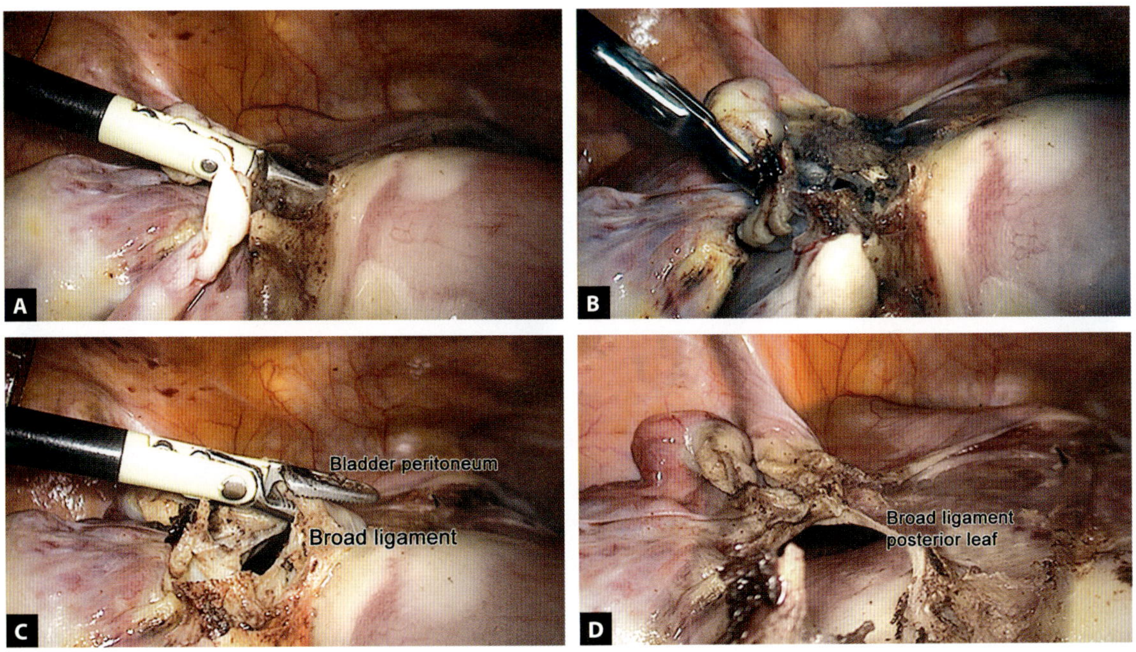

Figs. 35.55A to D: (A to D) Dissection of the bladder peritoneum as well as the anterior and posterior leaf of the broad ligament on the left side; The bladder peritoneum has already been opened from the right side and the posterior leaf of the broad ligament serves as an anatomic landmark for the uterine vessels.

the contralateral side and ensures that all parts of the endopelvic fascia (vesicouterine, cardinal and sacrouterine ligaments) are connected (Figs. 35.75 to 35.77).

Step 6: Vaginal closure: The remaining vaginal opening in the middle can now be closed with two U- or Z-sutures. These ensure both vertical and horizontal compression of the tissue, and minimize the risk of a vaginal stump hematoma. Neither peritonealization nor drainage is necessary (Figs. 35.78 and 35.79). Physiological reperitonealization occurs during the first 2 weeks after the operation. Any

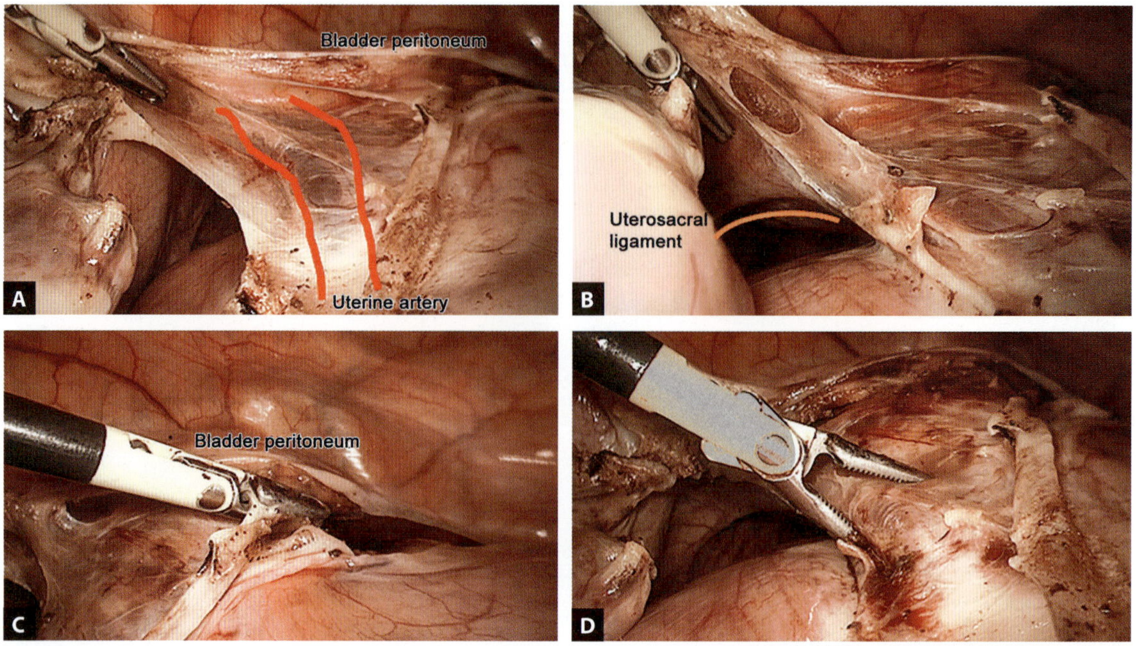

Figs. 35.56A to D: (A to C) Further opening of the bladder peritoneum and the broad ligament; (D) Commencement of coagulation of the left uterine vessels; (A) The uterine artery functions as an anatomic landmark leading downward. An intermediate glance at the back of the uterus shows that the cutting edge is above the conjunction of the sacrouterine ligaments.

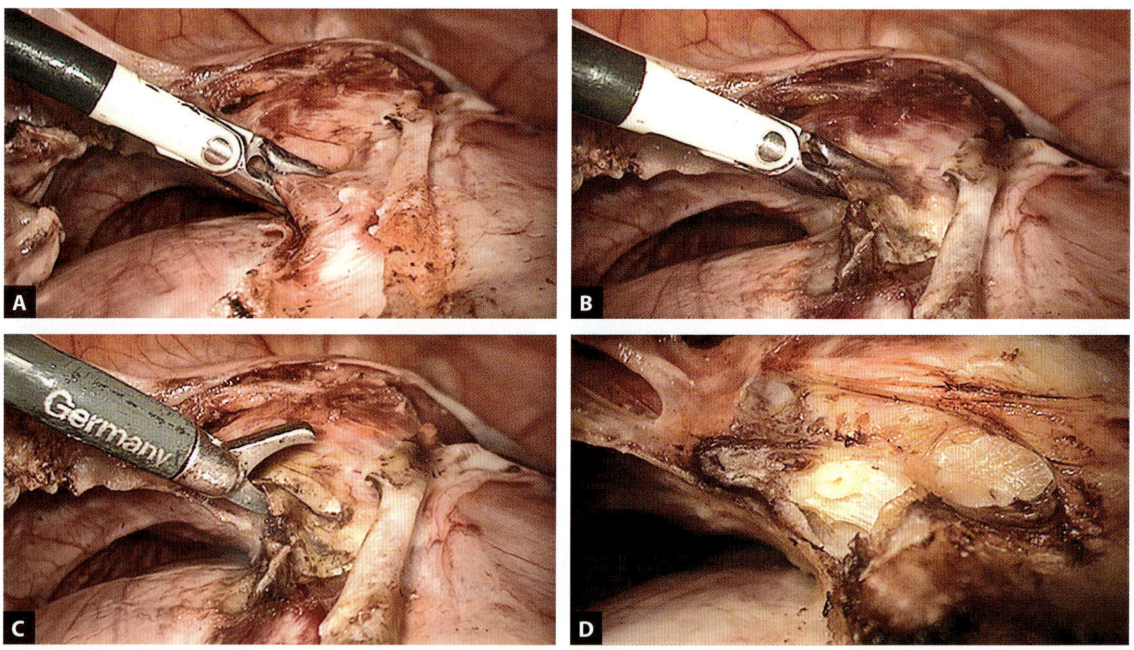

Figs. 35.57A to D: (A) Bipolar coagulation and separation of the uterine vessels on the left side; (B) The area of coagulation should include the upper parts of the artery to avoid any retrograde bleeding after dissection of the vessel. The color of the uterus changes to whitish/grey; (C and D) A deeper cut can be avoided by using the hook scissors; the uterine artery is dissected in two steps. This allows further coagulation of the tissue lying just behind the artery and avoids cumbersome venous bleeding.

additional peritoneal suturing might cause encapsulation of seroma or hematoma and increase the likelihood of postoperative infection as well as pain. If still inside, the uterus or the swab-filled glove is now taken out of the vagina. Figures 35.80A to D provides an overview of the procedure.

LAPAROSCOPIC SUBTOTAL HYSTERECTOMY

In laparoscopic supracervical hysterectomy, resection of the uterine corpus is performed at this stage of surgery. The preceding steps are very similar except

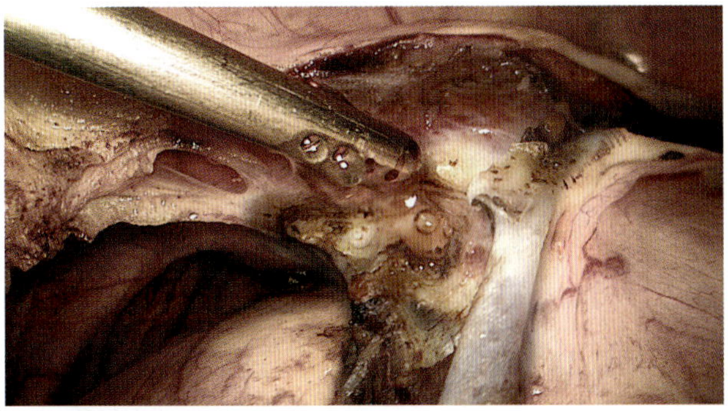

Figs. 35.58: Visualization of the separated left uterine pedicles. A few drops of physiological saline solution render the bipolar coagulation more effective because of better electrolyte flow, especially when the field of operation is very dry.

for the fact that a manipulator is not needed because uterus is elevated by traction. The corpus of the uterus is cut with a monopolar loop and the cervical channel is coagulated to prevent spotting. The cervical channel should be closed because of the high risk of ascending infection. Simultaneously, cervix can be suspended with a strong monofilament suture and extracorporeal knotting. The remaining uterine corpus needs to be morcellated intraabdominally (Figs. 35.81 to 35.86).

Figures 35.87A to D shows the outcome of supracervical and total hysterectomy.

Special Situations

The traditional technique of laparoscopic hysterectomy must be modified in cases of severe adhesions or concomitant deep infiltrating endometriosis. The surgical steps are quite similar to those for oncologic surgery; radical pelvic exposure is essential (Figs. 35.17, 35.18 and 35.40). After adhesiolysis, which may be very extensive in severe endometriosis or adenomyosis, the retroperitoneum is opened (Figs. 35.52, 35.88 and 35.89). Ureter and major vessels are localized, and the crossover of uterine artery is visualized and exposed (Figs. 35.89A to D). In some cases, clipping of the uterine artery just behind its point of departure from the internal iliac artery (Figs. 35.90 to 35.93) is useful for the following reasons:

- More distal preparation and skeletonization of uterine artery may be difficult or even impossible.
- Endometriotic scars and nodules are liable to modify the anatomy of the region. This may lead to unexpected bleeding, especially in cases of a larger uterus. Clipping of the initial portion of the uterine artery will minimize intraoperative bleeding.
- The proximity of the uterine artery to the ureter and the thermal spread of bipolar instruments may cause secondary coagulation defects of the ureter, which can be avoided by using vessel clips.

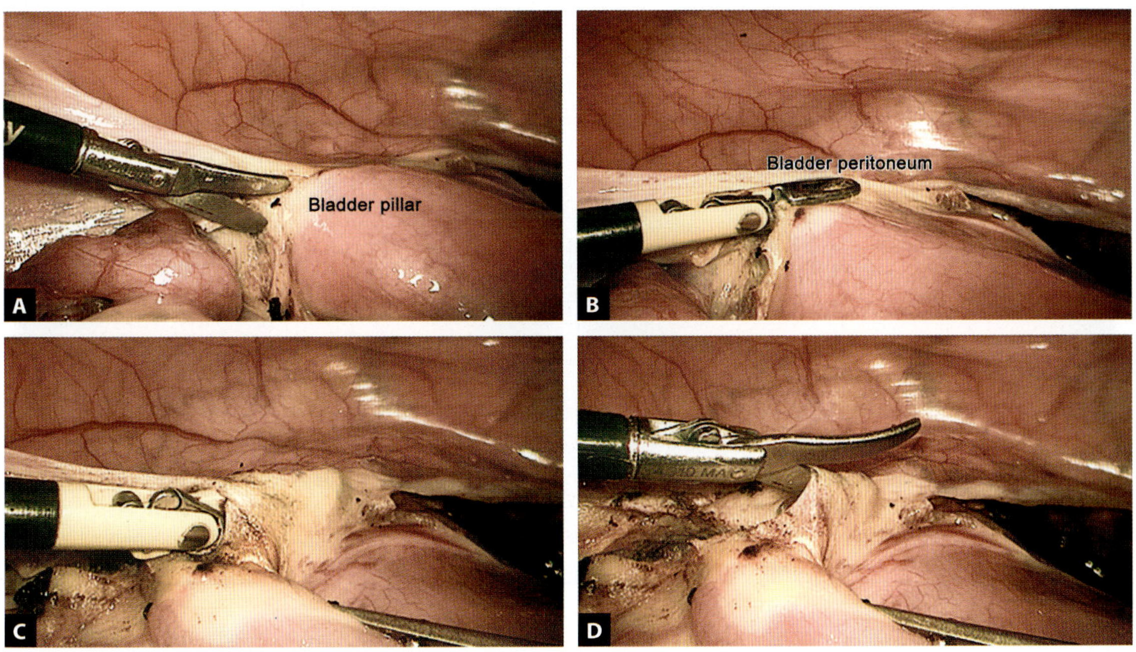

Figs. 35.59A to D: Final dissection of the bladder pillar and the bladder peritoneum from left to right, allowing the CO_2 distension medium to show the way. The bladder is pushed safely downward from the field of operation and the peritoneal line of the vesicouterine fold is easily recognized.

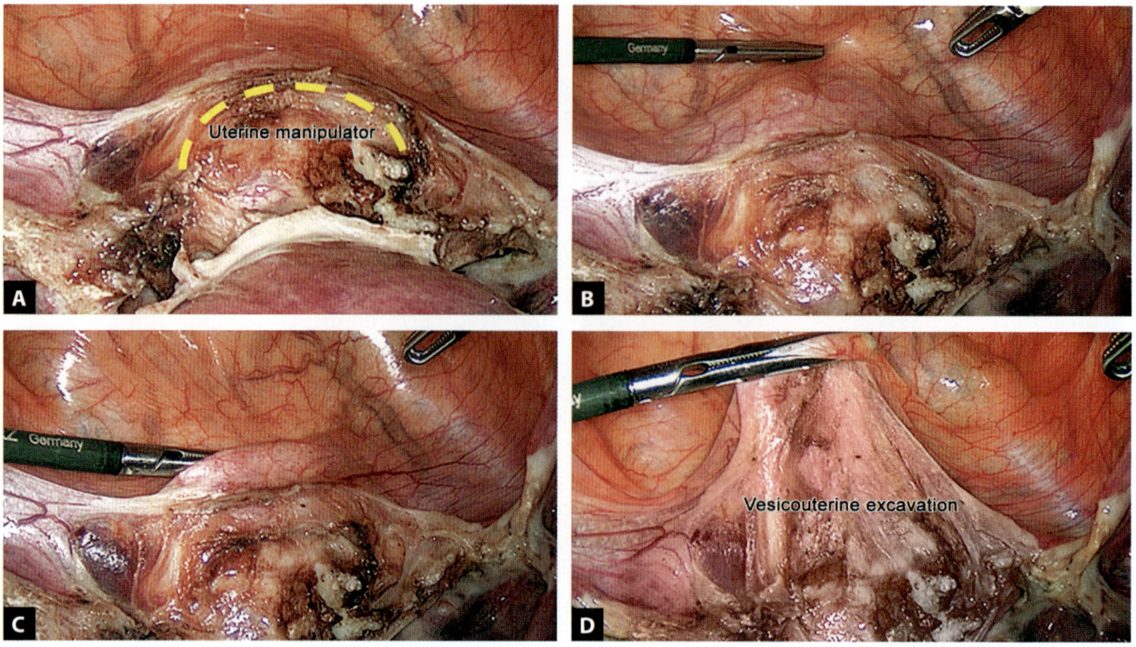

Figs. 35.60A to D: (A) Visualization of the intrauterine manipulator, if inserted; (B and C) The bladder cannot be identified immediately in all cases and is safely avoided. The bladder can be localized exactly when a blunt instrument is used to push the suspected bladder towards the cervix from the balloon of the Foley catheter. Once the bladder has been identified, it is elevated. Vesicouterine excavation can be used to push the bladder further downward (D).

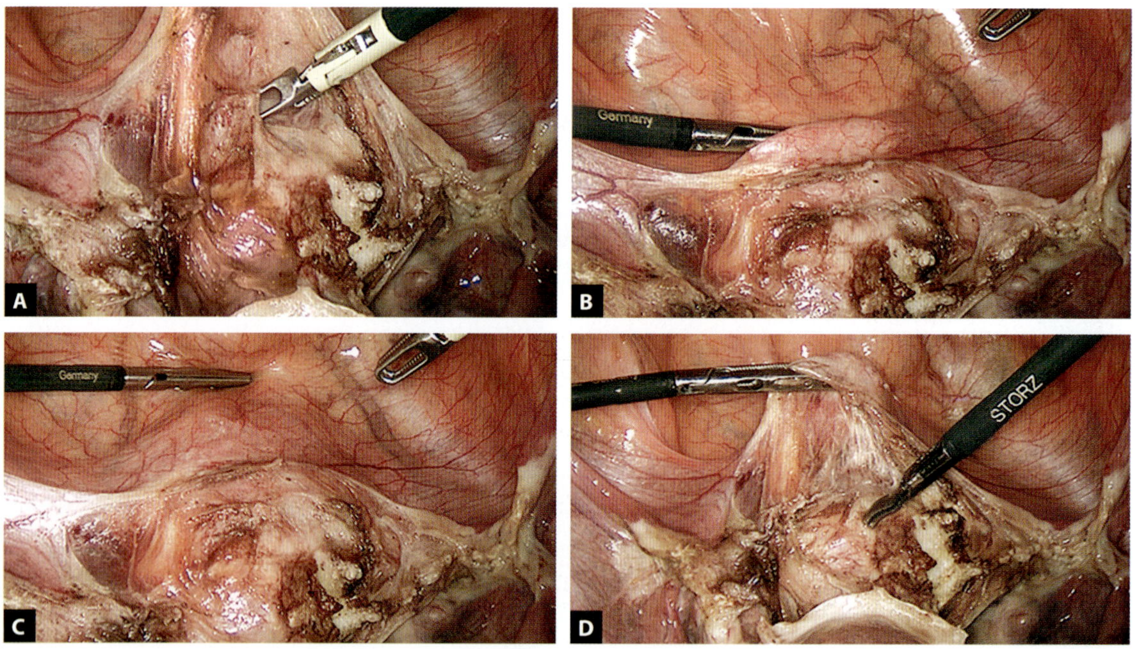

Figs. 35.61A to D: Minimal dissection of the bladder peritoneum by about 1 cm for LSH and 2–3 cm for LTH, by opening the vesicouterine excavation. This is easier when a manipulator is inside the vagina and the cervix is pushed upward; the step can also be performed by traction alone. Once the vesicouterine space has been opened, exposure is easily achieved with a blunt instrument while avoiding bleeding.

At the end of the procedure the abdominal cavity is irrigated with physiological saline solution and drained. Usually no drains are left in situ (Fig. 35.89).

We established this suture technique because it provides stable fixation of the vaginal end in addition to other safety advantages:

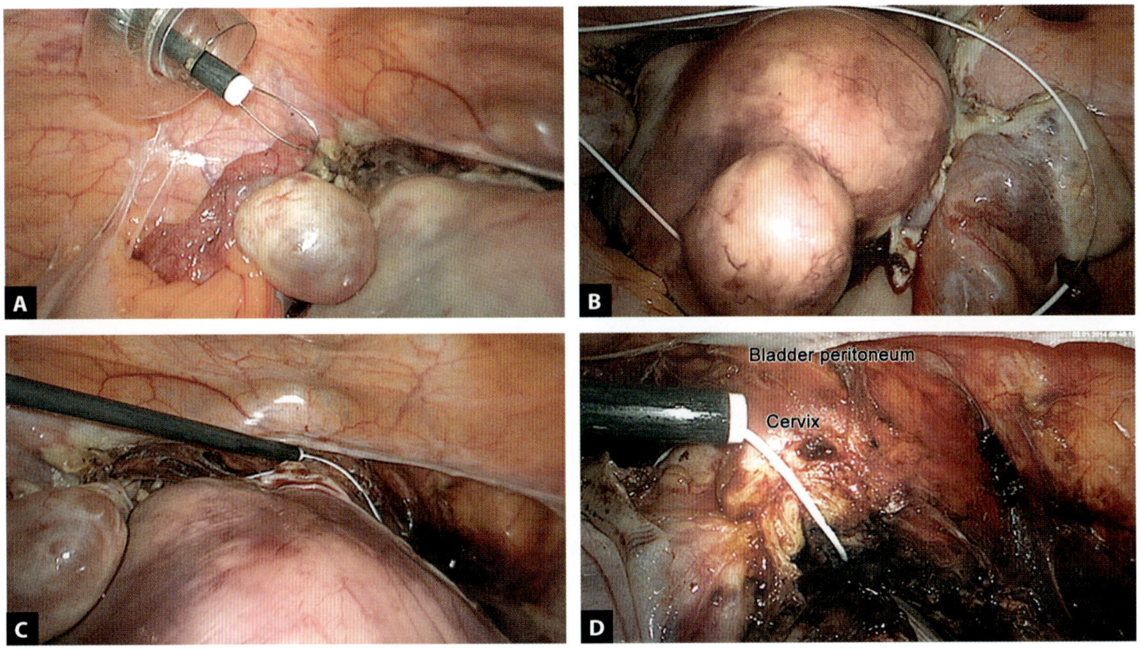

Figs. 35.62A to D: Introduction of a monopolar cutting loop for the cervix and exact placement prior to activation. The whitish uterus is lifted over the loop and the loop is tightened gently. Correct placement between the stumps of the uterine artery and above the conjunction of the sacrouterine ligaments is checked.

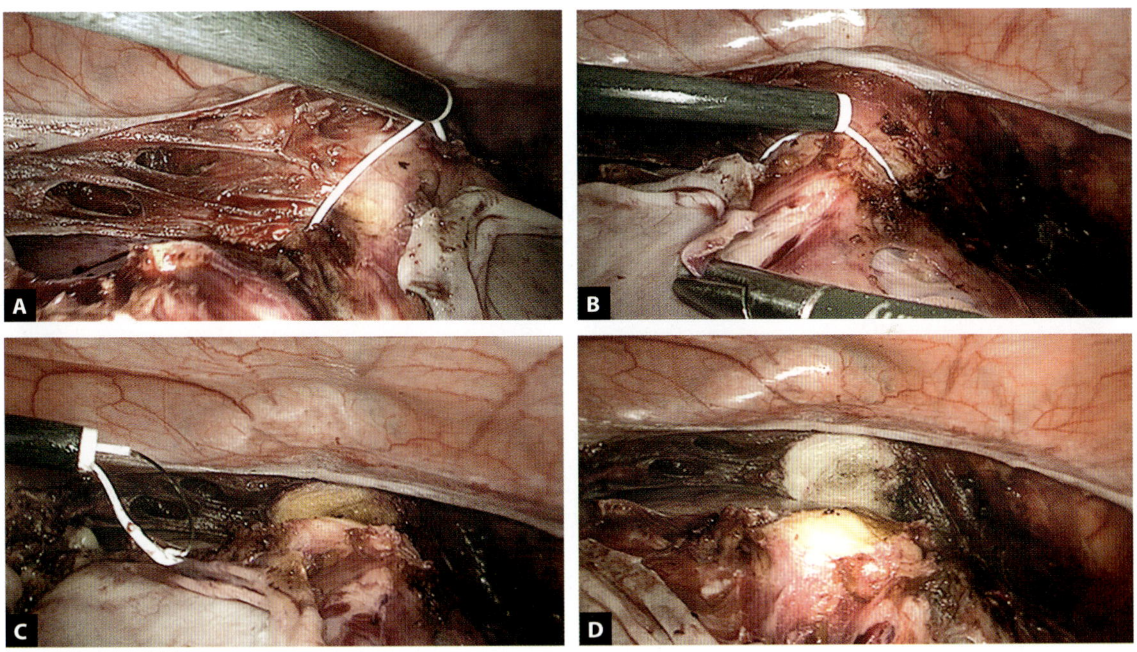

Figs. 35.63A to D: (A and B) Resection of the uterine corpus from the cervix after placing the cutting loop with the cutting point on the posterior cervix. Correct placement between the stumps of the uterine artery and above the conjunction of the sacrouterine ligaments is monitored; (C and D) Dissection of the cervix and the uterus is performed, in this case LSH by monopolar current only in the non-isolated field. When cutting; (B and D) the uterine corpus is pulled upward to achieve a retrograde conus.

- As the suture is applied parallel to the urethra, kinking of the ureters is avoided. The thread is led through the medial part of the cardinal ligament, along the anterior-posterior access.
- Compression of small vessels between the vaginal wall and uterine artery within the cardinal ligament minimizes the risk of bleeding.

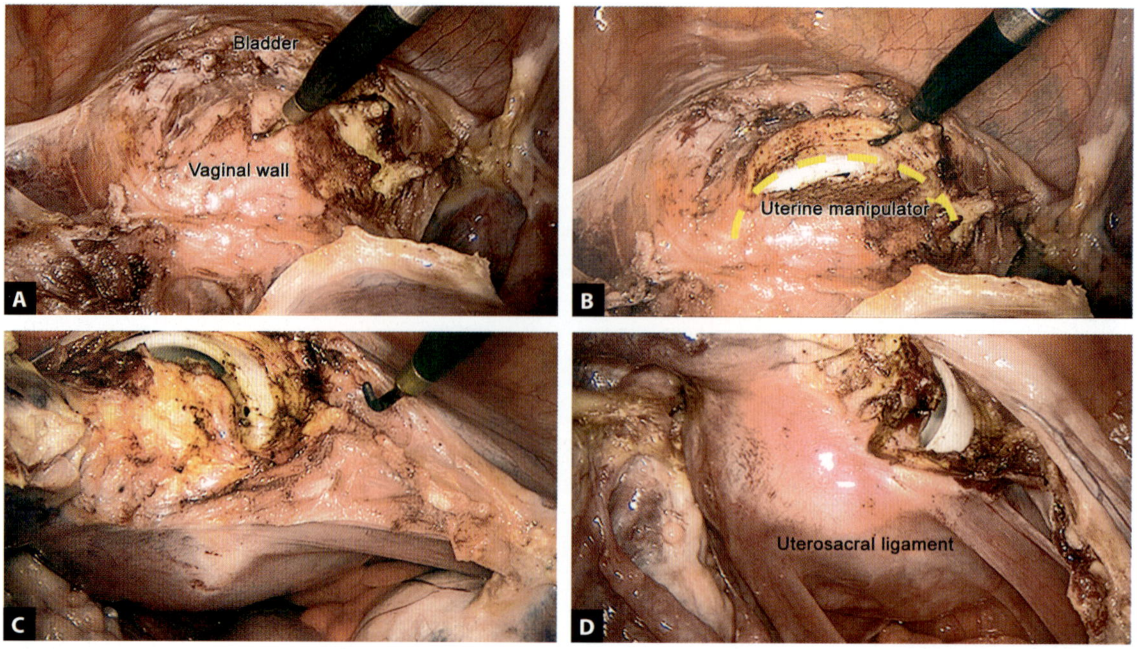

Figs. 35.64A to D: (A) In this case of LTH, the distance between the vagina and the bladder is increased because of exposure of the bladder peritoneum; (B to D) The intrauterine manipulator is firmly placed in the abdomen and dissection of the uterus from the vagina is performed in a stepwise manner. The conjunction of the sacrouterine ligaments is left in place.

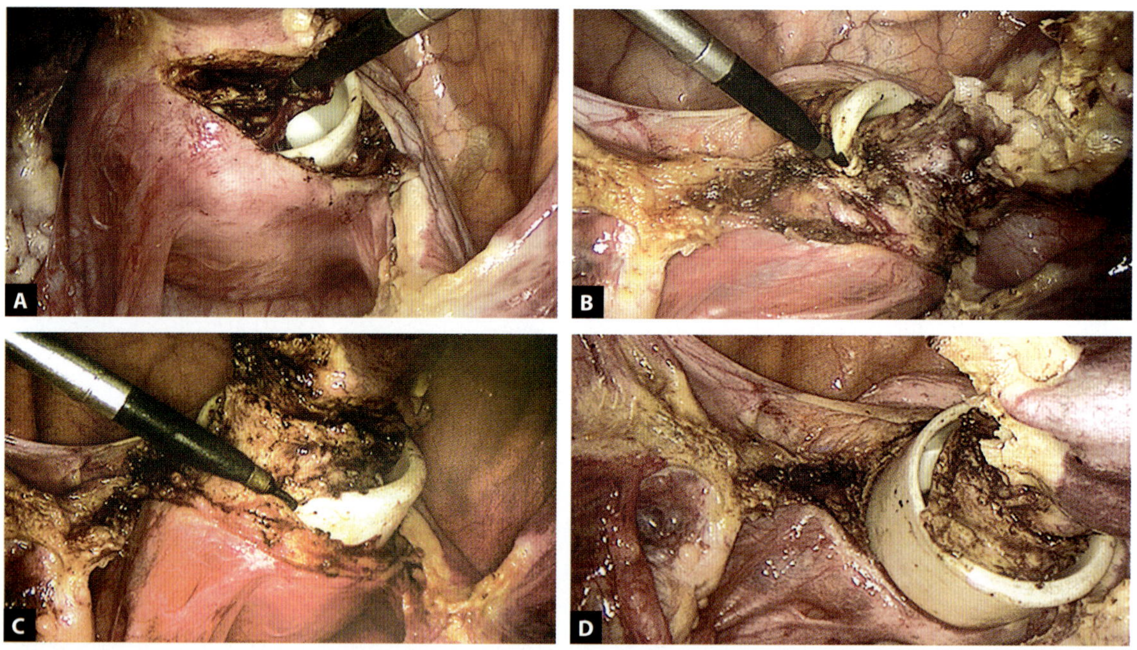

Figs. 35.65A to D: (A to C) Completion of the dissection of the vagina from the cervix and commencement of retraction of the uterine cervix, still grasped by the manipulator forceps, transvaginally. Excessive lens fogging caused by the monopolar current and the sharpness of the monopolar hook make it necessary to perform precise exposure under full vision. This can be done during simultaneous retraction/manipulation with the use of the 30° optic device. The surgeon's vision may worsen immediately when CO_2 gas leaks through the colpotomy. Visibility may then become extremely poor and the use of monopolar energy hazardous (D).

- Despite good suspension there is no relevant displacement of the vaginal access dorsally, which might increase the risk of a cystocele.

Posthysterectomy Inspection

The pedicles, bladder, ureters and bowel must be inspected under continuous irrigation with Ringer's

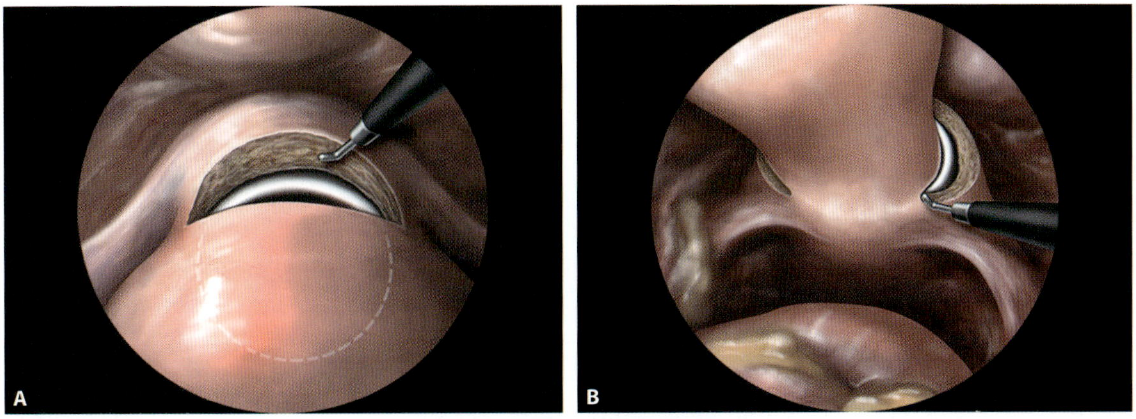

Figs. 35.66A and B: Schematic illustration of uterine dissection. (A) Colpotomy is usually started in the anterior part, on the palpable manipulator cap; (B) The intrafascial hysterectomy can be completed with the sacrouterine ligaments in view.

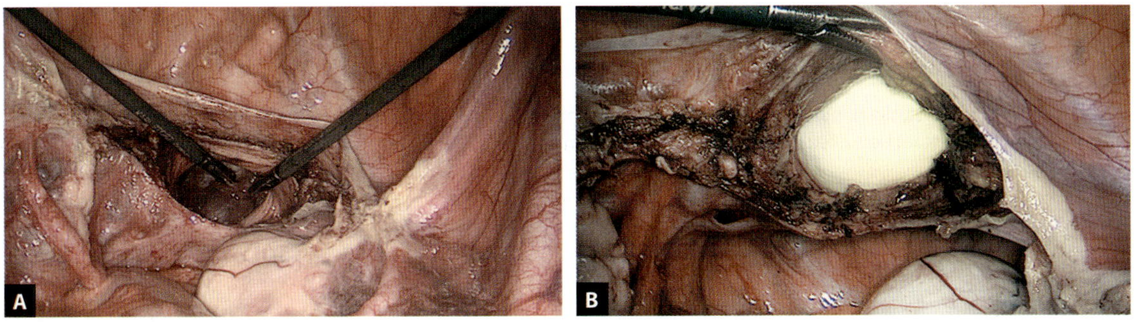

Figs. 35.67A and B: (A) Retraction of uterus through the vagina; (B) Introduction of a cotton swab-filled glove transvaginally to hinder breakdown of the CO_2 pneumoperitoneum.

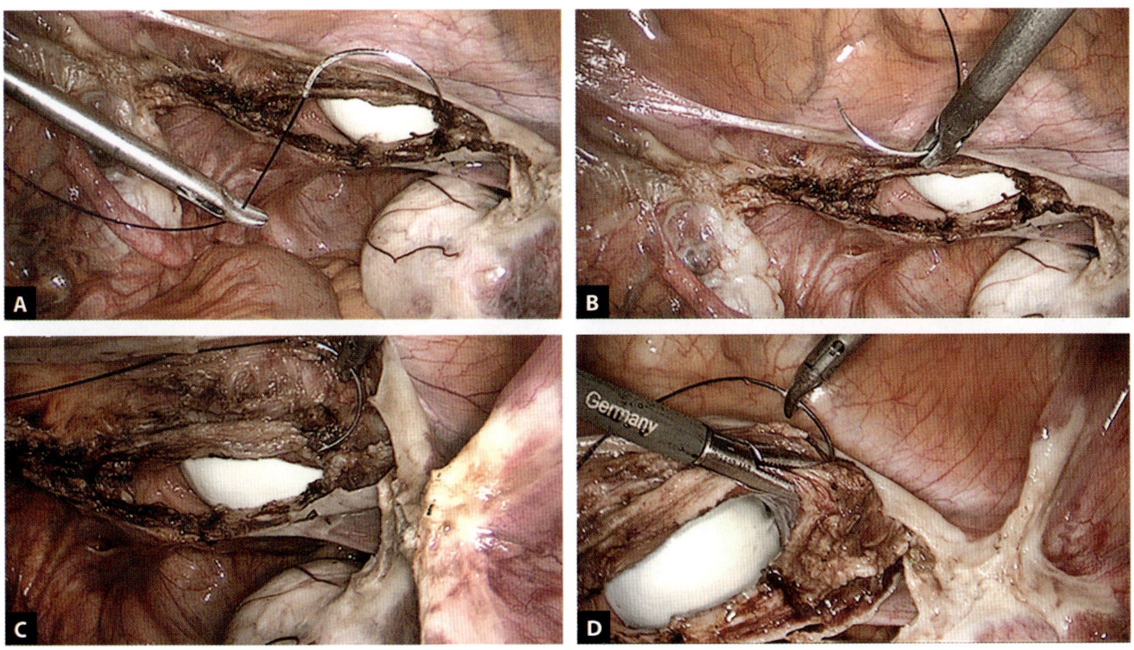

Figs. 35.68A to D: LTH: Right corner suture uniting the anterior and posterior vaginal wall, the posterior peritoneum, and the right sacrouterine ligament. The bladder can be omitted under sight. The forceps must be sharp in order to securely grab the vaginal epithelium. When the suture incorporates the vaginal wall alone and omits the epithelium, there is a high likelihood of postoperative granulomas.

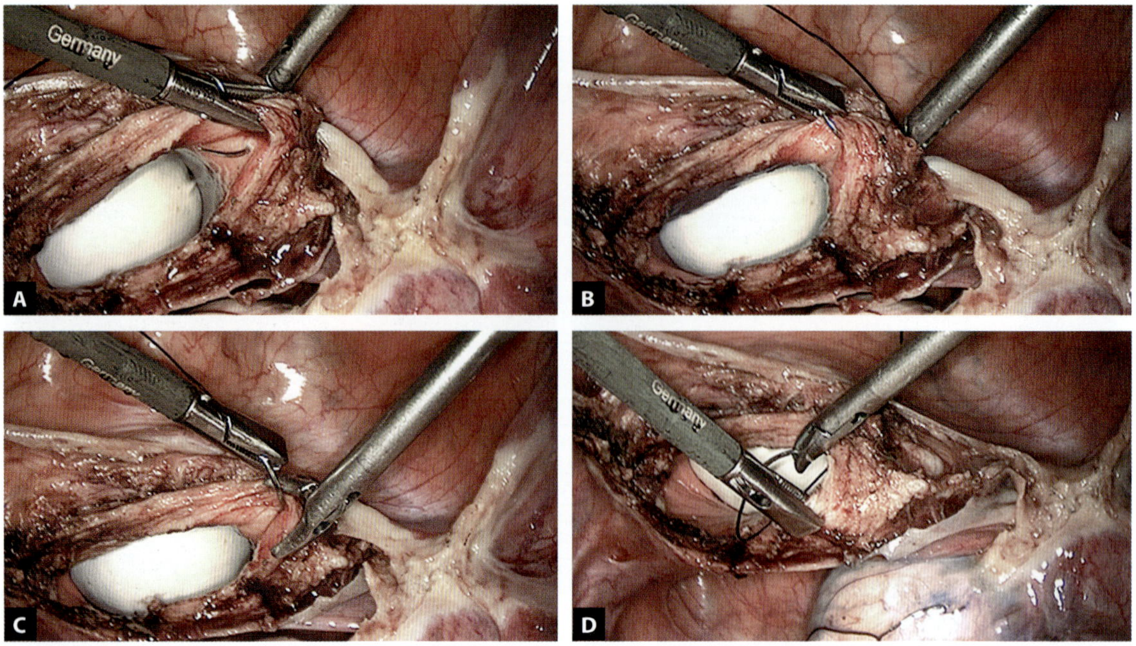

Figs. 35.69A to D: LTH: Continuation of the right corner suture. The 30° optic device helps to look into the vagina from below and above. The strong paravaginal tissue is grasped in large units.

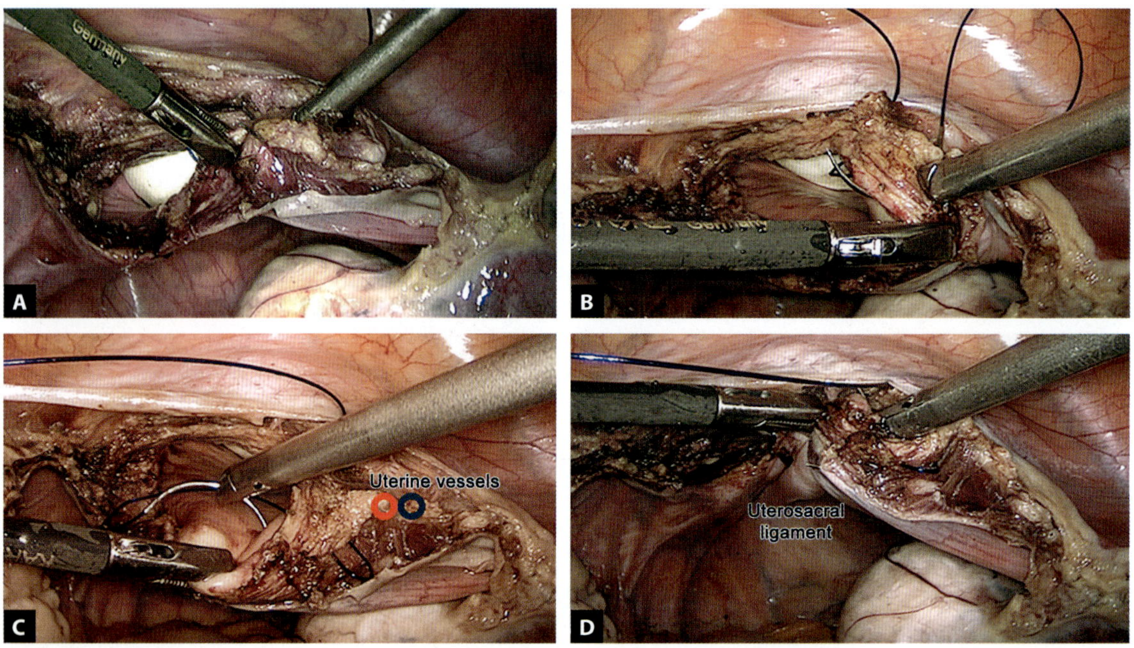

Figs. 35.70A to D: LTH: Continuation of the right corner suture while grabbing the right sacrouterine ligament. The vessel stumps are omitted and lateralized. When using this type of suture, the vessels are compressed mechanically.

lactate or Adept (Baxter). Ureter movement is no proof of integrity. In cases of suspected damage to the ureter or kinking of the ureter while closing the vagina, ureter must be visualized by opening the retroperitoneum and ureterolysis performed until ureter enters the parametria (Fig. 35.93). Alternatively, methylene blue can be injected. If no dye is seen intraabdominally, severe damage is unlikely. In critical cases the integrity of ureter can be proven by performing an intravenous pyelogram 2–3 days after the operation.

Postoperative Management

Urinary catheter is removed; it remains in place only in specific cases. A postoperative cystoscopy is

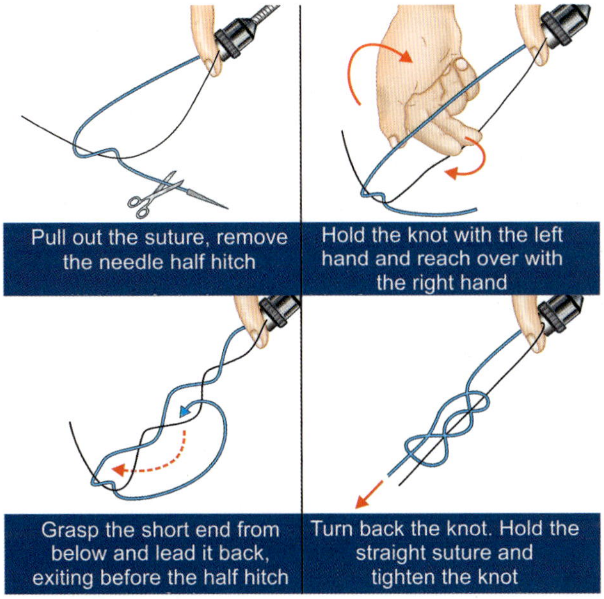

Fig. 35.71: LSH: Finalizing the extracorporeal knot of the PDS suture by using the "von Leffern knot".

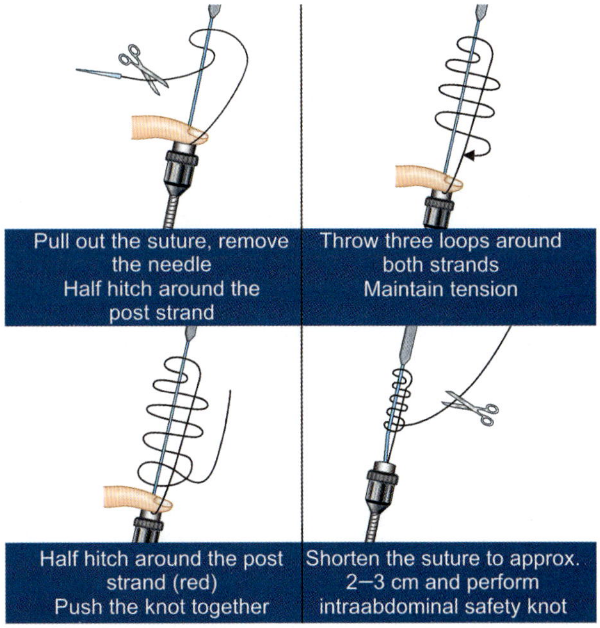

Fig. 35.72: LSH: Finalizing the extracorporeal knot of the PDS suture by using the "The Roeder" knot.

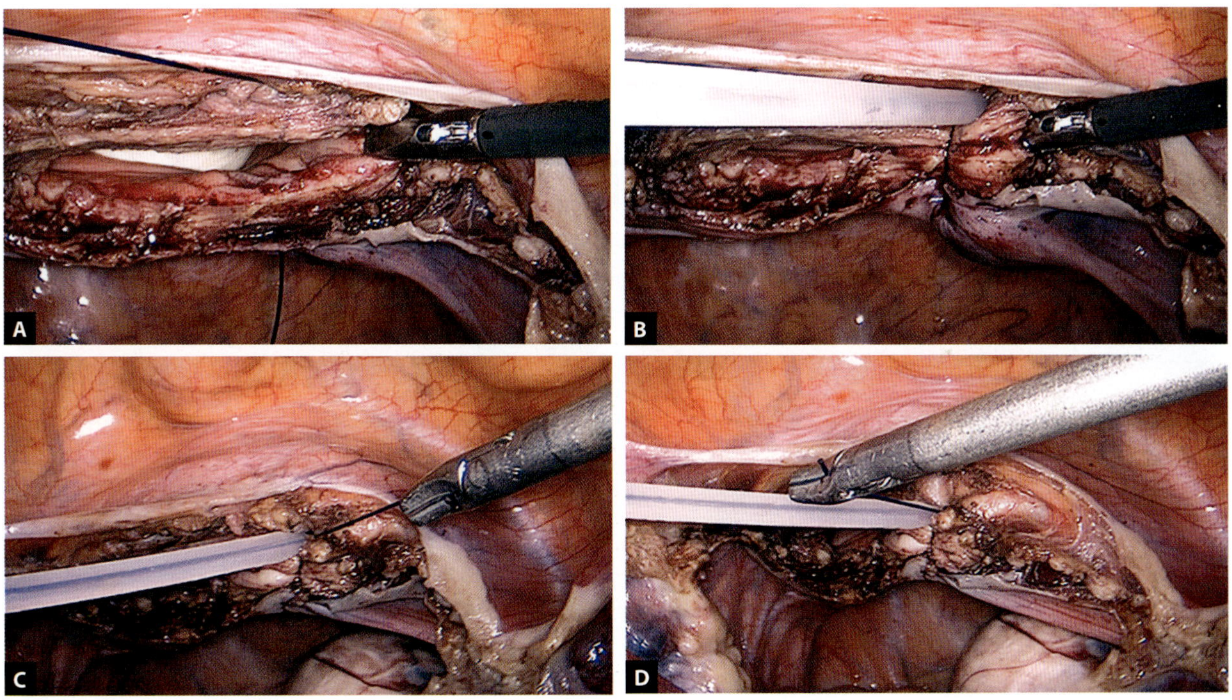

Figs. 35.73A to D: LTH: Completion of the extracorporeal "Roeder" or "von Leffern" knot by pushing it down with a plastic pushrod. The edge is pulled into the abdomen to avoid disturbance of intravaginal sensitivity.

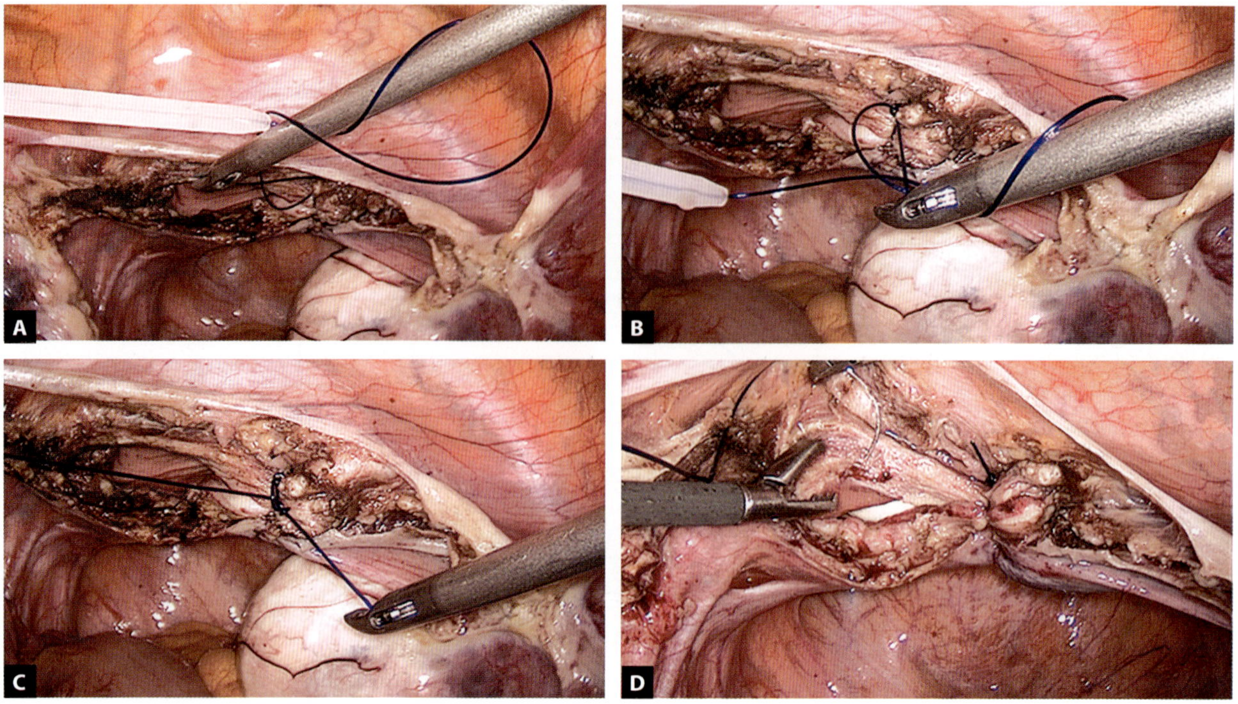

Figs. 35.74A to D: LTH: Placing an intracorporeal safety knot on the right corner stitch and cutting the thread.

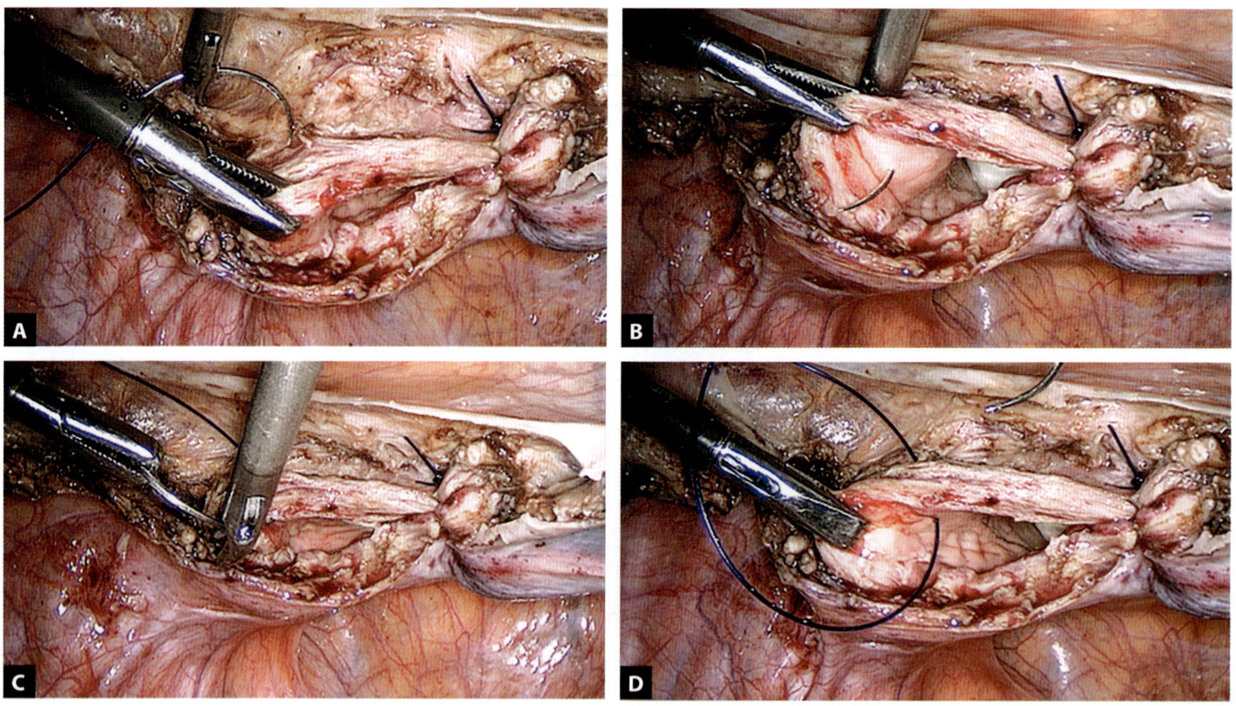

Figs. 35.75A to D: LTH: Left corner suture uniting the anterior and posterior vaginal wall, the posterior peritoneum, and the left sacrouterine ligament. The bladder can be omitted under sight. The forceps must be sharp in order to securely grasp the vaginal epithelium. When the suture incorporates the vaginal wall alone and omits the epithelium, there will be a high likelihood of post-operative granuloma or bleeding.

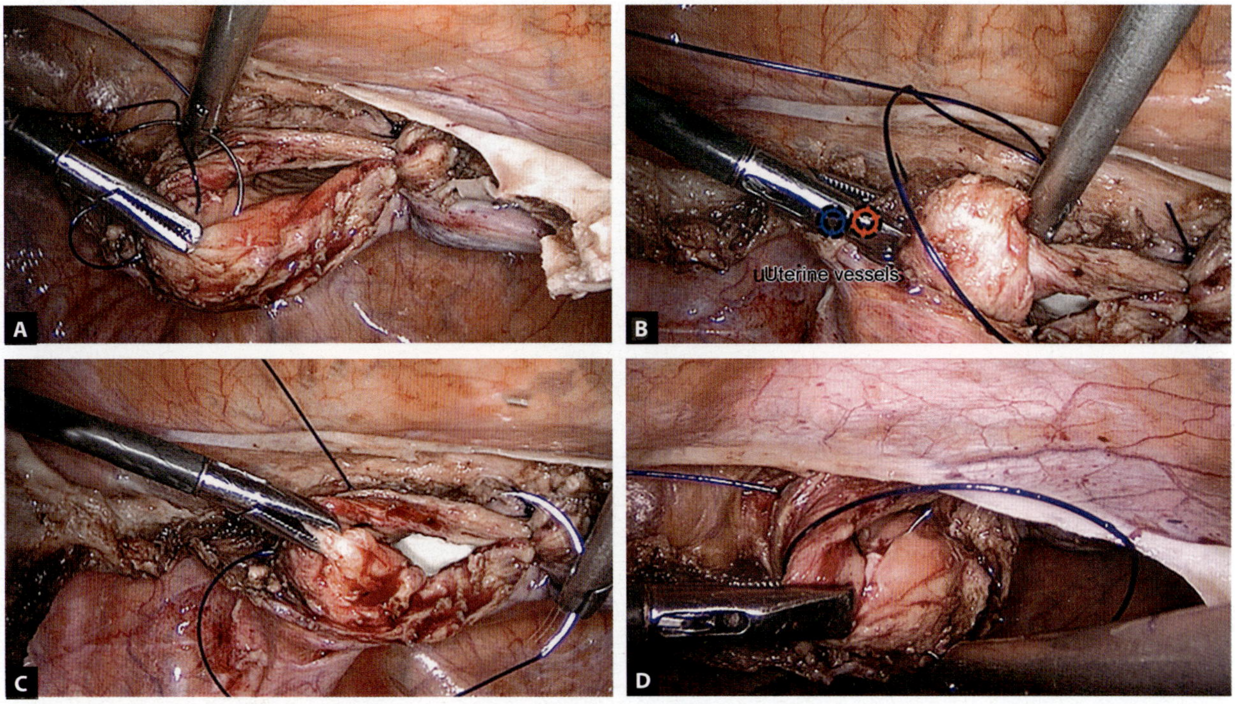

Figs. 35.76A to D: LTH: Continuation of the left corner suture. When using this type of suture, the vessel stump is omitted and compressed mechanically. Approximately 1 cm of the vaginal wall should be included in the suture.

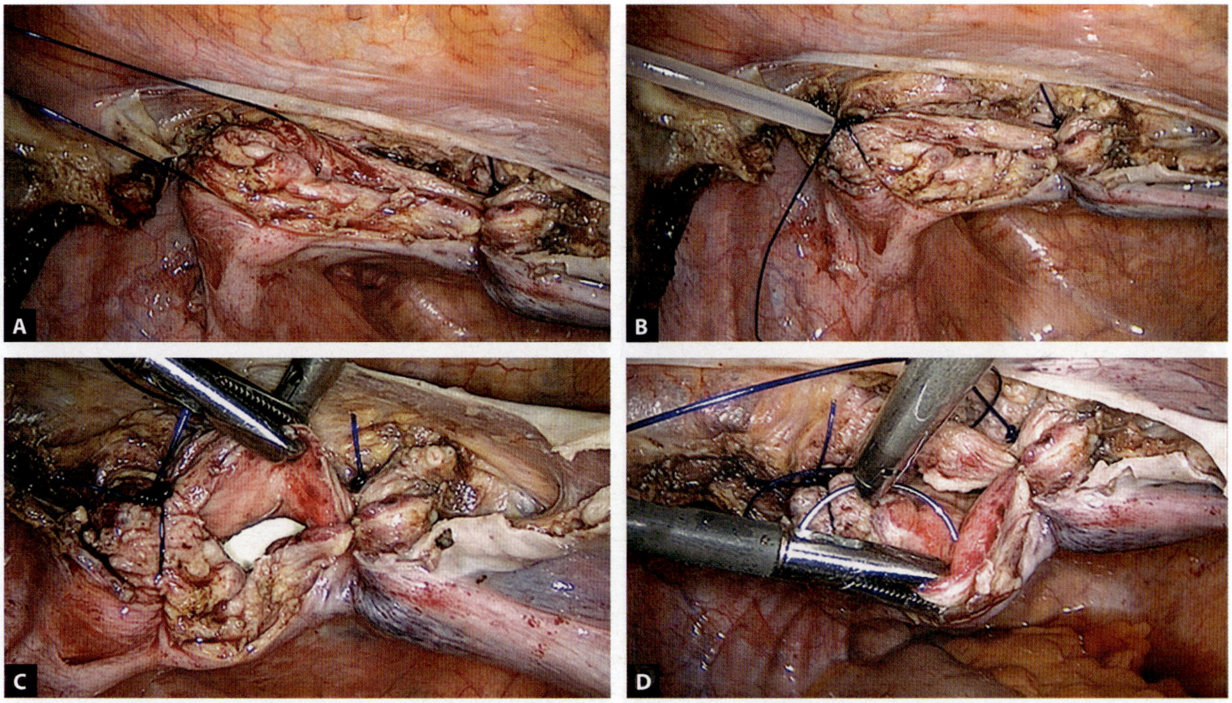

Figs. 35.77A to D: LTH: Completion of the left corner suture. (A to C) The extracorporeal knot is pushed down by the pushrod; (D) Commencement of a U-stitch or a Z-stitch in the middle. When the vaginal cuff is not entirely dry, it will be easier to close the edges first. A large part of the bleeding then stops automatically and further coagulation will not be necessary. Severe coagulation on the vaginal wall might increase the risk of vaginal stump infection or dehiscence.

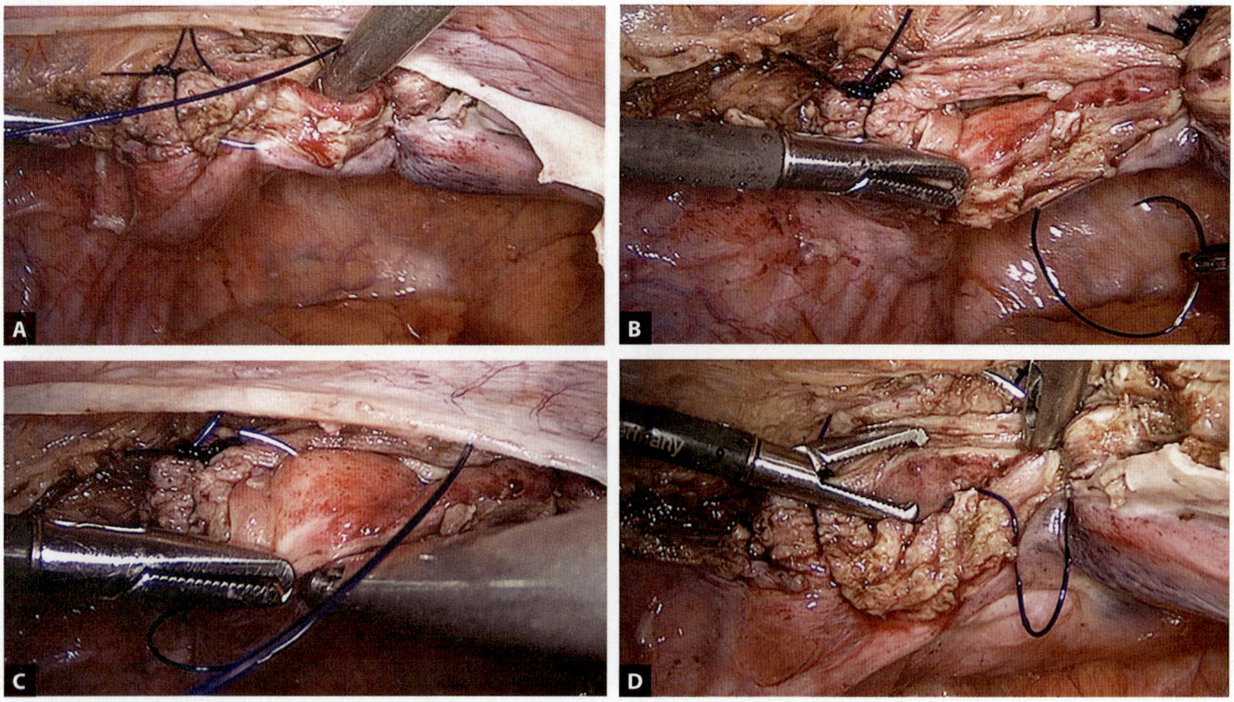

Figs. 35.78A to D: LTH: Final closure of the remaining vaginal opening with a U-suture or a Z-suture. When using the U-suture, the suture end should reach the bladder to prevent bowel damage.

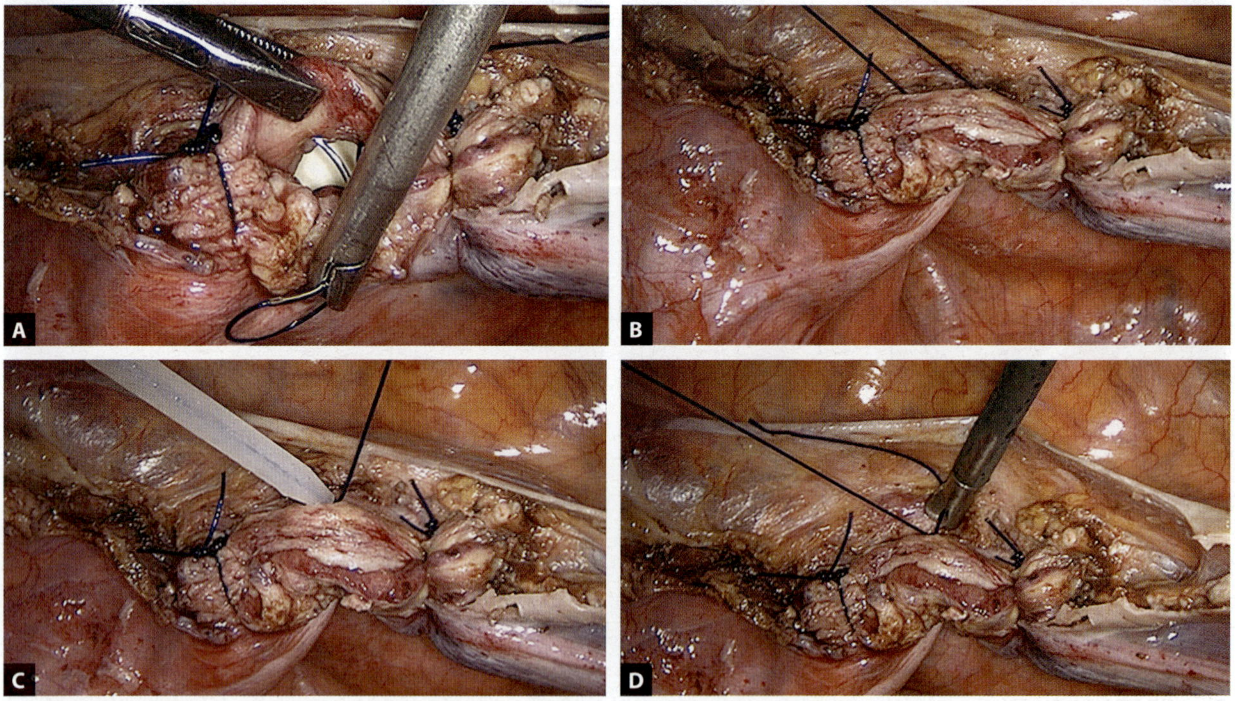

Figs. 35.79A to D: LTH: Completion of the central suture with a U-stitch or a Z-stitch. There is no need for extracorporeal suturing because the suture is set ideally and the tissue mass is adequate.

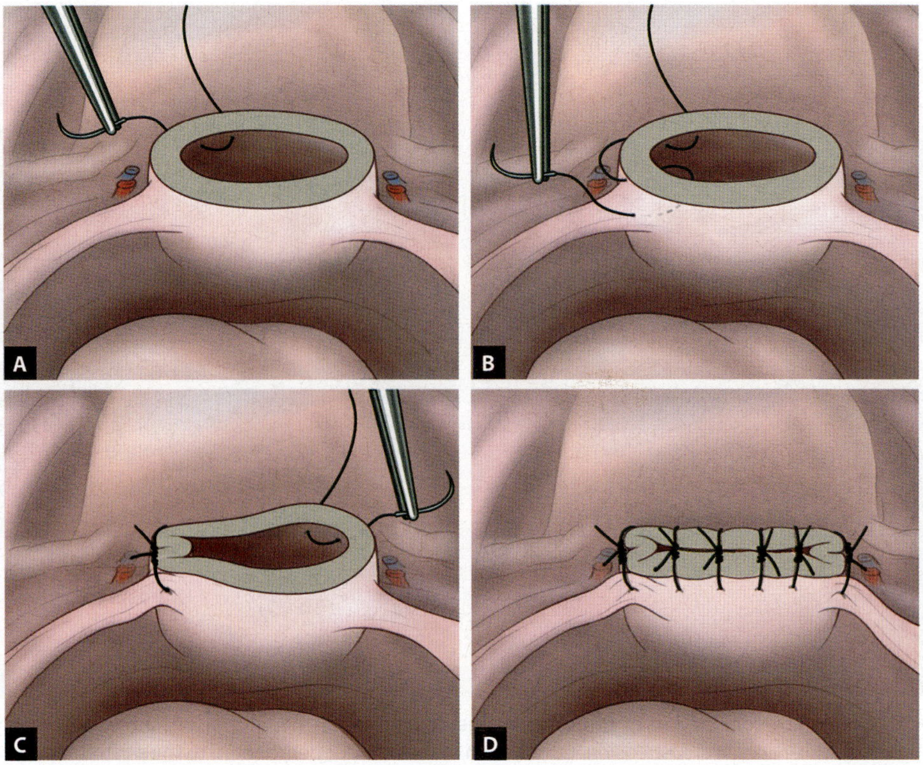

Figs. 35.80A to D: Schematic illustration of vaginal closure after LTH modified by Schollmeyer. A suture is passed through the endopelvic fascia, 1 cm below the cephalad edge of the vaginal epithelium. The needle is pushed from the vaginal lumen through the vaginal wall, passed between the uterine vessels (median part of the broad ligament), and returned through the vaginal lumen. The sacrouterine ligament is identified before the suture is passed through. The needle is pushed from the vaginal lumen through the vaginal wall and the rectovaginal septum, and pierces the sacrouterine ligament. Closure of the vaginal vault with single stiches, U-stiches or Z-stitches. The stitch is drawn through the endopelvic fascia and the vaginal wall, and then out of the vaginal wall and the endopelvic fascia.

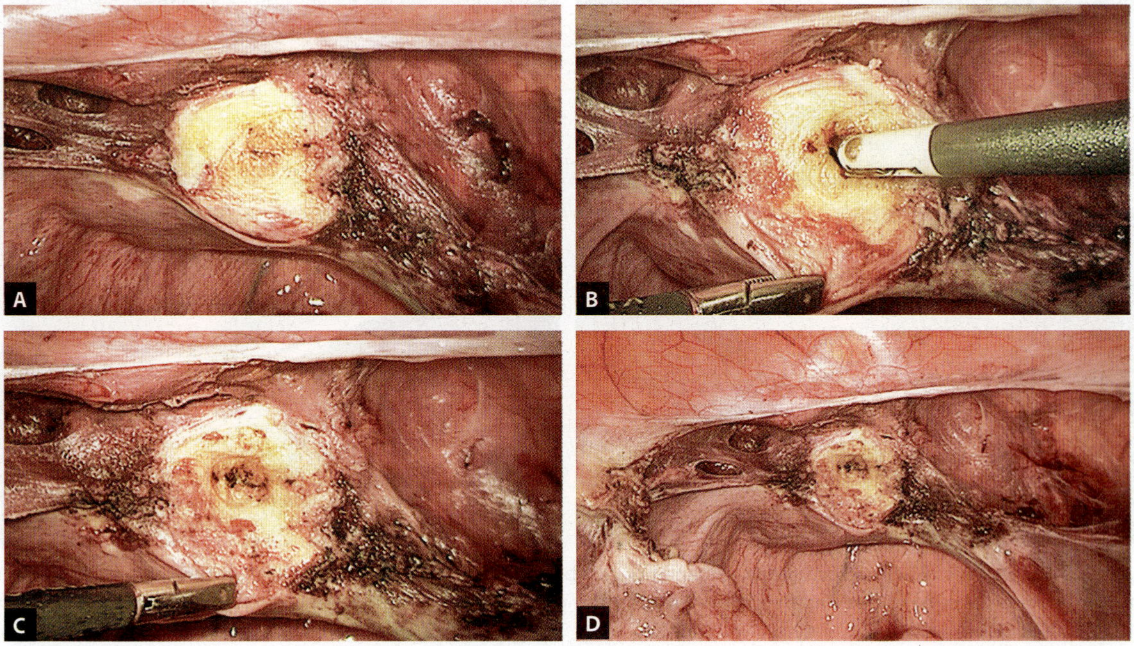

Figs. 35.81A to D: (A to C) The remaining cervical stump. Especially in cases of bleeding disorders, adenomyosis of the uterus or endometriosis, extended coagulation of the remaining cervical channel should be performed; (D) By pulling the uterus upward when cutting the cervix, resection if performed in the shape of an inverse cone.

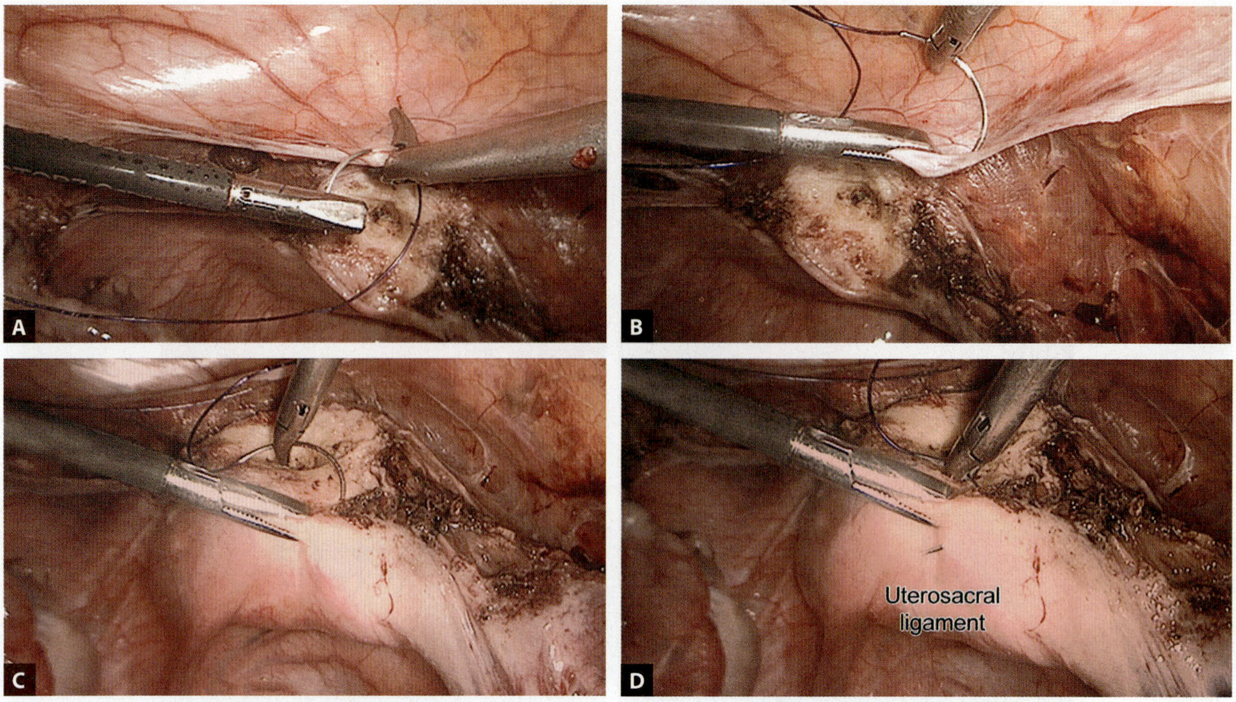

Figs. 35.82A to D: LSH: As the conjunction of the sacrouterine ligaments has been omitted, the two ligaments are grabbed; Included in the suture to achieve cervical suspension. Connection of the bladder peritoneum to the posterior peritoneum by means of a purse-string suture.

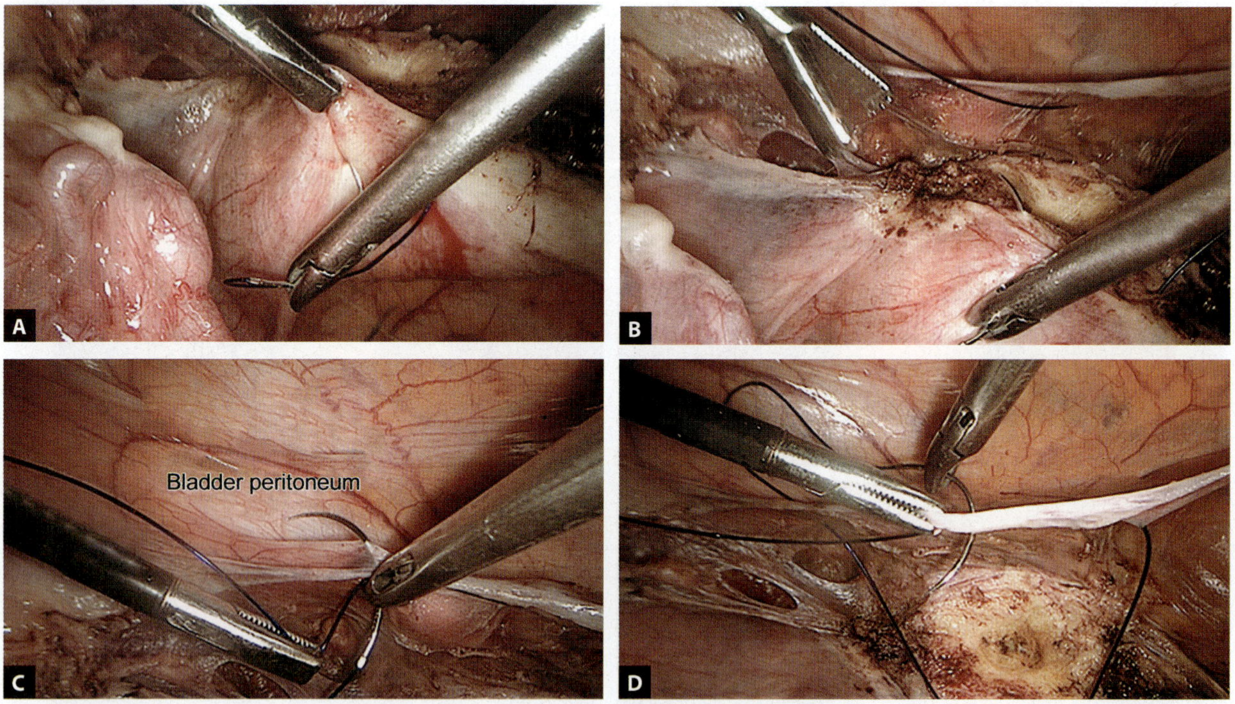

Figs. 35.83A to D: (A and B) The sacrouterine ligaments can be identified and included in the closure of the cervical stump; (C and D) As the bladder has been slightly exposed during the procedure, there is now enough tissue to functionally close the cervical channel.

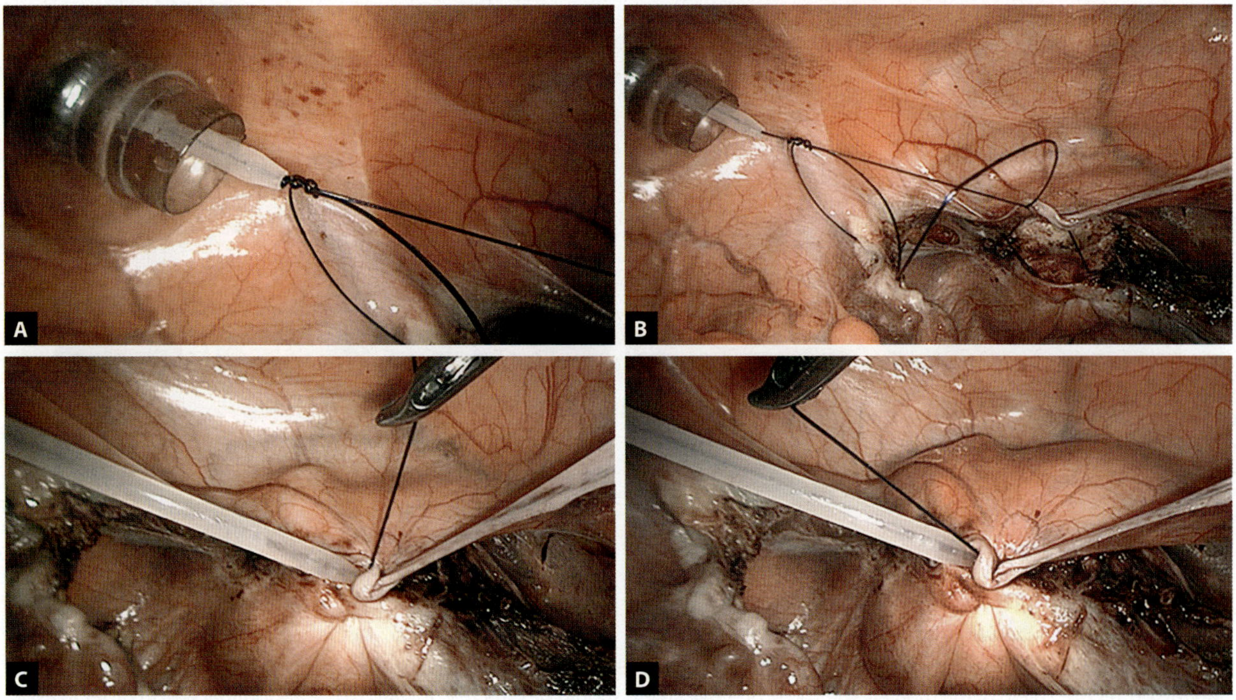

Figs. 35.84A to D: When using the extracorporeal knot, the peritoneum closes the cervical channel functionally and this leads to cervical suspension. The omitted sides still permit drainage if necessary.

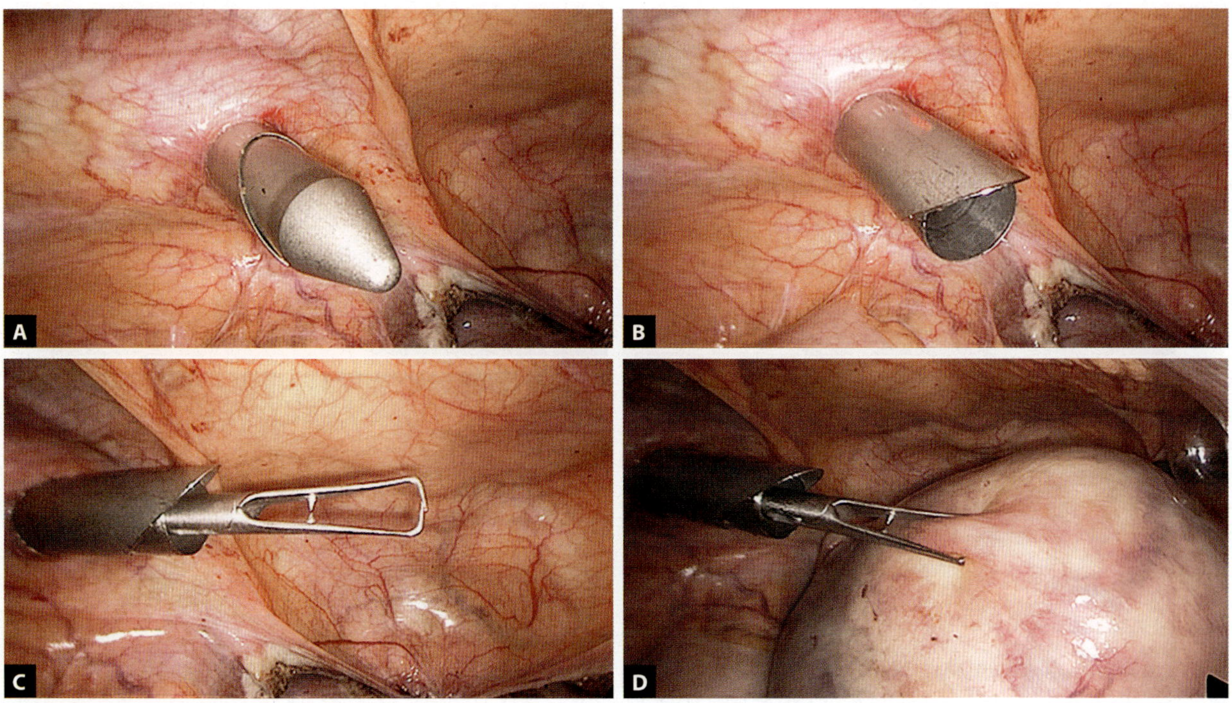

Figs. 35.85A to D: Introduction of the Roto-Cut morcellator, which is available in diameters of 12 mm and 15 mm. The knife should be protected by the shield and the tenaculum should be used under direct vision, regardless of the size of the uterus.

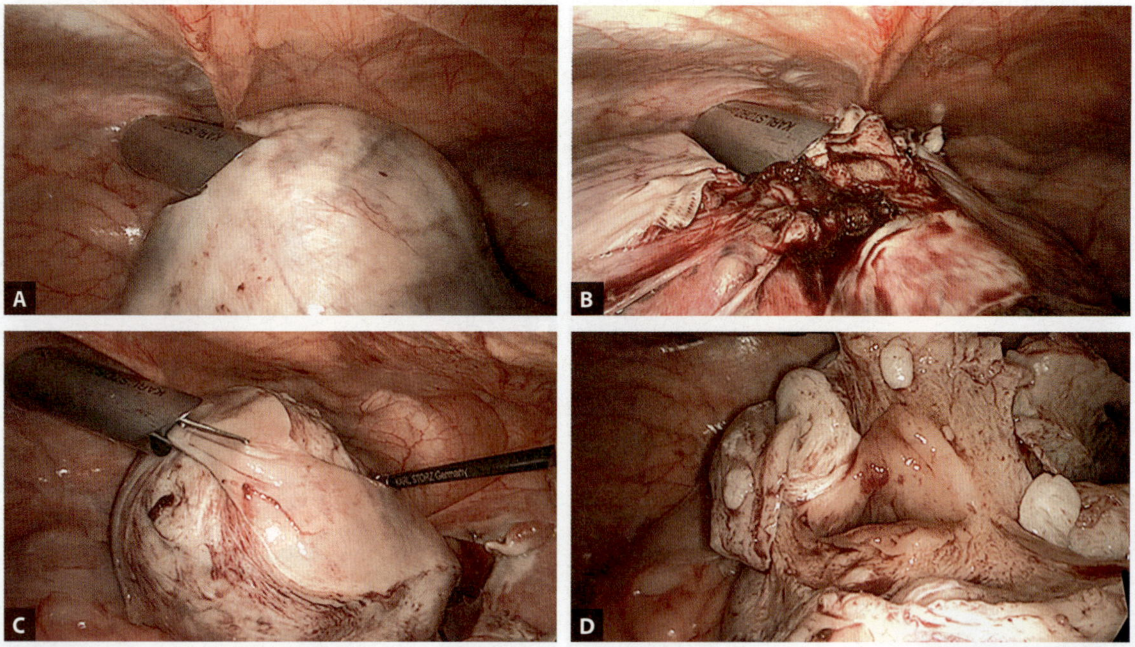

Figs. 35.86A to D: LSH: Morcellation of the myomatous uterus (850 g) under continuous observation of the rotating cutting edge and the protective shield of the morcellator. The protective shield should be directed upward to the abdominal wall in order to avoid cutting the vessels of the abdominal wall. Nevertheless, the lower part, especially the small bowel, must be exposed and kept out of the field of operation. The surgeon must be patient and observant in order to avoid cutting into the bowel, which is one of the major complications in the LSH procedure.

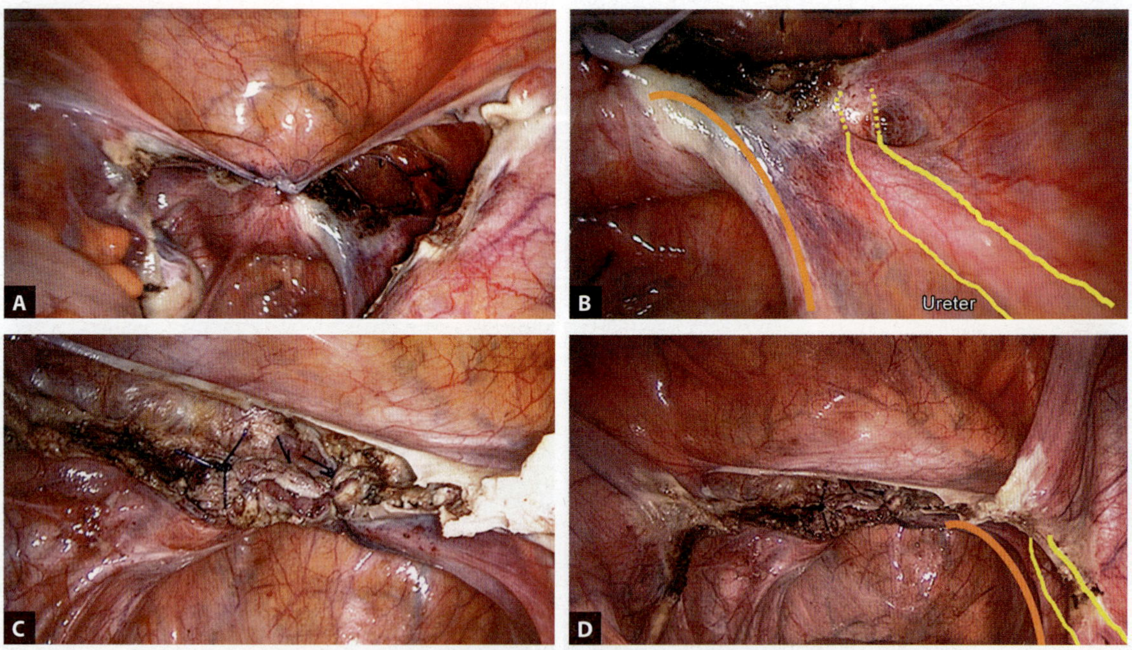

Figs. 35.87A to D: (A and B) Final situs after LASH. The cervical channel is covered by peritoneum and both sacrouterine ligaments are under slight tension, thus fixing the middle compartment and the cervical ring; (C and D) Final situs after LTH. Closure of vaginal stump has been performed; the sacrouterine ligaments have been elevated by 2 corner sutures. The peritoneum closes the cervical channel, and drainage can be effected on both sides. Both sacrouterine ligaments are under slight tension, thus ensuring colposuspension. Reperitonealization will occur approximately two weeks after the operation. The PDS suture allows safe closure and healing of the vaginal cuff because absorption occurs only after about 6 months. The sacrouterine ligaments and the ureter can be clearly identified. Since the anatomy of the ureter has not been affected, opening of the retroperitoneum and its visualization are not necessary.

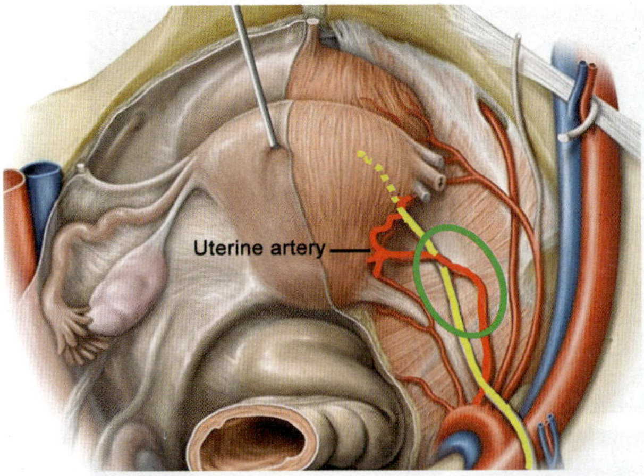

Figs. 35.88: Any uterine pathology may cause major difficulties in exposing the lateral uterine wall and the ascending branch of the uterine artery. Furthermore, all radical hysterectomies include the parametrium and imply a distal resection margin. This might make it necessary to expose the retroperitoneum and localize the departure of the uterine artery from the internal iliac artery.

performed in cases of severe endometriosis or adhesions in the upper part of the bladder. Early ambulation a few hours after surgery is good practice. Clear fluids can be ingested 6 h postsurgery, followed by a light diet. Thromboprophylaxis (mechanical and medical) must be used in appropriate cases. The patient can be discharged after 8–12 h. A post-operative ultrasound scan of the renal pelvis should be performed. Ordinary light activities are permitted and the patient may return to work after 4–5 days. Sexual activity, intensive sports and heavy work should be avoided for 6–8 weeks.

ANTICIPATED PROBLEMS

Vital symptoms, pain and temperature must be carefully monitored during the first 8 h. A patient who is discharged early must be given a phone number she may call in case of distress or pain. The insertion of a drain is not necessary. Fever, early pain, abdominal distension, delirium, decreased urine output, the shock index and hypotension must be recognized and attended to immediately, as these may be signs of complications.

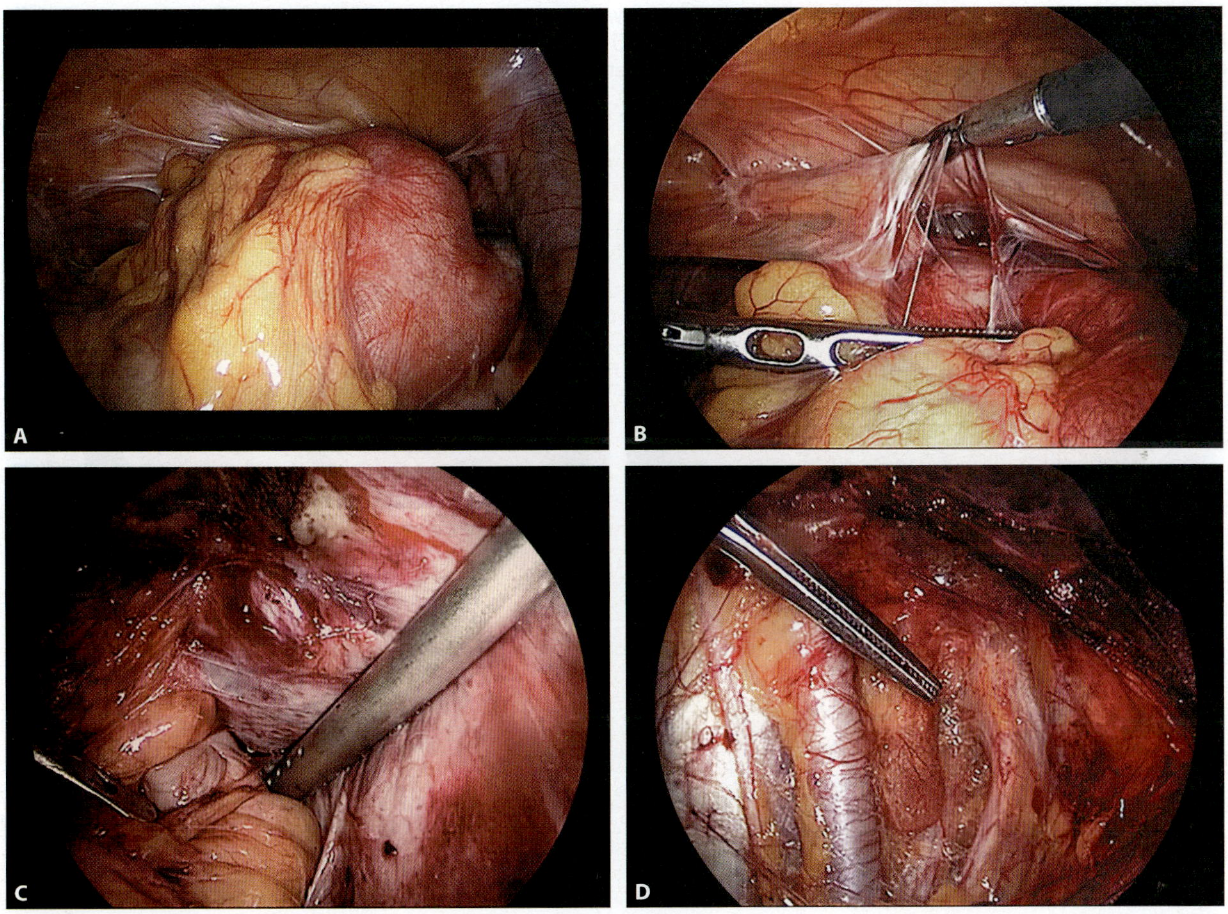

Figs. 35.89A to D: (A) A case of severe adenomyosis of the uterus with subsequent adhesions of the bowel; (B) The bladder; (C) Peritoneum. Access to the lateral aspect of the uterus is closed; (D) Retroperitoneal access is necessary.

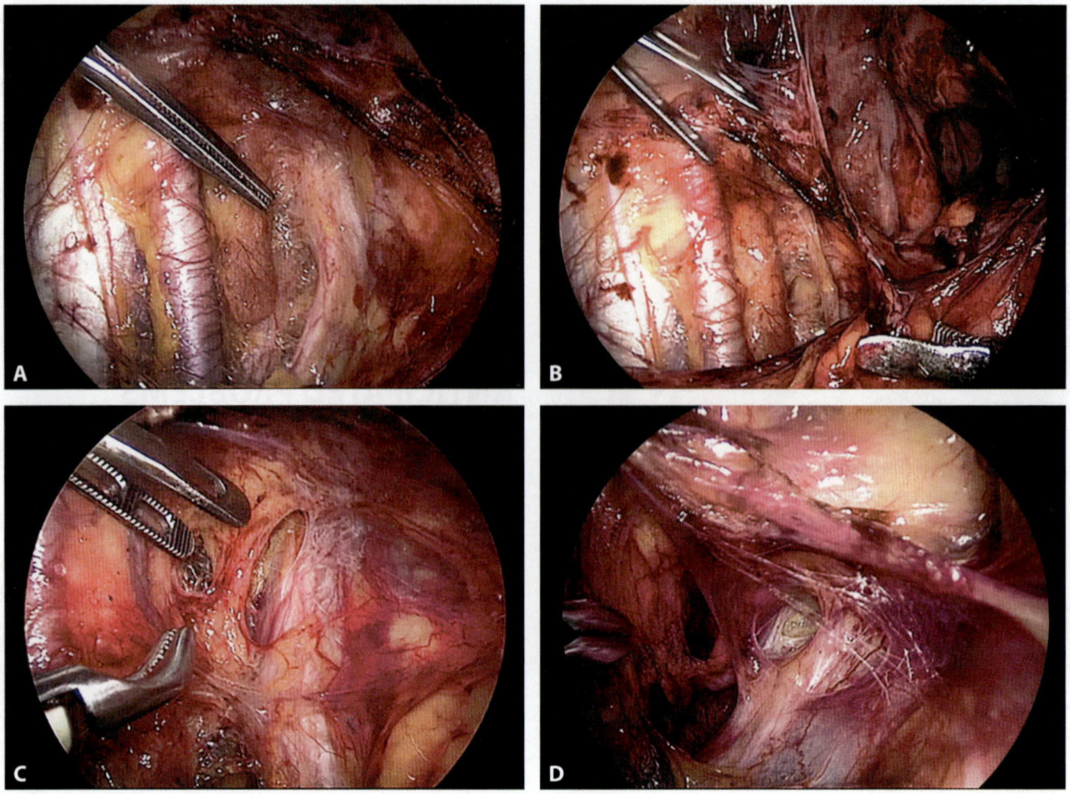

Figs. 35.90A to D: (A) After localization of the external iliac artery, the ureter is usually found adherent to the peritoneum. A major lymph node lies in between; (B) Opening of the pararectal; and (C) The paravesical fossa; (D) The crossing point of the uterine artery is demarcated, and the ureter is left in its adventitia to avoid skeletonizing and denudation.

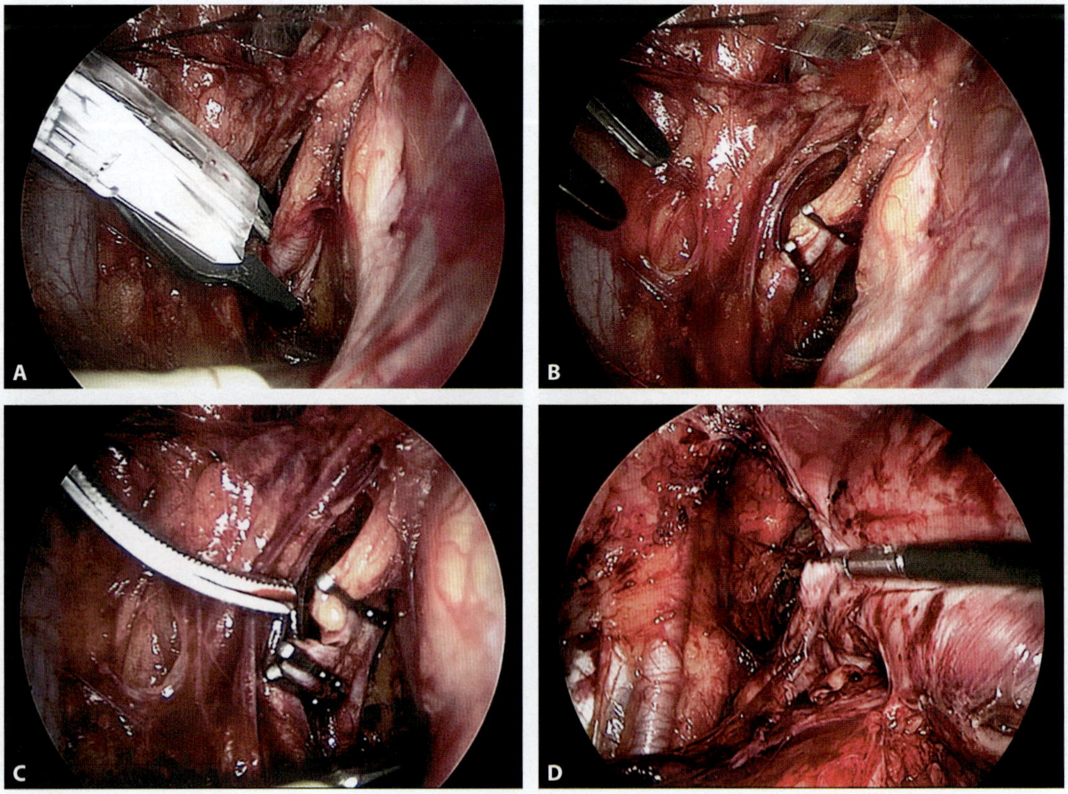

Figs. 35.91A to D: (A and B) Clips can be inserted and the artery can be closed and cut; (C) The uterine vein (deep) is seen just beneath the cut artery; (D) Overview of the exposed situs. To the right you see the uncolored uterus after closure of both arteries.

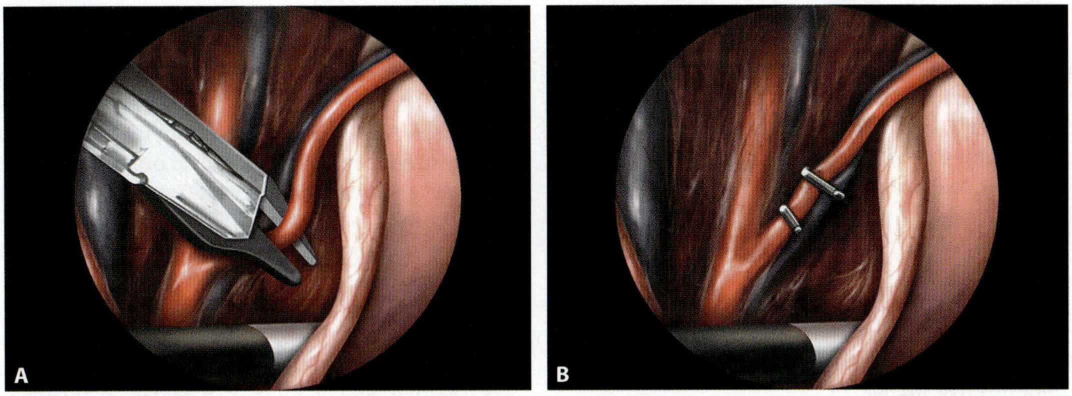

Figs. 35.92A and B: Schematic illustration of the retroperitoneal area where the ureter is undercrossing the uterine artery. The uterine vain is usually divided into a superficial part and a deep part. Clips can be set after medializing the ureter.

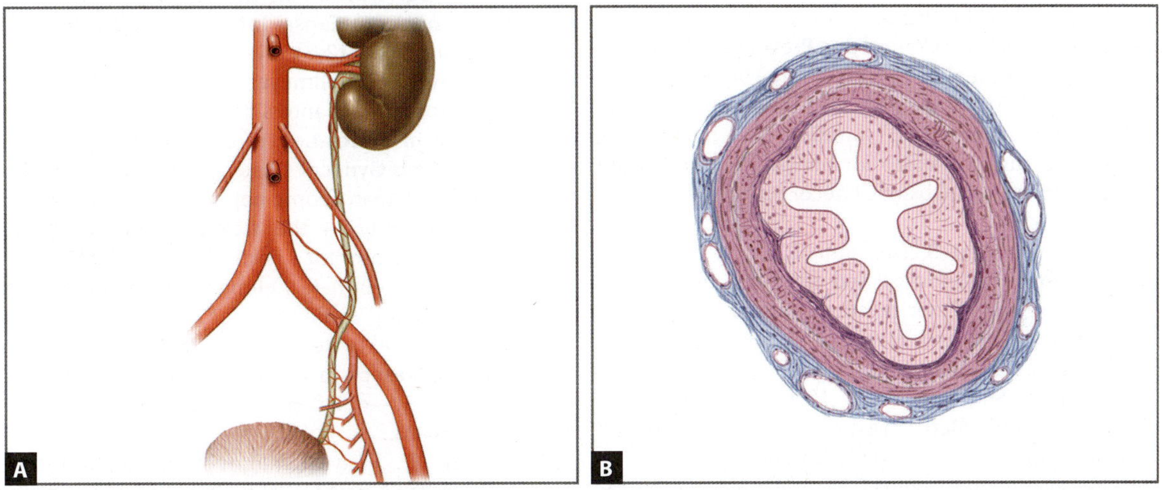

Figs. 35.93A and B: The anatomy of the ureter provides crucial information. (A) Vascularization is effected from the upper part: the renal artery, the ovarian artery, and the aorta. In the lower part the ureter is supplied by lateral vessels: the iliac vessels and the uterine artery. Blunt dissection causes minor bleeding at the respective location; (B) The histological cross-section shows that vascular supply is located in the adventitia. Therefore, electricity or manipulation causing destruction of the adventitia may lead to secondary fistulas and/or leakage.

SUMMARY

In addition to well-known laparoscopic techniques for myomectomy and hysteroscopic techniques for submucous fibroidectomy, laparoscopic subtotal and total hysterectomy are surgical options for the treatment of multiple fibroids. The surgical procedure is decided upon jointly by the patient and the doctor. The individual steps described in this chapter help the gynecological surgeon to perform a satisfactory operation and eliminate the onerous burden of multiple fibroids in patients who have completed planning their families.

CONCLUSION

- The transformation of classic intrafascial hysterectomy into laparoscopic hysterectomy, or even total atraumatic intrafascial laparoscopic hysterectomy (TAIL), is the first step for the prevention of a descensus. The uterine manipulator and structured procedure have made laparoscopic hysterectomy a much safer option.[28]
- In a comparison of various methods to avoid prolapse during vaginal hysterectomy, McCall culdoplasty proved to be the most effective technique in the short term and after three years.[39] A similar procedure is used for abdominal hysterectomy.[40,41] The method was modified by Harry Reich and adapted for laparoscopic procedures. One of its disadvantages is the unification of two lateral sutures in the midline, which results in an unphysiological narrowing of the apical pole of vagina. As transposition of the ureters bears the risk of kinking it would be advisable to use van Herendael's modified suture technique, which avoids this risk.[37]

REFERENCES

1. Kovac SR. Route of hysterectomy: an evidence-based approach. Clin Obstet Gynecol. 2014;57(1):58-71.
2. Schollmeyer T, Elessawy M, Chastamouratidhs et al. Hysterectomy trends over a 9-year period in an endoscopic teaching center. Int J Gynaecol Obstet. 2014;126(1):45-9.
3. Lefebvre G, Allaire C, Jeffery J, et al. SOGC clinical guidelines. Hysterectomy. J Obstet Gynaecol Can. 2002;24(1):37-61; quiz 74-6.
4. Stang A, Merrill RM, Kuss O. Hysterectomy in Germany: a DRG-based nationwide analysis, 2005–2006. Dtsch Arztebl Int. 108(30):508-14.
5. Brummer TH, Seppala TT, Harkki PS. National learning curve for laparoscopic hysterectomy and trends in hysterectomy in Finland 2000–2005. Hum Reprod. 2008;23(4):840-5.
6. Centers for Disease Control and Prevention. Women's Reproductive Health: Hysterectomy Fact Sheet.
7. Hanstede MM, Burger MJ, Timmermans A, et al. Regional and temporal variation in hysterectomy rates and surgical routes for benign diseases in the Netherlands. Acta Obstet Gynecol Scand. 2012;91(2): 220-5.
8. Alkatout I, Bojahr B, Dittmann L, et al. Precarious preoperative diagnostics and hints for the laparoscopic excision of uterine adenomatoid tumors: two exemplary cases and literature review. Fertil Steril. 2011;95(3):1119.e5-8.
9. Alkatout I, Schollmeyer T, Hawaldar NA, et al. Principles and safety measures of electrosurgery in laparoscopy. JSLS. 2012;16(1):130-9.
10. Hughes E, Brown J, Collins JJ, et al. Ovulation suppression for endometriosis. Cochrane Database Syst Rev. 2007;(3):CD000155.
11. Lethaby A, Ivanova V, Johnson NP. Total versus subtotal hysterectomy for benign gynaecological conditions. Cochrane Database Syst Rev. 2006;(2):CD004993.
12. Thakar R, Ayers S, Clarkson P, et al. Outcomes after total versus subtotal abdominal hysterectomy. N Engl J Med. 2002;347(17):1318-25.
13. Gorlero F, Lijoi D, Biamonti M, et al. Hysterectomy and women satisfaction: total versus subtotal technique. Arch Gynecol Obstet. 2008;278(5):405-10.
14. Roovers JP, van der Bom JG, van der Vaart CH, et al. Hysterectomy and sexual wellbeing: prospective observational study of vaginal hysterectomy, subtotal abdominal hysterectomy, and total abdominal hysterectomy. BMJ. 2003;327(7418):774-8.
15. Ascher-Walsh CJ, Tu JL, Du Y, et al. Location of adenomyosis in total hysterectomy specimens. J Am Assoc Gynecol Laparosc. 2003;10(3):360-2.
16. Sarmini OR, Lefholz K, Froeschke HP. A comparison of laparoscopic supracervical hysterectomy and total abdominal hysterectomy outcomes. J Minim Invasive Gynecol. 2005;12(2):121-4.
17. BMI, Demography Report: Report of the German federal government on the demographic situation and future development of the country 2011. German Federal Ministry of the Interior.
18. Nygaard I, Bradley C, Brandt D, Women's Health Initiative. Pelvic organ prolapse in older women: prevalence and risk factors. Obstet Gynecol. 2004; 104(3):489-97.
19. Olsen AL, Smith VJ, Bergstrom JO, et al. Epidemiology of surgically managed pelvic organ prolapse and urinary incontinence. Obstet Gynecol. 1997;89(4):501-6.
20. Symmonds RE, Pratt JH. Vaginal prolapse following hysterectomy. Am J Obstet Gynecol. 1960;79:899-909.
21. Toozs-Hobson P, Boos K, Cardozo L. Management of vaginal vault prolapse. Br J Obstet Gynaecol. 1998; 105(1):13-7.
22. Marchionni M, Brocco GL, Checcucci V, et al. True incidence of vaginal vault prolapse. Thirteen years of experience. J Reprod Med. 1999;44(8):679-84.
23. Swift SE, Pound T, Dias JK. Case-control study of etiologic factors in the development of severe pelvic organ prolapse. Int Urogynecol J Pelvic Floor Dysfunct. 2001;12(3):187-92.
24. Elessawy M, Schollmeyer T, Mettler L, et al. The incidence of complications by hysterectomy for benign disease in correlation to an assumed preoperative score. Arch Gynecol Obstet. 2015;292(1): 127-33.
25. Reich H. Laparoscopic oophorectomy and salpingo-oophorectomy in the treatment of benign tubo-ovarian disease. Int J Fertil. 1987;32(3):233-6.
26. Mettler L, Semm K, Lehmann-Willenbrock L, et al. Comparative evaluation of classical intrafascial-supracervical hysterectomy (CISH) with transuterine mucosal resection as performed by pelviscopy and laparotomy—our first 200 cases. Surg Endosc. 1995; 9(4):418-23.
27. Semm K. [Hysterectomy via laparotomy or pelviscopy. A new CASH method without colpotomy]. Geburtshilfe Frauenheilkd. 1991;51(12):996-1003.
28. Hohl MK, Hauser N. Safe total intrafascial laparoscopic (TAIL) hysterectomy: a prospective cohort study. Gynecol Surg. 2010;7(3):231-9.
29. Schüssler B, Scheidel P, Hohl MK. Hysterektomie Update. Frauenheilkunde aktuell, 2008;3:4-12.
30. Veress J. Neues Instrument zur Ausführung von Brust- und Bauchpunktionen und Pneumothorax-behandlung. Deutsche medizinische Wochenschrift. 1938;64:1480-1.
31. Alkatout I, Mettler L, Maass N, et al. Abdominal anatomy in the context of port placement and trocars. J Turk Ger Gynecol Assoc . 2015;16(4):241-51.
32. Kramer L. Mixed reviews on removing fallopian tubes to prevent ovarian cancer. CMAJ. 2013;185(9):E391-2.
33. Kurman RJ, Shih Ie M. Molecular pathogenesis and extraovarian origin of epithelial ovarian cancer—shifting the paradigm. Hum Pathol . 2011;42(7):918-31.
34. Caceres A, McCarus SD. Fallopian tube prolapse after total laparoscopic hysterectomy. Obstet Gynecol. 2008;112(2 Pt 2):494-5.
35. Altman D, Falconer C, Cnattingius S, et al. Pelvic organ prolapse surgery following hysterectomy on benign indications. Am J Obstet Gynecol. 2008;198(5): 572.e1-6.
36. Thompson JD, Warshaw J. Hysterectomy. In: Rock JA, Thompson JD (Eds). Te Linde's Operative Gynecology.

Philadelphia, PA: Lippincott Raven; 1996. pp. 771-854.

37. van Herendael B. Strategies to prevent vaginal vault descent during hysterectomy. In: Mettler L, editor. Manual of New Hysterectomy Techniques. New Delhi: Jaypee Brothers Medical Publishers (P) Ltd; 2007. pp. 82-85.
38. Hur HC, Guido RS, Mansuria SM, et al. Incidence and patient characteristics of vaginal cuff dehiscence after different modes of hysterectomies. J Minim Invasive Gynecol. 2007;14(3):311-7.
39. Cruikshank SH, Kovac SR. Randomized comparison of three surgical methods used at the time of vaginal hysterectomy to prevent posterior enterocele. Am J Obstet Gynecol. 1999;180(4):859-65.
40. Wall LL. A technique for modified McCall culdeplasty at the time of abdominal hysterectomy. J Am Coll Surg. 1994;178(5):507-9.
41. Ostrzenski A. A new, simplified posterior culdoplasty and vaginal vault suspension during abdominal hysterectomy. Int J Gynaecol Obstet. 1995; 49(1):25-34.

KIEL SCHOOL

36 of Gynaecological Endoscopy

Hysterectomies

Laparoscopic **Subtotal** Hysterectomy (**LSH**)

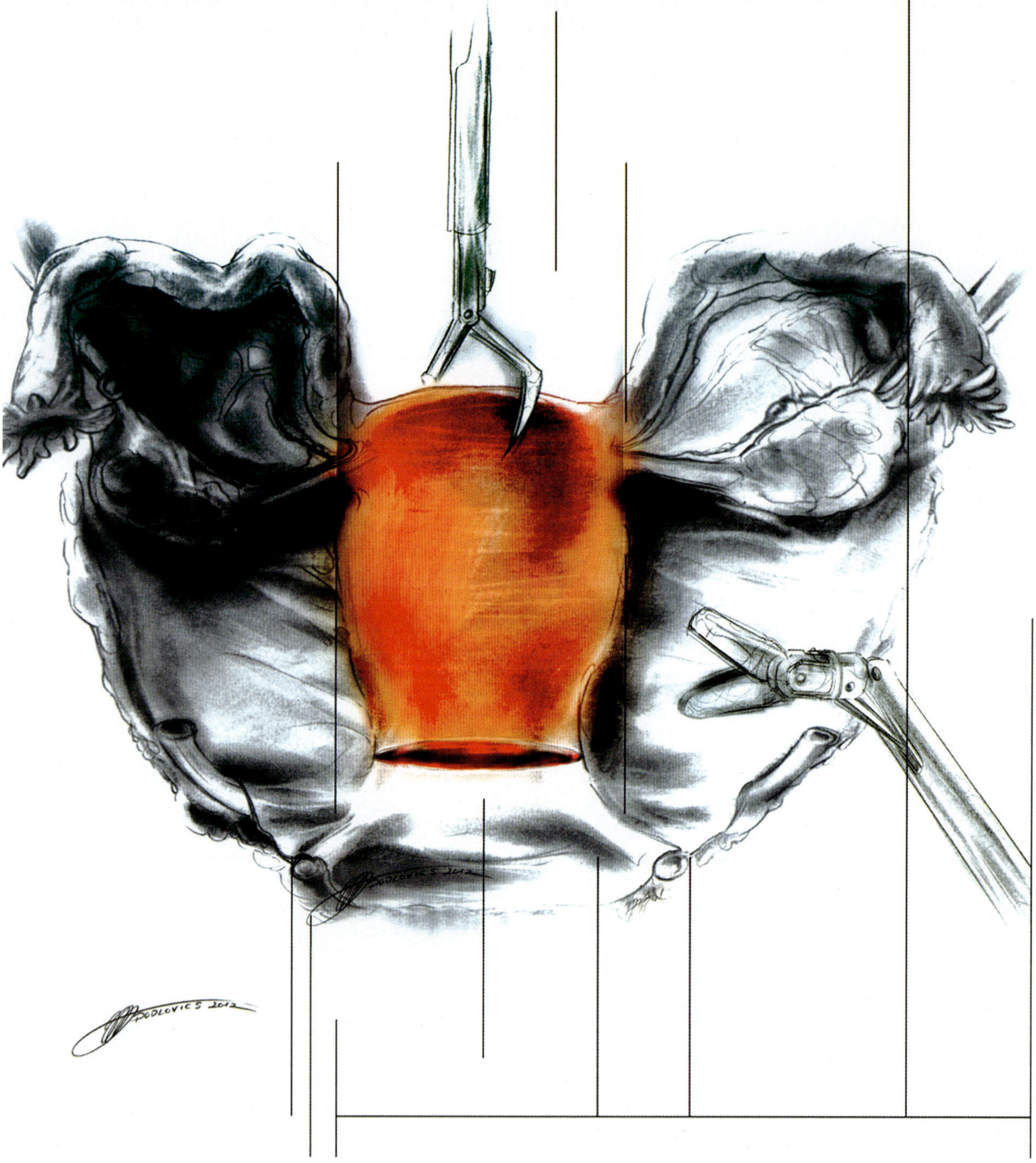

Chapter 36

Hysterectomies: Laparoscopic Subtotal Hysterectomy

Bernd Bojahr Pasacica, Garri Tchartchian, Khulkar Abdusattarova

INTRODUCTION

The aim of this chapter is to demonstrate a standardized, safe and minimal invasive technique of laparoscopic subtotal hysterectomy (LSH) developed at the Clinic for Minimal Invasive Surgery (MIC Klinik) in Berlin, Germany. Based on the experience of 11,598 LSH operations, the tips and tricks should help prevent complications even in difficult case situations of very enlarged uteri. The "change-over technique" is one way to prevent an abdominal hysterectomy in such cases. Our results regarding complication rates with the described surgical technique are compared with the literature and discussed.

The advantages of laparoscopic hysterectomy compared to abdominal hysterectomy were confirmed by a meta-analysis of 47 prospective randomized trials.[1] Moreover, several studies have demonstrated that LSH and total laparoscopic hysterectomy (TLH) are both effective procedures, but in the LSH group the mean operating time and the hospital stay were shorter, and the hemoglobin level and the complication rates were lower than in the TLH group.[2,3-5] For nonmalignant conditions LSH represents an alternative to total hysterectomy, with a low level of intraoperative and postoperative morbidity.[6] Various benign gynecological conditions, such as symptomatic uterine fibroids, menstrual disorders, adenomyosis of the uterus, endometriosis and excessive menstrual loss not responding to medical therapy, are indications for LSH.[7-9]

LSH may be favored over TLH as it is technically easier to leave the cervix intact. With this technique the two pitfalls of TLH, namely, uterine vessel hemorrhage and ureteric injury, can be avoided. LSH also results in lower levels of sexual, bladder and bowel dysfunction and offers superior protection of the integrity of the pelvic floor compared to total hysterectomy.[9,10]

Although laparoscopic surgery is well accepted by gynecologists worldwide, laparoscopic hysterectomy in Germany is still only performed by a few specialists as it is a highly skilled technique. At the MIC Klinik in Berlin, Germany, the surgeons are leading experts in LSH. Of the 11,598 LSH procedures performed at the clinic between 1998 and December 2014, 909 of the extirpated uteri had a weight of more than 500 g, with the largest removed uterus weighing 4,065 g. This chapter describes and illustrates in detail the surgical technique of LSH, comments on complications and offers tips and suggestions for implementation.

SURGICAL PROCEDURE

After bladder catheterism and vaginal disinfection, the patient is placed in a horizontal position, with stretched legs (Fig. 36.1). The surgeon, assistant, surgical nurse and instrument tables are positioned on the left side of the patient, facing the monitors and the endoscopic tower, with the electronic equipment on the right side (Figs. 36.2A and B). A uterine manipulator is not required. A CO_2 pneumoperitoneum to an intra-abdominal pressure of 15 mm Hg is established utilizing a Veress needle, which is placed through an incision in the inferior umbilical fossa. A 5 mm trocar is used for the laparoscopy with a 30° optic.

Tip: The excellent image quality provided by the Karl Storz digital three-chip camera and the 30° telescope is of great advantage, particularly in the case of large multimodal myomatous uteri or when the situs is obscure.

The patient is then placed in a Trendelenburg position, a maximum (steep) position. A further two 5 mm puncture sites in the lower abdomen are required (Fig. 36.3), the location of which depends

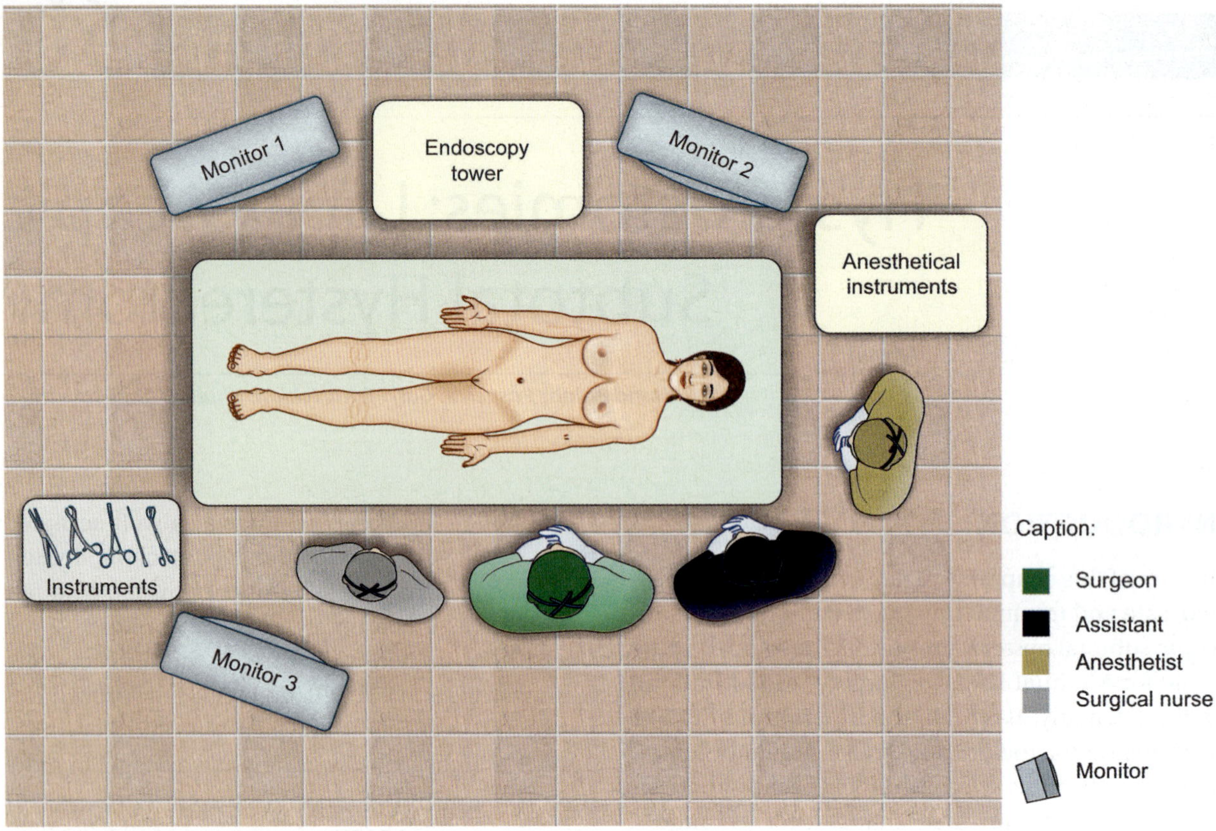

Fig. 36.1: Patient positioning and operating room equipment at the MIC Klinik in Berlin.

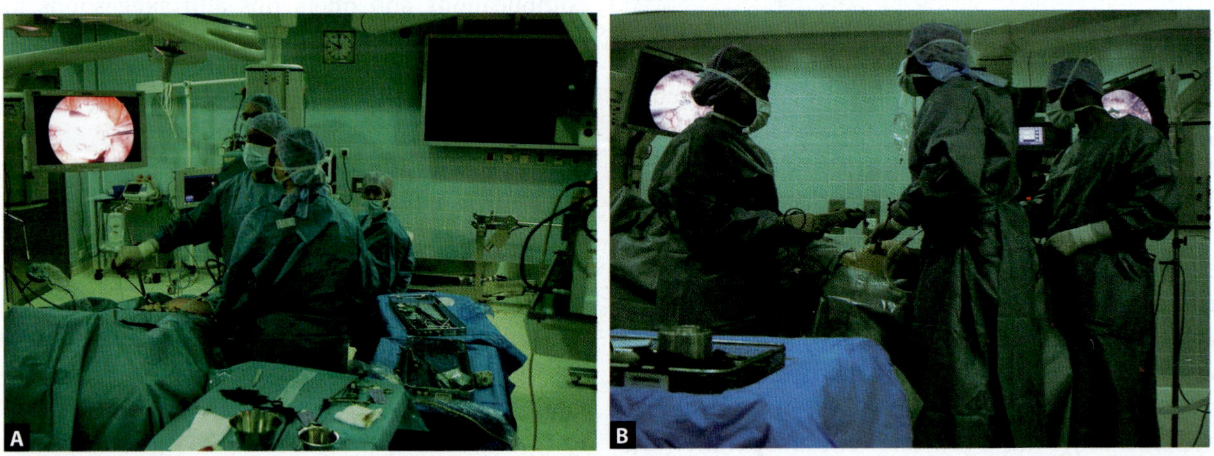

Figs. 36.2A and B: Surgeon, assistant, scrub nurse and instrument table are positioned on the left side of the patient.

on the size of the uterus. Two additional trocars are introduced left and right, lateral to the epigastric vessels in the region of pubic hair line, in the case of a normal-sized uterus. The larger the uterus, the further above the symphysis pubis the lateral trocars need to be positioned. In the case of uterus extension as far as the umbilicus, insufflation is performed on the left, below the costal arch with trocar introduction there or in the umbilicus. Correspondingly higher, additional trocars are positioned according to the size of the uterus, to enable the adnexa to be dissected (Fig. 36.4).

Tip: With a large myomatous uterus (Figs. 36.5A and B), localization of the two trocars in the lower abdomen depends on the size of uterus. They are then usually placed 2–3 cm above the pubic hair border. A fourth trocar should be introduced on the left, below the costal arch or above the umbilicus, to obtain a better overview of the uterus. From there, visualization can be performed with the telescope (Fig. 36.6).

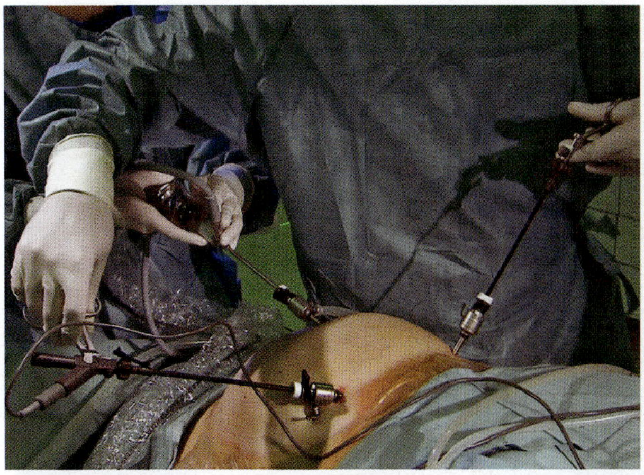

Fig. 36.3: Trocar placement for a LSH (normal-sized uterus).

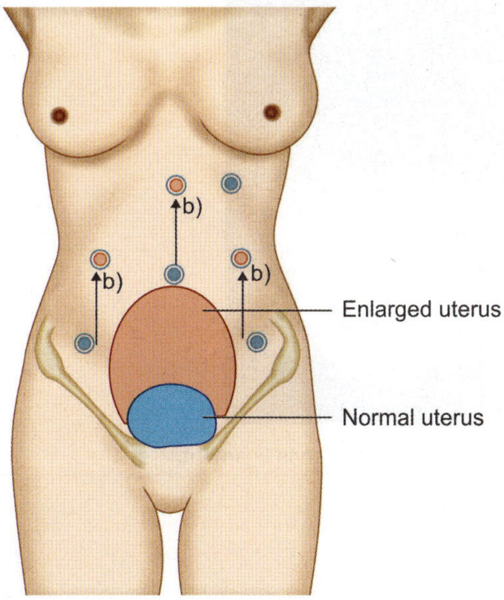

Fig. 36.4: Variations of trocar placement in cases of enlarged uteri.

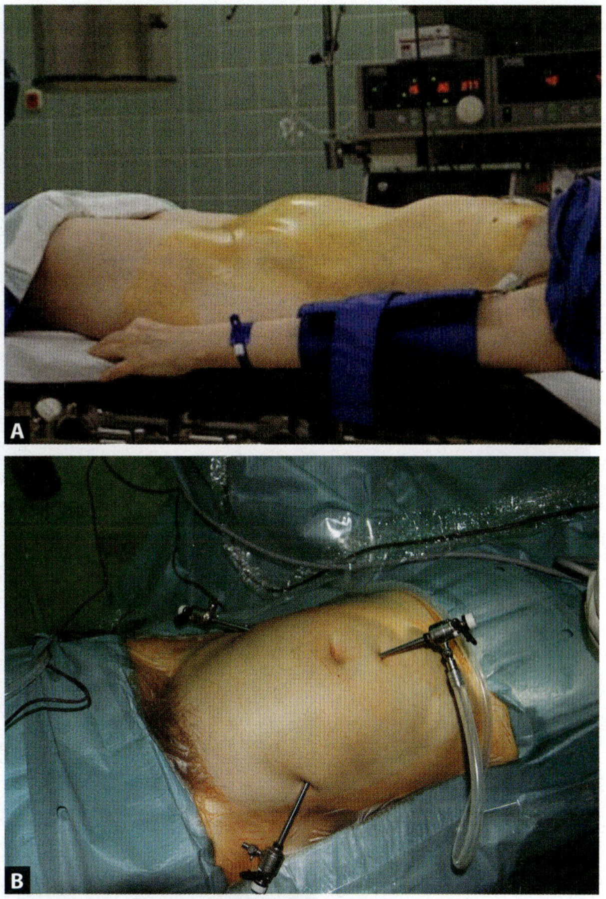

Figs. 36.5A and B: Uterus weighing 1107 g. (A) View from outside; (B) Trocar placement.

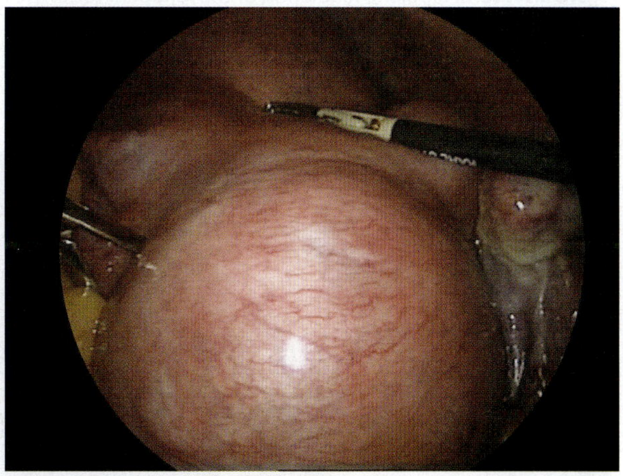

Fig. 36.6: Uterus weighting 1107 g—view from inside.

The uterus can then be pressed to the right or left using a palpation probe, so as to remove the adnexa laterally. With such large findings, good visualization of the anatomic structures with the 30° telescope is essential to avoid unnecessary bleeding.

The only additional reusable instruments needed for LSH include a bipolar coagulation clamp, Metzenbaum scissors, three various grasping forceps, a needle holder, a unipolar hook and a suction-irrigation system. Round ligaments, fallopian tubes and the ovarian ligaments are coagulated using bipolar forceps for mobilization of the uterus (Figs. 36.7A to C) and subsequently dissected using endoscopic Metzenbaum scissors (Figs. 36.8A and B).

Tip: Mobilization of the uterus can also be performed with the ultracision harmonic scalpel. Less frequent instrument changing is then required. The use of ultracision instruments, monopolar scissors and unipolar loops for the dissection of the corpus uteri has also been described.[11,12] Safety, precision

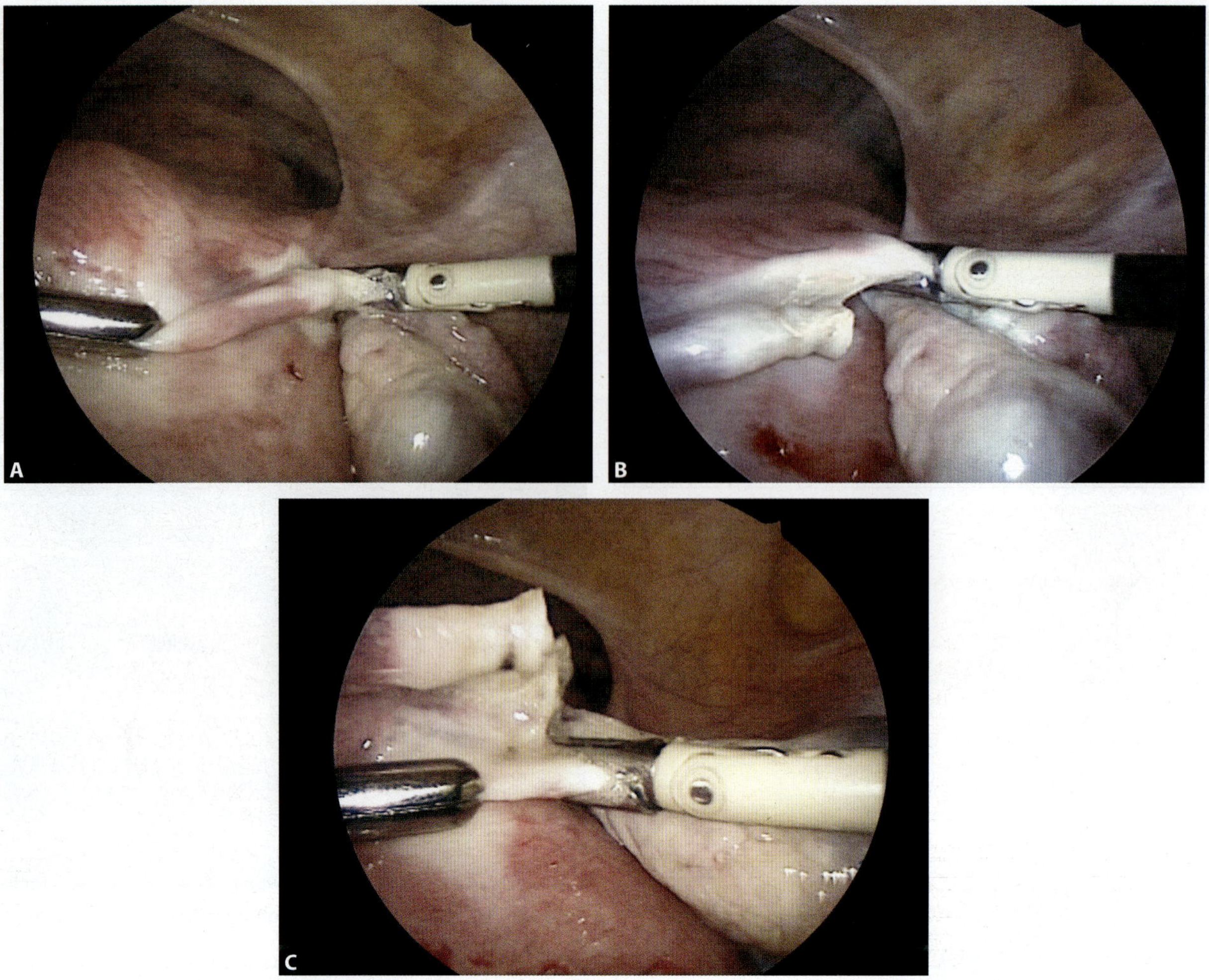

Figs. 36.7A to C: Bipolar coagulation of the fallopian tube, the round ligament and the ovarian ligament.

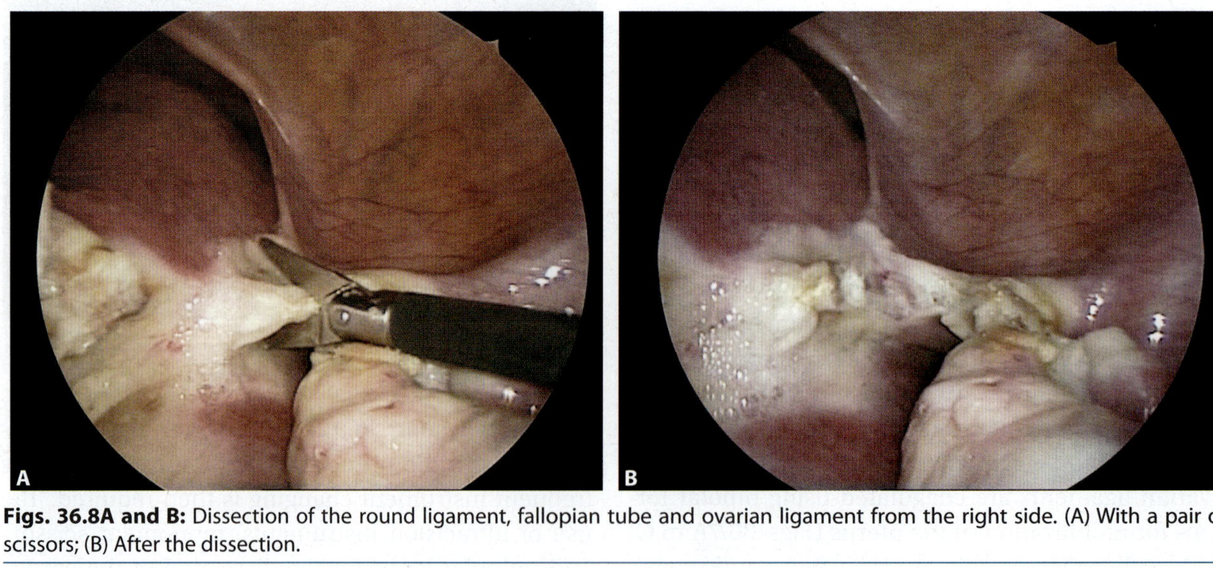

Figs. 36.8A and B: Dissection of the round ligament, fallopian tube and ovarian ligament from the right side. (A) With a pair of scissors; (B) After the dissection.

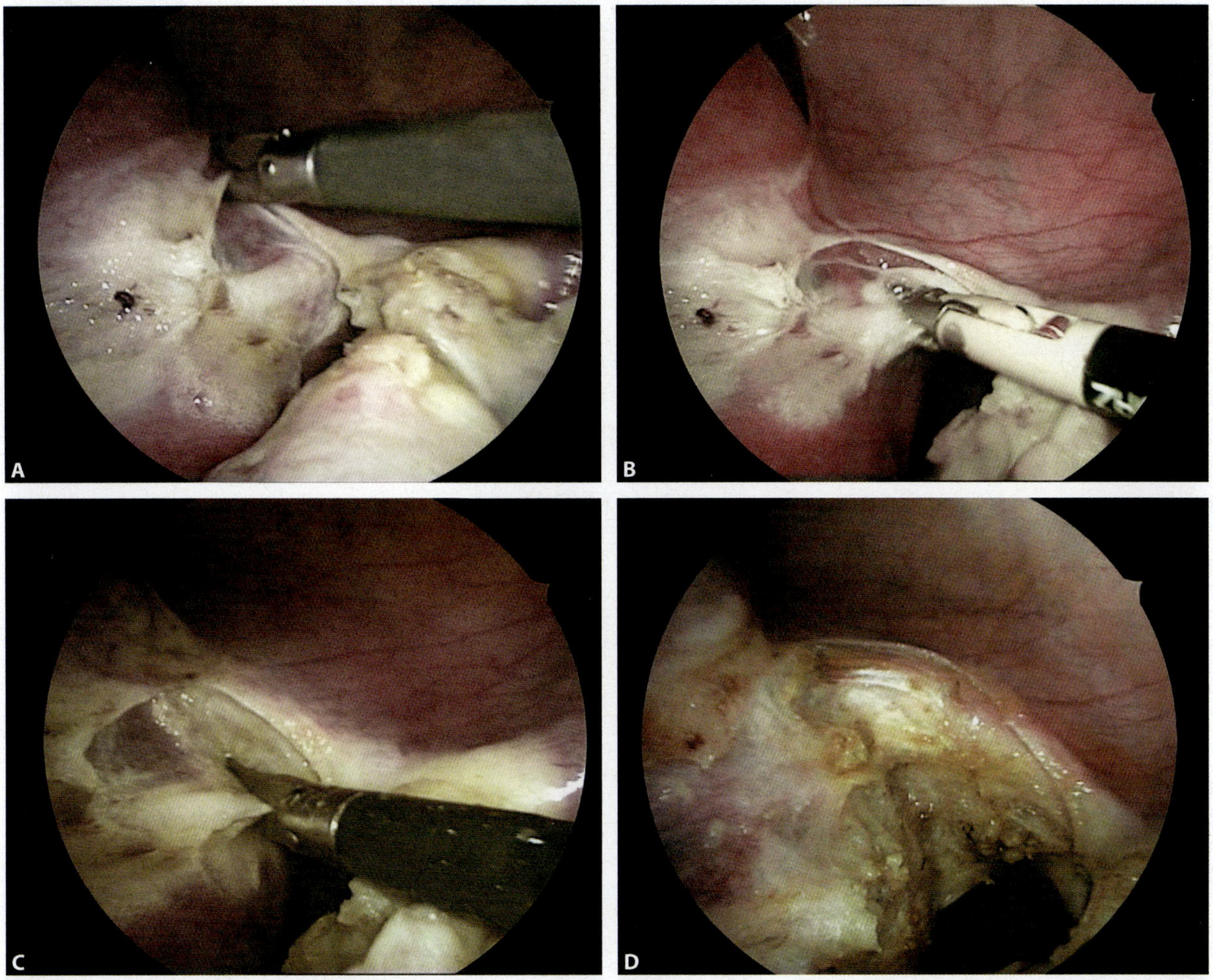

Figs. 36.9A to D: Identification and skeletonization, bipolar coagulation and dissection of uterine vessels on the right side.

of the cut and shortage of operating time are definite advantages of the unipolar loop.[13]

Tip: In the case of intraligamentous myomas the essential requirements are, on the one hand, sufficient hemostasis and, on the other hand, dissection close to the myoma. The majority of myomas can be mobilized with a blunt instrument. If the myomas extend as far as the pelvic wall, it is necessary for the ureter to be visualized during and after the removal. If endometriosis foci are present, irrespective of whether they are located in the Douglas, in the area of the round ligaments or in the area of the bladder peritoneum, it is important to also resect these foci completely to ensure that the symptoms complained of before the operation do not persist afterward.

After identification and skeletonization of the uterine vessels, bleeding is controlled by bipolar coagulation and the vessels are dissected using Metzenbaum scissors on the right side (Figs. 36.9A to D). Grasping forceps are used to pull the uterus to the contralateral side. After separation of the uterus from the ovaries and fallopian tubes and dissection through the round ligaments on the left side (Figs. 36.10A and B), the uterine vessels are coagulated and dissected (Figs. 36.11A and B) and a bipolar coagulation zone is placed on bladder peritoneum for delineation of the planned direction of incision to open the bladder peritoneum (Figs. 36.12A and B). Once the bladder peritoneum has been separated from the dissected round ligaments using scissors, it can be opened and the bladder pushed slightly caudally. Contrary to total hysterectomy, it is not necessary to push away the bladder. This is because dissection of the uterine body with a unipolar hook or with a pair of scissors (Figs. 36.13A and B) is done in the upper third, cranial to where the uterosacral ligaments leave the cervix.

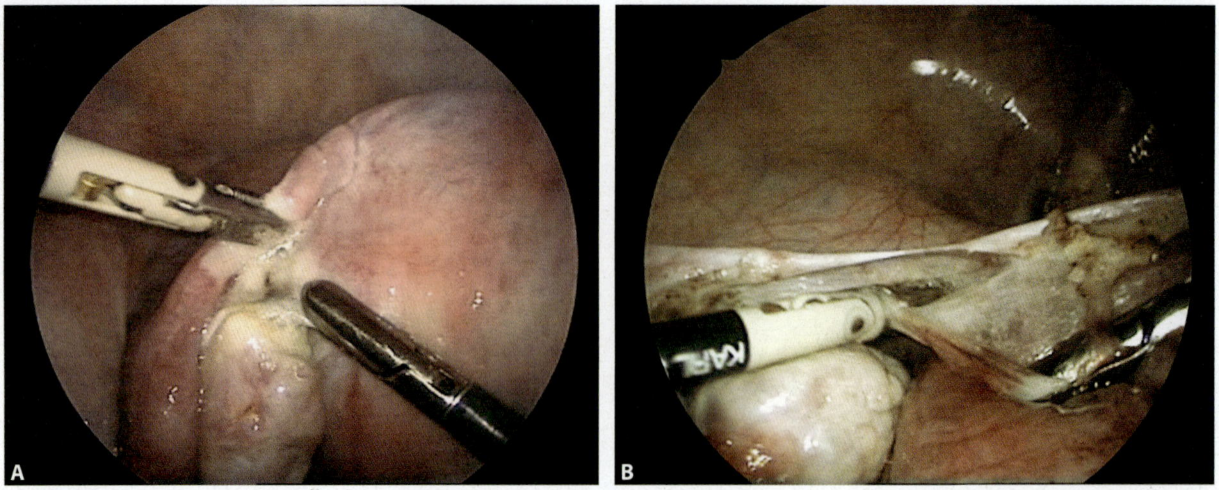

Figs. 36.10A and B: Bipolar coagulation and dissection of round ligament, fallopian tube and ovarian ligament from left side.

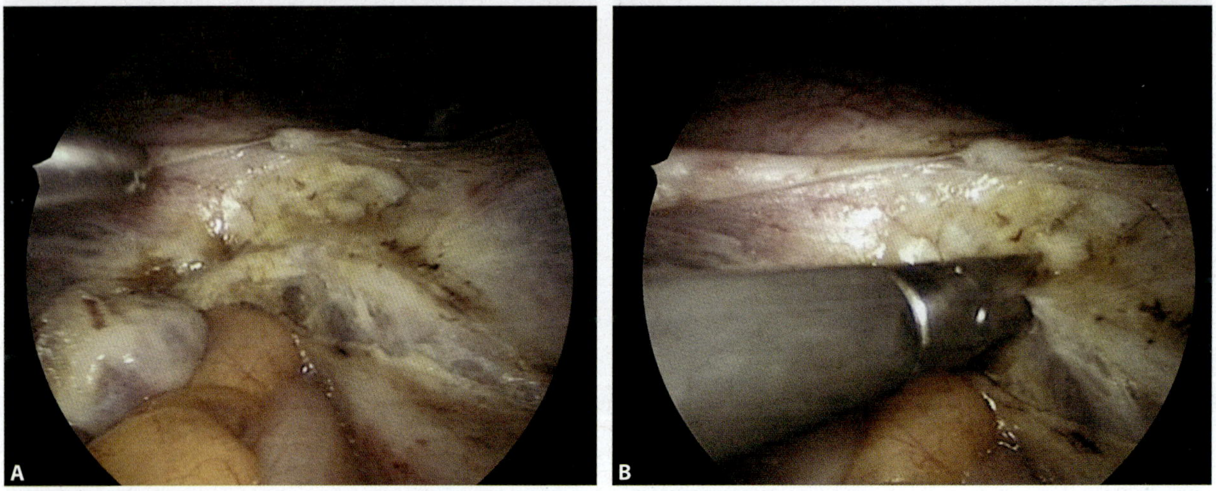

Figs. 36.11A and B: Identification and skeletonization, bipolar coagulation and dissection of uterine vessels on the left side.

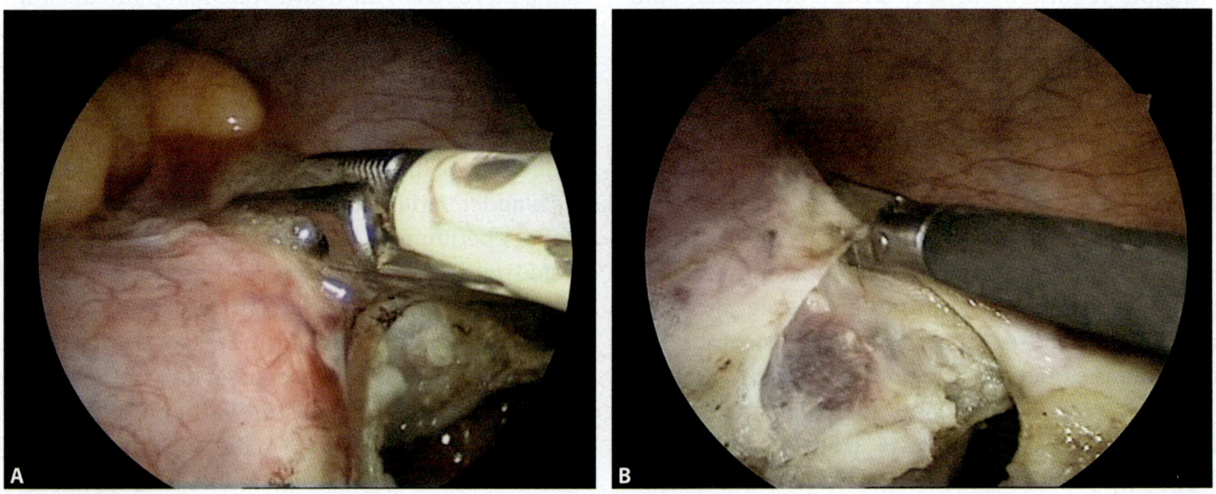

Figs. 36.12A and B: (A) A coagulation zone is made on the bladder peritoneum; (B) Undermining and opening of the bladder peritoneum.

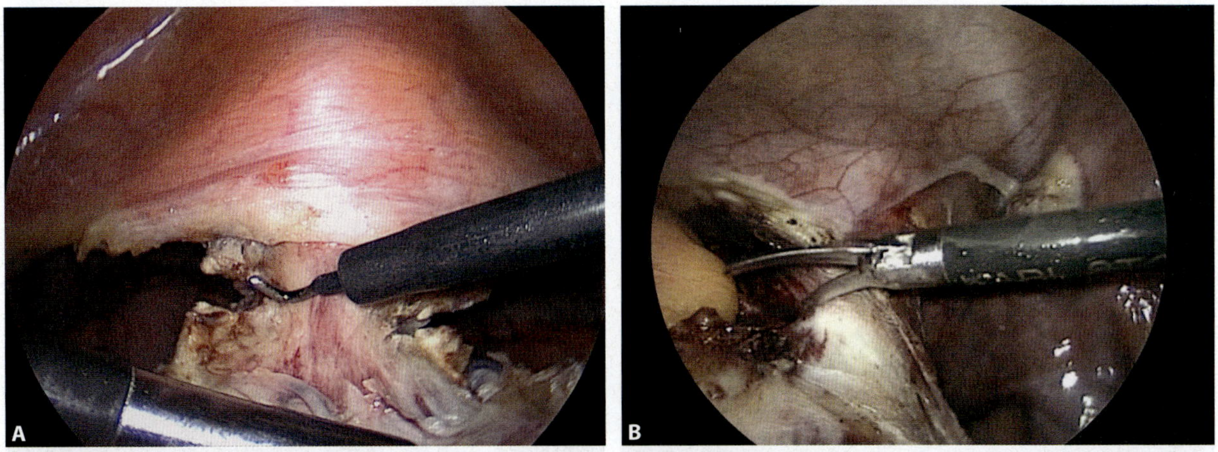

Figs. 36.13A and B: Transection of corpus uteri. (A) With unipolar hook; (B) With a pair of scissors.

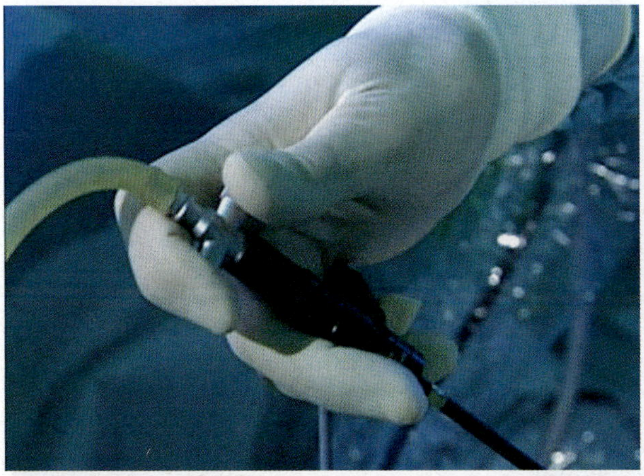

Fig. 36.14: Suction device connected to the unipolar hook.

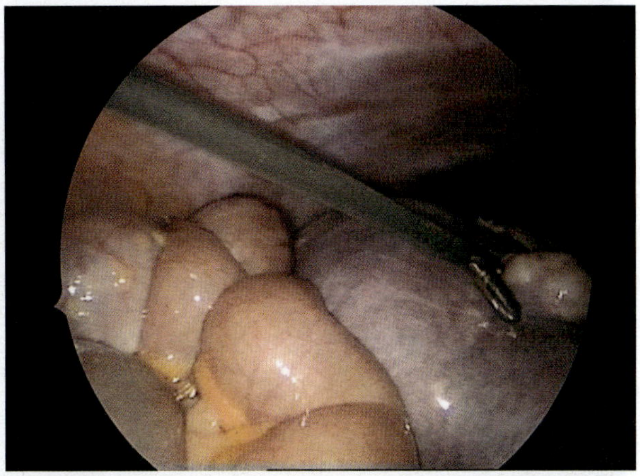

Fig. 36.15: Positioning of the transected corpus in the right-hand mesogastrium.

If dissection starts from the left side, uterus is held against the anterior wall using grasping forceps and pulled in a cranial direction. Due to the traction of uterus to the opposite side (where the dissection is to be performed), space can be created to identify uterine vessels in the cervical area and ureter. If coagulation and dissection of the uterine vessels are performed close to cervix, we do not visualize ureter. In cases of cervical myomas, the traction of uterus to the contralateral side is very helpful for visualizing ureter.

Dissection is done step by step starting from the right using the unipolar hook. In this phase of surgery the surgeon needs a clear vision to prevent injury to the adjacent organs; the development of excessive smoke can be prevented by actuating the suction on the hook (Fig. 36.14). The dissected body of uterus is positioned in the right-hand mesogastrium to enable hemostasis in the wound area (Fig. 36.15), followed by bipolar coagulation of the cervical canal (Fig. 36.16) after efficient hemostasis (Figs. 36.17A and B) in the area of cervix stump.

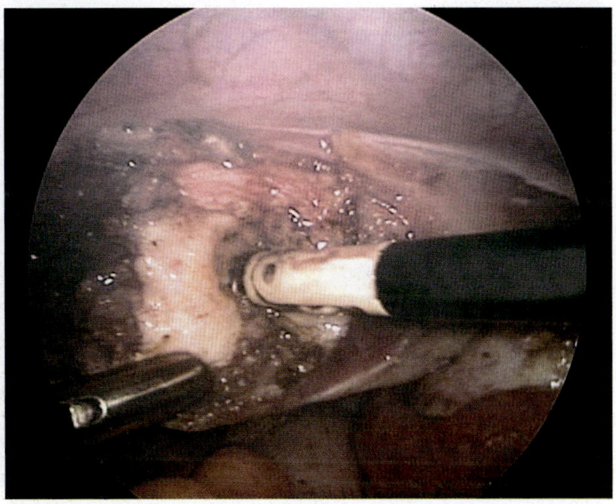

Fig. 36.16: Bipolar coagulation of the cervical canal.

Tip: If identification of the cervical canal is difficult, cervix can be held from the left using grasping forceps while searching for the entrance into cervical canal with a palpation probe or bipolar forceps.

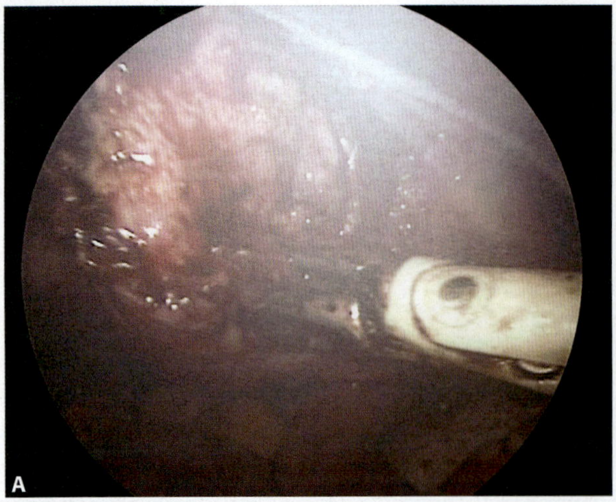
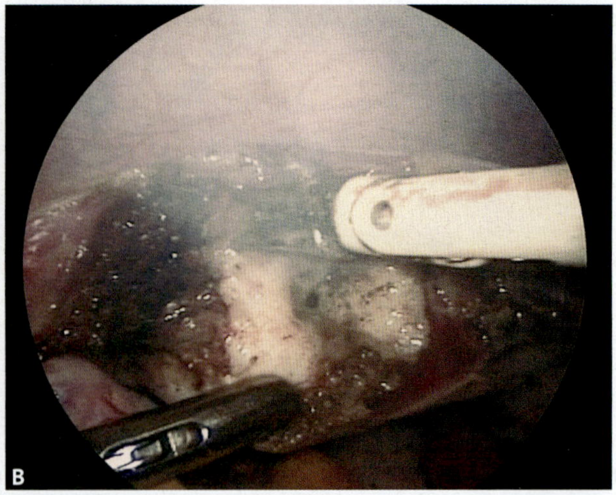

Figs. 36.17A and B: Hemostasis in the area of the cervical stump.

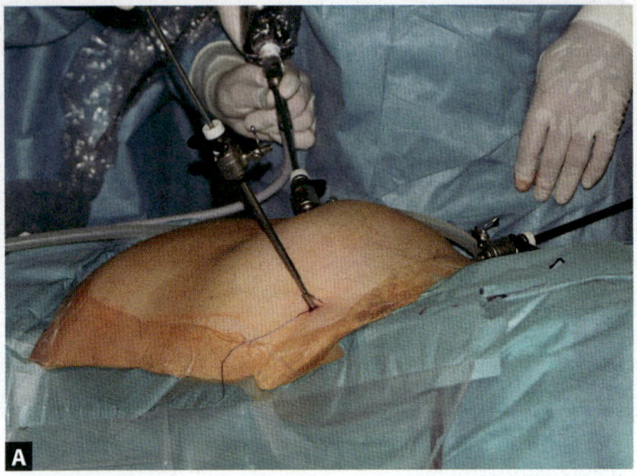
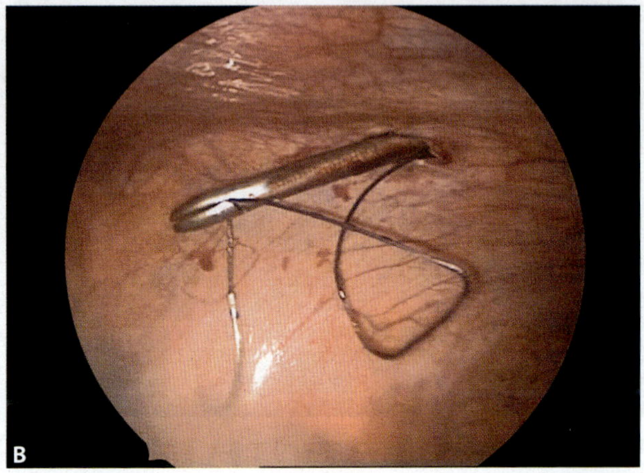

Figs. 36.18A and B: Introduction of a round needle. (A) Endoscopic view; and (B) View from outside.

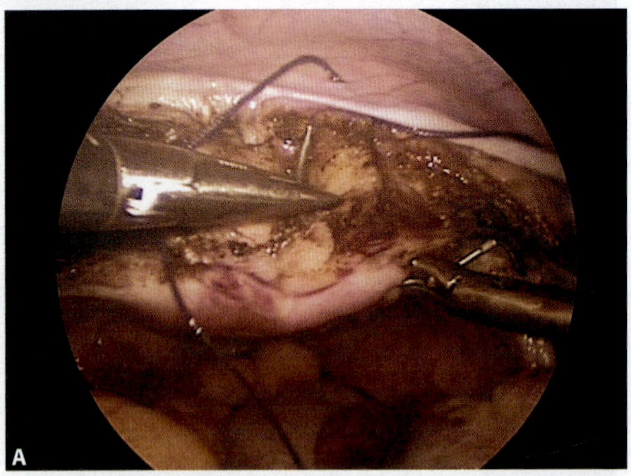
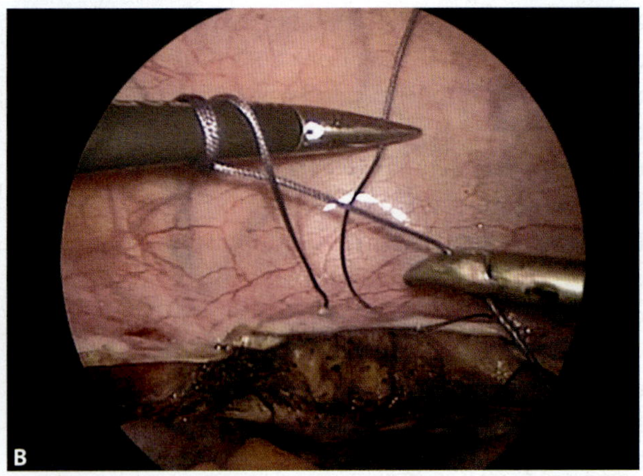

Figs. 36.19A and B: Continuous purse-string suture.

Coagulation is performed by opening and simultaneously rotating the damp in the cervical canal.

A Vicryl thread, shortened to approximately instrument length, is used for peritonealization of the cervical stump. Under vision, the round needle is introduced through the 5-mm incision (Figs. 36.18A and B). Cervix stump is then covered with peritoneum using a continuous purse-string suture, including both uterosacral ligaments (Figs. 36.19A and B). Following the preparation of a triple knot, peritoneum is pulled together with a fourth knot to secure the suture (Fig. 36.20). The incision is widened to 10–20 mm in the left-hand lower abdomen to remove uterus. Following injection of a local anesthetic beneath the wound area of the left-hand incision, an electric morcellator (STORZ® or WISAP®) (Figs. 36.21A to C) is introduced under direct vision. Uterus is then gripped from the left and pulled into the morcellator, which is activated by hand or foot pedal. It is of utmost importance to keep the sharp rotating blade continuously in view at the center of the laparoscopic image to avoid injuries (Figs. 36.22A and B). To remove a large section of tissue in a single piece, it is helpful to assist the process of morcellation with the right-handed grasping forceps so that the blade is always visible on the surface of the uterus (Figs. 36.23A and B). Morcellation is performed around the exterior of uterus. Then uterus is effectively peeled like a potato.

Tip: It is particularly important to ensure a good overview during morcellation and in the case of large uteri a 20 mm morcellator can also be used. This leads to a considerably shorter operation as the sections of uterus removed in this way are far larger. After removal of the uterus remaining smaller pieces of the uterus or the myoma are retrieved using 10 mm spoon grasping forceps (Figs. 36.24 and 36.25).

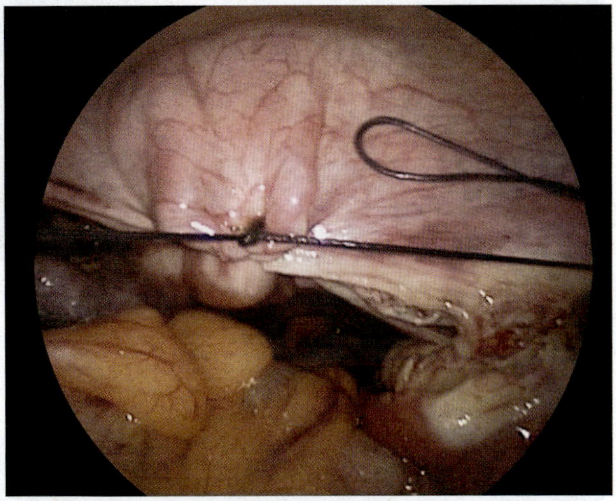

Fig. 36.20: Peritonealization of the cervical stump.

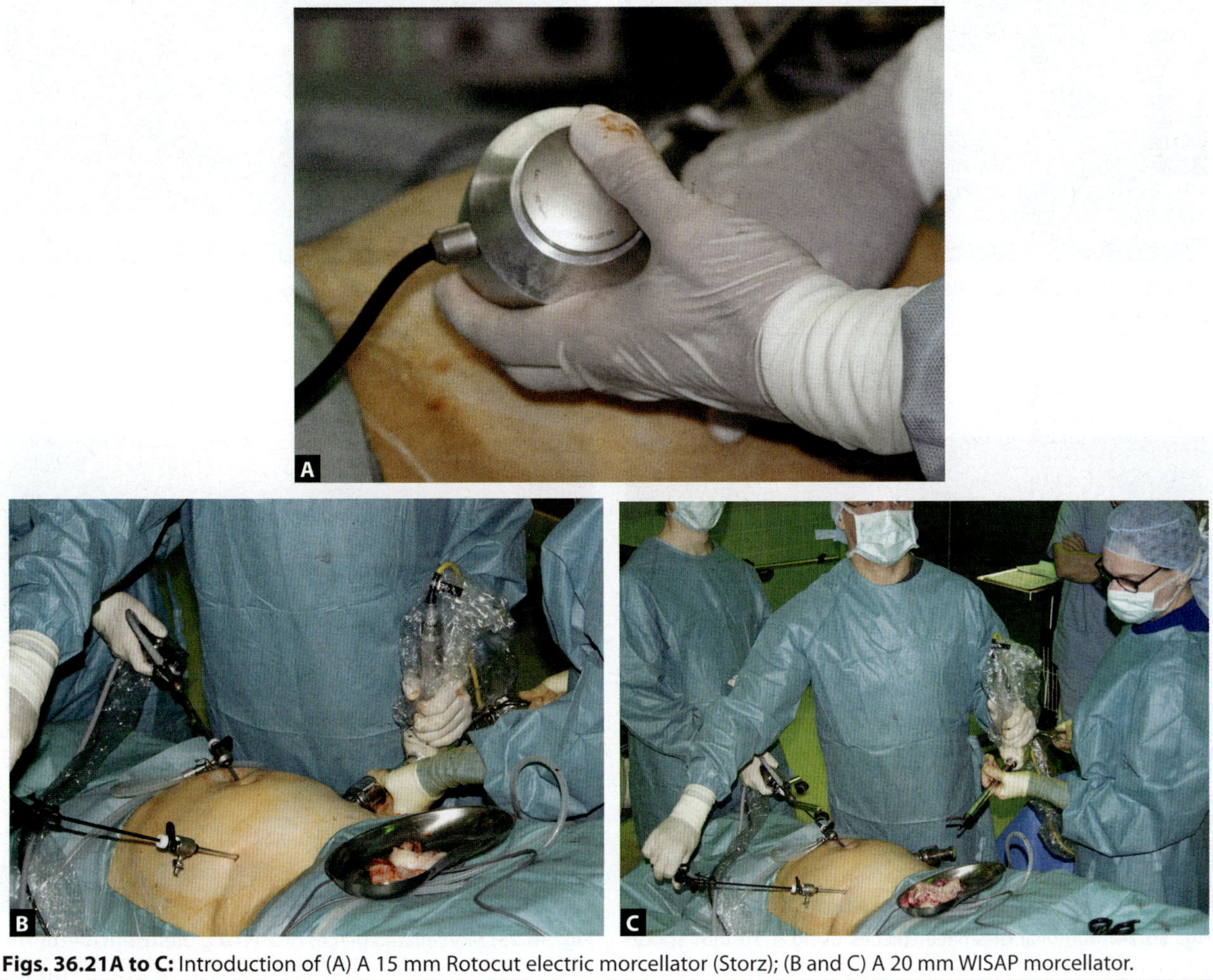

Figs. 36.21A to C: Introduction of (A) A 15 mm Rotocut electric morcellator (Storz); (B and C) A 20 mm WISAP morcellator.

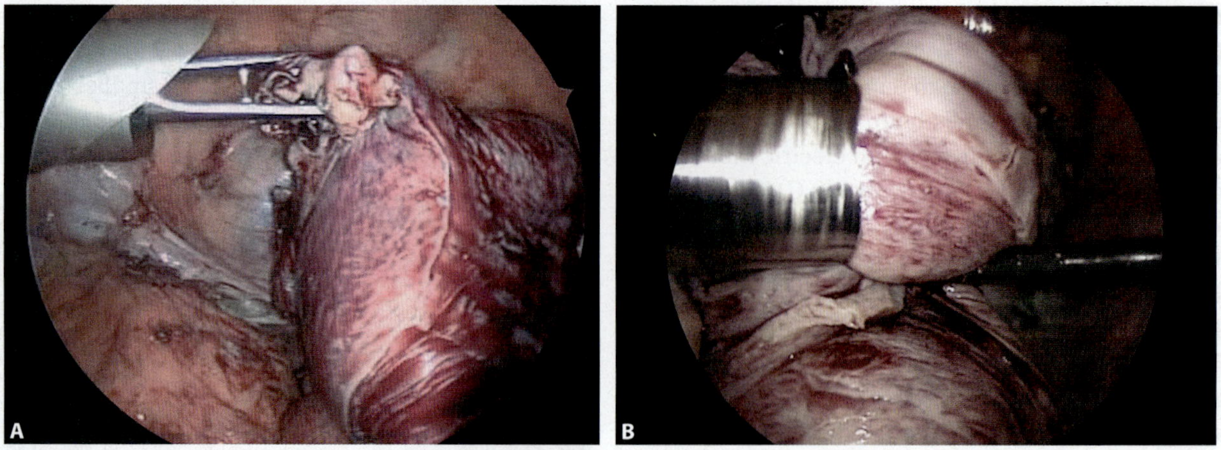

Figs. 36.22A and B: The sharp rotating blade of the morcellator is visible during morcellation. (A) Rotocut electric morcellator (Storz); (B) WISAP electric morcellator.

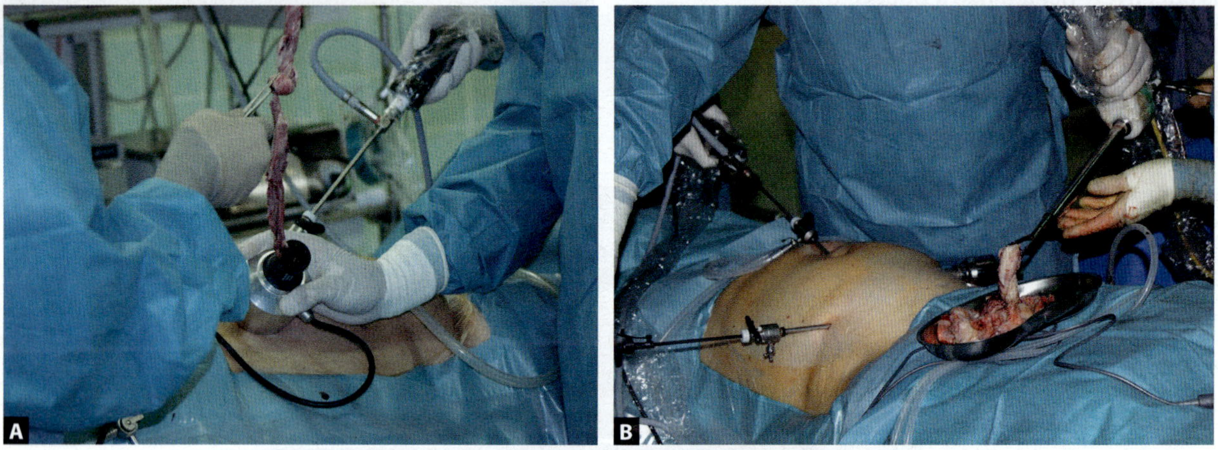

Figs. 36.23A and B: Morcellation—view from outside. (A) With the Rotocut electric morcellator (Storz); (B) With the WISAP electric morcellator.

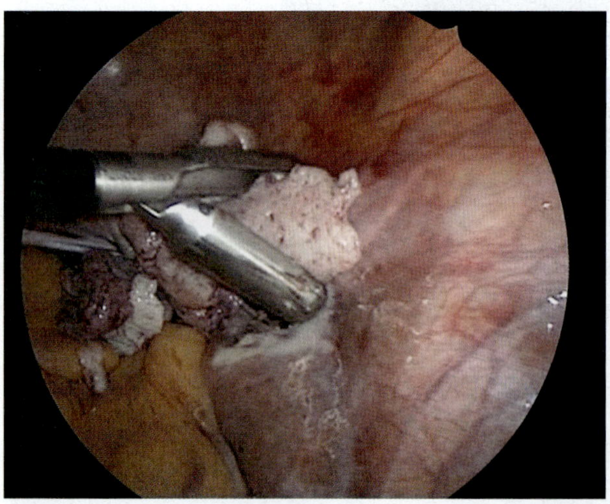

Fig. 36.24: Removal of smaller pieces using a 10 mm spoon grasping forceps.

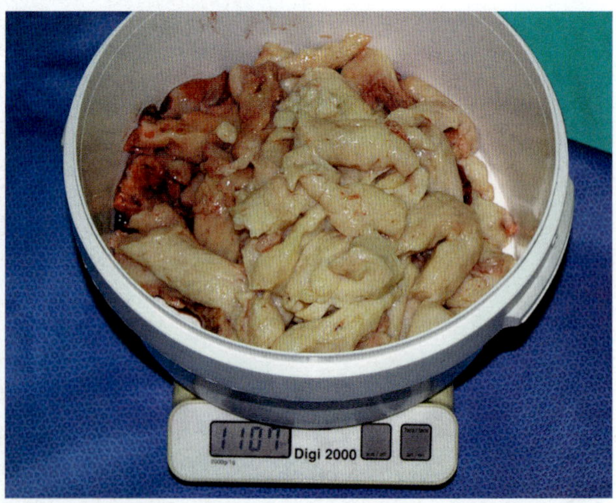

Fig. 36.25: Morcellated pieces of a 1107 g uterus.

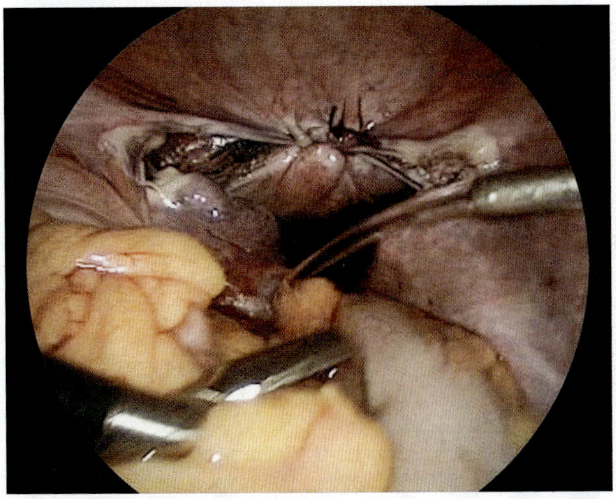

Fig. 36.26: Rinsing of the abdomen.

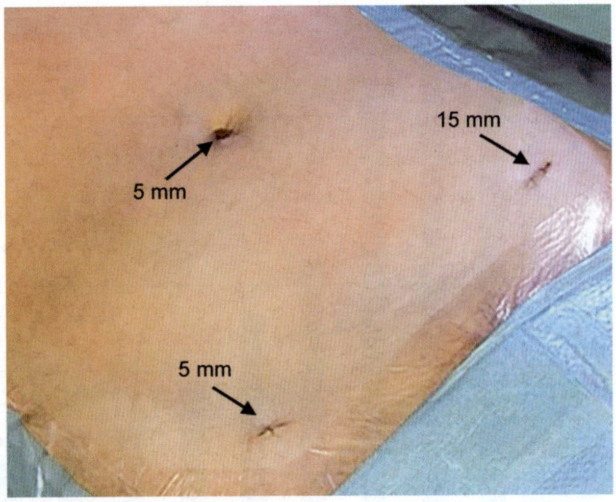

Fig. 36.27: Final abdominal situs.

The operation is completed with lavage and a final checking of the cervical stump (Fig. 36.26). Peritoneum in the area of 15 or 20 mm incisions is closed from the inside using bipolar coagulation. To avoid incision hernias, closure of the fasciae is also necessary. The skin is then closed using single-button sutures. The final abdominal situs for a normal-sized uterus shows two 5 mm incisions, one in the umbilicus and one on the right side of the lower abdomen, and a 15 mm incision on the left (Fig. 36.27). If the uterus is noticeably enlarged, an additional 5 mm and a 20 mm incision for the morcellation may become necessary.

COMPLICATIONS

Perioperative and Short-term Postoperative Complications

In our review of 18 studies, the total number of women who underwent LSH to treat benign uterine disease was 11,616[2-6,9,14-25] (Fig. 36.28). The overall incidence of intraoperative complications ranged from 0% to 6.56%. Moreover, the most frequently reported intraoperative complications, such as bladder injuries and ureteral injury, ranged from 0% to 1.84% and from 0% to 0.37%, respectively. Bladder injury most often occurred during dissection of the bladder from cervix due to the extensive adhesions between the bladder and the isthmic portion of uterus in patients who had a history of previous cesarean section. The frequency of intestinal injuries ranged from 0% to 1% and was observed only in five studies. Vascular injuries were documented in three studies and the incidence ranged from 0 to 0.48%. Furthermore, the majority of intraoperative complications were treated directly during the initial surgery. The rate of short-term postoperative complications, such as cervical stump infection, abdominal wound infection, uterine retention, ileus, abscess and secondary hemorrhage, ranged widely from 0 to 13.6%. However, in two large single-center studies, comprising 1,706 and 1,658 patients, the short-term postoperative complications were 1.18% and 1.4%, respectively (Fig. 36.29). The rate of intraoperative conversion to laparotomy ranged from 0 to 4.62%. The risk factors for conversion were extensive adhesions and the large size and weight of the uterus, which cause a lack of mobility and limited vision during laparoscopic procedures (Fig. 36.30).

Cervical Stump Symptoms after Subtotal Hysterectomy

Cervical stump symptoms, such as vaginal bleeding and pelvic pain, can be observed after subtotal hysterectomy whether an open or a laparoscopic operation is performed. However, these risk factors do not seem to affect patient satisfaction following the LSH in the long-term outcome analysis.[25,26]

The incidence of postoperative cervical stump bleeding was 21.4% among the 2,334 patients who underwent LSH at the MIC Klinik, Berlin, between 1998 and 2004.[27] To date, the predictive factors for postoperative cyclical bleeding after LSH are still controversial. There is an opinion that residual endometrial tissue in the upper cervix after LSH can be a reason for recurrent bleeding episodes after LSH. Berner et al. (2013) compared the rate of vaginal bleeding after LSH with and without excision of

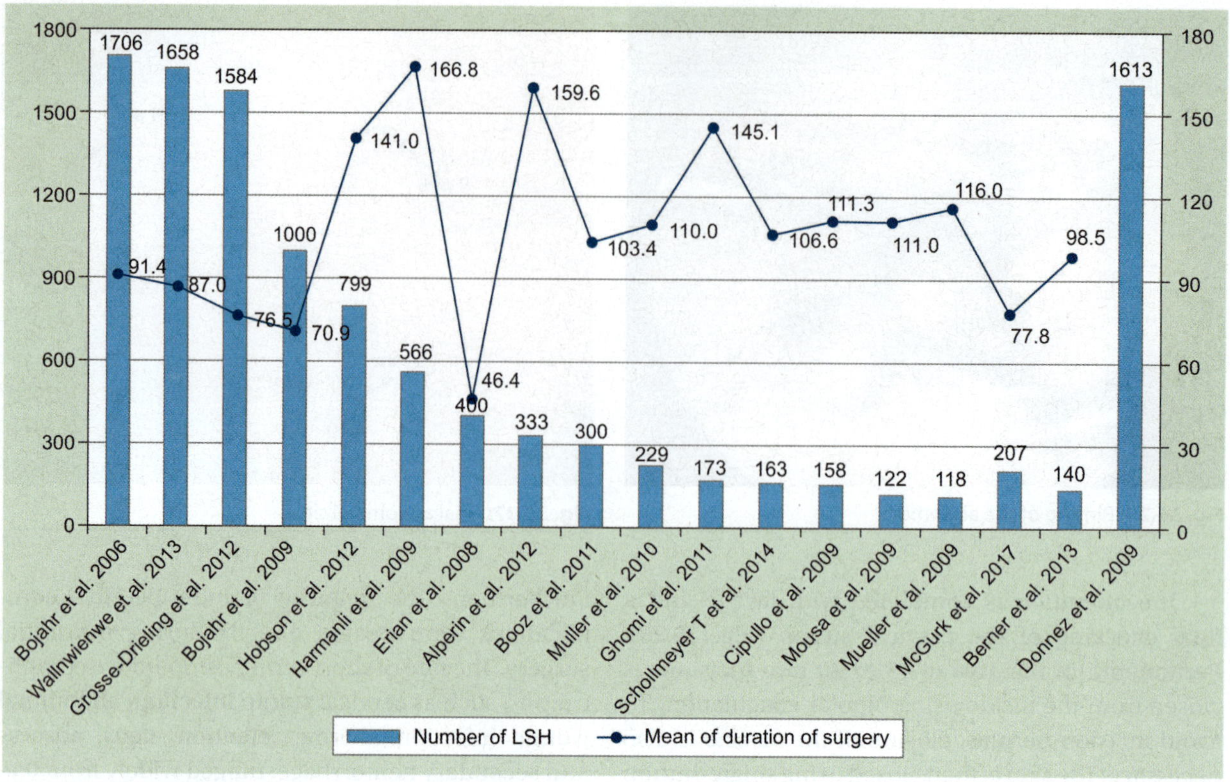

Fig. 36.28: Total number of laparoscopic subtotal hysterectomies (LSH) and the mean duration of the surgery by different studies.

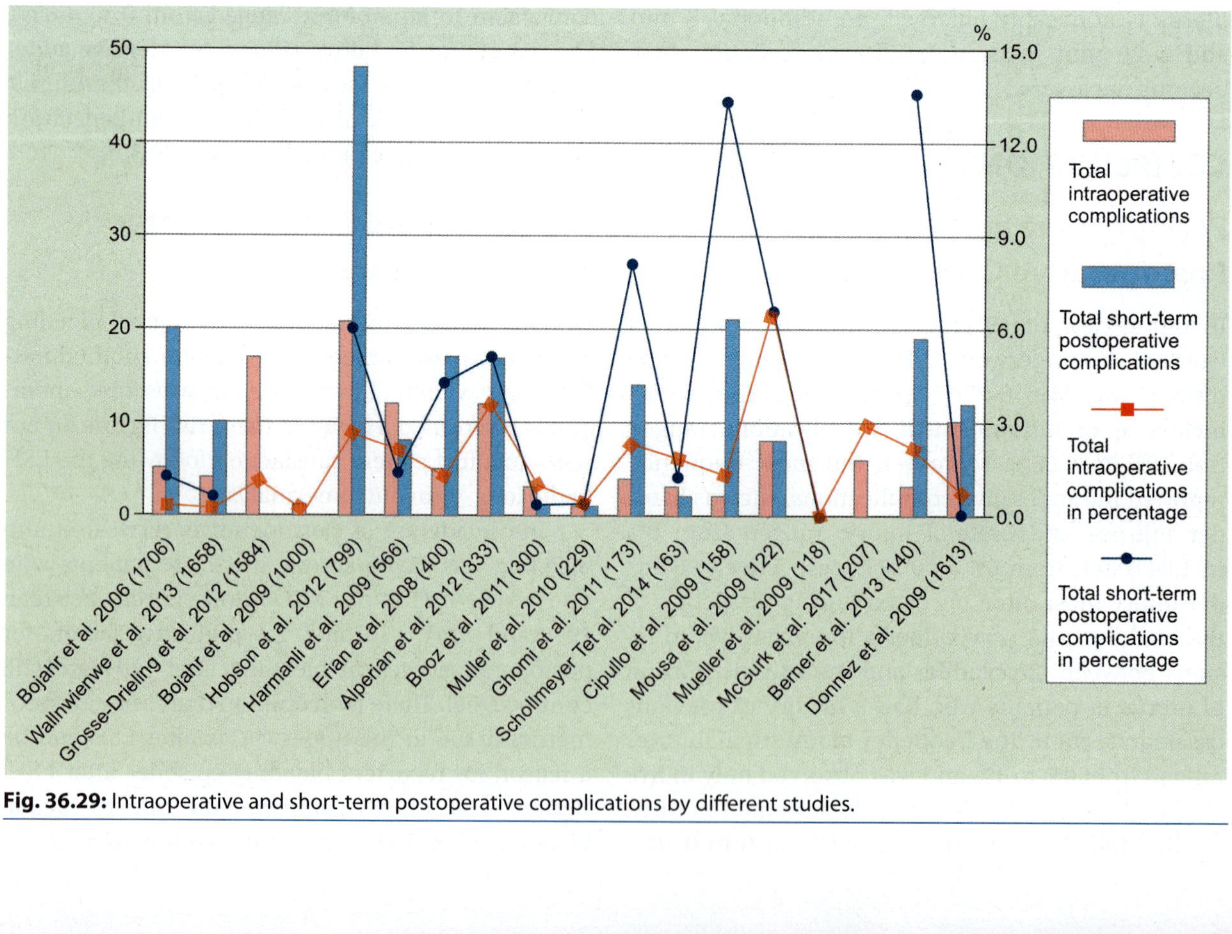

Fig. 36.29: Intraoperative and short-term postoperative complications by different studies.

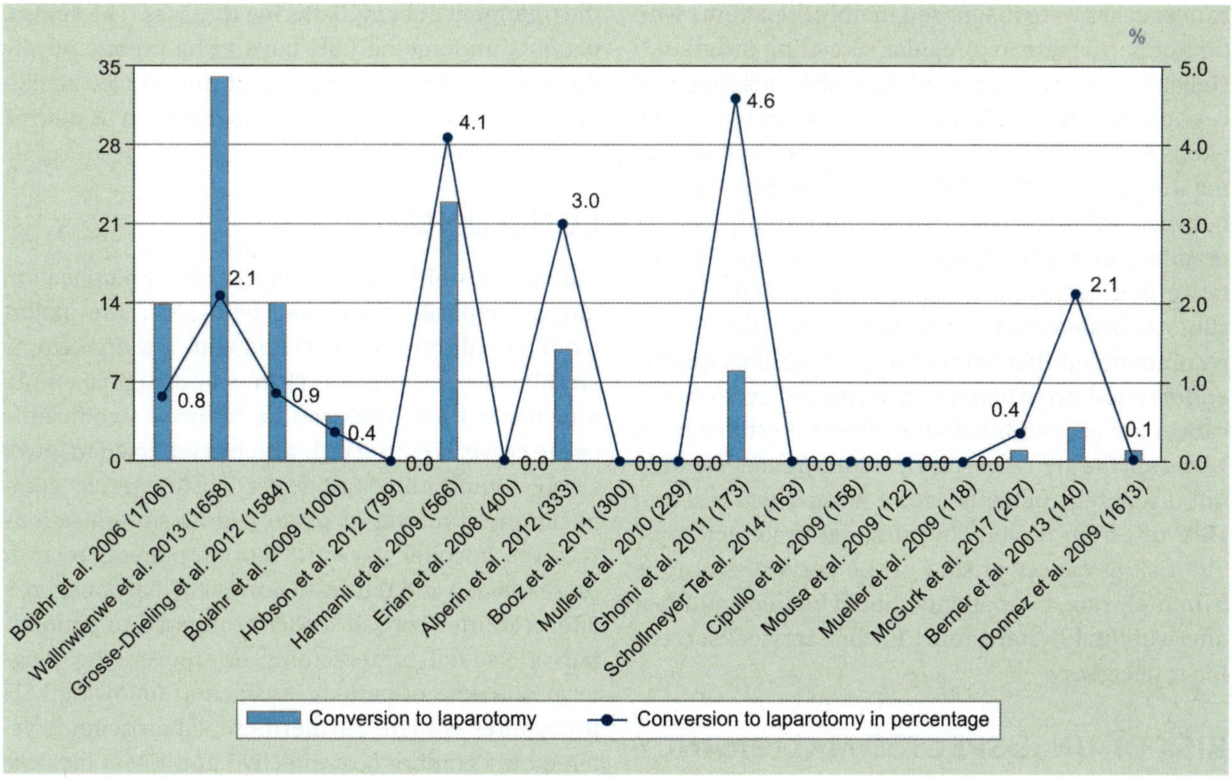

Fig. 36.30: Laparoscopic subtotal hysterectomy conversion to laparotomy by different studies.

endocervix. The removal of endocervix was performed by reverse conization. The study could not find any significant differences between the two treatment groups regarding the occurrence of vaginal bleeding after LSH within a 12-month period.[24] However, Schmidt et al. (2011) demonstrated that the postoperative bleeding episodes in patients who underwent excision of the endocervix was significantly reduced compared with the control group (1.4% vs 10.7%).[28] Currently, there is no evidence regarding the superiority of one particular surgical technique for the prevention of postoperative bleeding after LSH.[12] One probable reason for the bleeding could be an endometrial regeneration under the hormonal cyclical changes in the cervical canal.[29]

The impact of retained cervical stump on pain outcome in women with a history of subtotal hysterectomy is a subject of discussion as the reasons and exact mechanisms of developing cervical stump pain after subtotal hysterectomy are unclear. Berner et al.[30] analyzed the occurrence, intensity and reduction of cyclic pelvic pain and patient satisfaction 12 months after LSH. All 113 study patients, including women with endometriosis or adenomyosis, had suffered from cyclic pelvic pain preoperatively. Postoperative results showed that cyclic pelvic pain was observed in 34 (32.4%) cases; however, the intensity of pain was reduced significantly.[30] Additionally, Berner et al.[31] demonstrated that there were no differences between TLH and LSH in reducing cyclical pelvic pain at 12 months following surgery in women complaining of this symptom preoperatively.[31] Yunker et al.[32] studied the nerve fiber density in the removed cervical stump. Their results demonstrated that nerve fiber density was significantly increased in cervical stump, which was removed because of pain indications compared to non-pain indications and controls. They also reported that endometriosis can be an independent risk factor for postoperative pelvic pain due to the increase of nerve fiber density in the cervical stump.[32] Therefore, endometriosis lesions should be completely resected as further surgery might otherwise become necessary.[33]

RISK OF CERVICAL STUMP CANCER

In 2012 about 4,600 women were diagnosed with cervical cancer, representing an age-standardized incidence rate of 11.3 per 100,000 women in Germany. The most frequent type of invasive cancer of the cervix was squamous cell carcinoma, followed by adenocarcinoma.[34] The new cervical cancer cases were diagnosed mainly in patients who do not participate in a regular screening program.[35] Hellström et al.[36] reported that the incidence of cervical stump carcinoma was 2% among 8,028 women treated for invasive cervical carcinoma during the period 1959 to 2004. The mean time interval between subtotal hysterectomy and stump cancer manifestation was 17.6 years. It is of utmost importance that cervical screening is performed prior to subtotal hysterectomy.[36] An ACOG guideline (2014) recommended that women with cervical dysplasia, endometrial hyperplasia and suspected gynecologic cancer are not candidates for subtotal hysterectomy. However, the low risk of cervical stump cancer should not discourage patients with a normal Pap test and HPV test from undergoing subtotal hysterectomy.[37] The risk of cancer arising in the cervical stump is extremely rare, but patients should be informed that after subtotal hysterectomy further cervical screening is necessary.

RISK OF UNSUSPECTED MALIGNANCY

Since 2014 there remains Food and Drug Administration (FDA) concern regarding the safety of power morcellation due to the risk of unexpected malignancy among patients who underwent laparoscopic procedures.[38] Therefore, we conducted a retrospective study to evaluate the incidence of occult uterine malignancies after LSH in the period 1998 to 2014. The results revealed that the incidence of unsuspected uterine sarcoma was 0.06% and of endometrial carcinoma 0.07% among 10,731 women who underwent LSH to treat presumed benign uterine disease.[39] The risk of unsuspected malignancy is low; however, the concern over the risk of malignancy may decrease the frequency of laparoscopic surgery for patients with benign uterine pathology, which may negatively influence clinical outcomes.[40,41] Harris et al.[42] conducted a comparative analysis of 18,299 hysterectomies performed in the 15 months leading up to and the 8 months after the FDA safety communication in April 2014. The results show that the application of abdominal (1.7%) and vaginal hysterectomy (2.4%) increased whereas a 4.1% decline in laparoscopic hysterectomy occurred. An overall higher rate of complications, from 2.2 to 2.8%, was observed after the date of the FDA safety communication and the rate of hospital readmission within 30 days also increased from 3.4 to 4.2%.[42] The German Society of Obstetrics and Gynecology underlines that in many cases electric morcellation is important for the treatment of benign uterine diseases.[43] Moreover, patients undergoing LSH have to be preoperatively informed of the minimal risk of unexpected malignancy in the case of a rare pathology such as uterine sarcoma.

CONCLUSION

Minimal morbidity and an equally low complication rate are typically associated with LSH. The majority of complications associated with a hysterectomy are bladder and ureteral lesions and vaginal stump infections. These risks can be reduced significantly as the cervix is conserved, which is reflected in lower surgical morbidity and fewer postoperative complications. The rate of postoperative complications is lower, hospital stays are shorter, patients recover more quickly and return to normal activity and work after a shorter convalescence compared to abdominal or vaginal hysterectomy. Moreover, the long-term outcome of patient satisfaction following LSH procedures is high. Furthermore, laparoscopic hysterectomy is more cost-effective and a less invasive alternative than abdominal hysterectomy.[44]

REFERENCES

1. Aarts JW, Nieboer TE, Johnson N, et al. Surgical approach to hysterectomy for benign gynaecological disease. Cochrane Database Syst Rev. 2015;(8): CD003677.
2. Wallwiener M, Taran FA, Rothmund R, et al. Laparoscopic supracervical hysterectomy (LSH) versus total laparoscopic hysterectomy (TLH): an implementation study in 1,952 patients with an analysis of risk factors for conversion to laparotomy and complications, and of procedure-specific re-operations. Arch Gynecol Obstet. 2013: 288(6):1329-39.
3. Hobson DT, Imudia AN, Al-Safi ZA, et al. Comparative analysis of different laparoscopic hysterectomy procedures. Arch Gynecol Obstet. 2012;285(5):1353-61.
4. Boosz A, Lermann J, Mehlhorn G, et al. Comparison of re-operation rates and complication rates after total laparoscopic hysterectomy (TLH) and laparoscopy-assisted supracervical hysterectomy (LASH). Eur J Obstet Gynecol Reprod Biol. 2011;158(2):269-73.
5. Mueller A, Renner SP, Haeberle L, et al. Comparison of total laparoscopic hysterectomy (TLH) and laparoscopy-assisted supracervical hysterectomy (LASH) in women with uterine leiomyoma. Eur J Obstet Gynecol Reprod Biol. 2009;144(1):76-9.
6. Bojahr B, Raatz D, Schonleber G, et al. Perioperative complication rate in 1706 patients after a standardized laparoscopic supracervical hysterectomy technique. J Minim Invasive Gynecol. 2006;13(3):183-9.
7. Neis KJ, Zubke W, Römer T, et al. Indications and route of hysterectomy for benign diseases. Guideline

of the DGGG, OEGGG and SGGG (S3 Level, AWMF Registry No.015/070, April 2015). Geburtshilfe Frauenheilkd. 2016;76(4):350-64.

8. Desai VB, Guo XM, Fan L, et al. Inpatient laparoscopic hysterectomy in the united states: trends and factors associated with approach selection. J Minim Invasive Gynecol. 2017;24(1):151-8.e1.
9. Bojahr B, Tchartchian G, Ohlinger R. Laparoscopic supracervical hysterectomy: a retrospective analysis of 1000 cases. JSLS. 2009;13(2):129-34.
10. Mettler L, Ahmed-Ebbiary N, Schollmeyer T. Laparoscopic hysterectomy: challenges and limitations. Minimally Invasive Therap Allied Technol. 2005;14(3);145-59.
11. Brucker S, Rothmund R, Krämer B, et al. Cervical detachment using monopolar supra loop™ electrode versus monopolar needle in laparoscopic supracervical hysterectomy (LSH): an interventional, comparative cohort study. Geburtshilfe Frauenheilkd. 2013;73(11):1121-7.
12. Nesbitt-Hawes EM, Maley PE, Won HR, et al Laparoscopic subtotal hysterectomy: evidence and techniques. J Minim Invasive Gynecol. 2013;20(4):424-34.
13. Erian J, El-Shawarby SA, Hassan M, et al. Laparoscopic subtotal hysterectomy using the plasma kinetic and lap loop systems: an alternative approach in the surgical management of women with uterine fibroids. Eur J Obstet Gynecol Reprod Biol. 2008;137(1):84-7.
14. Grosse-Drieling D, Schlutius JC, Altgassen C, et al. Laparoscopic supracervical hysterectomy (LASH), a retrospective study of 1,584 cases regarding intra- and perioperative complications. Arch Gynecol Obstet. 2012;285(5):1391-6.
15. Harmanli OH, Tunitsky E, Esin S, et al. A comparison of short-term outcomes between laparoscopic supracervical and total hysterectomy. Am J Obstet Gynecol. 2009;201(5):536.e1-7.
16. Erian J, Hassan M, Pachydakis A, et al. Efficacy of laparoscopic subtotal hysterectomy in the management of menorrhagia: 400 consecutive cases. BJOG. 2008;115(6):742-8.
17. Alperin M, Kivnick S, Poon KY. Outpatient laparoscopic hysterectomy for large uteri. J Minim Invasive Gynecol. 2012;19(6):689-94.
18. Müller A, Thiel FC, Renner SP, et al .Hysterectomy—a comparison of approaches. Dtsch Arztebl Int. 2010;107(20):353-9.
19. Ghomi A, Cohen SL, Chavan N, et al. Laparoscopic-assisted vaginal hysterectomy vs laparoscopic supracervical hysterectomy for treatment of non-prolapsed uterus. Minim Invasive Gynecol. 2011; 18(2):205-10.
20. Schollmeyer T, Elessawy M, Chastamouratidhs B, et al. Hysterectomy trends over a 9-year period in an endoscopic teaching center. Int J Gynaecol Obstet. 2014;126(1):45-9.
21. Donnez O, Jadoul P, Squifflet J, et al. A series of 3190 laparoscopic hysterectomies for benign disease from 1990 to 2006: evaluation of complications compared with vaginal and abdominal procedures. BJOG. 2009;116(4):492-500.
22. Mousa A, Zarei A, Tulandi T. Changing practice from laparoscopic supracervical hysterectomy to total hysterectomy. Obstet Gynaecol Can. 2009;31(6):521-5.
23. McGurk L, Oliver R, Odejinmi F. Laparoscopic supracervical hysterectomy for the larger uterus (>500 g): a case series and literature review. Arch Gynecol Obstet. 2017;295(2):397-405.
24. Berner E, Qvigstad E, Langebrekke A, et al. Laparoscopic supracervical hysterectomy performed with and without excision of the endocervix: a randomized controlled trial. J Minim Invasive Gynecol. 2013;20(3):368-75.
25. Cipullo L, De Paoli S, Fasolino L, et al. Laparoscopic supracervical hysterectomy compared to total hysterectomy. JSLS. 2009;13(3):370-5.
26. Brucker SY, Taran FA, Bogdanyova S, et al. Patient-reported quality-of-life and sexual-function outcomes after laparoscopic supracervical hysterectomy (LSH) versus total laparoscopic hysterectomy (TLH): a prospective, questionnaire-based follow-up study in 915 patients. Arch Gynecol Obstet. 2014;290(6):1141-9.
27. Tchartchian G, Gardanis K, Bojahr B, et al. Postoperative patient satisfaction after laparoscopic supracervical hysterectomy. JSLS. 2013;17(1):107-10.
28. Schmidt T, Eren Y, Breidenbach M, et al. Modifications of laparoscopic supracervical hysterectomy technique significantly reduce postoperative spotting. J Minim Invasive Gynecol. 2011;18(1):81-4.
29. Mutlu L, Hufnagel D, Taylor HS. The endometrium as a source of mesenchymal stem cells for regenerative medicine. Biol Reprod. 2015;92(6):138.
30. Berner E, Qvigstad E, Myrvold AK, et al. Pelvic pain and patient satisfaction after laparoscopic supracervical hysterectomy: prospective trial. J Minim Invasive Gynecol. 2014;21(3):406-11.
31. Berner E, Qvigstad E, Myrvold AK, et al. Pain reduction after total laparoscopic hysterectomy and laparoscopic supracervical hysterectomy among women with dysmenorrhoea: a randomised controlled trial. BJOG. 2015;122(8):1102-11.
32. Yunker A, Curlin H, Banet N, et al. Does the uterine cervix become abnormally reinnervated after subtotal hysterectomy and what is the association with future trachelectomy? J Minim Invasive Gynecol. 2015;22(2):261-7.
33. Tsafrir Z, Aoun J, Papalekas E, et al. Risk factors for trachelectomy following supracervical hysterectomy. Acta Obstet Gynecol Scand. 2017;96(4):421-5.
34. Association of Population-Based Cancer Registries (GEKID) and the Robert Koch Institute (RKI). Cancer in Germany 2011/2012. http://www.krebsdaten.de.
35. Schneider V. Cervical cancer screening in Germany. Current status. Pathologe. 2012;33(4):286-92.
36. Hellström AC, Hellman K, Pettersson BF, et al. Carcinoma of the cervical stump: fifty years of experience. Oncol Rep. 2011;25(6):1651-4.
37. AAGL practice report: practice guidelines for laparoscopic subtotal/supracervical hysterectomy (LSH). J Minim Invasive Gynecol. 2014;21(1):9-16.
38. Barron KI, Richard T, Robinson PS, et al. Association of the U.S. food and drug administration morcellation

warning with rates of minimally invasive hysterectomy and myomectomy. Obstet Gynecol. 2015;126(6):1174-80.
39. Bojahr B, De Wilde RL, Tchartchian G. Malignancy rate of 10,731 uteri morcellated during laparoscopic supracervical hysterectomy (LASH). Arch Gynecol Obstet. 2015;292(3):665-72.
40. Kho KA, Lin K, Hechanova M, Richardson DL. Risk of occult uterine sarcoma in women undergoing hysterectomy for benign indications. Obstet Gynecol. 2016;127:468-73.
41. Pritts EA, Vanness DJ, Berek JS, et al. The prevalence of occult leiomyosarcoma at surgery for presumed uterine fibroids: a meta-analysis. Gynecol Surg. 2015;12(3):165-77.
42. Harris JA, Swenson CW, Uppal S, et al. Practice patterns and postoperative complications before and after US food and drug administration safety communication on power morcellation. Am J Obstet Gynecol. 2016;214(1):98.e91-98.e13.
43. Beckmann M, Juhasz-Böss I, Denschlag D, et al. Surgical methods for the treatment of uterine fibroids—risk of uterine sarcoma and problems of morcellation: position paper of the DGGG. Geburtshilfe Frauenheilkd. 2015;75(2):148-64.
44. Rutstein SE, Siedhoff MT, Geller EJ, et al. Cost-effectiveness of laparoscopic hysterectomy with morcellation compared with abdominal hysterectomy for presumed myomas. J Minim Invasive Gynecol. 2016;23(2):223-33.

KIEL SCHOOL

37 of Gynaecological Endoscopy

Transvaginal Natural Orifice Transluminal Endoscopic Surgery

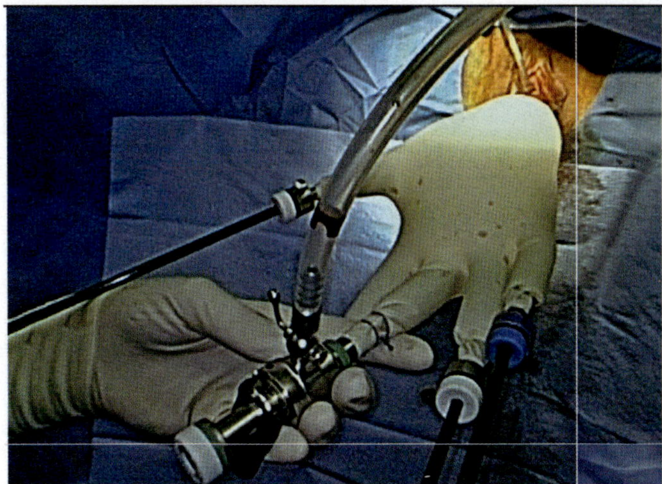

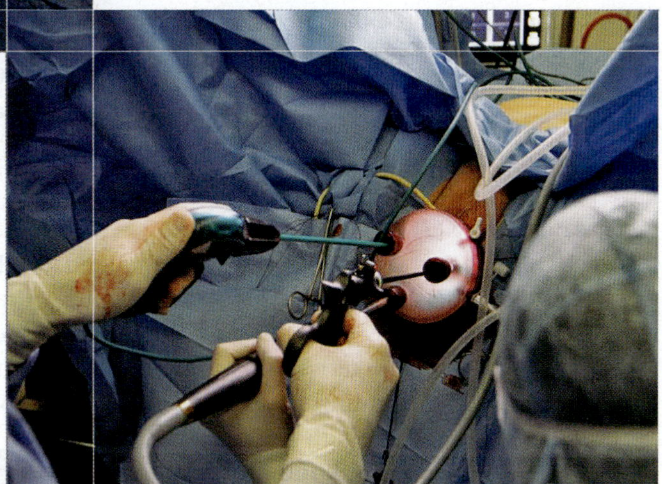

Chapter 37

Transvaginal Natural Orifice Transluminal Endoscopic Surgery

Jan F Baekelandt

INTRODUCTION

This chapter discusses techniques for gynecological surgery by pure transvaginal natural orifice transluminal endoscopic surgery (NOTES).

NOTES refers to endoscopic operations performed without leaving visible scars via a natural orifice. In pure NOTES no abdominal incisions are made, whereas in hybrid NOTES one or more abdominal incisions are made. Different natural orifices can be used for NOTES access; the most common are the vagina, anus, mouth and urethra. For gynecological surgery transvaginal access to the pouch of Douglas (POD) is most frequently used, but some procedures have been performed transgastrically.[1] This chapter focuses on pure vNOTES.

In vNOTES access to peritoneal cavity is obtained through the POD. Different trocars or ports can be used, but most commonly ports designed for single-incision laparoscopic surgery (SILS) are used off-label for vNOTES.[2] Depending on the procedure, the port can be placed in three different positions: in the POD for most procedures; in introitus of vagina for total vaginal NOTES hysterectomy (TVNH)[3]; around the cervix for vaginally assisted NOTES hysterectomy (VANH).[2]

In a first world setting commercially available ports such as Gelpoint (Applied Medical) are most commonly used. It is however possible to perform all vNOTES in a low-resource setting as well; the poor man's NOTES approach uses a self-constructed gloveport and only reusable endoscopic instruments. The gloveport is constructed by inserting reusable trocars into the fingers of a surgical glove and rolling the glove onto a wound protector[4,5] (Fig. 37.1).

PROCEDURES

Fertility Exploration

Introduction

D Von Ott is the forefather of vNOTES; he published the first "ventroskopie" in 1902 as a diagnostic procedure with access through the POD.[6] More recently, fertility surgeons were pioneers in introducing transvaginal laparoscopy in daily practice. S Gordts described the technique of transvaginal hydrolaparoscopy (THL) as a diagnostic procedure for fertility exploration.

Technique

THL can be performed under local or general anesthesia. With the patient is in lithotomy position, a speculum is placed and the cervix grasped with a tenaculum. Using a sprung needle system, a 3-mm trocar in inserted into the POD. A 30° 2.9 mm optic

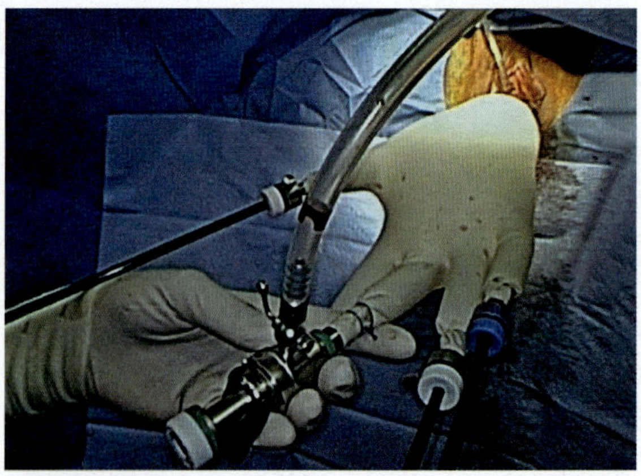

Fig. 37.1: Image of a self-constructed gloveport used for a poor man's NOTES approach.

scope is introduced through the trocar while saline solution is infused into the POD. The peritoneal cavity is visualized and the pelvic organs are inspected. Tubal patency is assessed by injecting methylene blue dye into the uterus through an additional catheter. Salpingoscopy can be performed by inserting the 2.9 mm optic scope into the lumen of Fallopian tubes. Through the same narrow trocar port peritoneal biopsies can be taken for endometriosis and ovarian drilling can be performed by laser or monopolar electrode. At the end of the procedure saline solution is drained and trocar is removed. The small perforation in the POD does not require suturing.

Evidence

THL is a viable alternative to a hysterosalpingography (HSG) for exploration of fertility. The combination of hysteroscopy, THL and chromoperturbation takes longer to perform than HSG, but can uncover more pelvic abnormalities and causes less post-procedure pain.[7] THL is as accurate as laparoscopy in discovering pelvic abnormalities such as endometriosis and adhesions.[8] For fertility exploration laparoscopy could be avoided in 93% of females by performing THL.[9] THL is effective enough to be used as a first-line study for fertility exploration; abdominal laparoscopy can be used as a supplement in patients for whom THL reveals abnormal findings.[10]

Conclusion

In many fertility centers THL has become the standard for fertility exploration. It is often combined with hysteroscopy, chromoperturbation and (micro-) salpingoscopy and then named fertiloscopy.[9] Due to transvaginal axis of the scope, it provides easy access for salpingoscopy. Adhesiolysis, ovarian drilling and ablation of endometriosis can be performed via THL. As no abdominal incisions are made, THL is more cosmetically appealing than laparoscopy. As we will see in the next chapter, THL can be used as a first step to make a diagnosis, before extending the opening in the POD from 4 mm to 2.5 cm to perform multi-instrument surgery via vNOTES.

Ectopic Pregnancy

Introduction

Transabdominal laparoscopy is still the gold standard for the diagnosis and treatment of ectopic pregnancy. In recent years, vNOTES has become a less invasive alternative to perform a salpingostomy or salpingectomy for ectopic pregnancy.[11-13] In cases of pregnancy of unknown location (PUL) the least invasive approach is to perform a THL through a 4 mm perforation in the POD and when an ectopic pregnancy is confirmed, extend the incision in the POD to 2.5 cm to treat the ectopic pregnancy by vNOTES[14] (Fig. 37.2).

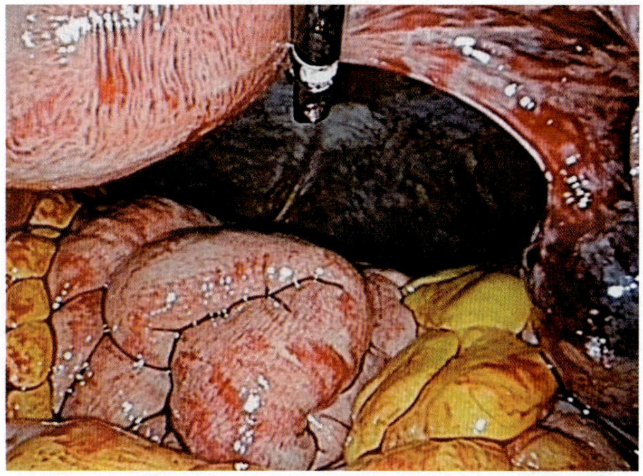

Fig. 37.2: The view through a vNOTES port is opposite to a standard laparoscopic view. This image shows the posterior aspect of the uterus and a left-sided ectopic pregnancy.

Technique

In case of a diagnosis of ectopic pregnancy on ultrasound, the patient is placed in lithotomy position under general anesthesia. The posterior lip of the cervix is grasped with a tenaculum and a 2.5 cm transverse incision is made in the posterior vaginal fornix. The POD is opened and a NOTES port (Gelpoint Mini or self-constructed gloveport for poor man's NOTES approach) is placed in the POD. The patient is placed in the Trendelenburg position, CO_2 is insufflated, and an endoscope is inserted. Hemoperitoneum is aspirated and rinsed. The tubal pregnancy is identified. The decision is made to perform salpingectomy or salpingostomy. In case of salpingectomy, the meso of the Fallopian tube is coagulated and transected from distally to proximally using a bipolar forceps and endoscopic scissors. The Fallopian tube is then transected at its origin and removed through the NOTES port. In case of a salpingostomy, an anti-mesenterial incision is made in the Fallopian tube and saline solution is used to dissect the ectopic pregnancy out of the Fallopian tube. At the end of the procedure the NOTES port is removed and the vaginal wall is closed using a resorbable suture.

Flowchart 37.1: The IMELDA approach to ectopic pregnancy.

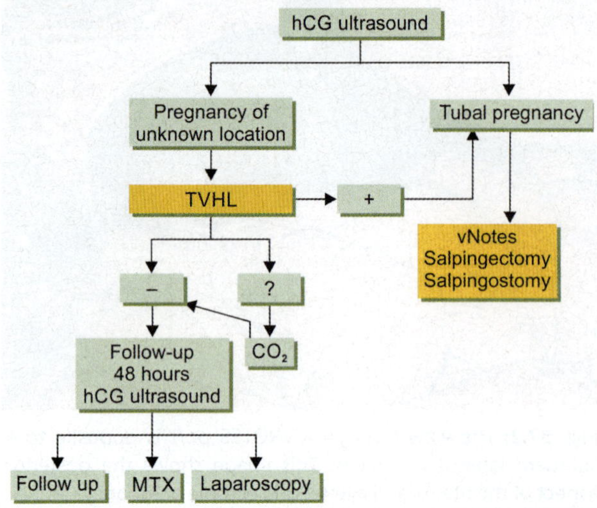

hCG, human chorionic gonadotropin; TVHL, transvaginal hydrolaparoscopy; MTX, methotrexate.

In case of a PUL on ultrasound, a THL as described in the section "Technique (of Fertility Exploration)" is used for investigation. If an ectopic pregnancy is confirmed, the THL port is removed and the incision in the POD is extended to 2.5 cm for a vNOTES approach as described above. If THL exploration is negative, the procedure is stopped and the patient is followed up further. If THL exploration is inconclusive, the saline solution is drained and CO_2 insufflated through the 4 mm THL port. Again, if the exploration is negative the procedure is stopped and the patient is followed up; if an ectopic pregnancy is diagnosed it is treated by vNOTES as described above (Flowchart 37.1).

Evidence

Four studies,[11-14] including 41 patients in total, have been published on the treatment of ectopic pregnancy via NOTES. One study was a prospective randomized study;[12] the others were case series. They demonstrate that vNOTES treatment for ectopic pregnancy is feasible and has the potential advantages of being less invasive than conventional laparoscopy, while offering a better cosmetic outcome.

Conclusion

These preliminary studies indicate that ectopic pregnancy can be treated by vNOTES but the evidence is limited to four small studies. The IMELDA transvaginal approach to ectopic pregnancy[14] enables surgeons to explore PUL and treat ectopic pregnancies without any abdominal incisions. It demonstrates that THL and vNOTES are complementary minimally invasive techniques: a negative THL investigation only leaves a 4-mm perforation in the POD that does not require suturing, and a vNOTES treatment for ectopic pregnancy only leaves a 2.5 cm incision in the POD.

Adnexal Surgery

Introduction

Transabdominal laparoscopy is the standard approach for benign adnexal surgery. vNOTES has become a potentially less invasive alternative for ovarian cystectomy and salpingo-oophorectomy (or adnexectomy) in recent years.

Technique

The patient is placed in lithotomy position under general anesthesia. The posterior lip of the cervix is grasped with a tenaculum and a 2.5 cm transverse incision is made in the posterior vaginal fornix. The POD is opened and a NOTES port (Gelpoint Mini or self-constructed gloveport for poor man's NOTES approach) is placed in the POD. The patient is placed in the Trendelenburg position, CO_2 is insufflated, and an endoscope and endoscopic instruments are inserted.

For ovarian cystectomy, the ovarian cortex is incised and the cyst is dissected using standard endoscopic instruments. Hemostasis of the ovary is achieved using a standard bipolar forceps.

For adnexectomy the ureter is first identified and when necessary dissected. Adnexectomy is performed by dissection of the infundibulopelvic and ovarian ligament, and the Fallopian tube using a standard bipolar forceps and cold scissors.

Small specimens can be retrieved in toto through the NOTES port, and larger specimens are placed in an endobag.

The colpotomy is closed using a resorbable suture.

Evidence

Six studies have been published on vNOTES for adnexal surgery: three case series on adnexectomy[5,15,16] including in total 30 patients; one case series including four ovarian cystectomy patients;[11] one case-matched study including 34 cystectomies.[17] One study focused on adnexectomy at the time of vaginal hysterectomy and includes six cadaver cases and two live cases.[18]

Conclusion

vNOTES for adnexal surgery is feasible and has the potential benefits of less postoperative pain, better cosmetic outcome and superior operative efficiency. The evidence however is limited. A prospective randomized controlled trial (NOTABLE trial, registered at National Institutes of Health at ClinicalTrials.gov NCT 02630329) comparing vNOTES adnexectomy with laparoscopic adnexectomy is currently underway.

Hysterectomy

Introduction

According to the Cochrane database, the first choice of hysterectomy is vaginal hysterectomy. When a vaginal hysterectomy is not possible, a laparoscopic hysterectomy has significant advantages over an abdominal hysterectomy (less pain, blood loss, febrile episodes and infections, improved quality of life, earlier discharge and quicker return to normal activities) but at a cost of more urinary tract injuries and longer operating time.[19]

New hysterectomy techniques via vNOTES make use of the advantages of endoscopic surgery to broaden the indications for vaginal hysterectomies.

In this chapter we will discuss four new hysterectomy techniques by pure vNOTES:

- *VANH:* vaginally assisted NOTES hysterectomy
- *TVNH:* total vaginal NOTES hysterectomy
- *RVANH:* robotic vaginal NOTES hysterectomy
- *RTVNH:* robotic total vaginal NOTES hysterectomy

VANH

Technique

A circular incision is made around the cervix using a cold knife. The POD and then the vesico-uterine peritoneum are opened using cold scissors. Both uterosacral ligaments are transected using cold scissors and tied off using a Vicryl-1 suture. A NOTES port is inserted into the peritoneal cavity, and CO_2 used to inflate it (Fig. 37.3). An optic is inserted and the peritoneal cavity is inspected. The patient is now placed in the Trendelenburg position and the small intestine lifted out of pelvis.

Ureter is identified, but not routinely dissected. The uterine artery is coagulated using a bipolar grasper and is transected. The ovarian artery and the meso of the Fallopian tube are coagulated using a bipolar grasper and transected. In patients requiring an adnexectomy, the infundibulopelvic ligament is coagulated using a bipolar grasper and is transected. Hemostasis is checked and the peritoneal cavity is rinsed. The NOTES port and the uterus are removed transvaginally and pneumoperitoneum is deflated.

Colpotomy is closed using a resorbable suture.

Evidence

Seven studies on VANH have been published, including a total of 731 patients.[20] In these studies different names are used to describe similar procedures. There are no randomized controlled trials. There is one preclinical study describing the technical feasibility of transvaginal NOTES hysterectomy on a female cadaver.[21] There is one prospective cohort study[22] and two studies retrospective comparative studies.[23,24] Three studies are case series.[25-27]

These studies confirm the feasibility of hysterectomy for benign diseases by vNOTES, but conclude that there is a need for further prospective studies.

Conclusion

These studies demonstrate the feasibility of a VANH. There is a lack of prospective randomized studies to recommend this technique as an alternative for a total laparoscopic hysterectomy, even though the preliminary studies seem to indicate that this may become so in the future.

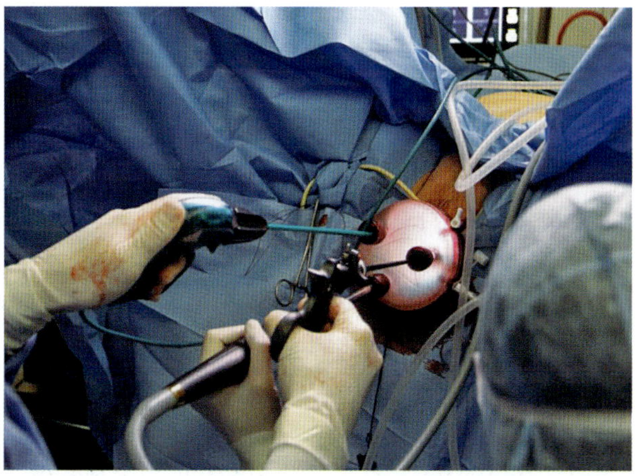

Fig. 37.3: Gelpoint (Applied Medical) is a suitable port for VANH.

TVNH

Technique

A vNOTES port is inserted into the vagina, and CO_2 is insufflated to create pneumovagina. An optic is inserted into pneumovagina. A circular incision is made around the cervix using a monopolar laparoscopic hook, and the POD is opened using laparoscopic scissors. Vesicouterine peritoneum is opened using laparoscopic scissors. Both uterosacral ligaments are coagulated using a laparoscopic bipolar grasper and transected. The patient is now placed in the Trendelenburg position and small intestine is lifted out of pelvis.

Ureter is identified, but not routinely dissected. It is only dissected if it cannot be identified transperitoneally. Uterine artery and ovarian artery are coagulated using a bipolar grasper and transected. The meso of the Fallopian tube is coagulated using a bipolar grasper and is transected. In patients requiring an adnexectomy, the infundibulopelvic ligament is coagulated using a bipolar grasper and is transected. Hemostasis is checked and peritoneal cavity is rinsed. The NOTES port and the uterus are removed transvaginally and the pneumoperitoneum is deflated.

Colpotomy is closed using a resorbable suture.

The major difference between TVNH and a VANH lies in the opening of the anterior and posterior peritoneum and the transection of the uterosacral ligaments. This is performed entirely endoscopically in the TVNH, whereas it is performed by classical vaginal surgery in a VANH. The TVNH technique can therefore also be used in nulliparous patients, patients without uterine prolapse and patients with a narrow vagina where classical vaginal surgery can be more challenging.[22,28]

Evidence

One case series, including 10 patients, demonstrated the feasibility of TVNH both in parous a nulliparous women. A self-constructed NOTES port and conventional reusable laparoscopic instruments were used. There were no conversions to transabdominal laparoscopy or laparotomy; no major complications and the operation times were reasonable.

Conclusion

The current evidence only indicates the feasibility of a TVNH. There is need for further prospective randomized studies before it can be considered as a standard alternative for total laparoscopic hysterectomy. This technique seems promising for nulliparous patients with a narrow vaginal access and without descensus, in whom a conventional vaginal hysterectomy and a VANH can be very challenging.

RVANH

Jan Baekelandt presented the first case report on transvaginal robotic surgery at the 7th Annual SERGS Meeting on Robotic Gynaecological Surgery in June 2015.[29] RVANH is similar to the VANH technique, but the endoscopic part is performed robotically instead of by conventional laparoscopic instruments.

Technique

The patient is placed in the lithotomy position as for a classical vaginal hysterectomy. The circumcision of the cervix, the opening of anterior and posterior peritoneum, and transection of both sacrouterine ligaments is performed by classical vaginal surgery. A NOTES port is constructed by assembling a surgical glove, a wound protector, four Da Vinci 8-mm trocars and one reusable 5 mm trocar. The ring of the wound protector is inserted transvaginally into peritoneal cavity to create pneumoperitoneum. A Da Vinci Xi surgical robot is side-docked between the legs of the patient and three arms are connected to the trocars in the NOTES port (Fig. 37.4). The fourth arm is not used. Using a 30° optic, a fenestrated bipolar grasper and a vessel sealer, hysterectomy is performed via transvaginal NOTES using the

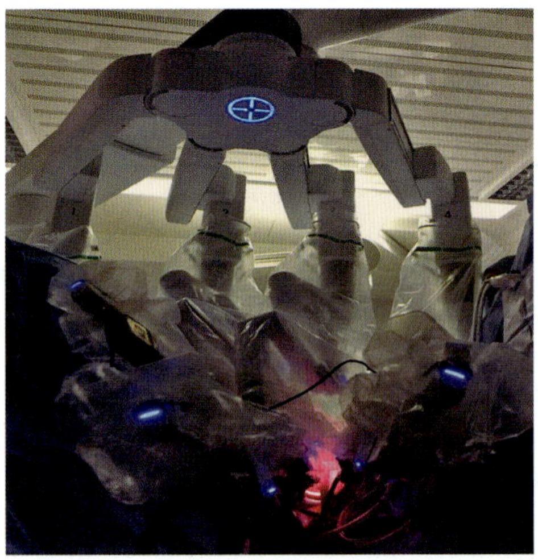

Fig. 37.4: A Da Vinci Xi surgical robot is side-docked between the legs of the patient to perform a RVANH.

surgical robot. Subsequently bilateral adnexectomy is performed using the same method. Once hysterectomy and bilateral adnexectomy are completed, the robot and gloveport are removed. When uterus is too large to extract in toto, it is manually morcellated so that it can be removed vaginally. Colpotomy is closed as in classical vaginal surgery. No abdominal incisions are made.

Evidence

One case series, including five patients, demonstrated that transvaginal robotic surgery is feasible and that hysterectomy can be performed using this technique.[30]

Conclusion

The current evidence only indicates the feasibility of RVANH.[30] Further prospective randomized studies are needed to validate the technique before it can be considered as a standard alternative for a laparoscopic or transabdominal robotic hysterectomy. The potential advantages of better camera control, improved ergonomics and articulated wrist motion will need to be weighed against the higher cost and longer setup time when compared to a VANH. The current problem of robotic arm collision will need to be overcome by further developments in robotic technology.

RTVNH

The technique of robotic TVNH was developed and first performed by Jan Baekelandt in 2015.

Technique

A NOTES port is constructed by assembling a surgical glove, a wound protector, three Da Vinci 8-mm trocars and one reusable 5-mm trocar. The ring of wound protector is inserted into the vagina to create pneumovagina. A Da Vinci Xi surgical robot is side docked between the legs of the patient and three arms are connected to trocars in the gloveport. The fourth arm is not used. Using a 30° optic, a fenestrated bipolar grasper and monopolar scissors, hysterectomy is performed via transvaginal NOTES using the surgical robot. Fallopian tubes are removed with uterus. When indicated, the ovaries are removed as well. Once the hysterectomy is completed, robot and gloveport are removed. When uterus is too large to extract in toto, it is manually morcellated so that it can be removed vaginally. Colpotomy is closed as in classical vaginal surgery. No abdominal incisions are made.

Evidence

Only one case series has been published, comparing eight RTVNH with eight RVANH.[31]

Conclusion

The current evidence only indicates the feasibility of a RTVNH.[31] Further prospective randomized studies are needed to validate the technique before it can be considered as a standard alternative for laparoscopic or transabdominal robotic hysterectomy. The potential advantages of improved ergonomics, better camera control and wristed instruments will need to be weighed against the higher cost and longer setup time when compared to a TVNH. This technique seems promising for nulliparous patients with a narrow vaginal access and without descensus, in whom conventional vaginal hysterectomy and a (R)VANH can be very challenging.

Discussion of vNOTES Hysterectomy

When planning hysterectomy, we have a choice of different techniques. Cochrane database tells us to choose conventional vaginal hysterectomy when possible. In cases where vaginal hysterectomy is not an option, laparoscopic approach can help avoid performing an abdominal hysterectomy.[19] It has been demonstrated that even large uteri can be removed by vaginal hysterectomy[32] and that vaginal hysterectomy can be safely performed in nulliparous women.[28] In recent years however, there has been a decrease in the incidence of vaginal and abdominal hysterectomy, while the incidence of laparoscopic and robotic hysterectomy has increased.[33] The choice of hysterectomy approach is patient and surgeon dependent: when choosing the route of hysterectomy, important determining factors are the surgeon's experience, the accessibility of vaginal passage and the disease of the uterus.[34] The proportion of hysterectomies performed by different techniques varies markedly across countries, within countries and between surgeons, depending largely on surgeons' training and patient expectations. The introduction of vNOTES hysterectomy adds other (four) options when deciding which technique would suit a specific patient best (Table 37.1). It shares the advantage

Table 37.1: Types of hysterectomy.

Abbreviation	*Name*	*Description*
TAH	Total abdominal hysterectomy	Total hysterectomy performed through a laparotomy under direct vision using conventional surgical instruments.
H	Vaginal hysterectomy	Total hysterectomy performed entirely through vaginal access under direct vision using conventional surgical instruments.
LASH	Laparoscopic supracervical hysterectomy	Subtotal hysterectomy performed by transabdominal laparoscopy.
LAVH	Laparoscopic-assisted vaginal hysterectomy	Total hysterectomy where first the cranial part of the uterus is dissected via transabdominal laparoscopy and afterwards the caudal part of the uterus (including ligating the uterine vessels) is dissected under direct vision using conventional instruments.
LH	Laparoscopic hysterectomy	Total hysterectomy where first the cranial part of the uterus is dissected via transabdominal laparoscopy (including ligating the uterine vessels) and afterwards part of the operation is performed vaginally under direct vision using conventional instruments.
TLH	Total laparoscopic hysterectomy	Total hysterectomy where the entire uterus is dissected via transabdominal laparoscopy.
RH	Robotic hysterectomy	Total hysterectomy where the entire uterus is dissected transabdominally using a surgical robot.
VANH	Vaginally assisted NOTES hysterectomy	Total hysterectomy where first the caudal part of the uterus is dissected vaginally under direct vision and afterwards the rest of the hysterectomy is performed via transvaginal NOTES using an endoscopic camera and endoscopic instruments.
RVANH	Robotic vaginally assisted NOTES hysterectomy	Total hysterectomy where first the caudal part of the uterus is dissected vaginally under direct vision and afterwards the rest of the hysterectomy is performed via transvaginal NOTES using a surgical robot.
TVNH	Total vaginal NOTES hysterectomy	Total hysterectomy where the entire uterus is dissected via transvaginal NOTES using an endoscopic camera and endoscopic instruments.
RTVNH	Robotic total vaginal NOTES hysterectomy	Total hysterectomy where the entire uterus is dissected via transvaginal NOTES using a surgical robot.

of no visible scarring with conventional vaginal hysterectomy.

In nulliparous women the risk of complications from vaginal hysterectomy is higher.[28] Vaginal hysterectomy becomes more challenging in women with a narrow vaginal access.[33,34] TVNH and RTVNH may help overcome the challenges of a narrow vagina due to the pneumovagina and therefore broaden the indications for transvaginal surgery. The improved visualization and CO_2 pressure help identify and dissect the surgical planes and facilitate the anterior and posterior colpotomy in nulliparous patients and after cesarean section.

In VANH the uterine vessels are ligated before dissecting the rest of the uterus. Removing very large uteri via VANH leads to less blood loss than a transabdominal laparoscopic approach where the occlusion of the feeding vessels is only achieved after more manipulation.[22,27] When compared to a laparoscopic approach, VANH also avoids the need for adhesiolysis to access the pelvis in patients with previous abdominal surgery.

Without making incisions to the abdominal wall and thus increasing the invasiveness of surgery, vNOTES provides the surgeon the comfort of operating under good endoscopic vision. The endoscopic vision of vNOTES hysterectomy also facilitates the removal of Fallopian tubes (and ovaries when indicated), which can be challenging in a conventional vaginal hysterectomy.

A potential risk of vNOTES hysterectomy could be infection due to insufflation of CO_2 through the vagina. Studies have demonstrated however that when prophylactic antibiotics are used, the risk of post-operative pelvic infection is unlikely.[22,35] The risk of dyspareunia after vNOTES hysterectomy is not expected to differ from a vaginal hysterectomy, as the vault is closed in the same way.

vNOTES broadens the indications of vaginal hysterectomy by using the advantages of endoscopic surgery. Further potential advantages are quicker recovery and less postoperative pain. Current studies prove the feasibility of these four vNOTES hysterectomy techniques but further studies are needed to validate them. The first prospective randomized controlled trial (HALON trial, registered at National Institutes of Health at ClinicalTrials.gov NCT02631837) comparing vNOTES hysterectomy with total laparoscopic hysterectomy is currently underway and the results are expected to be presented by the end of 2017.[36]

CONCLUSION

Gynecological surgery has traditionally been performed by laparotomy or in the case of hysterectomy, also by conventional vaginal surgery. At the end of the 1980s and during the 1990s the first major paradigm shift occurred with the introduction of laparoscopic surgery. The use of a camera allowed better visualization and, in combination with endoscopic instruments, enabled us to perform gynecological procedures through several small incisions instead of through one large one. This approach proved to be less invasive and allowed for a quicker recovery and more appealing cosmetic result. It has now, after an initial period of skepticism, become commonplace in most first world gynecology departments.

Pioneers and early adopters of transvaginal laparoscopy now see vNOTES as the next paradigm shift. In the last five years a lot of small IDEAL (Idea, Development, Exploration, Assessment, Long-term study) stage 1 and 2a studies have been published.[37] Since the end of 2015 prospective randomized controlled trials (such as the HALON and NOTABLE trial) have moved the research on vNOTES into IDEAL stage 2b. The number of vNOTES surgeons is increasing and important data are being collected in the prospective complication database of the International NOTES Society: vNOTES surgeons can register all their different vNOTES procedures prospectively and take part in validating this new technique according to the principles of the IDEAL collaboration. By following these IDEAL principles for the introduction of new surgical techniques correctly, vNOTES is gradually becoming a realistic alternative for abdominal and laparoscopic gynecological surgery.

In a low-resource setting vNOTES techniques such as poor man's NOTES[4,5] and iHysterectomy[38] may offer significant reduction of the invasiveness of surgery by making transvaginal endoscopic surgery accessible as an alternative for a laparotomy in areas where the necessary investment in conventional laparoscopic equipment is not available.

vNOTES offers obvious aesthetic advantages by leaving no visible scars. Simultaneously it maintains the superior endoscopic visualization and has many other potential advantages: less postoperative pain, fewer trocar related complications, no abdominal wall hernias, easier access in patients with previous abdominal surgery, less wound infections, shorter operating times, quicker recovery and shorter hospitalization.

Even though the early studies look very promising, the results of prospective randomized controlled trials need to be awaited to validate the value of vNOTES compared to laparoscopy.

Current evidence indicates that vNOTES procedures are safe in the hands of the few experts that perform these procedures. Gynecologists intending performing vNOTES should be skilled both in laparoscopic and in conventional vaginal surgery. Previous experience with single incision laparoscopic surgery (SILS) will help shorten the learning curve. The importance of training with an experienced vNOTES surgeon before performing your first vNOTES cases cannot be stressed enough.

REFERENCES

1. Hornemann A, Suetterlin M, Trunk MJ, et al. Pure natural orifice transluminal endoscopic surgery (NOTES) involving peroral endoscopic salpingo-oophorectomy (POESY). Int J Gynecol Obstet. 2014;125(1):86-88.
2. Baekelandt J, Cavens D. GelPOINT (Applied Medical) is a suitable port for transvaginal NOTES procedures. J Gynecol Surg. 2016;32(5):257-62.
3. Baekelandt J. Total vaginal NOTES hysterectomy: a new approach to hysterectomy. J Minim Invasive Gynecol. 2015;22(6):1088-94.
4. Baekelandt J. Poor man's NOTES: can it be a good approach for adhesiolysis? A first case report with video demonstration. J Minim Invasive Gynecol. 2015;22(3):319.

5. Reynders A, Baekelandt J. Adnexectomy by poor man's transvaginal NOTES. Gynecol Surg. 2015;12(3):900.
6. Von Ott D. Die Beleuchtung der Bauchhohle (Ventroskopie) als Methode bei Vaginaler Coeliotomie. Abl Gynakol. 1902;231:817-23.
7. Cicinelli E, Matteo M, Causio F, et al. Tolerability of the mini-pan-endoscopic approach (transvaginal hydrolaparoscopy and minihysteroscopy) versus hysterosalpingography in an outpatient infertility investigation. Fertility Steril. 2001;76:1048-51.
8. Campo R, Gordts S, Rombauts L, et al. Diagnostic accuracy of transvaginal hydrolaparoscopy in infertility. Fertil Steril. 1999;71(6):1157-60.
9. Watrelot A, Nisolle M, Chelli H, et al. Is laparoscopy still the gold standard in infertility assessment? A comparison of fertiloscopy versus laparoscopy in infertility: Results of an international multicentre prospective trial: The "FLY" (Fertiloscopy-Laparoscopy) study. Hum Reprod. 2003;18(4):834-9.
10. Hu X, Xu H, Wang D, et al. [Application of fertiloscopy in infertile women]. Zhonghua Fu Chan Ke Za Zhi. 2005;40(12):840-3.
11. Lee CL, Wu KY, Su H, et al. Transvaginal natural-orifice transluminal endoscopic surgery (NOTES) in adnexal procedures. J Minim Invasive Gynecol. 2012;19(4):509-13.
12. Xu B, Liu Y, Ying X, et al. Transvaginal endoscopic surgery for tubal ectopic pregnancy. J Soc Laparoendosc Surg. 2014;18(1):76-82.
13. Van Peer S, Baekelandt J. Natural orifice transluminal endoscopic surgery (NOTES) salpingectomy for ectopic pregnancy: a first series demonstrating how a new surgical technique can be applied in a low-resource setting. Gynecol Surg. 2015;12(4):299-302.
14. Baekelandt J, Vercammen J. IMELDA transvaginal approach to ectopic pregnancy: Diagnosis by transvaginal hydrolaparoscopy and treatment by transvaginal natural orifice transluminal endoscopic surgery. Fertil Steril. 2017;107(1):e1-2.
15. Yang YS, Hur MH, Oh KY, et al. Transvaginal natural orifice transluminal endoscopic surgery for adnexal masses. J Obstet Gynaecol Res. 2013;39(12):1-6.
16. Ahn KH, Song JY, Kim SH, et al. Transvaginal single-port natural orifice transluminal endoscopic surgery for benign uterine adnexal pathologies. J Minim Invasive Gynecol. 2012;19(5):631-5.
17. Wang CJ, Wu PY, Kuo HH, et al. Natural orifice transluminal endoscopic surgery-assisted versus laparoscopic ovarian cystectomy (NAOC vs. LOC): a case-matched study. Surg Endosc Other Interv Tech. 2016;30(3):1227-34.
18. Jallad K, Siff L, Thomas T, et al. Salpingo-oophorectomy by transvaginal natural orifice transluminal endoscopic surgery. Obstet Gynecol. 2016;128(2):293-6.
19. Aarts JWM, Nieboer TE, Johnson N, et al. Surgical approach to hysterectomy for benign gynaecological disease. Cochrane database Syst Rev. 2015; 8:CD003677.
20. Baekelandt J, De Mulder PA, Le Roy I, et al. Postoperative outcomes and quality of life following hysterectomy by natural orifice transluminal endoscopic surgery (NOTES) compared to laparoscopy in women with a non-prolapsed uterus and benign gynaecological disease: a systematic review and meta-analysis. Eur J Obstet Gynecol Reprod Biol. 2017;208:6-15.
21. Atallah S, Martin-Perez B, Albert M, et al. Vaginal access minimally invasive surgery (VAMIS): a new approach to hysterectomy. Surg Innov. 2015;22(4):344-7.
22. Lee CL, Wu KY, Su H, et al. Hysterectomy by transvaginal natural orifice transluminal endoscopic surgery (NOTES): a series of 137 patients. J Minim Invasive Gynecol. 2014;21(5):818-24.
23. Wang CJ, Huang HY, Huang CY, et al. Hysterectomy via transvaginal natural orifice transluminal endoscopic surgery for nonprolapsed uteri. Surg Endosc Other Interv Tech. 2014;29(1):100-7.
24. Yang YS, Kim SY, Hur MH, et al. Natural orifice transluminal endoscopic surgery-assisted versus Single-port laparoscopic-assisted vaginal hysterectomy: a case-matched Study. J Minim Invasive Gynecol. 2014;21(4):624-31.
25. Chen Y, Yen M, Tsai H, et al. Transvaginal natural orifice transluminal endoscopic surgery (NOTES) hysterectomy and bilateral salpingoovariectomy for female-to-male transsexuals. J Minim Invasive Gynecol. 2012;19:S123-50.
26. Lee C-L, Wu K-Y, Su H, et al. Natural orifice transluminal endoscopic surgery in gynecology. Gynecol Minim Invasive Ther. 2012;1(1):23-6.
27. Su H, Yen CF, Wu KY, et al. Hysterectomy via transvaginal natural orifice transluminal endoscopic surgery (NOTES): feasibility of an innovative approach. Taiwan J Obstet Gynecol. 2012;51(2):217-21.
28. Agostini A, Bretelle F, Cravello L, et al. Vaginal hysterectomy in nulliparous women without prolapse: a prospective comparative study. BJOG An Int J Obstet Gynaecol. 2003;110(5):515-8.
29. Baekelandt J. Transvaginal robotic surgery: the first case reports of robotic NOTES hysterectomy. SERGS. Conference: 7th Annual SERGS Meeting on Robotic Gynaecological Surgery, At Istanbul, Turkey, 2015.
30. Baekelandt J. Robotic vaginally assisted NOTES hysterectomy: the first case series demonstrating a new surgical technique. Gynecol Surg. 2016;13(1): 57-62.
31. Baekelandt J. Robotic vaginal NOTES hysterectomy: two new surgical techniques. J Gynecol Surg. 2016;32(5):270-7.

32. Hwang J-L, Seow K-M, Tsai Y-L, et al. Comparative study of vaginal, laparoscopically assisted vaginal and abdominal hysterectomies for uterine myoma larger than 6 cm in diameter or uterus weighing at least 450 g: a prospective randomized study. Acta Obstet Gynecol Scand. 2002;81(12):1132-8.
33. Wasson MN, Hoffman MK. Impact of a robotic surgical system on hysterectomy trends. Del Med J. 2015;87(2):45-50.
34. Chakraborty S, Goswami S, Mukherjee P, et al. Hysterectomy...which route? J Obstet Gynecol India. 2011;61(5):554-7.
35. Zornig C, Mofid H, Siemssen L, et al. Transvaginal NOTES hybrid cholecystectomy: feasibility results in 68 cases with mid-term follow-up. Endoscopy. 2009;41(5):391-4.
36. Baekelandt J, De Mulder PA, Le Roy I, et al. HALON—hysterectomy by transabdominal laparoscopy or natural orifice transluminal endoscopic surgery: a randomised controlled trial (study protocol). BMJ Open. 2016;6(8):e011546.
37. McCulloch P, Altman DG, Campbell WB, et al. No surgical innovation without evaluation: the IDEAL recommendations. Lancet. 2009;374(9695): 1105-12.
38. Baekelandt J, Bosteels J. Hysterectomy through the looking glass: iHysterectomy frugal by iPhone. BMJ Innov. Online. February 14, 2017.

Overview of Endoscopic Pelvic Floor Defect Corrections

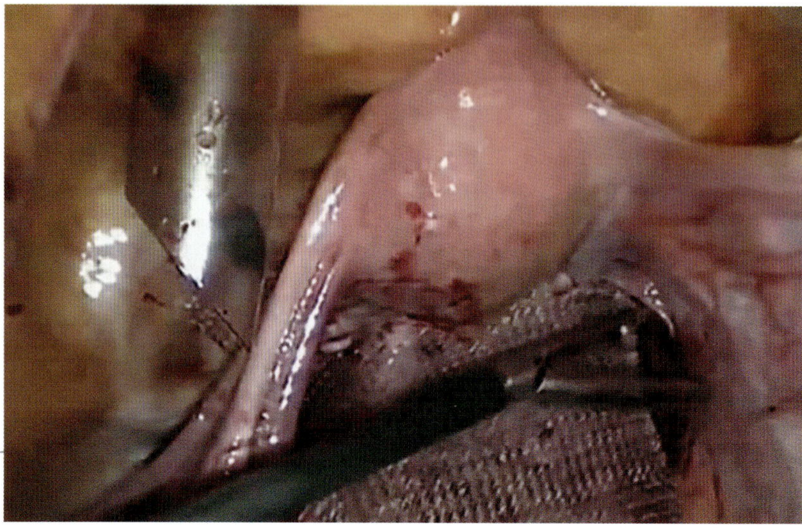

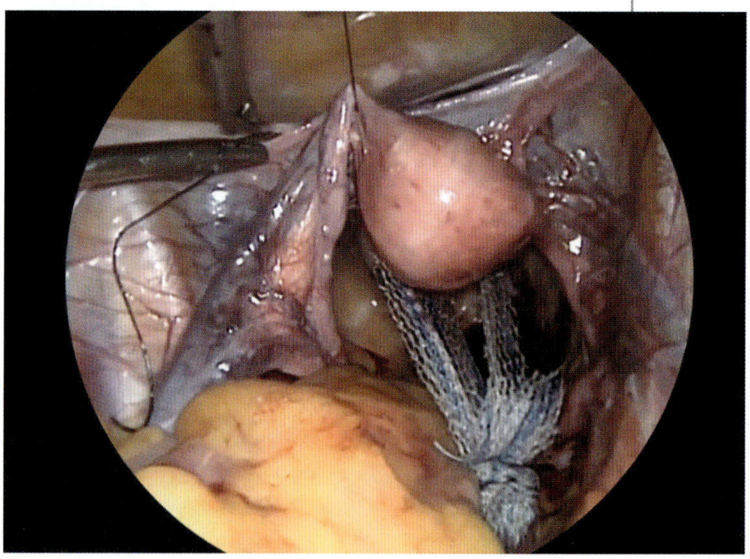

Chapter 38

Overview of Endoscopic Pelvic Floor Defect Corrections

Guenter K Noé

INTRODUCTION

As the traditional repair techniques like Manchester-Fothegill, sacrospinous fixation, vaginal native tissue repair and others show a poor long-term outcome an industry-driven mesh technique began to find wide application in the beginning of the third millennium. Most of the published new approaches referred to the integral theory of Petros and Ulmsten.

The problem was that Petros and Ulmsten tried to describe the load vectors in the pelvic floor that have influence on the function of pelvic organs but the theory tells nothing about the vectoring in the pelvic fascia itself. Replacing the fascia by polypropylene mesh can work from the anatomical point of view but cannot replace the dynamic function of the native tissue. The meshes have been placed in multiple techniques without long-term data and clearly worked out risk profiles. At the end this led to huge complication rate and caused the Food and Drug Administration (FDA) warning for mesh implantation.

The discussion around mesh application is still going on. As the discussion and legal issues are increasing the interest in laparoscopic approaches is growing rapidly.

Laparoscopic repairs are based on the traditional sacral fixation, which is referred to be the "gold standard" as you can find a high number of monocentric studies for decades. On the other hand, there is no standardization and a high variation in the approach.

As in the field of laparoscopic approaches we again find an extended number of techniques based on the experience of single centers without randomized trials. I want to give an overview of the different techniques available. As the number is permanently increasing I do not claim completeness of data or approaches.

SACRAL FIXATION

One of the first to describe the laparoscopic sacral vault fixation were Nezaht and Dorsey.[1] They adapted the traditional open approach technique and defined the cranial fixation point to be at the sacral vertebra 1–2. The sacral vertebra 1–2 lies in the direction of the vaginal axis. This approach avoids a deviation of vaginal axis.

Additionally in this area the surgeon has to deal with crossing vessels, which can lead to serious bleedings. Therefore, most surgeons use the promontory as fixation area today. To complete the procedure faster many of them use tackers for cranial fixation.

In the last years bilateral techniques were introduced. Some of them are using tunneling techniques, some use standard instruments and some have developed tunneling devices.

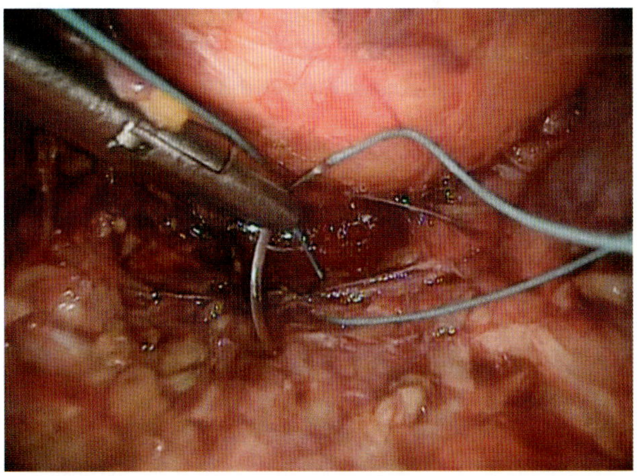

Fig. 38.1: Suture on the level of sacral vertebra one. Tackers are difficult to place as the longitudinal ligament is thin and the angle instrument to sacrum is inconvenient.[2]

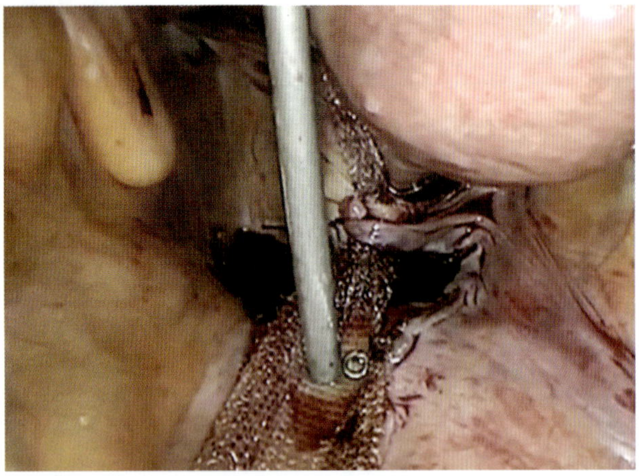

Fig. 38.2: Fixation to the promontory by tacker.

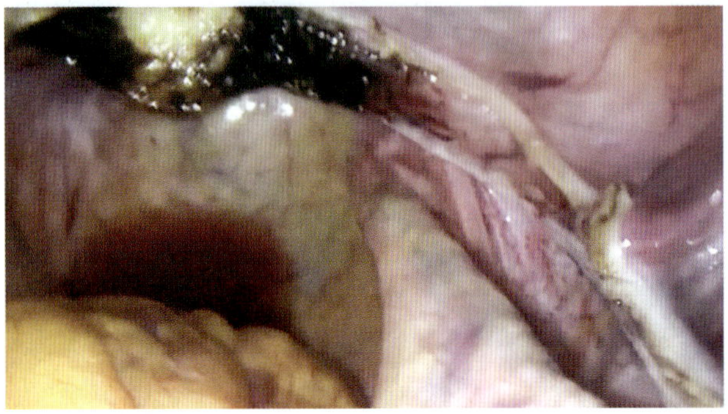

Fig. 38.3: Retroperitoneal tunneling by a grasper.

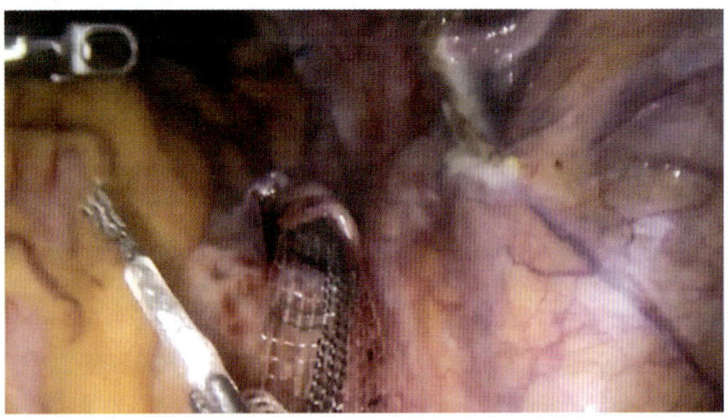

Fig. 38.4: Mesh arm is pulled through the tunnel

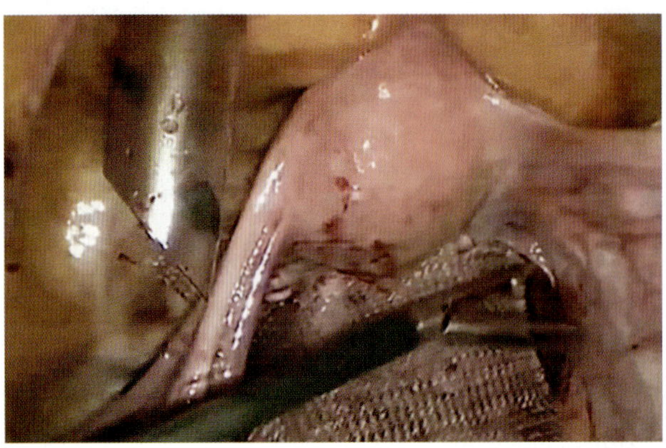

Fig. 38.5: The mesh arms are pulled through the peritoneum bilateral.

This approach reduces suturing after mesh placement but until today there are no reliable data about embarrassment of the ureter or the hypogastric nerve. A bilateral technique also bares the risk that the arms close the space for the rectum when they are under traction like a closing glottis.

You often find the sacral fixation performed as a hysteropexy. The variation rate is also high. Many surgeons perform the fixation of the uterus by

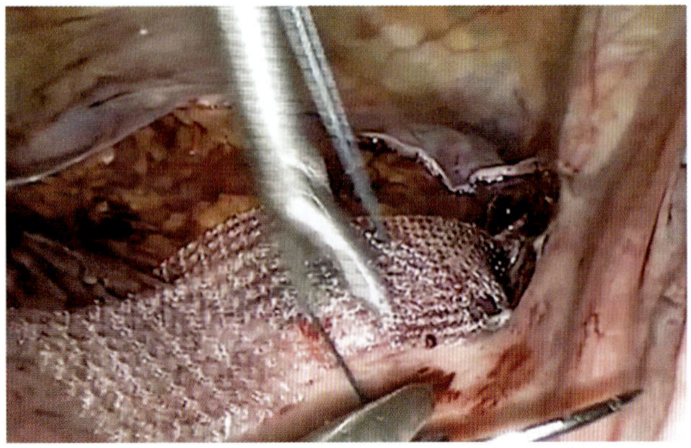

Fig. 38.6: The arms are fixed anteriorly by overlapping above the cervix.

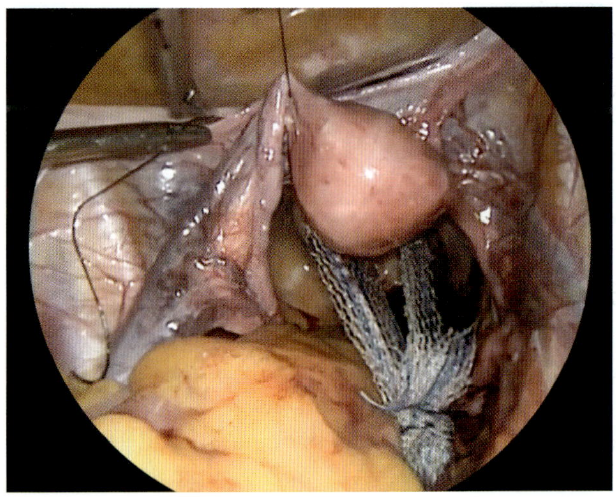

Fig. 38.7: Combination of rectopexy and hysteropexy.

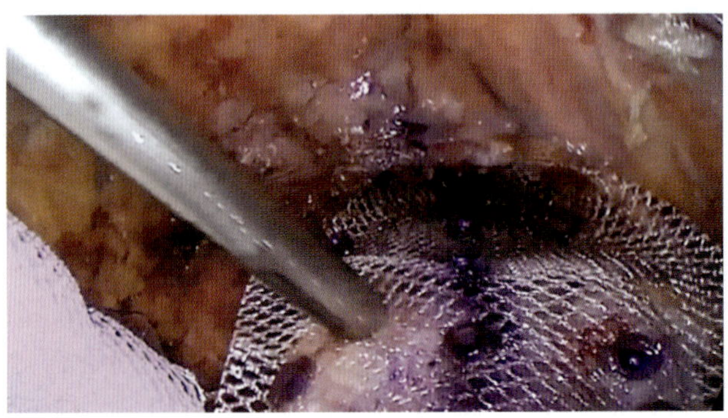

Fig. 38.8: Attachment of the mesh to the anterior tunneling.

putting a mesh like a necklace around the cervix. Others attach a mesh posteriorly to the uterosacral ligaments ore directly to the cervix itself.

Another strategy is to combine hysteropexy with a rectopexy. This extensive use of mesh material can cause concomitant risks. These techniques are performed on congresses and published but yet without dependable data.

BILATERAL SUSPENSION

In the past years many techniques have been introduced that use a bilateral approach without the sacrum. One group fixes a mesh to the apical structures and pulls two arms bilaterally extra peritoneal to the abdominal wall. This approach is a variation of the technique published by Williams and Richardson in the 1950s.[3]

Dubuisson published this technique in 2008[4] using a mesh to cover the whole vagina anteriorly and posteriorly. Others have meanwhile adapted this approach with different meshes and materials. No reliable data are available today.

The technique appears to be performable very easily. Long-term data are not available and the direction of the arms seems to be quite high that a vaginal lifting is to be estimated comparable to the result of the technique by Williams and Richardson.

The use of the pectineal ligament was reported by Joshi in 1993 as an open procedure for hysteropexy. Meanwhile long-term data have been reported. Unfortunately, the data do not have details about concomitant defects and additional treatment. Some surgeons have adapted his technique for laparoscopy.

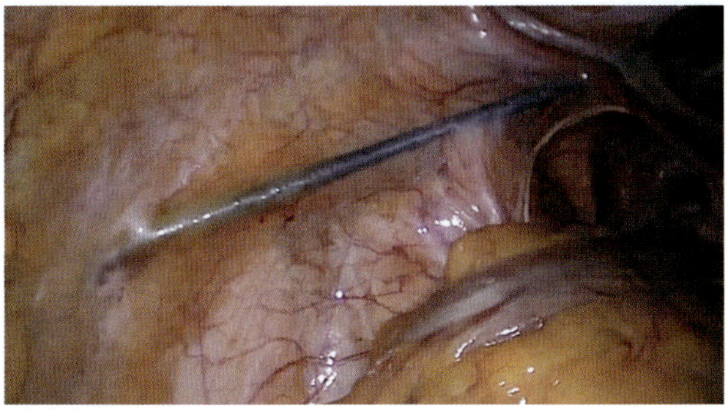

Fig. 38.9: Retroperitoneal grasper for wall of the vagina.

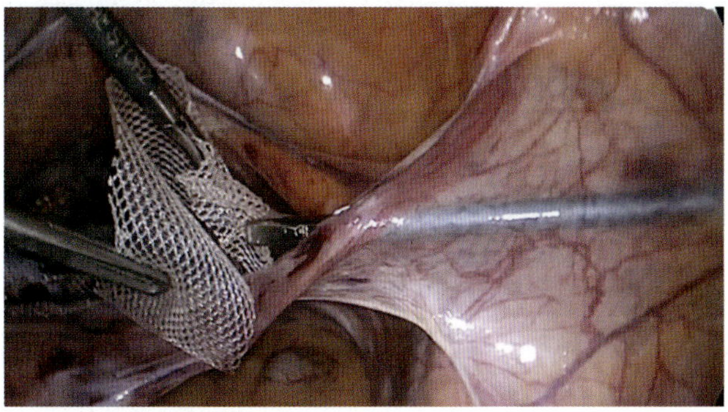

Fig. 38.10: Placement of the mesh arm.

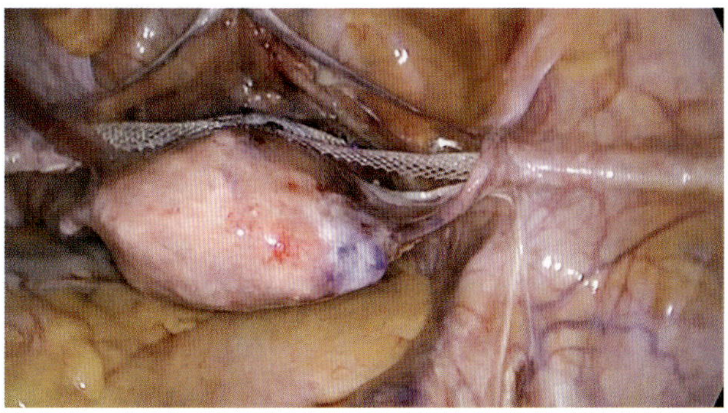

Fig. 38.11: Final position.

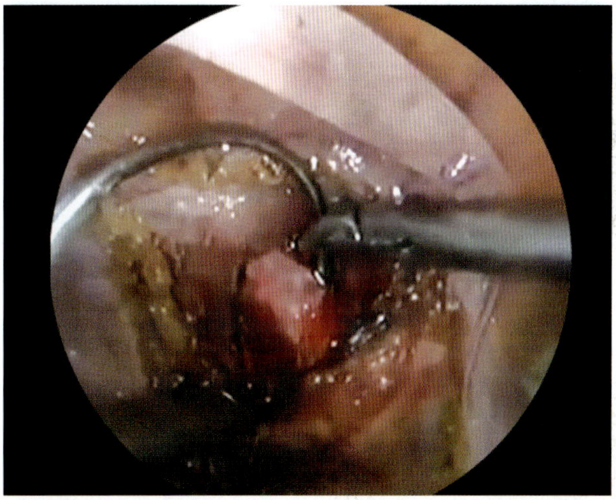

Fig. 38.12: Attachment to the right pectineal ligament.

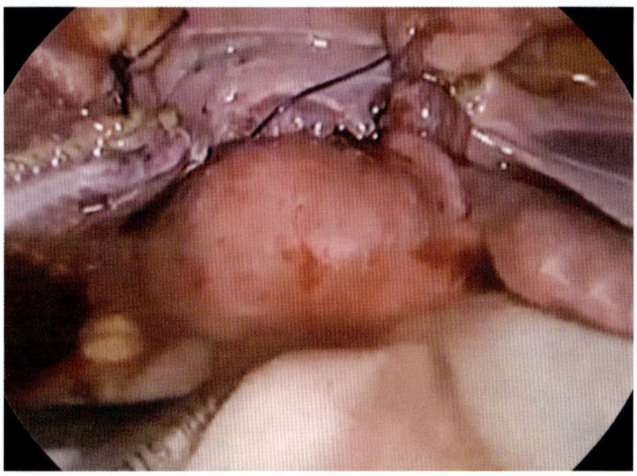

Fig. 38.13: Final situs.

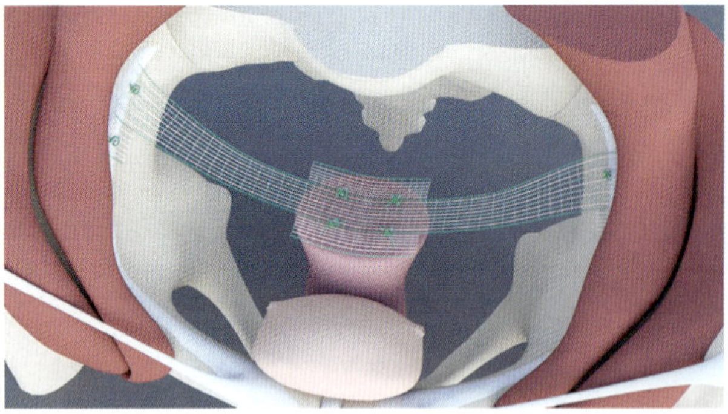

Fig. 38.14: PVDF Tape fixed bilateral at the pectineal ligament.

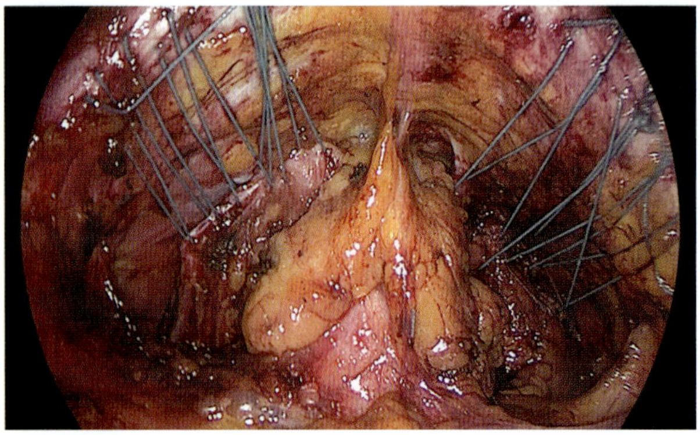

Fig. 38.15: Bilateral colposuspension extraperitoneal/lateral repair.

The pectineal ligament is cleared caudally from the medial umbilical ligament. A non-absorbable tape is used to fix the uterus bilaterally. The lateral fixation point lies close to the level of the apex. A close attachment can lead to a deviation of the apex.

In 2007, we have developed the laparoscopic pectopexy on the level of the psoas muscle. This provides an attachment on the level of sacral vertebra 1 and a hammock-like position of the PVDF tape.

NATIVE TISSUE REPAIR

Colposuspension

Colposuspension can be used for incontinence therapy as well as for the treatment of lateral defect. The early approach in the 1950s was described as a suturing of the lateral pelvic fascia to the "white line."[5] The "white line" structure is controversial in the literature discussion. Most of the time rest for a week of the pelvic fascia is recommended. Therefore, the attachment of pelvic fascia to pectineal ligament provides the highest effectiveness of lateral stabilization.[6]

By laparoscopy the anatomy can be explored extraperitoneal or transperitoneal. The technique is a mesh-free alternative especially for younger patients.

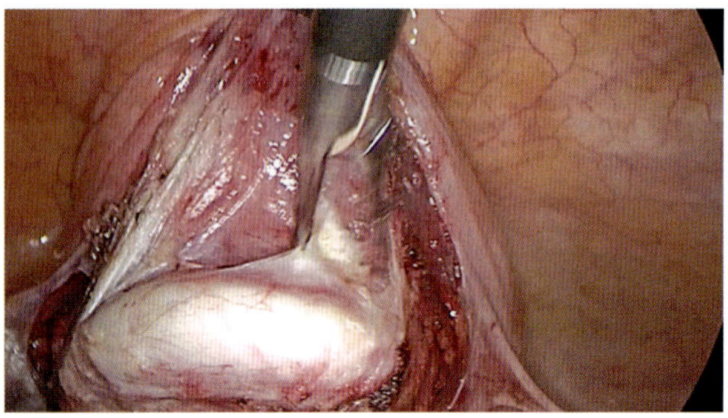

Fig. 38.16: Preparation of the anterior vaginal wall.

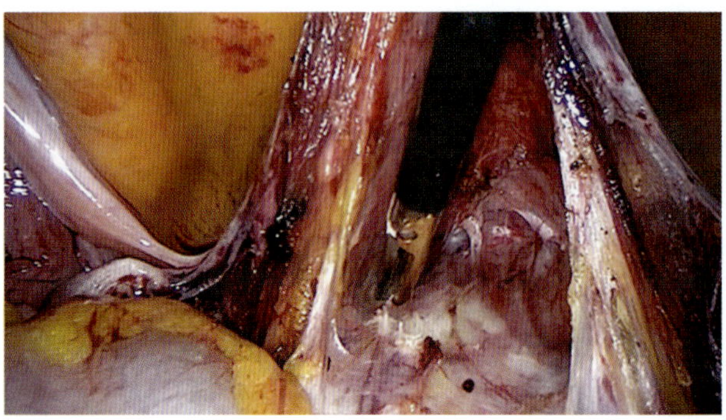

Fig. 38.17: The tissue is cleared until the urethra is reached.

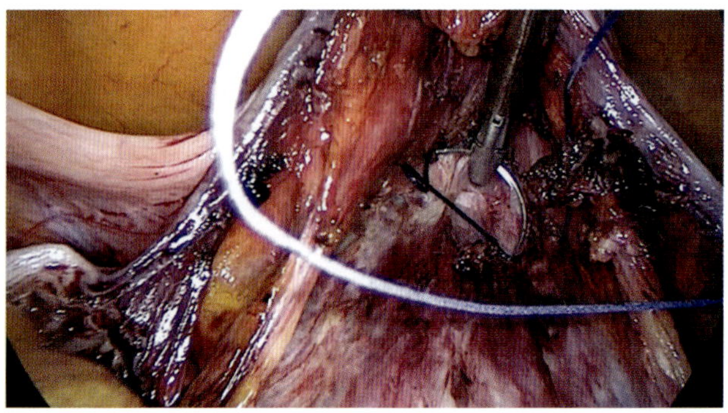

Fig. 38.18: First layer of the compressive suture.

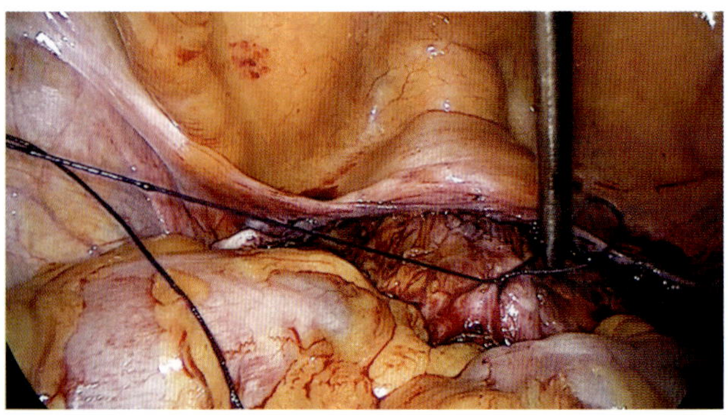

Fig. 38.19: Fully compressed fascia by a running suture.

Colporrhaphy Anterior

Since 2015 we performed a laparoscopic reconstruction of pelvic fascia. The fascia is cleared and the adapted by a running suture or single sutures. The fascia is stitched five to seven times and then compressed. The advantage compared to the vaginal approach is that the vaginal mucosa is not divided from the fascia. The results are promising but not yet ready to be published.

Figures 38.1 to 38.19 demonstrate the described pelvic floor repair steps.

REFERENCES

1. Nezhat CH, Nezhat F, Nezhat C. Laparoscopic sacral colpopexy for vaginal vault prolapse. Obstet Gynecol. 1994;84(5):885-8.
2. Banerjee C, Noé KG. Die laparoskopische Sakropexie—eine unterrepräsentierte Methode der Deszensus-Chirurgie. Geburtshilfe Frauenheilkd. 2008;68(5):492-6.
3. Williams GA, Cullen Richardson A. Transplantation of external oblique aponeurosis: an operation for prolapse of the vagina following hysterectomy. Am J Obstet Gynecol. 1952;64:552-8.
4. Dubuisson JB, et al. Treatment of genital prolapse by laparoscopic lateral suspension using mesh: a series of 73 patients. J Minim Invasive Gynecol. 2008;15(1):49-55.
5. Richardson AC, Edmonds PB, Williams NL. Treatment of stress urinary incontinence due to paravaginal fascial defect. Obstet Gynecol. 1981;57(3):357-62.
6. Banerjee C, Noé GK. Endoscopic cystocele surgery: lateral repair with combined suture/mesh technique. J Endourol, 2010;24(10):1565-9.

Critical Evaluation of
Mesh-supported Vaginal and Endoscopic Pelvic Floor Surgery

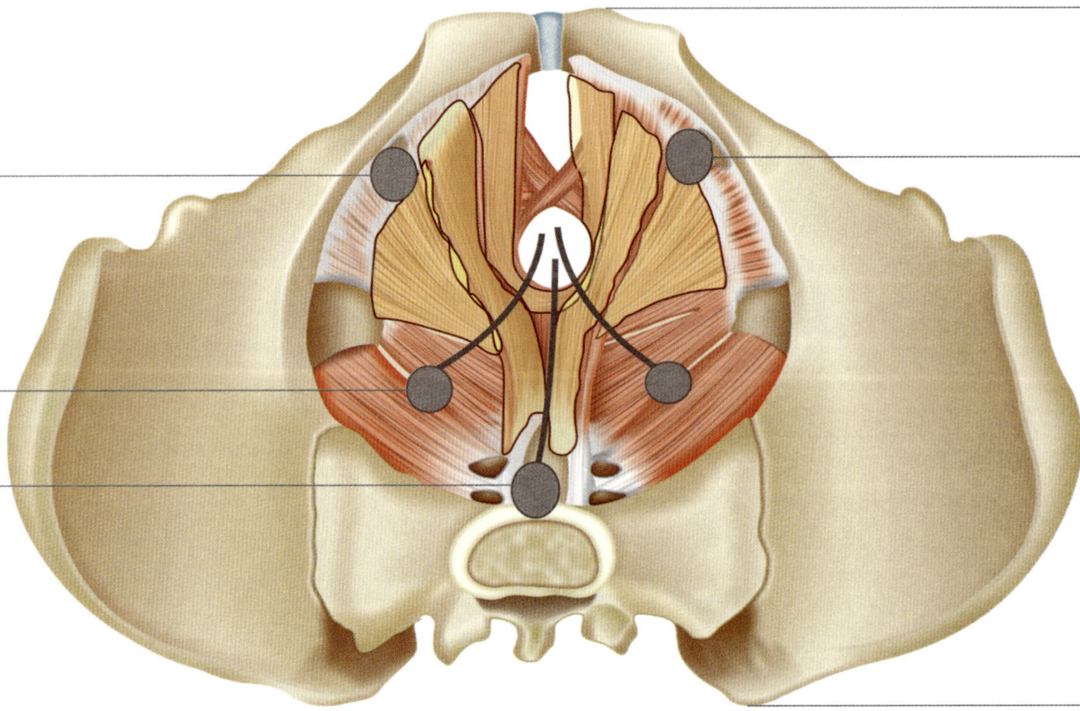

Chapter 39

Critical Evaluation of Mesh-supported Vaginal and Endoscopic Pelvic Floor Surgery

Bernd Holthaus, Haytham Elmeligy

A woman's estimated lifetime risk of pelvic organ prolapse (POP) is 30–50%, with 2% of women becoming symptomatic.[1] In total, women have an estimated 11% lifetime incidence of surgery to repair POP or stress incontinence.[2] Following the Food and Drug Administration (FDA) warnings regarding the safety of vaginal meshes surgical treatment for POP underwent significant changes.

SYMPTOMS

Pelvic organ prolapse may seriously influence the physical, psychological and social well-being of affected individuals and is associated with considerable resource implications for the health service.[3] Generalized symptoms of prolapse include pelvic heaviness; bulge, lump or protrusion coming down from the vagina; a dragging sensation in the vagina; or backache. Symptoms of bladder, bowel or sexual dysfunction are frequently present (Fig. 39.1).

DIAGNOSIS

History taking is mostly underestimated this must include patients' main complain and how is this affecting her quality of life, as well as her expectations after treatment.

The diagnosis is mainly based on the clinical examination. Where all compartments are to be assessed (Fig. 39.2).

Quantification of the prolapse can be done according to one of the available systems e.g., POP-Q system (Fig. 39.3).

Transvaginal ultrasound and introitus ultrasound are cheap, available and interactive tools. That help in assessment for bladder neck and urethral reaction during different situations (e.g., Cough, Pushing, etc. ...). It has also a role during biofeedback treatment that the patients understand better the pelvic floor muscles.

Urodynamic and MRI are helpful tools.

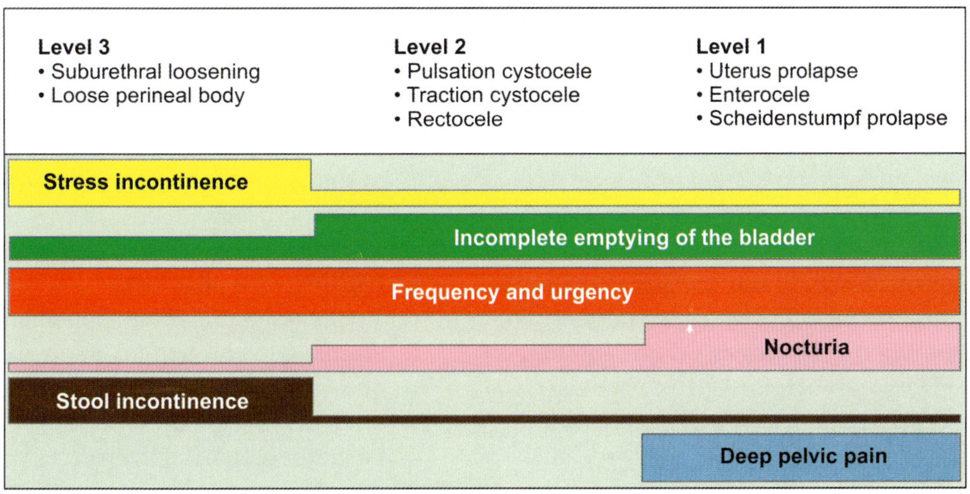

Fig. 39.1: Symptoms of pelvic organ prolapse.

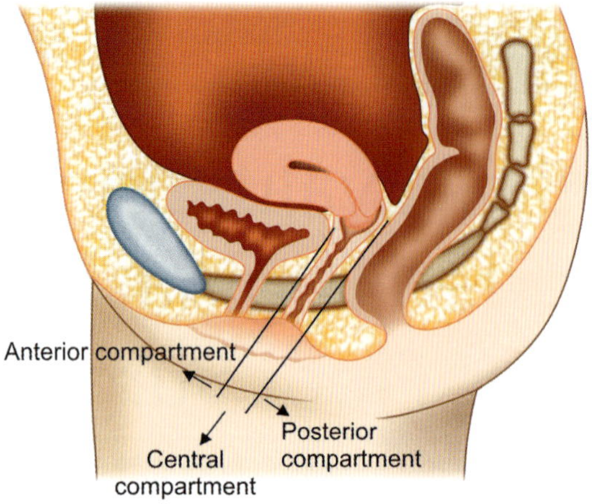

Fig. 39.2: Compartments to be assessed.

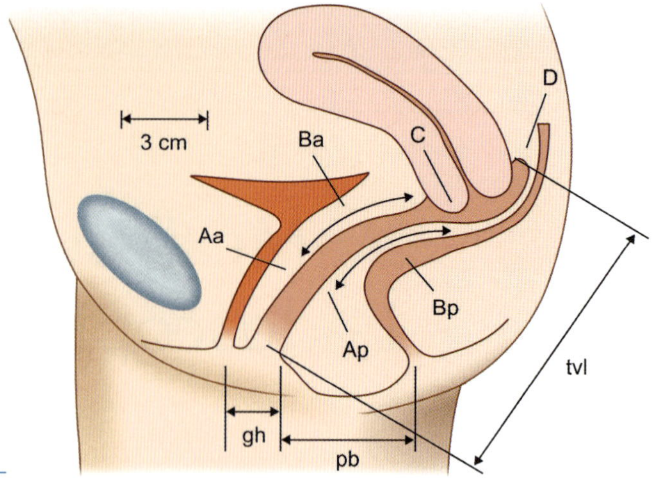

Fig. 39.3: Points and landmarks for POP-Q system examination. Aa: Point A anterior; Ap: Point A posterior; Ba: Point B anterior; Bp: Point B posterior; C: Cervix or vaginal cuff; D: Posterior fornix (if cervix is present); gh: Genital hiatus; pb: Perineal body; tvl: Total vaginal length.[4]

MANAGEMENT

The patients' expectations, including disappearance of symptoms, better function of the included organs (bladder, vagina, rectum and urethra), minimum side effects and complications, long-term anatomical and functional correction and no new problems for example; de novo stress incontinence or dyspareunia must be considered.

Treatment of prolapse depends on the severity of the prolapse, its symptoms, the woman's general health, and surgeon preference and capabilities. Options available for treatment are:

- **Conservative** e.g., pelvic floor training or Biofeedback. Pelvic floor muscle exercise may result in regression of POP stage, but mainly improves associated functional symptoms.[5,6]
- **Mechanical** like pessary, rings or tampons. The most common side effects are malodorous vaginal discharge, bleeding, erosions and ulcers, de novo incontinence and interference with sexual intercourse, this leads to preference of surgery by some women.[7]

SURGICAL INTERVENTION

Technical development and better knowledge of the female pelvis functional anatomy is enabling today a more precise understanding of its physiopathology, so it facilitates the design of site-specific operations. Various surgical approaches and techniques are offered depending on the defect, where combined procedures give good solutions. It is necessary to have an appropriate surgical training to obtain the better competence, and a safe and correct repair.[8]

- *Anterior compartment:*
  - Anterior colporrhaphy with or without Mesh
  - Lateral repair.
    For the repair of paravaginal defect. Here the vaginal fascia is sutured to the arcus tendineus fasciae pelvis using nonabsorbable sutures. This can be performed through an extraperitoneal endoscopy or abdominal as described originally by Richardson.[9]
- *Central compartment (Fig. 39.4):*
  - Vaginal sacrospinous fixation.
  - Laparoscopic sacropexy/hysteropexy.
    Is considered the gold standard for the repair of central compartment defect
  - Laparoscopic sacropexy with anterior repair.
    Combining the repair of anterior compartment defect with central support reduces the rate of recurrence
  - Laparoscopic sacropexy with posterior repair.
    Laparoscopic posterior compartment repair using a tension free posterior fixation through the levator ani as well as central fixation at the sacral promontory. This gives a good support to the posterior vagina without touching the vaginal mucosa.
  - Laparoscopic bilateral sacropexy (slim sling)
  - Laparoscopic pectopexy.
    The lateral parts of the iliopectineal ligament are used for a bilateral mesh fixation of the descended structures.[10]
- *Posterior compartment:*
  - Posterior colporrhaphy with or without Mesh
- *Incontinence operations:*
  - Colposuspention Burch

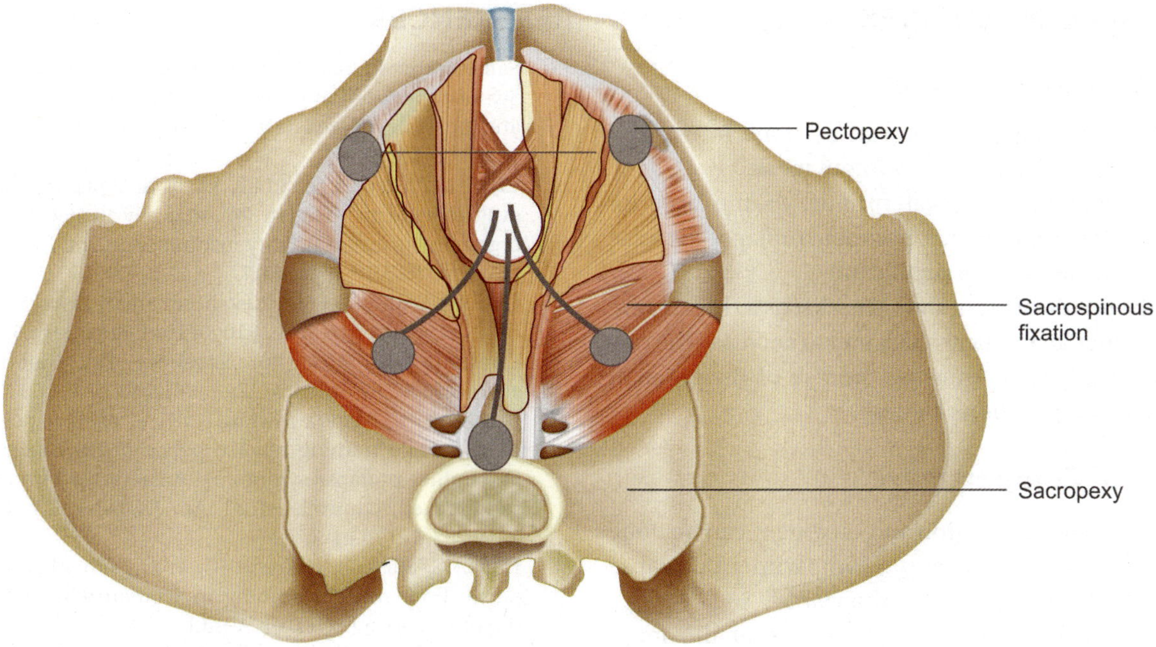

Fig. 39.4: Central compartment surgeries and fixation points.
Courtesy: Alkatout I.

An extraperitoneal endoscopic approach improves visualization, less risk of bleeding, and faster recovery but requires high training.

- TVT sling operation

EVALUATION OF MESH

Surgical meshes have been used in abdominal POP repair (sacrocolpopexy) for decades. Their use in transvaginal POP surgery has increased over the last decade, but their safety has been questioned. A choice has to be made between native tissue repairs with standard vaginal surgery, and mesh associated repairs either through the vaginal or the abdominal route.[7]

Anterior Compartment

Awareness of prolapse: This was probably more likely after native tissue repair suggesting that if 13% of women were aware of prolapse after mesh repair, 18%–30% would be aware of prolapse after native tissue repair.

Repeat surgery for prolapse: This was probably more likely after native tissue repair.

Recurrent anterior compartment prolapse: This was probably more likely after native tissue repair.

Repeat surgery for prolapse, stress urinary incontinence SUI or mesh exposure: Evidence suggests that if 10% of women require repeat surgery after polypropylene mesh repair, 4% to 8% would do so after native tissue repair.

De novo SUI: No evidence suggested a difference in rates of repeat surgery for SUI.

Dyspareunia (de novo): Evidence suggested few or no differences between groups.[11]

Central Compartment

There is consistent and reproducible evidence that abdominal sacrocolpopexy using mesh has a higher success rate than vaginal surgery as well as less post-operative dyspareunia. A few randomized controlled trials compared abdominal sacropexy with vaginal surgery, and all of the trials demonstrated significantly improved anatomical but also functional outcomes.[12,13]

The current recommendation of the Canadian urological association does not support the routine use of transvaginal mesh for prolapse repair. This recommendation does not apply to the use of transabdominal mesh used during a minimally invasive or open sacrocolpopexy.[11]

Posterior Compartment

So far, no studies have shown any benefit of mesh in posterior compartment repair. Traditional midline fascial plication has a high anatomical cure rate of between 80% and 90%.[7]

GERMAN GUIDELINES

Anterior Compartment

- Anterior colporrhaphy can be done in the primary situation with or without mesh.
- Combining an apical fixation to the anterior repair by anterior compartment prolapse increase the rate of success significantly.
- The option of Mesh should be discussed to achieve a better anatomical result and to decrease the rate for recurrence knowing the risk of Reoperation and complications of mesh.

Central Compartment

- Sacrospinous fixation and sacropexy can be done as a treatment to central compartment prolapse with success rates more than 90%.
- The abdominal sacropexy is one of the long-term evaluated operations and the laparoscopic approach has comparable success rates.
- Uterus conserving surgeries can be discussed.

Posterior Compartment

- Posterior colporrhaphy can be done in the primary situation.
- There are no randomized controlled studies to support adding a Mesh in the primary situation.
- The available retrospective und prospective uncontrolled studies show less recurrence but higher erosion and pelvic pain rates.[14]

CONCLUSION

Informed decision making is the key to successful management of the prolapse. The patient must understand her option including benefits and risks of every method and should share in the decision making.

Laparoscopy offers a lot of options for pelvic floor repair, due to high technology, detailed view and better dissection we can achieve a better defect oriented surgery.

Higher training and more randomized controlled studies are still needed to assess the laparoscopic use of mesh in treatment of anterior and posterior compartment defects.

REFERENCES

1. Samuelsson EC ea. Signs of genital prolapse in a Swedish population of women 20 to 59 years of age and possible related factors. Am J Obstet Gynecol. 1999:299-305.
2. Clark AL, Gregory T, Smith VJ, et al. Epidemiologic evaluation of reoperation for surgically treated pelvic organ prolapse and urinary incontinence. Am J Obstet Gynecol. 2003;189(5):1261-7.
3. Giarenis I, Robinson D. Prevention and management of pelvic organ prolapse. F1000Prime Rep. 2014;6:77.
4. Danforth TL, Aron M, Ginsberg DA. Robotic sacrocolpopexy. Indian J Urol. 2014;30(3):318-25.
5. Braekken IH, Majida M, Engh ME, et al. Can pelvic floor muscle training reverse pelvic organ prolapse and reduce prolapse symptoms? An assessor-blinded, randomized, controlled trial. Am J Obstet Gynecol. 2010;203(2):170.e1-7.
6. Hagen S, Stark D, Glazener C, et al. Individualised pelvic floor muscle training in women with pelvic organ prolapse (POPPY): A multicentre randomised controlled trial. The Lancet 2014;383(9919):796-806.
7. Dällenbach P. To mesh or not to mesh: a review of pelvic organ reconstructive surgery. Int J Womens Health 2015;7:331-43.
8. González-Enguita C, Gennaro-DellaRossa N, López-López E, et al. Estado actual de la Colposacropexia Laparoscópica (CSPL) en la corrección del Prolapso de Órganos Pélvicos (POP). Arch Esp Urol. 2017;70(4):400-11.
9. Chinthakanan O, Miklos JR, Moore RD. Laparoscopic Paravaginal Defect Repair: Surgical Technique and a Literature Review. Surg Technol Int. 2015;27:173-83.
10. Banerjee C, Noé KG. Laparoscopic pectopexy: a new technique of prolapse surgery for obese patients. Arch Gynecol Obstet. 2011; 284(3):631-5.
11. Welk B, Carlson KV, Baverstock RJ, et al. Canadian Urological Association position statement on the use of transvaginal mesh. Can Urol. Assoc. J 2017; 11(6Suppl2):S105-7.
12. Nygaard IE, McCreery R, Brubaker L, et al. Abdominal sacrocolpopexy: a comprehensive review. Obstet Gynecol. 2004;104(4):805-23.
13. Roovers J-PWR, van der Vaart CH, van der Bom JG, van Leeuwen JHS, Scholten PC, Heintz APM. A randomised controlled trial comparing abdominal and vaginal prolapse surgery: effects on urogenital function. BJOG 2004;111(1):50-6.
14. Baessler K. Diagnosis and treatment of the pelvic organ prolaps. Guideline of the German society of Gynecology and Obestetrics: S2e level, AAWMF registry N0. 015/006. April 2016 [cited 2017 Aug 15].

Surgery for Pelvic **Floor Defects**

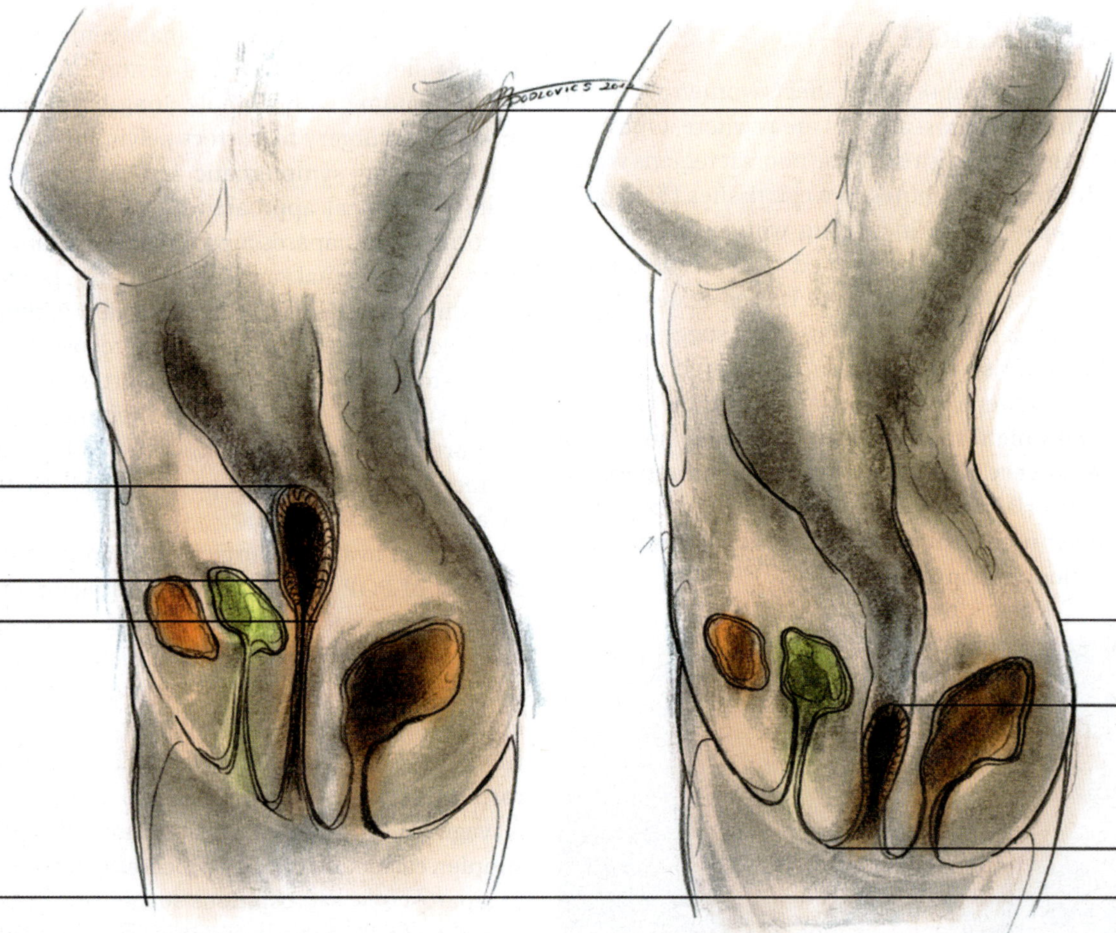

Chapter 40

Surgery for Pelvic Floor Defects

Shanti I Mohling, CY Liu

INTRODUCTION

Pelvic organ prolapse (POP) affects women across the world, from the most affluent areas where large birth weights increase the risk to the poorest regions where malnutrition contributes to weak tissues (Fig. 40.1). Rates appear to be increasing with nearly 300,000 surgical procedures performed for POP or urinary incontinence each year in the United States alone.[1] Early seminal work by Olsen et al. suggested that the lifetime risk for a woman to undergo a surgery for prolapse repair was estimated at 11.1%, however up to 30% of those women will ultimately undergo a repeat surgery.[2] The pathophysiology is complex and multifactorial with genetic predisposition overlapping with medical history and childbirth resulting in pelvic floor prolapse.[3]

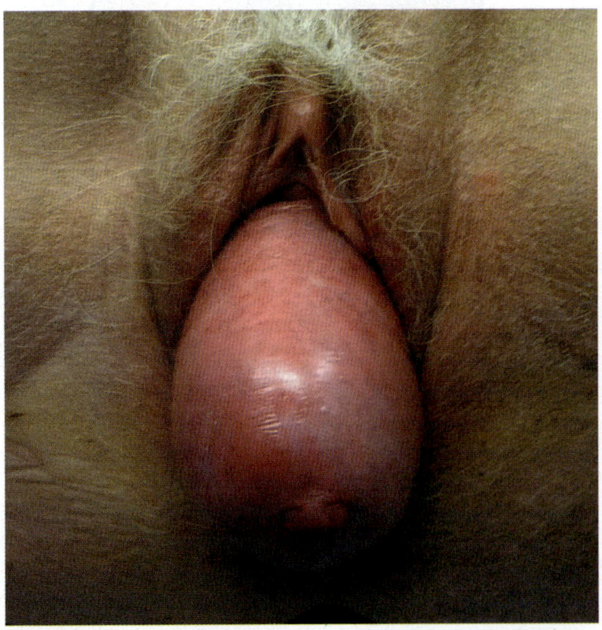

Fig. 40.1: Complete uterovaginal prolapse.

The goals for surgical management of POP are to relieve symptoms and restore normal functional anatomy with durable, long-term outcomes. In general, surgery to correct pelvic floor defects is performed on symptomatic individuals. Although multiple surgical approaches have been described to correct POP, laparoscopy provides certain advantages over vaginal and laparotomic procedures, including an enhanced, magnified view of the operative field, less blood loss, and rapid recovery.

Restoration of the apical support is the keystone for a successful POP surgery, without adequate support at the vaginal apex; even the best surgical correction of anterior and posterior walls is doomed to fail.

Current available surgical techniques for apical support of POP include uterosacral ligament (USL) suspension, sacrocolpopexy and sacrospinous fixation; all these three surgical techniques can be performed laparoscopically. While each of these approaches to repair POP may have specific merit, we would not recommend using laparoscopic sacrospinous suspension for vaginal apical support. A vaginal sacrospinous suspension is actually a simpler, easier and quicker procedure in comparison to laparoscopic sacrospinous suspension and also is associated with a lower operative complication rate. However, in our experience, the laparoscopic USL suspension is a superior procedure to vaginal sacrospinous suspension.

The focus of this chapter is on laparoscopic USL suspension with native tissue, a technique that does not require the use of mesh. Therefore, we will not discuss laparoscopic surgeries that would require the use of synthetic mesh such as laparoscopic sacrocolpopexy or laparoscopic perineo-colpo-hysterosacropexy.

ANATOMY

The functional dynamic anatomy of pelvic organ support is complex; however, the visualization afforded by laparoscopy allows for an amplified perspective of internal anatomic defects visually as well as providing laparoscopic guidance while performing vaginal digital palpation.

Pelvic organ prolapse surgery, in essence, is to repair, reconstruct and restore the integrity of endopelvic fascia. The key to a successful pelvic floor prolapse repair is a deep understanding of the surgical anatomy of endopelvic fascia; it is structure and the specific role of each individual segment of endopelvic fascia in the pelvic floor support, their precise locations and their relationship to the important anatomic landmarks in the pelvis.

Following is a brief description of the anatomy of endopelvic fascia; however, readers are encouraged to study more in depth about endopelvic fascia elsewhere. The cardinal ligament originates from the anterior border of the greater sciatic foramen. In a standing woman, the cardinal ligament follows internal iliac vessels in a 90° fashion toward the ischial spine. Therefore, cardinal ligament is actually the perivascular connective sheath of internal iliac vessels. At the level of ischial spine, cardinal ligament continues with uterine vessels toward the cervix and upper vagina where it merges with USL, forming the uterosacro-cardinal ligament complex (Fig. 40.2). This complex wraps and circles around cervix and upper part of vagina and becomes the structure of the pericervical ring supporting cervix and upper vagina. Anteriorly, pericervical ring becomes pubocervical fascia, which supports anterior vaginal wall, bladder and urethra in their proper position. Pubocervical fascia attaches to the pelvic sidewall at the level of arcus tendineus fascia pelvis (white line) laterally. After passing symphysis pubis caudally, it merges with urogenital diaphragm (perineal membrane). Posteriorly, pericervical ring becomes rectovaginal septum, which supports the posterior vaginal wall. Rectovaginal septum attaches to pelvic sidewall on the medial fascia of the levator ani muscle and arcus tendineus fascia pelvis (white line) and caudally it fuses with perineal body. Therefore, from the anterior border of greater sciatic foramen to introitus, endopelvic fascia is a continuous sheath of tough and strong fascia that passively supports the female pelvic floor. The active support of pelvic floor comes from the dynamic function of levator ani muscles. It is beyond the scope of this chapter for us to discuss the dynamic functional support of levator ani muscle. Readers are encouraged to further study this important subject elsewhere.

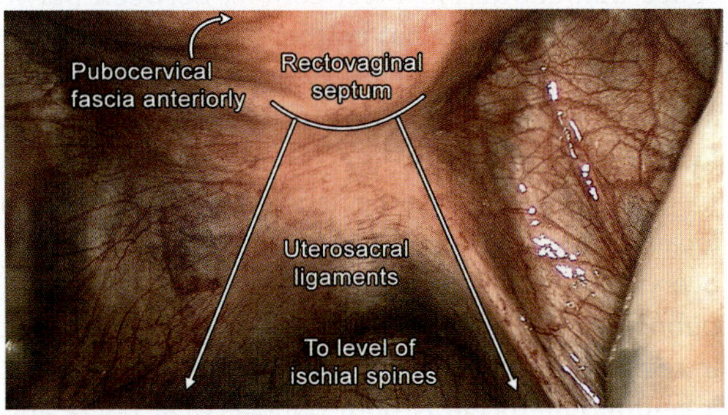

Fig. 40.2: Pericervical ring in a healthy woman without prolapse. This image captures the relationship of intact fascia in a woman without prolapse. The concept of a confluence of fascia of the uterosacral ligaments merging with the rectovaginal fascia at the level of the cervix and the level of the ischial spines can be appreciated here.

During reparative surgery for POP, one must pay special attention to the pericervical ring. This is the pivotal structure that supports vaginal apex and cervix and its location is at the level of the ischial spines.

Many recent studies underscore the key role of apical suspension in pelvic organ support. Lowder et al. demonstrated in a population of women with stage II or greater prolapse that simulated apical support resulted in the reduction of prolapse to stage 0 or stage I in 55% of patients in the context of anterior prolapse and in 30% of patients in the context of posterior prolapse.[4] Employing dynamic magnetic resonance scans to evaluate women with known POP at rest and during Valsalva; Summers et al. concluded, "Half of the observed variation in anterior compartment support may be explained by apical support."[5] Thus, achieving a well-supported vaginal apex during pelvic floor reconstruction is of paramount importance and crucial for a satisfactory long-term result.

Restoration of the pericervical ring will not only restore the normal vaginal length, but most likely the vaginal axis as well. Anatomically, the confluence of the pubocervical fascia, rectovaginal septum and USL complex at the level of the ischial spines constitutes the pericervical ring. Surgically, one should broaden one's concept about "pericervical ring." Instead of thinking of it as a "ring"-shaped structure, one must have the image that the pericervical ring actually is a band of strong connective tissue and muscles that spans in between two ischial spines. Therefore, from surgical point of view, it would be wise for surgeons to include the coccygeus muscle and the sacrospinous ligament in their concept of "pericervical ring." This pericervical ring constitutes the strongest part of the endopelvic fascia and is located in the narrowest space of the pelvis (bi-ischial space). During the labor and delivery, particularly in the second stage of labor, as the fetal head negotiates its passage through the narrowest part of the pelvis, the tough fascia of the pericervical ring will invariably and ultimately be damaged, weakening the pelvic floor support and consequently contributing to future pelvic organ prolapse.

In summary, from a surgical anatomy point of view, the two most crucial aspects that contribute to a successful and long-lasting POP surgery are the following:

- A precise knowledge with deep understanding of the anatomy of the pericervical ring
- The surgeon's ability to know how to correctly identify the individual segments of the endopelvic fascia and their defects during surgery and to adequately repair the defects to restore the integrity of the fibromuscular vaginal tube.

PREOPERATIVE EVALUATION

Evaluation begins with a comprehensive in-office assessment. A complete patient history is obtained with attention given to the detailed past obstetrical history, medical conditions, surgical procedures (particularly female pelvic reconstructive cases), current medications and supplements, and urinary, defecatory and sexual complaints. A complete physical examination is performed with the patient examined in both erect and supine positions to map out pelvic floor defects appropriately. Pelvic examination should include bimanual and rectovaginal examinations, evaluation of the pelvic floor muscle strength and objective documentation of the POP using either the Baden–Walker or the pelvic organ prolapse quantification (POP-Q) systems. Stress urinary incontinence is evaluated clinically and the post-void residual volume must be measured. Laboratory testing should include complete blood count, serum creatinine and electrolytes, urinalysis and, if indicated, a urine culture. Ancillary testing, such as multichannel urodynamics, pelvic floor electromyography, transvaginal and anal ultrasonography, and dynamic magnetic resonance imaging, may be ordered if clinically needed to clarify atypical cases of POP.

After the evaluation is completed, medical and surgical options are presented to and discussed with the patient. If surgical intervention is elected, risks and alternatives to surgery are reviewed and consent for surgery is obtained. As POP is not a life-threatening condition, the surgeon should emphasize that surgical repair of POP is an elective procedure that is performed in the attempt to restore the normal anatomy and to potentially relieve bothersome symptoms. While this chapter focuses on prolapse repair without the use of mesh, if synthetic mesh, especially transvaginal mesh is to be used, careful counseling regarding the associated risks must occur with the patient verbalizing a clear understanding. Finally, the surgeon should counsel the patient regarding reasonable expectations for surgical outcomes and never guarantee that surgery will satisfactorily restore anatomy or relieve symptoms.

RECOGNIZE ENTEROCELE PRIOR TO SURGERY FOR PELVIC ORGAN PROLAPSE

A significant and frequent cause of a failed POP surgery is the missed diagnosis and repair of an existing enterocele. Vagina is a fibromuscular tube encapsulated by the endopelvic fascia, and this tube is entirely lined by vaginal epithelium. In the normal condition, between vaginal epithelium and pelvic peritoneum, there should be intervening endopelvic fascia throughout the entire vagina. Pelvic peritoneum and vaginal epithelium are separated by fascia and do not have direct contact with each other; there should always be fascia in between them.

The components of endopelvic fascia are smooth muscle, fibrin, collagen and elastin. This kind of structure is biomechanically fragile cannot be overstretched; it will break under constant tension or pressure. On the other hand, both pelvic peritoneum and vaginal epithelium can be stretched endlessly under tension or pressure. An enterocele is formed when there is a break in vaginal fascia, creating a space that allows for direct contact between pelvic peritoneum and vaginal epithelium. At this broken area, under tension or pressure, both peritoneum and vaginal epithelium stretch and bulge into vagina forming an enterocele.

An enterocele can be labeled according to its location; an anterior enterocele is a break of pubocervical fascia from the pericervical ring or a tear in pubocervical fascia. A posterior enterocele is a break in rectovaginal septum from the pericervical ring and a central enterocele is both pubocervical fascia and rectovaginal septum detached from USLs at the vaginal apex. Other classifications of enterocele, such as pulsion or traction enterocele, may be based on the degree, shape, and other coexisting associated prolapse.

All enterocele must be detected and adequately repaired. Missing and failing to repair small and medium-sized enterocele during the POP surgery is common and is one of the major reasons for poor surgical outcome.

LAPAROSCOPIC UTEROSACRAL LIGAMENT SUSPENSION FOR PELVIC ORGAN PROLAPSE

Overview

In 2004, John DeLancey's group at the University of Michigan published a paper on "Quantitative Analysis of Uterosacral Ligaments: Origin and Insertion Points by MRI." The study tracked uterosacral ligaments on 62 nulliparous women using magnetic resonance imaging (MRI) and found that more than 82% of USLs inserted into the sacrospinous ligament/coccygeus muscle, 11% into the ischial spines and piriformis muscle and only 7% to sacrum. This study and subsequent other studies point to the fact that at the level of ischial spine, USL and sacrospinous ligament/coccygeus muscle merge together and form part of pericervical ring to support the vaginal apex and the cervix.[6] Subsequent studies on USLs all point to the insertion site of uterosacral ligaments to fascial muscular tissue at the level of ischial spine.

Suspension of the vaginal apex in patients with POP to the USLs at the level of ischial spine is a simple and effective procedure to address apical support without the use of mesh. A review of 133 patients with symptomatic prolapse of grade II or greater by Lin et al. demonstrated an objective success rate of 87% over a follow-up period of 2.0–7.3 years.[7] Similarly, Seman et al. demonstrated an objective success rate of 90% at 2 years in 47 patients with symptomatic POP who underwent laparoscopic USL suspension. Additionally, high patient satisfaction rates were reported, noting that 85% of their cohort would recommend the procedure to a friend.[8]

The following is a summary of essential steps for laparoscopic USL vaginal vault or uterine suspension for POP:

- Restore the integrity of fibromuscular vaginal tube by identify and repairing the coexisting enterocele.
- Suspend the apex of vagina or cervix to USLs bilaterally at the level of ischial spines.
- Repair the paravaginal defect laparoscopically, if needed, by entering retropubic space to repair paravaginal defects and perform a Burch colposuspension if necessary.
- Perform a vaginal midurethral sling for urinary incontinence if laparoscopic Burch and paravaginal repair was not performed.
- Repair the low rectocele and perineorrhaphy vaginally if indicated.
- Cystoscopic examination.

TECHNIQUE

Patient Preparation

The patient undergoes general endotracheal anesthesia, and an orogastric or nasogastric tube is introduced. She is placed in dorsolithotomy position with legs well supported in stirrups. An examination under anesthesia is performed, and the findings are compared to the preoperative evaluation. Abdomen, perineum and vagina are prepped, and the patient is draped in sterile fashion. A Foley catheter is placed. It is important for the surgeon to have access to the perineum during the procedure so as to be able to perform frequent digital vaginal or rectal examinations, adjust the uterine manipulator or adjust the vaginal or rectal probes.

Laparoscopic entry into the abdomen is accomplished per the surgeon's preference. A 10–12 mm port is placed at the umbilicus, and under direct visualization, two 5 mm ports are placed lateral to the inferior epigastric vessels in the lower quadrants, and additional one or two 5 mm ports lateral to the rectus muscles at the level of the umbilicus. The abdominal and pelvic cavities are then carefully inspected. In steep Trendelenburg position, the small bowel is retracted cephalad and toward the right paracolic gutter, and the rectosigmoid is retracted cephalad. In some cases, especially with obese patients, the sigmoid colon may need to be sutured to the abdominal sidewall to enhance the exposure of the deep pelvis.

Step 1: Identification and Exposure of Pelvic Ureters

The rate of ureteral injury or kinking has been estimated at 2–11% in vaginal USL suspension procedures;[9] identification and dissection of both ureters for all laparoscopic USL suspension procedures is recommended to prevent ureteral injury.

Transperitoneal ureteral dissection is preferred to retroperitoneal technique to prevent injury or tethering of the ureter during the suspension. The ureters

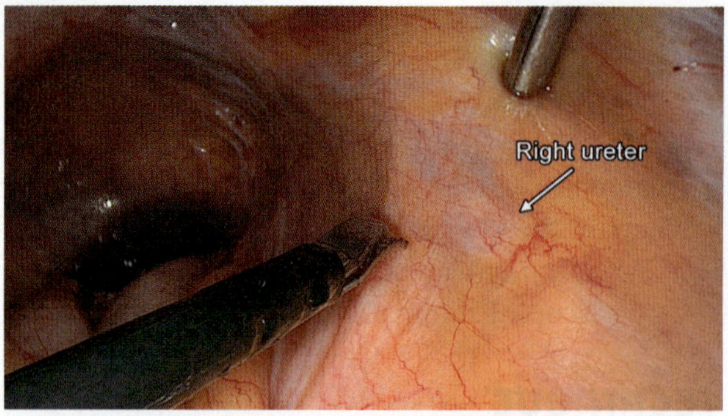

Fig. 40.3: Transperitoneal view of right ureter coursing through pelvis.

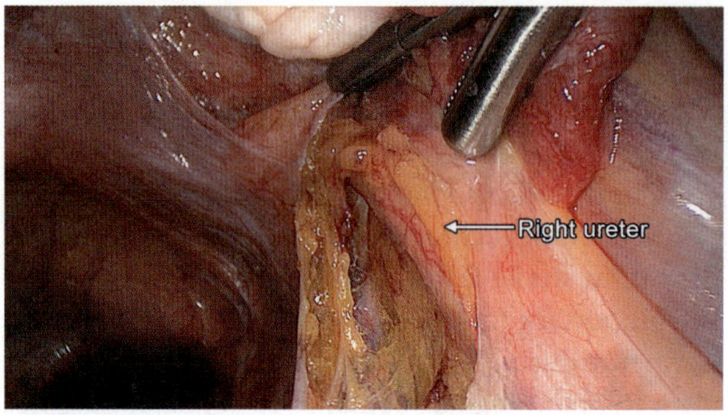

Fig. 40.4: Transperitoneal exposure of right ureter.

on both sides are visualized through the laparoscope (Fig. 40.3). An incision on the overlying peritoneum of the ureter on the pelvic sidewall is made and the ureter is dissected caudally to expose the ureter to the level of the ureteric tunnel where anatomically it is at the level of ischial spine on both sides (Fig. 40.4). This simple procedure performed at the very beginning of the procedure can help us to avoid the ureter being compromised by the suspension stitches. Over the past 25 years, we have not had a single ureteral injury or kinking with our USL suspension procedures. This attests to the value of doing this simple procedure done at the beginning of each repair.

Step 2: Exposure of the Rectovaginal Septum and Pubocervical Fascia

The enterocele must be identified and repaired after the ureters are adequately exposed. The integrity of the fibromuscular vaginal tube must be restored first by exposing both rectovaginal septum and pubocervical fascia. The use of vaginal probe is an excellent way to identify small enteroceles, which may be missed in the preoperative pelvic examination. A bright snow-white tip vaginal probe is especially useful (Fig. 40.5). With the vaginal probe inside the

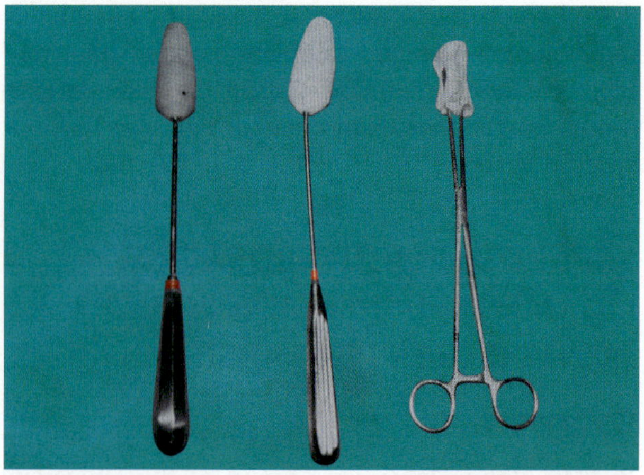

Fig. 40.5: Vaginal probes may be used to reveal and demonstrate an enterocele.

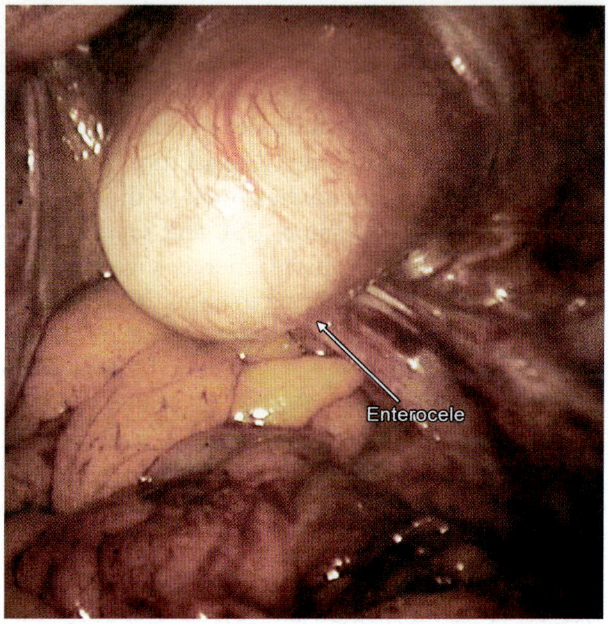

Fig. 40.6: Vaginal enterocele with vaginal probe demonstrating the thin tissues of peritoneum and vaginal mucosa, but no fascia.

vagina, the enterocele has a translucent appearance when viewed laparoscopically (Fig. 40.6). As the peritoneum of the enterocele sac is opened and dissected back, the broken edge of the endopelvic fascia can be easily delineated (Fig. 40.7). The small enterocele sac can then be excised and both fascial edges reapproximated in double layers with permanent non-absorbable sutures (Fig. 40.8).

Rectovaginal septum is usually exposed first (Fig. 40.9). A rectal probe or an end-to-end anastomosing (EEA) sizer may be placed in the rectum to help to identify the rectum and to deviate it away from the operative field. A longitudinal incision is made in the peritoneum overlying

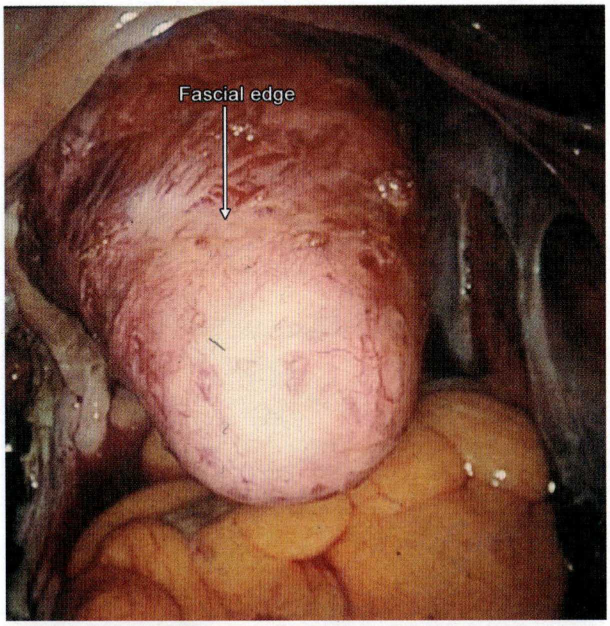

Fig. 40.7: The peritoneum has been dissected away to reveal the vaginal mucosa surrounded by the torn surrounding fascia.

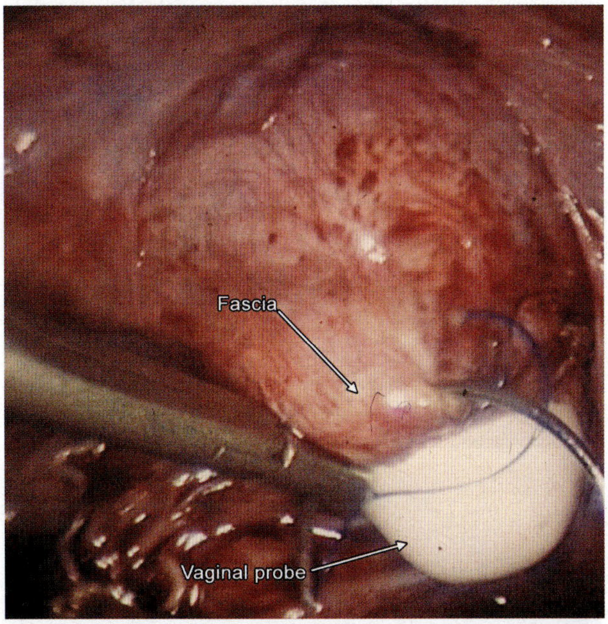

Fig. 40.8: The fascia must be reapproximated by taking large bites with a nonabsorbable suture.

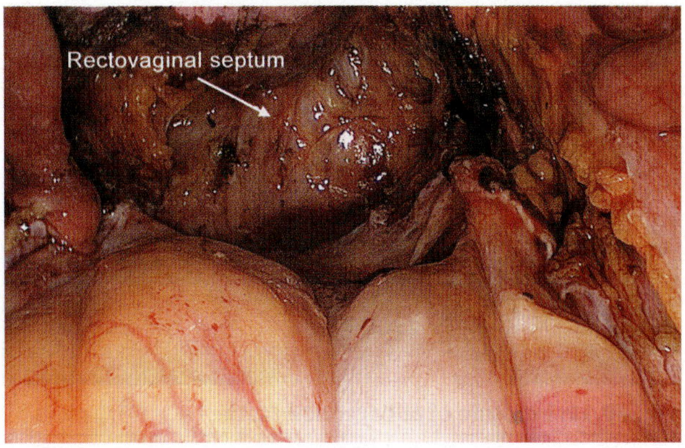

Fig. 40.9: Exposure of rectovaginal septum.

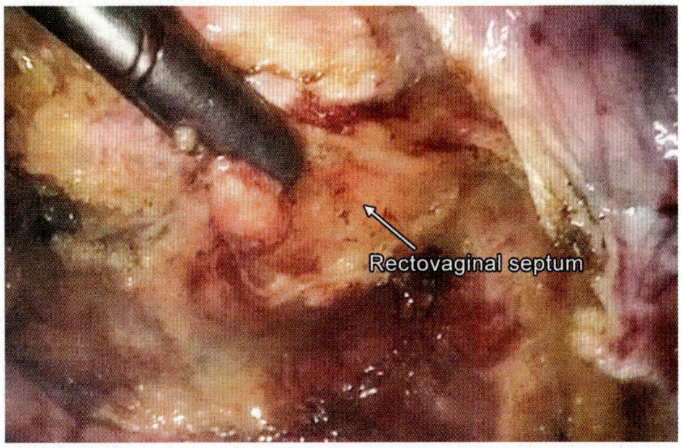

Fig. 40.10: Laparoscopic tugging on rectovaginal septum to confirm healthy and intact tissue.

the right pararectal space, and this is extended caudally toward the rectovaginal space. The same procedure is repeated on the left side. The placement of rectal probe is important for inexperienced surgeons, but not a necessity for those who are experienced laparoscopists. Such surgeons are usually quite familiar and competent working within the cul-de-sac and entering and dissecting the rectovaginal space as in the case of severe endometriosis. After entering the rectovaginal space, it must be dissected wide laterally and down toward the introitus until the broken edge of rectovaginal septum is adequately exposed and identified. The rectovaginal septum can be verified first by grasping it and tugging on it laparoscopically to be certain that it is tough and strong (Fig. 40.10).

Rectovaginal septum can be further confirmed by placing the surgeon's index and middle fingers on the posterior vaginal wall transvaginally and noting the entire posterior vaginal wall being pulled up while simultaneously tugging and pulling on the assumed rectovaginal septum laparoscopically. The pubocervical fascia can be verified in the same way, after entering wide and dissecting deep into the vesicocervical and vesicovaginal space (Fig. 40.11).

Special attention must be paid to the course of ureter in the repair of an anterior enterocele, as ureter curves across anterior lateral vaginal fornix to enter into the bladder. The surgeon's two fingers can be placed on the anterior vaginal wall to feel the strong pulling up of the entire anterior vaginal

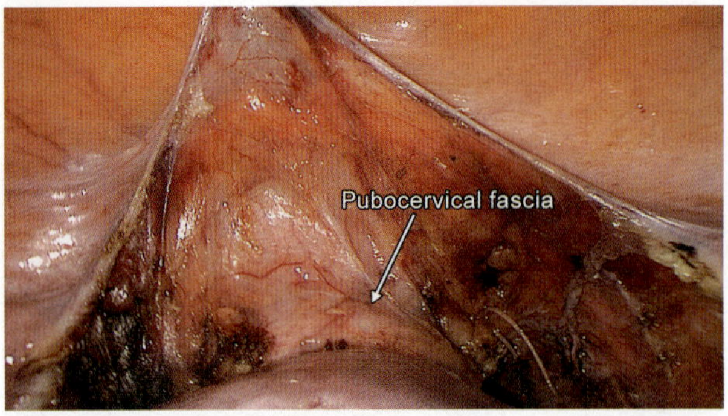

Fig. 40.11: Exposure of pubocervical Fascia.

wall during the simultaneous tugging and pulling of the assumed pubocervical fascia laparoscopically. If heavy bleeding is encountered during dissection of the bladder away from the cervix and upper part of vagina, it is likely that the dissection has deviated from the proper plane, as usually the space between the bladder and pubocervical fascia is relatively avascular. The integrity of the bladder may be ascertained by backfilling 200–300 mL of dyed saline if excessive bleeding is noted or there is any suspicion of possible bladder injury. A cystoscopic examination at the end of surgery can confirm that the bladder is intact and has not been compromised.

Pubocervical fascia and rectovaginal septum must be reattached back to the cervix or to each other (posthysterectomy patient). This will restore the integrity of the fascial vaginal tube. Big bites of the fascial tissue of at least with 0.5–1 cm with permanent non-absorbable sutures must be employed.

Step 3: Reconstruct and Resuspend Pericervical Ring: Uterosacral Ligament Suspension

After integrity of fibromuscular vaginal tube is restored, the cervix or apex of the vagina (in posthysterectomy patient) is suspended to the USLs, bilaterally, at the level of the ischial spines.

The surgeon palpates the ischial spines transvaginally, while viewing the finger movements at the ischial spine laparoscopically, to identify the location of ischial spines (Figs. 40.12A and B). A rectal probe is placed, and the rectum is deviated contralaterally. Using a large gauge nonabsorbable suture (such as 0-Ethibond or CV-0 Gore-Tex), a double-bite of the USL is taken 1.5–2 cm medial and posterior to the ischial spine (Figs. 40.13A and B).

The bites must be deep and sutures must be tugged and pulled to ensure adequate strength of

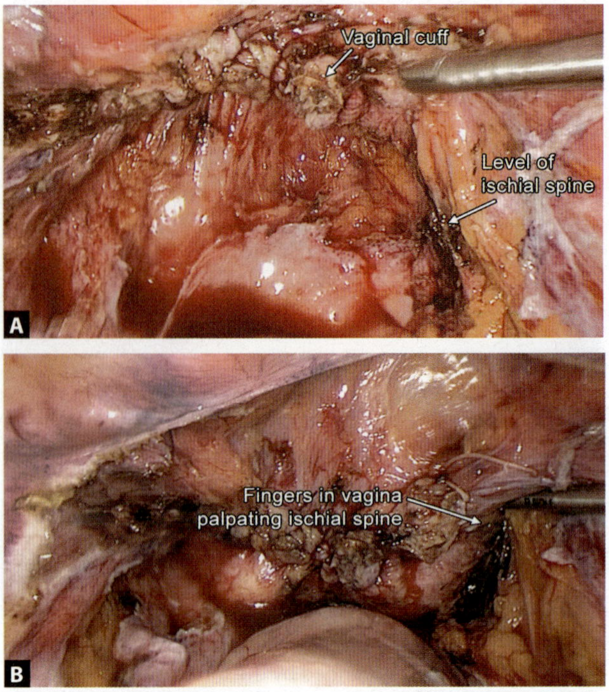

Figs. 40.12A and B: (A) Vaginal cuff without fingers palpating the ischial spines; (B) Vaginal cuff with fingers palpating the right ischial spine in order to determine the initial suture placement through the proximal uterosacral ligament.

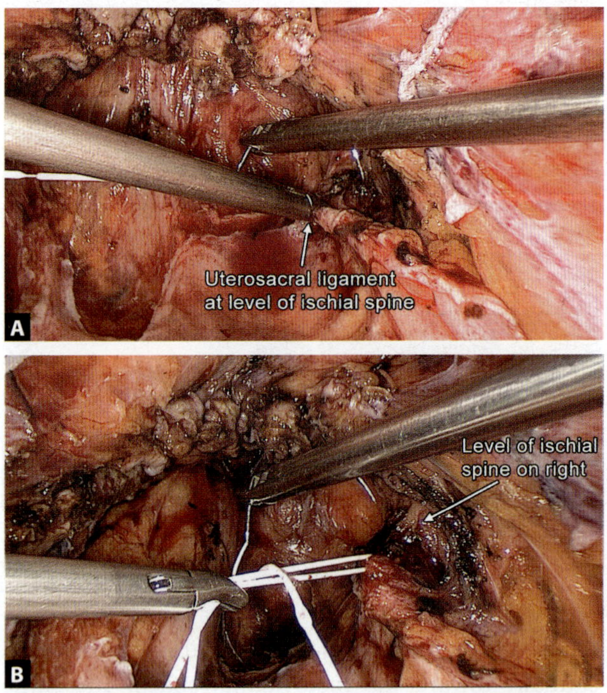

Figs. 40.13A and B: (A) Suturing the right uterosacral ligament with the first tissue purchase; (B) Suturing the right uterosacral ligament by lifting up on the initial suture placement to secure a deeper bite of the ligament.

the USL tissue. Note that if the suspension is taken too high above the level of the ischial spines, there is a risk of catching the piriformis muscle, which has some branches of sciatic nerve, causing bothersome postoperative symptoms of buttock pain, which radiates down to patient's posterior thigh and leg. If this occurs, the patient will have to return to the operating room for removal of the nerve-entrapping stitches immediately after the appearance of symptoms. In this event, the location of the ischial spines is reassessed and a new replacement suspension suture is placed. There is no risk of nerve entrapment when the suspension stitches are placed no higher than the level of the ischial spines. The apex of the vagina is sutured to the suspension stitches on both sides by incorporating the anterior and posterior fascia of the vagina or the posterior lateral cervix (Figs. 40.14 and 40.15). Special care must be paid to take sufficiently deep fascial bites at the vaginal apex, yet avoid penetration into the vaginal canal. The permanent nonabsorbable stitches in the vaginal canal through the epithelium can cause protracted granulation tissues and produce undesirable and troublesome vaginal discharge. The steps are then repeated on the contralateral side. The suspension stitches are tied without undue tension on the tissue. The tissue must be approximated without leaving any suture gaps. Additional sutures may be needed to accomplish this goal of approximating the tissue without undue tension and without suture gaps (Fig. 40.16).

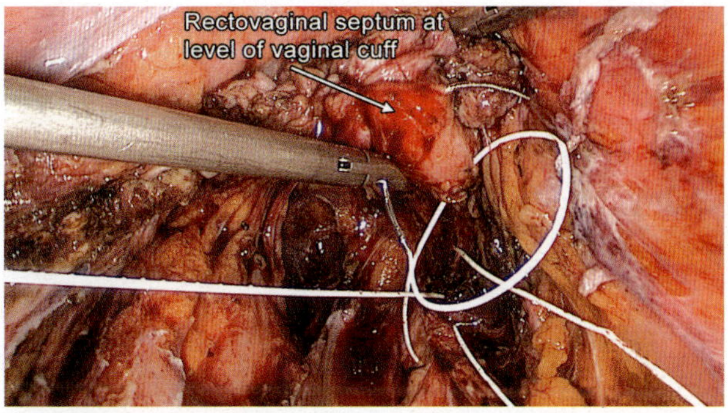

Fig. 40.14: Incorporating the rectovaginal septum at apex of vagina into the suspension.

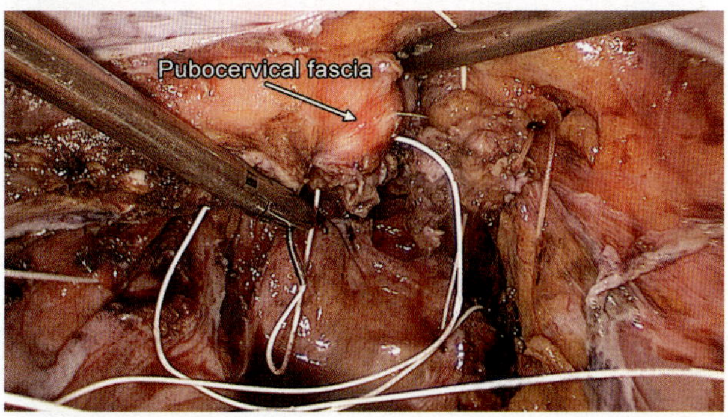

Fig. 40.15: Incorporating the pubocervical fascia at apex of vagina into the suspension.

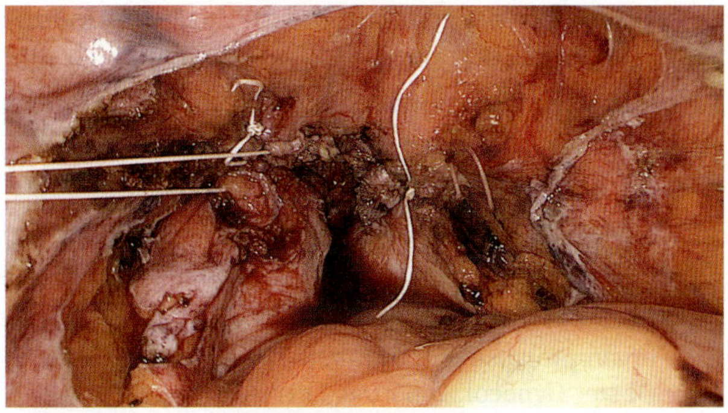

Fig. 40.16: Completing the suspension with extracorporeal sutures incorporating bilateral uterosacral ligaments, rectovaginal septum and pubocervical fascia.

Step 4: Reassessment of Pelvic Floor Support

A vaginal examination is performed to confirm that the vaginal apex is well supported and to ensure that no suture material is palpable within the vagina.

Cystoscopy

Cystoscopy is performed following completion of the suspension. A cystoscope is introduced into the bladder, and the urothelium is examined closely for any evidence of cystotomy and foreign suture material. Indigo carmine dye may be administered intravenously. Jetting of indigo carmine stained urine from the ureteric orifices confirms ureteral patency. However, other options for visualization of ureteral patency have been described, such as use of fluorescein dye, D50 dextrose, or phenazopyridine. Simple observation of concentrated urine in saline may suffice.

POSTOPERATIVE CONSIDERATIONS

Patients generally tolerate the laparoscopic USL suspension well and discharge is expected the same day or the first postoperative day. Specific complaints of pain and numbness radiating from the buttock to the posterior thigh in the postoperative period are concerning for entrapment or injury to the pudendal and/or sciatic nerves, and warrant immediate revision of the USL sutures. A voiding trial may be necessary prior to discharge to evaluate for urinary retention, particularly if a continence procedure was concurrently performed.

Patients are asked to adhere to lifting restrictions and pelvic rest for 6–8 weeks. In general, they should report that they feel better each day following surgery. Patients are evaluated in the office in 6 weeks, 3 and 6 months and annually thereafter.

REFERENCES

1. Boyles SH, Weber AM, Meyn L. Procedures for pelvic organ prolapse in the United States, 1979-1997. Am J Obstet Gynecol. 2003;188(1):108-15.
2. Olsen AL, Smith VJ, Bergstrom JO, et al. Epidemiology of surgically managed pelvic organ prolapse and urinary incontinence. Obstet Gynecol. 1997;89(4): 501-6.
3. Weber AM, Richter HE. Pelvic organ prolapse. Obstet Gynecol. 2005;106(3): 615-34.
4. Lowder JL, Park AJ, Ellison R, et al. The role of apical vaginal support in the appearance of anterior and posterior vaginal prolapse. Obstet Gynecol. 2008;111(1):152-7.
5. Summers A, Winkel LA, Hussain HK, et al. The relationship between anterior and apical compartment support. Am J Obstet Gynecol. 2006; 194(5):1438-43.
6. Umek WH, Morgan DM, Ashton-Miller JA, et al. Quantitative analysis of uterosacral ligament, origin and insertion points by MRI. Obstet Gynecol, 2004; 103(3):447-51.
7. Lin LL, Phelps JY, Liu CY. Laparoscopic vaginal vault suspension using uterosacral ligaments: a review of 133 cases. J Minim Invasive Gynecol. 2005;12(3): 216-20.
8. Seman EI, Cook JR, O'Shea RT. Two-year experience with laparoscopic pelvic floor repair. J Am Assoc Gynecol Laparosc. 2003;10(1):38-45.
9. Shull BL, Bachofen C, Coates KW, et al. A transvaginal approach to repair of apical and other associated sites of pelvic organ prolapse with uterosacral ligaments. Am J Obstet Gynecol. 2000;183(6):1365-73; discussion 1373-4.

41 Laparoscopic **Pectopexy**

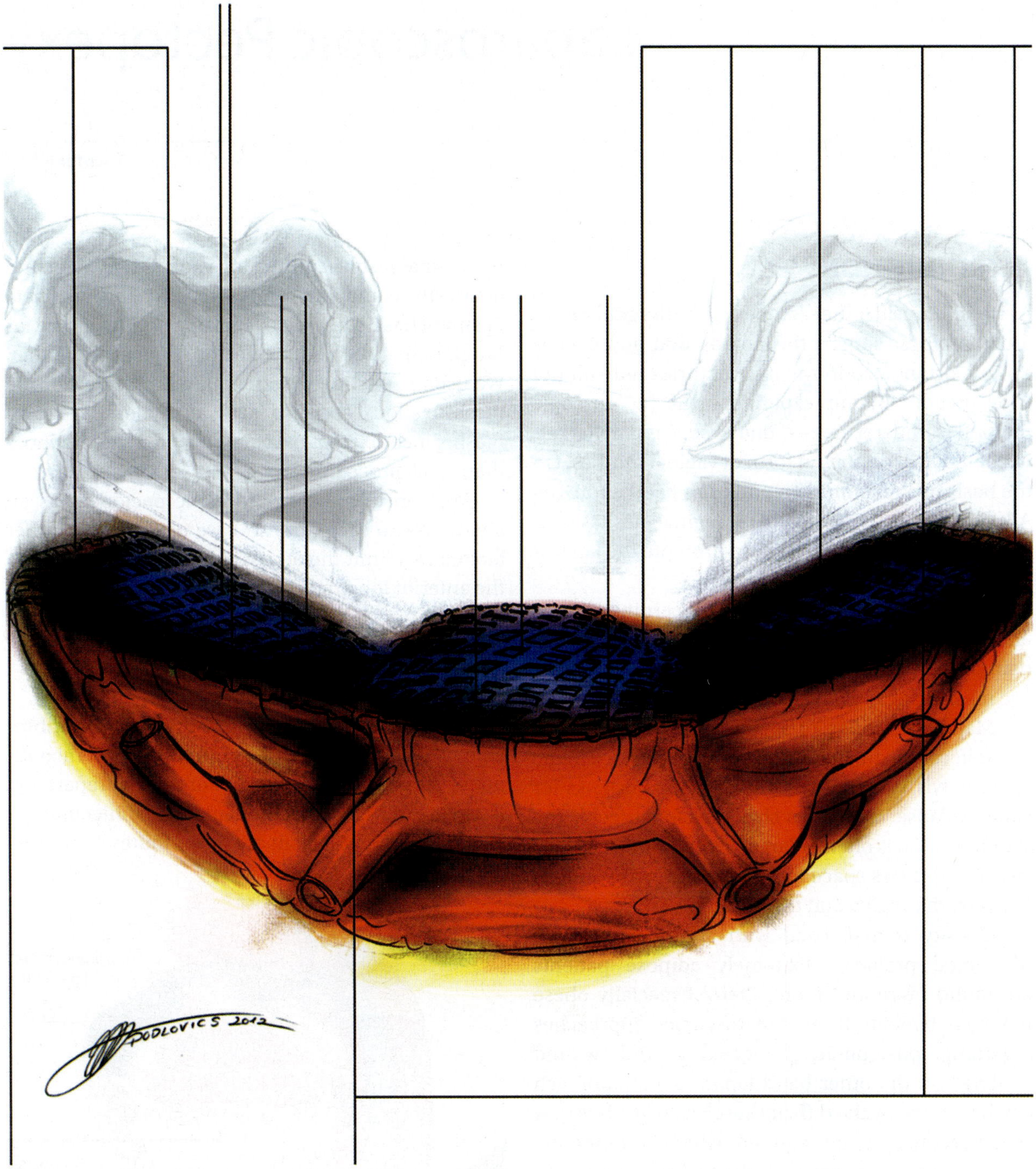

Chapter 41

Laparoscopic Pectopexy

Guenter K Noé

INTRODUCTION

As we still consider the sacropexy to be the gold standard in prolapse surgery the laparoscopic approach is the important step in the last centuries but still not widespread.[1-5] In our experience the laparoscopic method is underestimated due to successful marketing of medical devices in form of vaginal meshes. On the basis of a recommendation from Food and Drug Administration (FDA) not to use vaginal meshes first-line, it seems to be important to promote the laparoscopic procedures.

They offer several advantages concerning postoperative comfort, recovery time, scars, postoperative pain and duration of hospitalization.[6] We generally use meshes for less tension at the fixation points.[5,6]

Major difficulties of sacral colpopexy are ileus and defecation difficulties caused by less space in the lower pelvis. As obesity is one of the major risks for vault prolapse, it can be a challenge for surgery. The sigmoid colon is often enlarged by fatty tissue. In this case there is less space for the placement of a mesh between the vagina and the sacrum.

Obesity is associated with an increasing risk of genital prolapse. Extremely adipose patients are found more and more often.[7] Especially obese patients benefit from laparoscopic approaches regarding postoperative morbidity and wound healing. On the other hand laparoscopic approach can be limited by the difficult surgical field. Thus new repair techniques are required, which combine the benefits of laparoscopy with the unfavorable conditions we find in case of obesity.

In the following we describe a new approach of prolapse surgery using the lateral parts of pectineal ligament (Fig. 41.1). The new method is easier and more secure in patients with difficult surgical field. Functional results concerning vaginal size, slant and depth are comparable to sacropexy. The pectineal ligament has been used over a long period of time for Burch operation[8] and the pectopexy does this either. We use the pectineal ligament on both sides for the mesh fixation[10] so there is no restriction caused by mesh. Since 2007 we have now experience with more than 1,000 procedures.

We consider the laparoscopic pectopexy as an alternative to sacropexy in case of obesity or other factors that limit the access to the lesser pelvis or to the anterior longitudinal ligament. The indication for the pectopexy is the same as for a sacropexy.

PREOPERATIVE CONSIDERATIONS

As the technique uses its own pathways it is combinable with most techniques in prolapse and incontinence surgery. No special diet or bowel preparation is necessary. Low-dose subcutaneous injections of an antithrombosis agent are given routinely starting

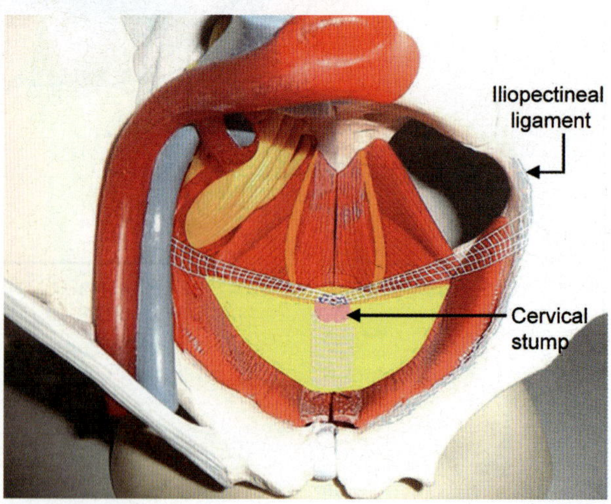

Fig. 41.1: Mesh position in the pelvis.

one evening before operation. Single-shot antibiotics (cefuroxime 1.5 g and metronidazole 0.5 g intravenously) should be applied routinely 20 min before starting surgery.

PROCEDURE

Step 1: Patient Preparation

The patient is placed in a dorsal lithotomy position with both arms tucked to her side. Depending on the expected operation time (longer than 1 h) or a second procedure (e.g., colposuspension) a 16 F catheter with a 10 mL balloon tip is inserted into the bladder and attached to a continuous drainage. Operation is done under general anesthesia.

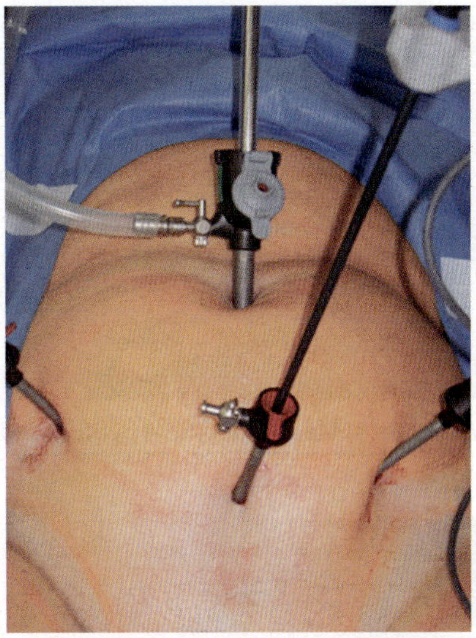

Fig. 41.2: Access port position.

Step 2: Insertion of Endoscope

Routinely we prefer to perform an incision in the middle of the umbilicus and insert a 12 mm access port to introduce the laparoscope. The abdomen is insufflated with CO_2 up to 12 mm Hg intra-abdominal pressure. Three additional 5 mm access ports are placed 2–4 cm medial and inferior the anterior superior iliac spine at both sides and 2–3 cm superior to symphysis (Fig. 41.2).

Step 3: Preparation of Iliopectineal Ligaments

The round ligament of uterus is used as first anatomic landmark. As a second landmark we identify the medial umbilical ligament. These two structures in general form a triangle, which fills the lateral part of the pectineal ligament under the peritoneum (Figs. 41.3A and B).

The preparation of ligament is started with a superficial incision of the peritoneum next to the round ligament (Fig 41.4A and B). A strict superficial preparation reduces the danger of an accidental injury of nerves and vessels.

After blunt preparation of the soft tissue of pelvic wall pectineal ligament can be identified. Some lymph nodes may be identified; in this case they should be pushed off. Coagulation of lymphatic vessels is required.

The iliac external vessels are visualized and pushed off. The ligament will be uncovered over 3.5 cm. This procedure is repeated on the left side. The psoas muscle is exposed (Figs. 41.5 to 41.7).

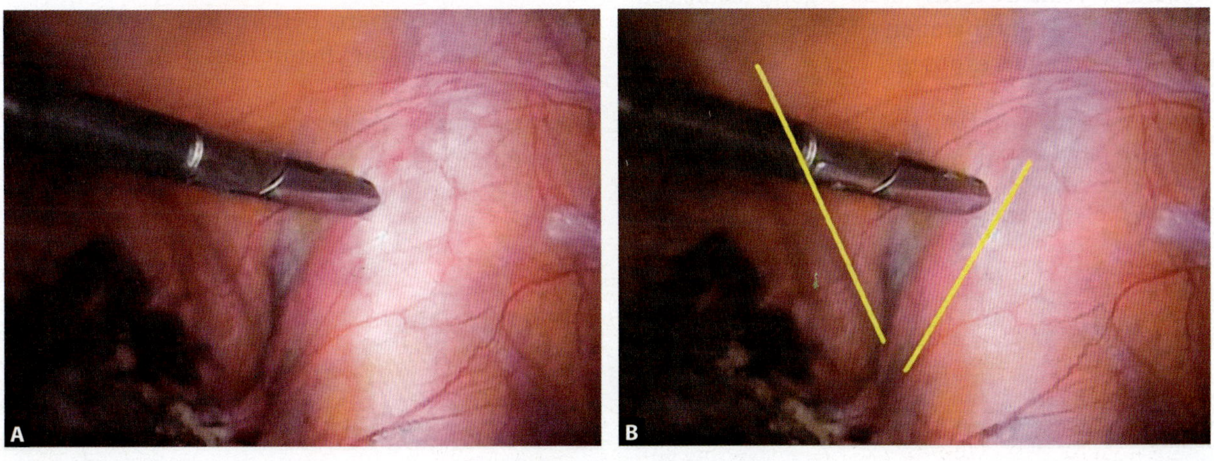

Figs. 41.3A and B: (A) Round ligament; (B) Medial umbilical and round ligaments.

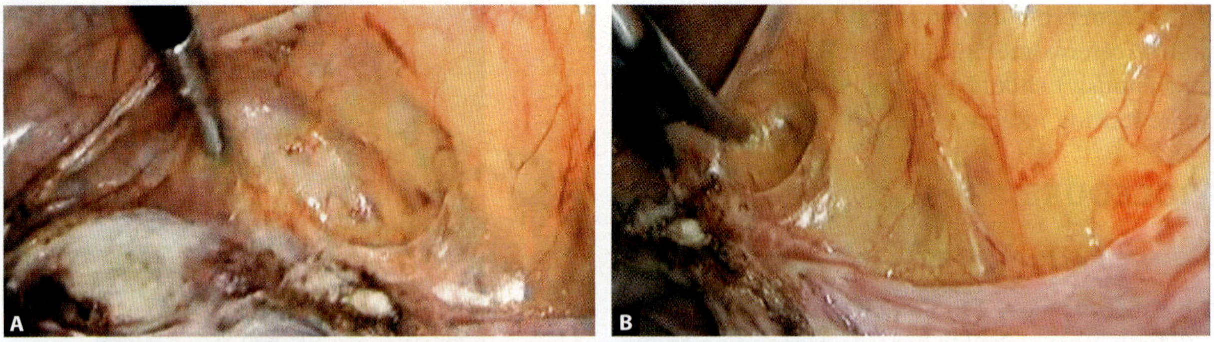

Figs. 41.4A and B: (A) Medial superficial peritoneal dissection; (B) Lateral superficial dissection.

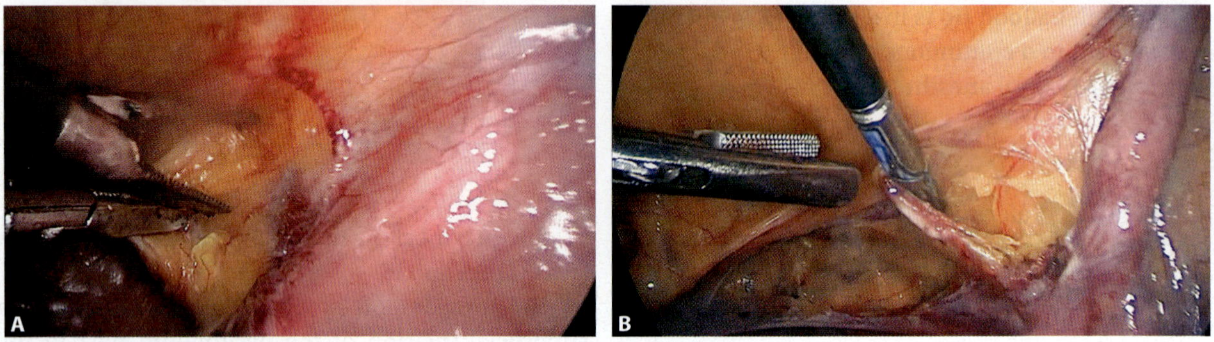

Figs. 41.5A and B: (A) Superficial incision fatty; (B) Pulling the umbilical ligament.

Step 4: Peritoneal and Vaginal Apex/ Cervical Stump Preparation

If peritoneum is not opened during hysterectomy, it has to be opened to the middle. If possible we would prefer to fix the mesh at the remaining cervical stump. The anterior and posterior brim of the cervical stump provides a good tissue for a stable fixation.

Patients who have undergone a complete hysterectomy receive a fixation directly to the apical vagina. Therefore the vagina is armed with a "Breisky vaginal speculum." It makes it easy to have good tactile sensation to do the preparation of vaginal stump. An area of 4 × 4 cm gets exposed.

Step 5: Mesh Fixation

We use a polyvinylidene fluoride (PVDF) monofilament mesh (e.g. DynaMesh® PRP, 3 × 15 cm). It is fixed with non-absorbable suture (0 with attached needle). Needle and mesh are inserted via the 12 mm port.

One end of the mesh is fixed with two stitches first at the right iliopectineal ligament.

The procedure is repeated at the left side. The positioning of mesh should be as cranial as possible. The assistant therefore has to extend the operation field by pushing the iliac vein while the stitch is performed.

All four knots are performed by intracorporal knot tying technique. Before continuing the needle

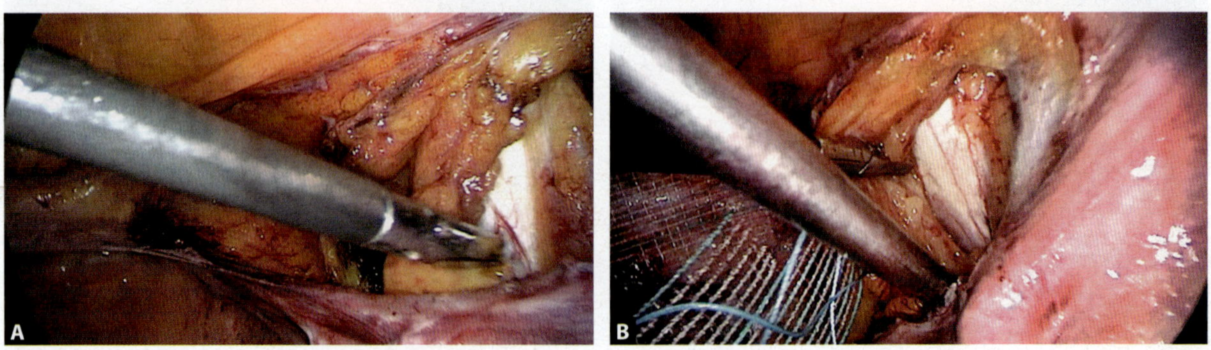

Figs. 41.6A and B: (A) Dissection of the lymphatic trunk; (B) Ligament, Psoas, iliacac vessel.

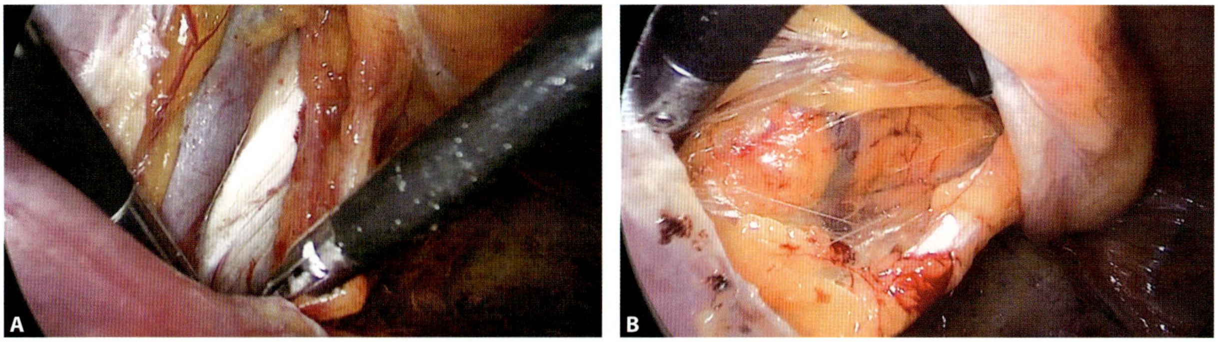

Figs. 41.7A and B: (A) Pectineal ligament on the left; (B) Med umbilical ligament left side under traction.

rest suture is removed. Central fixation will be done by a non-absorbable suture in case of a remaining cervical stump. Otherwise a polydioxanone suture PDS® (2-0) has proven to be feasible. It is important to use a monofilament suture to fix vagina. It is difficult to avoid penetration of the vaginal tissue because after hysterectomy it measures only 1–2 mm. In case of penetration a polyfilamental suture could accelerate an infection because of wicking.

The vaginal apex or cervical stump respectively is elevated to the intended tension-free position and fixed with a running suture in two rows to avoid wrinkling. The mesh will lie flat on the support base (Figs 41.8A and B).

If the mesh is too long it can easily be shortened by "darts" on both sides. Therefore the non-absorbable suture is recommended. Very rarely the mesh can be too short. In that case you should cut the mesh in the middle and suture it with a patch of another mesh. After fixing the mesh we recommend to close peritoneum properly to avoid hernia or adhesions. This can be achieved by a running suture starting on the right side (Vicryl 2-0; 35 cm) (Figs. 41.9 to 41.11).

After removing needle, suture rest and continuous urinary drainage CO_2 is released. We completely pass on any kind of intraabdominal drainage.

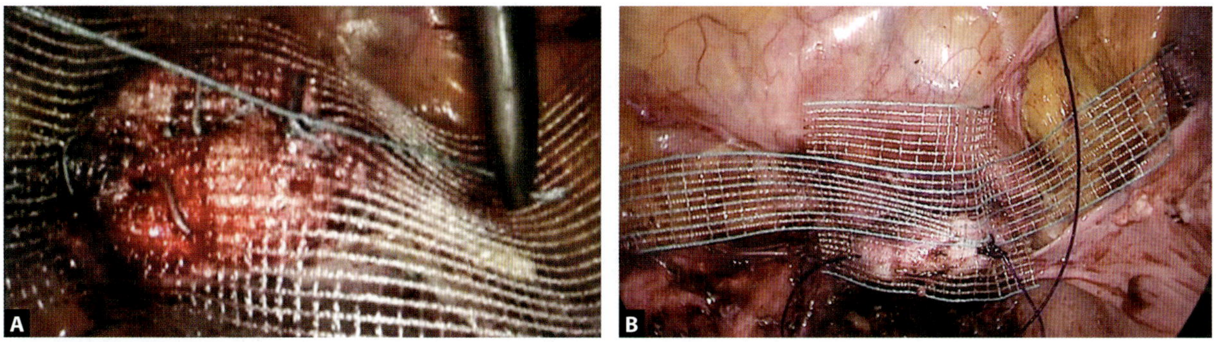

Figs. 41.8A and B: (A) Fixation at the cervical stump; (B) Fixation at the vagina.

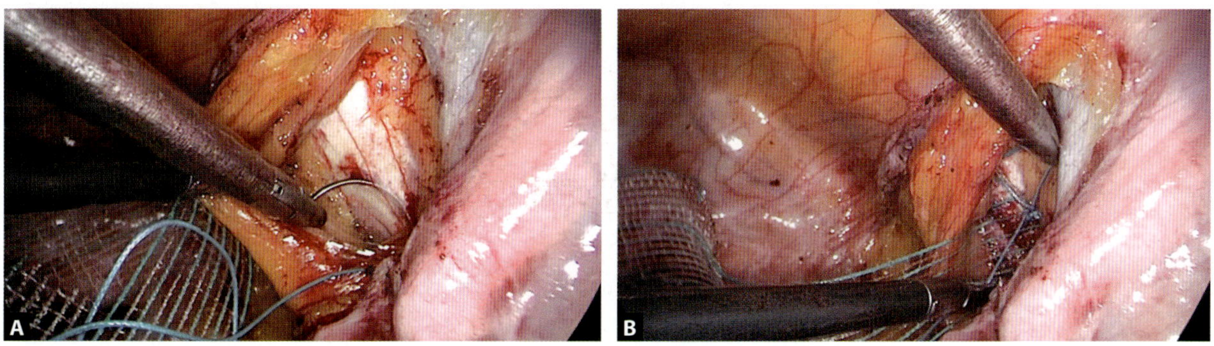

Figs. 41.9A and B: (A) First stich right pectineal ligament; (B) knot tying after second stich.

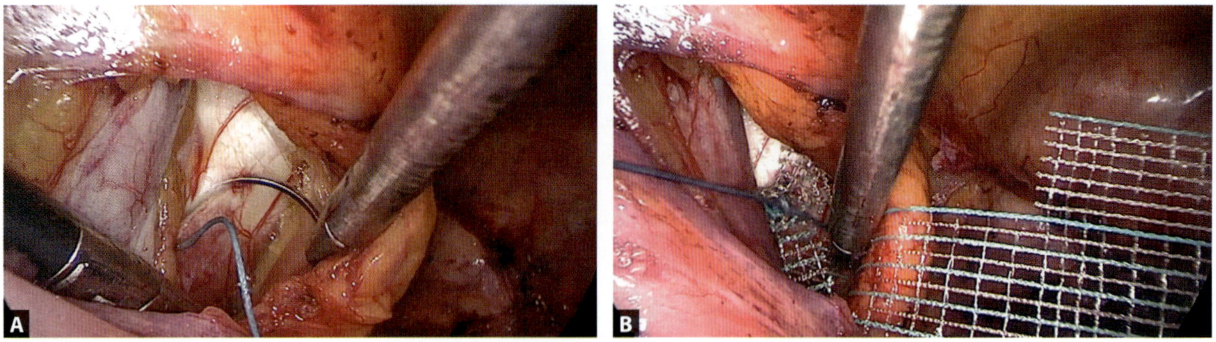

Figs. 41.10A and B: (A) First stich left pectineal ligament; (B) Knot tying left side.

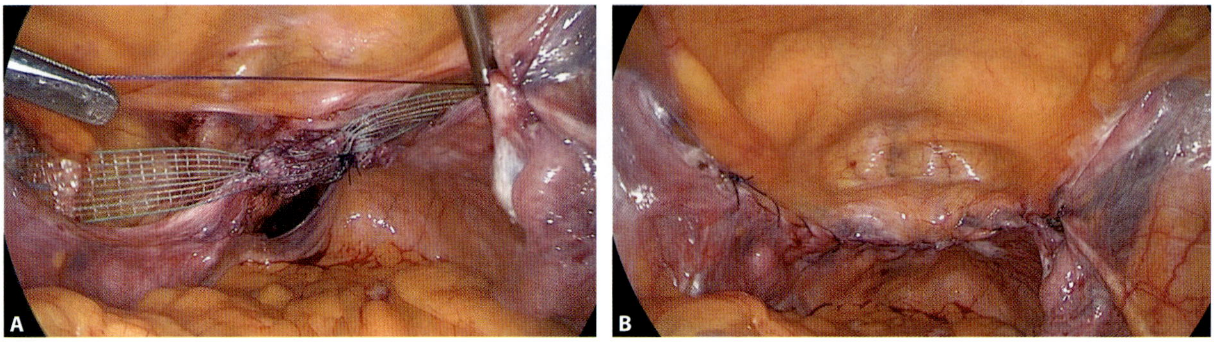

Figs. 41.11A and B: (A) Closure of the peritoneum; (B) Final result after closure of the peritoneum.

POSTOPERATIVE TREATMENT

Hospital stay is 3–5 days depending on the health conditions of the patient. Patients start with a mild form of pelvic floor exercise on the second day after surgery. Nonsteroidal antiphlogistics will be sufficient to reduce postoperative pain. It is not required to purge the bowels or to continue antibiotics.

EQUIPMENT

Full HD Camera 0°	
Access ports:	2–3 × 5 mm, 1 × 12 mm
Instruments:	1 scissor, 2 × universal (blunt) grasping forceps, 1 bipolar forceps,
1 needle holder	
PVDF mesh	15 cm × 3 cm (e.g. Dynamesh® PRP)
Lateral fixation:	2 suture (2-0 non-absorbable suture of 15 cm length with attached needle, and six knots with a short tale)
Caudal fixation:	Cervical stump fixation: 1 suture (2-0 non-absorbable suture of 25 cm Length with attached needle)
	Vaginal apex fixation: 1 PDS suture (2-0, 25 cm length with attached needle)
Peritoneum:	1 suture (2-0 absorbable suture of 35 cm length with attached needle)

According to our assessment pectopexy is a technique that is easily to learn by an experienced surgeon. So, it extends the portfolio of surgical options especially in difficult surgical fields.

Laparoscopic pectopexy provides a stable replacement of descended vaginal or uterine parts in combination with a good tension control to avoid over correction and the resulting negative side effects. The high acceptance of patients due to reduced morbidity by laparoscopic surgery increases having a new option in difficult cases. The long-term follow-up has to define the indication independently from surgical conditions.

As Cosson et al. showed that the pectineal ligament is statistically significantly stronger than the sacrospinous ligament and arcus tendineus of pelvic fascia[9] we expect a stable fixation at the ligament.

A superficial preparation of the peritoneum leads to bleedings and organ damage. Blunt dissection in the triangle cannot cause heavy bleedings, which are not manageable. Two structures should be handled carefully. Iliac vein should be protected during stitching. As it is a big structure this is good performable for an experienced surgeon. The obturator nerve lies at the deep end of the triangle. There is no need for such a deep preparation but if you want to go the same way the nerve can be uncovered bluntly with low risks. Other structures like bladder and ureter are not touched by the technique so that there is no need for special precautions.

The surgeon should be trained in laparoscopic suture and knotting techniques and have knowledge of anatomic retroperitoneal structures.

To date no major complications were seen. Some smaller complications like urinary infections or other postoperative urinary dysfunctions only were found in cases with combined surgery (vaginal approach or colpo-suspensions). Among more than 1,000 procedures we had four cases we had to re-operate for a seroma at the fixation points.

In a prospective randomized, controlled trial we could show that there are now new risks for the patients. In the pectopexy group no de-novo defecation disorders were seen, and in the sacropexy group it was 19%. Pectopexy also seems to be protective for de-novo lateral defects.[11,12]

TIPS AND TRICKS

- In case of a supracervical hysterectomy it can be useful to adjust the position of cervical stump by depositing a sponge or small sterile towel filling the vagina carefully. It makes it much easier to find the correct intraabdominal position (Fig. 41.12).

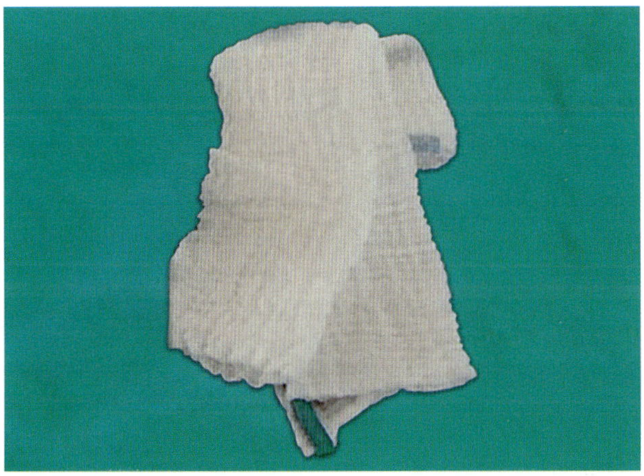

Figs. 41.12: Small towel to fill the vagina to esthimated length.

- In women who have had hysterectomy the margin at the vaginal stump is thin. It is no problem to penetrate while stitching. A mono filamental, absorbable suture can avoid infection (PDS).
- High tension (cranial) on the vaginal stump while dissecting the peritoneum and bladder makes it easier to find the layers.
- The most important landmark is the round ligament. In case of heavy fatty tissue you cannot feel out the symphysis. After superficial preparation along the ligament push the fatty tissue begins at the most lateral point of the ligament.
- The optimal angle for mesh can be achieved if the first stitch is positioned underneath the iliac vein. The tip of the needle should point inward to reduce the risk of injuring the vein.
- Training on model facilitates orientation and reduces stress during the first surgeries. We have a simple wooden model for our pelvitrainer. Ligaments are simulated by plaster.
- All suturing is done using the middle access port. I would suggest not deviating from this procedure until the first 10 surgeries are done successfully.
- The fixation of the PRP mesh can also be started in the middle. This provides the direct determination of the correct length.

REFERENCES

1. Nygaard IE, McCreery R, Brubaker L, et al., Pelvic Floor Disorders Network. Abdominal colpopexy: a comprehensive review. Obstet Gynecol. 2004; 104(4): 805-23.
2. David-Montefiore E, Barranger E, Dubernard G, et al. Functional results and quality of life after bilateral sacrospinous ligament fixation for genital prolapse. Eur J Obstet Gynecol Reprod Biol. 2007;132(2): 209-13.
3. Maher C, Baessler K, Glazener C, et al. Surgical management of pelvic organ prolapse in women. Cochrane Database of System Rev. 2004;4:233-46.
4. Beer M, Kuhn A. Surgical techniques for vault prolapse: a review of the literature. Eur J Obstet Gynecol. 2005;119(2):144-55.
5. Rivoire C, Botchorishvili R, Canis M, et al. Complete laparoscopic treatment of genital prolapse with meshes including vaginal promontofixation and anterior repair: a series of 138 patients. J Min Invas Gynecol. 2007;14(6):712-8.
6. Gadonneix P, Ercoli A, Salet-Lizeé D. Laparoscopic sacrocolpopexy with two separate meshes along the anterior and posterior vaginal walls for multicompartment pelvic organ prolapse. J Am Assoc Gynecol Laparosc. 2004;11(1):26-35.

7. Irvine L, Shaw R. The effects of patient obesity in gynaecological practice. Curr Opin Obstet Gyn. 2003;13:179-84.
8. Miklos J, Kohli N. Laparoscopic paravaginal repair plus Burch colposuspension: review and descriptive technique. Urology. 2000;56(6 Suppl 1):64-9.
9. Cosson M, Boukerrou M, Lacaze S, et al. A study of pelvic ligament strength. Eur J Obstet Gynecol Reprod Biol. 2003;109(1):80-7.
10. Banerjee C, Noé KG. Laparoscopic pectopexy: a new technique of prolapse surgery for obese patients Arch Gynecol Obstet. 2011;284(3):631-5.
11. Noe KG, Spuntrup C, Anapolski M. Laparoscopic pectopexy: a randomised comparative clinical trial of standard laparoscopic sacral colpo-cervicopexy to the new laparoscopic pectopexy. Short-term post-operative results. Arch Gynecol Obstet. 2013; 287(2): 275-80.
12. Noe KG, Schiermier S, Alkaout I, et al. Laparoscopic pectopexy: a prospective, randomized, comparative clinical trial of standard laparoscopic sacral colpocervicopexy with the new laparoscopic pectopexy-postoperative results and intermediate-term follow-up in a pilot study. J Endourol. 2015;29(2): 210-5.

Esthetic Aspects of Pelvic Floor Repair

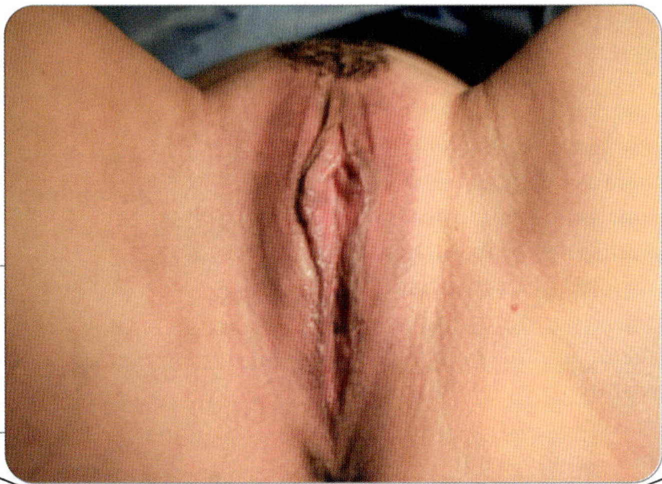

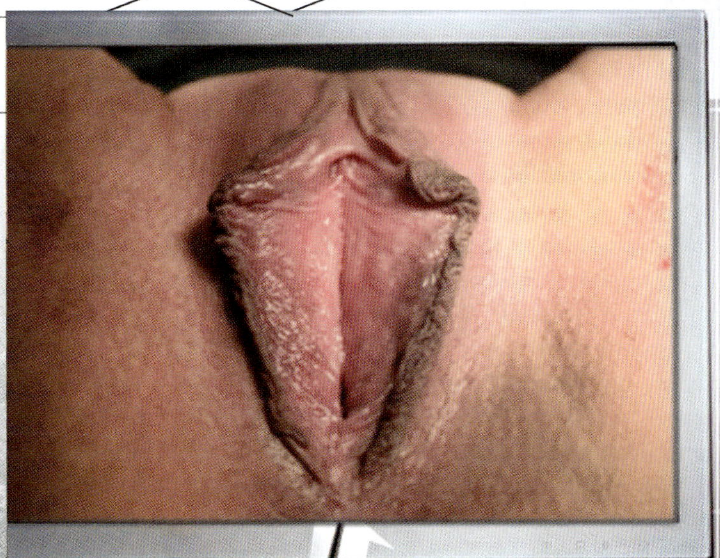

Chapter 42

Esthetic Aspects of Pelvic Floor Repair

Rupinder Kaur Ruprai, Alexandros Bader

INTRODUCTION

As women age, physiologic changes in genital region occur. In an aging vagina, there is laxity and loss of tone in pelvic floor. The mons pubis progressively enlarges through fat deposits and sags, whereas there is loss of volume in labia majora, further enhancing the visual sagging impact. Hypertrophy of labia minora occurs that may be secondary to mechanical irritation by intercourse/masturbation, childbirth, lymph-statis, myelodysplastic disease, irritation from chronic dermatitis/urinary incontinence; hereditary factors may also play a role.

Vagina and its supportive tissues are actively remodeled in response to different environmental stimuli. Not only synthesis of structural proteins, but also balance between activity of major proteolytic enzymes that degrade them, and inhibitors of proteolysis are important components to consider in the pathogenesis of pelvic organ prolapse (POP), which is estimated to affect almost 50% of women above the age of 50 years, and has a lifetime prevalence of 30–50%.[1]

The esthetic and functional procedures that compromise female genital cosmetic surgery (FGCS) include traditional vaginal prolapse procedures as well as cosmetic vulvar and labial procedures. The distinction between cosmetic and therapeutic procedures is not well defined. While significant advances have been made in the minimally invasive field that offers the added advantage of cosmesis, the same momentum has not been generated for pelvic floor repair (PFR). Often, repairs employ traditional suturing techniques, and more often than not, tissue scarring and/or esthetic appearance of tissues is ignored. Women seeking FGCS need to be evaluated for pelvic support disorders (POP and stress urinary incontinence [SUI]), and should act autonomously without coercion from partners or surgeons. This chapter attempts to address esthetic aspects of PFR, means to ensuring optimal results during and following PFR, and gives an overview of current understanding of biomolecular changes during tissue remodeling.

PELVIC FLOOR AND TISSUE REMODELING

Pelvic Floor Connective Tissue

Vaginal wall is composed of four layers: superficial layer of stratified squamous epithelium, subepithelial dense connective tissue layer (composed primarily of collagen and elastin), layer of smooth muscle (muscularis) and adventitia (composed of loose connective tissue). Vaginal subepithelium and muscularis together form a fibromuscular layer beneath the vaginal epithelium, providing longitudinal and central support.

The connective tissue underlying vagina contains relatively a few cells: mainly fibroblasts producing components of extracellular matrix (ECM), besides fat cells and mast cells. All elements are embedded in an ECM, composed of fibrillar elements (collagen and elastic fibers) embedded in non-fibrillar viscoelastic matrix/ground substance (proteoglycans, glycoproteins and hyaluronan). These tissues contain significant amount of smooth muscle cells (with exception of arcus tendinous fasciae pelvis).[2] The fibrillar component contributes the most to the biomechanical behavior of these tissues in the vaginal wall, and passive tissue strength is provided by ECM. Collagen and elastin are the two major ECM components of pelvic floor connective tissues, providing resistance to stretching and other tensile forces, and elasticity and resilience to the tissues, respectively, whereas structural glycoproteins create tissue cohesiveness. The ECM of vaginal tissue largely determines its tissue tensile strength, and its mechanical stability is remodeled and maintained by fibroblasts. It is the delicate balance between production and degradation of ECM proteins in connective tissue that is critical to the pelvic floor integrity.[3]

Collagen

There are 28 types of collagen. Collagens I, III and V, present in the vagina, and its supportive tissues are thought to be the principal determinants of soft tissue strength. Collagen I fibers are universally present and are large, high-tensile strength fibers and offer strength and great resistance to tension. Collagen III forms smaller fibers of lower tensile strength, are predominant in tissues that require increased flexibility and distension and that are subject to periodic stress, and is the major collagen subtype in vagina.[4] It is the primary collagen subtype in vagina and supportive tissues. Type V collagen forms small fibers of low tensile strength, and its role in the vagina and supportive tissue has not been elucidated yet. Type III and V collagen fibers copolymerize with type I collagen to form fibrils with controlled diameters and tensile strength. These fibrils influence the biomechanical characteristics of a given tissue. Higher higher I/III ratio results in higher tensile strength. An increase in collagen III and V decreases the mechanical strength of connective tissue by decreasing fiber size.[5] Cross-linking of tropoelastin and procollagen to form mature functional collagen and elastin fibers is by lysyl oxidase (LOX) family of enzymes.[6]

Mature, slowly metabolizing collagen is susceptible to non-enzymatic cross-linking, known as glycation/Maillard reaction. These advanced glycated end products (AGEs) of collagen accumulate with age. The "over mature" collagen is stiffer and more fragile.[7] This mechanism is the major cause of substantial dysfunction of collagenous tissues and is responsible for complications of connective tissues seen at older age.

Elastin

Elastin, an insoluble polymer, is formed by assembly of tropo-elastin monomers by lysyl oxidases (LOX). Elastin allows the tissue to stretch and return to its original shape without energy input. In most organs, elastin biosynthesis is limited to a brief period of development. The assembly of elastic fibers is complete by maturity when tropo-elastin synthesis ceases. In undisturbed tissues, elastic fibers produced in the third trimester of fetal life last the rest of life.[7] In the female reproductive tract, however, elastic fiber turnover is continuous. The LOX is essential for elastic fiber homeostasis.[8] Fibulin-5 (elastic binding protein crucial for elastic fiber assembly[9]) acts as a bridge between cells and tropo-elastin for effective cross-linking and assembly of tropo-elastin into mature elastic fibers. Increased synthesis of tropo-elastin and fibulin-5 may be necessary to counteract for disruption of elastic fibers and to regenerate elastic fibers in the vaginal wall. Synthesis and assembly of elastic fibers are crucial for recovery of pelvic organ support after damage.

The quantity and quality of collagen and elastin are regulated through a precise equilibrium between synthesis, maturation and degradation, and this process results in a dynamic process of constant remodeling is important for maintaining tissue integrity and tensile strength. They remodel their surrounding matrix in response to mechanical and biochemical stimuli. Precursor collagens and elastin are synthesized by fibroblasts and are then secreted into ECM as raw material of fibril assembly. These mechanosensitive cells produce anabolic proteins such as collagens, and activate catabolic/ proteolytic enzymes, such as matrix metalloproteinases (MMPs). Degradation depends upon combined activity of MMPs and their regulation of release, activation or sequestration of growth factors, growth factor binding proteins, cell surface receptors and cell–cell adhesion molecules.[7] MMPs degrade ECM components (collagen, elastin, proteoglycans and glycoproteins) and are responsible for loss of strength of fibrous collagen and hence loss of tissue integrity. Activity of MMPs is antagonized by tissue-derived inhibitors of metalloproteinases (TIMPs).[7]

Transforming growth factor-β1 (TGF-β1), as an important regulator of fibrotic metabolism, and is involved in fibrosis and degenerative fibrotic disease[10] that induces fibroblast differentiation, promotes collagen and elastin synthesis and reduces degradation by inhibiting MMPs and upregulating TIMPs.[11] The TGF-β1 reduces the level of collagenase mRNA and increases the level of TIMP mRNA.[12]

Alpha-2 macroglobulin (a2-M) is an extracellular panproteinase inhibitor with a broad-specificity proteinase inhibitory ability in ECM.[13] The quantity and quality of collagen, elastin and other components in the pelvic supporting tissues are maintained through a precise balance between proteolytic and a2-M inhibitory activity in ECM. Decreased a2-M expression and protease inhibitory activity result in higher proteolytic activity. The a2-M is also a carrier of tissue repair growth factors, such as TGF-β1.[14]

BIOMOLECULAR CHANGES AND CLINICAL IMPACTS

Physiological ovarian hormones variation[6] modulates expression of specific groups of enzymes responsible for formation and degradation of collagen and/or elastin fibers in human vagina. Estrogen receptors (ERs) are present in structures that support pelvic organs, including vagina, corroborate for ovarian hormones modulation of pelvic floor. Decreased levels of estrogen and progesterone receptors are seen in postmenopausal POP women. Estrogen and progestogen may control vaginal collagen metabolism, and estrogen environment is protective against collagen degradation via MMP1/TIMP1 homeostasis. There is an estrogen-mediated increase in TIMP1 expression in cultured fibroblasts from human vagina,[15] and increased overall collagen metabolism during proliferative phase of menstrual cycle. There is significant increase in LOXL4 mRNA expression during estrogen-dominant proliferative phase compared to secretory phase.[16] Genes responsible for vaginal ECM metabolism are modulated by the hormonal fluctuation during the menstrual cycle.[6]

The synthesis of components of ECM by fibroblasts is influenced by stretch. Mechanical stretch disturbs fibroblasts' ability to maintain the cytoskeleton architecture. Estrogens do not reverse the process or protect cells from the effect of stretch, but significantly increase the rate of fibroblast proliferation, suggesting their role in the healing process.[7]

Causes/Influencers: Age, Genetic, Radiation, Diet, Exercise, Surgery[7,17]

Pelvic floor defects are visible as a bulge on anterior and/posterior vaginal walls with resultant SUI, incomplete defecation/fecal incontinence, chronic pelvic pain, vaginal relaxation, sexual dysfunction and social isolation. In some cases, the only complaint may be the appearance.

Factors contributing to development of POP can be divided into genetic and acquired factors. Acquired factors include pregnancy and parity as well as myopathy and neuropathy. Obesity, smoking, pulmonary disease and obstipation are examples of POP-promoting factors. Patients with these risk factors tend to develop POP in a higher frequency with aging and menopause as superimposing decompensation factors.

Where pelvic floor muscles are weakened, decrease in pelvic connective tissue resilience—related to age and menopause—may facilitate progression to symptomatic POP. Age is a risk factor for POP. There is a 10% increased risk for each decade of life.[18] The cumulative incidence of primary operation for POP and incontinence increase from 0.1% in age group 20–29, up to 11.1% in age group 70–79.[19] Among types of POP, cystocele has the greatest incidence.[20] POP is one of the most common reasons for gynecological surgery in women after the fertile period. The failure rate is relatively high: an estimated 30% of women require re-operation.[19] The biomechanical microenvironment may be further compromised if non-resorbable polymeric meshes are used to replace tissue function.[21]

Genetic predisposition may play a role as well. When a mother has POP, the relative risk for the daughter of developing POP is 3.2. With a sister's positive medical history, this relative risk is 2.4.

Parity is the strongest factor in development of POP. After an injury such as childbirth, supporting connective tissue of vaginal wall will remodel itself in order to adapt to the tensile stress. During childbirth, neuromuscular damage occurs. Not only direct injury to levator ani muscle resulting in mechanical disruption, but also damage to nerve supply, especially pudendal nerve, can lead to their inability to contract. When pelvic floor muscles relax or are damaged, suspensory ligaments sustain the load of pelvic organs for short periods of time, connective tissues stretch and eventually fail if pelvic floor muscles do not close the pelvic floor in time. The increased flexibility and decreased tensile strength associated with an increase in collagen III, together with decrease in elastin levels, likely contribute to progression of POP. Other childbirth-related factors associated with prolapse include high infant birth weight, prolonged second stage of labor, and maternal age less than 25 years at first delivery.

Pelvic surgery: Retropubic urethropexy or needle suspension procedures may result in more anterior deviation of anterior vaginal wall, which alters the distribution of force on all of vaginal walls. As a result, apex and posterior vaginal wall may become prone to development of support defects, including enterocele or rectocele.

Elevated intra-abdominal pressure: Women who are laborers/factory workers, chronic constipation, chronic obstructive pulmonary disease, may cause stretch injury to pudendal nerve.

Increasing body mass index (*BMI*): Women with BMI >25 kg/m^2 have a threefold higher risk of having POP compared to nonobese women. Women with joint hypermobility have a significant higher prevalence of POP; connective tissue factor is involved. With collagen abnormality, women may metabolize collagen such that there is a decrease in type I collagen and an increase in type III collagen.

Pelvic Floor Connective Tissue in POP

The tissue that supports vagina and pelvic organs can be divided into suspensory system part (De Lanceys' level I and II) and supportive part (level III).[22] Quantity, type and organization of collagen, elastin and smooth muscles cells vary within different tissues.[23] Para-colpium and uterosacral and cardinal ligaments have a different composition when compared to the vaginal tissue.[24]

Pelvic floor tissues in POP/ SUI have decrease in total collagen content, with higher rate of immature collagen more susceptible to rupture,[23] and deficiency of ECM components.[13,24] Accelerated remodeling of ECM is observed in pelvic supporting tissues in women with SUI and/or POP. The relative activity of MMPs is increased and their respective inhibitors (TIMP-1) is decreased in vaginal wall tissues of women with POP/ SUI.[13] Dysregulation of balance of ECM synthesis/ degradation, in parallel with changes in mature collagen fiber composition, compromise the quality of connective tissue leading to prolapse. There is reduced total collagen content, with relatively high content of immature collagen cross-links. The newly formed collagen is degraded more easily than older glycated material, resulting in bulk of deficient glycated old, brittle collagen that is difficult to degrade and susceptible to rupture with impaired mechanical tissue strength.[7] The bulk of this deficient glycated old collagen, which is brittle and susceptible to rupture, is an important etiologic factor in POP.

Collagen Synthesis and Subtypes in POP

There is an increase in type III,[7] resulting in decreased I/III ratio. Increase in collagen III in combination with increase in MMP-9 is typical of tissue that is remodeling after injury or a tissue that is remodeling to accommodate a progressively increasing mechanical load.[25] Increased type III collagen within muscularis layer appears to result from phenotypic switch from SMCs to myofibroblasts, in the absence of apoptosis.[26] An increase in MMP-9 specifically in women with POP is associated with tissue remodeling.[7]

Inhibitor of MMP

Increased metabolic turnover of collagen (higher MMP-2 and MMP-9) in prolapse tissue is seen that accelerates degradation of connective tissue in vagina and supportive tissue in POP (increased MMP expression and decreased TIMP-1 expression).[7]

Elastin Metabolism in POP

A deficient synthesis and degradation of elastic fibers may be associated with POP.[7,24]

Fibroblast in POP

The quantity (cellularity) of supporting and contractile cells, fibroblasts, and quality (functionality of fibroblast), in connective tissue may be disturbed in POP. It is not related to defects in capacity of vaginal fibroblasts to synthesize/process procollagen. The contractibility of vaginal (myo)fibroblasts is decreased in POP, which may result in deficient collagen.[7]

Differences in stress loads can upregulate different proteins. The expression of collagen III is upregulated in women with POP.[11] Mechanical stress during birthing process, with predisposing risk factors, could result in reduced SMC contractile function in muscularis of anterior wall of vagina concomitant with acquisition of synthetic phenotype, resulting in deposition of an excessive quantity of ECM that eventually compromises the function of pelvic floor.

Morphological alterations of anterior vaginal wall are characterized by disorganization of architecture of the *muscularis* in POP.[26] Collagen fibers are loosely dispersed among the poorly organized muscle bundles. In vaginal *muscularis*, there is increased expression of type III collagen (thinner) and reduced expression of type I collagen (thicker more robust). Smooth muscle cells are more disorganized and disrupted in POP. Collagen III deposition and rare elastic fibers are seen, distinguished by typical wave-like aspect, interspersed among muscular fiber bundles, resulting in alteration of normal architecture of *muscularis propria*. These cell type, driven by platelet-derived growth factor β (PDGF β), can lead to phenotypic modulation (aberrant transition from quiescent contractile phenotype to myofibroblast-like proliferative synthetic state). During transition to synthetic phenotype, activated myofibroblasts synthesize ECM causing tissue remodeling.[26]

Platelet-derived growth factor (PDGF) is overexpressed in POP samples and may be involved in this metaplastic smooth muscle cell to myofibroblast trans-differentiation. Its expression is low under normal conditions but is increased in several pathological conditions. Mechanical and physical stress activates PDGF signaling pathway in smooth muscle cells, resulting in muscle remodeling. The PDGF promotes fibroblast migration and is responsible for excessive deposition of ECM leading to aberrant organ fibrosis with significant local and systemic consequences.[26] Abnormal levels of connective tissue within the *muscularis* of anterior wall of vagina in POP is associated with an increased MMP expression and may be implicated in remodeling of this excessive matrix.[27]

Together with increased type III collagen and MMP activity and decreased TIMP activity is linked to a stress mechanism activated by overstretching of pelvic connective tissue results in consequent tissue remodeling and adaptation.[3,6,26] There is also a reduction in concentration of elastin and rise in elastinolitic activity in endopelvic fascia and vaginal wall.[26,28]

Decreased expression of a2-M mRNA and protein and protease inhibitory activity in vaginal wall tissues may contribute to the development of SUI. Low level of a2-M causes decreased synthesis of ECM components through a decrease in TGF-b1. As a result, the weakened connective tissues lose their tensile strength and mechanical stability, accelerating the development of SUI.[13]

The molecular mechanisms underlying POP in women after menopause are different from the ones observed in premenopausal women. Pelvic tissue from women with SUI and POP show a genetic predisposition to abnormal ECM remodeling, which is modulated by reproductive hormones, trauma, mechanical stress load and aging. Positive family history of POP and incidence of concomitant SUI are significantly higher in POP patients, suggesting a possible familial inheritance of genes involved in pathophysiology. The ECM metabolisms are modulated by reproductive hormones and selective estrogen receptor modulators.[10] Physiological ovarian hormones variation can regulate ECM degrading proteins.

Ovarian hormone deficiency and aging are known to influence the quality of pelvic floor tissue. Molecular mechanisms involving vaginal ECM deficiency in POP differ between women before and after menopause. Age and menopause influence the expression of genes involved in ECM biogenesis and remodeling in vaginal tissues of older women with POP. There is an alteration in expression of genes coding for MMPs, TIMPs and LOXs enzymes.

Expression of all MMPs is dramatically downregulated in women after menopause. All TIMPs are decreased in vaginal biopsies of postmenopausal POP patients indicating that mechanism of their regulation is independent of menopausal status. The protective effect of ovarian hormones on ECM-regulating enzymes seen in asymptomatic women during proliferative phase as compared to secretory phase of menstrual cycle is lost in POP,[6] possibly due to acquired effects or risk factors associated with increased mechanical loading of pelvic floor that can cause POP.[3]

Expression of LOX, LOXL1 and LOXL3 genes and proteins is diminished in premenopausal POP.[6] LOXL2 enzyme is significantly upregulated in postmenopausal compared to premenopausal women without POP. The LOX enzymes and their substrate elastin expression also diminish with age. This correlation reflects an increased incidence of pelvic floor diseases in the elderly. LOXL2 gene is significantly downregulated in vagina of the postmenopausal with severe POP.[6]

HISTOLOGICAL CHANGES WITH TISSUE REMODELING[29]

Premenopausal vaginal mucosa is characterized by squamous stratified nonkeratinized epithelium and lamina propria protruding into undersurface of epithelium, with papillae rich in small blood vessels. The connective tissue is rich in fibrillar and nonfibrillar components (as described above), and in blood vessels, that penetrate as small capillaries inside the papillae, providing metabolic support (nutrients, oxygen and other molecules) to intermediate and superficial cell layers. The high permeability of the matrix permits easy diffusion of water, ions, nutrients and signaling molecules, through the ECM maintaining tissue hydration. Epithelial cells proliferate from the basal layer, as they differentiate and move toward the mucosal surface and eventually shed off. Glycogen synthesized by the intermediate cells is stored in the superficial cells from where it is eventually released and utilized by Lactobacilli, maintaining the acidic pH of vagina.

Postmenopausal vaginal mucosa is characterized by tissue atrophy, with significant thinning with reduction of epithelial layers, renewal dynamics and absence of superficial cell desquamation. The epithelium-connective tissue interface effaces smooth due to reduction and/or absence of papillae and blood vessels. There is significant reduction in fibrillar components quantity and quality. Fibroblasts are characterized by smaller cytoplasm. Cells exhibit lower number of organelles, especially the rough endoplasmic reticulum (RER) and Golgi apparatus, both of which are involved in synthesis and turnover of molecular components of ECM.

TRADITIONAL UNDERTAKING OF PELVIC FLOOR REPAIR: ADDRESSING REPAIRS OF DEFECTS, VAGINAL LENGTH

Traditional undertaking of PFR has been to repair with closest possible anatomical correction, which has typically involved anterior colporrhaphy and/or posterior colpoperineorrhaphy and lateral vaginal wall/site-specific defects. Repairs have often involved steps to ensure adequate vaginal length with the aim to not just address the vaginal length for structural support, but also to ensure sexual functionality. Often, little importance is given to sexual functionality, where vaginal caliber is not tested during repair and the resultant outcome is a tight introitus leading to dyspareunia, or even as a result of tissue fibrosis where tissue handling for optimal results has been overlooked.

EXTERNAL GENITALIA: BRIEF ON ANATOMY AND VASCULAR LANDMARKS[30]

With increasing demand for labiaplasty, vaginoplasty and vaginal rejuvenation procedures it is fundamental to have a complete knowledge of local anatomy to avoid inadvertent injury to neurovascular structures and to obtain an optimal outcome and normal physiological changes occurring within the anatomy. The intimate relationship between the muscles, ligaments and fascia that provide support is critical to restore during surgery for correction of prolapse or esthetic surgeries. The internal and external genitalia are closely related to muscles and fascia, and work as one functioning unit. The external female genitalia include mons pubis, labia majora and minora, clitoris, vestibular bulbs with glands, perineal body, and muscles and fascia surrounding these structures. Through the perineal membrane and perineal body, these structures are structurally related to deep pelvic muscle levator ani with its fascia. Levator ani along with coccygeus forms pelvic floor and provides support and stability to the perineum. The endopelvic fascia, surrounding the pelvic organs, is continuous with paraurethral and paravaginal fascia attached to perineal membrane. The vagina, urethra and rectum pass through the pelvic diaphragm formed by levator ani to open into vestibule. The remnants of hymen surround the vaginal opening. Vestibule is surrounded by labia minora and majora on each side and perineal body posteriorly. Perineal body is the meeting point of superficial perineal muscles, levator ani and perineal membrane providing stability to the area. The perineal membrane is a triangular fibromuscular structure that extends from ischial tuberosities laterally to pubic bone anteriorly.

External Genitalia

The blood supply is through multiple collaterals from the internal and external pudendal artery.

- *Anatomy and histology*: The skin of external genitals is comprised of epidermis, dermis and subcutaneous tissue. Epidermis has stratified squamous epithelium containing basal cells (that form keratinocytes) and keratinocytes. Cells divide in the basal layer and move up, resulting in continuous replacement of cells in the epidermal layer. Keratinocytes synthesize insoluble protein and becomes the stratum corneum. The dermis has an upper, thin papillary layer, composed of thin randomly arranged collagen fibers and a deeper reticular layer, with thick collagen fibers arranged parallel to the surface of the skin surface.[31] The lateral aspect of labia majora is covered with dry, keratinized, hair-bearing skin. The medial aspect and the entire labia minora display moist, modified mucous membrane, comprised of partially keratinized epithelium that contains subtle hair follicles, apocrine sweat glands and sebaceous glands. A distinct line of demarcation,

"Hart's line," is seen at the base of medial aspect of each labium minus, separating the modified mucous membranes of labia minora from that of the vestibule. The tissue medial to Hart's line is an unkeratinized, non-hair bearing epithelium with mucous secreting glands.

- Mons pubis is an inverted triangular area that extends from glans clitoris inferiorly to pubic hairline (base of triangle). It consists of loose adipose tissue overlying fascia, that is a continuation of Colles and Scarpa's fascia.
- Labia majora are prominent cutaneous folds between mons pubis and perineum consisting of adipose tissue, hair follicles and sebaceous glands. They unite anteriorly to form anterior commissure and posteriorly to form posterior commissure. The outer surface is covered with pigmented skin containing glands and pubic hair. The inside is smooth, pink and hairless. Camper's fascia with predominance of fat is superficially located. The thicker Colles' fascia forms the deeper layer and corresponds to Scarpa's fascia in abdominal wall. Colles' fascia is inferiorly attached to ischiopubic rami, posteriorly to urogenital diaphragm and lacks anterior attachment. This prevents spread of hematomas and infections to the thigh, but spread can occur to the anterior abdominal wall. The round ligament of uterus and obliterated processus vaginalis terminate in the labia majora.
- Labia minora are fat devoid skin folds, rich in sebaceous glands lying medial to labia majora with a core of connective tissue and vascular erectile tissue with sensory nerve endings. Each labia minora splits anteriorly around clitoris, uniting with the contralateral side to form the prepuce above, and frenulum under, the clitoris. Lloyd et al. measured and mapped the external and internal female genitalia and reported a large variation between 7 mm and 5 cm, with mean width of 2 cm.[32] Hypertrophy with maximum distance from the base to the edge >4 cm is an indication for corrective surgery.
- Clitoris, embryonic equivalent of male penis, a highly neurovascular erectile structure with over 8,000 nerve endings, is derived from undifferentiated phallus and consists of paired corpora, vestibular bulbs and glans. The corpora diverge to form the crura on each side along the ischiopubic rami. The glans is the most richly innervated part of the clitoris. Clitoris is suspended by superficial and deep suspensory ligaments that provide stability during intercourse. The superficial suspensory ligament is attached to the deep fascia of the mons, glans and body of clitoris further extending into the labia majora. The deep suspensory ligament originates from symphysis pubis and attaches to the body, bulbs and glans of the clitoris. Accurate knowledge of its relations, and neurovascular supply is important in performing surgeries to achieve normal morphology without affecting sexual function. It is important to preserve the bulbs with erectile tissue related closely to ventral aspect for sexual function, and suspensory ligaments to maintain the anatomic position.[33]
- Vestibule extends from clitoris to posterior fourchette between the two labia minora and contains vaginal orifice, external urethral meatus, vestibular bulbs, opening of two vestibular glands and many mucous, lesser vestibular glands. A shallow vestibular fossa nests between vaginal orifice and frenulum of labia minora. Bulbs of vestibule are paired elongated erectile tissue located along sides of the vaginal ostium under bulbospongiosus muscles, about 3 cm in length. Bartholin's/ greater vestibular glands are present on either side of vaginal ostium with openings through ducts 2 cm in length, in the groove between hymen and labia minora.

Neurovascular Supply of External Genitalia

Improper surgical techniques result in failure largely due to denervation/ devascularization that results due to lack of anatomical knowledge. Arterial supply of vulva is derived from external and internal pudendal arteries. The vessels follow the course of pudendal nerve and supply the superficial perineal muscles and external genitalia. Inferior rectal artery supplies the anal canal; perineal artery supplies superficial perineal muscles, posterior labial branch, artery to bulb of vestibule, dorsal and deep arteries of clitoris; and urethral artery supplies the respective structures. Superficial and deep external pudendal arteries (branches of femoral artery) distribute into labia majora and anastomose with branches of internal pudendal artery. Anastomosis between branches of these arteries is seen throughout the external genitalia.

Perineal nerve supplies bulbocavernosus, ischiocavernosus, superficial transverse perineal muscles, and skin of medial portion of labia majora, labia minora and vestibule. Inferior rectal nerve supplies perianal skin and external anal sphincter. Pudendal nerve is the main sensory and motor nerve of perineum that arises from ventral rami of S2–S4, runs underneath piriformis and exits pelvis through greater sciatic foramen, runs just behind ischial spines and reenters pelvis through lesser sciatic foramen. It then runs in Alcock's (pudendal) canal in obturator fascia ventral to sacrotuberous ligament. As it enters the perineum, it lies on lateral wall of ischiorectal fossa and divides into three branches: inferior rectal, perineal and dorsal nerve of clitoris. Dorsal nerve of clitoris lies on perineal membrane along ischio-pubic ramus and anterolateral surface of clitoris, one on each side, supplying the clitoris. In addition, innervation is also from cutaneous branch of ilioinguinal nerve, genital branch of genitofemoral nerve, and perineal branch of posterior femoral cutaneous nerve.[34]

Fascia and Muscles of the Pelvis

Pelvic floor is formed by pelvic diaphragm consisting of levator ani and coccygeus muscles with their fasciae, and perineal membrane with superficial and deep perineal muscles along with perineal body.

Fascia

Fascia is a loosely organized combination of elastin, collagen, adipose tissue and neurovascular tissue. The endopelvic fascia (condensation of visceral fascia around pelvic organs) connects the organs to lateral pelvic wall. Paravaginal connective tissue that attaches anterior vaginal wall to arcus tendinous fascia pelvis and posterior vaginal wall to levator ani is an extension of endopelvic fascia.

Muscles

The muscles within the pelvis form two groups. Levator ani and coccygeus muscles form pelvic diaphragm with urethra, vagina and rectum passing through the urogenital hiatus, while piriformis and obturator internus muscles form lateral walls of pelvis. The fascia covering the levator is continuous with endopelvic fascia above, perineal fascia below, and obturator fascia laterally.

- Arcus tendinous fascia pelvis (ATFP) is the thickening in obturator fascia and extends from pubis anteriorly to ischial spine and provides attachment to paravaginal connective tissue.
- Arcus tendinous levator ani, thickening of levator ani fascia, arises from a similar location on pubis but extends superior to ATFP.

Levator ani muscle provides the main support and has three components: pubococcygeus, iliococcygeus and puborectalis. Pubococcygeus is further subdivided into puboperinealis, pubovaginalis and puboanalis. Pubococcygeus originates on inner side of pubic bone anteriorly and inserts into perineal body, mid-urethral level of vaginal wall and intersphincteric groove between internal and external anal sphincter in anal skin. It elevates the respective structures and provide a constant tone to pelvic floor. Puborectalis originates from pubic bone and forms a sling around rectum, playing a role in anal incontinence. Iliococcygeus originates from arcus tendinous levator ani and fuses with its counterpart in anococcygeal raphe (levator plate) to form a supportive diaphragm between anus and coccyx. Levator fascia covers the levator muscle and fuses inferiorly with perineal membrane. Levator ani is supplied by inferior gluteal artery, inferior vesical artery and pudendal artery. Innervation is from ventral nerve roots of S2–S4.

Perineum, diamond-shaped area lying superficial to perineal membrane that includes the vulva and anus and is bound by pubic symphysis, ischiopubic rami, sacrotuberous ligaments and coccyx. An arbitrary line between two ischial tuberosities divides the perineum into two triangles: anterior urogenital and posterior anal triangle. Urogenital triangle located anteriorly includes female external genitalia, with perineal membrane, which divides it into superficial and deep perineal spaces. Anal triangle contains anal orifice and posterior part of perineum. Clinically, perineum is the area between vaginal introitus and anus.

Perineal membrane (urogenital diaphragm) consists of dense fibromuscular tissue that attaches laterally to ischiopubic rami, posteriorly to perineal body, medially to lateral walls of vagina and urethra and apically to arcuate pubic ligament. The female striated urogenital sphincter (deep transverse perinei) consists of sphincter urethrae, urethrovaginal sphincter and compressor urethrae. These muscles lie superior to perineal membrane in deep perineal space continuous with pelvic cavity. The superior fascia of these muscles is continuous with endopelvic fascia. The superficial perineal space lies between perineal membrane and subcutaneous tissues and contains clitoris, bulbocavernosus (bulbospongiosus), ischiocavernosus muscles and the vestibular bulbs.

The superficial Colles' fascia of urogenital triangle forms a clear plane beneath the skin of anterior perineum and is firmly attached posteriorly to the fascia over superficial transverse perineal muscle and posterior limit of perineal membrane. Laterally, it is attached to margins of ischiopubic rami till ischial tuberosities and then runs superficially to the skin of urogenital triangle, lining the external genitalia before running anteriorly into skin of lower abdominal wall where it is continuous with membranous Scarpa's fascia.

Perineal membrane consists of ventral and dorsal components. The ventral component is continuous with paraurethral and paravaginal connective tissues and ATFP and provides attachment to female-striated urogenital sphincter muscles and vestibular bulbs. Clitoris fuse to its inferior surface. The dorsal component attaches laterally to ischiopubic rami on each side, medially to vagina and perineal body. Levator ani attaches to its superior surface and to perineal body. Disruption of perineal body during childbirth leads to separation of perineal membrane, displacement of levator ani and widening of genital hiatus. Anatomic restoration of perineal body during posterior repair reestablishes perineal muscles and levator ani.

Superficial transverse perineal muscles are narrow strips of muscles originating from ischial tuberosity and inserting on perineal body (central tendon). Ischiocavernosus arises from ischial tuberosity and clitoral crura along inferior portion of ischiopubic ramus and inserts on body of clitoris. Bulbocavernosus runs on either side of vagina and attaches to perineal body posteriorly and body of clitoris anteriorly. Blood supply is through internal and external pudendal vessels; innervation is via perineal branch of pudendal nerve from below and sacral plexus and pelvic splanchnic nerves from above.

Perineal body (central perineal tendon) is an aggregation of fibromuscular tissue located in midline between posterior fourchette and anus, originally believed to be an insertion point for bulbospongiosus, external anal sphincter, vaginal muscularis, superficial transverse perineal muscle, perineal membrane and pubovisceral part of levator ani. It is an area where perineal muscles cross from one side to another without insertion at a particular site.

SURGICAL CORRECTION: OBJECTIVES OF PELVIC FLOOR REPAIR

Looking beyond Just Anatomical Repair: Look Good, Feel Good (Functionality, Esthetics)

Esthetic surgery of female genitalia is designed to improve the appearance subjectively, and potentially provide psychological and functional improvement in sexual stimulation and satisfaction. In modern times, physical discomfort or unsightly esthetic appearance is a growing complaint of women seeking surgical correction. With growing trend toward lifestyle and antiaging medicine, cosmetic vaginal surgery (with PFR as mainstay) is emerging and offered as a means to not just enhance the appearance but also improve the sexual function. Women seek FGCS for both esthetic and functional reasons including pain with intercourse or sports, vulvar irritation, chafing and discomfort with underclothing. Feelings of embarrassment with sexual dysfunction including strong desire to improve strained relationships are commonly cited as reasons for FGCS. The current trend of pubic hair removal allows for easier vulvar visualization and many may perceive their own genitalia as abnormal. Perception of the ideal female external genitalia differs from country to country and the ideal genital may differ historically and cross-culturally. In in parts of Africa elongated labia minora are considered attractive and believed to optimize sexual intercourse and are deliberately stretched from a young age (Kudenga), whereas in Mozambique they are seen as a sign of modesty; butterfly appearance is considered sexually desirable in Japan, and in the western society, these are considered less attractive.[35,36]

General Principles

There is not always a clear distinction between esthetic and reconstructive genital surgery. In majority, the indication is partially reconstructive (for functional/medical indication) as well as esthetic. As the levator drops, a more vertical vaginal axis is produced, this produces effects relating to orgasm and sexual enjoyment, which are ignored. Also ignored is the fact that a woman's sexual enjoyment is mediated by her genital self-image.[37,38] What seems straightforward to diagnose and treat surgically is actually unpredictable with regard to symptom relief for patients when the entire focus is on the bulge. In traditional repairs, sexual or body image issues have not been considered or addressed. Assessment of sexual function and body image are key areas to address in evaluation, therapeutic options, and goals for successful treatment. The impact of colpoperineorrhaphy on sexual function has shown improvement in several series, despite increased dyspareunia.[39] When caring for women with posterior compartment prolapse, its impact on her sexual function and body image should be discussed. Clinicians need to pay closer attention to the rehabilitation of sexual function, esthetics and muscular strength and personalize the repair technique to achieve a greater success rate.[40]

For functional symptoms, surgical repair involves reconstruction of vaginal anatomy and corrective procedures for urinary and/or defecation disorders, termed pelvic floor repair (PFR), which also improves the appearance of external genitalia and perhaps sexual function. Vaginoplasty per se is not intended to correct floor defects; however, these repairs are modifications of traditional colporrhaphy and are frequently performed in conjunction with reconstructive procedure for prolapse and involve techniques to anatomically modify the vaginal caliber by reducing the diameter of lower third of vagina and reconstructing the perineal body. Full-length vaginoplasty involves lower two-thirds of the vagina as far up as the ischial spines. The desired outcomes of these procedures include improvement in both esthetic external appearance and an increase in frictional forces during intercourse. Labiaplasty is often undertaken that can either involve surgical alteration to either reduce or enhance with silicon/fat injections. Occasionally coupling it with hymenoplasty (as maybe desired in certain cultures), and augmentation of G-spot/O-spot, these procedures are collectively termed vaginal rejuvenation.[35]

Indications

- Genital hypertrophy or significant discrepancy
- Discomfort with sports activities or clothing, or vaginal entrapment with coitus
- Genital changes due to childbearing/obstetrical injury affecting appearance and pleasurable coital sensation/functionality.

The indication for surgery should be made in mutual understanding. Current gynecological disease, smoking, unrealistic expectations and sexual dysfunction are relative contraindications. Patients should be made aware that FGCS carries inherent risks and complications that eventually may result in a diminished function.

COMMON ESTHETIC SURGICAL CORRECTIONS

Preoperative Details

Patients are evaluated while standing and marked in lithotomy position. They should not shave immediately prior to operation to avoid increased infection risks. Communication regarding the patient's expectations is critical. Planning and drawing of incision lines on the patient's genitalia is one of the most important parts of the procedure. This is done on dry skin, with a sterile marking pen at the beginning of the case, prior to injecting local anesthesia, utilizing gentle traction. "Dots" may be used rather than drawing a "line" in the presence of skin redundancy.

Labiaplasty

Labiaplasty broadly refers to reduction of labia minora or majora, and/or to augmentation (injection of bulking agents/ autologous fat transfer). "Barbie look" is a colloquial term for external genitalia characterized by minimal labia minora tissue that may extend beyond the labia majora and the vaginal orifice appears as a fine vertical line (Figs. 42.1A and B).

Labia minora protect the vagina from drying out and play a significant role in micturition by funneling the urine stream, therefore minimal labial width should be 1 cm.[41] Labia are considered hypertrophic if maximum distance from base to edge is greater than 4 cm.[31,42] Hormonal changes during puberty result in growth of external genitals; inner labia become "longer" than outer labia.

The following grading system by Davison and West to objectively measure labia minora hypertrophy has been used clinically:[43]

- *None*: labia minora extends no farther than the labia majora
- *Mild/moderate*: labia minora extends 1–4 cm beyond the labia majora
- *Severe*: labia minora extends greater than 4 cm beyond the labia majora.

Reduction of Labia Minora

Reduction labiaplasty has been reported in medical literature since 1971. Labia minora plasty involves techniques to reduce size and/ or alter the shape

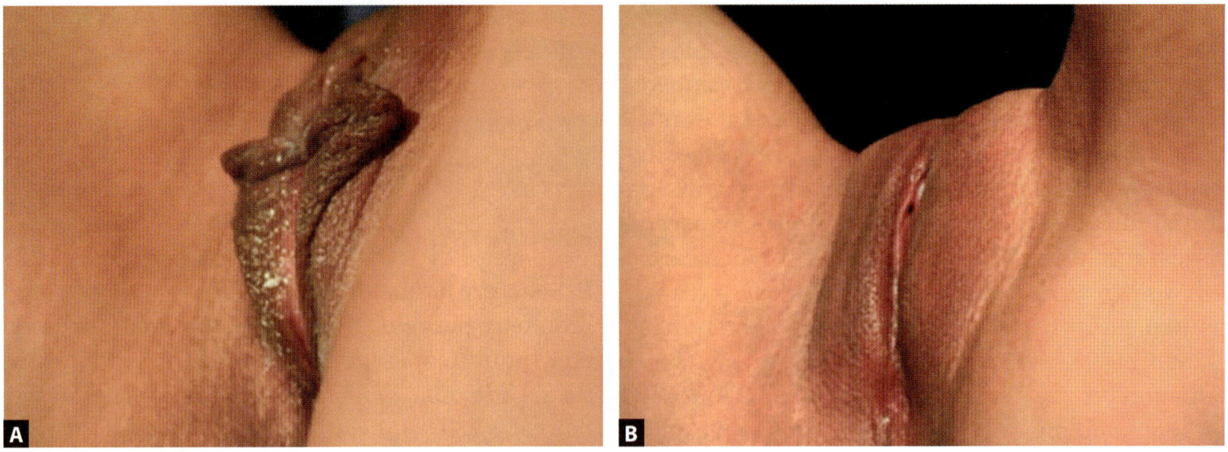

Figs. 42.1A and B: Labia minora plasty with extended labial tissues reduction "Barbie look." Confocal CO_2 laser tip was used to perform the procedure.

for esthetic or functional purposes. Women seek labiaplasty for different reasons.[44,45] A growing number seek this purely for esthetic reasons, and more so as they are becoming more conscious with the increasing trend of pubic hair removal. Functional indications include discomfort in clothing or during sports, dyspareunia due to invagination of labia on penetration.

Standard techniques include curved linear excision/amputation, central/posterior wedge resection, de-epithelialization, and W-shaped labial resection. Laser/radiofrequency tools are found beneficial due to their precision cut and safety in clitoral area. The vulvar epithelium of labia minora is highly innervated and sensitive. During sexual arousal, labia evert and contribute to erotic sensation and pleasure. Surgical manipulation could compromise this sensitivity. Neuroma-like hypersensitivity has been reported after surgery.[31,41] De-epithelialization attempts to preserve the natural free edges and neurovascular supply of the labia minora. Reduction of excess prepuce is required in >90% of cases.

Labial curved linear edge excision/amputation (Figs. 42.2A and B) is the simplest one: complete excision of excess labial tissue over its entire length is performed with edges then sutured using absorbable sutures, usually in a running technique. The disadvantage is that the natural contour of free edge is lost, and pink visible color visible gives an unnatural appearance. One must limit the excision level keeping a minimal margin width of at least 1 cm. Smaller minimal width can result in unesthetic scarring too close to the introitus with resultant dyspareunia, sensory loss or chronic pain.[41]

De-epithelialization technique involves de-epithelializing central part on both sides of labia sparing the labial vessels or nerves, and then re-approximating edges of defect on both sides. This preserves sensitivity of free border and reduces vertical dimension; however, it fails to shorten length of

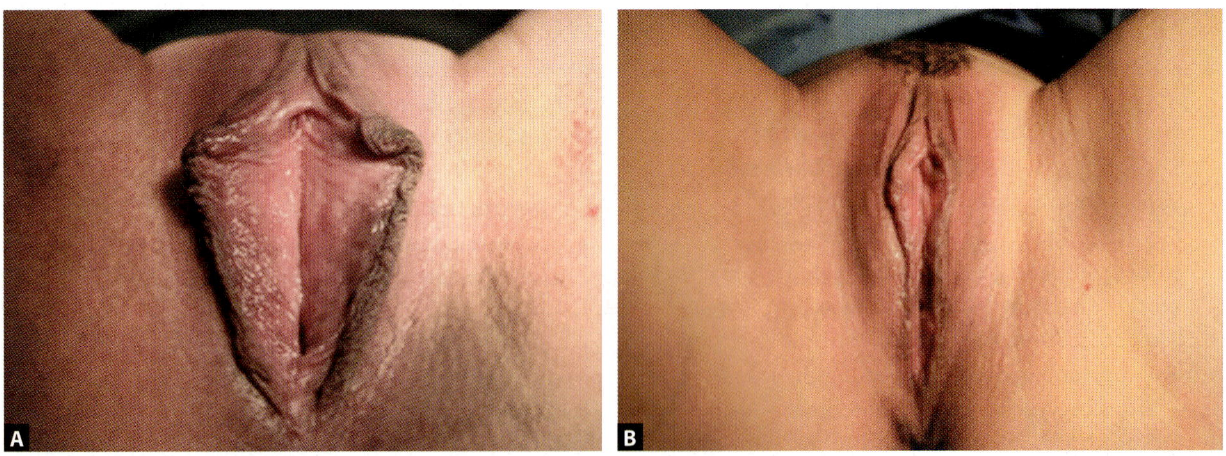

Figs. 42.2A and B: Labia minora plasty using the modified curved line technique. RF tip was used to perform the procedure.

free border that can give a redundant appearance. The increased labial thickness with centrally retained parenchyma and abrupt color change at suture line are other drawbacks.[41,46] This is more suitable for patients with thinner labia and not those with bulk hypertrophy. The de-epithelialization technique in combination with clamp resection is used for patients with considerable excess skin.

Wedge resection labiaplasty consists of wedge excision either central or posterior/anterior part of labia minora. It preserves the natural outline, pigmentation of free edge and neurovascularity, although there is a potential sensory loss at the top of labium.[46,47] There are three described techniques for central wedge. The first involves de-epithelialization of central wedge and preserving the underlying submucosa. The second involves full-thickness resection of V-shaped wedge of excess labial tissue. This maintains the natural edge and minimizes scar. The third approach is 90° Z-plasty that reduces tension on suture line, minimizing the scar. In inferior wedge resection, wedge is taken in inferior part of labia, using superior large remnant as a flap to reconstruct the labia.[48]

Intraoperative Details

Labiaplasty surgery can be successfully performed under local anesthesia (LA), sedation or general anesthesia (GA). LA should be used during GA and sedation anesthesia for added vasoconstriction and postoperative pain control. First mark the resection line and then infiltrate underneath external skin and internal mucosal layer marking. Resection of outer and inner lining is done to preserve as much of subcutaneous layer as possible because it usually retracts. Avoid undue traction and maintain equal tension on suture line. Wet 4 × 4 gauze are placed behind the labia minora prior to laser usage to prevent excess heat transfer to surrounding tissue. Start superiorly 1 cm below the frenulum and distal to outlining mark.

Conservative trimming: Care should be taken not to extend labial resection to fourchette and to keep labial width to 1 cm.[45] The most common complication is taking too much off because attachment of labia minora laterally (interlabial fold) is far shorter than from the mucosal aspect, and, any stretch on the labia further distorts the anatomy. Cutting with only medial/mucosal view, without marking and moving interior to Hart's line medially leads to unfavorable outcomes. Mark the lateral side, without tension 1/2–1 cm from the interlabial fold and continually assess the margins laterally during excision. Attempt the larger, more difficult side first then match the smaller side to larger one. It's prudent to take less off rather than more.

No one technique is ideal for all patients; therefore, specific or a combination of techniques may have to be used. Any excess tissue remaining on the transition from the clitoral hood to the labia minora is amputated. It is important to attain perfect hemostasis since a hematoma will result in traction on suture lines with a risk of wound dehiscence, asymmetry of labia and/or suboptimal esthetic results. As postoperative bleeding is a risk, handheld electrocautery coagulation is highly recommended to reduce bleeding risk from resected mucosal edges.

Meticulous suturing of subcutaneous layer is important to prevent wound dehiscence and fistula formation.[41,48] The deep planes are closed with 4.0 or 5.0 Monocryl sutures and labial edge is approximated with a 5.0 Vicryl Rapide if needed; else, the option of using dermal glue is a great alternative to achieve the approximation. Skin closure is performed with 5.0 Vicryl Rapide subcuticular or 5.0 fast-absorbing suture. A subcuticular suture line is difficult for V-wedge closure and risks separation. With interrupted sutures, care must be taken to avoid inward rolling of edges. Periodic mattress sutures minimize this risk. Running sutures externally can lead to esthetically poor results on the free edge of labia minora in linear resections while buried running suture can create a smooth free edge. This scalloped look to free edge is esthetically unappealing and is hard to correct. Feathering technique using monopolar radiofrequency has been described by Dr. Alinsod to correct the same.[49]

Some swelling immediately postoperatively is expected. The first postoperative visit is usually scheduled around 1 week, or sooner in case of swelling, pain or hematoma. Patients can return to work after 3–4 days. Sexual intercourse, bicycling and intensive sports should be avoided until complete healing of the wounds has occurred, about 6 weeks.

Adverse effects reported include bleeding, infection, iatrogenic asymmetry, poor wound healing and under-/overcorrection that may require revision surgery, or medical intervention, unpleasing esthetic results after surgery and even secondary dyspareunia.[46] If there is a color discrepancy between the mucosal and lateral surfaces of the labum, a "color line" will be present along the line of resection. Usually this fades and merges within a year.

Reduction of Labia Majora

The problems of labia majora can be twofold: (1) atrophy of the fat and (2) excess skin. A distinction should be made between primary labia majora hypertrophy (volume excess) and secondary labia majora hypertrophy due to volume loss (skin excess). The solutions are fat grafting and surgical resection, respectively.[50] When there is a true volume excess, enlarged labia majora can be reduced by liposuction. However, this might create sagging and skin excess.

Majora reduction is effected by a vertical elliptical wedge excision labial dermis, on inner edge of labia minora along its length.[51] to place the final closure into the labial crease with/without a portion of underlying adipose tissue within Colles' fascia, with subcutaneous imbricating sutures (monofilament 3-0 to 5-0 subcuticular sutures/interrupted nylon skin closure). If found to be torn, Colles' fascia may be repaired with fine synthetic nonreactive absorbable sutures. The suture line may be partially hidden in interlabial fold. It may also be accomplished by injection of autologous fat transplantation/synthetic bulking agents. The RF energy applied externally to heat and potentially denature/shrink underlying collagen with resultant modest minimization of redundancy can be used at monthly intervals with touch up session after 18 months.

Preparation/setup/anesthesia: Trimming, shaving or other hair removal technique should be performed >1 week prior to surgery, or immediately preoperation (to avoid possible folliculitis). Patients are generally advised to undergo permanent laser hair removal as this prevent any possible hair growth toward the vaginal introitus. Evaluation and planning is done in the adducted position. After appropriate skin prep, incision lines are drawn with a sterile marking pen. If LA, 0.5% bupivacaine with an absolute limit of 30 mL is preferred. Buffer with 0.15–0.2 mL sodium bicarbonate/10 mL anesthetic, administered with a 1.5 inch 25 G needle, beginning with a skin wheal at the nadir of incisional ellipse, proceeding with small ribbon of anesthetic just outside of incision lines. The epithelium in this area is relatively fibrous and has a rich nerve supply.

Incision and excision: Draw incision lines starting medially, placing "inner" line vertically at junction of hair-bearing and hairless area just lateral to interlabial fold. Outer portion of incision line, extends in a curvilinear manner to include majority of redundant labial epithelium. Start the incision (2–3 mm in depth) line from the bottom, progressing to the top, to avoid blood flow from obscuring incision lines. Superficial skin removal is done using dissection scissors/surgical fiber on fulguration/hemostatic wave form. Take care to not breach the Colles' fascia. In cases where follicular removal is intended, the procedure can be performed either by using the surgical scalpel, shaving the follicles with the sharp edge, or by cauterizing the follicles directly with the common electrocautery tip.

Repair: Hemostasis is mandatory. Small venous and tiny arterial bleeders are controlled with focal electrocautery; larger vessels and arterial bleeders are controlled with suture ligation (4-0 or 5-0 multi- or monofilament delayed absorbable). Any rent in Colles' fascia should be repaired. Place a subcutaneous layer (either an interrupted/continuous 4-0 braided/monofilament inverting suture line), taking care to include subepithelial fascia and little or none of the fatty layer to provide tension-free approximation and minimize dead space. Skin closure is done (5-0 Monocryl subcuticular/interrupted 5-0 mattress sutures, with removal in 7–10 days). For subcuticular closure, place interrupted (5-0 Vicryl Rapide) skin sutures. Steri-Strips/Dermabond® may be used.

Postoperative complications are bleeding and transient hypersensitivity for 4–6 weeks.[42] Full activities may be resumed at 1 month; it will take 6–12 months before the incision line is esthetically mostly undetectable.

Augmentation Labia Majora Plasty (Figs. 42.3A and B)

If a patient has atrophy of fat in the labia majora, inject 10–15 mL of fat into each side of labia majora, of which approximately 40–60% survives.[52] When performing a lipofilling of labia majora, minor hypertrophy of labia minora can be masked. The procedure consists of augmentation through autologous fat injections or lipofilling. Fat can be harvested from the abdomen or inner thigh.[51]

Vaginoplasty

Up to 76% of women experience decreased vaginal sensation, most commonly with a feeling of a widened vagina/vaginal laxity. Decreased vaginal sensation comes from a widened vagina, causing less friction.[53] Vaginal tightening surgery has been around since the mid-1950s, where vaginal entrance was tightened with an extra stitch while repairing vaginal and perineum tears or episiotomies after

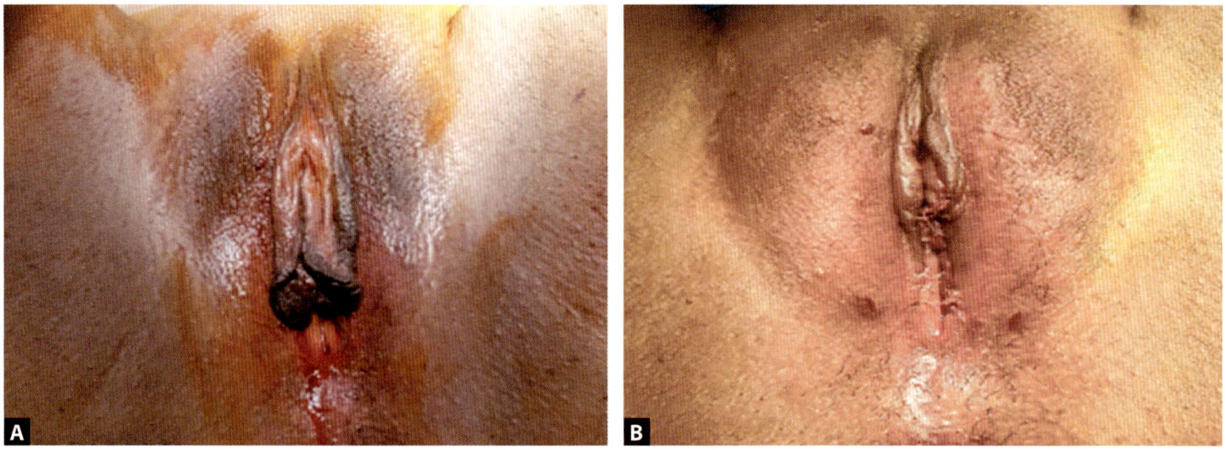

Figs. 42.3A and B: Labia majora augmentation by autologous fat transfer; 20 cc of pure fat was used each side after centrifugation.

giving birth (husband's stitch/knot).[54] The goal is to narrow the lower third of vaginal introitus and perineal body. Vaginoplasty differs from the traditional posterior colporrhaphy where in the levator plication is not undertaken, and instead includes several steps undertaken in order to reach better esthetic results of the perineal area.

Vaginoplasty: Surgical Technique

Esthetic vaginoplasty includes anterior colporrhaphy, posterior colporrhaphy, excision of lateral vaginal mucosa or a combination, via scalpel, needle electrode or laser.[55] Posterior colporrhaphy involves plication of rectovaginal muscularis, creating a narrower diameter. Sometimes, levator ani plication is also performed, but this may cause significant dyspareunia and is not recommended for cosmetic surgery. Lateral removal of mucosal strips from vaginal fornices (lateral colporrhaphy) allows reduction of vaginal canal diameter as well as the introitus and perineum. It causes less scarring but does not adequately address pelvic defects. In most cases, a mucosa strip is simply excised and primarily closed with an absorbable running suture. Several studies suggest the lateral colporrhaphy to be a more effective technique in reducing the size of the vagina without placing scars within the areas of highest sensitivity, thereby causing less dyspareunia.

Ninety-five percent of patients treated with lateral colporrhaphy reported an improvement in sexual sensitivity, as well as greater vaginal tightness at the 6 months follow-up.[54-56] Known complications are localized infection and vaginal bleeding. Risk of vaginal tightening procedures include dyspareunia, wound disruption and de novo incontinence.

Single-thread vaginal tightening (Figs. 42.4A and B) is a novel technique (first described by Dr. Alexander Bader) performed using a single thread of barbed monofilament suture with two needles at each end. The barbed thread usually is 30 cm long. This technique minimizes the necrotic tissues in

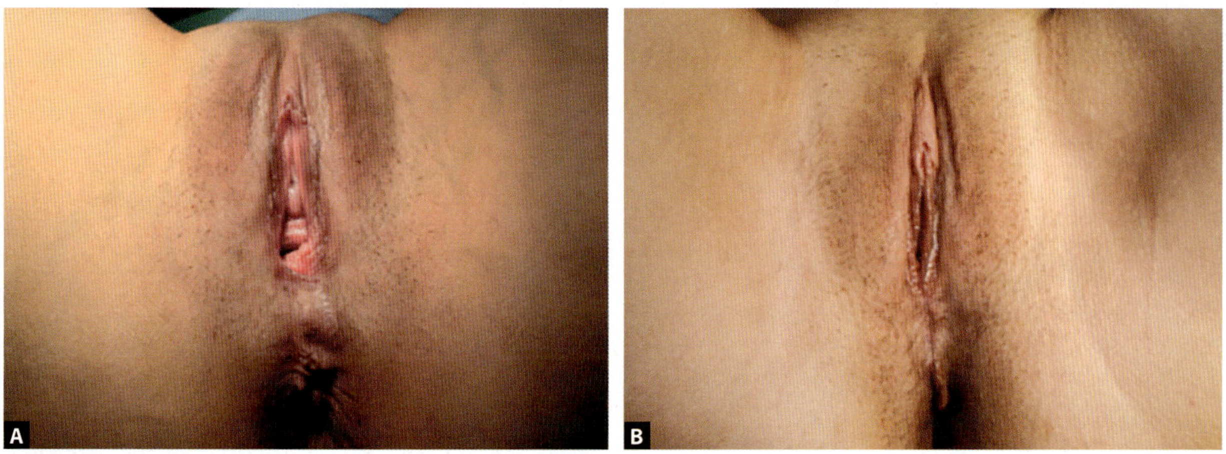

Figs. 42.4A and B: Vaginoplasty using single thread of monofilament suture.

the fascial and mucosal layer by approximating the layers without lock, and employs full-length approximation of the vaginal wall. The thread absorbs in 120 days. Using a single thread minimizes the total procedure time to 30 min. It is remarkable to mention that the surgeon is able to correct also the introital defect and the perineal scar (if any) with the same thread.

Laser vaginal rejuvenation (LVR) (trade-marked term) refers to traditional posterior and anterior colporrhapies carried out to treat a "wide" vagina using a 980-nm diode contact fiber laser to alter the vulva and vagina. Designer laser vaginoplasty (DLV) (trade-marked term) refers to reshaping and re-sculpting of external vulva including clitoral unhooding, labiaplasty of labia minora and majora, augmentation labiaplasty of labia majora and liposuction of vulva and mons pubis.

There are several reports on injection of autologous fat or bulking agents such as hyaluronic acid for vaginal tightening. Hyaluronic acid resorbs over time; multiple injections may be necessary for the desired result. While there may be a on mucosal trophicity, there is also a risk of granuloma formation.[57]

Hymenoplasty is surgical suturing of hymenal remnants with absorbable interrupted sutures to narrow the vaginal orifice. In some cultures, intact hymen emblematic of family honor; however, the absence of hymen is not a sign of lost virginity.[58] It can remain intact in as many as 52% of adolescent girls who have had sexual intercourse. It is a relatively bloodless membrane and is unlikely to bleed significantly even if torn. Promoting the concept of intact hymen as a sign of virginity is nothing but perpetuation of myth.

Clitoroplasty

Clitoral hood reduction is designed to exposure more of the clitoral body for improved sexual stimulation and to improve the appearance of genital area. Women request this either because the clitoris is "buried" under prepuce, leading to little direct stimulation or because women find their preputial folds unsightly/source of embarrassment.[44,51] This is usually performed via simple skin excision using lateral preputial or central croissant-formed excision. Excisions are avoided in midline because of possible scarring and subsequent dysfunction. This procedure can be combined with labiaplasty. The resection line should never be close to border of the clitoris because scars close to the clitoris can result in sexual dysfunctioning.

Composite reductions of labia (Figs. 42.5A and B) are performed to ensure a symmetrical result and is combined with clitoral unhooding.[59] Excessive exposure leads to hypersensitivity, as well as the appearance of the microphallus.[60] The classic clitoral unhooding is a modified Y-to-V technique. The clitoral hood is incised and the excess tissue on either side of the Y can be amputated.

An alternative to clitoral unhooding is clitoral tightening.[50] In conjunction with a central wedge, wings of anterior labia are advanced posterior and clitoris is tightened posteriorly into the cleft.

Clitoropexy

Clitoropexy involves V-to-Y plasty, moving the clitoris and its attached labia minora in an anterior and superior direction. A deep holding suture from suspensory ligament of clitoris to fascia/periosteum of pubis is used at the medial and lateral side of

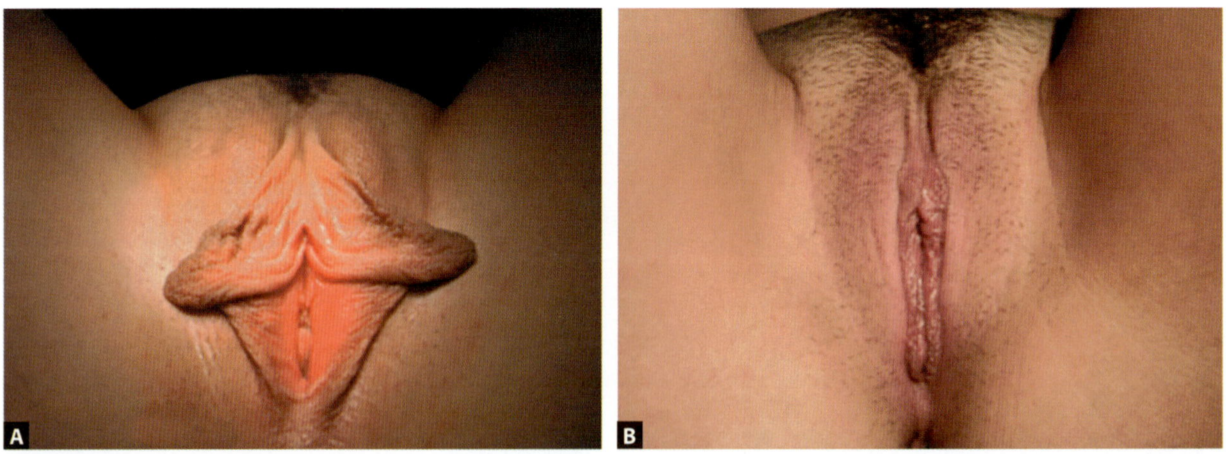

Figs. 42.5A and B: Labia minora reduction with modified linear technique combined with clitoral hood reduction. CO_2 laser and RF were used for this procedure.

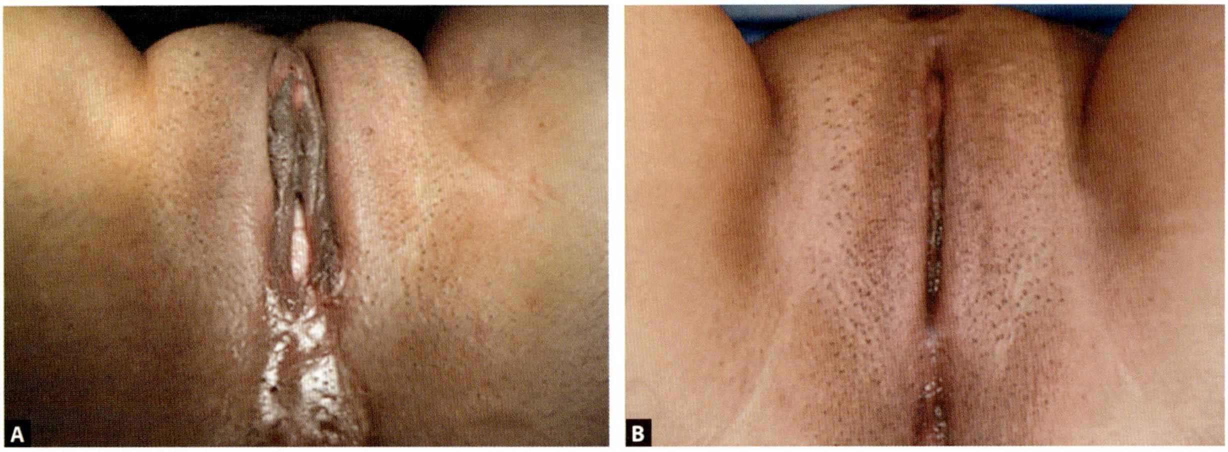

Figs. 42.6A and B: Perineoplasty. The procedure was performed using confocal CO_2 laser tip. Diamond-shaped wedge and closer with self-dissolvable sutures.

clitoris and never in the midline where the neurovascular pedicle is located.[41]

Clitoral Reduction

Clitoral hypertrophy may be primary or secondary to hormonal or genetic abnormalities (disorders of sex development [DSD]). Clitoral reduction differs from clitoropexy in that it truly reduces the length of clitoral shaft and/or head, with preservation of sensitivity. This is often more a reconstructive functional procedure rather than cosmetic procedure.

Perineoplasty (Figs. 42.6A and B) involves reconstruction of vaginal introitus, with minor low-posterior compartment repair and reapproximation of levator ani musculature to effect an elevated perineum and strengthened perineal body with resultant improved sexual function.[44] A diamond-shaped wedge of tissue is removed, with apex in posterior one-third of vagina and nadir on perineum superior to the anus.

PUBIC ENHANCEMENT

Monsplasty

The mons has been an increasing region of focus in FGCS. Using a wedge excision method, wide mons is reduced.[43] The procedure can be done in combination with labiaplasty and/or abdominoplasty in patients who have had massive weight loss.

Pubic Lifting

Reduction of mons pubis for ptosis or excess tissue usually is done by wedge excision in transverse direction and is usually either combined with or part of an abdominoplasty procedure.[51]

Pubic Liposuction

Liposuction of mons pubis is effective in patients without skin excess. During abdominoplasty, wedge resection of fat pad through lower abdominal incision is done.[51]

PRACTICE TIPS DURING COMMON SURGICAL REPAIRS

The end result with pleasing results is dependent on preoperative "marking," fine blepharoplasty delicate instruments, 4-0 and 5-0 "eye" sutures, exacting suturing techniques, meticulous attention to detail during surgery and explicit postoperative care by patients with training and teaching prior to surgery.

Tissue Handling

Handling, cutting and re-approximating tissue with absolute minimal trauma is one of the major keys to success.

Preparation

Patient is draped in dorsal lithotomy position. Vagina and vulva are prepared with betadine solution. For postoperative pain control, pudendal block (5 cc of 0.5% Marcaine with epinephrine) is placed bilaterally prior to starting the procedure. Local infiltration along resection lines may also be utilized.

Operative Procedure Marking

The tissue is dried to allow for drawing. Utilizing a sterile marking pen, incision lines are drawn, taking into account the patient's desires and individual anatomy. For labiaplasty, take care to be conservative and stay outside Hart's line on mucosal surface and well medial to the interlabial fold on lateral surface. Take care to not put the labum on stretch when drawing markings, and remember to curve the line, leaving more tissue in situ at cephalad portion. Bevel the line into the descending clitoral hood fold, or incorporate the fold into the incision line.

Instruments

Short-handled equipment (~5") is preferable: 5" needle driver; Adson forceps; baby Metzenbaum/ Kaye scissors serrated supercut scissors, 4-1/2" curved; suture scissors; two mosquito clamps; Allis clamps; towel clips or clamps to secure draping; sterile fine-tipped marking pen; 50 mL medicine cup for drawing up anesthetic agent; and #11 blade is used for resection. For vaginal tightening procedures, add two to four Allis-Adair or T-type clamps, heavier Metzenbaum/Mayo dissecting scissors. Heany-curved jaw needle holder.

Suture Material and Needles

Labia Minora Plasty and Clitoral Hood Reduction

- 5-0 Monocryl on PC-5 needle; 5-0 or 4-0 Vicryl on a SH-1 needle for sub-cutaneous closure
- 5-0 Vicryl Rapide or 5-0 Vicryl on PC-3 needle for skin (subcuticular or interrupted/ mattress).

Labia Majora Plasty

- 4-0 Vicryl, 4-0 Monocryl, or 4-0 PDS on SH or SH-1 needle for subcutaneous layer
- 5-0 Monocryl on PC-5 needle for subcuticular closure, or 5-0 nylon on PS-3 needle for skin closure.

Perineo- and Vaginoplasty

- 2-0 Monocryl on CT-2 needle for deep layers (levators; perineal body)
- 3-0 or 4-0 Monocryl on SH or CT-2 needle for second (rectovaginal fascia) layer
- 3-0 or 4-0 Vicryl on SH-I needle for vaginal mucosa and perineal closure.

Cutting and cautery may be effected with scalpel, electrosurgical needle electrode, fine plastic scissors (baby-Metzenbaums, Kaye, etc.), laser or RF needle electrode; elctrosurgical units for needle-point cutting and cautery capability. Both RF and laser are precise cutting tools. The surgical concepts remain the same with scissors, laser, or RF.

Laser

Both erbium and carbon dioxide (CO_2) lasers can be used. Proposed benefits are reduced blood loss and enhanced healing. Limitations of this technique include higher risk for epidermal inclusion cysts. Compared with conventional surgery, LVR using contact CO_2 lasers is reportedly associated with reduced morbidity, scarring and favorable outcomes in vaginal caliber in combination with standard cautery and achieves similar results, but no studies have confirmed superiority of laser or radiofrequency dissection compared with traditional scalpel, scissors or electrocautery.

Radiofrequency (RF) device[61] allows incision, microsmooth cutting and resurfacing. It is effective in ironing rough surfaces, smoothing uneven edges, excising tissue and sealing small blood vessels. Compared to lower frequency electrosurgery instruments, monopolar RF treatment is associated with decreased tissue resistance and maximum control in precision cutting as well as tissue tightening to smooth wrinkled skin. The RF unit cuts and coagulates soft tissue using either monopolar or bipolar energy and enables precise microsurgical manipulation required to seal off open small blood vessels with minimal lateral thermal damage of 20–40 μm. The fine wire cutting tip is available as straight and 30° curved. By stimulating coagulation, attachable ball electrode tips promote soft tissue shrinkage and skin tightening. Monopolar RF surgery is associated with less thermal with negligible thermal dispersal into tissue, thereby reducing burning or charring during techniques to excise or smoothen vulvar skin.

To Aid in Skin Analgesia Prior to Injection

4% Emla cream or 5% lidocaine gel to the area and occluding with plastic film an hour prior to procedure, or ethyl chloride spray or, LA spray just prior to local injection. The time and effort do not appear to offer any advantage. By the time the patient is evaluated, prepped, and markings drawn, the analgesia wears off. Buffering the anesthetic with sodium bicarbonate offers the best reduction of injection pain.

Local Anesthesia

(a) Injection Solution

Technique for labia minora/clitoral hood local injection

- 0.25%, 0.5% bupivacaine with/ without 1:100,000 epinephrine, or 1–2 cc of 0.25% Marcaine with epinephrine, or 1% lidocaine with epinephrine or 1% xylocaine with epinephrine 50/50 with 1% Marcaine plain, buffered with 0.15–0.2 mL sodium bicarbonate/10 mL
- Application of topical anesthetic (BLT cream: benzocaine (20%), lidocaine (6%) and tetracaine (4%)) can also be undertaken as the thin mucosa of labia allows rapid penetration followed by injection of LA; maintains LA for up to 2 h.[50]
- Syringe with 18 or 20 G needle for drawing solution and 1.5 inch 25 or 27 G needle for injecting
- *Volume*: 6–10 mL total for both sides: If using any more local than necessary, tissue plane dissection, and small vessel hemostasis will distort and/ or disrupt the surgical site.
- Labia minora are infiltrated at base. All injections are done medial to proposed lines of dissection. This minimally distorts surgical dissection lines, provides anesthesia, hemostasis, and tissue planes.
- Individual injections may be limited to 20-s intervals. Incision lines are tested with a forceps prior to skin incision. At least 5 min should be allowed to elapse for the epinephrine to take effect and induce vasoconstriction.

Technique for Labia Majora Local Injection

- Needles <25 G is difficult secondary to resistance of labia majora epithelium.
- *Total volume*: 8–10 mL usually suffices for both sides.
- Injection is made just outside of the incision lines.

Technique for Perineoplasty and Hymenoplasty Local Injection (Office Cases, Local Tumescent Anesthesia)

- *Total volume*: 20–30 mL, averaging 15–25 mL for perineoplasty and 4–5 mL for hymenoplasty
- *For perineoplasty alone*: 0.5% bupivacaine; if combining procedures: mix 0.5% with 0.25% bupivacaine 50/50, giving a 0.375% solution, (maximal volume: 45 mL), or use 0.25% bupivacaine.

(b) Injection Technique

Initial injection: skin wheal at base of incision line. All subsequent needle entries are via this wheal or into previously anesthetized areas. Injection is slow minimum ribbon of anesthetic just inside of incision lines. Test anesthetic effect with forceps prior to commencing incision.

Excision and hemostasis: Excision may be effected with either dissecting scissors, laser, RF or electrical current. Meticulous attention to hemostasis is imperative. Even a small hematoma can stretch the area of repair and compromise surgical outcome. Meticulous hemostasis is assured with a needle point electrocautery. All venous bleeders must be cauterized in as localized manner. Arteriolar bleeders should always be isolated and ligated (4-0 Vicryl interrupted mattress sutures), minor ones may be grasped and fulgurated. It is important to leave a dry field and avoid "spray" hemostasis. Venous bleeders in inferior portion of labia minora usually are controlled with skin sutures, locking where necessary.

Skin closure: The key to closure is eliminating all dead space with tension free sutures, taking tension off edge closure, everting the edge and closing. Absorbable monofilament or polyfilament (never chromic) subcutaneous sutures (3-0 to 5-0) is used to diminish dead space and provide additional support. Subcutaneous suture must be nonreactive and of small caliber (4-0 or 5-0 multifiber/monofiber absorbable sutures). 5-0 Monocryl is difficult to see and work with; PDS may be substituted (4-0 or 5-0).

In labia minoraplasty, subcuticular closure works well for linear technique, but is technically difficult for V-wedge. A series of interrupted 5-0 Vicryl Rapide sutures placed 2–3 mm apart, with generous use of mattress sutures to prevent edge inversion is preferred. A continuous suture line should not be used on the labial edge. More scalloped appearance follows if the edge is closed by running or tightly placed sutures (occasionally with scarring and disfigurement), hypersensitivity of the edge, and if resection is performed close to the frenulum or clitoris, pain with genital excitation.

Dressing: The incision is coated with antibacterial ointment and covered with a nonstick dressing (Telfa, etc.), gauze and disposable panties. Care is taken with immediate postoperative ambulation, and it is done slowly and in stages to avoid hypotension in a premedicated patient who has been in dorsal lithotomy for 1–2.5 h.

At 4–6 weeks initial results may be appreciated, and full activities, including sexual activities, may be resumed. However, it will be 3–6 months before final results are manifested.

Postoperative Care

Topical antibiotic ointment is applied to incision immediately following surgery and continued for first 5 postoperative days. Sanitary pad may be used at all times until the incisions have healed. Postoperative pain occasionally requires moderate narcotics.

For labial procedures, it is important in postoperative period to reduce edema as it may result in wound dehiscence by placing excess tension on wound closures and may compromise esthetic results. Icing the labia in in the postoperative period 15–20 min of every hour for the initial 48–72 h after surgery is advised. Patients are instructed to wear loose-fitting underclothing, to avoid touching the operative area, and to refrain from sexual intercourse and placing anything in the vagina and only to shower (no submersion) for a period of 6 weeks. Patients should expect pruritus upon suture hydrolysis. Once candida is excluded, reassuring the patient that this situation is temporary and counseling that she may take an antihistamine to ease these symptoms is helpful.

For vaginoplasty, vaginal packing is left postoperatively and removed prior to discharge. Routine instructions for vaginal surgery are given to the patient and she is seen for follow-up at 4 weeks postoperatively or sooner as indicated. The vaginal introitus and caliber are assessed.

Follow-up

Patients are seen postoperatively at 1 week and 1 month following their procedure. The patient may return to normal work in 3–4 days. It is recommended to avoid tampons or tight clothing, and sexual intercourse for 4 weeks.

Postoperative Instructions

Patients are given all pre- and postoperative instructions in written form, which they read preoperatively and *sign.*

- Q-Tip instructions are given for first 48 h with Neosporin or peroxide to keep labia edges from sticking to each other.
- Showering instructions, allowing soaping water to "drip" and how to pat dry.
- Application of local estradiol cream (0.01–0.02%) in addition to, or mixed with a copper peptide cream (Cu-3), applied sparingly to edges for patients who are over 42 or 43 years old.
- Advise patients to not frequently look at the surgical area and to never pull up to visualize.
- Apply ice-pack for first 48–72 h and continue if necessary. Heat is advised after 72 h if swelling persists.
- No running, jumping, aerobics, lower body exercising or swimming for 3 weeks.
- Tampax use is discouraged until 28 days.
- Soaking is fine after day 21.
- Sexual activity is not advised for 5–6 weeks.

Revisions

A revision should not be undertaken in most cases until a minimum of 3–4 months (and in many cases 6 months) from the primary procedure as it takes atleast 3 months until the tissue has healed sufficiently. Prior to this, "softening" and other tissue changes continue to occur. Also, revascularization takes a minimum of 3–6 months to expect a normal healing process in the area.

Perineoplasty Overtightening

Overtightening in distal one-third to one-half of the vagina is seen in 10–15% of cases (more common when V-wedge labiaplasty is performed with perineo- or vagino-plasty). Usually this can be resolved over 2–4 weeks with use of progressive dilators, beginning at ~2.5–3 cm. For peri- or postmenopausal women, best results are obtained after pre-treating with 2–3 weeks of vaginal estradiol applications, and continuing through the dilating process.

For overtightening with overvigorous plication of levator in mid-vagina or at junction of mid- and distal vagina, correction is done making an incision over the area where the suture may be palpated, carefully dissecting down and separating the suture. An alternative is to wait until complete suture absorption (8–10 weeks) and begin careful progressive dilatations.

The "touch-up" rate is less than 6% with 92% overall satisfaction.

BRIDGING THE GAP FROM ESTHETICS TO FUNCTIONALITY: TISSUE REMODELING MANIPULATION

Role of Energy-based Devices[29]

When absorbed in sufficient amounts, light energy can induce changes in the skin and mucosal matrix.

Lasers devices allow for delivery of light to the skin in a controlled manner. The past decade has seen a surge in technological advancements of energy-based devices (EBD) (fractional laser and radiofrequency) that work on vaginal wall to reverse its age-related tissue remodeling. Thermal energy delivered on vaginal wall stimulates neovascularization, and collagen formation and proliferation of glycogen-enriched epithelium leading to improved natural lubrication and urinary continence.

The wavelengths across the electromagnetic spectrum are differentially absorbed by different tissue chromophores, including hemoglobin, melanin and water.[62] Distinct physiological characteristics of the target tissue and technical parameters of energy-based devices influence the tissue interactions at cellular level. These include laser wavelength, energy density, pulse duration, spot diameter, tissue absorption, hydration, and oxygenation, blood supply, degree of keratinization and insulating properties (adipose tissue).

Controlled power of the energy source must be used in vaginal tissue that varies in its water content and cellular component with age, and under hormonal influence, among other factors.[63]

Skin Optics[64]

A thorough understanding of interactions between light and biologic tissue is critical for selection of a laser device as well as effective and safe use of the equipment. Molecules that absorb light are called chromophores. Melanin, oxyhemoglobin and water are examples of biologic chromophores that are frequently targeted. Light absorbed into a target chromophore is converted to thermal energy, leading to heating and destruction of the chromophore.

THERAPEUTIC PARAMETERS

Wavelength and pulse duration are the most important laser parameters that govern effects of laser light on skin. Fluence, irradiance and spot size are additional laser settings that influence clinical outcomes.

- *Wavelength*: Emitted light determines its depth of penetration into skin. Long wavelengths of light penetrate more deeply into skin than shorter wavelengths. Chromophores absorb light most effectively at different wavelengths. To exert the greatest effect, wavelength should be near the maximum absorption of target chromophore and should be of sufficient length to penetrate to the depth of target. Because light scattering decreases with increasing wavelength, greater penetration is achieved with longer wavelengths of light. In contrast, high absorption of light by water molecules in epidermis markedly limits the depth of penetration of light emitted from mid-infrared (2,940 nm erbium: yttrium aluminum garnet (Er:YAG)) and far infrared (10,600 nm carbon dioxide, CO_2) lasers.
- *Pulse duration*: Setting is determined by the thermal relaxation time of the target chromophore.
- *Thermal relaxation time*: It is defined as amount of time it takes temperature of a target to return to the ambient temperature following heating.[65] If an object is heated for a period equal to or shorter than its thermal relaxation time, accumulated heat and resultant damage is confined to target object alone. This selective photothermolysis dramatically reduces the risk of scarring. The CO_2 laser penetrates skin to a depth of 0.05 mm, and thermal relaxation time of this thickness of tissue is approximately 1 ms.[66,67]
- *Fluence*: It is a measurement of amount of energy delivered or unit area.
- *Irradiance*: Power describes the rate of energy delivery and is measured in J/second (watts). Irradiance relates this measurement to size of the treated area and describes the rate of energy delivery/ unit area (watts/cm^2).[68] Irradiance is calculated from laser power output and spot size. It is a measurement of intensity of energy delivery. Very high irradiance achieves much faster heating than low irradiance. Decreasing the pulse duration of a laser device without changing the energy results in higher level of irradiance. Slow heating (low irradiance) coagulates tissue while fast heating (high irradiance) can vaporize tissue.
- *Spot size*: It is the diameter of beam of light emitted that hits the skin surface. Light delivered through a small spot size is more susceptible to scattering than light delivered through large spot sizes. Larger spot sizes are preferred when targeting structures in the mid or deep dermis. Spot size is less important for superficial targets.

There are essentially three variables one can control, namely power (watts), spot size (mm^2/cm^2) and, exposure time or pulse duration (fractions of seconds). Power may be kept constant with widely varying effects, depending on spot size and duration of exposure. Irradiance (W/cm^2) is a more useful measure of intensity of beam at focal point because it considers surface area of spot. One can vary the amount of energy delivered to target tissue (and hence proportional to depth of penetration) by varying the exposure time (pulse width). Depth of penetration is determined by fluence that allows for broad-based superficial pattern of ablation limited to epidermis and superficial papillary dermis. By manipulating number of pulses, density and energy per pulse, degree of thermal injury to tissue can be controlled.[69]

Selective photothermolysis describes use of light energy to selectively destroy specific structures in skin while minimizing damage to other tissues. The following principles compose the theory of selective photothermolysis:[65]

- Wavelength of light should be absorbed preferentially by target chromophore and penetrate the skin sufficiently to reach its depth.
- Light must be delivered in a period of time that is short enough to prevent transfer of excessive heat to adjacent structures.
- Energy delivered per unit area (fluence) must be sufficient to exert desired therapeutic effect, but at a level that minimizes collateral tissue damage.

Fractional photothermolysis is a method of maintaining tight control over extent of laser light injury. The technique involves use of infrared light, which is well absorbed by water, to coagulate/ablate narrow columns of tissue called microthermal zones (MTZs).[70] A pattern of thousands of MTZs (approximately 0.1 mm in diameter) is laid down. In general, proportion of injured tissue represents 10–50% of skin or mucosal surface. Skin between the columns is spared from injury (Fig. 42.7). The reservoir of undamaged skin adjacent to sites of laser injury allows for rapid reepithelialization after treatment through the migration of viable cells into wounded areas. As healing occurs, remodeling of the affected epidermis and dermis contributes to changes in the appearance or texture of the skin.[71]

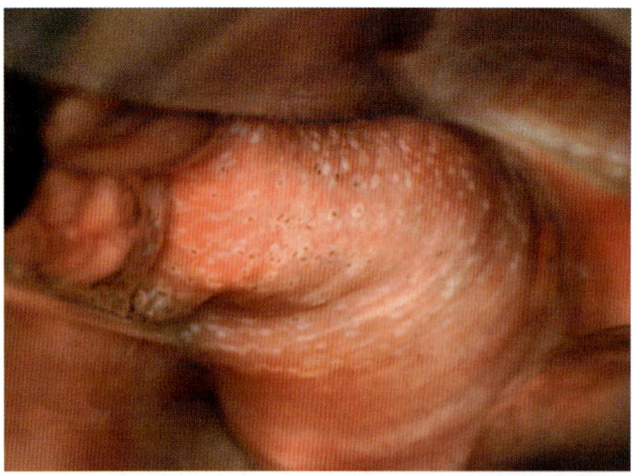

Fig. 42.7: Fractional CO_2 laser application to the upper vaginal wall. This picture was taken immediately after the energy application.

CLASSIFICATION OF DEVICES

The three major categories include continuous wave lasers, pulsed lasers and fractionated lasers.

Continuous and quasi-continuous wave lasers emit continuous laser beam as long as foot or finger switch is depressed. Scanning devices are not always effective in preventing cutaneous damage. As a result, continuous wave lasers have been mostly supplanted by pulsed lasers.

Pulsed Lasers

Pulsed lasers produce a laser beam that is emitted in short pulses with long period (0.1–1 s) between pulses. Pulsed ablative CO_2 and Er:YAG lasers are used for laser skin resurfacing.[66] They are useful for precisely ablating superficial skin lesions while leaving behind a very narrow zone of thermal damage.

Fractionated Lasers

For fractional photothermolysis most commonly are used for skin resurfacing and the treatment of scars.[72,73] They are divided into nonablative and ablative devices:

- *Nonablative fractionated lasers*: Thermally coagulate narrow vertical columns of epidermis and variable portions of dermis. This is achieved with near infrared lasers (1,320, 1,440, 1,540, 1,550 and 1,927 nm). These lasers emit light that is absorbed by water in skin to a lesser extent than light from mid and far infrared lasers, which are used for fractional ablation. Following treatment, thermally coagulated epidermis is rapidly sloughed off and reepithelialization is completed within 2–3 days. The thermally coagulated dermis is gradually replaced with new collagen deposition and collagen remodeling. A series of treatments usually is necessary to gradually remodel the entire skin surface.
- *Ablative fractionated laser*: Delivery creates ablative MTZs in skin that extend into the dermis. This is achieved with mid infrared (2,940 or 2,790 nm) and far infrared (10,600 nm) lasers, which emit light that is strongly absorbed by water.[74,75] A zone of thermally coagulated tissue also occurs around the ablated zone. With

Er:YAG (2,940 nm) laser, peripheral coagulated zone is very narrow, which accounts for frequent appearance of pinpoint bleeding during treatment. The CO_2 (10,600 nm) laser yields a thicker coagulated zone, which reduces bleeding. Reepithelialization usually occurs around 4 days after treatment with fractionated Er:YAG laser and after about 7 days following fractionated CO_2 laser therapy. This relatively short time course to reepithelialization is an advantage over traditional laser resurfacing with pulsed CO_2 or Er:YAG lasers, which requires a healing period of around 7–10 days.

Blue or red light-emitting diode (LED) sources, a variety of visible light lasers, and intense pulsed light (IPL) devices all have been utilized as light sources for photodynamic therapy. Photodynamic therapy has been used for the treatment of actinic keratoses, skin cancer and acne, as well as for photorejuvenation.[76,77]

CLINICAL APPLICATIONS OF ENERGY-BASED DEVICES ON FEMALE GENITALIA

Indications and Applications

- Vaginal dryness, burning/ itching
- Loss of elasticity and tone (laxity/ vaginal relaxation syndrome)
- Urinary incontinence
- Thrush and bladder infections
- Painful intercourse
- Vaginal or vulva pain
- Mild Prolapse
- Reduced sensitivity and sexual arousal
- Lichen sclerosus
- Vulval skin resurfacing for scars, tissue laxity or skin rejuvenation.

Vaginal Atrophy

Many patients with chronic urinary tract infections (UTI), or urinary symptoms find improvement after CO_2 microablative laser with reductions in urgency, frequency and UTIs. Ideal patient is postmenopausal female with dyspareunia or vaginal dryness, plus or minus lower urinary tract symptoms, and particularly breast cancer patients who are not really candidates for traditional therapies such as vaginal estrogen. Breast cancer patients who have taken anti-neoplastics such as aromatase inhibitors suffer severe debilitating atrophy of genital tissues. Most breast cancer patients suffer doubly from genitourinary syndrome of menopause (GSM) due to lack of estrogen and an exacerbation from medications they take to prevent recurrence of their breast cancer.[78] EBDs are a very fast, relatively painless way to induce changes in vaginal skin. Lubricants are not a treatment option; they are a symptom reliever. Lubricants and vaginal moisturizers do have place to combat dyspareunia.

Laser vaginal application focuses on restoring functionality by reversing the age or mechanical stress-related vaginal remodeling that results in vaginal laxity. Surgical techniques for vaginal tightening aim to modify the caliber of the vaginal canal but do not alter the quality of vaginal mucosa and/ or its functionality. Microablative fractional lasers, RF and high-intensity focused ultrasound (HiFU) devices induce superficial tissue shrinkage as well as deep stimulation of ECM layer of submucosa.[79-82] Histologically evident alterations in postmenopausal atrophic vaginal mucosa following fractional CO_2 laser treatment has provided an understanding the underlying molecular mechanisms responsible for tissue remodeling.[83-85] Neocollagenesis, production of ground substance components within ECM and glycogen and acidic mucins within epithelium and on epithelial surface, transform the mucosa from an atrophic state to a healthy premenopausal state (Figs. 42.8A to D).[85] Robust data is available on impact of laser treatment on human skin, studied using reverse transcriptase real-time polymerase chain reaction (rt-PCR) technology and Immunohistochemistry (IHC).[86]

Mucosal Responses Following Fractional Laser Treatment

Following fractional CO_2 laser treatment stratified squamous epithelium is thicker and comprised of 20–40 cell layers that provide cells for differentiation and superficial shedding. Basal layer cells are closely packed and appear stratified. Increased papillary projections with blood capillaries, of basal layer, protruding onto undersurface of epithelium with indentations is seen. Intermediate layer cells appear enlarged, with nucleus surrounded by a wide cytoplasm rich in glycogen. Shedding of superficial epithelial cells with exposure to glycogen into the vaginal lumen is seen. *Lactobacilli vaginalis* dependent on glycogen from shedding of superficial epithelial cells acidify the vaginal transudate at mucosal surface, and restore the vaginal pH to acidic premenopausal state,

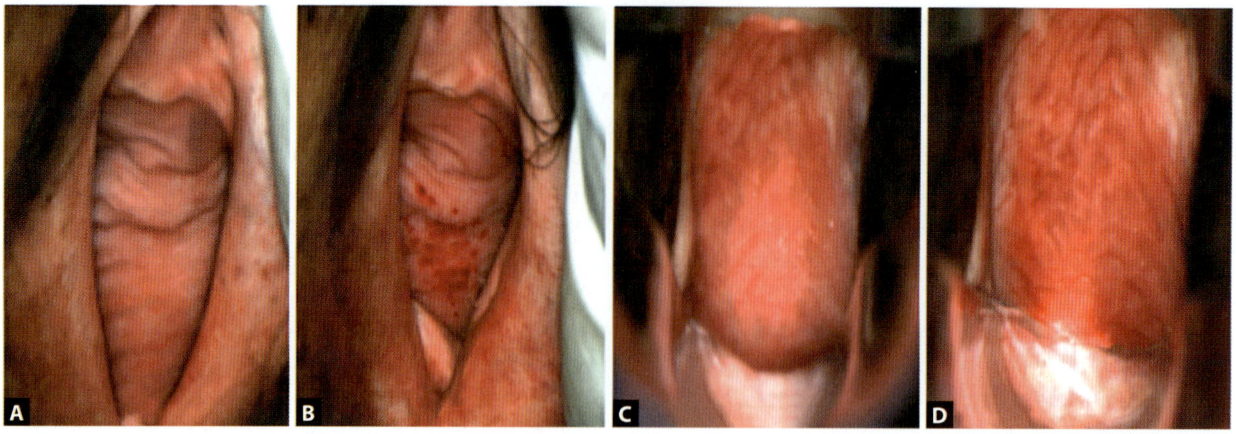

Figs. 42.8A to D: The efficacy of fractional CO_2 laser applied on atrophic anterior vaginal wall. The serial of the pictures shows the vaginal tissue before the application, immediately after the application, 3 months after application and 6 months after the application.

preventing colonization of pathogens.[87,88] Increased vascularity (capillaries penetrating newly formed papillae underneath the epithelium) in connective tissue supports the renewed activity of fibroblasts and provides the metabolic support for epithelial cell proliferation and differentiation.

Biomolecular Effects of EBD Application on Vaginal Mucosa

The epithelial restorative changes, with new active epithelial cells with increased layers and desquamation, are a consequence of activation of cytokines or growth factors in connective tissue that further stimulates new collagen synthesis and ground substance rich in fibrillar and nonfibrillar components and increases angiogenesis that improve the hydration and permeability of ECM. This increases the molecular traffic inside the connective tissue, and between the newly formed vessels and the epithelium, with resultant restoration of related epithelial functions (proliferation, differentiation, renewed glycogen synthesis and desquamation).

Lamina propria fibroblasts have high organelle content, RER (site of procollagen synthesis) and well-developed Golgi (site of synthesis of polysaccharides and of glycosylation of protein components of ground substances (glycoproteins, proteoglycans, and adhesive glycoproteins)).[89,90] These structures provide for synthesis of both fibrillar and ground substance components of ECM. Collagen I induction is the most direct predictor of clinical efficacy. The significant increase in mRNA levels of procollagen, MMPs, interleukin-1b (IL-1b), tumor necrosis factor-a (TNF-a) and TGF-b1 following laser (that are fluence dependent) suggests stimulation of tissue renewal mechanisms:

- Stimulation of connective tissue remodeling by fibroblasts has been correlated with activation of heat shock protein (HSP) response persisting at least 3 months following treatment.[91] The HSP get activated and other growth factors come into play to induce type 1 versus type 3 collagen. The HSP47 in RER plays an important role in early stages of post-treatment collagen biosynthesis.[92-97]
- Acute inflammation is largely an expression of innate immunity, which involves induction of cytokines, chemokines and antimicrobial peptides that stimulate influx and activation of monocytes and neutrophils. Local increase in different cytokines, particularly TGF-b (stimulating collagen), basic fibroblast growth factor (bFGF; stimulates angiogenetic activity with endothelial cell migration and proliferation), epidermal growth factor (EGF; stimulates re-epithelization), PDGF (stimulates fibroblasts to produce ECM components), TNF-a and vascular endothelial growth factor (VEGF; regulates vasculogenesis and angiogenesis) is seen. Their expression is initiated in the suprabasal layers of epithelium (glycogen synthesis) and in connective tissue with stimulation of fibroblast activity and formation of new vessels.[98]
  - Neutrophils and macrophages are prominent cell types that participate in the initial stage of wound repair. Influx of both cells types is observed within 24 h after treatment. At 3 days, substantial accumulation of neutrophils and macrophages is observed throughout the dermis. By 7 days after treatment, presence of both cell types is substantially lower in treated skin.
  - IL-1b (primary cytokine) is significantly increased 1 day after treatment and returns

to near baseline levels within 3 days after treatment.
  - Chemokine IL-8 (potent neutrophil chemoattractant that plays an important role in innate immunity) is significantly increased within 1 day after treatment and returns to baseline within 1 week after treatment.
  - Antimicrobial peptides (AMP) play an important role in innate immune responses to protect against cutaneous infection. Gene expression of AMP is significantly induced after treatment, with maximal induction during first week.
  - Inflammatory infiltrate including CD3+ and CD20+ cells are important in clearance of thermally altered tissue as dermal remodeling occurs.
- Inflammatory mediators induce enzymes (MMP-1, MMP-3 and MMP-9) that degrade the dermal collagen-rich ECM significantly within 1 day. This degradation facilitates motility of immune cells within dermis and sets the stage for production of new ECM during remodeling phase. MMP-1 initiates cleavage of collagen fibrils, which are further degraded by MMP-3 and MMP-9. MMP-1 and MMP-3 (observed throughout the upper dermis) remain high during first week after treatment and then fall sharply by second week, whereas MMP-9 expression remain high for at least 2 weeks. MMP-9 gene (stored within secretory granules in neutrophils) expression is increased in a more delayed fashion, with maximal staining of observed within first week after treatment, and consistent with neutrophil elastase, and peaks at 2 to 3 weeks after treatment.[98]

After inflammatory phase of wound healing, dermal fibroblasts produce new ECM, primarily composed of type I and type III collagen fibrils. Fractionated laser treatment significantly induces type I procollagen mRNA and protein. Significant induction of type I and type III procollagen mRNA is observed at 2 weeks and remains high for at least 5 weeks after treatment. Average peak induction after with fractionated CO_2 laser is 8.4-fold.[98] In addition, dermal wound repair involves increased vascularization. Fractionated CO_2 laser treatment increases density of CD31-positive vessels and endothelial cells at 3 and 5 weeks after laser treatment.[98]

Long pulse, nonablative modes have been evaluated for their ability to induce deep thermal effects on vaginal mucosa. Deep coagulation by stacking repetitive Er:YAG laser pulses on the same tissue site has been described.[99] This mode generates a thermal change in deeper layers, with only minor superficial ablation (5 µm) on surface, but with enough caloric effect to thermally alter the chromophore. Using a large spot size (> 5 mm), heating can be achieved and with repetition of exposures (stacking), this deepens the heat effect in lamina propria to a depth of at least 500–1,000 µm (depending on degree of tissue hydration), inflicting the "Joule effect" (photothermal and thermochemical effect) on vaginal mucosa. With local rise in temperature, bradykinin and histamine are released with relaxation of precapillary arteriolar sphincters, and vasodilation, an effect called "phenomenon of thermal reperfusion."[100-102]

Stress Urinary Incontinence

Urethral support can be improved by inducing thermal effects on suburethral tissue using energy-based devices. Numerous studies[103-109] confirm improvement in urinary control following treatment with Er:YAG laser, CO_2 laser and RF all of which trigger a photo-thermal effect, as deep as 0.5 mm inside the anterior vaginal wall, and results in 30% reduction in tissue volume. The thermally induced neocollagenesis improves thickness, elasticity and firmness of the vaginal wall, and acts locally at the suburethral plexus level.[104,105]

Application of EBD on External Genitals

Indications

- Aging skin
- Scarred tissue following trauma, perineal repairs
- Cosmesis
- Lichen sclerosus
- Vulvodynia.

Skin Changes with Aging

Chronologic aging contributes to changes in skin, such as dyschromia, rhytides, textural alterations and skin laxity. Skin starts showing its first signs of aging in late twenties to early thirties. Chronic exposure to ultraviolet light (photodamage) also promotes damage to dermis, which manifests clinically as rhytides and skin laxity and histologically as disorganized collagen fibrils and abnormal elastotic material.[110]

Characteristics of aging: Loss of dermal substrates (collagen, elastin and ground substances). The epidermis tends to thicken and there is general loss of subcutaneous fibrous connectivity with loss of soft tissue volume, and ptosis of soft tissues. Superficial epidermal–dermal changes include dyschromias, brown discoloration, hyperpigmentation, erythema, telangiectasia, rosacea and dark melanin dyschromia, especially in photodamaged skin.[81]

Common histologic and molecular-level features include reduction in the amount of collagen, fragmentation of collagen fibers, degeneration of elastic fibers, upregulation of MMPs (especially MMP-1 and MMP-2), dilated and tortuous dermal vessels and atrophy and disorientation of epidermis.[111,112]

Several modalities have been developed in order to reverse dermal and epidermal signs of photo- and chronological aging. The main concept is removing epidermis and inducing controlled form of skin wounding to promote collagen biosynthesis and dermal matrix remodeling. Most commonly used interventions as of today are retinoic acid, dermabrasion, chemical peels and ablative laser resurfacing with CO_2 or Er:YAG lasers or combination of these wavelengths.[113-115] Nonablative skin rejuvenation aims to improve photoaged and aging skin without destroying epidermis.[116,117]

Vulvodynia and Provoked Vestibulodynia

Provoked, localized vestibulodynia (PVD), previously called vulvar vestibulitis syndrome, shows a significantly favorable response to fractional microablative CO_2 laser treatment after three sessions.[118] Fractional CO_2 laser has also shown to be effective in cases of postpartum dyspareunia and perineal pain.[119]

Lichen Sclerosus

Lichen sclerosus (LS) in genital area can lead to vulvar scarring, loss of portions or all of the labia minora (resorption), clitoral adhesion and narrowing of introitus. If left untreated, it can lead to progressive destruction of vulvar architecture, or less commonly to vulvar squamous cell carcinoma (SCC).[120] Superficial ablation of LS by fractional CO_2 laser using very low energy, three sessions (three passes each session) at 4–6 week intervals has been described[121-125] with a healing period of several weeks. Symptomatic improvement along with visible improvement of skin color, elasticity and vascularity is seen after the third session and maintained beyond 6 months. Histological evaluations after laser treatment confirm healing changes.

Laser Skin Resurfacing and Rejuvenation

Lasers rely on differing techniques to produce thermal damage to epidermis and dermis, resulting in tissue ablation and collagen proliferation. Each laser varies in intensity of treatment, efficacy, and side-effect profile.

Choice of laser: For a given device, degree of ablativeness depends on multiple factors, including fluence, repetition rate, degree of coverage of the device and patient skin types and anatomic sites, whether the treatment is ablative, partially ablative or non-ablative. Ablative lasers include continuous wave CO_2 lasers, short-pulse, high peak-power CO_2 lasers, rapidly scanned, focused-beam CO_2 lasers, and normal-mode Er:YAG lasers. Traditional Er:YAG laser requires more laser passes (retreatment of same area during a single treatment session) than traditional CO_2 lasers to achieve a similar depth of ablation.[126,127] Er:YAG also appears to have lower risk for scarring than CO_2 laser. Nonablative fractional lasers have also been used for skin rejuvenation, but are less effective for this indication.[128]

The high-energy, short-pulsed lasers offer controlled ablation of skin and are based on selective photo-thermolysis, with CO_2 and Er:YAG laser systems targeting epidermal and dermal water leading to effective cutaneous ablation with minimal surrounding collateral tissue damage. Absorption of light energy by water in epidermis leads to rapid accumulation of heat and consequent vaporization of epidermis. Thermal damage extends beyond penetration of light known as residual thermal damage (RTD). Both amount of tissue ablation and zone of RTD play an important role in the efficacy of ablative laser resurfacing.[129-131] Residual thermal damage represents the true depth of injury and is the primary factor leading to effectiveness.[132] It is increased with higher fluence,[133,134] whereas increased density results in greater depth of ablation. The RTD reaches depths of 100–150 μm with traditional CO_2 lasers and 10–40 μm with traditional ER:YAG lasers.[23] The heat transferred to underlying dermal collagen is believed to contribute to collagen contraction and remodeling as well as clinically evident skin tightening.[132,135-138]

The CO_2 lasers target water by emitting a 10,600-nm light pulse that leads to vaporization of intra- and extracellular water, resulting in tissue ablation. Absorption coefficient for CO_2 laser is 770/cm in liquid water, and is comparable in nearly all biological substances; its scattering coefficient in any histologic material is negligible by comparison. It has small minimum focal-spot diameter and achieves hemostasis in vessels of 0.5 mm or smaller.[139] To achieve ablation without excessive thermal damage, a fluence of 5 J/cm^2 must be delivered within a pulse duration of < 1 ms, the generally agreed upon thermal relaxation time of skin. At a setting of 5 J/cm^2 and pulse duration of <1 ms, light from CO_2 laser penetrates to depth of 20–30 μm. Depending on duration and intensity of exposure, depth of dermal ablation, and damage to surrounding tissue is varied.[140]

Fluence levels of 5–15 J/cm^2 are commonly used for ablative resurfacing with Er:YAG lasers. Water molecules have greater affinity for light emitted from Er:YAG lasers, and therefore a shallower absorption depth, which reaches depths of only 1–3 μm per J/cm^2. This leads to less RTD and faster healing, but Er:YAG is less effective for dermal collagen remodeling because laser does not affect the dermis as significantly as CO_2 laser. The most effective Er:YAG lasers use longer pulse durations to increase residual thermal damage depth.[141]

The size of vessels in the dermis increases with increasing depth of penetration. The zone of collagen denaturation around the zone of vaporization assists in sealing off some of these vessels to limit the bleeding. This might provide a significant advantage as compared to Er:YAG ablative resurfacing, which lacks a significant zone of coagulation to promote hemostasis.[142] The smaller zone of RTD would also limit the efficacy of Er:YAG resurfacing compared to CO_2.[143]

Heat in Laser Resurfacing

Thermal Shrinkage of Collagen by Lasers

Heat generated in the skin by absorption of laser light causes shrinkage of collagen fibers. Thermal shrinkage of collagen occurs between 55°C and 58°C. Denaturing of collagen occurs between 60°C and 70°C.[132] Once denatured, it rapidly contracts to one-third of their length.[144] The shrinkage of collagen is the primary mechanism of skin tightening, although vaporization of intracellular water and ablation contribute as well. The shrinkage observed when a laser beam strikes skin is shrinkage caused by desiccation, i.e., when water content of epidermis is reduced from 70% to lower values, the histologic structural matrix contracts.[139] A wound-healing phase is then initiated characterized by high levels of MMP.[145] Rapid reconstitution of epidermis from adjacent epidermal cells contrasts with healing after traditional resurfacing in which new epidermis is derived from cells that migrate from adnexal structures. A prolonged period of dermal neocollagenesis of up to at least 6 months follows.[86]

Excessive transfer of heat to dermis can lead to adverse effects such as scarring and permanent hypopigmentation. To minimize this risk, the time the laser beam is in contact with skin (pulse duration) should be shorter than the tissue thermal relaxation time. High-energy pulsed CO_2 laser (pulse duration <1 ms) and short-pulsed Er:YAG laser (pulse duration 250–350 μs) induce ablation, while maintaining tight control over duration of light delivery and reducing risk for inadvertent damage. Rapidly scanning CO_2 lasers utilize computerized scanning mechanism to limit duration of contact of laser beam with any given site on skin and are an alternative to pulsed devices.

In darker skin, laser-induced dyspigmentation is a major concern, as risk rises with increasing baseline skin pigmentation. Hyperpigmentation and hypopigmentation may occur with all forms of ablative laser resurfacing, but is most likely after treatment with traditional CO_2 lasers.[126,146-148] Fractional ablative lasers may be a preferable alternative in this population.[146,148]

Fractionated lasers have become the cornerstone of laser skin rejuvenation. Fractional laser treatments have been shown to cause collagen remodeling and thickening of dermal collagen. There is clinical evidence of improvement of dyspigmentation and textural abnormality after fractional resurfacing. Histologic studies suggest that thermal injury to dermis initiates a cascade of inflammatory events, including fibroblastic proliferation and upregulation of collagen expression. Collagen deposition then assumes a horizontal orientation parallel to the plane of epidermis, leading to appearance of dermal thickening.[149]

Fractional erbium (Er:YAG) and CO_2 lasers are ablative fractional resurfacing systems widely used to improve the skin appearance and atrophic scars. Efficacy of fractional ablative lasers for skin tightening exceed that of traditional ablative lasers, plus relatively short recovery period and reduced risk for adverse effects associated with fractional ablative lasers have contributed to them as preferred devices for ablative laser resurfacing.[71] The proportion of surface area that is fractionated is not comparable across devices. It is also not the case that if a set of parameters is said to affect 10% of the skin surface, then

10 passes would lead to complete ablation; far fewer passes are likely to cause focal thermal burns.[150]

Mechanism of Fractional Ablative Lasers

Ablative fractional resurfacing producing zones of ablation and coagulation.[151] Target chromophore for fractional lasers is water. Microscopic arrays of ablative and thermal coagulation zones are generated using a range of laser parameters. Microlesions involving a tapering ablative zone in skin lined by a thin layer of eschar surrounded by a thermal coagulation zone, together constitute the MTZ. Fractional lasers deliver MTZs that are usually less than 400 μm in diameter and up to 1300 μm deep; the type of fractional laser and specific laser settings determine the size of MTZ.[152] The microscopic treatment zones form the building blocks for a macroscopic treatment effect. Microepidermal necrotic debris (MEND) is a spheroid or button-shaped collection of necrotic debris located just below an intact stratum corneum overlying each dermal wound (i.e., over each MTZ). Photothermal tissue necrosis involving epidermal and dermal compartments down to the mid-reticular dermis is clinically well tolerated when MTZ grid spacing is above twice the diameter of individual MTZs (i.e., >200 μm).[70] Ablative fractional resurfacing demonstrates much more rapid re-epithelialization, whether powered by erbium or CO_2 lasers. By 48 h, complete reepithelialization with restoration of basement membrane is apparent no later than 7 days post-treatment. Erythema subsides within 4-7 days after treatment.[91]

Heat Shock Proteins (HSP)

- hsp72 is an early (hours) responder to thermal damage in skin.[153] hsp72 expression is upregulated significantly at 48 h post-treatment and peaks between 2 and 7 days later. There is persistence of spindle cells in dermis consistent with an ongoing fibroblastic response.
- Increased hsp47 expression is delayed, first apparent at 7 days post-treatment and remains elevated at least for 3 months. It appears to play a more important role in long-term wound healing by acting as a procollagen chaperone[154] promoting neocollagenesis. Expression of hsp47 is diffuse in dermis at 3 months post-treatment, indicating that activation of fibroblasts is occurring in both treated and untreated tissue. Diffuse upregulation of hsp47 expression provides conclusive evidence that neocollagenesis is persistent for minimum of 3 months post-treatment.
- The dermal component of MTZ repair involves removal and replacement of necrotic cellular materials and denatured ECM in a relatively prolonged process that does not appear to involve a classical "inflammatory" phase of wound repair. Remodeling of matrix components is apparent by 3 months. Increased undulating rete ridge patterns in treated skin is seen.[70] Ablative fractional resurfacing treatment leads to long-term dermal remodeling with increased collagen synthesis.

Ablative fractional resurfacing also removes a relatively large volume of dermal tissue to depths that conventional CO_2 and Er:YAG laser resurfacing were previously incapable of reaching without causing untoward side effects. Dermal tissue as deep as 659 ± 69 μm at 30 mJ can be removed through ablative fractional resurfacing with a general trend toward greater increases in depth than width with increasing pulse energy.[91] This implies that the aspect ratio of ablative zone (i.e., ablative depth-to-width ratio) increases with rising pulse energies, a phenomenon not observed with nonablative fractional resurfacing treatment.[155] Thus, an advantage is its potential to remove more unwanted and deep dermal material post-fractional resurfacing.[151] A skin tightening effect also occurs after treatment with ablative fractional lasers; both immediate and delayed collagen contraction and collagen remodeling may contribute to improvements in skin laxity.[156]

Adverse Effects

The risk of developing complications after cutaneous laser resurfacing is influenced by number of laser passes performed, energy densities used, degree of pulse/scan overlap, preoperative skin condition, skin type and anatomic areas to be resurfaced. Virtually all patients initially experience intense erythema, edema, serous discharge and crusting. These are more intense and prolonged after CO_2 because of slower rate of re-epithelization (8.5 vs 5.5 days, CO_2 vs Er:YAG laser).[78]

Adverse effects range from mild to severe. Mild reactions include prolonged erythema, acne or milia formation, contact dermatitis or pruritus. Moderate complications include viral, bacterial or fungal infections; postinflammatory hyperpigmentation (PIH); and delayed onset hypopigmentation. The rare and most serious complications include hypertrophic scarring, ectropion formation and disseminated infection.

Traditional ablative laser resurfacing is contraindicated in patients with a history of keloidal scarring, recent history oral isotretinoin therapy and sclerotic disorders involving the site to be treated. Compared with traditional ablative laser resurfacing, complications of fractional ablative laser resurfacing are less severe and less frequent.

Treatment-induced erythema is expected and usually resolves within a few days. Prolonged erythema (lasting more than one month) occurs in approximately 12% of patients[157] and usually resolves within three months.

Transient postinflammatory hyperpigmentation (PIH) occurs in approximately 30% of patients and is more likely to occur in those with skin phototypes III or higher.[158-160] Risk of PIH rises with increasing baseline skin pigmentation. However, duration and severity tend to be less in patients treated with fractional lasers.[157] Longer treatment intervals and adjustments to the energy and density settings may be beneficial for reducing the incidence of hyperpigmentation.[157,146] Hypopigmentation is rare after fractional laser resurfacing.

Hypopigmentation, more common in light-skinned individuals, may not be evident until several months after procedure.[149] Dyschromia is more likely to occur with CO_2 laser resurfacing than other forms of laser.

Scarring is uncommon, but can be devastating when it occurs.[161,162] Initial signs of scarring include a focal, persistent area of erythema or induration that appears a few weeks after therapy.

Viral, bacterial, or fungal infections can follow treatment. The risk for herpes simplex virus (HSV) infection after fractional laser resurfacing is lower than for traditional laser resurfacing (0.3–2% versus 2–7%).[157] Patients with HSV infection may present only with nonspecific superficial erosions in the treated area. One day prior to treatment, prophylactically administer either acyclovir 200 mg BID, valacyclovir 500 mg BID or famciclovir 500 mg BID, and should be continue for 5–7 days after treatment.

Other complications of fractional ablative laser resurfacing include transient acneiform eruptions, milia and ectropion. Ectropion may be most likely to occur in patients with a history of eyelid surgery or reduced skin elasticity in this area at baseline.[157]

Patient Evaluation

Selection of appropriate patient is of critical importance in laser skin resurfacing. The patient should be thoroughly informed of the expected treatment outcome, anticipated recovery period and treatment risks. A variety of factors influence the selection of the appropriate laser resurfacing technique, including the severity and location of photodamage, the patient's skin color and patient preference regarding the length of time required for healing. In most cases, treatment results in mild to moderate improvements in cutaneous signs of photoaging.

Preoperative Considerations

- Priming with estrogen once a week for 2 weeks may be done prior to intiating laser treatment.
- Retinoids may be stopped 1 week prior to treatment as they can blunt the heat shock response, which assists with rapid reepithelialization following tissue injury.[149]
- Topical anesthesia is often sufficient for treatment with fractional non-CO_2 devices. The CO_2 fractional laser typically produces more discomfort than non-CO_2 lasers, caused by greater tissue-heating effect on type C pain fibers.[62] Nerve blocks may be achieved using lidocaine 1–2% with 1:100,000 or 1:200,000 epinephrine, and can be enhanced using bupivacaine 0.5%, 1:10 $NaHCO_3$ 8.4%, and hyaluronidase.[135] Fanning or radially spacing subcutaneous injections from a single entry site techniquue is useful.
- The risk of dyspigmentation, PIH, rises with increasing skin pigmentation.[163] It is the most common complication in patients with dark skin (IV–VI). Patients with ethnic skin are at high risk of hyperpigmentation with fractional CO_2, and even with non-CO_2 fractional devices should be treated with less aggressive settings to minimize this risk. The rate of PIH has been found to be directly proportional to both energy and more to density of treatment.[146] Thus, it is important to start with conservative settings—low density and intensity—on such patients (even when using nonablative resurfacing techniques). Because the risks for dyspigmentation are greatest with CO_2 laser, generally avoid CO_2 laser resurfacing for skin rejuvenation in patients with skin phototypes IV or higher and prefer fractional ablative or traditional Er:YAG lasers. Pretreatment with topical tretinoin is recommended to improve

healing time.[164-170] To reduce the incidence of PIH, many advocate pre- and postoperative use of hydroquinone, tretinoin and/ or glycolic acid (although studies are inconclusive on their efficacy for prevention).[163,171] Skin lightening products (10% glycolic acid cream, or hydroquinone 4% cream plus tretinoin 0.025% cream) are of no benefit in the pretreatment phase,[170] but can be utilized in the post-treatment setting. In combination with nonablative devices, these agents may be of more use in preventing and treating hyperpigmentation.

- Scarring may occur with fractional CO_2 resurfacing. Fractional resurfacing has been used to treat many types of scars (acne, surgical, traumatic). Certain areas are especially prone to scarring because of the decrease in vascularity and thinness of the skin. To reduce this risk use low fluences, coupled with reduced surface area coverage, and avoid multiple passes and heat stacking by applying numerous repeat treatments to the same location, as these approaches can cause injury to the deep dermis. Patient- and device-specific factors should be considered. Some patients may be "poor healers," and it is important to elicit this in their medical history. Underlying collagen vascular diseases, and prior resurfacing procedures may predispose to scarring with fractional laser. For example, previous phenol peels or dermabrasion may make the patient's skin more sensitive, and fractional resurfacing may go deeper than anticipated, even with moderate settings. A 5% coverage with one device may be equivalent to 15% coverage with another, which may impact treatment results.[149]

Intraoperative

Clinician familiarity with the device utilized is essential. In general, use of higher energies with small spot sizes increases the depth of laser injury. Increasing pulse duration widens the diameter of MTZ and may increase the depth of ablation.[172] The density setting (amount of space between MTZs) can also be altered. It is advisable to reduce density in areas at greater risk for complications. Deeper penetrating MTZs of fractional injury associated with higher laser fluence (i.e., greater depth) may be better at inducing dermal collagen coagulation and neocollagenesis, which may lead to skin tightening and improving acne scarring,[173] whereas shallower but more extensive coverage (i.e., greater density) with lower fluences may be better for improving fine photodamage and dyspigmentation.[71] Variations in fractional laser device settings can significantly affect posttreatment outcomes, and settings may be selected based on the desired effect.[149]

It is important to remember that a patient's true Fitzpatrick type may not always be clinically apparent based on casual inspection of their skin color.[149] In darker-skinned patients, photodamage may be better treated with intense, lower density treatments because this may mitigate the risk of PIH. For instance, Asian patients with photodamage that receive a high-energy, low-density treatment (average fluence 16.3 mJ, density 1000 MTZ/cm^2) have lower prevalence of hyperpigmentation than those who received a low-energy, high-density session (fluence 8.2 mJ, density 2000 MTZ/cm^2).[146]

Skin should be cleansed thoroughly with a gentle cleanser. Ablative laser therapy is painful. Topical anesthetic is applied one hour prior to treatment and cold air is used to further improve patient comfort during treatment session.[174] Many advocate removal of epidermis by several sequential passes of laser beam, at low to moderate fluence, with mechanical debridement of desiccated epidermal debris gently between one pass and the next. The beneficial role of heat, generated by absorption of laser light in avascular epidermis, is to create a field of miniature, localized explosions caused by ultrarapid flashing of histologic water into steam that strip away the epidermis precisely. When CO_2 laser is used, dehydrated residue must be removed because it strongly absorbs the laser light at 10,600 nm but has no water remaining to hold the temperature at 100°C. This is not necessary with Er:YAG laser unless a buildup of eschar is noted, because absorption at 2,940 nm in this cutaneous debris is much lower.[139]

Postoperative

Proper wound management during immediate postoperative period is vital to success of laser resurfacing. Short-term recovery process may be hastened by frequent application of thick, healing ointments with cold, wet compresses and ice packs several times daily for first 48 h. Immediately after treatment, apply ice-cold wet compresses. Home care involves gentle skin cleansing and repeated application of ointment to maintain constant skin moisture until crusting ceases (usually by day 3).[135] For pruritus, prescribe a mid-potency topical corticosteroid for application twice daily for a few days. Itching most commonly begins on the third postoperative day. Desquamation for several days after treatment is normal. Scratching or rubbing of the skin should be avoided. Most patients can return to work 4–10 days after fractional CO_2 laser resurfacing depending on the extent and intensity of treatment. After fractional Er:YAG laser resurfacing, the recovery period is between 1 and 3 days. Daily application of topical hydroquinone cream, retinoids, and/or peeling agents such as low-potency glycolic acid can be prescribed to accelerate resolution.[126,160] Topical retinoids are added if tolerated.

Postoperative Considerations

Although adverse events are uncommon with fractional resurfacing, early detection can mitigate the risks of delayed healing, infection, and pigmentary abnormality.

- Erythema and edema are expected consequences of fractional resurfacing. Prolonged erythema, pigmentary alternation and scarring can be avoided by using lower energy density setting. However, delayed healing (more than 3 or 4 days for nonablative devices per month with ablative resurfacing) may be a sign of latent infection.[175] To facilitate wound healing, corticosteroids, cold compresses and persistent use of vinegar soaks followed by petrolatum may be used.
- Although complications caused by viruses, bacteria and fungi are rare, antibacterial and antiviral prophylaxis 2 days before and continuing for 5 days afterward affords protection during the perioperative period. Herpes simplex virus infection (0.3–2% of cases) is the most common following fractional resurfacing.[157]. Bacterial infection accounts for 0.1% of the infections. Extreme pruritus may be caused by *Candida*.[176] Vinegar soaks can be a useful adjunct that soothe the skin and provide protection from pseudomonal species.

Treatment Scheduling

Multiple treatments are required for a clinical significant result, with six or more non-CO_2 fractional treatments being a relatively common regimen. Although degree of clinical improvement depends on a variety of factors, including type of device, operative techniques, skin type, proportion of surface area treated and fluence, multiple treatments are usually necessary for significant improvement.[149]

External Genitals Scarring

CO_2 fractional laser is a potentially effective and safe modality for the treatment of hypertrophic scars, particularly in terms of pliability.[177] Fractional ablative CO_2 laser is employed in selective collagen remodeling by targeting the skin water (chromophore) content in abnormal collagen to improve, thickness, pliability, pain, pruritus and tightness.[69]

Anesthesia for small scars can be achieved with a combination of topical and injected local anesthetic agents. Grafted and traumatized sites are often insensate and pain is quite often limited to the deeper treatment of normal border skin, which is treated for 5 mm as often the tightness of scars can extend subclinically into these regions.[69] Larger more confluent areas of burn scars necessitate GA. Fractional CO_2 laser therapy parameters should be selected to avoid bulk heating of the scar tissue.

General principles include a minimum ablation threshold of 5 J/cm^2, a short pulse width to approximate the thermal relaxation time of skin (<1 ms) and a relatively narrow beam (<500 μm) to maintain ablation but limit excessive collateral thermal injury and thus potentially delayed healing with the risk of further scarring. Isolated areas of textural, pigment abnormalities or atrophy can be treated with lower pulse energies and higher densities whereas thicker scars require higher pulse energies and lower treatment densities.[69] Immediately post-treatment erythema lasts for a few hours only. Treatment interval is normally 3 months. Postoperative care regimen includes daily wash with antimicrobial and emollient lotion and application of petrolatum- or petroleum-based ointment until the treatment site is fully epithelialized, normally within 5 days of treatment. Viral prophylaxis and antibiotics are given to those patients at risk of infection and 1% hydrocortisone is given if pruritus is a feature. Normal activities can resume immediately postoperatively with avoidance of hot water, due to wound sensitivity.

Fractional technology operates via ultrafast pulses of energy to produce tissue ablation and minimize heat deposition allowing rapid re-epithelialization and deeper ablated columns of disorganized elastotic dermal type III collagen is also disrupted allowing replacement of the older injured collagen matrix with new organized type I collagen in a controlled manner.[91] There is an upregulation of type III collagen specific MMP-1 and microRNAs expression with associated alteration of type I and III procollagen mRNA levels and of TGF-β1-3 and basic fibroblast growth factor (bFGF) along with isolated MTZ fibroblastic apoptosis.[178-180] As a result, microperforations in may also cause weakening of adhesions between the scar and underlying tissue aiding functional recovery.[181]

Application of fractionated light therapy to a burn injury theoretically avoids excessive thermal injury, prolonged erythema, hypopigmentation and the potential of severe scarring.[158,182-188] Improvement in scar characteristics as well functionality and symptoms are most marked within first 2 weeks following the first session, with more modest improvements following subsequent treatments. Treatment carries inherent risks, most notably related to delayed wound healing, which include worsening of existing scarring or development of new scars or permanent hypopigmentation.

Skin Rejuvenation for Tissue Laxity

Ablative Chemical and Dermabrasion Techniques

In standard chemical ablation, chemical agents result in nonthermal chemical dissolution and coagulation of associated dermal proteins and wound healing that occurs over several weeks results in new collagen, elastin and skin tightening. Older chemical ablative techniques and macro-dermabrasion gave way to ablative laser resurfacing, including CO_2 and Er:YAG lasers.[183,189] Wavelengths and energies from IPL, pulse dye, IR diodes and IR heating lamps result in a nonablated, intact epidermal-dermal junction, whereas dermal water was the principal chromophore for IR devices. Hemoglobin and melanin were chromophores for very near IR and invisible skin-tightening light devices. Multiple treatments are often required with nonablative techniques and long-term results of skin tightening, and texture irregularities are often subtle at best.[81] These nonablative laser and light devices work by a photon interaction with a dermal chromophore. These nonablative laser and light devices, selective photothermolytic remodeling process will often result over several months, in some subtle to moderate tightening or texture improvements, and, depending on device, improvements in melanin and/or vascular discoloration. Examples of these devices include early infrared devices as well as IPL and pulse-dye laser technology. Often, combined with Botox, soft tissue fillers, microdermabrasion and other minimally invasive techniques to achieve quite pleasing esthetic results.[81]

If energy source, either laser-based or RF-based device, is placed in immediate subdermal space, significant soft tissue skin contraction and correction of laxity can be induced without an epidermal-dermal ablation. All of these devices will interact with dermal water, resulting in a photothermalytic thermal response. Generally, more ablative the laser or photon device, better the tightening results will be.[191] One can divide skin-tightening devices into two broad categories: transepidermal delivery of energy and subdermal delivery of energy (Table 42.1).

Ablative resurfacing with pulsed CO_2 (10,600 nm) and Er:YAG (2,940 nm) lasers, with photothermolytic process involving the photons being attracted to dermal water, are highly effective treatment options for severe photodamage and tissue laxity, resulting in ablative and nonablative coagulative disruption.[131,183,189] They have more selective depth control and precision injury. Significant tissue tightening is achieved with immediate collagen shrinkage followed by long-term collagen remodeling. Immediate disruption of collagen triple helix accounts for immediate, "on-table" skin-tightening effects and then a secondary tightening effect over 6 months from secondary neocollagenesis, elastin, and ground substance production.[189,190] A safer and

Table 42.1: Classification of energy-based skin-tightening devices.

Transepidermal energy delivery	IR lamp technology, 700 and 2000 nm Monopolar RF energy Bipolar RF energy in combination with other light sources Multipolar transepidermal skin-tightening RF devices IPL
Transepidermal fractional energy delivery	Transepidermal fractional CO_2 resurfacing Transepidermal fractional delivery of IR wavelengths Fractional IR delivery of Er YAG Er:YSGG (Yttrium–scandium–gallium–garnet) Fractional transepidermal RF energy
Subdermal delivery of energy	Subdermal delivery of fiberoptic laser energy Subdermal delivery of RF energy

less invasive treatment approach known as fractional deep dermal ablation (FDDA™) has been developed. Volume reduction through deep dermal ablation of tissue leads to clinically observed skin tightening. Histologic collagen remodeling and rapid histologic re-epithelialization occurs by 48 h. Two important risks that are associated with traditional ablative resurfacing, scarring and hypopigmentation, are not reported for up to 2 years.[143] This results in improvement in skin texture with high patient and physician satisfaction.

Radiofrequency Skin Tightening

Significant tissue tightening without disrupting the epidermal–dermal junction is seen with nonablative RF skin-tightening technologies. Through minimal to no epidermal–dermal ablation, RF energy is delivered into the dermis, where, rather than targeting traditional chromophores (hemoglobin, melanin or water), all molecules in RF pathways are oscillated 1–6 million times/s.[190,191] It is resistance to RF traveling through tissue that results in molecular oscillation and thermal energy. RF, either fractional/nonfractional, can be selective and targeted in different depths of dermis and combined with other energy sources.[190,191] Linear contractions of 15% to more than 30% over 3 months can be achieved and area contractions averaging 40–60% have been reported.[192-195] Keeping epidermal temperatures at 40–42°C and subreticular dermal temperature of 50–55°C, the result is nonablative, coagulative disruption of deep reticular collagen fibers and biopsy proven neocollagenesis occurs over subsequent 3–6 months with significant measurable and quantitative skin and tissue tightening. Almost 90% of patients observed immediate tightening and that more than 90% of patients had visible and measurable moderate skin tightening 6 months after treatment. More than 94% find the treatment meets their expectations.[192] New devices delivering RF energy and therapeutic effect with multiple RF electrodes (tripolar, quadripolar and octopolar) have been developed.[192-200] The transepidermal RF procedures can be delivered in presence of neurotoxin and can be combined with IPL sources, either during same treatment session or at subsequent dates and as well as microdermabrasion to enhance synergistic esthetic results.[81]

Laser Tightening for Vulval Laxity[201]

As with any other aging human tissue, the natural course of labia majora often involves tissue atrophy and poor circulation, which is associated with loss of hormonal support, or following pregnancy, delivery and significant weight loss in younger women with resultant loss of labia volume, flaccidity and ptosis. On the other hand, protuberant labia majora can lead to functional difficulties in sexual stimulation and satisfaction, complicate hygiene maintenance, influence choice of undergarments and sportwear and negatively impact self-confidence and self-image. Severe skin laxity is often best managed with interventions, such as injectable cosmetic fillers and surgery. Surgical labia majora plasty may be associated with nerve-ending damage, significant anatomical deformities, scarring and hair growth toward the vaginal entrance, which can further exacerbate patient discomfort and dissatisfaction. As an alternative to surgery, dermal rejuvenation of lax labia majora using EBD are is preferred that uses either fractional laser (Figs. 42.9 and 42.10), or RF that

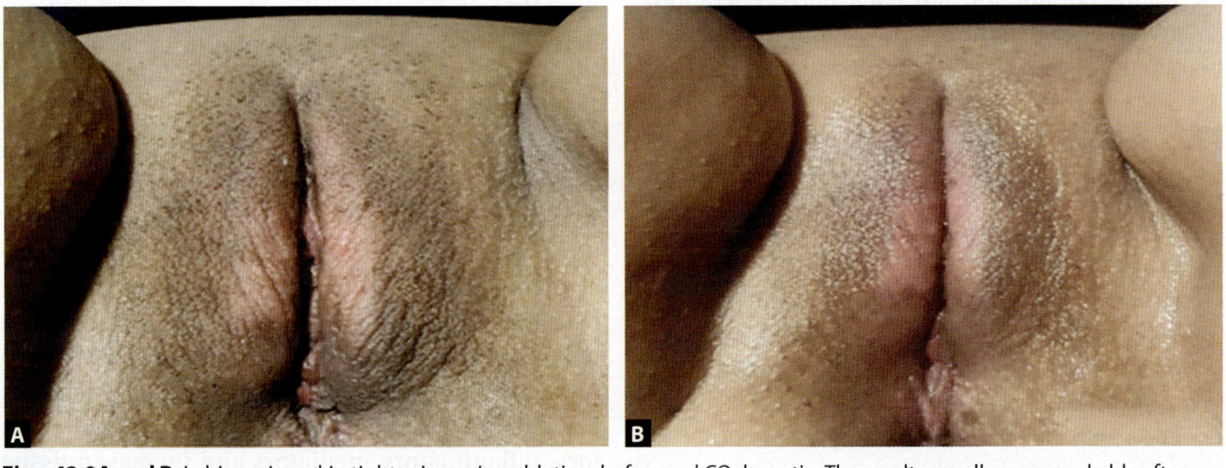

Figs. 42.9A and B: Labia majora skin tightening using ablative de-focused CO_2 laser tip. The results usually are remarkable after one single session.

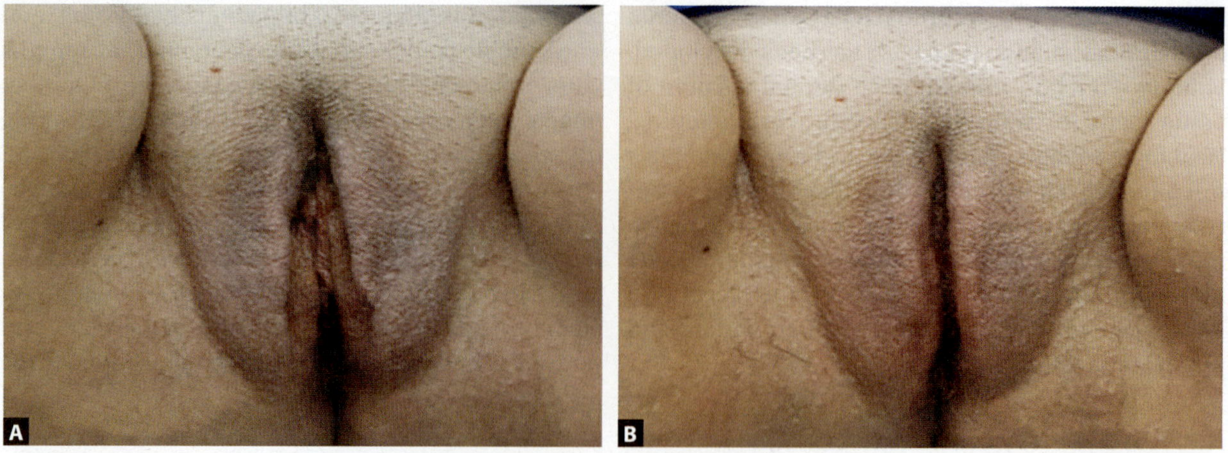

Figs. 42.10A and B: Labia majora skin tightening using ablative de-focused CO_2 laser tip. The results usually are remarkable after one single session. The technique frequently would improve also the perineal body skin with important impact for functional enhancement alongside with the aesthetic aspect.

deliver heat gently and cause tissue remodeling by neocollagenogenesis.[200]

Procedure

A local anesthetic (lidocaine 2% mixed with N/S 0.9% (1:1)) is injected using 27 G needle and the area is cleaned with an iodine-free antiseptic solution and dried. A thin layer of oil is applied over the target area. The device probe is then moved over the skin in circular movements ensuring the temperature does not exceed 42°C (as indicated by the device monitor) for more than 5 s. The human tissue is tolerant of temperatures up to 45°C. Beyond these levels, irreversible reduction in cell viability occurs. Rehydration cream is applied immediately after the treatment and continued for 5 days. Patient tolerates the procedure well with no downtime. Results may be visible immediately after the session, but continuous improvement over the 3–6 months following treatment is seen, which is the estimated time for new collagen regeneration.[98] Follow-up after 6 months is advised. A maintenance treatment session every year is recommended.

TIPS AND TRICKS WITH LASER

- Use anesthetic gel at introitus few minutes before the treatment and then wipe off prior to inserting the probe.
- Lubricate the vaginal probe with oil (mineral/baby oil) and not with water/water-based gel, in order to avoid laser energy loss due its high absorption in water.
- For vaginal reejuvenation, make sure that the probe reaches the top of vagina so that it comes in contact with vaginal vault/cervix.
- The withdrawal of the probe is intended to be at 1 cm intervals.
- Many patients have more severe atrophy in the introital area due to combination of vulvar atrophy as well as vaginal atrophy, or following radiation. Use mild settings. Treat the vestibule from three o'clock to nine o'clock, entire posterior fourchette, and upper part of perineum.
- In patients with excessive pubic hair, recommend trimming this hair prior to placement of the anesthetic cream.
- Ensure to perform the treatment in an laser-authorized room.
- Always ensure all safety measures including, wearing of proper laser designated goggles by all personnel, and patient, in the room.

Photobiomodulation, or Low-level Light Therapy for Skin Rejuvenation

Photobiomodulation, also known as low-level light therapy (LLLT), is a noninvasive, painless treatment using light-emitting diodes (LEDs) to stimulate cellular function. The photons are absorbed by mitochondrial chromophores in skin cells. Consequently, electron transport, adenosine triphosphate (ATP) nitric oxide release, blood flow, reactive oxygen species increase and diverse signaling pathways get activated. Stem cells can be activated allowing increased tissue repair and healing. to increase ATP production and various transcription factors.[202] Ultimately, it increases protein synthesis and modulation of growth factors, inflammatory mediators and increased tissue oxygenation and repair.

As a light source for nonthermal, nonablative skin rejuvenation, it is effective for improving wrinkles and skin laxity.[203-213] The application of heat has a twofold effect on connective tissue. On a macro-tissue level, heat increases circulation and metabolism, whereas on a micro-tissue level, dimensional changes are induced in collagen molecule itself. At tissue temperatures elicited by device (40–42°C), denaturing and reconfiguring of these bonds occurs, which increases the elasticity and strength of collagen fibers. Increase in production of pro-collagen, collagen, basic fibroblast growth factors (bFGF) and proliferation of fibroblasts after exposure to LLLT is seen. It increases microcirculation, vascular perfusion in skin, alters PDGF, transforming growth factor (TGF-β1) and inhibits apoptosis.[202] Histologic and ultrastructural changes following LED phototherapy:[214]

- Alteration in MMPs and TIMPs
- mRNA levels of proinflammatory cytokines IL-1β, TNF-α increase (and may further induce MMP), whereas IL-6 levels decreases
- Increase in amount of collagen seen.

Treatments can induce physiological reactions with healing benefits, including tissue repair and regeneration, improved nerve function, wound healing and reduced inflammation or chronic pain. Intravaginal application of LLLT, heat and therapeutic vibration improves incontinence symptoms and sexual function by positive adaptations to connective tissue and ECM, in addition to increasing micro-circulation and exerting anti-inflammation properties. The LLLT utilizes light in 662 nm (red) and 855 nm (infrared) spectrums, two parts of normal broad spectrum light profile to upregulate functions of muscles, nerves and connective tissues that helps with lubrication, collagen and elastin production, nerve healing and increased voluntary muscle control. LLLT enhances feedback loop in nerves for maintaining involuntary (baseline) tone to pelvic floor muscles and provides users better voluntary control over those muscles and have a positive impact on bladder control.

LLLT for Hypertrophic Scars and Keloids

Hypertrophic scars and keloids: Fibroblastic proliferation and excess collagen deposits are the two main characteristics[215] and imbalance between rates of collagen biosynthesis and degradation superimposed on individual's genetic predisposition have been implicated in their pathogenesis. Poor regulation of interleukin (IL)-6 signaling pathways and TGF-βI expression have a significant role. LLLT decreases IL-6 mRNA levels, modulates PDGF, TGF-β, interleukins (IL-13 and IL-15) MMPs.[202] Use of LLLT as a prophylactic method to alter wound healing process to avoid or attenuate formation of hypertrophic scars or keloids has been reported, where following scar revision, a single scar was treated daily by the patient at home.[215] For scar prevention and healing, treatments are recommended at least 1 day before surgery, and 3 or more consecutive days after.[202]

OPTIMIZING ESTHETIC RESULTS

Adjuncts to Improvise or Augment Results

Dermal Fillers[215]

Soft tissue fillers reduce contour defects through replacement of tissue volume lost due to aging, trauma or other events. They can be used alone or in combination with other esthetic procedures. Dermal fillers (injectable implants/soft tissue fillers) are medical device implants injected or placed into dermis for increasing the tissue volume. A wide variety of implants are available, including biodegradable products (hyaluronic acid, collagen, calcium hydroxylapatite, and poly-L-lactic acid), products that remain indefinitely in tissue (polymethylmethacrylate microspheres, hydrogel polymers and silicone) and viable autologous fat. As opposed to permanent fillers, which persist indefinitely, temporary fillers are eventually resorbed by the body. Some agents, such as injectable collagen and hyaluronic acids, function primarily through a volume-filling effect. Others, including calcium hydroxylapatite and poly-L-lactic acid fillers, act as scaffolds for endogenous collagen formation.

Hyaluronic acid, a naturally occurring glycosaminoglycan, is an essential component of extracellular matrix of dermis. It plays a key role in maintenance of skin structure and function, and its high water-binding capacity is of value for maintenance of moisture in skin. The clinical effects of treatment typically persist for 6 to 12 months.[216] Naturally occurring or uncross-linked hyaluronic acid is degraded in skin within a few days. Therefore, most preparations are altered through cross-lining that allows the molecule to resist rapid degradation by hyaluronidase and other factors in the skin. The amount of uncross-linked (soluble) and cross-linked (insoluble) hyaluronic acid in a gel influences gel

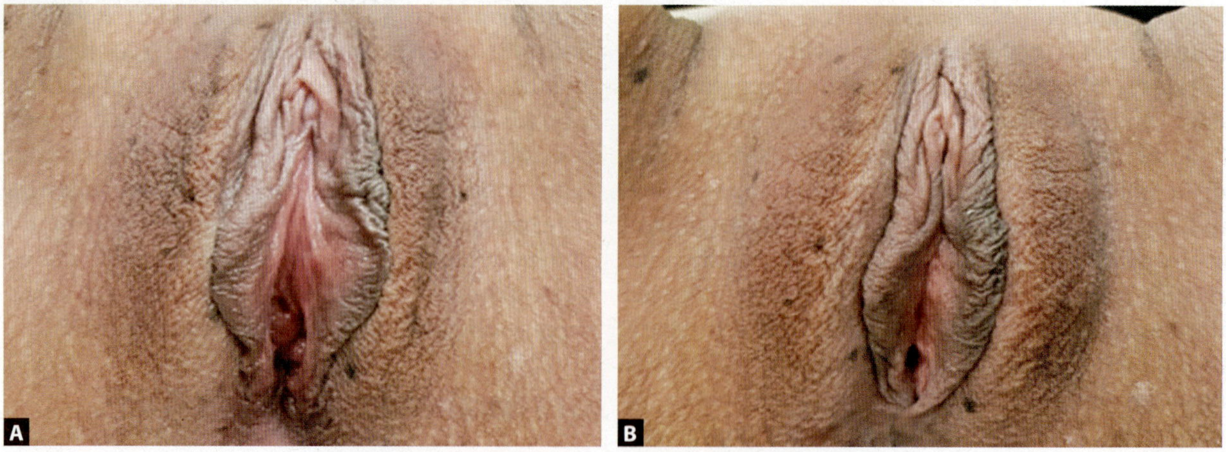

Figs. 42.11A and B: Labia majora augmentation by hyaluronic acid. The material was injected with linear technique following the normal anatomy of the area. The improvement of the perineal body is remarkable.

viscosity. Decreasing proportion of cross-linked contributes to less viscous product and smoother flow during injection and reduces hardness of gel, but may contribute to a shorter duration of effect. Stimulation of collagen synthesis may contribute to treatment efficacy as mechanical tension on fibroblasts is associated with regulation of collagen synthesis, and may contribute to clinical effect of filler.[217]

After skin preparation with an antiseptic solution, the filler is injected using either the linear (Figs. 42.11A and B), fanning or cross-hatching technique. Post procedure, the area is massaged to ensure uniformity of filler distribution and avoid clumping of filler material. Patient is advised to avoid heavy exercise or tight underclothing and intercourse for 24 h.

Adverse Effects

Most frequent adverse effects associated with hyaluronic acid filling agents are transient and mild, and include pain bruising, edema and erythema at injection site. Fan-like needle use, rapid injection (>0.3 mL/min) and high-volume injections have been associated with increased rates of adverse effects. Noninflammatory nodules or bluish discoloration of skin can occur when injections are placed too superficially. Delayed hypersensitivity and granulomatous reactions to hyaluronic acid filling agents are rare, i.e., 0.02% of treatments. Delayed reactions typically manifest as inflammatory papules or nodules that appear weeks to months after injection. Complications such as bacterial and mycobacterial infections or vascular occlusion resulting in tissue necrosis are also uncommon.

Reversal[218]

Misplacement or excessive injection of hyaluronic acid fillers can be treated with injection of hyaluronidase. It is well tolerated; local injection site reactions occur infrequently, and urticaria, angiedema or anaphylaxis rarely occur. Due to potential for anaphylaxis, patients should be tested to evaluate for immediate hypersensitivity reactions prior to injection. Optimum dosing of hyaluronidase has not been established; doses from less than 5 units to 75 units per injection site. Doses of 10 units is effective. Hyaluronidase can also be used in filler-induced granulomatous reactions, in failed improvement with intralesional and topical corticosteroids, and with hyaluronic acid embolic event.

Collagen is no longer recommended as they are associated with a relatively shorter duration of effect, and skin testing is required prior to the use of bovine-derived agents.

Calcium hydroxylapatite is composed of synthetic, uniform and smooth calcium hydroxylapatite microspheres suspended in an aqueous carboxymethylcellulose gel carrier.[218] Once injected, carrier gel is gradually resorbed and remaining calcium hydroxylapatite microspheres stimulate local production of endogenous collagen. Eventually, microspheres are degraded into calcium and phosphate ions and are excreted. It exhibits greater duration of effect when compared with hyaluronic acid and human collagen fillers. It supplied as gel in prefilled syringe; use of 25–27 G needle is recommended. Premix with lidocaine prior to injection to reduce patient discomfort. Depth of injection is subdermal. Overcorrection of defects should be avoided. Massage of treatment site immediately after injection facilitates even distribution of product.

Large particle calcium hydroxylapatite (Coaptite):[219] FDA approval for Coaptite is limited to the treatment of urinary incontinence, and additional studies are necessary to explore the efficacy and safety of this agent as a cosmetic filler. It is generally well tolerated. Injection-site reactions, including transient erythema, edema, ecchymosis, pain on injection and pruritus are most frequently reported side effects. Noninflammatory nodules secondary to aggregation of filling agent can occur after treatment. Nodules can resolve over time; there is no injectable product that can be used to dissolve the product after injection. Massage, needle disruption or surgical excision can be utilized to accelerate resolution. Vascular occlusion resulting in skin necrosis and ocular ischemia is rare.

Poly-L-lactic acid contains microparticles of poly-L-lactic acid (PLLA), biocompatible and biodegradable synthetic polymer.[220] It does not "fill" the skin. Once injected, PLLA induces subclinical inflammatory response that stimulates fibroblast proliferation and collagen formation, leading to progressive increase in the volume of dermis. PLLA is gradually degraded over the course of 9–24 months.[217] The duration of effect exceeds that of hyaluronic acid and collagen fillers. It must be reconstituted with sterile water at least 2 h prior to injection to ensure complete hydration of product. The injection should be placed in deep dermis or subcutaneous fat with a 26 G or larger needle. Because treatment results progressively improve over time, under-correction of defect is the goal. Transient tissue edema may develop immediately after injection, resulting in appearance of full correction. Subsequent treatments should be spaced by at least 3 weeks to allow for assessment of response. Treatment should also be avoided in patients with history of keloidal or hypertrophic scarring and patients with known hypersensitivity to any of product components. Potential adverse effects of injection include hematoma, bruising, edema, discomfort, inflammation and erythema. Another common complication is the occurrence of asymptomatic, subcutaneous papules weeks to months after treatment. Proper dilution of product, avoidance of poor injection technique (e.g., superficial injections, overcorrection) and manual tissue massage immediately after injection may decrease the risk for this adverse effect nodule formation. Nodules typically resolve spontaneously without intervention. Nodules that fail to resolve may require subcision (disruption of papules with a needle), excision or intralesional corticosteroid therapy. Delayed appearance of granulomatous reactions has also been reported in a few patients.

Autologous fat:[221] The main advantage of autologous fat in comparison to other soft tissue fillers is lack of risk for hypersensitivity or foreign body reactions. Retention of fat has been estimated to range from 20 to 80%.[222-224] A variety of factors, including harvesting technique, type of fat implanted, treatment site and injection technique can influence efficacy of treatment. The advent of new harvesting and processing techniques, such as the addition of platelet-rich plasma or adipose-derived stem cells to transplanted fat, may lead to improved viability.[225-229] Fat transfer procedures can be complicated by morbidity in donor site, prolonged edema, infections, contour irregularities and necrosis or calcification of injected fat. Fat emboli leading to stroke and vision loss have been reported.[230-239]

Discussion on other permanent soft tissue filler is outside the scope of this chapter.

G-spot Amplification

The G- or Grafenberg-spot, first described in 1950s, is a highly erogenous zone inside the vagina that enlarges when directly stimulated. It can be found on anterior wall of vagina along the course of urethra, like the corpora cavernosa of penis. Although the location varies, it is typically located half way between pubic bone and cervix, 2–5 cm into vagina.[240,241] Many refute its existence, while others claim its validity using ultrasound scans.[242]

G-spot Alteration

Both fat grafting and fillers can be applied to the anterior vaginal wall to enhance the perceived G-spot. G-spot amplification (G-shot™ first described by Matlock, 2001)[243] focuses on functional improvement to enhance sexual stimulation by increasing the prominence of the G-spot (3–5 mm). In nonaugmented state, G-spot lies beneath the surface of vaginal wall, when projected into the vagina it is more accessible for direct stimulation. Injections of fillers and/or collagen to the G-spot enhance the size, which should, in turn, increase sexual pleasure. This is achieved by collagen or hyaluronan injections (patient first indicates the right zone to be augmented by palpation). The effect is not permanent and lasts for 4–6 months.

Known complications include hypersensitivity, urinary infection or retention, urethral irritation, periurethral pseudocyst formation, urethrovaginal fistulas, postoperative bleeding and erosion of the G spot with open sores and scars, and rarely embolism if inadvertently injected in to veins.

ROLE OF HORMONES AS TISSUE MODULATORS

Sex steroid hormones are important modulators of tissue parameters that may ultimately affect vaginal hemodynamics and arousal. Ovariectomy or menopause produces a dramatic effect in vaginal morphology, and these changes are reversed by administration of estradiol. Decreases in ovarian steroids following menopause induces structural changes in vagina and contribute to genital pathophysiology.[244,245] Shortening and narrowing of vagina accompanied by pale, thin, less elastic and progressively smooth vagina with loss of vaginal folds. Epithelial surface becomes flattened and keratinized. There is a reduction of number of layers in vaginal epithelium, including a loss of intermediate cells, which results in an overall reduction in epithelial height.[246] There is reduced collagen content and hyalinization, decreased elastin, altered appearance and function of smooth muscle cells, and density of connective tissue and fewer blood vessels. Blood flow reduces and secretions diminish, elasticity of the vaginal vault decrease, resultant tissues become more friable and vaginal flora shifts from lactobacillus-dominant flora to an anaerobic gram-negative rods and gram-positive cocci flora, and increase in pH. In POP, vaginal smooth muscle content is most diminished in menopausal women not on estrogen replacement.[247]

There is a dose-dependent response to estradiol, with subphysiological doses producing hyperplasia of epithelium and nonvascular smooth muscle. There is a differential role of sex steroid hormones in the vagina. Testosterone administered stimulates production of mucus but not keratin in superficial cells. Estrone, on the other hand, causes superficial layer of epithelium to disappear, with a concurrent increase in basal cells and keratinization.[248] Higher doses of estrone (100 g/d) cause only an increase in basal cells and keratin formation, whereas combining testosterone (1 mg) and estrone (1 g) cause epithelial stratification with decrease in mucoprotein formation and cessation of keratin production.[248]

Sex steroids affect vaginal tissue structure and play a role in neurotransmitter expression.[249] Nerve fibers within the epithelium are seen only in introitus, with most fibers ending after penetrating two-thirds the height of epithelium. Networks of smaller fibers just below the epithelium are seen and these are more prevalent in distal regions, and are more numerous in anterior versus posterior walls. Innervated blood vessels are seen in deep submucosal layers of all regions.[250] Although progesterone and testosterone do not appear to have a great influence on vaginal morphology, a unique effect of testosterone is the increase in small adrenergic nerve fibers.

Role of Estrogen in Collagen Metabolism in POP

Estrogen receptors (ER) have been identified in nuclei of connective tissue and of smooth muscle cells of bladder trigone, urethra, vaginal mucosa, levator ani stromal and uterosacral ligament. These receptors participate in maintaining the supportive system of pelvis by increasing synthesis or by decreasing breakdown of collagen and other ECM proteins.[251] Lower estrogen receptor expression in patients with POP have been found in combination with lower serum concentrations of estrogen.[252,253] Estrogen replacement therapy has been used to improve structural integrity of pelvic tissue with favorable effects on urinary incontinence.[254-256] Increase in mRNA expression for collagen I and III in estrogen replacement therapy has been reported.[257-259] This suggests that estrogen increases the turnover of connective tissues of pelvic floor and restores the collagen metabolism to a premenopausal state.[7]

In postmenopausal women with SUI treated with estradiol (E_2), the immature cross-links are increased, indicating newly synthesized collagen. However, ratio of type I/III collagen is unchanged, and total collagen content is significantly decreased. Also, elevation of both MMP-2 and MMP-9 is found. This results in a decrease in total collagen content.[260] Also, combination of upregulation of MMPs and suppression of TIMP by estrogen results in an increase of ECM breakdown.[261] Inhibition of MMP by estrogen therapy is also reported.[262,263] Only E_2 combined with progesterone decreases the active form of MMP-1, which suggests that both hormones are necessary to maintain the integrity of pelvic floor.

Estrogens and Fibroblasts

17β-Estradiol may have a suppressive effect on proliferation of fibroblasts in POP. Therefore, it may have a role in inducing POP by negatively affecting the concentration of fibroblasts in pelvic organ connective tissue.[264] Estrogen therapy, thus, induces turnover of collagen. An increased mRNA expression of collagen types I and III as a reaction to hormone replacement therapy, with a concomitant increased synthesis of these collagen types is seen. However, an increased activity of MMP, resulting in an increase in collagen degradation, is also seen.[7]

ROLE OF REGENERATIVE MEDICINE: STEM CELLS, PRP

There has been a recent surge in the use of regenerative medicine and their advances and technologies for applications in esthetics and functional medicine. Platelet-rich plasma (PRP) and stem cells (adipose derived or bone marrow derived) are being used with dramatic improvement in esthetic results.[225-229] The use of PRP or stem cell procedure has been extended to also cover lichen sclerosus, to rejuvenate the vulvar and vaginal mucosa. These procedures can be used alone or in combination with other esthetic procedures. Often, these are being combined following the use of an energy based device to augment the rejuvenative effects.

Cell-based tissue engineering strategies provide alternatives to current surgical reconstruction of POP.[266] Combining biomaterials with autologous cells (fibroblasts or stem cells), or induced pluripotent stem cell lines from vaginal tissue,[266] can stimulate vaginal tissue repair. Changes in ECM composition of those tissues is an acquired defect in POP.[267] Therefore, autologous cell-based therapies could be considered as alternative treatments for most cases.[21]

It has been suggested to treat POP with autologous stem cells. These stem cells are stimulated to differentiate into fibroblast-like cells producing collagen and can be seeded on biocompatible material serving as a "bioactive scaffold."[7] Stem cells have been used to create striated sphincter muscle in vitro; autologous myoblasts and fibroblasts have been injected lateral from urethra to treat urinary incontinence.[268-270] It should be possible to develop a biocompatible and bioresorbable scaffold with appropriate mechanical properties in which stem cells are able to contribute to tissue regeneration by proliferation and differentiation into (myo) fibroblasts and by formation of appropriate connective tissue.[7]

CUV Complex Amplification (O-Shot[tm])

The O-shot employs the use of PRP to augment the clito-urethral vaginal complex,[271] a procedure first described by Charles Runels.[272] This procedure has revolutionized the sexual esthetic practice and addresses the female sexual dysfunction with a reported success rate of over 85% in ongoing trials (www.oshot.org).

CONCLUSION

Female genital surgery mostly consists of labiaplasty or vaginal tightening. These procedures have acceptable and reasonable outcomes. More than 90% of patients are satisfied with results of their surgery after a 6- to 42-month follow-up. Significant subjective enhancement in sexual functioning for both women and their sexual partners is seen.

With the rapid pace of change occurring in our field, it is important to have readily available resources and innovations that are critical to the advancement of our specialty. It is of tremendous benefit to be able to provide our patients with a variety of treatment options with the best possible solution to their functional and esthetic needs. It is up to each of us to be our own investigator and our own judge of what is appropriate in our practice. That requires ascertaining whether a given procedure or technology has been truly validated as safe and effective. Any decision made by a competent woman regarding her own body and medical treatment should be respected. As for every new specialty, guidelines need to be set up and long-term studies undertaken.

Declaration of Conflicting Interests

The authors declared no potential conflicts of interest with respect to the research, authorship, and/or publication of this chapter.

Ethical Approval

The authors confirm that the necessary written, informed consent was obtained from patients for this chapter.

REFERENCES

1. Subak LL, Waetjen LE, van den Eeden S, et al. Cost of pelvic organ prolapse surgery in the United States. Obstet Gynecol. 2001;98(4):646-51.
2. Goh JT. Biomechanical and biochemical assessments for pelvic organ prolapse. Curr Opin Obstet Gynecol. 2003;15(5):391-94.
3. Alarab M, Kufaishi H, Lye S, et al. Expression of extracellular matrix-remodeling proteins is altered in vaginal tissue of premenopausal women with severe pelvic organ prolapse. Reprod Sci. 2014; 21(6): 704-15.

4. Bailey AJ. Molecular mechanisms of ageing in connective tissues. Mech Ageing Dev. 2001;122(7):735-55.
5. Birk DE, Fitch JM, Babiarz JP, et al. Collagen fibrillogenesis in vitro: interaction of types I and V collagen regulates fibril diameter. J Cell Sci. 1990;95(Pt 4):649-57.
6. Shynlova O, Bortolini MAT, Alarab M. Genes responsible for vaginal extracellular matrix metabolism are modulated by women's reproductive cycle and menopause. Int Braz J Urol. 2013;39(2):257-67.
7. Kerkhof MH, Hendriks L, Brölmann HAM. Changes in connective tissue in patients with pelvic organ prolapse—a review of the current literature. Int Urogynecol J Pelvic Floor Dysfunct. 2009;20(4):461-74.
8. Alperin M, Debes K, Abramowitch S, Meyn L, Moalli PA. LOXL1 deficiency negatively impacts the biomechanical properties of the mouse vagina and supportive tissues. Int Urogynecol J Pelvic Floor Dysfunct 2008;19:977-986.
9. Nakamura T, Lozano PR, Ikeda Y, et al. Fibulin-5/DANCE is essential for elastogenesis in vivo. Nature. 2002;415(6868):171-5.
10. Chen B, Yeh J. Alterations in connective tissue metabolism in stress incontinence and prolapse. J Urol. 2011;186(5):1768-72.
11. Liu et al. TGF-β1 Is a potential therapeutic target for pelvic organ prolapse. Int J Molec Med. 2017;40:347-56.
12. Overall CM, Wrana JL, Sodek J. Transcriptional and post-transcriptional regulation of 72-kDa gelatinase/type IV collagenase by transforming growth factor-beta 1 in human fibroblasts. Comparisons with collagenase and tissue inhibitor of matrix metalloproteinase gene expression. J Biol Chem. 1991;266(21):14064-71.
13. Wen et al. Is a2-macroglobulin important in female stress urinary incontinence? Hum Reproduc. 2008;23(2):387-93.
14. Ma H, Li R, Zhang Z, et al. mRNA level of alpha-2-macroglobulin as an aging biomarker of human fibroblasts in culture. Exp Gerontol. 2004;39(3):415-21.
15. Chen B, Wen Y, Wang H, et al. Differences in estrogen modulation of tissue inhibitor of matrix metalloproteinase-1 and matrix metalloproteinase-1 expression in cultured fibroblasts from continent and incontinent women. Am J Obstet Gynecol. 2003;189(1):59-65.
16. Mogami H, Keller P, Acevedo JF, et al. Differential regulation of lysyl oxidases in uterine and cervical tissues during pregnancy, parturition, and the puerperium. Reprod Sci. 2010;17(Suppl 3):76A.
17. Amy JP, Tristi WM, Marie FRP. Clinical manifestations, diagnosis, and nonsurgical management of posterior vaginal defects. UpToDate. September 8, 2015.
18. Swift S, Woodman P, O'Boyle A, et al. Pelvic Organ Support Study (POSST): the distribution, clinical definition, and epidemiologic condition of pelvic organ support defects. Am J Obstet Gynecol. 2005;192(3):795-806.
19. Olsen AL, Smith VJ, Bergstrom JO, et al. Epidemiology of surgically managed pelvic organ prolapse and urinary incontinence. Obstet Gynecol. 1997;89(4):501-6.
20. Lensen EJM, Withagen MIJ, Kluivers KB, et al. Surgical treatment of pelvic organ prolapse: a historical review with emphasis on the anterior compartment. Int Urogynecol J. 2013;24(10):1593-602.
21. Ruiz-Zapata AM, Kerkhof MH, Zandieh-Doulabi B, et al. Functional characteristics of vaginal fibroblastic cells from premenopausal women with pelvic organ prolapse. Molec Hum Reprod. 2014;20(11):1135-43.
22. Delancey JO. The anatomy of the pelvic floor. Curr Opin Obstet Gynecol. 1994;6(4):313-6.
23. Moalli PA, Shand SH, Zyczynski HM, et al. Remodeling of vaginal connective tissue in patients with prolapse. Obstet Gynecol. 2005;106(5 Pt 1):953-63.
24. Karam JA, Vazquez DV, Lin VK, et al. Elastin expression and elastic fibre width in the anterior vaginal wall of postmenopausal women with and without prolapse. BJU Int. 2007;100(2):346-50.
25. Chiquet M. Regulation of extracellular matrix gene expression by mechanical stress. Matrix Biol. 1999;18(5):417-26.
26. Vetuschi A, D'Alfonso A, Sferra R, et al. Changes in muscularis propria of anterior vaginal wall in women with pelvic organ prolapse. Eur J Histochem. 2016;60(1):2604.
27. Shapiro SD. Metalloproteinase degradation of extracellular matrix: biological consequences. Curr Opin Cell Biol. 1998;10(5):602-8.
28. Landsheere L, Blacher S, Munaut C, et al. Changes in elastin density in different locations of vaginal wall in women with pelvic organ prolapse. Int Urogynecol J. 2014;25(12):1673-81.
29. Tadir Y, Gaspar A, Lev-Sagie A, et al. Light and energy based therapeutics for GSM: consensus and controversies. Lasers Surg Med. 2017;49(2):137-59.
30. Yavagal S, de Farias TF, Medina CA, et al. Normal vulvovaginal, perineal, and pelvic anatomy with reconstructive considerations. Semin Plastic Surg 2011;25(2):121-9.
31. Mirowski GW, Edwards L. Geniatl anatomy. In: Edwards L (Ed). Genital Dermatology Atlas. Philadelphia, PA: Lippincott Williams and Wilkins; 2004. pp 1-8.
32. Lloyd J, Crouch NS, Minto CL, et al. Female genital appearance: "normality" unfolds. BJOG. 2005;112(5):643-6.
33. Lean WL, Hutson JM, Deshpande AV, et al. Clitoroplasty: past, present and future. Pediatr Surg Int. 2007;23(4):289-93.
34. Shafik A, el-Sherif M, Youssef A, et al. Surgical anatomy of the pudendal nerve and its clinical implications. Clin Anat. 1995;8(2):110-5.
35. Dobbeleir JM, Landuyt KV, Monstrey SJ. Aesthetic surgery of the female genitalia. Semin Plastic Surg. 2011;25(2):130-41.

36. Miklos J, Moore R. Vaginal reconstruction and rejuvenation surgery: is there data to support improved sexual function? Am J Cosmetic Surg. 2012;29:97-113.
37. Pujols Y, Meston CM, Seal BN. The association between sexual satisfaction and body image in women. J Sex Med. 2010;7(2 Pt 2):905-16.
38. Shick VR, Calabrese SK, Rima BN, et al. Genital appearance dissatisfaction: implications for women's genital image self-consciousness, sexual esteem, sexual satisfaction, and sexual risk. Psychol Women Q. 2010;34(3):394-404.
39. Azar M, Noohi S, Radfar S, et al. Sexual function in women after surgery for pelvic organ prolapse. Int Urogynecol J Pelvic Floor Dysfunt. 2008;19(1):53-7.
40. Goodman MP, Bachmann G, Johnson C, et al. Is elective vulvar plastic surgery ever warranted, and what screening should be conducted preoperatively? J Sex Med. 2007;4(2):269-76.
41. Choi HY, Kim KT. A new method for aesthetic reduction of labia minora (the deepithelialized reduction of labioplasty). Plast Reconstr Surg. 2000;105(1):419-22; discussion 423-4.
42. Di Saia JP. An unusual staged labial rejuvenation. J Sex Med. 2008;5(5):1263-7.
43. Davison SP, Baker CL, West JE. Labiaplasty and labia minora reduction. Medscape Reference. Available at http://reference.medscape.com/article/1372175-overview.
44. Goodman MP, Placik OJ, Benson RH III, et al. A large multicenter outcome study of female genital plastic surgery. J Sex Med. 2010;7(4 Pt 1):1565-77.
45. Miklos JR, Moore RD. Labiaplasty of the labia minora: patients' indications for pursuing surgery. J Sex Med. 2008;5(6):1492-5.
46. Paarlberg KM, Weijenborg PT. Request for operative reduction of the labia minora: a proposal for a practical guideline for gynecologists. J Psychosom Obstet Gynaecol. 2008;29(4):230-4.
47. Giraldo F, Gonzalez C, de Haro F. Central wedge nymphectomy with a 90-degree Z-plasty for aesthetic reduction of the labia minora. Plast Reconstr Surg. 2004;113(6):1820-5; discussion 1826-7.
48. Munhoz AM, Filassi JR, Ricci MD, et al. Aesthetic labia minora reduction with inferior wedge resection and superior pedicle flap reconstruction. Plast Reconstr Surg. 2006;118(5):1237-47; discussion 1248-50.
49. Alinsod R. Radiofrequency resurfacing and revision of deepithelialized labia minora labiaplasty: review of literature and case study. Pelviperineology. 2013;32: 106-9.
50. Gress S. Composite reduction labiaplasty. Aesthetic Plast Surg. 2013;37(4):674-83.
51. Kolb S. Plastikos Surgery Centre, Atlanta. Aesthetic female genital surgery: expanding your practice. Available at: http://www.labiaplastysurgeon.com/sexual-enhancement.html.
52. Coleman SR. Fat augmentation of the anterior vaginal wall: a novel use of fat augmentation in enhancing the female sexual experience. Am J Plast Surg. 28: 171-6.
53. Schultz W, vande Wiel H, Klatter J, et al. Vaginal sensitivity to electric stimuli: theoretical and practical implications. Arch Sex Behav 1989;18(2):87-95.
54. Green FJ. From clitoridectomies to "designer vaginas": The medical construction of heteronormative female bodies and sexuality through female genital cutting. Sexualities Evol Gender. 2005;7(2):153-87.
55. Goodman MP. Female cosmetic genital surgery. Obstet Gynecol. 2009;113(1):154-9.
56. Ciro A, Corvi M. Cosmetic mucosal vaginal tightening (lateral colporrhaphy): improving sexual sensitivity in women with a sensation of wide vagina. Plast Reconstr Surg 2009;123(6):212-3.
57. Brambilla M. Intramuscular-submucosal lipostructure for the treatment of vaginal laxity. Paper presented at Congresso Internazionale di Medicina Estetica, October 10, 2008, Milan, Italy.
58. Raveenthiran V. Surgery of the hymen: from myth to modernization. Indian J Surg. 2009;71:224-6.
59. Hamori CA. Postoperative clitoral hood deformity after labiaplasty. Aesthet Surg J. 2013;33(7):1030-6.
60. Alter GJ. A new technique for aesthetic labia minora reduction. Ann Plast Surg. 1998;40(3):287-90.
61. Alinsod R. Awake In-Office Barbie Labiaplasty, Awake In-Office Labia Majora Plasty, Awake In-Office Vaginoplasty, Awake In-Office Labial Revision. Congress on Aesthetic Vaginal Surgery (CAVS), Tucson, AZ, November 2011.
62. Alexiades-Armenakas MR, Dover JS, Arndt KA. The spectrum of laser skin resurfacing: nonablative, fractional, and ablative laser resurfacing. J Am Acad Dermatol. 2008;58 (5):719-37, quiz 738-40.
63. Lev-Sagie A. Vulvar and vaginal atrophy: physiology, clinical presentation, and treatment considerations. Clin Obstet Gynecol. 2015;58(3):476-91.
64. Hruza GJ. Laser and intense pulsed light for cutaneous lesions. UpToDate. March 13, 2017.
65. Anderson RR, Parrish JA. Selective photothermolysis: precise microsurgery by selective absorption of pulsed radiation. Science. 1983;220(4956):524.
66. Lowe NJ, Lask G, Griffin ME, et al. Skin resurfacing with the ultrapulse carbon dioxide laser. Observations on 100 patients. Dermatol Surg. 1995;21(12):1025.
67. Teikemeier G, Goldberg DJ. Skin resurfacing with the erbium:YAG laser. Dermatol Surg. 1997;23(8):685.
68. Nelson JS, Berns MW. Basic laser physics and tissue interactions. Contemp Dermatol. 1988;2:1.
69. McGoldrick RB, Theodorakopoulou E, Azzopardi EA, et al. Lasers and ancillary treatments for scar management. Scars Burns Healing. 2017;2:1-7.
70. Manstein D, Herron GS, Sink RK, et al. Fractional photothermolysis: a new concept for cutaneous remodeling using microscopic patterns of thermal injury. Lasers Surg Med. 2004;34(5):426-38.
71. Tierney EP, Eisen RF, Hanke CW. Fractionated CO_2 laser skin rejuvenation. Dermatol Ther. 2011;24(1):41-53.
72. Kono T, Chan HH, Groff WF, et al. Prospective direct comparison study of fractional resurfacing using different fluences and densities for skin rejuvenation in Asians. Lasers Surg Med. 2007;39(4):311.

73. Sherling M, Friedman PM, Adrian R, et al. Consensus recommendations on the use of an erbium-doped 1,550-nm fractionated laser and its applications in dermatologic laser surgery. Dermatol Surg. 2010; 36(4):461.
74. Hunzeker CM, Weiss ET, Geronemus RG. Fractionated CO_2 laser resurfacing: our experience with more than 2000 treatments. Aesthet Surg J. 2009;29(4):317.
75. Mahmoud BH, Srivastava D, Janiga JJ, et al. Safety and efficacy of erbium-doped yttrium aluminum garnet fractionated laser for treatment of acne scars in type IV to VI skin. Dermatol Surg. 2010;36(5):602.
76. Alster TS, Tanzi EL, Welsh EC. Photorejuvenation of facial skin with topical 20% 5-aminolevulinic acid and intense pulsed light treatment: a split-face comparison study. J Drugs Dermatol. 2005;4(1):35.
77. Kawada A, Aragane Y, Kameyama H, et al. Acne phototherapy with a high-intensity, enhanced, narrow-band, blue light source: an open study and in vitro investigation. J Dermatol Sci. 2002; 30(2):129.
78. Alster TS, Lupton JR. Treatment of complications of laser skin resurfacing. Arch Facial Plast Surg. 2000;2(4):279-84.
79. Gaspar A, Addamo G, Brandi H. Vaginal fractional CO_2 laser: a minimally invasive option for vaginal rejuvenation. Am J Cosmetic Surg. 2011;28(3):156-162.
80. Millheiser LS, Pauls RN, Herbst SJ, et al. Radio-frequency treatment of vaginal laxity after vaginal delivery: nonsurgical vaginal tightening. J Sex Med. 2010;7(9):3088-95.
81. Mulholland RS. Radio frequency energy for non-invasive and minimally invasive skin tightening. Clin Plast Surg. 2011;38(3):437-48.
82. Alinsod RM. Transcutaneous temperature controlled radio-frequency for orgasmic dysfunction. Lasers Surg Med. 2016;48(7):641-5.
83. Salvatore S, Leone Roberti Maggiore U, Athanasiou S, et al. Histological study on the effect of microablative fractional CO_2 laser on atrophic vaginal tissue: an ex vivo study. Menopause. 2015;22(8):845-9.
84. Zerbinati N, Serati M, Origoni M, et al. Microscopic and ultrastructural modifications of postmenopausal atrophis vaginal mucosa after fractional carbon dioxide laser treatment. Lasers Med Sci. 2015;30(1): 429-36.
85. Salvatore S, Nappi RE, Zerbinati N, et al. A 12-week treatment with fractional CO_2 laser for vulvovaginal atrophy: a pilot study. Climacteric. 2014;17(4):363-9.
86. Orringer JS, Kang S, Johnson TJ, et al. Connective tissue remodeling induced by carbon dioxide laser resurfacing of photodamaged human skin. Arch Dermatol. 2004;140(11):1326-32.
87. Mac Bride MB, Rhodes DJ, Shuster LT. Vulvovaginal atrophy. Mayo Clin Proc. 2010;85(1):87-94.
88. Athanasiou S, Pitsouni E, Antonopoulou S, et al. The effect of microablative fractional CO_2 laser on vaginal flora of postmenopausal women. Climacteric. 2016; 19(5):512-8.
89. Stephens DJ. Cell biology: collagen secretion explained. Nature 2012;482(7386):474-5.
90. Alberts B, Johnson A, Lewis J. Transport from the ER through the Golgi apparatus. Molecular Biology of the Bell, 4th edition. New York: Garland Science; 2002. pp. 775-81.
91. Hantash BM, Bedi VP, Kapadia B, et al. In vivo histological evaluation of a novel ablative fractional resurfacing device. Lasers Surg Med. 2007;39(2):96-107.
92. Ishida Y, Nagata K. Hsp47 as a collagen-specific molecular chaperone. Methods Enzymol. 2011;499: 167-82.
93. Tasab M, Batten MR, Bulleid NJ. Hsp47: a molecular chaperone that interacts with and stabilizes correctly-folded procollagen. EMBO J. 2000;19(10):2204-11.
94. Dafforn TR, Della M, Miller AD. The molecular interactions of heat shock protein 47 (Hsp47) and their implications for collagen biosynthesis. J Biol Chem. 2001;276(52): 49310-9.
95. Prignano F, Campolmi P, Bonan P, et al. Fractional CO_2 laser: a novel therapeutic device upon photobiomodulation of tissue remodeling and cytokine pathway of tissue repair. Dermatol Ther. 2009;22(Suppl 1): S8-15.
96. Nowak KC, McCormack M, Koch RJ. The effect of superpulsed carbon dioxide laser energy on keloid and normal dermal fibroblast secretion of growth factors: a serum-free study. Plast Reconstr Surg. 2000;105(6):2039-48.
97. Manolis EN, Kaklamanos IG, Spanakis N, et al. Tissue concentration of transforming growth factor b1 and basic fibroblast growth factor in skin wounds created with a CO_2 laser and scalpel: a comparative experimental study, using an animal model of skin resurfacing. Wound Repair Regen. 2007;15(2):252-7.
98. Orringer JS, Sachs DL, Shao Y, et al. Direct quantitative comparison of molecular responses in photodamaged human skin to fractionated and fully ablative carbon dioxide laser resurfacing. Dermatol Surg. 2012;38:1668-77.
99. Reinisch L. Scatter-limited phototherapy: a model for laser treatment, of skin. Lasers Surg. Med. 2002;30(5):381-8.
100. Lukao M, Mqjaron B, Rupnik T. Ablative and thermal effects of Er:YAG laser on human tissue. In: Waidelich W, Waidelich R, Waldschmidt J, editors. Lasers in Medicine. Berlin: Springer; 1998. pp. 566-72.
101. Majaron B, Plesteniak Lukaĉ M. Thermo-mechanical laser ablation of soft biological tissue: modeling the micro explosions. Appl Phys B. 1999;69(1):71-80.
102. Gaspar A, Brandi H, Gomez V, et al. Efficacy of erbium: YAG laser treatment compared to topical estriol treatment for symptoms of genitourinary syndrome of menopause. Lasers Surg. Med. 2016;49(2):160-8.
103. Fistonic N, Fistonic I, Lukanovic A, et al. First assessment of short term efficacy of Er:YAG laser treatment on stress urinary incontinence in women: Prospective cohort study. Climacteric. 2015;18(Sup 1): 37-42.
104. Ogrinc BU, Sencar S. Novel minimally invasive laser treatment of urinary incontinence in women. Lasers Surg Med. 2015;47:689-97.

105. Fistonic N, Fistonic I, Findri Gustek SS, et al. Minimally invasive, non-ablative Er:YAG laser treatment of stress urinary incontinence in women—a pilot study. J Laser Med Sci. 2016;31(4):635-43.
106. Pardo J, Sola V, Morales A. Treatment of female stress urinary incontinence with erbium YAG laser in non-ablative mode. Eur J Obstet Gynecol Reprod Biol. 2016;204:1-4.
107. Tien YW, Hsiao SM, Lee CN, et al. Effects of laser procedure for female urodynamic stress incontinence on pad weight, urodynamics, and sexual function. Int Urogynecol J. 2016;28(3):469-76.
108. Pitsouni E, Grigoriadis T, Tsiveleka A, et al. Microablative fractional CO_2-laser therapy and the genitourinary syndrome of menopause: an observational study. Maturitas. 2016;94:131-6.
109. Leibaschoff G, Izasa PG, Cardona JL, et al. Transcutaneous temperature controlled radiofrequency (TTCRF) for the treatment of menopausal vaginal/genitourinary symptoms. Surg Technol Int. 2016;26(XXIX):149-59.
110. Alexiades M. Nonablative skin resurfacing for skin rejuvenation. UpToDate. Aug 15, 2017.
111. Kligman LH. Photoaging. Manifestations, prevention, and treatment. Clin Geriatr Med. 1989;5(1):235-51.
112. Takema Y, Yorimoto Y, Kawai M, et al. Age-related changes in the elastic properties and thickness of human facial skin. Br J Dermatol. 1994; 131(5):641-8.
113. Branham GH, Thomas JR. Rejuvenation of the skin surface: chemical peel and dermabrasion. Facial Plast Surg. 1996;12(2):125-33.
114. Airan LE, Hruza G. Current lasers in skin resurfacing. Facial Plast Surg Clin North Am. 2005;13(1):127-39.
115. Paasch U, Haedersdal M. Laser systems for ablative fractional resurfacing. Expert Rev Med Devices. 2011;8(1):67-83.
116. Weiss RA, McDaniel DH, Geronemus RG. Review of nonablative photorejuvenation: reversal of the aging effects of the sun and environmental damage using laser and light sources. Semin Cutan Med Surg. 2003; 22(2):93-106.
117. Hardaway CA, Ross EV. Nonablative laser skin remodeling. Dermatol Clin. 2002;20(1):97-111.
118. Murina F, Karram M, Salvatore S, et al. Fractional CO_2 laser treatment of the vestibule for patients with vestibulodynia and genitourinary syndrome of menopause: A pilot study. J Sex Med. 2016; 13(12):1915-7.
119. Filippini M and Farinelli M: Use of the MonaLisaTouch® Treatment for post-partum dyspareunia. A pilot study. Social Security Institute San Marino, December 2014.
120. Cooper SM, Arnold SJ. Vulvar lichen sclerosus. UpToDate 2016. June 6, 2016.
121. Kartamaa M, Reitamo S. Treatment of lichen sclerosus with carbon dioxide laser vaporization. Br J Dermatol 1997; 136(3):356-9.
122. Windahl T. Is carbon dioxide laser treatment of lichen sclerosus effective in the long run? Scand J Urol Nephrol. 2006;40(3):208-11.
123. Peterson C, Lane J, Ratz J. Successful carbon dioxide laser therapy for refractory anogenital lichen sclerosus. Dermatol Surg. 2004;30(8):1148-51.
124. Lee A, Lim A, Fischer G. Fractional carbon dioxide laser in recalcitrant vulval lichen sclerosus. Australas J Dermatol. 2016;57(1):39-43.
125. Baggish M. Fractional CO_2 laser treatment for vaginal atrophy and vulvar lichen sclerosus. J Gynecol Surg 2016;32(6):309-317.
126. Alster TS, Lupton JR. Erbium:YAG cutaneous laser resurfacing. Dermatol Clin. 2001;19(3):453.
127. Riggs K, Keller M, Humphreys TR. Ablative laser resurfacing: high-energy pulsed carbon dioxide and erbium:yttrium-aluminum-garnet. Clin Dermatol. 2007;25(5):462.
128. Tierney EP, Kouba DJ, Hanke CW. Review of fractional photothermolysis: treatment indications and efficacy. Dermatol Surg. 2009;35(10):1445.
129. Ross VE, Miller C, Meehan K, et al. One-pass CO_2 versus multiple-pass Er:YAG laser resurfacing in the treatment of rhytides: a comparison side-by-side of pulsed CO_2 and Er:YAG lasers. Dermatol Surg. 2001;27(8):709-15.
130. Tanzi EL, Alster TS. Single-pass carbon dioxide versus multiple-pass Er:YAG laser skin resurfacing: a comparison 24. of postoperative wound healing and side-effect rates. Dermatol Surg. 2003;29(1):80-4.
131. Sapijaszko MJ, Zachary CB. Er:YAG laser skin resurfacing. Dermatol Clin. 2002;20(1):87-96.
132. Ross EV, McKinlay JR, Anderson RR. Why does carbon dioxide resurfacing work? A review. Arch Dermatol 1999;135(4):444-54.
133. Bernstein EF, Brown DB, Kenkel J, et al. Residual thermal damage resulting from pulsed and scanned resurfacing lasers. Dermatol Surg. 1999;25(10):739-44.
134. Saluja R, Khoury J, Detwiler SP, et al. Histologic and clinical response to varying density settings with a fractionally scanned carbon dioxide laser. J Drugs Dermatol. 2009;8(1):17-20.
135. Brightman LA, Brauer JA, Anolik R, et al. Ablative and fractional ablative lasers. Dermatol Clin. 2009; 27(4):479-89.
136. Fulton JE Jr, Barnes T. Collagen shrinkage (selective dermaplasty) with the high-energy pulsed carbon dioxide laser. Dermatol Surg. 1998;24(1):37.
137. Ross EV, Yashar SS, Naseef GS, et al. A pilot study of in vivo immediate tissue contraction with CO_2 skin laser resurfacing in a live farm pig. Dermatol Surg. 1999;25(11):851.
138. Walia S, Alster TS. Prolonged clinical and histologic effects from CO_2 laser resurfacing of atrophic acne scars. Dermatol Surg. 1999;25(12):926.
139. Study Guide for the Basic Laser Science, Tissue Interaction and Laser Safety. Written Examinations. Americal Board of Laser Surgery. 2012 edition.
140. Ramsdell WM. Fractional carbon dioxide laser resurfacing. Semin Plast Surg. 2012;26(3):125-30.
141. Ross EV, McKinlay JR, Sajben FP, et al. Use of a novel erbium laser in a Yucatan minipig: a study of residual thermal damage, ablation, and wound

healing as a function of pulse duration. Lasers Surg Med. 2002;30(2):93-100.

142. Papadavid E, Katsambas A. Lasers for facial rejuvenation: a review. Int J Dermatol. 2003;42(6):480.
143. Rahman Z, McFalls H, Jiang K, et al. Fractional deep dermal ablation induces tissue tightening. Lasers Surg Med. 2009;41(2):78-86.
144. Gardner ES, Reinisch L, Stricklin GP, et al. In vitro changes in non-facial human skin following CO_2 laser resurfacing: a comparison study. Lasers Surg Med. 1996;19(4):379-87.
145. Fisher GJ, Varani J, Voorhees JJ. Looking older: fibroblast collapse and therapeutic implications. Arch Dermatol. 2008;144(5):666-72.
146. Chan HH, Manstein D, Yu CS, et al. The prevalence and risk factors of post-inflammatory hyperpigmentation after fractional resurfacing in Asians. Lasers Surg Med. 2007;39(5):381-5.
147. Kim YJ, Lee HS, Son SW, et al. Analysis of hyperpigmentation and hypopigmentation after Er:YAG laser skin resurfacing. Lasers Surg Med. 2005;36(1):47-51.
148. Tan KL, Kurniawati C, Gold MH. Low risk of postinflammatory hyperpigmentation in skin types 4 and 5 after treatment with fractional CO_2 laser device. J Drugs Dermatol. 2008;7(8):774.
149. Shah S, Alam A. Laser resurfacing pearls. Semin Plast Surg. 2012;26(3):131-6.
150. Alam M, Dover JS, Arndt KA. To ablate or not: a proposal regarding nomenclature. J Am Acad Dermatol. 2011;64(6):1170-4.
151. Hantash BM, Bedi VP, Sudireddy V, et al. Laser-induced transepidermal elimination of dermal content by fractional photothermolysis. J Biomed Opt. 2006; 11(4):041115.
152. Bogdan Allemann I, Kaufman J. Fractional photothermolysis-an update. Lasers Med Sci. 2010; 25(1):137.
153. Keagle JN, Welch WJ, Young DM. Expression of heat shock proteins in a linear rodent wound. Wound Rep Reg. 2001;9(5):378-85.
154. Razzaque MS, Foster CS, Ahmed AR. Role of collagen-binding heat shock protein 47 and transforming growth factor-beta1 in conjunctival scarring in ocular cicatricial pemphigoid. Invest Ophthalmol Vis Sci. 2003;44(4):1616-21.
155. Bedi VP, Chan KF, Sink RK, et al. The effects of pulse energy variations on the dimensions of microscopic thermal treatment zones in fractional photothermolysis. Lasers Surg Med. 2007;39(2):145-55.
156. El-Domyati M, Abd-El-Raheem T, Abdel-Wahab H, et al. Fractional versus ablative erbium:yttrium-aluminum-garnet laser resurfacing for facial rejuvenation: an objective evaluation. J Am Acad Dermatol. 2013;68(1):103-12.
157. Metelitsa AI, Alster TS. Fractionated laser skin resurfacing treatment complications: a review. Dermatol Surg. 2010;36(3):299-306.
158. Ross EV, Grossman MC, Duke D, et al. Long-term results after CO_2 laser skin resurfacing: a comparison of scanned and pulsed systems. J Am Acad Dermatol. 1997;37(5 Pt 1):709-18.
159. Shah S, Alster TS. Laser treatment of dark skin: an updated review. Am J Clin Dermatol. 2010;11(6):389-97.
160. Alster TS, Garg S. Treatment of facial rhytides with a high-energy pulsed carbon dioxide laser. Plast Reconstr Surg. 1996;98(5):791.
161. Fife DJ, Fitzpatrick RE, Zachary CB. Complications of fractional CO_2 laser resurfacing: four cases. Lasers Surg Med. 2009;41(3):179-84.
162. Ross RB, Spencer J. Scarring and persistent erythema after fractionated ablative CO_2 laser resurfacing. J Drugs Dermatol. 2008;7(11):1072-3.
163. W, Triwongwaranat D, Varothai S, Eimpunth S, et al. Efficacy and safety of a carbon-dioxide ablative fractional resurfacing device for treatment of atrophic acne scars in Asians. J Am Acad Dermatol. 2010;63(2):274-83.
164. Orringer JS, Kang S, Johnson TM, et al. Tretinoin treatment before carbon-dioxide laser resurfacing: a clinical and biochemical analysis. J Am Acad Dermatol. 2004;51(6):940-6.
165. Hevia O, Nemeth AJ, Taylor JR. Tretinoin accelerates healing after trichloroacetic acid chemical peel. Arch Dermatol. 1991;127(5):678-82.
166. Mandy SH. Tretinoin in the preoperative and postoperative management of dermabrasion. J Am Acad Dermatol. 1986;15(4 Pt 2):878-9.
167. Vagotis FL, Brundage SR. Histologic study of dermabrasion and chemical peel in an animal model after pretreatment with Retin-A. Aesthetic Plast Surg. 1995;19(3):243-6.
168. Mandy SH. Dermabrasion. Semin Cutan Med Surg. 1996;15(3):162.
169. Drake LA, Dinehart SM, Goltz RW, et al. Guidelines of care for chemical peeling. Guidelines/Outcomes Committee: American Academy of Dermatology. J Am Acad Dermatol. 1995;33(3):497-503.
170. West TB, Alster TS. Effect of pretreatment on the incidence of hyperpigmentation following cutaneous CO_2 laser resurfacing. Dermatol Surg. 1999;25(1):15-7.
171. Sriprachya-anunt S, Marchell NL, Fitzpatrick RE, et al. Facial resurfacing in patients with Fitzpatrick skin type IV. Lasers Surg Med. 2002;30(2):86-92.
172. Tierney EP, Hanke CW, Petersen J. Ablative fractionated CO_2 laser treatment of photoaging: a clinical and histologic study. Dermatol Surg. 2012; 38(11):1777.
173. Alam M, Hsu TS, Dover JS, et al. Nonablative laser and light treatments: histology and tissue effects—a review. Lasers Surg Med. 2003;33(1):30-9.
174. Tierney EP, Hanke CW. The effect of cold-air anesthesia during fractionated carbon-dioxide laser treatment: prospective study and review of the literature. J Am Acad Dermatol. 2012;67(3):436-45.
175. Fisher GH, Geronemus RG. Short-term side effects of fractional photothermolysis. Dermatol Surg. 2005;31(9 Pt 2):1245-9, discussion 1249.
176. Alam M, Pantanowitz L, Harton AM, et al. A prospective trial of fungal colonization after laser

resurfacing of the face: correlation between culture positivity and symptoms of pruritus. Dermatol Surg. 2003;29(3):255-60.

177. Choi, JE, Oh, GN, Kim JY, et al. Ablative fractional laser treatment for hypertrophic scars: comparison between Er:YAG and CO_2 fractional lasers. J Dermatolog.Treat. 2014:25(4):299-303.
178. Qu L, Liu A, Zhou L, et al. Clinical and molecular effects on mature burn scars after treatment with a fractional CO_2 laser. Lasers Surg Med. 2012;44(7):517-24.
179. Grunewald S, Bodendorf M, Illes M, et al. In vivo wound healing and dermal matrix remodeling in response to fractionated CO_2 laser intervention: clinicopathological correlation in non-facial skin. Int J Hyperthermia. 2011;27(8):811-8.
180. Helbig D, Bodendorf M, Grunewald S, et al. Immunohistochemical investigation of the wound healing response to fractional photothermolysis. J Biomed Opt. 2009;14(6):064044.
181. Kroonen L, Shumaker PR, Kwan JM, et al. Treatment of split-thickness skin graft-related forearm scar contractures with a carbon dioxide laser protocol: 3 case reports. J Hand Surg Am. 2013 38(11):2164-8.
182. Schwartz RJ, Burns AJ, Rohrich RJ, et al. Long-term assessment of CO_2 facial laser resurfacing: aesthetic results and complications. Plast Reconstr Surg. 1999;103(2):592-601.
183. Fitzpatrick RE. CO_2 laser resurfacing. Dermatol Clin. 2001;19(3):443-51, viii.
184. Duke D, Khatri K, Grevelink JM, et al. Comparative clinical trial of 2 carbon dioxide resurfacing lasers with varying pulse durations: 100 microseconds vs 1 millisecond. Arch Dermatol. 1998;134(10):1240-6.
185. Apfelberg DB, Smoller B. UltraPulse carbon dioxide laser with CPG scanner for deepithelialization: clinical and histologic study. Plast Reconstr Surg. 1997;99(7):2089-94.
186. Trelles MA, Rigau J, Mellor TK, et al. A clinical and histological comparison of flashscanning versus pulsed technology in carbon dioxide laser facial skin resurfacing. Dermatol Surg. 1998;24(1):43-9.
187. Taub AF. Fractionated delivery systems for difficult to treat clinical applications: acne scarring, melasma, atrophic scarring, striae distensae, and deep rhytides. J Drugs Dermatol. 2007;6(11):1120-8.
188. Alster TS, Tanzi EL. Hypertrophic scars and keloids: etiology and management. Am J Clin Dermatol. 2003;4(4):235-43.
189. Fitzpatrick RE, Goldman MP, Satur NM, et al. Pulsed carbon dioxide laser resurfacing of photo-aged facial skin. Arch Dermatol. 1996;132(4):395-402.
190. Sukal SA, Geronemus RG. Thermage: the nonablative radiofrequency for rejuvenation. Clin Dermatol. 2008;26(6):602-7.
191. Dover JS, Zelickson BD. Results of a survey of 5,700 patient monopolar radiofrequency facial skin tightening treatments: assessment of a low-energy multiple-pass technique leading to a clinical end point algorithm. Dermatol Surg. 2007;33(8):900-7.
192. Blugerman G, Shavelzon D, Paul M. A safety and feasibility study of a novel radiofrequency-assisted liposuction technique. Plast Reconstr Surg. 2010;125(3):998-1006.
193. Paul M, Mulholland RS. A new approach for adipose tissue treatment and body contouring using radiofrequency assisted liposuction. Aesthetic Plast Surg. 2009;33(5):687-94.
194. Paul M, Blugerman G, Kreindel M, et al. Three-dimensional radiofrequency tissue tightening: a proposed mechanism and applications for body contouring. Aesthetic Plast Surg. 2011;35(1):87-95.
195. Mulholland RS. An in-depth examination of radiofrequency assisted liposuction (RFAL). J Cosmetic Surg Med. 2009;4:14-8.
196. Kreindel M, Mulholland RS. Radiofrequency energy. Body Language. 2009;29:23-4.
197. Paul MD. Radiofrequency assisted liposuction comes of age: an emerging technology offers an exciting new vista in nonexcisional body contouring. Plastic Surgery Pract. 2009;2:18-9.
198. Mulholland RS. The latest technologies to fight the bulge. Healthy Aging. 2009;4:7-11.
199. Brightman L. RFAL Arm study Am Society Lasers Med and Surg annual meeting. Kissimmee (FL), June 2010.
200. Vicariotto F, Raichi M. Technological evolution in the radiofrequency treatment of vaginal laxity and menopausal vulvo-vaginal atrophy and other genitourinary symptoms: first experiences with a novel dynamic quadripolar device. Minerva Ginecologica. 2016;68(3):225-36.
201. Bader A. Non-invasive labia majora tightening and skin rejuvenation with CO_2 laser femitight Alma Surgical.
202. Avci P, Gupta A, Sadasivam M, et al. Low-level laser (light) therapy (LLLT) in skin: stimulating, healing, restoring. Semin Cutan Med Surg. 2013;32(1):41-52.
203. Dierickx CC, Anderson RR. Visible light treatment of photoaging. Dermatol Ther. 2005;18(3):191-208.
204. Weiss RA, Weiss MA, Geronemus RG, et al. A novel non-thermal non-ablative full panel LED photomodulation device for reversal of photoaging: digital microscopic and clinical results in various skin types. J Drugs Dermatol. 2004;3(6):605-10.
205. Weiss RA, McDaniel DH, Geronemus RG, et al. Clinical experience with light-emitting diode (LED) photomodulation. Dermatol Surg. 2005;31(9 Pt 2): 1199-1205.
206. Weiss RA, McDaniel DH, Geronemus RG, et al. Clinical trial of a novel nonthermal LED array for reversal of photoaging: clinical, histologic, and surface profilometric results. Lasers Surg Med. 2005; 36(2):85-91.
207. Bhat J, Birch J, Whitehurst C, et al. A single-blinded randomised controlled study to determine the efficacy of Omnilux Revive facial treatment in skin rejuvenation. Lasers Med Sci. 2005;20(1):6-10.
208. Russell BA, Kellett N, Reilly LR. A study to determine the efficacy of combination LED light therapy (633 nm and 830 nm) in facial skin rejuvenation. J Cosmet Laser Ther. 2005;7(3-4):196-200.
209. Barolet D, Roberge CJ, Auger FA, et al. Regulation of skin collagen metabolism in vitro using a pulsed 660 nm

LED light source: clinical correlation with a single-blinded study. J Invest Dermatol. 2009;129(12):2751-9.
210. Abergel RP, Lyons RF, Castel JC, et al. Biostimulation of wound healing by lasers: experimental approaches in animal models and in fibroblast cultures. J Dermatol Surg Oncol. 1987;13(2):127-33.
211. Yu W, Naim JO, Lanzafame RJ. The effect of laser irradiation on the release of bFGF from 3T3 fibroblasts. Photochem Photobiol. 1994;59(2):167-70.
212. Schindl A, Heinze G, Schindl M, et al. Systemic effects of low- intensity laser irradiation on skin microcirculation in patients with diabetic microangiopathy. Microvasc Res. 2002;64(2):240-6.
213. Ben-Dov N, Shefer G, Irintchev A, et al. Low-energy laser irradiation affects satellite cell proliferation and differentiation in vitro. Biochim Biophys Acta. 1999;1448(3):372-80.
214. Lee SY, Park KH, Choi JW, et al. A prospective, randomized, placebo-controlled, double-blinded, and split-face clinical study on LED phototherapy for skin rejuvenation: clinical, profilometric, histologic, ultrastructural, and biochemical evaluations and comparison of three different treatment settings. J Photochem Photobiol B. 2007;88(1):51-67.
215. Uitto J, Kouba D. Cytokine modulation of extracellular matrix gene expression: relevance to fibrotic skin diseases. J Dermatol Sci. 2000;24(Suppl 1):S60-9.
216. Duranti F, Salti G, Bovani B, et al. Injectable hyaluronic acid gel for soft tissue augmentation. A clinical and histological study. Dermatol Surg. 1998;24(12):1317-25.
217. Alastair Carruthers. Injectable soft tissue fillers: temporary agents. UpToDate. January 19, 2017.
218. Radiesse® Injectable Implant: Instructions for Use. Franksville, WI: BioForm Medical, Inc.; 2008.
219. Alam M, Havey J, Pace N, et al. Large-particle calcium hydroxylapatite injection for correction of facial wrinkles and depressions. J Am Acad Dermatol. 2011;65(1):92-6.
220. Sculptra® (injectable poly-L-lactic acid) Prescribing Information. Bridgewater, NJ: Dermik Laboratories; 2006.
221. Alastair Carruthers. Injectable soft tissue fillers: Permanent agents. July 7, 2017.
222. Coleman SR. Long-term survival of fat transplants: controlled demonstrations. Aesthetic Plast Surg. 1995;19(5):421-5.
223. Fulton JE, Suarez M, Silverton K, et al. Small volume fat transfer. Dermatol Surg. 1998;24(8):857-65.
224. Fournier PF. Fat grafting: my technique. Dermatol Surg. 2000;26(12):1117-28.
225. Cervelli V, Palla L, Pascali M, et al. Autologous platelet-rich plasma mixed with purified fat graft in aesthetic plastic surgery. Aesthetic Plast Surg. 2009;33(5):716-21.
226. Alexander RW. Use of platelet-rich plasma to enhance effectiveness of autologous fat grafting. In: Shiffman MA, editor. Autologous Fat Transfer: Art, Science, and Clinical Practice. Heidelberg: Springer; 2010. p. 87.
227. Yoshimura K, Sato K, Aoi N, et al. Cell-assisted lipotransfer for facial lipoatrophy: efficacy of clinical use of adipose-derived stem cells. Dermatol Surg. 2008; 34(9):1178-85.
228. Sterodimas A, de Faria J, Nicaretta B, et al. Cell-assisted lipotransfer. Aesthet Surg J. 2010;30(1):78-81.
229. Sterodimas A, de Faria J, Nicaretta B, et al. Tissue engineering with adipose-derived stem cells (ADSCs): current and future applications. J Plast Reconstr Aesthet Surg. 2010;63(11):1886-92.
230. Teimourian B. Blindness following fat injections. Plast Reconstr Surg. 1988;82(2):361.
231. Dreizen NG, Framm L. Sudden unilateral visual loss after autologous fat injection into the glabellar area. Am J Ophthalmol. 1989;107(1):85-7.
232. Egido JA, Arroyo R, Marcos A, et al. Middle cerebral artery embolism and unilateral visual loss after autologous fat injection into the glabellar area. Stroke. 1993;24(4):615-6.
233. Feinendegen DL, Baumgartner RW, Schroth G, et al. Middle cerebral artery occlusion and ocular fat embolism after autologous fat injection in the face. J Neurol. 1998;245(1):53-4.
234. Yoon SS, Chang DI, Chung KC. Acute fatal stroke immediately following autologous fat injection into the face. Neurology. 2003;61(8):1151-2.
235. Thaunat O, Thaler F, Loirat P, et al. Cerebral fat embolism induced by facial fat injection. Plast Reconstr Surg. 2004;113(7):2235-6.
236. Mori K, Ohta K, Nagano S, et al. [A case of ophthalmic artery obstruction following autologous fat injection in the glabellar area]. Nippon Ganka Gakkai Zasshi. 2007;111(1):22-5.
237. Park SH, Sun HJ, Choi KS. Sudden unilateral visual loss after autologous fat injection into the nasolabial fold. Clin Ophthalmol. 2008;2(3):679-83.
238. Gleeson CM, Lucas S, Langrish CJ, Barlow RJ. Acute fatal fat tissue embolism after autologous fat transfer in a patient with lupus profundus. Dermatol Surg. 2011;37(1):111-5.
239. Park YH, Kim KS. Images in clinical medicine. Blindness after fat injections. N Engl J Med. 2011; 365(23):2220.
240. The Esybron Institute 2007. The female genital system. Available at: http://www.esybron.org/index.phtml?p=female.
241. Goldstein I, Meston C, Davis S. Women's Sexual Function and Dysfunction: Study Diagnosis and Treatment. London: Taylor and Francis; 2006.
242. Burri AV, Cherkas L, Spector TD. Genetic and environmental influences on self-reported G-spots in women: a twin study. J Sex Med. 2010;7(5):1842-52.
243. Physician info, the G-shot: overview. Available at: www. thegshot.com.
244. Forsberg JG. A morphologist's approach to the vagina-age-related changes and estrogen sensitivity. Maturitas. 1995;22(Suppl):S7-15.
245. Park K, Ahn K, Lee S, et al. Decreased circulating levels of estrogen alter vaginal and clitoral blood flow and structure in the rabbit. Int J Impot Res. 2001;13(2):116-24.
246. Zaino R. Diseases of the vagina. In: Kurman, RJ, editor. Blaustein's Pathology of the Female Genital Tract. New York: Springer-Verlag; 2002. pp. 132-6.

247. Boreham MK, Wai CY, Miller RT, et al. Morphometric analysis of smooth muscle in the anterior vaginal wall of women with pelvic organ prolapse. Am J Obstet Gynecol. 2002;187(1):56-63.
248. Huggins C, Jensen EV, Cleveland AS. Chemical structure of steroids in relation to promotion of growth of the vagina and uterus of the hypophysectomized rat. J Exp Med. 1954;100(3):225-40.
249. Pessina MA, Hoyt RF Jr, Goldstein I, et al. Differential effects of estradiol, progesterone, and testosterone on vaginal structural integrity. Endocrinology. 2006;147(1):61-9.
250. Hilliges M, Falconer C, Ekman-Ordeberg G, et al. Innervation of the human vaginal mucosa as revealed by PGP 9.5 immunohistochemistry. Acta Anat (Basel). 1995;153(2):119-26.
251. Da Chung J, Bai SW. Roles of sex steroid receptors and cell cycle regulation in pathogenesis of pelvic organ prolapse. Curr Opin Obstet Gynecol. 2006; 18(5):551-4.
252. Bai SW, Chung DJ, Yoon JM, et al. Roles of estrogen receptor, progesterone receptor, p53 and p21 in pathogenesis of pelvic organ prolapse. Int Urogynecol J. 2005;16(6):492-6.
253. Lang JH, Zhu L, Sun ZJ, et al. Estrogen levels and estrogen receptors in patients with stress urinary incontinence and pelvic organ prolapse. Int J Gynaecol Obstet. 2003;80(1):35-9.
254. Savvas M, Bishop J, Laurent G, et al. Type III collagen content in the skin of postmenopausal women receiving oestradiol and testosterone implants. Br J Obstet Gynaecol. 1993;100(2):154-6.
255. Brincat M, Moniz CF, Kabalan S, et al. Decline in skin collagen content and metacarpal index after the menopause and its prevention with sex hormone replacement. Br J Obstet Gynaecol. 1987;94(2):126-9.
256. Brincat M, Kabalan S, Studd JW, et al. A study of the decrease of skin collagen content, skin thickness, and bone mass in the postmenopausal woman. Obstet Gynecol. 1987;70(6):840-5.
257. Clark AL, Slayden OD, Hettrich K, et al. Estrogen increases collagen I and III mRNA expression in the pelvic support tissues of the rhesus macaque. Am J Obstet Gynecol. 2005;192(5):1523-9.
258. Falconer C, Ekman-Ordeberg G, Ulmsten U, et al. Changes in paraurethral connective tissue at menopause are counteracted by estrogen. Maturitas. 1996;24(3):197-204.
259. Rizk DE, Hassan HA, Al Marzouqi AH, et al. Combined estrogen and ghrelin administration restores number of blood vessels and collagen type I/III ratio in the urethral and anal canal submucosa of old ovariectomized rats. Int Urogynecol J Pelvic Floor Dysfunct. 2008;19(4):547-52.
260. Jackson S, James M, Abrams P. The effect of oestradiol on vaginal collagen metabolism in postmenopausal women with genuine stress incontinence. Br J Obstet Gynaecol. 2002;109(3):339-44.
261. Helvering LM, Adrian MD, Geiser AG, et al. Differential effects of estrogen and raloxifene on messenger RNA and matrix metalloproteinase 2 activity in the rat uterus. Biol Reprod. 2005;72(4):830-41.
262. Brincat M, Versi E, Moniz CF, et al. Skin collagen changes in postmenopausal women receiving different regimens of estrogen therapy. Obstet Gynecol. 1987; 70(1):123-7.
263. Moalli PA, Klingensmith WL, Meyn LA, et al. Regulation of matrix metalloproteinase expression by estrogen in fibroblasts that are derived from the pelvic floor. Am J Obstet Gynecol. 2002;187(1):72-9.
264. Liu YM, Choy KW, Lui WT, et al. 17beta-estradiol suppresses proliferation of fibroblasts derived from cardinal ligaments in patients with or without pelvic organ prolapse. Hum Reprod. 2006;21(1):303-8.
265. Boennelycke M, Gras S, Lose G. Tissue engineering as a potential alternative or adjunct to surgical reconstruction in treating pelvic organ prolapse. Int Urogynecol J. 2013;24(5):741-7.
266. Wen Y, Wani P, Zhou L, et al. Reprogramming of fibroblasts from older women with pelvic floor disorders alters cellular behavior associated with donor age. Stem Cells Transl Med. 2013;2(2): 118-28.
267. Kerkhof MH, Ruiz-Zapata AM, Bril H, et al. Changes in tissue composition of the vaginal wall of premenopausal women with Prolapse. Am J Obstet Gynecol. 2013;210(2):168.e1-9.
268. Cannon TW, Lee JY, Somogyi G, J et al. Improved sphincter contractility after allogenic muscle-derived progenitor cell injection into the denervated rat urethra. Urology. 2003;62:958-63.
269. Strasser H, Marksteiner R, Margreiter E, et al. Stem cell therapy for urinary incontinence. Urologe A. 2004;43(10):1237-41.
270. Strasser H, Marksteiner R, Margreiter E, et al. Autologous myoblasts and fibroblasts versus collagen for treatment of stress urinary incontinence in women: a randomised controlled trial. Lancet. 2007; 369(9478): 2179-86.
271. Puppo V. Anatomy and physiology of the clitoris, vestibular bulbs, and labia minora with a review of the female orgasm and the prevention of female sexual dysfunction. Clin Anat. 2013;26(1):134-52.
272. Runels C, Melnick H, Debourbon E, et al. A pilot study of the effect of localized injections of autologous platelet rich plasma (PRP) for the treatment of female sexual dysfunction. J Women Health Care. 2014;3:169.

KIEL SCH•OL

43 of Gynaecological Endoscopy

Oncologic Surgery on the Ovary

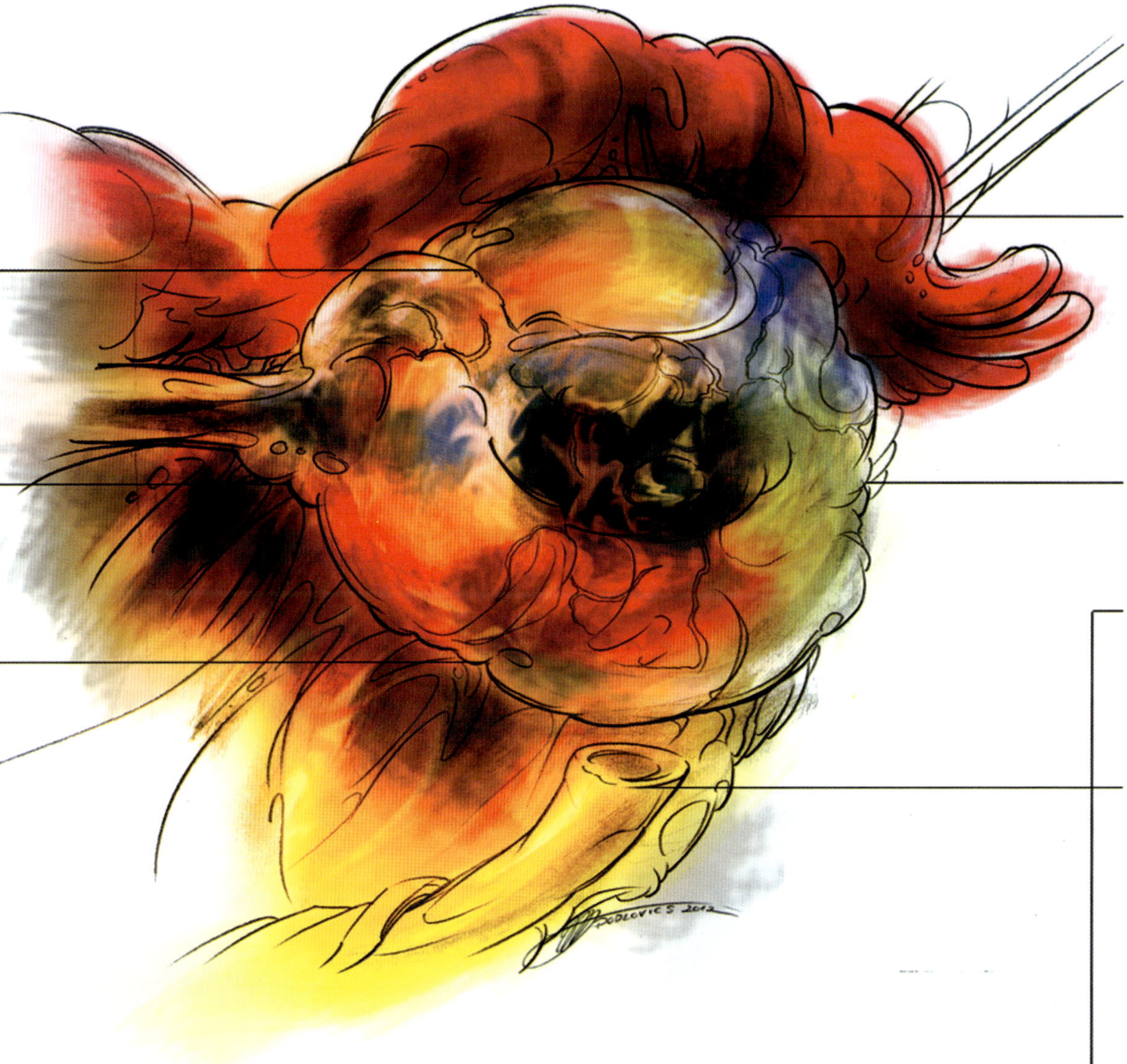

Chapter 43

Oncologic Surgery on the Ovary

Ivo Meinhold-Heerlein

INTRODUCTION

The use of laparoscopy to diagnose and treat gynecological cancers emerged during the 1960s. Zoeckler and Hegstrom[1] reported about the peritoneoscopy in malignant lesions of the abdomen, Miniconi et al.[2] about the value of laparoscopy in the diagnosis of peritoneal carcinosis and Lacey et al.[3] about laparoscopy in the evaluation of gynecologic cancer where 60 patients with a variety of known or suspected gynecologic neoplasms were evaluated. His group performed both staging laparoscopy before treatment and surveillance laparoscopy for the evaluation of treatment success. The latter type of operation was later called second look laparoscopy and performed until the 1990s to evaluate the response of advanced ovarian cancers to cytostatic drugs. It was a rocky road from the pure diagnostic use of laparoscopy to laparoscopic surgery of gynecological malignancies. Certain inventions like the automated CO_2 insufflator, laparoscopic suturing techniques and energy sources and devices for coagulation laid essential foundations to operate gynecological malignancies. Finally, Canis et al.[4] published his study on first radical hysterectomy. Besides this milestone in endoscopic surgery, Canis et al. cautiously stated in 1994:[5] "More clinical research is required before this approach can be proposed as an alternative to laparotomy." Eleven years later he concluded: "All the procedures, which may be required to treat a gynecologic cancer, can be performed endoscopically."[6] Confirming this statement several groups have successfully shown the feasibility to stage gynecological cancers endoscopically and established their own surgical procedures.[7-17] The repertoire of surgeons with oncological and endoscopic expertise includes:

- Total laparoscopic hysterectomy (TLH)
- Laparoscopic radical hysterectomy (LRH, laparoscopic Wertheims)
- Salpingectomy, oophorectomy
- Pelvic (iliac) and para-aortic lymphadenectomy
- Omentectomy
- (Anterior/posterior) exenteration.

Although results of prospective randomized trials to compare laparoscopy and laparotomy with respect to patient's outcome (overall survival, disease-free survival) are lacking, advantages of laparoscopy (e.g., shorter duration of surgery, shorter hospital stay, less blood loss, better quality of life, less postoperative pain, less intra- and postoperative complications) have been shown for thousands of patients in certain randomized trials and also many case series, cohort studies and case-control studies. The comparable oncological safety (number of lymph nodes, resection margins) demonstrated in these studies suggest that for certain indications—such as early-stage cervical and endometrial cancer as well as borderline tumors of the ovary—laparoscopy will be safe to replace laparotomy in the future.[18]

Ovarian cancer carries the worst prognosis among all gynecological malignancies, because most cases (>75%) are diagnosed in an advanced stage due to the lack of early symptoms and the lack of an effective screening method for an early detection of the disease. Early stage cancers are often found by chance and have a far better prognosis than advanced stage cancers. Ultrasonographically suspicious ovarian cysts often turn out to reflect histologically early stage cancers or borderline lesions of the ovary. Most suspicious adnexal masses are operated laparoscopically, if there are no clear signs of malignancy. If such a mass turns out to be malignant the questions arises how to complete the surgical staging procedure: endoscopically or open?

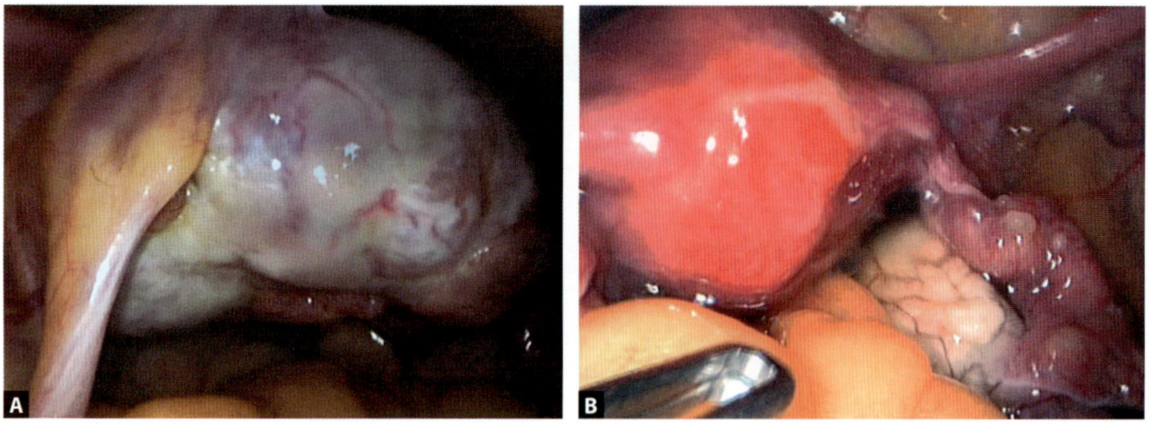

Figs. 43.1A and B: Ovarian cancer of the left ovary. A 47-year-old patient with a history of hereditary breast cancer presented with clinical normal ovaries to undergo a prophylactic adnexectomy. The histological result revealed a high-grade serous ovarian cancer of the left ovary (A) left ovary and (B) right ovary. In case of a prophylactic adnexectomy for hereditary breast cancer patients or mutation carriers, the fallopian tubes have to be removed completely since malign tumors of these patients arise in the fallopian tube rather than on the ovarian surface.

This question cannot be answered conclusively, because no randomized clinical trial has been performed to compare laparoscopy and laparotomy for the treatment of ovarian cancer, neither for early stage nor for advanced stage invasive tumors, nor for non-invasive borderline lesions. It is, however, widely accepted to utilize laparoscopy for diagnostic and prophylactic procedures. For the treatment of invasive cancers an open approach is preferable.[18]

The purpose of this chapter is to illuminate difficulties of laparoscopic surgery with ovarian malignancies and to:

- *Summarize knowledge and published data on laparoscopy for ovarian malignancies:*
  - prophylactic operations
  - diagnosis and treatment of borderline tumors
  - diagnosis and treatment of early stage invasive cancers
  - diagnosis and treatment of early stage invasive cancers
- Give advice on the adequate indication to choose a laparoscopic approach including a preoperative workup
- Describe the appropriate laparoscopic procedures systematically
- Show how to avoid and handle typical complications.

LAPAROSCOPY FOR OVARIAN MALIGNANCIES

Prophylactic Operations

Women carrying an increased risk to develop ovarian cancer—for example in case of BRCA1/2 mutations or a hereditary nonpolyposis colorectal cancer (HNPCC) syndrome known also as Lynch syndrome—may undergo prophylactic laparoscopic bilateral salpingo-oophorectomy. This operation reduces the risk for women with BRCA1/2 mutations at about

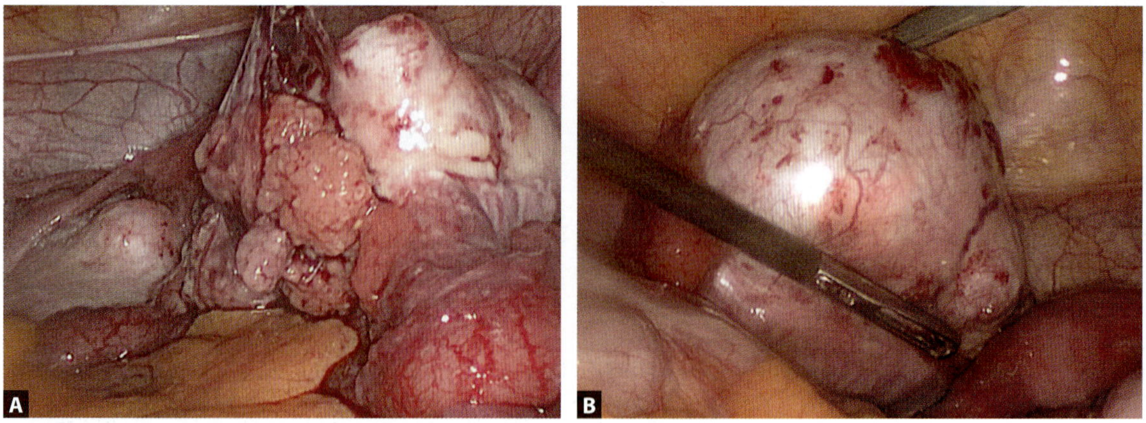

Figs. 43.2A and B: Serous borderline tumor of both ovaries: (A) right ovary and (B) left ovary

50% for breast cancer and about 80% for Fallopian tube or ovarian cancer. It has been shown that the adnexal malignancies of BRCA1/2 mutation carriers rather originate from the Fallopian tube than from the ovarian surface. Therefore, it has to be evaluated in the future if the prophylactic removal of the Fallopian tubes may be sufficient. Today, the laparoscopic bilateral salpingo-oophorectomy with complete resection of the Fallopian tubes at the age of 40 and after completion of family planning represents the gold standard to prevent women with an increased risk from developing adnexal malignancies.[19,20]

Borderline Tumors

Most of the published case series of early stage ovarian malignancies include also ovarian tumors of low malignant potential (LMP), so-called borderline tumors. Many groups have shown the feasibility to operate LMP tumors laparoscopically. The procedures include bilateral adnectomy, hysterectomy, infracolic omentectomy and peritoneal biopsies.[17,21-23] Some authors have described port site metastases after laparoscopic surgery for LMP tumors; most of these cases were associated with tumor morcellation, which is contraindicated in any case of ovarian tumor, and with tumor spillage, which has to be avoided during the surgical procedure.[24] Like early-stage invasive cancer, LMP tumors are rare and prospective randomized trials to compare the surgical and survival outcome are lacking. However, the data and our own experience suggest to manage LMP tumors laparoscopically provided that the necessary expertise in advanced laparoscopic surgery is ensured and the procedure meets the same oncological criteria like in open surgery.[24-26] In case of a premenopausal patient with desire to have children, fertility-conserving surgery can be performed. This may include cyst enucleation or (partial or complete) unilateral adnectomy, infragastric omentectomy, peritoneal biopsies and peritoneal washings. The patient then needs to be informed about the higher relapse risk, which is associated with

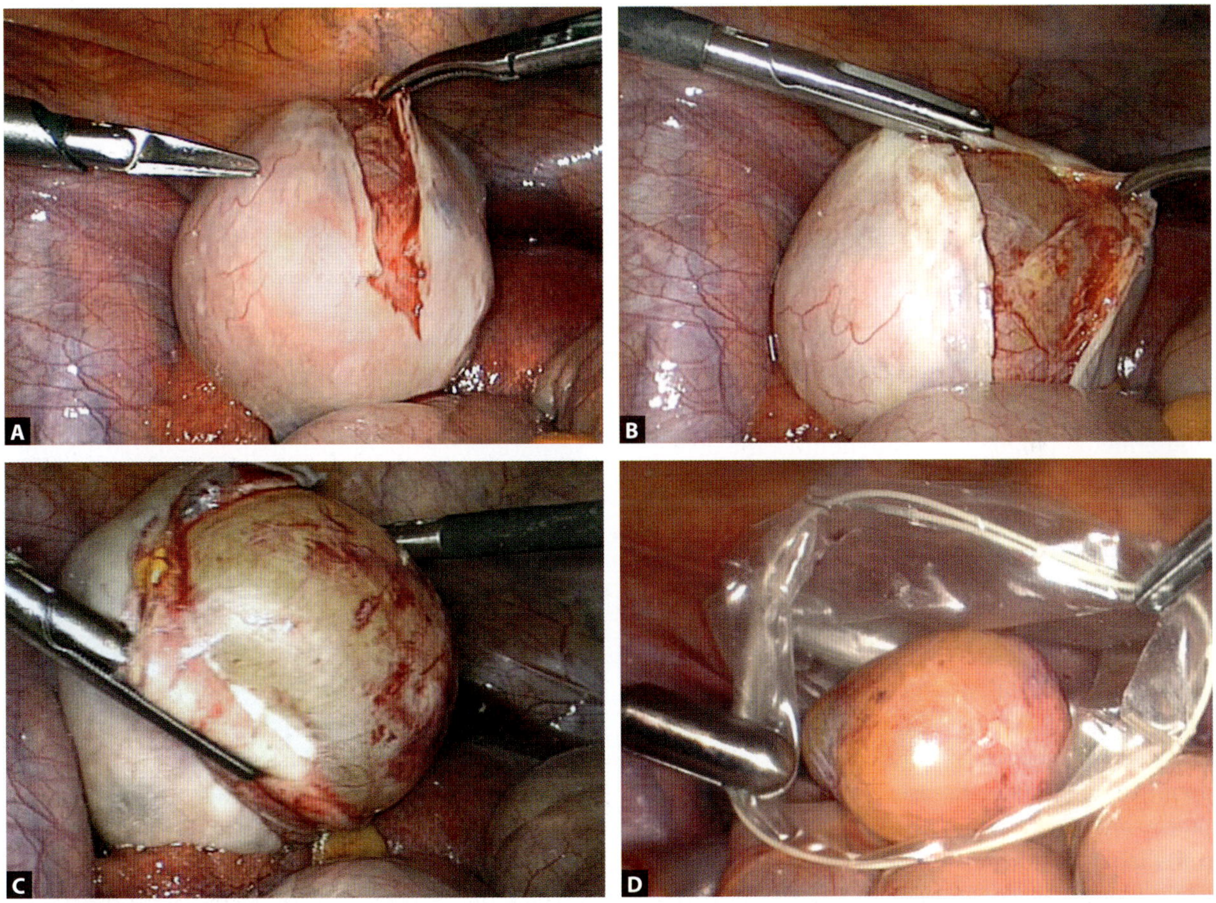

Figs. 43.3A to D: Dermoid cyst enucleation out of the left ovary. A sequence is shown: (A) The ovarian capsule is coagulated and cut preventing a cyst rupture; (B) The ovarian tissue is separated from the cyst carefully. It is always necessary to use both hands; (C) It helps to peel the ovarian tissue while twisting the grasper around its own axis; (D) The specimen is inside a retrieval bag. Even cysts with a benign clinical appearance should—if possible—be prevented from rupturing since sometimes the histological result reveals a malign result.

fertility-conserving operations of borderline tumors.[27] Recently, the Arbeitsgemeinschaft Gynäkologische Onkologie (AGO) study group (Germany) has conducted a cohort study (ROBOT study) showing that the relapse rate and the prognosis of ovarian borderline tumors depend on the accuracy of surgical. The authors also showed that there is no significant difference, if the staging is performed laparscopically or with open surgery. Thus, when respecting the oncological principles, laparoscopy is safe and beneficial to treat borderline tumors.[28]

Early-Stage Invasive Tumors

The operation of early-stage invasive tumors has—regardless of open or endoscopically—to include hysterectomy, bilateral adnectomy, omentectomy, pelvic and para-aortic lymphadenectomy, peritoneal washings and biopsies. A recently published Cochrane analysis evaluating 706 published studies from 1990 until 2007 identified just three valuable observational studies addressing the comparison of laparoscopy and laparotomy for ovarian cancer surgery.[23,29-31] The cohort study published by Tozzi et al.[23] described the experience with 24 patients suffering from ovarian cancer FIGO IA-B who underwent laparoscopic surgery as primary treatment (13/24) or as secondary operation to complete the surgical staging (11/24). The mean operation time was 182 min for the primary operation and 166 min for completion of staging operation. No major intraoperative complication and no trocar metastasis occurred. Five patients received adjuvant chemotherapy after a median of 7 days. Two patients developed a relapse. After a median follow-up of 46 months, the disease-free survival was 91.6% and the overall survival 100%.

Ghezzi et al. performed a case–control study comparing laparoscopic staging of early ovarian cancer with conventional surgical staging via laparotomy; 15 patients undergoing laparoscopic staging were compared with 19 historical controls who have had conventional staging with open surgery. There were no significant differences between the two groups with regard to median number of lymph nodes and likelihood of identifying metastatic disease. No conversion to laparotomy and no intraoperative complication occurred in the laparoscopy group. Operative time was significantly longer in the laparoscopy group when compared with the laparotomy group (377 ± 47 vs. 272 ± 81 min, $P = 0.002$). One patient in the laparoscopy group had a retroperitoneal hematoma recognized in the postoperative period, and this required laparotomy. Minor postoperative complications occurred in one patient in the laparoscopy group and in eight patients in the laparotomy group ($P = 0.047$). Hospital stay was significantly shorter in the laparoscopy group (3 [2–12] vs. 7 [4–14] days, $P = 0.001$). The median follow-up was 16 (4–33) and 60 (32–108) months in the laparoscopy and laparotomy group, respectively. Eleven laparoscopically treated patients and 13 conventionally operated patients received adjuvant treatment. Even although the postoperative follow-up of the laparoscopy group is just 16 months and therefore hard to compare to historical controls, the authors suggest that laparoscopic surgical staging of early stage ovarian cancer is as safe and adequate as the standard surgical staging performed via laparotomy.[30]

An actual review article investigated the efficacy and safety of minimally invasive surgery for the treatment of early-stage epithelial ovarian cancer. 3,065 patients were included, 1,450 operated with laparoscopy and 1,615 with laparotomy, respectively. Survival outcome did not differ significantly between the two groups and pooled data suggested that the minimally invasive approach may be equivalent. However, the authors admit that the included studies contain a low level of evidence and further randomized trials are warranted.[32]

Thus, the Cochrane analysis published in 2008 remains valid: this analysis revealed that the value of laparoscopy to manage early stage ovarian cancer cannot be assessed to date. The standard for staging remains the laparotomy via midline incision, until randomized controlled trials have shown the similarity of both surgical techniques.[31]

The most recent analysis was published by Nezhat et al.[17] who compared surgical and survival outcome of 36 patients with early stage ovarian malignancies including 20 invasive epithelial tumors, 11 borderline tumors and five nonepithelial tumors. The mean number of pelvic nodes was 12.23 and of para-aortic nodes 14.84, respectively; 83% underwent a laparoscopic omentectomy; 7 patients had to be upstaged. Postoperative complications included one small bowel obstruction, two pelvic lymphoceles and one lymphocele cyst. Within the follow-up of 55.9 months, no recurrence occurred. The authors conclude the feasibility and safety of laparoscopic management when the operation is performed by a gynecologic oncologist experienced with advanced laparoscopy.[17]

Since several authors had described port site metastases after laparoscopic surgery of ovarian cancers[33-35] it has been questioned if tumor cell implants inside the abdominal wall may be more frequent in port sites after laparoscopy than in wound incisions after laparotomy. It has indeed been shown that the rate of port site metastases increases with tumor stage and amount of ascites. The overall rate is estimated between 0 and 2.3%.[17] Some authors suggest that CO_2 insufflation may damage the integrity of the peritoneum, thus inducing angiogenic effects (such as vascular epithelial growth factor (VEGF)) and attracting tumor cells to attach at the abdominal wall. In this regard, surgeons carefully closing the peritoneal incision and the abdominal wall did not recognize port site metastases.[17] In addition, an intraoperative paclitaxel treatment may reduce the ascites level of VEGF and subsequently the risk of port site metastases as shown in a nude mice model.[36] However, although there are controversial results of several studies, port site metastases have not been correlated with overall survival or progression-free survival.[25] It is self-evident that a careful handling of the specimen in an endo-bag preventing tumor cell spillage has highest priority. Zivanovic et al.[37] evaluated the rate of port-site tumor implantation after 2,251 laparoscopic procedures in women with malignant disease and concluded that it is low and almost always occurs in the setting of synchronous, advanced intraabdominal or distant metastatic disease. They confirmed the presence of port-site implantation as a surrogate for advanced disease and suggest that port site metastases should not be used as an argument against laparoscopic surgery in gynecologic malignancies.[36]

Advanced-Stage Invasive Tumors

There is an international consensus that advanced stage tumors should be treated with a midline laparotomy enabling a complete open staging procedure and tumor removal before adjuvant chemotherapy. If an advanced ovarian cancer is detected by chance during a laparoscopic operation, the surgeon should convert and complete the operation in an open fashion. If the setting does not allow a complete open staging operation, the laparoscopic operation should be terminated and the reoperation to complete the staging should follow within one week.

During the last years, several groups have used laparoscopy successfully to assess the feasibility to achieve an optimal or even a suboptimal debulking (tumor rest <1 cm). Rutten and coauthors[38] conclude from their randomized controlled trial that laparoscopy may reduce the number of futile laparotomies in patients with advanced-stage ovarian cancer.

With the increasing number of clinical trials applying preoperative neo-adjuvant chemotherapy, a staging laparoscopy becomes the method of choice to take ascites samples and tissue biopsies for histological confirmation of malignancy. If this type of systemic treatment will be performed routinely as it is for locally advanced breast cancer, primary laparoscopy might gain an impact for the management of metastasized and advanced ovarian cancer. Laparoscopy is then, however, preferable over open surgery because the neoadjuvant systemic treatment can be started earlier due to the small incisions. Apart from the treatment standard, several groups perform a laparoscopic staging operation following neoadjuvant chemotherapy. A retrospective cohort study comparing interval debulking after neoadjuvant chemotherapy included 3,071 patients, of whom 450 underwent laparoscopic surgery. This study revealed no significant difference between both groups regarding suboptimal debulking or survival.[39]

In addition, a diagnostic laparoscopy is indicated in case of a CUP syndrome (current unknown primary) where metastases are detected at extra-abdominal sites and the primary tumor is missing.[40]

INDICATION AND PREOPERATIVE WORKUP

If the diagnosis of a suspicious ovarian tumor is made via gynecologic investigation and transvaginal ultrasound, the question arises whether the operation should be performed laparoscopically or open. The following aspects may help to ease this decision:

Laparoscopy may be the preferred procedure, if:

- The diameter of the tumor is less than 5 cm.
- Unilateral or bilateral tumors are mobile and it is assumed that the tumor(s) can be removed without spilling.
- The tumor marker CA 125 is negative.
- There is no or little ascites.
- The tumor has been monitored for months without major change in size and morphology.
- A possible additional MRI or CT scan or PET-CT has not revealed a suspicion of malignancy and/or (lymph node or distant) metastases.
- A biopsy needs to be taken before neoadjuvant chemotherapy.
- The operation serves as a staging procedure in case of a CUP syndrome and
- An early stage borderline tumor is suspected or confirmed and the setting and knowledge of the

surgeon allows a complete staging operation for borderline tumors.

Laparotomy may be the preferred procedure, if:

- The tumor is highly suspicious to represent an invasive cancer and the tumor marker CA 125 is elevated more than 100 U/L.
- A high tumor burden is suspected.
- There is much ascites.
- The tumor/the cyst is greater than 5 cm.
- Peritoneal carcinosis is palpable (transabdominal, rectal) or seen in ultrasound, MRI, or CT scan.
- The tumor has grown rapidly and
- A borderline tumor has been histologically confirmed already, but the FIGO stage is advanced.

LAPAROSCOPIC PROCEDURES

The procedures to operate for ovarian malignancies include salpingo-oophorectomy (adnectomy), omentectomy, peritoneal washings and biopsies, hysterectomy, pelvic and para-aortic lymphadenectomy and, for mucinous tumor types, appendicectomy. The latter four procedures are omitted in this paragraph since they are described in additional chapters of this book.

Whenever an oncological entity is operated laparoscopically, the preparation and the stage for optimal surgical conditions have to be set. This includes a complete bowel preparation (3 L KleanPrep, peglec or similar). An epidural catheter is recommended, because (a) sympathicolysis keeps the bowel contracted and after Trendelenburg bedding the small bowel remains cephalad outside the pelvis, (b) the need of opiates intra- and postoperatively is less and therefore the risk of bowel constipation is reduced, (c) the use of analgesics postoperatively is less.

Salpingo-oophorectomy (Adnectomy)

Basically, the operation can be performed with three trocars: optic trocar subumbilical and two working trocars below the cephalad margin of the pubic hairs (in the line between superior iliac spine and symphysis and lateral from the epigastric artery which can be visualized with the laparoscope). We prefer the 10 mm telescope over the 5 mm telescope because it brings more light and a broader view and therefore a more comfortable situation to operate. The operation starts with the inspection of the whole abdominal cavity, including the liver, the stomach, the spleen (if visible), the omentum and all peritoneal surfaces, the diaphragm, the appendix and—finally and after bringing the patient in Trendelenburg position—the organs of the pelvis. Uterus, both ovaries and Fallopian tubes, the pouch of Douglas, and the bladder region have to be inspected. Besides malignant tissues one has to pay attention to endometriosis. It is important to keep in mind that in case of endometriosis the tumor marker CA125 can be mildly elevated (mostly up to 150 U/L) and that ovarian endometriosis is associated with endometrioid ovarian cancer! Aspiration of fluid from the pouch of Douglas has to be taken. It is best to aspirate the fluid with a blunt suction device. If there is no fluid, a peritoneal washing is performed with approximately 10–20 mL NaCl solution. Given that the surgeon and the scrub nurse both stand on the left side of the patient, the left trocar should be used to introduce the coagulation device and the scissors. It is easier for the nurse to change the instruments (e.g., bipolar coagulation device and scissors) through the left trocar, if she stands on the left side. The following description applies to a lift-side adnexectomy. In this setting, a blunt grasper will be introduced through the right trocar to pull the adnexa away from the left pelvic side wall. This is important, because pulling the adnexa from the side wall allows more distance from the ureter, which can normally be seen with peristalsis. In addition, this prepares the distance of several centimetres used to coagulate the IP (infundibulopelvic) ligament, which carries the ovarian artery. If it is impossible to properly see IP ligament and ureter, embryonic adhesions of the sigmoid colon need to be cut (at least partially) with scissors. Then, at least three coagulation steps next to each other should be taken for the IP ligament, because the ovarian vessels tend to bleed. The coagulation-cutting sequence is performed several times until the round ligament is reached. Then, the grasper pulls the adnexa cephalad and exposes the isthmic part of the fallopian tube as well as the ovarian ligament, which carries the ovarian branch of the uterine artery. These two structures are coagulated carefully and cut. The specimen is kept in the pouch of Douglas. The left 5 mm working trocar is replaced by a 10 mm working trocar and a retrieval bag (alternatively a bag made from a sterile glove) is introduced for the specimen. It is very important to avoid any spilling of the tumor! For a bigger specimen, it may be necessary to enlarge the skin incision with the knife and also the fascia and the peritoneum with the index finger. Do not pull too much since the bag may rupture! Also in case of a benign condition like a dermoid cyst spilling should be avoided. There are two options in this setting to remove the contralateral right adnexa: using the right trocar to introduce a grasper, which pulls the adnexa medial and keep the left trocar for coagulating and cutting. Or the left trocar is used to introduce the manipulating grasper and the right trocar is used for coagulating and cutting. Both options may reveal an optimal result. If the operation is finished, peritoneal tissue is closed with bipolar coagulation. This may reduce the risk of any port site metastasis in case of an invasive tumor. The fascia should be closed with a 0 vicryl suture. All other steps to finish the operation are according to the routinely performed procedures.

Omentectomy

While it is hardly possible to perform an infragastric omentectomy laparoscopically, it is feasible to perform an infracolic omentectomy. The indication for the latter type of operation is usually given for the operation of a borderline tumor of the ovary. For this operation, the surgeon needs two assistant surgeons: one camera person and one assisting surgeon. It is recommendable to use the same trocar placement as described by S. Puntambekar in the chapter "Oncologic Surgery on the Uterus." Nevertheless, there is some difference in the setting: the surgeon stands between the legs. The 10 mm working trocar in the lower abdomen is used for the telescope. If the working trocar is in the left lower abdomen, the surgeon uses the lower right and the paraumbilical left trocar to operate. The assistant surgeon uses subumbilical and right paraumbilical trocar to elevate transverse colon. Omentectomy is much easier if a vessel sealing device—either bipolar or ultrasound-based—is used. Then, the surgeon can use one hand to pull the omentum and one hand to coagulate and cut in one. It is easier to start the preparation in the medial section of the transverse colon and step by step separating the infracolic part of the omentum majus from the transverse colon to both sides. The coagulation must not be too close to the bowel wall to avoid thermal damage. When omentum is separated from the bowel, it should be brought to the pelvis. Then, the team rearranges according to standard setting. A retrieval bag is introduced as described in the previous paragraph. If hysterectomy is performed during the same operation, the specimen can be retrieved vaginally. If the uterus has been taken previously or a fertility-conserving operation of a borderline tumor is performed, retrieval should be performed as described in the section before.

Peritoneal Washings and Biopsies

Aspiration of peritoneal fluid, or peritoneal washings have to be taken from the pouch of Douglas at the beginning of the surgical procedure, for the reason that a later cyst rupture may falsify the cytologic result. Peritoneal biopsies should be taken from the paracolic abdominal wall, from the bladder peritoneum, from the ovarian fossa, and, if possible, from the lower part of the diaphragmal peritoneum. A grasper in one hand is used to pull the peritoneum and bipolar scissors or an ultrasound scalpel in the other hand is used to cut peritoneal biopsy. The camera has always to follow the specimen inside the grasper until the specimen is retrieved through trocar. Small bleeders of the peritoneal wound are coagulated bipolar.

COMPLICATIONS AND HANDLING

Cyst Rupture

Depending on the size and the strength of its capsule, potential adhesions and careful handling a cystic tumor may rupture. This needs to be avoided since tumor spilling may promote local tumor recurrence and may deteriorate the prognosis in case of invasive cancer. Therefore, rupture of cystic ovarian tumor should be avoided.

Bleeding

Different kinds of bleedings may complicate laparoscopic surgery. Epigastric artery may be damaged during trocar entry (especially when sharp trocars with blades to overwhelm fascia and abdominal wall are used). From intraabdominal, it is possible to visualize the inferior epigastric artery and therefore the lower trocars should be introduced under vision. Multiple arteries and veins of the abdominal wall may be damaged during trocar entry and during retrieval of the specimen. Therefore, trocars should be introduced under sight if diaphanoscopy reveals an area without blood vessels. The ovarian vessels (IP ligament and ovarian ligament) may bleed if cut without sufficient previous coagulation. A three-clamp technique—three coagulation steps adjacent to each other along the IP ligament—should be performed before cutting the ligament. Peritoneal vessels may bleed, if the patient's intraoperative blood pressure is too high. The anesthetist's attention need to be brought up to achieve an ideal blood pressure between RR 90/50 and RR 110/60. Omental vessels have a big diameter and tend to bleed, if they are not coagulated sufficiently. The omentum preparation should be performed slowly and with patience.

Accidental Detection of Invasive Cancer

If an invasive cancer is suspected or detected accidentally during a laparoscopic operation, a biopsy should be taken. If possible, an adnectomy can be performed. In addition, a peritoneal washing has to be taken. In any case, all movements should be performed with care to avoid any change of anatomy and to leave an almost virgin anatomical site for the open reoperation.

Accidental Detection of Deep-infiltrating Endometriosis

If a deep infiltrating endometriosis is found, the operation may be terminated. A detailed history has to be taken, the patient needs to be involved in the decision of a more advanced pelvic surgery, such as dissection of rectovaginal septum, pelvic deperitonealization or bowel resection. The preoperative evaluation for the laparoscopic reoperation includes rectoendosonography, sigmoidoscopy and bowel preparation before surgery. During surgery, an epidural catheter should be placed.

Bowel Perforation

This can occur during the abdominal entry (open or with Verress needle) in case of bowel adhesions due to previous surgeries or infections. If adhesions are suspected, the abdominal entry should be performed at Palmers point. A perforation can also occur when sharp graspers (which should be avoided) are used to move the bowel. If the anesthesia is not deep enough the patient may move and bring the bowel close to sharp instruments or coagulation devices. Therefore, the surgeon always needs to instruct the anesthetist how important his or her contribution to the operative anatomical site is.

Ureteric Lesions

Thermal damage to the ureter can occur during coagulation of the IP ligaments. The ureter needs to be seen before coagulating and cutting the ovarian vessels, because these structures are closely related to each other. If the ureter needs to be identified, one should remember that the ureter crosses the common iliac artery at the level of the sacral promontory. On the left side, it may be necessary to first remove the embryonic adhesions between sigmoid colon and pelvic side wall before the ureter can be identified. Furthermore, ureter may be damaged when adherent to an endometriotic lesion in the ovarian fossa. It needs to be identified and carefully distended before coagulating and cutting of any adjacent tissue.

Wound Infection

The same standards of disinfection and rules of sterility as used for open surgery have to be followed. Generally, the umbilicus needs to be washed and disinfected carefully. In obese patients, diabetes patients and patients with a suppressed immune system as well as in case of long surgeries (more than one hour) a single-shot antibiosis should be applied to prevent a wound infection.

TIPS AND TRICKS OF THE TRADE

- Use a retrieval bag! The bag has to be big enough for the specimen. If commercially available bags cannot be afforded, a sterile glove can be used as a bag. It may help to cut the glove and/or knot the tip of the bag with a suture. Never pull the bag too much because it may rupture. Rather enlarge the abdominal incision. If the specimen is big and difficult to place in the bag: use a third working trocar; one grasper may hold the specimen close to the lower abdominal wall while the two remaining graspers impose the bag on the specimen from dorsal to ventral.
- Save the ureter. Always identify the ureter when working on the adnexas. If an adnexal mass is big, use a retroperitoneal approach: open the retroperitoneal space, identify and separate the ureter from the ovary and then remove the adnexal mass via bipolar coagulation and dissection. If a thermal damage of the ureter is suspected, ask the urologist to put a DJ stent prophylactically, which may remain for 3–6 weeks. If a perforation with leakage is suspected, use intravenous Methylene Blue dye to identify any lesion. Then ask the urologist to help you managing the lesion. It may be sufficient to just put a DJ stent for a period of several weeks.
- Save the bladder! It may be difficult to always find the right plane for an adnexectomy if a hysterectomy was performed in a previous operation.

The difficulty lies in the lack of clear anatomical structures (e.g. ovarian ligament and isthmic part of the Fallopian tube). A manipulation of vagina with a swab pushed cephalad may ease to identify vagina and bladder. If a bladder perforation is suspected, the bladder should be filled with 200–300 mL NaCl solution dyed with Methylene Blue. A simple bladder leakage can be sutured in two layers endoscopically:3.0 vicryl running suture for the mucosal tissue and 2.0 vicryl interrupted sutures for the muscular tissue.

- Save the rectum! If a rectum perforation is suspected, air should be insufflated from the anal canal while NaCl solution is inside the pelvis. Air bubbles may confirm a rectum perforation. Then, you should ask the general surgeon to help you to manage the bowel complication.
- How to handle obese patients? Ask an experienced anesthetist to take care of the patient during the operation, since you will need good relaxation and Trendelenburg position. An epidural catheter should be placed. An intense bowel preparation (e.g., 3 L of solution) should be given the day before. The lower trocars should be placed a bit higher up (McBurneys point and opposite) to prevent the surgeon from fighting the abdominal wall when moving the instruments. Perform slow and very exact movements with the endoscopic instruments, since the space to perform the operation is limited!

SUMMARY

Laparoscopic management of gynecologic cancers has been discussed controversially for decades. Much progress has been achieved technically enabling an experienced endoscopic surgeon to perform most of the gynecologic oncologic procedures such as bilateral salpingo-oophorectomy, hysterectomy, radical hysterectomy, pelvic and para-aortic lymph node dissection, omentectomy, anterior, posterior, and total pelvic exenteration.

Although the value of laparoscopy with respect to oncological safety and patient's outcome has not been shown in prospective randomized clinical trials conclusively, many studies with altogether thousands of patients have revealed the feasibility and also similar oncologic results of laparoscopy when compared to laparotomy. In addition, when compared to open surgery, laparoscopy in oncology has been shown to be associated with a shorter hospital stay, less blood loss, less short-time morbidity and a faster return to work. Therefore, laparoscopic approach has become well accepted for certain oncological indications, especially when early stage cancer cases are treated.

REFERENCES

1. Zoeckler SJ, Hegstrom GJ. Peritoneoscopy in malignant lesions of the abdomen. J Am Med Assoc. 1953;152(17):1617-8.
2. Miniconi P, Salasc J, et al. [Value of laparoscopy in the diagnosis of peritoneal carcinosis.]. Alger Medicale. 1960;64:809-10.
3. Lacey, CG, Morrow CP, Disaia PJ, et al. Laparoscopy in the evaluation of gynecologic cancer. Obstet Gynecol. 1978;52(6):708-12.
4. Canis M, Mage G, Wattiez A, et al. [Does endoscopic surgery have a role in radical surgery of cancer of the cervix uteri?]. J Gynecol Obstet Biol Reprod (Paris). 1990;19(7):921.
5. Canis M, Mage G, Wattiez A, et al. The role of laparoscopic surgery in gynecologic oncology. Curr Opin Obstet Gynecol. 1994;6(3):210-4.
6. Canis M, Farina M, Jardon K, et al. [Laparoscopy and gynecologic cancer in 2005]. J Gynecol Obstet Biol Reprod (Paris). 2006;35(2):117-35.
7. Querleu D. Laparoscopic paraaortic node sampling in gynecologic oncology: a preliminary experience. Gynecol Oncol. 1993;49(1):24-9.
8. Querleu D. Laparoscopic radical hysterectomy. Am J Obstet Gynecol. 1993;168(5):1643-5.
9. Nezhat C, Nezhat F, Burrell MO, et al. Laparoscopic radical hysterectomy with paraaortic and pelvic node dissection. Am J Obstet Gynecol. 1994;170(2):699.
10. Nezhat C, Nezhat F, Teng NN, et al. The role of laparoscopy in the management of gynecologic malignancy. Semin Surg Oncol. 1994;10(6):431-9.
11. Pomel C, Canis M, Mage, G, et al. [Laparoscopically extended hysterectomy for cervix cancer: technique, indications and results. Apropos of a series of 41 cases in Clermont]. Chirurgie. 1997;122(2):133-6; discussion 136-7.
12. Possover M, Krause N, Künhe-Heid R, et al. Value of laparoscopic evaluation of paraaortic and pelvic lymph nodes for treatment of cervical cancer. Am J Obstet Gynecol. 1998;178(4):806-10.
13. Possover, M, Krause N, Plaul K, et al. Laparoscopic para-aortic and pelvic lymphadenectomy: experience with 150 patients and review of the literature. Gynecol Oncol. 1998;71(1):19-28.
14. Altgassen C, Possover M, Krause N, et al. Establishing a new technique of laparoscopic pelvic and para-aortic lymphadenectomy. Obstet Gynecol. 2000;95(3): 348-52.
15. Puntambekar SP, Palep RJ, Puntambekar SS, et al. Laparoscopic total radical hysterectomy by the Pune technique: our experience of 248 cases. J Minim Invasive Gynecol. 2007;14(6):682-9.

16. Nezhat F, Yadav J, Rahaman J, et al. Analysis of survival after laparoscopic management of endometrial cancer. J Minim Invasive Gynecol. 2008;5(2):181-7.
17. Nezhat FR, Ezzati M, Chuang L, et al. Laparoscopic management of early ovarian and fallopian tube cancers: surgical and survival outcome. Am J Obstet Gynecol. 2009;200(1):83.e1-6.
18. Mettler L, Meinhold-Heerlein I. The value of laparoscopic surgery to stage gynecological cancers: present and future. Minerva Ginecol. 2009;61(4): 319-37.
19. Kurman RJ, Shih IeM. Molecular pathogenesis and extraovarian origin of epithelial ovarian cancer—shifting the paradigm. Hum Pathol. 2011;42(7): 918-31.
20. Domchek SM, Rebbeck TR. Prophylactic oophorectomy in women at increased cancer risk. Curr Opin Obstet Gynecol. 2007;19(1):27-30.
21. Querleu D, Papageorgiou T, Lambaudie E, et al. Laparoscopic restaging of borderline ovarian tumours: results of 30 cases initially presumed as stage IA borderline ovarian tumours. BJOG. 2003;110(2): 201-4.
22. Camatte S, Morice P, Thoury A, et al. Impact of surgical staging in patients with macroscopic stage I ovarian borderline tumours: analysis of a continuous series of 101 cases. Eur J Cancer. 2004;40(12):1842-9.
23. Tozzi, R., C. Kohler, Ferrara A, et al. Laparoscopic treatment of early ovarian cancer:surgical and survival outcomes. Gynecol Oncol. 2004;93(1):199-203.
24. Vaisbuch E, Dgani R, Ben-Arie A, et al. The role of laparoscopy in ovarian tumors of low malignant potential and early-stage ovarian cancer. Obstet Gynecol Surv. 2005;60(5):326-30.
25. Schlaerth AC, Abu-Rustum NR. Role of minimally invasive surgery in gynecologic cancers. Oncologist. 2006;11(8):895-901.
26. Lee CL, Kay N, Chen HL, et al. The roles of laparoscopy in treating ovarian cancer. Taiwan J Obstet Gynecol. 2009;48(1):9-14.
27. Trillsch F, Mahner S, Ruetzel J et al. Clinical management of borderline ovarian tumors. Expert Rev Anticancer Ther. 2010;10(7):1115-24.
28. du Bois A, Ewald-Riegler N, de Gregorio N, et al. Borderline tumours of the ovary: a cohort study of the Arbeitsgemeinschaft Gynäkologische Onkologie (AGO) Study Group. Eur J Cancer. 2013;49(8):1905-14.
29. Hua KQ, Jin FM, Xu H, et al. (2005). [Evaluation of laparoscopic surgery in the early stage-malignant tumor of ovary with lower risk.]. Zhonghua Yi Xue Za Zhi. 2005;85(3):169-72.
30. Ghezzi F, Cromi A, et al. Laparoscopy versus laparotomy for the surgical management of apparent early stage ovarian cancer. Gynecol Oncol. 2007;105(2): 409-13.
31. Medeiros LR, Rosa DD, Bozzetti MC, et al. Laparoscopy versus laparotomy for FIGO stage I ovarian cancer. Cochrane Database Syst Rev 2008;(4):CD005344.
32. Bogani G, Borghi C, Leone Roberti Maggiore U, et al. Minimally invasive surgical staging in early-stage ovarian carcinoma: a systematic review and meta-analysis. J Minim Invasive Gynecol. 2017;24(4): 552-62.
33. Martinez J, Targarona EM, Balagué C, et al. Port site metastasis. An unresolved problem in laparoscopic surgery. A review. Int Surg. 1995;80(4):315-21.
34. Nagarsheth NP, Rahaman J, Cohen CJ, et al. The incidence of port-site metastases in gynecologic cancers. JSLS. 2004;8(2):133-9.
35. Ramirez, PT, Frumovitz M, Wolf JK, et al. Laparoscopic port-site metastases in patients with gynecological malignancies. Int J Gynecol Cancer. 2004;14(6): 1070-7.
36. Yen CF, Lee CL, Murk W, et al. Reducing peritoneal vascular endothelial growth factor concentration and inhibiting cancer scattering in a mouse model of laparoscopy. Am J Obstet Gynecol. 2008;198(4): 423.e1-7.
37. Zivanovic O, Sonoda Y, Diaz JP, et al. The rate of port-site metastases after 2251 laparoscopic procedures in women with underlying malignant disease. Gynecol Oncol. 2008;111(3):431-7.
38. Rutten MJ, van Meurs HS, van de Vrie R, et al. Laparoscopy to predict the result of primary cytoreductive surgery in patients with advanced ovarian cancer: a randomized controlled trial. J Clin Oncol. 2017;35(6): 613-21.
39. Melamed A, Nitecki R, Boruta DM 2nd et al. Laparoscopy compared with laparotomy for debulking ovarian cancer after neoadjuvant chemotherapy. Obstet Gynecol. 2017;129(5):861-9.
40. Gultekin M, Diribas K, Buru E, et al. Interval debulking in epithelial ovarian carcinomas: the past, present and the future. Eur J Gynaecol Oncol. 2008;29(3): 242-5.

KIEL SCHOOL

44 of Gynaecological Endoscopy

Oncologic Surgery on the Uterus

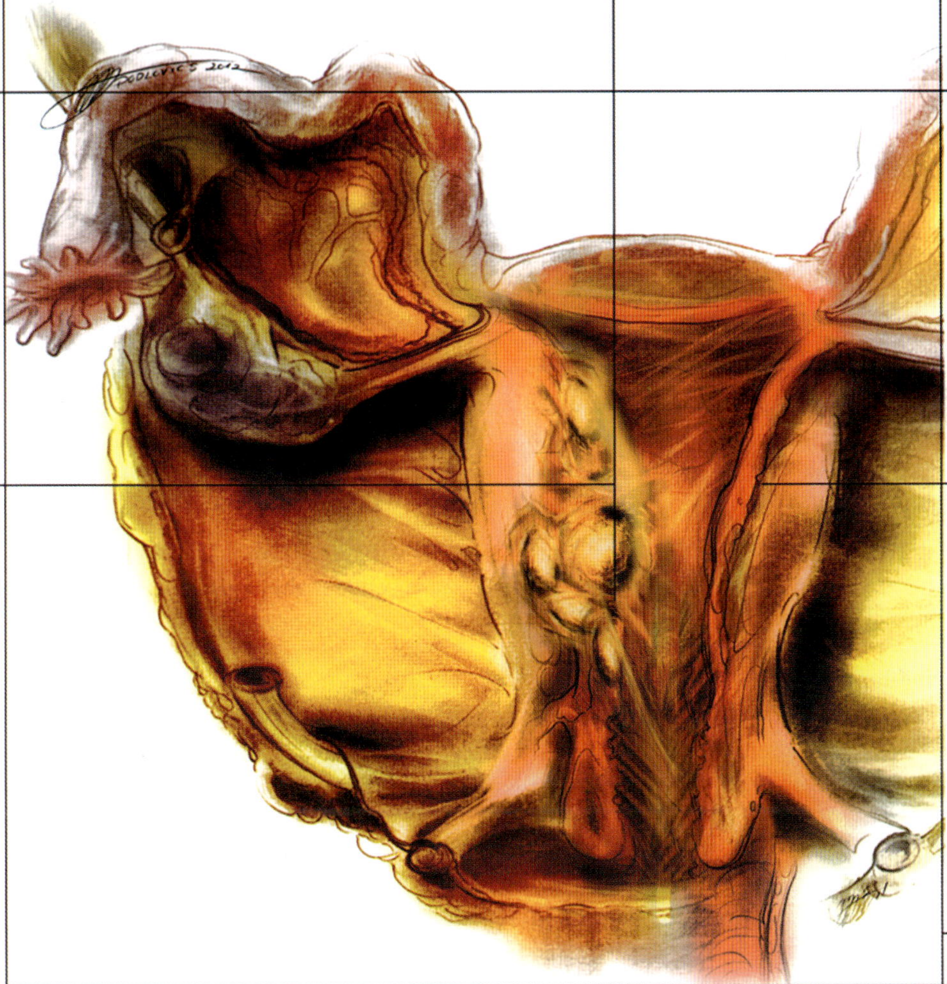

Chapter 44

Oncologic Surgery on the Uterus

Shailesh Puntambekar, Seema Puntambekar, RM Sathe, Sambit Nanda, Raviraj Tiruke, Tejashree Bakre, Meenakshi Chate, Aishwarya Puntambekar

INTRODUCTION[1,2]

Uterine malignancies are the second most common cause of cancer death in women worldwide. Its incidence appears to have risen in recent years because of increasing awareness and screening. The gold standard treatment of uterine cancer is radical hysterectomy. Since the first radical hysterectomy performed by Clark in 1895 and the advent of Wertheim's technique of radical hysterectomy in 1898, radical hysterectomy has evolved into a simpler procedure and the surgical approach has also transformed over a period of time into a highly specialized and minimally invasive modality. With technological advances, we can now perform the radical hysterectomy with minimally invasive techniques, such as laparoscopy and robotics. The mainstay of these procedures are less post-operative pain, an early recovery of the patient due to smaller incisions, allowing the patient to take up adjuvant treatment as early as possible and overall a good quality of life of the patient. Thus the acceptance of minimally access surgeries in recent years has increased.

In this chapter, the "Pune technique" of laparoscopic radical hysterectomy is described by the authors with operative steps that are standardized. This makes this technique universally acceptable as it is easily duplicable. Its application in robotic radical hysterectomy, pelvic exenterations and single-port surgeries are also covered.

LAPAROSCOPIC RADICAL HYSTERECTOMY[3-9,13]

Indications

1. Cervical cancers stage 1A2 to stage 2A. Cases of stage 1A1 with a high risk for lymph node spread are also included in the group.
2. Endometrial cancer up to stage 2

Preoperative irradiation is not a contra-indication for the laparoscopic procedure.

Contraindications

1. Tumor size of more than 4 cm at the largest diameter.
2. Evidence of peritoneal carcinomatosis or distant metastatic disease.
3. Evidence of grossly involved lymph nodes.

Preoperative

- Liquid diet one day prior to surgery.
- Polyethylene glycol the night before the operation to clear the bowels so as to keep them away from the operative field.
- Enema and bowel wash should be avoided as this leads to dilatation of sigmoid colon.

Anesthesia

A combined regional and general anesthesia is administered. Regional anesthesia, by blocking the sympathetic activity, contracts the small bowel and keeps it away from the operative field.

Patient Position

Patient is placed in a modified Lloyd Davis position. A bolster is placed at the level of the anterior superior iliac spine, which causes elevation of the pelvis and results in a drop of the intestines cephalad. A gauze piece is kept in the vagina to prevent loss of pneumoperitoneum after colpotomy.

Port Positions (Fig. 44.1)

A total of five ports are used.

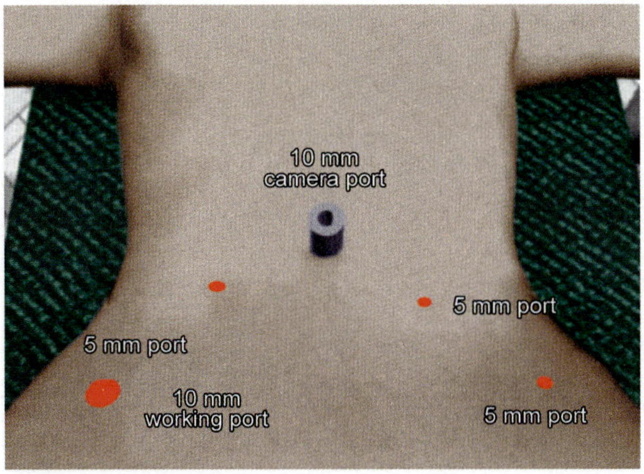

Fig. 44.1: Port positions.

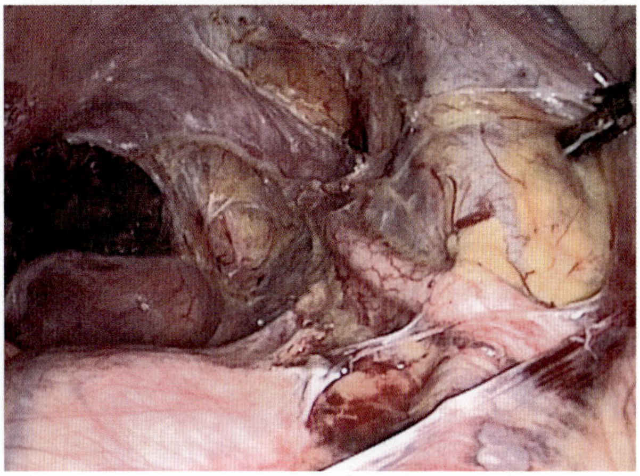

Fig. 44.3: Right ureter crossing the bifurcation of the common iliac at the level of the sacral promontory.

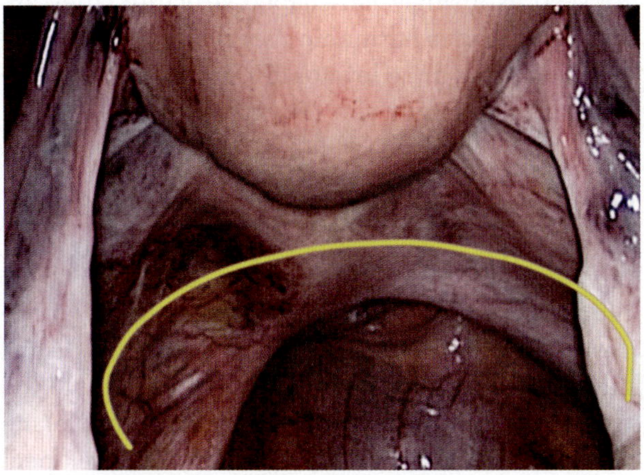

Fig. 44.2: Posterior "U Cut."

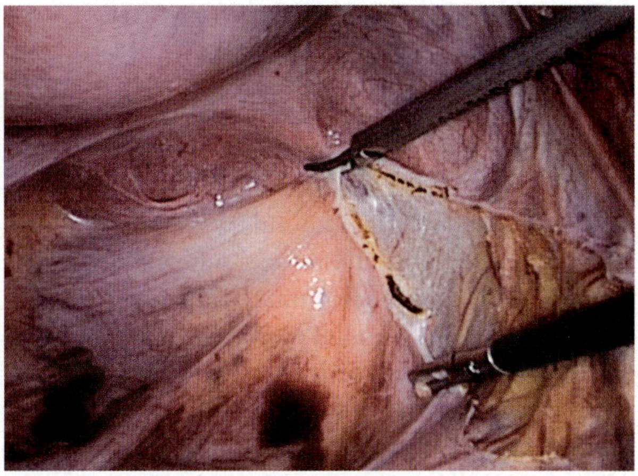

Fig. 44.4: Posterior cut extended toward the Pouch of Douglas.

- A 10 mm camera port at the umbilicus
- A 10 mm working port at the McBurney's point on the right side
- A 5 mm port pararectally at the midclavicular line at the level of the umbilicus
- A set of two 5 mm ports are inserted as a mirror image on the left side.

Procedure

The uterus is hitched in cases of endometrial malignancy. In cases of cervical malignancies a myoma screw is used and it is introduced from the upper left port and inserted into the fundus for uterine manipulation.

Step 1: Posterior U Cut (Fig. 44.2)

Uterus is anteverted. The right ureter is identified underneath the peritoneum at the level of sacral promontory. The peritoneum over it is excised with the help of harmonic shears to expose the ureter. This cut is extended down up to the pouch of Douglas keeping the ureters laterally and constantly under vision. The same steps are repeated on the left side and both the peritoneal cuts joined in the POD forming the posterior U cut (Figs. 44.3 and 44.4).

Step 2: Dissection of Rectovaginal Space (Figs. 44.5 and 44.6)

The peritoneum in the pouch of Douglas is pulled cephalad and incised with the help of harmonic shears. The dissection is carried out between the two layers of Denon Villiers fascia (Fig. 44.6). The plane between the fat and the posterior vaginal wall is dissected keeping in mind the dictum "fat belongs to the rectum,"(Fig. 44.5).

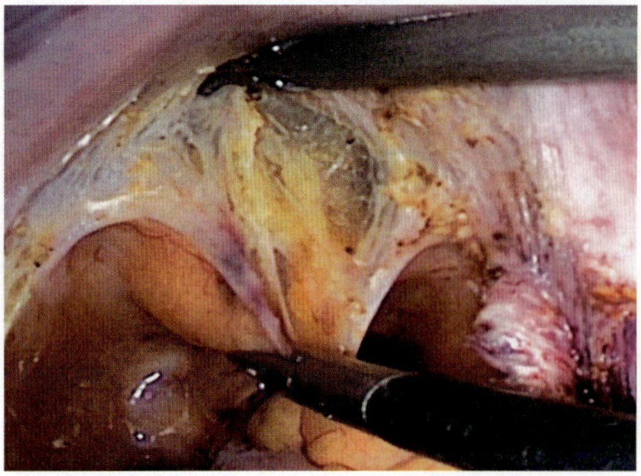

Fig. 44.5: Dissection in POD. Fat belongs to the rectum. Right plane and wrong plane.

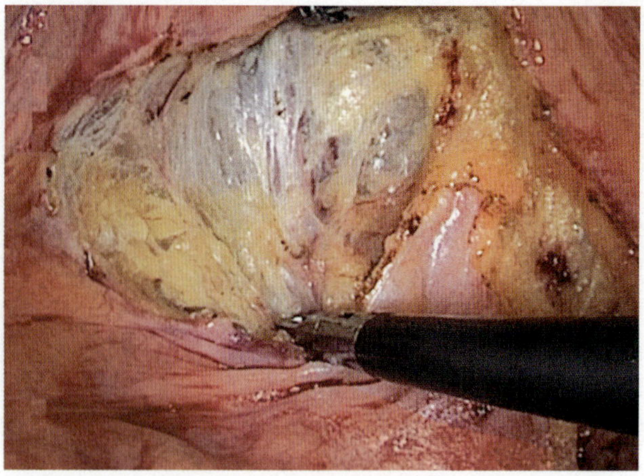

Fig. 44.6: Dissection in the POD. Two layers of the Denon Villers' fascia.

Step 3: Dissection of the Pararectal Space (Fig. 44.7)

The left ureter is retracted medially and the posterior leaf of broad ligament above the ureter is cut. The cut is extended downward toward the bladder. The ureter forms the medial boundary of the pararectal space and the internal iliac artery forms the lateral boundary. The ureter is retracted medially and the dissection is done parallel to the ureter to open the pararectal space. The uterine artery crosses the pararectal space transversely. The space anterior to the uterine artery and medial to the obliterated hypogastric artery is dissected. This dissection is continued to the paravesical space up to the levator ani. The uterine vein is seen below the artery. Both the artery and the vein are individually clipped or ligated and then cut. The ureter is retracted medially to expose the uteroscaral and Mackenrodt's ligaments, which are seen as a single fan-shaped structure. They are then cut with the harmonic shears in the downward direction toward the levator ani. The same steps are repeated on the right side (Fig. 44.8).

Step 4: Anterior U Cut (Figs. 44.9 and 44.10)

The uterus is retroverted. The peritoneum over the uterovesical fold is cut using the harmonic shears, starting from the round ligament on one side to the other, forming the anterior U cut. The fascial plane between the bladder and the uterus is developed, keeping in mind the dictum "fat belongs to bladder." The peritoneal cut is further extended up to the infundibulopelvic ligaments. A cut is made in the broad ligament and the ureter can now be seen through this broad ligament window.

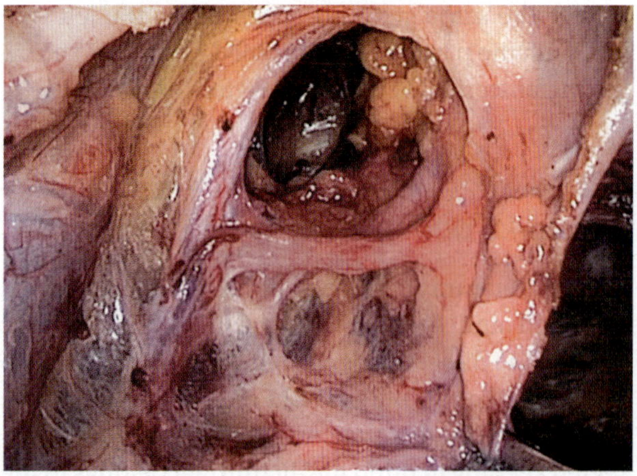

Fig. 44.7: Left pararectal space. Uterine artery and vein.

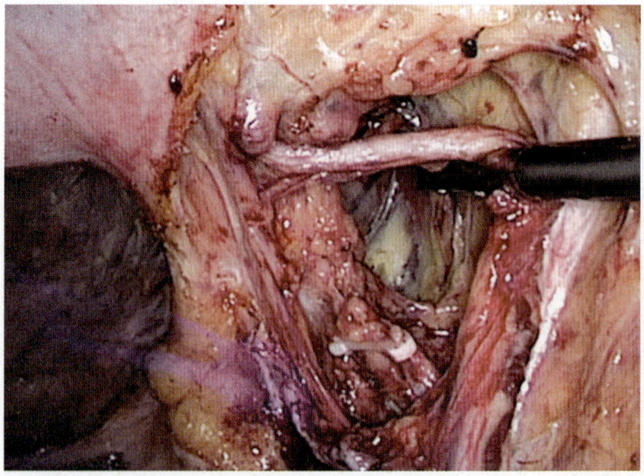

Fig. 44.8: Right cardinal ligaments seen as single fan-shaped structure.

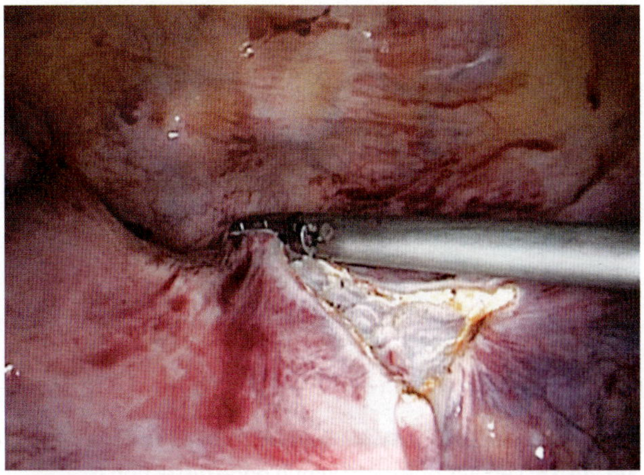

Fig. 44.9: Anterior U cut.

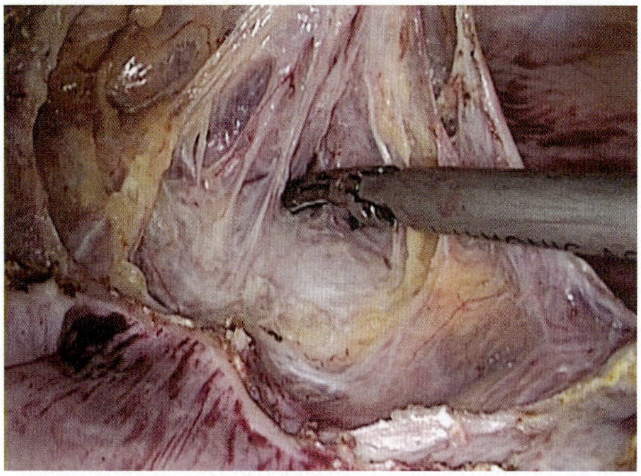

Fig. 44.10: Anterior U cut. Dissection up to the bladder pillar.

Step 5: Dissection of Ureteric Tunnel (Fig. 44.11)

The uterus is pulled to the right. The left ureter is traced along its entire course toward the bladder. The bladder peritoneum is held and the bladder is retracted upward. Thus the uretic tunnel is exposed. This tunnel is dissected with the help of Maryland's forceps. There are two veins in the roof of the tunnel, which can be clipped and then cut. This helps in pushing the ureter further laterally. The ureter can be seen as it enters the bladder at the uterovesical junction. The bladder is pushed further down to achieve a good vaginal cuff, below the growth. The paracolpos is then cut as laterally as possible. These steps ensure that we can obtain maximum amount of paracolpos and the vaginal margin. The same steps are repeated on the right side making the trigonal area visible. Colpotomy is done above this level with the help of harmonic shears (Figs. 44.12 and 44.13).

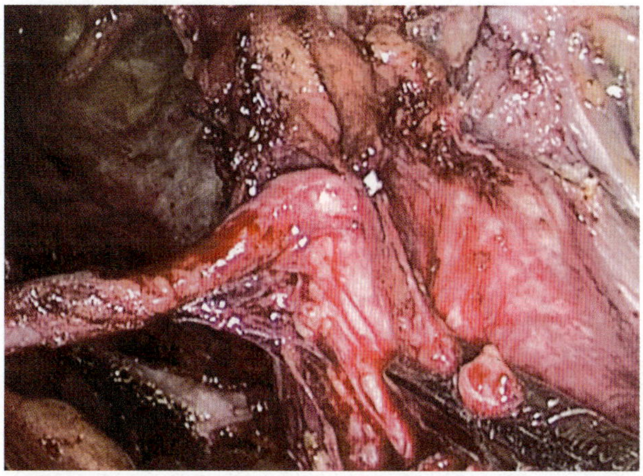

Fig. 44.11: Left ureteric tunnel dissection.

The infundibulopelvic ligaments are then cut and the entire specimen is separated and placed in an endobag (Fig. 44.15).

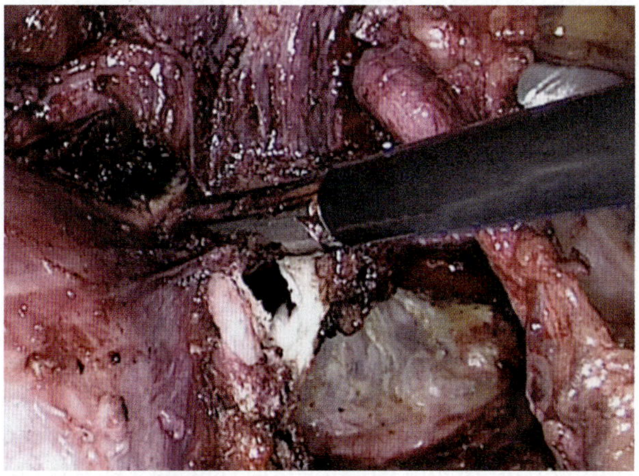

Fig. 44.12: Colpotomy.

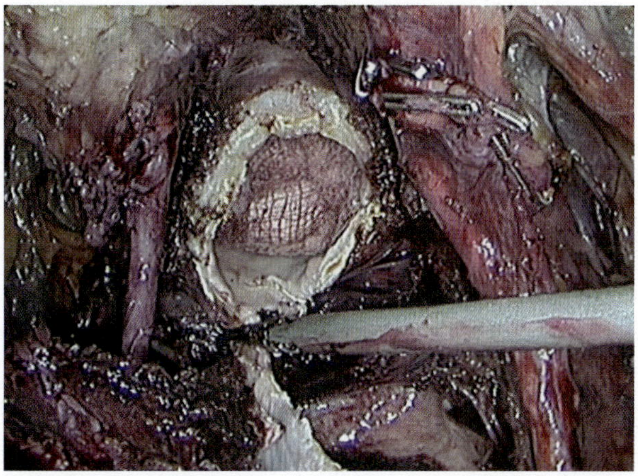

Fig. 44.13: Completed colpotomy.

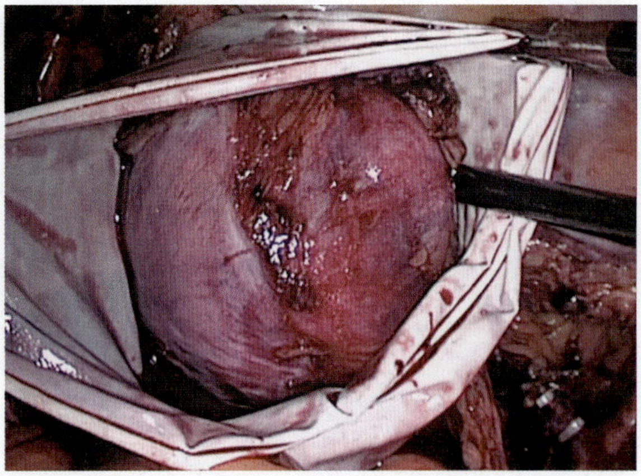

Fig. 44.14: Specimen put in an endobag.

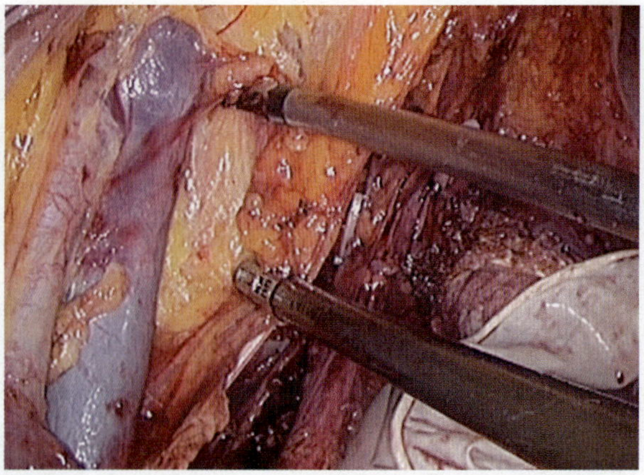

Fig. 44.15: Left ilio-obturator lymph node dissection.

Step 6: Lymph Node Dissection (Fig. 44.14)

Lymph node dissection is started at the bifurcation of the common iliac artery. The dissection is done with the help of suction cannula as it is relatively atraumatic. No energy source is used here. All the fibro fatty tissue along the external iliac vein is dissected, sweeping the cannula in a direction parallel to the vessels up to the iliac bone, which forms the lateral limit of the dissection. The medial limit is formed by the internal iliac artery and the lower limit is the obturator nerve. Similar dissection is done on both the sides (Fig. 44.16). The entire nodal tissue obtained is put in the endobag.

The endobag is removed vaginally. Hemostasis is achieved. The wound is irrigated with normal saline. The vault is closed with continuous locking intracorporeal suturing with vicryl 2-0, which is introduced through the 10 mm working port (Fig. 44.17). It is not necessary to use any intra-abdominal drain. The ports are removed under vision and the port sites closed.

The Specimen: This technique achieves a Pivers type III radical hysterectomy (TYPE C2 QUERLOW AND MOORE) with a paracervical clearance of more than 3cm, a distal vaginal margin of more than 2.5–3 cm and a nodal yield of at least 18–20 nodes (Fig. 44.18).

Complications

- Hemorrhage
- Bladder injury
- Ureteric injury
- Bowel injury
- Fistulas

LAPAROSCOPIC NERVE-SPARING RADICAL HYSTERECTOMY (Figs. 44.19 to 44.22)

The main disadvantage of laparoscopic radical hysterectomy is the bladder dysfunction. This is caused due to autonomic nerve disruption with loss of anatomical bladder neck support and over distension of

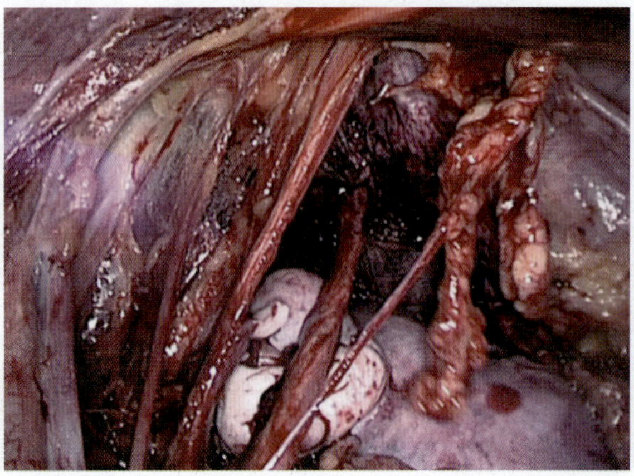

Fig. 44.16: Completed left ilio-obturator lymph node dissection.

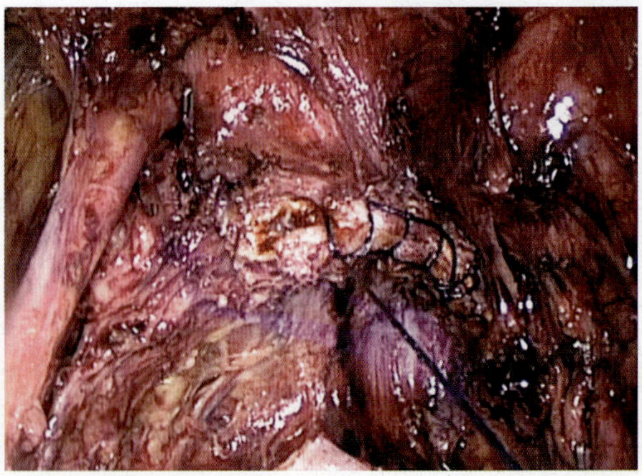

Fig. 44.17: Intracorporeal vault closure.

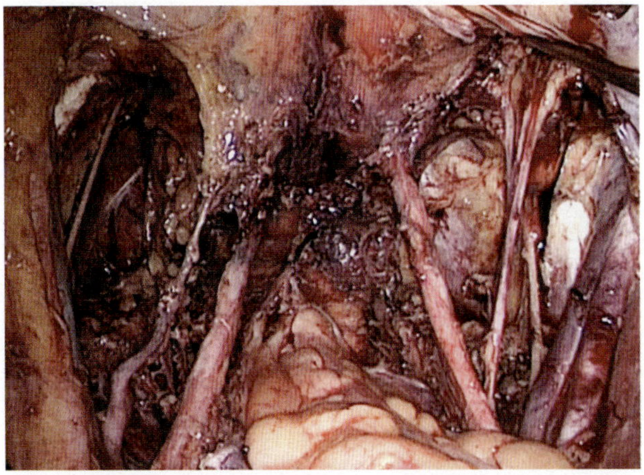

Fig. 44.18: Road map after completion of dissection.

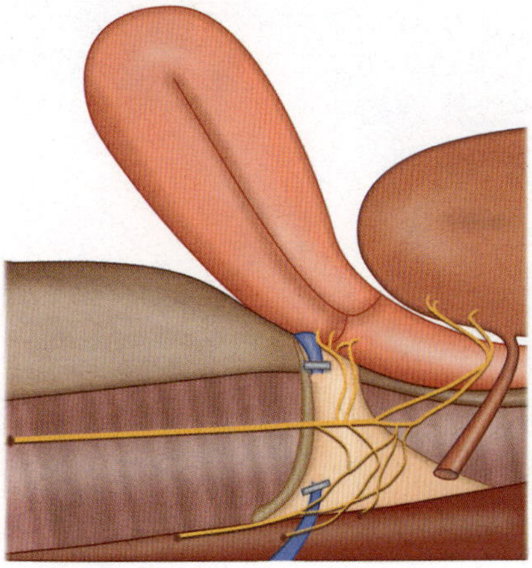

Fig. 44.19: Pelvic nerves schematic diagram.

the bladder. A nerve-sparing radical hysterectomy involves the preservation of the superior and inferior hypogastric and the pelvic splanchnic plexus, thus overcoming the complication of bladder dysfunction.

The procedure is similar to laparoscopic radical hysterectomy. The hypogastric plexus lies lateral to the uterosacral ligaments (Fig. 44.20). Thus the dissection at the level of uterosacrals is done carefully. The nerves are identified lateral to the uterosacrals and medial to the ureter. The branches of the hypogastric nerve going to the uterus are identified in the connective tissue just posterolateral to the vagina and these branches are selectively cut and the nerve plane is lateralized on the posterior side. The bladder branch of the inferior hypogastric plexus is spared by lateralizing the nerve plane and the ureter. The posterior leaf of the vesicouterine ligament contains vesical veins that drain into the deep uterine veins, which are individually clipped and cut. The bladder branch that passes just below the inferior vesical vein is also spared. The uterine and cervical branches of the inferior hypogastric plexus in the anterior part are also selectively cut. During colpotomy the nerve is lateral to ureter whereas in the initial stages of the dissection the hypogastric nerve and inferior hypogastric plexus were anatomically posteromedial to the ureter. The rest of the procedure is completed in the same way as the laparoscopic radical hysterectomy explained earlier.[10, 12, 15, 20]

Postoperatively the Foley catheter is removed after 48 hours. If urinary retention occurs, Foley catheterization is done again and patient is reassessed every 7 days.

ANTERIOR EXENTERATION (Figs. 44.24 to 44.40)[14, 22]

Currently it is offered as a curative procedure in patients with primary cancer who present in an advanced stage disease with or without

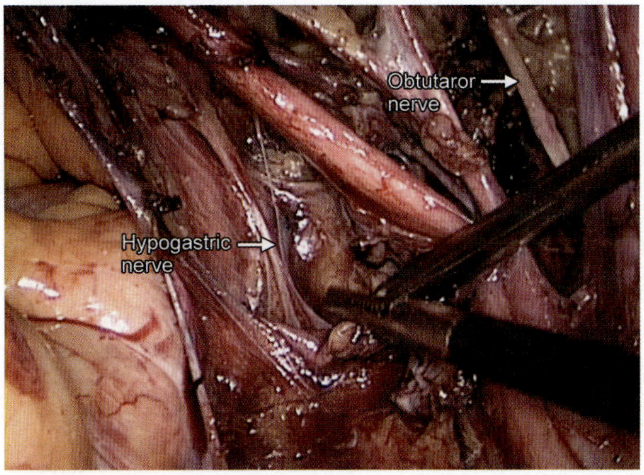

Fig. 44.20: Hypogastric nerve plexus.

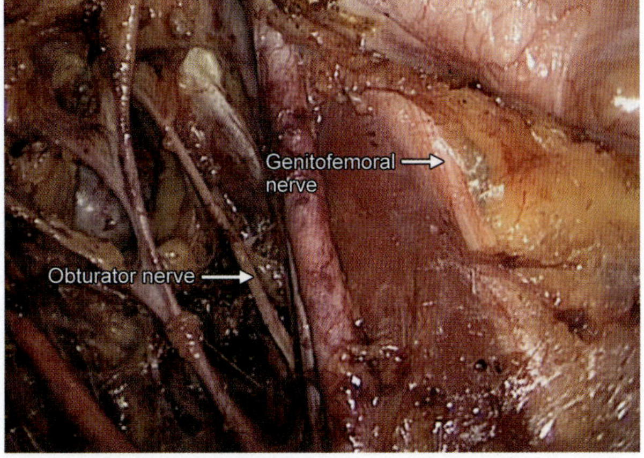

Fig. 44. 21: Pelvic nerves.

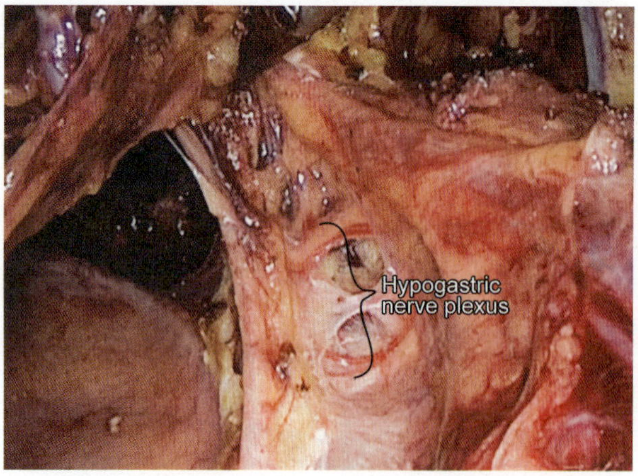

Fig. 44.22: Hypogastric nerve plexus.

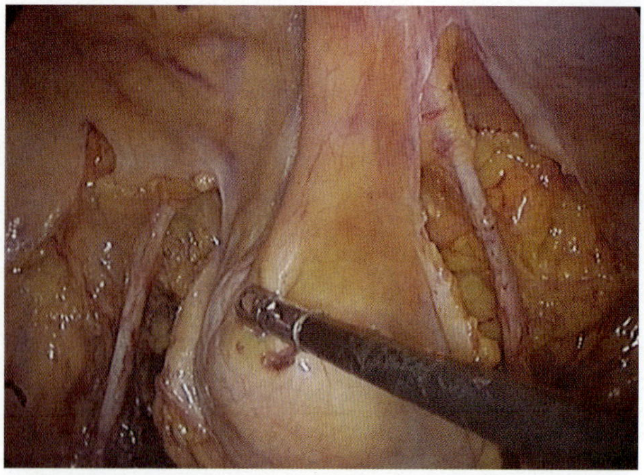

Fig. 44.23: Bladder is dissected down from the anterior abdominal wall to enter the Cave of Retzius.

complications. It was initially considered a palliative procedure but there have been reports of 5-year survival rates in the range of 40–60% of the patients. The advantages of laparoscopy in exenterations are minimal blood loss, a quick recovery, less postoperative pain, a lower rate of adhesion formation and early application of adjuvant chemoradiation following laparoscopy as there is no incision.

The anterior exenteration involves removal of bladder, lower ureters, perivesical stump, uterus, ovaries and lymph nodes up to the pelvic brim.

Patient selection is important before offering such an extensive and morbid surgery as a treatment modality. The following criteria should be used to decide the operability.

- Histological documentation of cancer in the palpable mass.
- Absence of tumor extension to parametrium or pelvic sidewalls.
- No involvement of the rectum by the growth.
- Absence of gross pelvic or para aortic lymph node enlargement.
- No peritoneal implants or bowel involvement.
- No evidence of distant metastasis.

Absolute contra indications for surgery are as follows:

- Unilateral or bilateral pedal edema.
- Sciatica or bone pain.
- Poor medical condition.

Preoperative investigations, such as a thorough general examination, examination under anesthesia (EUA) and cystoscopy, a CT scan or MRI, and ultrasound help to decide the operability of the patient.

Anesthesia, patient position and port position are the same as in laparoscopic radical hysterectomy.

Step 1: The uterus is manipulated with the help of a myoma screw. The right ureter is identified under the peritoneum at the level of the sacral promontory and the peritoneum over it is incised with the harmonic shears.

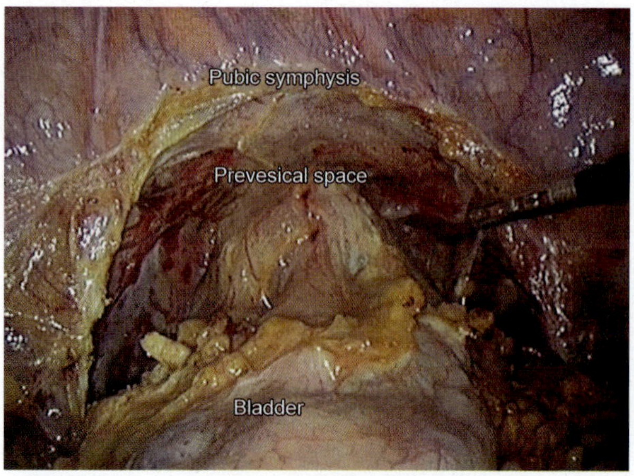

Fig. 44.24: Prevesical space or the Cave of Retzius.

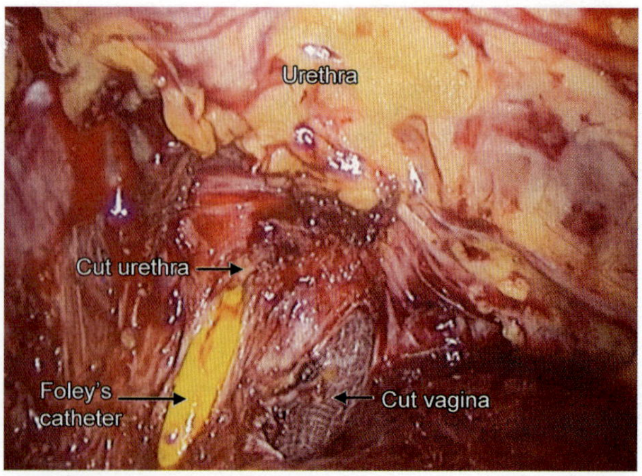

Fig. 44.25: Urethra being cut.

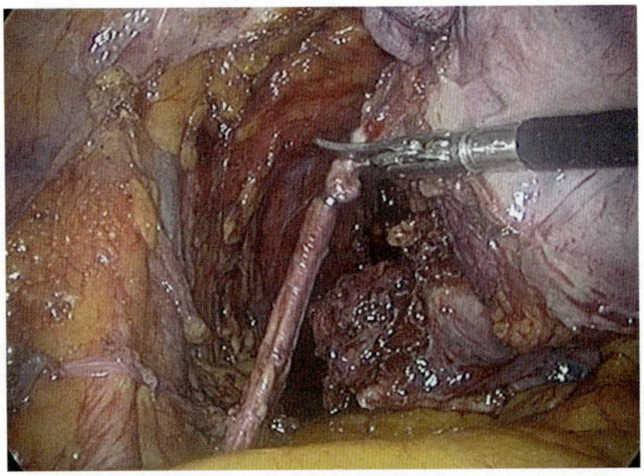

Fig. 44.26: Left ureter being clipped and cut.

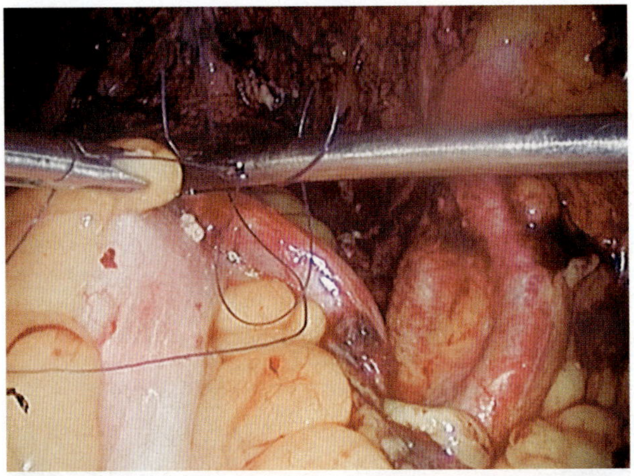

Fig. 44.27: Transfix the right ureter to the sigmoid colon anteriorly.

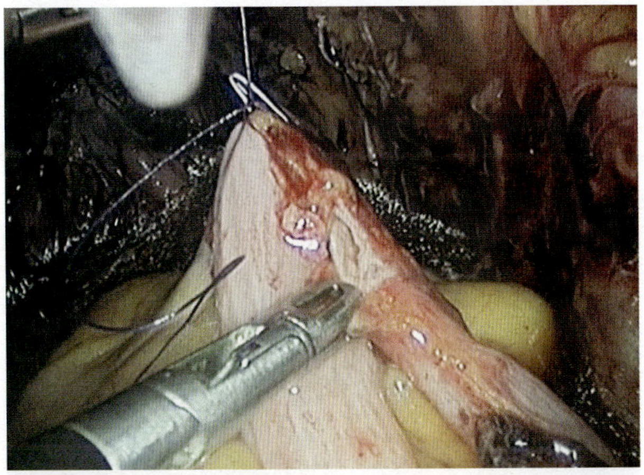

Fig. 44.28: Cut is made on the ureter and shaped into a fish mouth. The assistant holds up the suture.

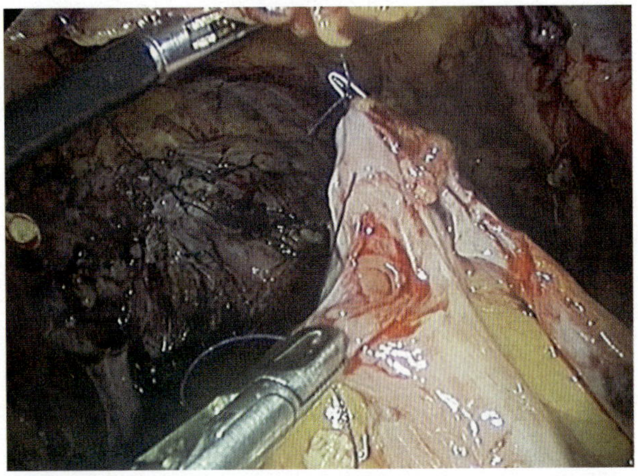

Fig. 44.29: Cut is made on the sigmoid.

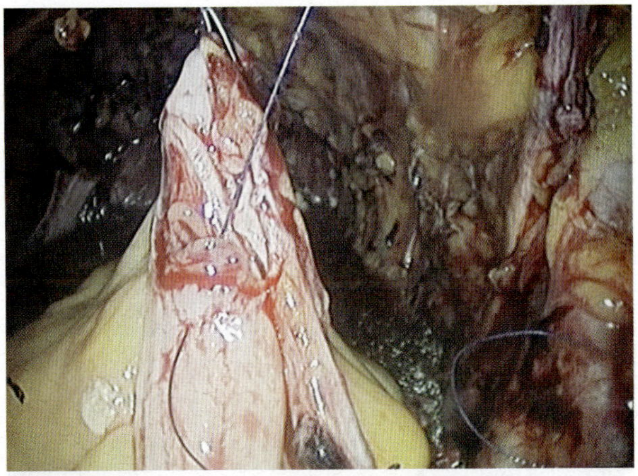

Fig. 44.30: A proximal full thickness stitch taken outside-in on colon and continued inside-out on the ureter.

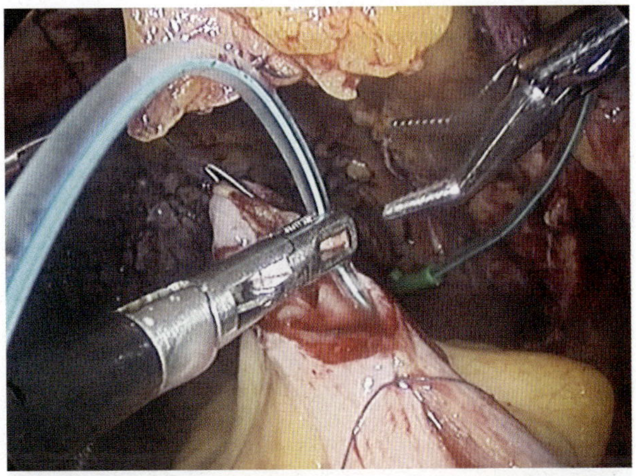

Fig. 44.31: A no. 5 or 6 infant feeding tube to act as a stent across the anastomosis. It is proximally put into the ureter, up to the renal pelvis. The distal end is put through the sigmoid colon.

The ureter is medialized and the pararectal space dissection is carried parallel to the ureter. The internal iliac artery is identified. The anterior division is clipped or ligated and then cut. The uterine artery and vein are identified, clipped and cut. The dissection

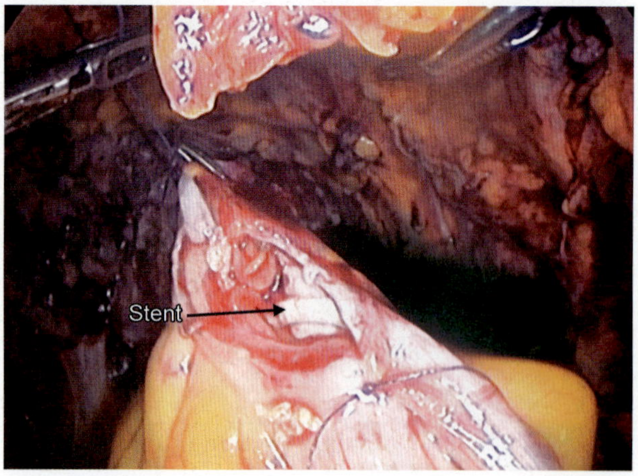

Fig. 44.32: Once the stent is in place, the ureter edges are sutured with a 3:0 Vicryl continuous suture.

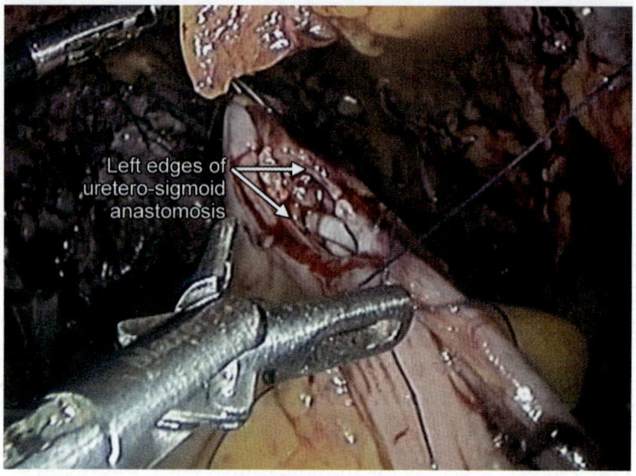

Fig. 44.33: Ureterosigmoid anastomosis.

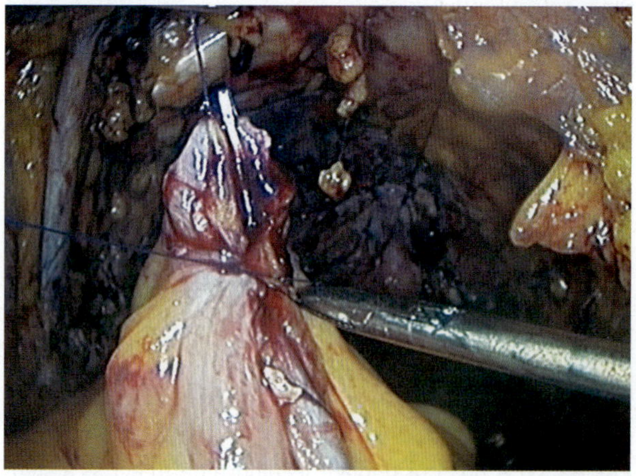

Fig. 44.34: Going round the apex of the ureterosigmoid anastomosis.

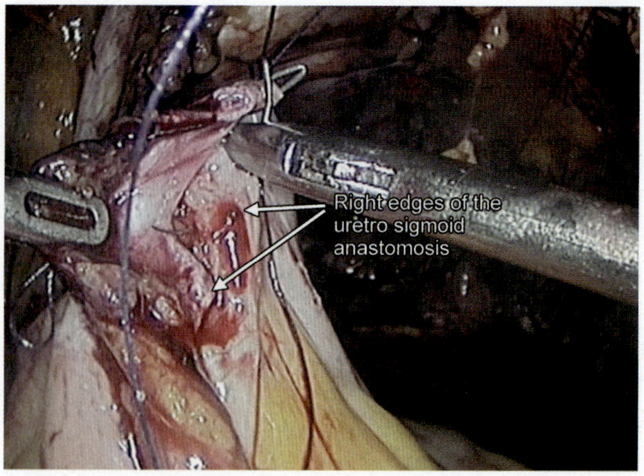

Fig. 44.35: Right edges of the ureterosigmoid anastomosis are sutured.

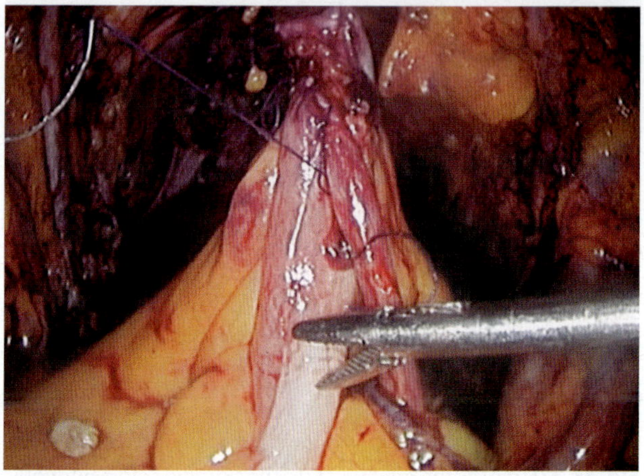

Fig. 44.36: The suture is brought around from below the ureter, to be tied to its tail on the left side.

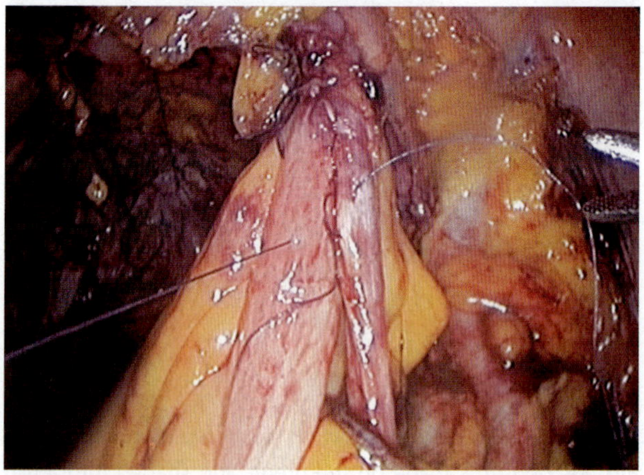

Fig. 44.37: Transfixation suture is taken.

is carried on to the paravesical space anteriorly and the levator ani caudally. Similar steps are repeated on the left side.[14]

Step 2: Posterior dissection in the pouch of Douglas is carried out in a similar to how it is done in laparoscopic radical hysterectomy. Thus, the rectum is separated from the posterior

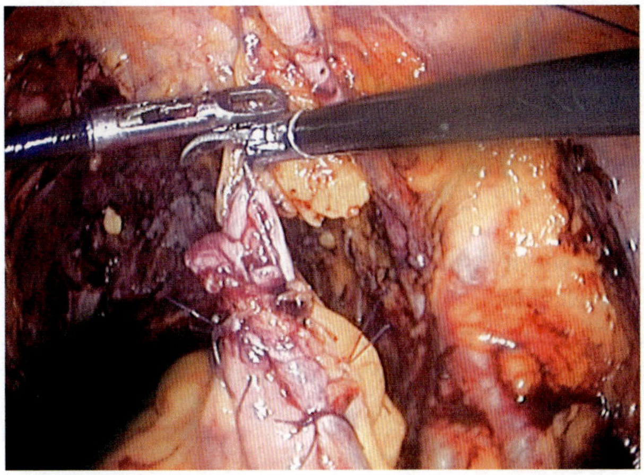

Fig. 44.38: Excess tip of ureter is trimmed.

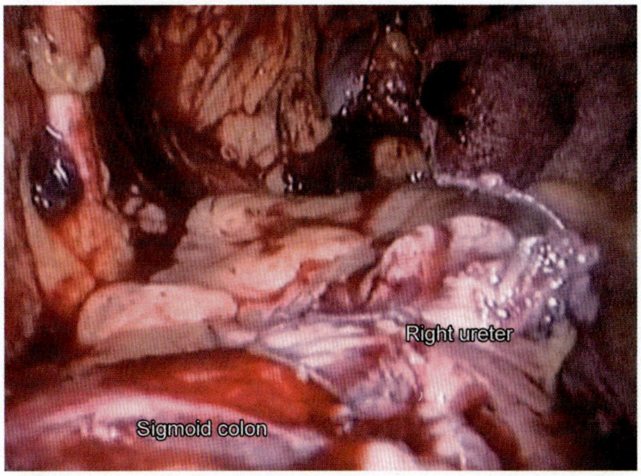

Fig. 44.39: Completed ureterosigmoid anastomosis.

vaginal wall. A posterior U cut is taken as explained in radical hysterectomy. The ureter is pushed medially to expose the cardinal ligaments and the uterosacrals, which are cut on both the sides. The caudal limit is the levator ani muscle.

Step 3: The anterior dissection is done by cutting the anterior leaf of the broad ligament and the round ligament on the right. The peritoneum medial to the obliterated hypogastric artery is cut and the peritoneal cut is extended to the anterior abdominal wall to separate the bladder from the anterior abdominal wall. Similar steps are repeated on the left side. (Fig. 44.23)

Step 4: The bladder is then brought down from the anterior abdominal wall to enter the retro-pubic space, i.e. the Cave of Retzius (Fig. 44.24). The tissue anterior and lateral to the urethra and vagina is cut. The urethra is accessed anteriorly. The posterior urethral wall and the anterior vaginal wall are cut. A good length of vagina below the growth is exposed. The aim is to have a distal vaginal cuff 2.5–3 cm.

Step 5: Colpotomy is performed. Ilio obturator nodal dissection is done on both sides and the tissue put into an endobag. The specimen is removed vaginally. The vagina is repacked to prevent air leak.

The type of urinary diversion plays an important role in the quality of life. The various types of urinary diversions that can be done are illeal conduit, uretero sigmoid, orthotropic ileal neobladders and Indiana pouch. Ureterosigmoidostomy and ileal conduit can be done entirely laparoscopically while Indiana pouch and neobladder have to be done by opening the abdomen. Here the author describes the ureterosigmoid anastomosis, which is a continent pouch.

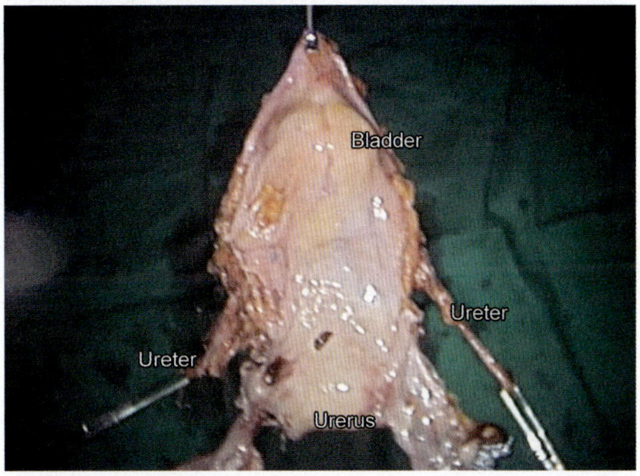

Fig. 44.40: Specimen of anterior exenteration.

Step 6: The right ureter is cut and transfixed to the sigmoid colon, anteriorly over the taenia coli (Fig. 44.27). The end of the suture is held up for better visualization. A cut is made on the ureter, which is fashioned into a fish mouth (Fig. 44.28). A cut is also made on the sigmoid, anteriorly, overlying the taenia coli (Fig. 44.29). A proximal full thickness stitch is taken, outside-in on the colon and continued inside-out on the ureter (Fig. 44.30). An infant feeding tube no. 5 or 6 is inserted into it to act as a stent across the anastomosis. It is proximally put into the ureter, up to the renal pelvis. A note is made of the presence of flowing urine in the tube to confirm proper placement. It is distally inserted into the opening made in the sigmoid colon. (Fig. 44.31). Once the stent is in place, the ureter edges are sutured with a 3:0 Vicryl continuous suture (Fig. 44.32). A full thickness continuous suture is taken on one side of the anastomosis, going from proximal to distal. The same suture is taken around and continued from distal to proximal end on the opposite side of the anastomosis. The right edge of the ureterosigmoid anastomosis is sutured (Fig. 44.35). The suture is brought around from below the ureter, to be tied to its tail on the left side (Fig. 44.36). A transfixation suture (hypnotic) is taken (Fig. 44.37). The excess tip of the ureter is trimmed (Fig. 44.38). The left ureter is brought under the colon and then to the right side (Fig. 44.39).

Step 7: The vagina is then sutured with 2:0 Vicryl continuous intracorporeal suturing. Hemostasis is achieved. An abdominal drain is placed through the right iliac fossa lower port. The ports are then removed under vision and closed.

POSTERIOR EXENTERATION[16-18]

Posterior exenteration is a morbid and extensive surgery done in cases of advanced carcinoma of the cervix with the involvement of rectum. It involves removal of the rectum, uterus, vagina and the vulva, if required, along with all the fibro-fatty lymphovascular tissue along the external iliac veins and the obturator nerves.

The operability criteria are as follows:

1. Histological documentation of cancer in the palpable mass.
2. Absence of tumor extension to parametrium or pelvic side walls or distant metastasis or para aortic lymph node involvement.

Preoperative investigations, such as a thorough clinical examination to determine the extent of rectal involvement, computed tomography (CT) scan of the abdomen and pelvis, chest X-ray, liver function tests, cystoscopy, proctoscopy and examination under anesthesia help to decide the operability.

The position of the patient and anesthesia is the same as in laparoscopic radical hysterectomy.

Port Positions

- A 10-mm camera port in the umbilicus
- A 10-mm working port in the McBurney's point on the right side
- A 5-mm port pararectally in the midclavicular line
- A set of 5-mm ports in the mirror images on the left side
- A 12-mm port about 2 cm above the pubic symphysis used for the endostapling device.

Procedure

Step 1: Uterus is hitched to the anterior abdominal wall.

Step 2: Ureter identified at the level of the sacral promontory. The pararectal spaces on both sides are dissected as in laparoscopic radical hysterectomy.

Step 3: The paravesical space anterior to the uterine artery is dissected to reach the levator ani, which is the distal limit of dissection. The uterine arteries and the veins are clipped or ligated. The cardinal ligaments on both sides are coagulated and cut.

Step 4: The anterior U cut is taken from one round ligament to other as in laparoscopic radical hysterectomy and the urinary bladder is separated and pushed downward.

Step 5: Remembering the dictum fat belongs to the rectum, the dissection is carried out in the avascular pre-sacral space between the rectum and the presacral fascia, i.e. the two layers of Denon Villiers' fascia. The plane is dissected distally up to the levator ani.

Step 6: The distal level of rectal involvement is the criteria to decide if rectal continuity can be achieved by performing a supra-levator resection or an infra-levator resection in case of extensive involvement of the rectum with involvement of the sphincter complex.

Step 7: A low colpotomy is performed. Following colpotomy, pneumoperitoneum is maintained by placing the pack in the vagina. The rectum distal to the tumor becomes visible, enabling transection with the endostapling device.

Step 8: The infundibulo-pelvic ligaments on both sides are coagulated and cut.

Step 9: The inferior mesenteric artery is clipped and cut at its origin.

Step 10: The proximal large bowel is then mobilized.

Step 11: A 12-mm port is inserted about 2 cm above the pubic symphysis through which an Echelon endostapler is introduced. After mobilization of the proximal colon the stapler is fired.

Step 12: There are two ways to perform a coloanal anastomosis. A lower midline mini-laparotomy can be done for specimen extraction, proximal bowel transection and placement of the anvil of the EEA stapler. The other method is to retrieve the specimen per vaginally. The proximal colon is brought out through the anal canal and the anvil of the stapler can thus be inserted.

Step 13: Circular stapled coloanal end-to-end anastomosis is performed.

Step 14: Bilateral ilio obturator lymph node dissection is done.

Step 15: A temporary transverse colostomy is performed. An abdominal drain is placed and the port sites closed.

TOTAL PELVIC EXENTERATION[11]

In cases of advanced cancer of the cervix with spread to the bladder or rectum, this surgery is offered as a method of palliation to improve the quality of life. The anesthesia, position of the patient and the port position remain the same as in the case of laparoscopic radical hysterectomy. (Fig. 44.41)

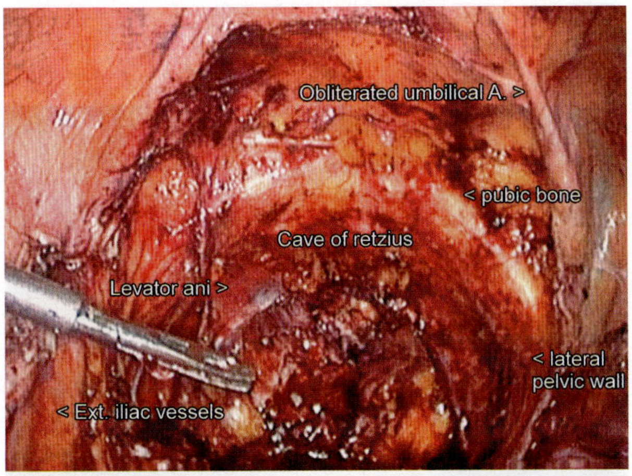

Fig. 44.41: The empty pelvis is seen after removal of the bladder, uterus with parametrium, paracolpos, upper half of the vagina and the rectum. The pubic bone anteriorly, levator ani inferiorly and the iliac vessels laterally show good regional clearance.

Procedure

Step 1: A scope is introduced through the 10-mm umbilical port. A staging laparoscopy is performed to assess the operability by observing the extent of the disease, the fixity of the tumor to the pelvic side walls and the involvement of the iliac vessels.

Step 2: The ureter on the right side is identified at the level of the sacral promontory and the peritoneum over it is incised with harmonic shears. The ureter is medialized and the pararectal space is dissected. The internal iliac artery is identified and its anterior division is clipped or ligated and cut. The uterine artery is identified.

Step 3: Dissection is done anterior to the uterine artery and medial to the obliterated umbilical artery in the paravesical space up to the levator ani. The ureter is medialized and the uterosacral and cardinal ligaments are coagulated and cut. The same steps are performed on the left side.

Step 4: The right-round ligament is cut and the cut is extended anteriorly, remaining medial to the obliterated umbilical vessels. The bladder is dissected off the anterior abdominal wall and the Cave of Retzius is entered. The paraurethral tissue and urethra are cut with the harmonic shears.

Step 5: Colpotomy is performed. The infundibulopelvic ligaments are cut.

Step 6: The ureters are clipped and cut. The sigmoid mesentery is opened to enter the presacral space posterior to the rectum. The inferior mesenteric vessels are ligated and cut. The dissection posterior to the rectosigmoid is continued until the levator ani is reached. The sigmoid colon is then dissected off the lateral pelvic wall and the rectum distal to the tumor is stapled with a linear stapler and cut. Proximally the colon is tied at two places and cut in between the ligatures. Splenic flexure mobilization is performed.

Step 7: Ilio-obturator nodal dissection is done. The specimen is placed in the endobag.

Step 8: The abdomen is opened by a small incision of 5–6 cm, either midline vertical or transverse muscle cutting. The mouth of the bag is brought out at the incision and the specimen is removed from the bag piece by piece, thus avoiding any contamination.

Step 9: The vagina is sutured intracorporeally with 2.0 Vicryl. Colorectal anastomosis is done by inserting the anvil of a circular stapler in the proximal cut end of the colon. The head of the stapler is introduced per rectally into the distal stump. The ureters are brought out through this incision and are implanted into the ileum extracorporeally. A temporary transverse colostomy is performed. The ureters can also be implanted into the sigmoid colon and a wet colostomy be performed instead.

ROBOTIC RADICAL HYSTERECTOMY (Figs. 44.42 to 44.50)[21]

As the modality of minimal access surgery in gynecological oncology is becoming more and more popular, new technologies are emerging. Robotic surgery for cervical cancer is one such landmark that has changed the whole outlook of minimal access surgery. It overcomes the difficulties and the restriction of laparoscopic surgery while giving the benefits of open surgery. Even though there are a few drawbacks, including the limited range of motion intra-abdominally (only four degrees of freedom), loss of tactile feedback, large bulky robotic arms, limited variety of instrumentation and cost, due to the three-dimensional view, dexterity of instruments and more rapid learning, even without any prior experience in laparoscopy, many surgeons are adapting to this minimally invasive technique. Here the author describes the procedure of robotic radical hysterectomy with the use of the 3-Arm Da Vinci robot system (Intuitive Surgical, Sunnyvale, CA, USA), applying the same Pune technique used for laparoscopic radical hysterectomy.

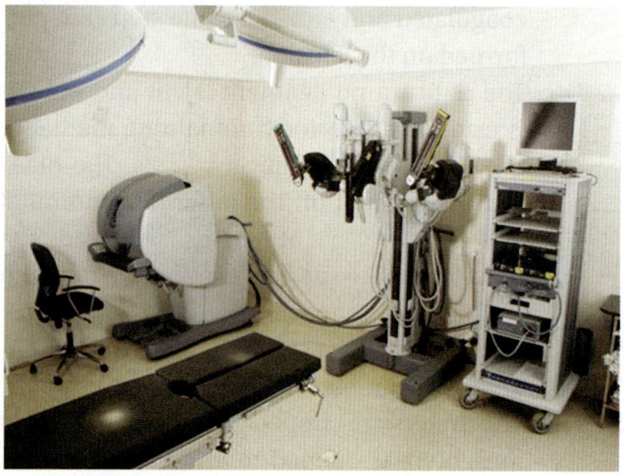

Fig. 44.42: Robotic setup.

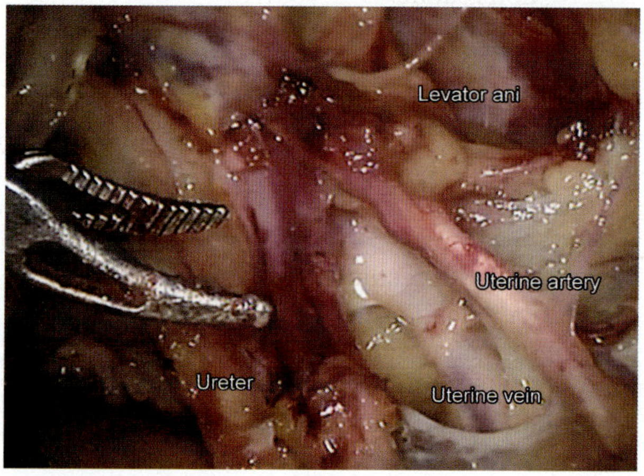

Fig. 44.44: Right pararectal space.

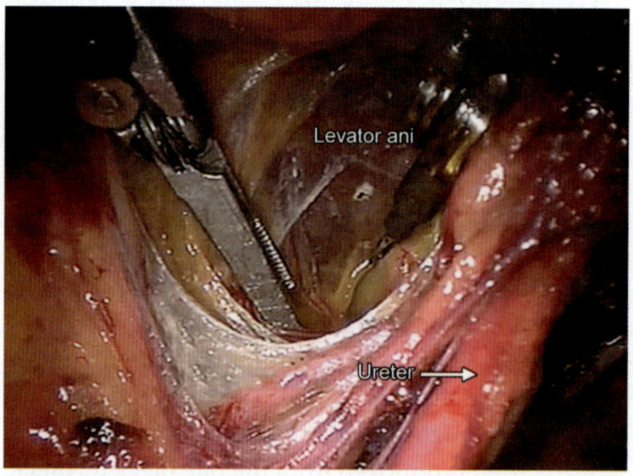

Fig. 44.43: Dissection of the pararectal space.

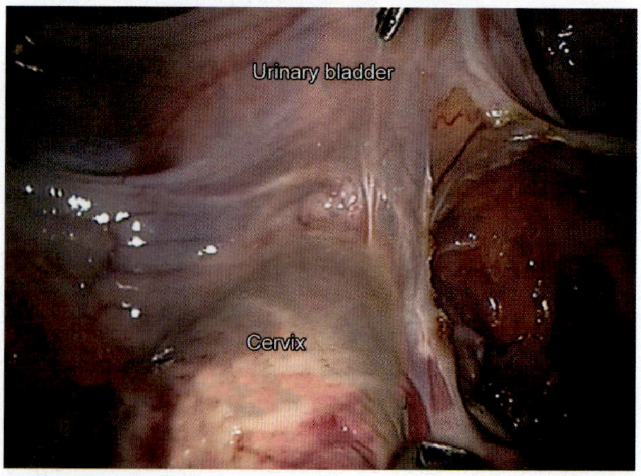

Fig. 44.45: Anterior U cut.

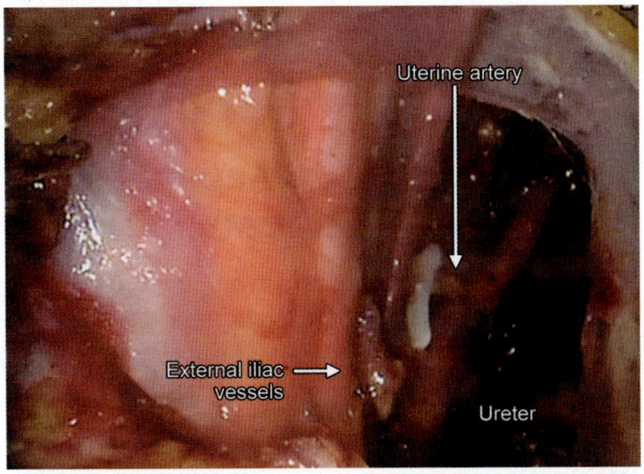

Fig. 44.46: Left pararectal space with left uterine artery clipped.

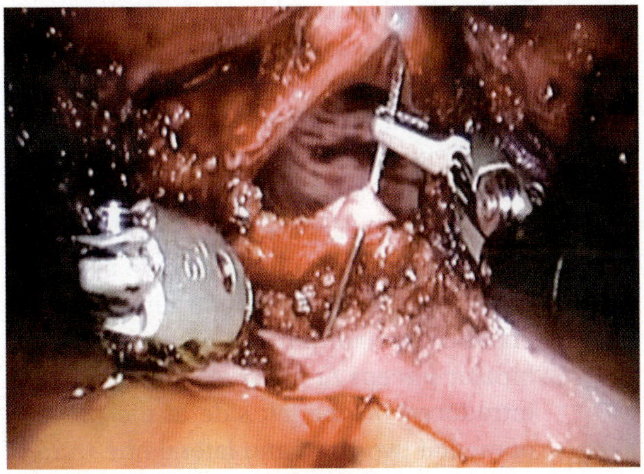

Fig. 44.47: Intracorporeal suturing of vault.

Indications, contraindications and the preoperative preparation of the patient remain the same as in laparoscopic radical hysterectomy.

Anesthesia: A combination of regional and general anesthesia.

Patient position: Modified Lloyd Davies position with a bolster placed at the anterior superior iliac spine. A gauze piece is kept in the vagina to prevent loss of pneumoperitoneum after colpotomy.

Port Positions

- A 12-mm camera port is placed just above the umbilicus.
- An 8-mm robotic port is placed on the left side, 10 cm lateral and 5 cm caudal to the camera port.
- The right-sided robotic port is a mirror image of the left robotic port.
- Two assistant 10-mm ports were placed pararectally at the level of the camera port.

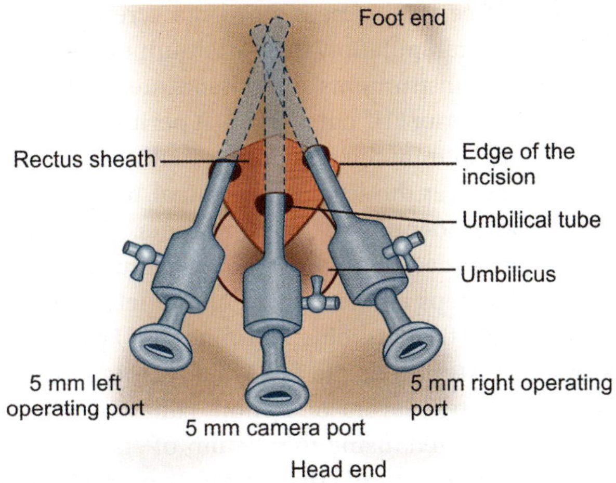

Fig. 44.48: Port position.

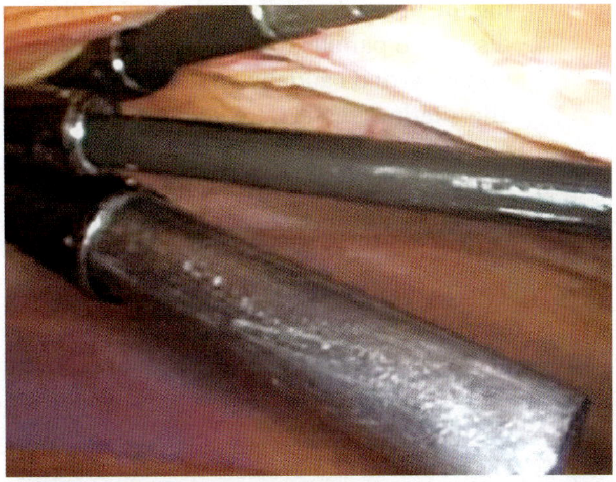

Fig. 44.49: Internal view of the ports.

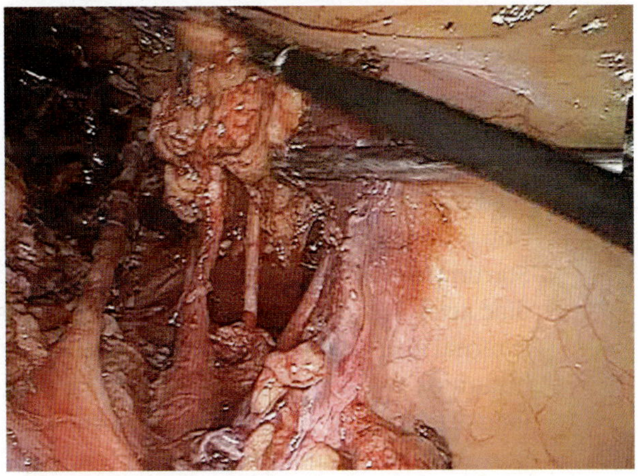

Fig. 44.50: Nodal dissection.

Procedure

The robotic cart is docked between the legs. The uterus is hitched in cases of endometrial carcinoma.

In cases of cervical cancer a myoma screw is used for uterine manipulation via the left upper assistant port. Bipolar instruments and scissors are used.

Step 1: Posterior "U" cut is taken. A peritoneal cut is taken from the right infundibulo-pelvic ligament at the level of the sacral promontory after identifying the right ureter. This cut is extended up to the Pouch of Douglas. Similar steps are performed on the left side and both the cuts joined forming the U cut.

Step 2: Dissection in the POD. The plane between the two layers of Denon Villiers' fascia is dissected, using the dictum of "fat belongs to the rectum." The rectum is pushed away from the posterior vaginal wall.

Step 3: The pararectal space is opened by retracting the ureter medially and carrying out the dissection parallel to the ureter. This dissection is carried caudally up to the levator ani. The uterine vessels are identified, clipped and cut.

Step 4: The Mackenrodt and the uterosacrals are then divided laterally. The same steps are repeated on the other side.

Step 5: The uterus is retroverted. An anterior peritoneal "U" cut was taken from one round ligament to the other round ligament. The entire bladder is then dissected away from the anterior vaginal wall.

Step 6: Dissection in the ureteric tunnel. The anterior leaf of the broad ligament is opened to expose the underlying ureter. The ureters are traced up to their entry into the bladder. The ureteric tunnel is exposed and divided, thus lateralizing the ureter further.

Step 7: Colpotomy is done after confirming a good distal vaginal margin.

Step 8: Bilateral ilio-obturator lymph nodal dissection is done the same way as in laparoscopy. Starting from the bifurcation of the common iliac artery, all the fibrofatty tissue along the external iliac artery and the nodes above the obturator nerve are cleared. The internal iliac artery is the medial limit and the iliac bone the lateral limit of our dissection.

Step 9: The separated specimen and the entire nodal tissue is put into an endobag and removed vaginally.

Step 10: The vault is closed with intracorporeal suturing, preferably with Vicryl 2-0.

Knowledge of these steps are the basis for any successful laparoscopic anterior exenteration[23] and uterine transplantation[24], which however demands the cooperation of a multi-specialty team and has been successfully performed in our institution, as well.

SINGLE-INCISION LAPAROSCOPIC RADICAL HYSTERECTOMY[19]

Minimal access surgeries are advancing toward more cosmetically apt surgeries, such as laparoendoscopic single-site surgery (LESS) and natural orifice transluminal endoscopic surgery (NOTES). Here the author describes single-incision laparoscopic radical hysterectomy.

Anesthesia and patient position is the same as described in laparoscopic radical hysterectomy.

Step 1: The vagina is incised 3 cm from the tumor margin to develop a vaginal cuff, and then sutured with Vicryl. This helps to know the extent of our dissection.

Step 2: The 5 mm primary port is introduced through the umbilicus for the telescope. Two 5-mm trocars are introduced on either side of the primary port, as shown in Fig. 48. The left port is used for nontraumatic graspers and the right port for harmonic shears, bipolar forceps or scissors. A 5 mm port is introduced on the left side at the junction of medial two-third and lateral one-third of the line joining umbilicus and the anterior superior iliac spine for bladder retraction.

Step 3: The uterus is hitched up to the anterior abdominal wall.

Step 4: The dissection is carried out in the same way as described in the radical hysterectomy performed with the Pune technique.

Step 5: The specimen is removed vaginally. Suturing of the vault can be done intracorporeally but is very cumbersome and time consuming due to the limited amount of maneuvering possible. It is recommended that the vault be sutured vaginally to avoid the same.

The postoperative recovery of the patient is similar to that after laparoscopic radical hysterectomy.

The advantages of single-incision surgery are now being recognized and are being applied to more and more gynecological procedures. The technique has many advantages over traditional minimally invasive surgery: cosmetic advantages and advantages relating to wound infection, postoperative pain and recuperation. There are disadvantages, such as the clashing of instruments, a limited working field, clashes between the operating surgeon's hand and the camera surgeon. This can be overcome by more experience.

REFERENCES

1. GLOBOCAN 2008 (IARC) Section of Cancer Information. Accessed March 7, 2012.
2. Canis M, Mage G, Wattiez A, et al. Does endoscopic surgery have a role in radical surgery of cancer of the cervix uteri? J Gynecol Obstet Biol Reprod (Paris). 1990;19:921.
3. Nezhat CR, Burrell MO, Nezhat FR, et al. Laparoscopic radical hysterectomy with para-aortic and pelvic node dissection. Am J Obstet Gynecol. 1992;166:864-5.
4. Ramirez PT, Slomovitz BM, Soliman PT, et al. Total laparoscopic radical hysterectomy and lymphadenectomy: The M.D. Anderson Cancer Center experience. Gynecol Oncol. 2006;102:252-5.
5. Gil-Moreno A, Diaz-Feijoo B, Roca I, et al. Total laparoscopic radical hysterectomy with intraoperative sentinel node identification in patients with early invasive cervical cancer. Gynecol Oncol. 2005;96: 187-93.
6. Pomel C, Atallah D, Le Bouedec G, et al. Laparoscopic radical hysterectomy for invasive cervical cancer: 8-year experience of a pilot study. Gynecol Oncol. 2003;91:534-9.
7. Abu-Rustum NR, Gemignani ML, Moore K, et al. Total laparoscopic radical hysterectomy with pelvic lymphadenectomy using the argon-beam coagulator: Pilot data and comparison to laparotomy. Gynecol Oncol. 2003;91:402-9.
8. Spirtos NM, Eisenkop SM, Schlaerth JB, et al. Laparoscopic radical hysterectomy (type III) with aortic and pelvic lymphadenectomy in patients with stage I cervical cancer: Surgical morbidity and intermediate follow-up. Am J Obstet Gynecol. 2002;187:340-8.
9. Kim DH, Moon JS. Laparoscopic radical hysterectomy with pelvic lymphadenectomy for early, invasive cervical carcinoma. J Am Assoc Gynecol Laparosc. 1998;5:411-7.
10. Krause N, Schneider A. Laparoscopic radical hysterectomy with para-aortic and pelvic lymphadenectomy. Zentralbl Gynakol. 1995;117: 346-8.
11. Brunschwig A. Complete excision of pelvic viscera for advanced carninoma, Cancer 1948;1:177-83.
12. Brunschwig A. What are the indications and results of pelvic exenteration? JAMA 1965;194:274.
13. Puntambekar S, Palep R, Puntambekar S, et al. Laparoscopic total radical hysterectomy by the Pune technique: Our experience of 248 cases. J Minim Invasive Gynecol. 2007;14:682-9.
14. Puntambekar SP, Kudchadkar RJ, Gurjar AM, et al. Laparoscopic pelvic exenteration for advanced pelvic cancers: a review of 16 cases. Gynecol Oncol. 2006;102(3):513-6.
15. Caceres A, Mourton SM, Bochner BH, et al. Extended pelvic resections for recurrent uterine and cervical cancer: out-of-the-box surgery. Int J Gynecol Cancer. 2008;18:1139-44.
16. Bannura GC, Barrera AE, Cumsille MA, et al. Posterior pelvic exenteration for primary rectal cancer. Colorectal Dis. 2006;8:309-13.
17. Tixier H, Fraisse J, Chauffert B, et al. Evaluation of pelvic posterior exenteration in the management of advanced-stage ovarian cancer. Arch Gynecol Obstet. 2010;281:505-10.
18. Costa SR, Antunes RC, Paula RP, et al. Pelvic exenteration for T4 rectal cancer: a series of 15 resectable cases. Arch Gastroenterol. 2007;44:284-8.
19. Puntambekar SP, Puntambekar SS, Patil MA, et al. Testing the limits of single incision laproscopy: First ever radical hysterectomy attempted through single incision-ABSTRACT PRESENTED AT AAGL 2014.
20. Puntambekar SP, Wagh GN, Puntambekar SS, et al. A novel technique of total laparoscopic hysterectomy for routine use: evaluation of 140 cases. Int J Biomed Sci. 2008;4(1):38-43.
21. Puntambekar SP, Agarwal GA, Joshi SN, et al. Robotic radical hysterectomy: applying principles of the laparoscopic Pune technique. J. ROBOTIC SURG. 2010 DEC (4):259-64.
22. Puntambekar S, Sharma V, Jamkar AV, et al. Our experience of laparoscopic anterior exenteration in locally advanced cervical carcinoma. J Minim Invasive Gynecol. 2016:396-403.
23. Puntambekar S, Telang M, Kulkarni P, et al. Laparoscopic-assisted uterus retrieval from live organ donors for uterine transplant. J Minim Invasive Gynecol. 2017. (Epub ahead of print) PMID 29133152.

KIEL SCH•OL

45 of Gynaecological Endoscopy

Robot-assisted Surgery in Gynecology

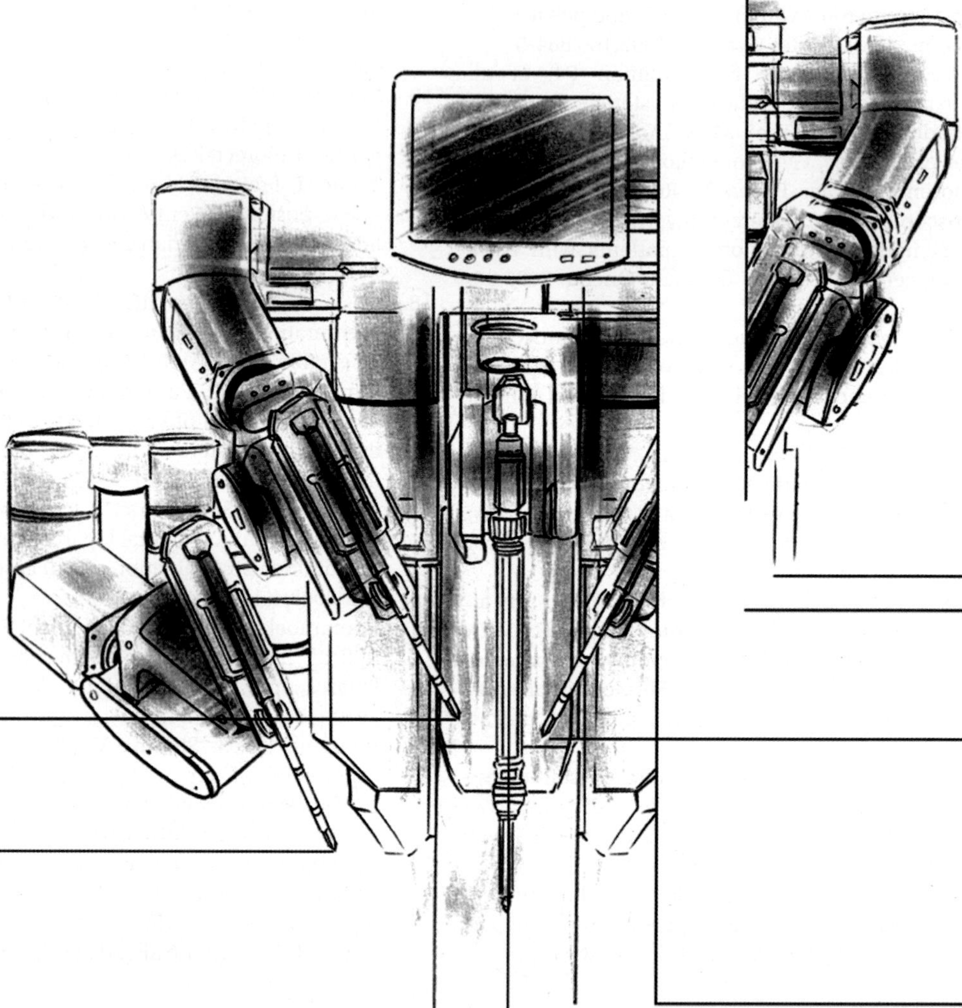

Chapter 45

Robot-assisted Surgery in Gynecology

Kubilay Ertan

AN OVERVIEW

After introduction of daVinci S® system 2006 and daVinci Si® system 2009, daVinci Xi® system was launched 2014 (Figs. 45.1 and 45.2).

In addition to several new functions like the integration of energy sources for HF surgery in the daVinci® vision system, the Crystal Clear 3D HD vision, the so-called Firefly® function and the possibility of integration for future advancements especially in the surgeon console (platform for future technologies) and enhancement or new development of the patient side cart (Figs. 45.3 and 45.4) constitutes the most significant innovation, because the robotic arms are docked now to the trocars from a vertically adjusted and rotatable platform, fixed at a gibbet, effectively hanging from above, tentacle-like, supported by a laser-guided sight device (target anatomy with laser precision, anatomical access from virtually any position).

This results in several advantages in the handling of patient side cart, both concerning the docking maneuver and the surgical procedure itself: the laser-guided placement of the robotic arms

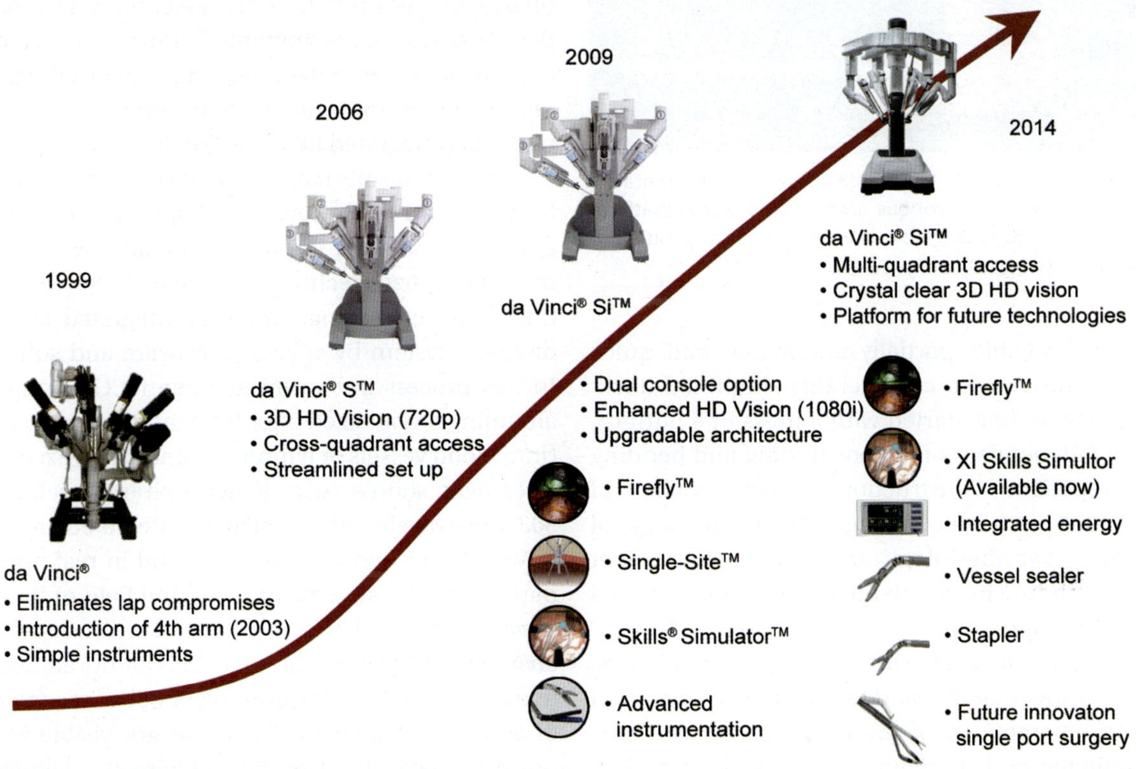

Fig. 45.1: Development of the daVinci® system from 1999 to 2014.
Source: Intuitive Surgical, Sunnyvale, CA.

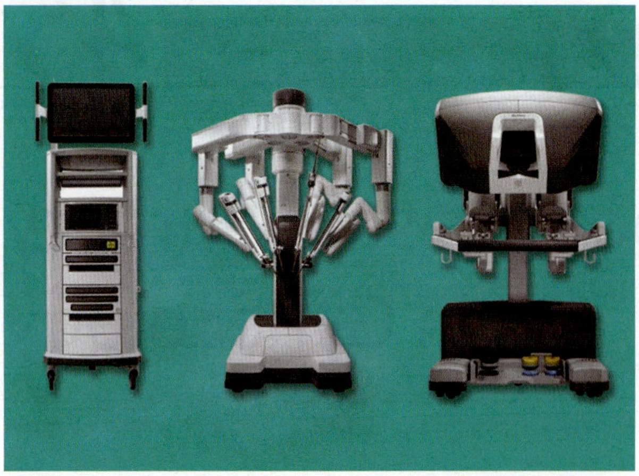

Fig. 45.2: The hardware components of the daVinci Xi® system; from left to right: vision system, patient side cart, surgeon console.
Source: Intuitive Surgical, Sunnyvale, CA.

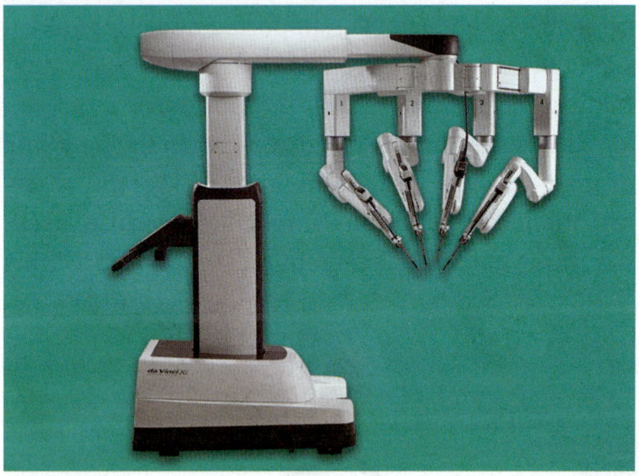

Fig. 45.3: Patient side cart of the daVinci Xi® system: tentacle-like arrangement of the robotic arms at a rotatable platform with a vertical adjustable gibbet-like device—home position.
Source: Intuitive Surgical, Sunnyvale, CA.

permits a reliable, partially automated and quick and, for this reason, considerably simplified docking maneuver (get started with a press of a button), largely independent of the positioning and bedding of the patient, constructional characteristics of the operating theater, arrangement of the surgical assistant, anesthesiology team and instrument tables including the scrub nurse and the target area of the operation.

The patient side cart also guarantees free choice of the anatomical target region of operation and an enlargement of the operating space intra-abdominally and therefore the surgical sites, thus increasing the accessibility of a larger region; this particularly plays a major role in oncological operations

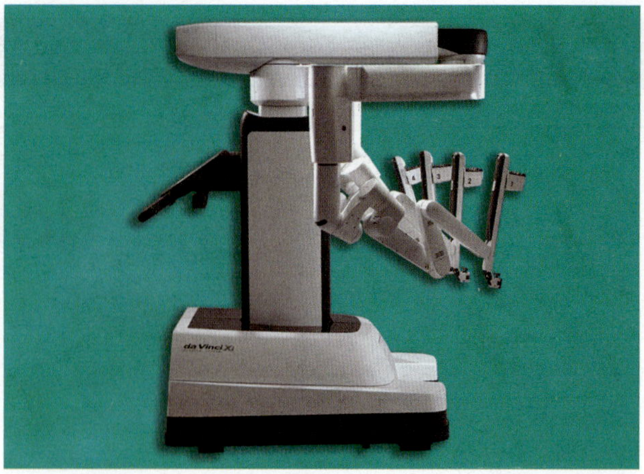

Fig. 45.4: Patient side cart of the daVinci Xi® system: tentacle-like arrangement of the robotic arms at a rotatable platform with a vertical adjustable gibbet-like device—docked position.
Source: Intuitive Surgical, Sunnyvale, CA.

(for instance, better accessibility of the para-aortic lymph drainage region and the mobilization of parts of the intestine in combined gynecological and visceral surgical operations with bowel resections and bowel anastomosis, that is, multiquadrant surgery in general (e.g., in ovarian cancer operations or other extended staging operations). Furthermore, intra-operative changes of positioning between different phases of the operation are essentially facilitated. Based on these developments, a future advancement of the system with integrated and concerted parallel motion or co-movement of the operating table is planned (integrated table motion function (ITM)).

With the term "image-guided surgery" additional functions are described, enabled by daVinci Xi® platform. The most important, already realized and routinely utilized technique, is the so-called real-time fluorescence imaging, which is integrated into the daVinci® system by specific hardware and software. In this process indocyanine green (ICG), bound to albumin, is visualized after intravascular application (into blood vessels or lymph streams) by an excitatory laser light source (use of near-infrared technique, 803 nm wavelength), which is integrated into the daVinci® endoscope. This is overlaid in real time by particular filter systems in the vision field of the surgeon console, and by activation and inactivation with an integrated switch (Fig. 45.5). This allows additional image information, for example a better recognition of anatomical structures that are not visible in the normal image, or that are not already delineated and exposed (e.g., presentation of the ureter, blood vessels, etc.; Fig. 45.6); tissue and organ borders can

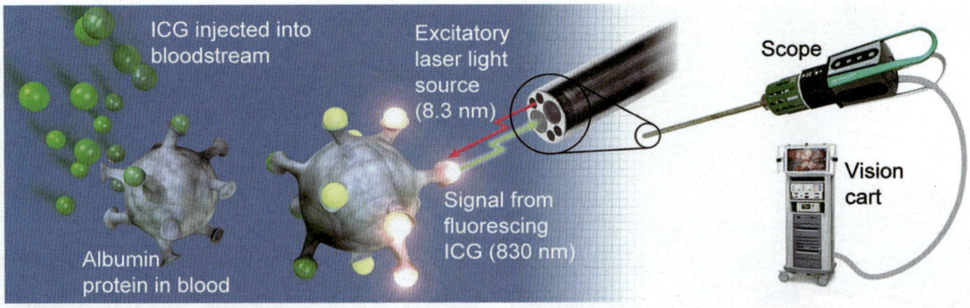

Fig. 45.5: Integrated fluorescence imaging with near-infraread wavelength (803 nm) with indocyanine green application.
Source: Intuitive Surgical, Sunnyvale, CA.

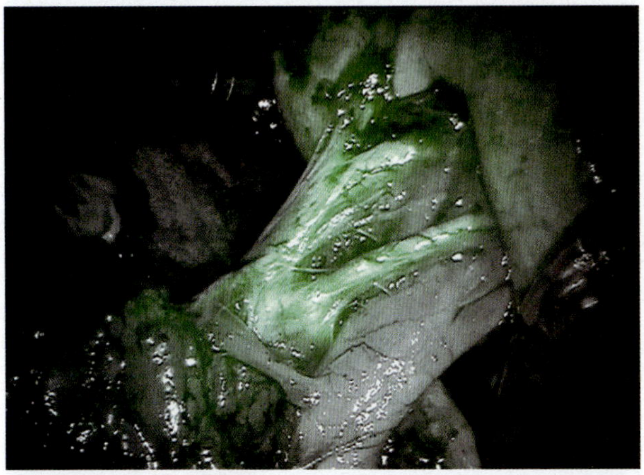

Fig. 45.6: Example of use of integrated fluorescence imaging with near-infrared wavelength (803 nm) after application of indocyanine green; here aspect of the renal hilus for vessel delineation in partial nephrectomy.
Source: Intuitive Surgical, Sunnyvale, CA.

be identified better, which could be greatly helpful for instance in compartment-based operations such as the total mesometrial resection in cervical cancer (TMMR). Furthermore, through this, lymph nodes and particularly sentinel lymph nodes can be detected easier, and, consequently, the selective extirpation can be facilitated. In addition, there is also a better visualization of tumor boundaries (Fig. 45.6).

Other possibilities of image-guided surgery are the superimposition of other image information into the vision field of the surgical console (such as, real-time ultrasound via intraoperative used transvaginal ultrasonic probes, or images of computed tomography and magnetic resonance tomography (MRI)), thus making it available directly to the surgeon (Figs. 45.7A and B).

Also important for further development of robot-assisted surgical techniques are the innovations of surgical instruments that guarantee a highest possible compatibility with the daVinci® system, and permit the surgeon a considerably greater flexibility and maximum exploitation of possible surgical techniques and features concerning tissue manipulation, dissection and preparation. This includes the launch of EndoWrist® instruments with suction and irrigation function, vessel sealer function, clip applicator and harmonic function (ultrasound energy systems); in addition, laser and argon plasma coagulation systems are also available (Figs. 45.8 to 45.12)

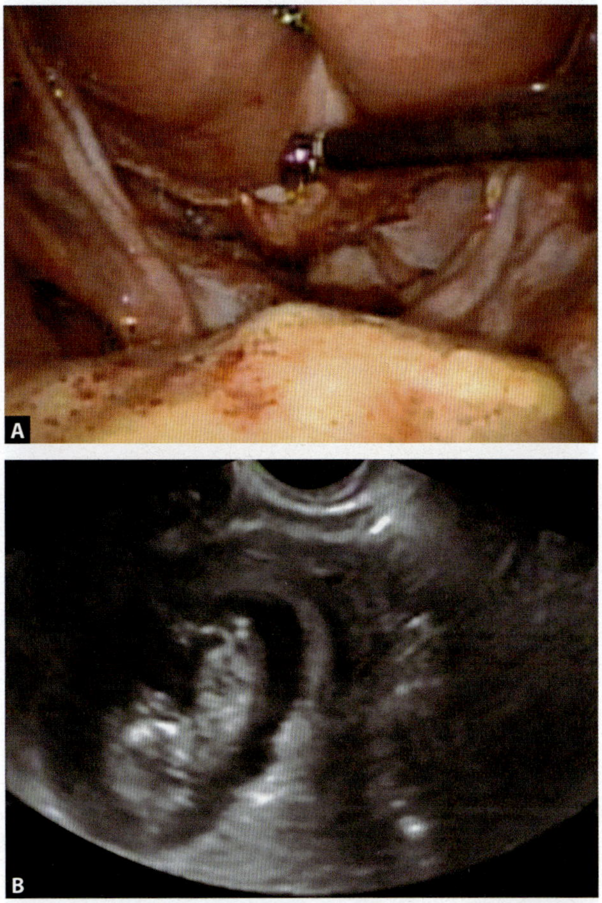

Figs. 45.7A and B: Vision panel at the surgeon console with superimposition of additional image infromation (here transvaginal ultrasound during robot-assisted laparoscopic cerclage).
Source: M Borahay, UTMB, Galveston, TX.

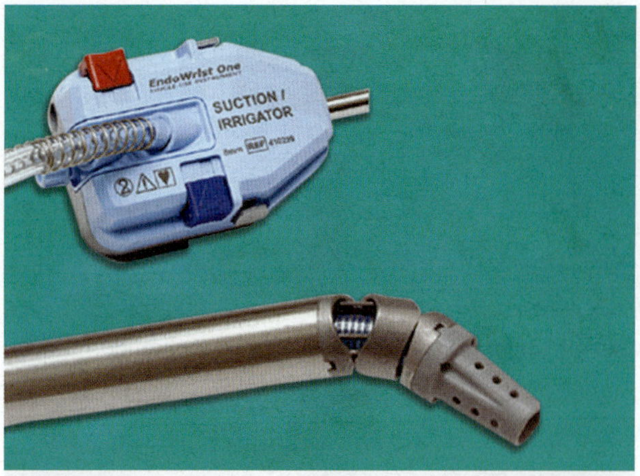

Fig. 45.8: Innovation of the EndoWrist® instruments: Suction and irrigation system.
Source: Intuitive Surgical, Sunnyvale, CA.

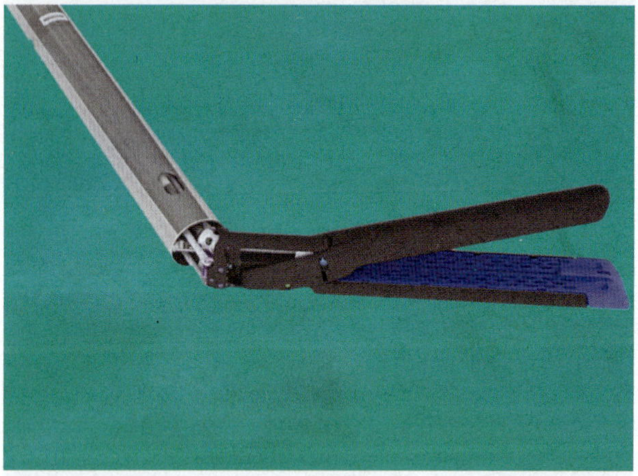

Fig. 45.9: Innovation of the EndoWrist® instruments: Linear stapler.
Source: Intuitive Surgical, Sunnyvale, CA.

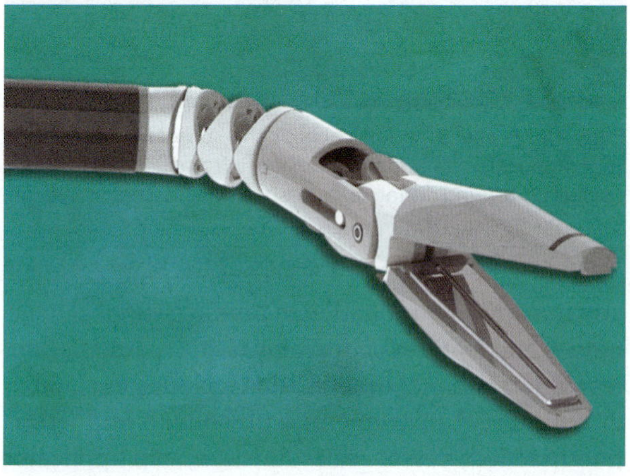

Fig. 45.10: Innovation of the EndoWrist® instruments: Sealing instrument.
Source: Intuitive Surgical, Sunnyvale, CA.

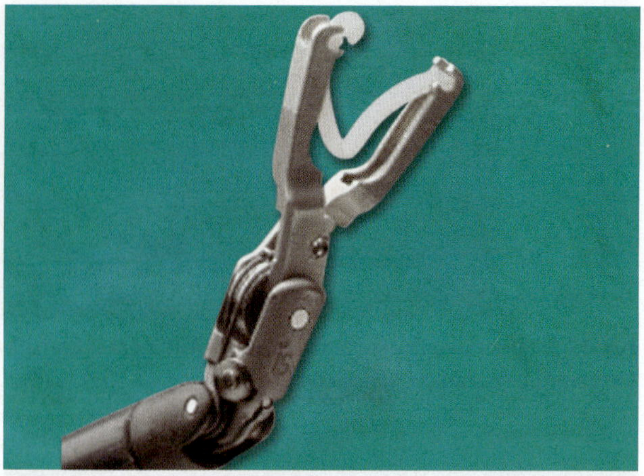

Fig. 45.11: Innovation of the EndoWrist® instruments: Clip applicator.
Source: Intuitive Surgical, Sunnyvale, CA.

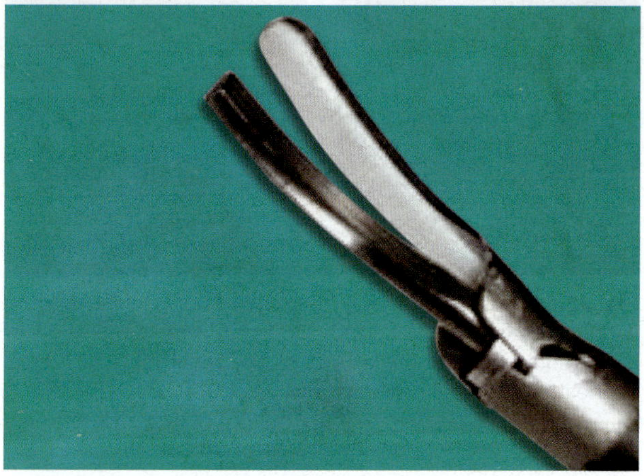

Fig. 45.12: Innovation of the EndoWrist® instruments: Ultrasound sealing and dissection instrument (Harmonic).
Source: Intuitive Surgical, Sunnyvale, CA.

Although the more conventional single-port technique of the daVinci® system (Fig. 45.13) is mainly suitable for simple gynecological procedures, and less for complex gynecological operations the upcoming commercial launch of an extended single site system, where a flexible 3D high-definition camera within a 25 mm cannula, together with three fully articulating instruments (Figs. 45.14 and 45.15), compatible with the latest daVinci Xi® robot, is representing a fascinating innovation, which allows also the realization of complex oncological procedures by a single port and which this technology puts it close to the NOTES philosophy.

Lack of tactile feedback of the daVinci® system, which is consistently advocated as a drawback of robot-assisted surgery, does not apply to current

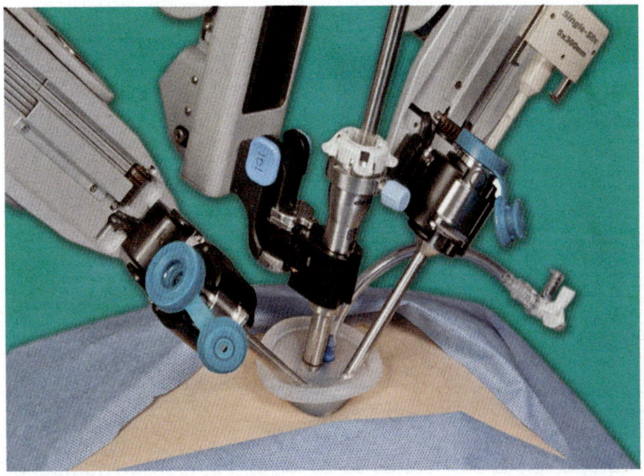

Fig. 45.13: daVinci® single port system; three robotic arms and three trocars in one umbilical access.
Source: Intuitive Surgical, Sunnyvale, CA.

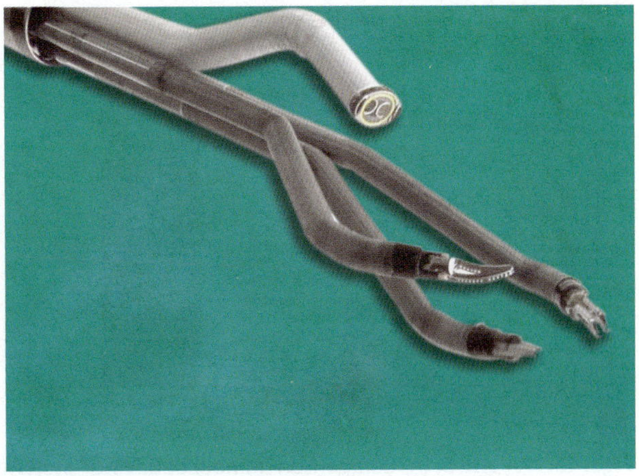

Fig. 45.15: daVinci Sp® single port robotic system—moved-out camera (at the top) and surgical instrument.
Source: Intuitive Surgical, Sunnyvale, CA.

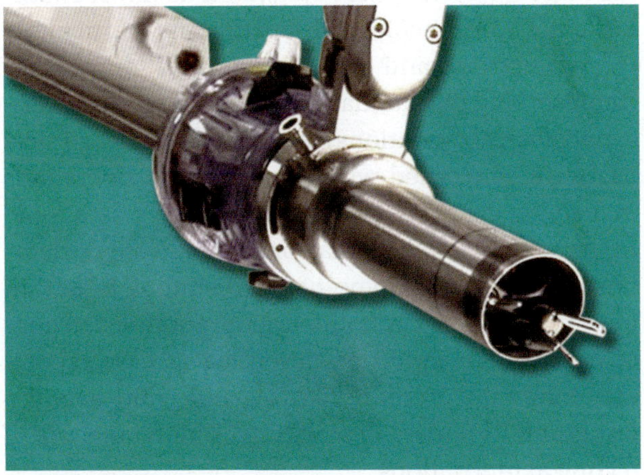

Fig. 45.14: daVinci Sp® single port robotic system.
Source: Intuitive Surgical, Sunnyvale, CA.

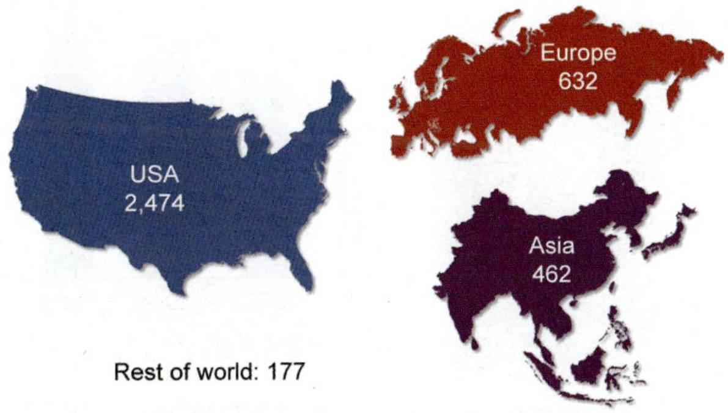

Fig. 45.16: Installed daVinci® systems, installierte daVinci-Systeme, status 06/2016.
Source: Intuitive Surgical, Sunnyvale, CA.

advancements of the daVinci® system. The efforts in improvement of visualization dominates in all technical innovations of the robotic system; this seems not only to compensate the missing haptics but appears to make it increasingly irrelevant.

GLOBAL APPLICATION OF THE DaVinci® SYSTEMS

Intuitive Surgical that developed daVinci® system was founded in 1995 and more than 3 million daVinci® procedures have been performed (as on June 2016). Approximately two-thirds of the daVinci® systems are used in the United States (2,474 in the United States; 1,271 systems outside the United States), but also in Europe the number of systems has more than doubled between 2011 and 2016 (Figs. 45.16 and 45.17). About the half of the daVinci® operations are carried out on the gynecological side; for the United States it has been revealed that the percentage of open abdominal operations in malignant diseases of the uterus was lowered from 90% to 10% between 2004 and 2015, whereas, more than 80% of operations in uterine cancer performed are robot-assisted. In Europe the number of surgical interventions are distributed otherwise, which can be ascribed to the traditionally more powerful approach of conventional laparoscopy. Nevertheless, the number of surgical interventions in robot-assisted operations outside the United States shows a continuous rise (Fig. 45.18). Therefore, the technique of robot-assisted laparoscopic operations with the daVinci® system leads the way in further developments and advancements in minimal invasive interventions, especially in gynecological surgery, where the largest spectrum of operations offering important advantages by robotic

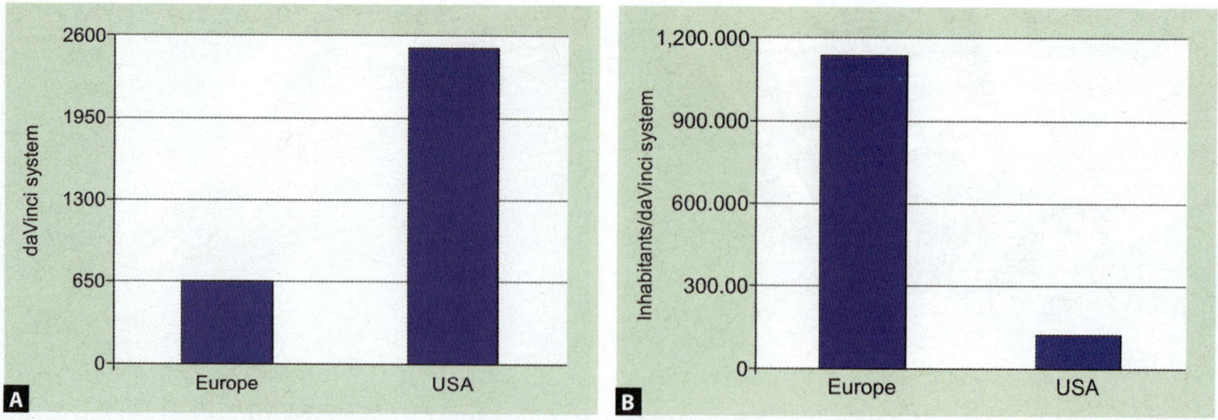

Figs. 45.17A and B: (A) Comparison number of daVinci® systems in Europe versus USA (status 06/2016); (B) Comparison number of daVinci® systems per population in Europe versus USA (status 06/2016).
Source: Intuitive Surgical, Sunnyvale, CA.

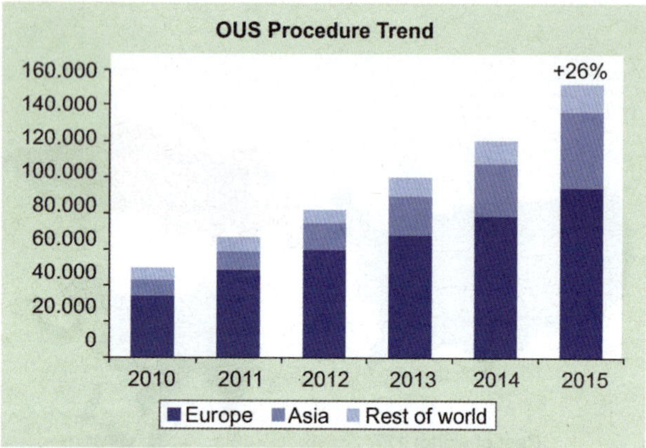

Fig. 45.18: Increase of robot-assisted interventions, 2010-2015 outside of the USA.
Source: Intuitive Surgical, Sunnyvale, CA.

assistance is provided. And, still, the different generations of daVinci® systems are the only available and efficient robotic systems, so that discourses in professional societies and in the specialist literature about robot-assisted operations refer substantially to daVinci® techniques in all medical disciplines.

RECENT LITERATURE ON DaVinci® OPERATIONS

Consequently, with augmentation of the used daVinci® systems in the past years the quantity of publications about robot-assisted operations in the gynecological field has increased significantly. At this juncture, the main part of publications refer to the topics of endometrial cancer, the complex of problems of obese patients, just related to endometrial malignancies, cervical cancer, in particular gyneco-oncological issues altogether, cost analysis, the impact on healthcare system on health economics and urogynecological operations, particularly colposacropexy and cervicosacropexy procedures (representing the standard abdominal access of urogynecological operations). Increasingly fewer clinical trials are concerned with robot-assisted operations in benign gynecological diseases (such as simple hysterectomies in myomas or myomectomy), demonstrating that this type of interventions is not an ideal indication for robotic surgery; another category of publications could be described as case reports about very uncommon diseases and entities, and a last group of papers deal with feasibility analysis of technical innovations.

Whereas cost analyses mostly demonstrate that robot-assisted interventions are obviously more expensive (current costs of the daVinci system: $1.85–2.3 million; instrument costs: $2200–3200 [each 10 uses]), the results of cost-effectiveness analyses depended on analysis of single-procedure costs or inclusion of overall robotic costs, costs incurred by robotic surgery by capital acquisition, limited use of instruments, team-training expenses, equipment maintenance and repair and operating room setup time. It works out to approximately $2,000 more per case than the same procedure performed by conventional laparoscopy. Elevated cost is the greatest detriment to continued implementation of robotic surgery, and industry competition has not yet emerged to instigate more affordable pricing, although estimate the lower and upper threshold at 100 and 250 procedures to reach a compromise between cost per procedure and overall costs. Thus almost all studies about robot-assisted operations in gynecology where larger number of cases are observed, and also reviews and meta-analyses, show exemplary weaknesses. These are retrospective and short-term observations (relating to operation time, length of hospital stay, blood loss, perioperative complications, etc.), with no randomized controlled trials and frequently no appropriate control groups, and data are scarce on about long-term outcomes. Also in meta-analyses only perioperative acquired data are compared, matched and summarized. Mostly, the question of does a patient feel better by a robot-assisted operation in the long term, or does she live longer, or longer and better than by an open abdominal or traditional laparoscopic operation is not answered.

A selection of 12 current publications should illustrate on the one hand the host of problems, and, on the other hand, depict a choice of exemplary topics.

Surgical Technical Considerations on Robot-assisted Operations

In the review paper of Tse et al.[1] (Queen Mary Hospital, Hong Kong) the authors deal with complications of robot-assisted operations and how to prevent them. They arrive at the conclusion that robot-assisted operations allow a more precise operation in patients with gynecological malignancies; the incidence of complications would be comparable or even lower than in traditional laparoscopy and laparotomy. The major prevention strategy of complications is good knowledge of abdominal and pelvic anatomy, handling of the robotic system, availability of an experienced team and a careful manipulation of the instruments. Continued analyses of surgical complications and long-term survival rates are demanded in order to improve the quality of treatment and to ensure appropriate oncological results. As practical items it is emphasized that robot-assisted operations in gynecological oncology are safe, the incidence of complications is low and complications essentially occur because of patient positioning, capnoperitoneum, trocar placement, inadequate instrument handling, isolation errors and poor communication between the surgeon (console surgeon) and the bedside assistant.

Vessel injuries are recognized as the main cause of death in the context of robot-assisted operations. An exhaustive knowledge about anatomy, utilization of fundamental surgical principles of traction force and counterforce and dissection along tissue borders would be the key to preventing complications; equally an experienced team is very important. A convincing evidence that a prophylactic preoperative ureteral stent insertion, open access techniques and mechanical bowel preparation could prevent ureteral, bowel and vessel injuries is not available. Moreover, there is no explicit scientific knowledge that the use of barbed sutures for vaginal cuff closure could prevent a vaginal cuff dehiscence.

For further investigation and trials the following need to be done: analysis of long-term survival data of patients with uterine, cervical and ovarian cancer compared to traditional laparoscopic and open abdominal procedures, use of prophylactic ureteral stent insertion previous to radical hysterectomy, use of mechanical bowel preparation in robotic surgery, significance, impact and consequences of port-site metastases after robot-assisted operations, especially in ovarian cancer patients, and the evaluation of patient-based results (so-called patient-reported outcomes, in question of quality of life, patient preferences and patient satisfaction) of robot-assisted surgery.

Robot-assisted Operations in Endometrial Cancer

In a meta-analysis in 2016[2] (Shanxi, PR China) about the comparison of robot-assisted versus traditional laparoscopic operations for staging of endometrial cancer there were no significant differences between both groups (robot-assisted operations, $n = 912$ patients; traditional laparoscopic operations, $n = 1,193$) concerning operation time and number of retrieved lymph nodes. There were significant differences with regard to hospital stay, total blood loss and conversion rate to laparotomy, each with better results in robot-assisted operations. Particularly, a mean intraoperative blood loss difference of about 80 mL seems to be unimportant. However, the presentation of this result is symptomatic and representative of many studies of this type, because a significant difference is suggested between diverse surgical procedures and technique; indeed, it is only a theoretical difference that has no influence on patient condition, prognosis, quality of life or long-term general health. The authors conclude in this meta-analysis that the robot-assisted alternative to the traditional laparoscopy is clinically safe and effective, and that further studies are necessary to concretely determine potential advantages or disadvantages of robot-assisted operations. Besides absence of data from prospective evaluations, most important analyses for long-term treatment quality and results (disease-free survival and overall survival) or the quality of life of these patients are ignored completely.

In a further meta-analysis by Park et al.[3] in 2016 (Seoul, South Korea) 24 studies for comparison of robot-assisted versus open hysterectomies in endometrial cancer and another 24 studies for comparison of robot-assisted versus traditional laparoscopic hysterectomies were considered. There were no significant differences in the results for survival data. Duration of hospital stay, blood loss, complication rates, transfusions and hospital readmissions were significantly lower and, in fact, more infrequent after robot-assisted operations. But overall operation time and the incidence of vaginal cuff dehiscence were higher. Patient-based results (i.e., patient-related outcomes) showed a significant benefit for robot-assisted operations, whereupon data from only one study in this meta-analysis were reported. Accordingly, the authors' conclusion fails by assuming that robot-assisted hysterectomies in patients with endometrial cancer would be, in generally, more safe and the better option compared to open abdominal or traditional laparoscopic hysterectomies. Further prospective trials with analysis of long-term data are required.

Another meta-analysis by Xie et al.[4] (Peking, 2016) that took into account 19 studies, consisting of 3,056 patients with endometrial cancer, in which only robot-assisted with traditional laparoscopic operations are compared, gives almost the same results. Superiority of robot-assisted hysterectomies is assumed, but a verification of this assumption is demanded by the authors in their conclusions. As weaknesses of this meta-analysis it is observed that no randomized, prospective and controlled trials are included and no relevant long-term follow-up data for survival rates were available. Only in three studies results for survival data were presented, in which the median follow-up time for robot-assisted operation was less than three years. Therefore an equivalent oncological safety in comparison to traditional laparoscopy for that much longer follow-up data are available is not proven at all ("long-term survival outcomes must be tracked to ensure that the cure rates are not compromised with robot-assisted surgery").

Robot-assisted Operations in Cervical Cancer

In the meta-analysis by Liu et al.[5] (2016, Peking, PR China) about robot-assisted operations in cervical cancer patients compared to traditional operations (open abdominal operations and traditional laparoscopies) 19 studies were included for analysis. As main results it was demonstrated that robot-assisted interventions in cervical cancer compared to open abdominal operations were beneficial with regard to length of hospital stay, frequency of complications, blood loss amounts and number of blood transfusions. Compared to traditional laparoscopic surgery there were longer operation times, higher blood losses and shorter hospital stays for robot-assisted operations. The quality of trials was denominated as poor. The included studies would be on a low level of evidence, and they would have a lower standard for reporting. Furthermore, the enrolled studies would have a risk of significant bias. Because in surgical field for prospective randomized controlled trials to be feasible they would need in future a better assessment, especially with regard to the measured methods of outcomes and the exact extent of surgeon experiences. There was also criticism that there were no reports about postoperative functional results such as bladder and sexual function after robotic surgery, "representing a missing opportunity to identify possible benefits which should be attributed to the minimally invasive surgical procedures." Moreover, a striking lack of relevant studies allowing a comparison of the prognosis of the disease subjected to the particular surgical modality was highlighted.

Obviously, a review of Mendivil et al.[6] (2015, Newport Beach, CA, USA) was not noticed in the aforementioned meta-analysis. Here, the 5-year survival rate of patients with cervical cancer was analyzed in a retrospective trial. Patients with cervical cancer were treated either by open abdominal, traditional laparoscopic or robot-assisted hysterectomy. However, this evaluation concerns a relative low case number with 49 laparoscopic (LRH), 58 robot-assisted (RRH) and 39 open abdominal (ORH) operated patients. After 60 months the progression-free survival was 89.8% (LRH), 89.7% (RRH), respectively 84.6% (ORH); the overall survival was 95.9% (LRH), 96.6% (RRH) and 92.3% (ORH). It was reasoned that patients with an early detection of cervical cancer treated with radical hysterectomy have comparable 5-year disease-free and overall survival rates independent of the surgical technique or, more accurately, surgical access. Low case number, heterogeneous comparison groups (e.g., concerning the treated FIGO stage) and the retrospective study design were mentioned as drawbacks of the study by the authors themselves.

In a review of 2017 surgeries, Park et al.[7] (Seoul, South Korea) come to the conclusion that robot-assisted operations have several advantages compared to open abdominal operations. They are successful with regard to usual listing of perioperative benefits. Compared to traditional laparoscopy robot-assisted interventions would have an equivalent effectiveness. The tentative assumption that by future advancements of robot-assisted platforms, robot-assisted operations would be without doubt the better surgical approach for treatment of cervical cancer than conventional laparoscopic surgery is not further substantiated, or rather is not proved on the basis of data. Neither here is it ascertained that there are good designed prospective studies comparing robot-assisted operations in cervical cancer patients with open abdominal and conventional laparoscopic procedures. In addition, long-term results as regards prognosis of cervical cancer (OS, DFS) are not available due to short-term implementation of robot-assisted techniques; therefore, further clinical trials should evaluate the long-term survival rates after robot-assisted surgery in cervical cancer ("research agenda: prospective, randomized trials comparing RRT with abdominal radical trachelectomy or LRT in cervical cancer; clinical trials evaluating long-term survival outcomes").

In a binational retrospective multicenter trial by Sert et al.[8] (2016, Oslo, Norway) data of 419 patients with early stage cervical cancer were analyzed; between 2005 and 2011 robot-assisted radical hysterectomy (RRH) was performed in 259 patients, and an open radical hysterectomy (ORH) in 232 patients. Perioperative parameters showed distinct advantages of robot-assisted radical hysterectomies, the overall complication rate between the two study groups was not significantly different, and intraoperative complications were clearly more unusual in the robotic group. There was no significant difference between both groups regarding recurrence and death rate within a median follow-up of 39 months. It was concluded that the present data "in the absence of randomised trials to compare clinical outcomes with open radical hysterectomy could be hypothesis generating and at least guide clinical management with some degree of uncertainty" and "results from this study should be further evaluated in a larger multi-centre setting with mature surgical experiences." At least, results from a randomized phase III trial, initiated in 2008, of laparoscopic or robotic radical hysterectomy versus abdominal radical hysterectomy in patients with early-stage cervical cancer is eagerly awaited in 2022[9].

Robot-assisted Operations in Ovarian Cancer

In a review[10] (2017) the application of the robot-assisted technique in the treatment of early ovarian cancer has been valued positively. Robot-assisted operations in the treatment or within the scope of surgical staging in patients with ovarian cancer would be underestimated. Certainly, the available data from literature would show a low level of evidence; comparisons with other techniques with respect to accesses (laparotomy, traditional laparoscopy) would suggest different advantages of robot-assisted operations without compromising the survival rate. It is underlined that a careful selection of patients who are appropriate for robot-assisted operations has to be made. Particularly in patients with an early ovarian cancer robot-assisted interventions would be a feasible alternative to traditional laparoscopy without relevant differences concerning perioperative and oncological outcomes. In cases of advanced ovarian cancer only a portion of highly selected patients would be eligible for robot-assisted operations; this concerns patients with limited peritoneal carcinomatosis or isolated and localized relapsing tumors. Prospective and randomized data are missing completely in this analysis. Nowadays, in ovarian cancer with diffuse peritoneal carcinomatosis and multiquadrant involvement, diffuse metastasis in the upper abdomen, etc., a robot-assisted operation is not indicated. However, in future, new robotic techniques could overcome the current limitations of robot-assisted operations in surgical treatment of advanced ovarian cancer.

Robot-assisted Laparoscopic Surgery in Urogynecological Diseases

In a review and meta-analysis of Pan et al.[11] (2016) the studies about robot-assisted and traditional laparoscopic sacrocolpopexies (RALSC versus LSC) were compared. Seven studies were included in this analysis with 264 RALSCs and 257 LSCs. The clinical results between RALSC and LSC were comparable and did not show significant differences; however, an inferior efficiency was observed for RALSC as regards costs and operation time. The authors recommend self-effacement and critical handling for the use robotic assistance in urogynecological operations. In particular, advantages of robot-assisted operations relating to complication rates and anatomical and functional results are still unclear. Notably, in studies where long-term results concerning prolapse relapse and patient satisfaction (evaluated by diverse methods and questionnaires) have been analyzed no differences between robot-assisted and traditional laparoscopic approaches were demonstrated.

Evaluation of Technical Innovations of the Robotic System

In a review by Rocha et al.[12] (2016, Oporto, Portugal) the technique of sentinel node biopsy in endometrial and cervical carcinomas with the aid of fluorescence imaging (with indocyanine green (ICG)) was investigated. Ten studies with a total of 422 patients were consulted for the review; 368 of these patients were treated by robot-assisted surgery, 39 by open abdominal surgery and 15 by traditional laparoscopy. The detection rate of the sentinel lymph node by ICG injection into the cervix uteri was 78–100%, hysteroscopic application technique resulted in a detection rate of 33–100%; the sensitivity and negative predictive value varied between 50–100% and 88–100%; with the injection in two quadrants of the cervix the highest detection rates were reported. Complications by ICG application did not appear. It was concluded that the fluorescence technique by ICG application is feasible both for robot-assisted intervention (the highly represented group in the available literature about this topic shows by itself that fluorescence-guided imaging is very practicable in the field of robot-assisted surgery) and open abdominal and traditional laparoscopic techniques, safe and time efficient, and it seems to be a reliable method for mapping of mainly pelvic and possibly para-aortic lymph nodes in early cervical and endome-trial cancer.

Randomized trials with higher patient numbers are needed. Nothing significant could be deduced out of the data and available literature for robot-assisted surgery performed for sentinel lymph node mapping and biopsy. Certainly, because of the high percentage of patients treated with robot-assisted ICG- and fluorescence-based lymph node biopsy it is demonstrated that this technique is already implemented on the surgical schedule of robot-assisted interventions as a sort of an algorithm.

Review of Robot-assisted Laparoscopic Operations in Gynecology

In a latest review from 2017[13] (Haifa, Israel) all applications of robot-assisted operations in gynecology are recapitulated and evaluated. Although the title of this publication, "The Future Is Here," - anticipates a positive assessment of the robot-assisted surgical technique no important and comparative data for long-term survival, relapse rates and quality of life in oncological diseases, and long-term success rates of robotic surgery in benign gynecological conditions (e.g., long-term success rate of urogynecological operations or after myomectomies, scientific knowledge about robotic surgical treatment of endometriosis is sparse and the advantages of the use of robot-assisted laparoscopy are very questionable) were presented. It is concluded that primarily randomized controlled clinical trials (RCTs) would be able to place robot-assisted operations in gynecology as the predominant technique and would be able to define clearly whose weight and preferential applications are in use in gynecological diseases. The authors denominate eleven indexed RCTs for different sectors and for several sets of questions in gynecological surgery.

In summary, data are needed for long-term follow-up; furthermore for oncological studies this means information about quality of life and especially about survival and relapse rates, and for non-oncological trials specifications of quality of life and long-term effectiveness of the performed surgical intervention (e.g., in prolapse surgery). The information regarding these parameters should preferably be acquired in prospective controlled and randomized trials.

CURRENT SITUATION OF ROBOT-ASSISTED LAPAROSCOPIC OPERATIONS IN GYNECOLOGY

In most European countries robotic surgery with the daVinci® system is well established. The density of systems is low in comparison to the United States. Generally, medical progress is expensive (e.g., cytotoxic drugs). Thus, additional costs for robotic surgery demonstrating decisive advantages in long-term patient health have to be accepted.[14]

The daVinci® system and technique is an advanced technique and is developed, enhanced and refined rapidly. Thus, no price competition exists, making reduction of costs unlikely in the near future (at least in the next decade). Optimization of the daVinci® operations is necessary (dedicated robotic surgeons, correct selection of complex cases, restriction of the number of used instruments, high degree of capacity utilization by a high number of cases, multidisciplinary use, reduction of hospital stay). Prospective RCTs are needed to compare costs between different surgical approaches and different procedures to determine operations where robotic surgery can be used cost effectively (e.g., obese patients). Furthermore, prospective studies must prove the efficacy of robotic surgery in long-term follow-up and quality of life observations so that maybe even higher costs would be justified if this approach provides the best possible care for patients (societal factor of costs).

For surgeons who are not comfortable with advanced laparoscopic procedures, robotic surgery could be an alternative in daily patient care as these surgeons may provide minimally invasive surgery to their patients in procedures formerly conducted with laparotomy. For experienced laparoscopic surgeons, robotic surgery may offer a further increase in precision and also a decrease of physical workload.

The future of robotics looks bright as robots will become even smaller and easier to handle, and surgeons will get better performing robotic surgery. The decision to adopt robotic surgery will have to take into account not only cost analyses but also technical characteristics and possible impact on patients, as well as hospitals' organizational framework. Rejecting robotic technology could be as risky as adopting it.

REFERENCES

1. Tse KY, Ngan HYS, Lim PC. Robot-assisted gynaecological cancer surgery and complications and prevention. Best Pract Res Clin Obstet Gynaecol. 2017. April 23. Online.
2. Chen SH, Li ZA, Huang R, et al. Robot-assisted versus conventional laparoscopic surgery for endometrial cancer staging: a meta-analysis. Taiwan J Obstet Gynecol. 2016;55(4):488-94.
3. Park DA, Lee DH, Kim SW, et al. Comparative safety and effectiveness of robot-assisted laparoscopic hysterectomy versus conventional laparoscopy and laparotomy for endometrial cancer: a systematic review and meta-analysis. Eur J Surg Oncol. 2016;42(9): 1303-14.
4. Xie W, Cao D, Yang J, et al. Robot-assisted surgery versus conventional laparoscopic surgery for endometrial cancer: a systematic review and meta-analysis. J Cancer Res Clin Oncol. 2016;142(10): 2173-83.
5. Liu Z, Li X, Tian S, et al. Superiority of robotic surgery for cervical cancer in comparison with traditional approaches: a systematic review and meta-analysis. Int J Surg. 2017;40:145-54.
6. Mendivil AA, Rettenmaier MA, Abaid LN, et al. Survival rate comparisons amongst cervical cancer patients treated with an open, robotic-assisted or laparoscopic radical hysterectomy: a five-year experience. Surg Oncol. 2016;25(1):66-71.
7. Park JY, Nam JH. Role of robotic surgery in cervical malignancy. Best Prac Res Clin Obstet Gynaecol. 2017. April 24. Online.
8. Sert BM, Boggess JF, Ahmad S, et al. Robot-assisted versus open radical hysterectomy: a multi-institutional experience for early-stage cervical cancer. Eur J Surg Oncol. 2016;42(4):513-22.
9. Obermair A, Gebski V, Frumovitz M, et al. A phase III randomized clinical trial comparing laparoscopic or robotic radical hysterectomy with abdominal radical hysterectomy in patients with early stage cervical cancer. J Minim Invasive Gynecol. 2008;15(5):584-8.
10. Lucidi A, Chiantera V, Gallotta V, et al. Role of robotic surgery in ovarian malignancy. Best Pract Res Clin Obstet Gynaecol. 2017. May 10. Online.
11. Pan K, Zhang Y, Wang Y, et al. A systematic review and meta-analysis of conventional laparoscopic sacrocolpopexy versus robot-assisted laparoscopic sacrocolpopexy. Int J Gynecol Obstet. 2016;132(3): 284-91.
12. Rocha A, Domínguez AM, Lécuru F, et al. Indocyanine green and infrared fluorescence in detection of sentinel lymph nodes in endometrial and cervical cancer staging—a systematic review. Eur J Obstet Gynecol Reprod Biol. 2016; 206: 213-9.
13. Lauterbach R, Matanes E, Lowenstein L. Review of robotic surgery in gynecology—the future is here. Rambam Maimonides Med J. 2017;8(2):e0019.

Section 3

Specific Hysteroscopic Procedures

KIEL SCH•OL

46 of Gynaecological Endoscopy

Diagnostic and **Office** Hysteroscopy

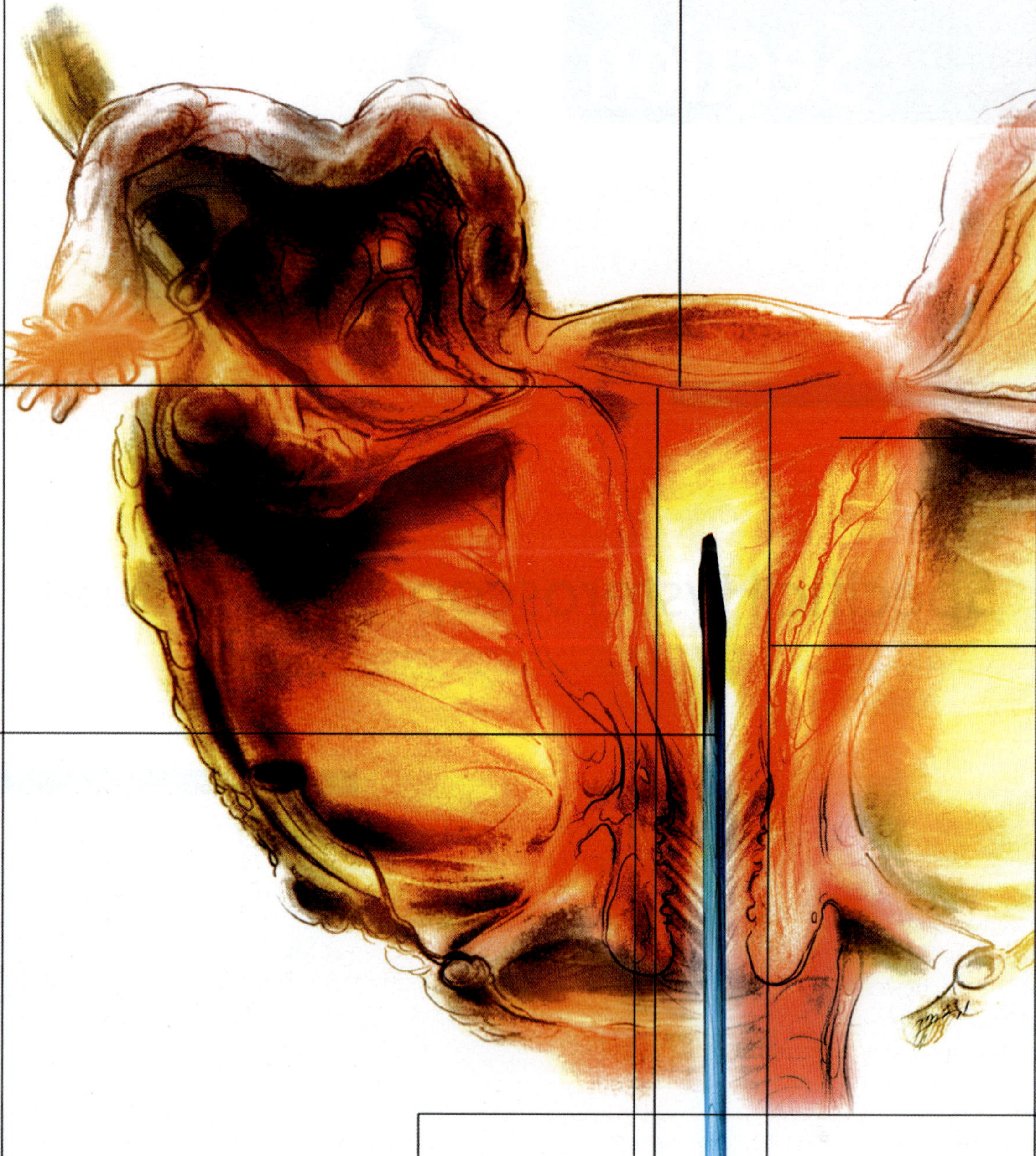

Chapter 46

Diagnostic and Office Hysteroscopy

Lotte Clevin

INTRODUCTION

This chapter discusses mini-hysteroscopy used for diagnostic purposes and for treatment of minor intrauterine pathology in an office setting.

INSTRUMENTS AND EQUIPMENT

Mini-hysteroscope

The literature does not clearly define the size limits for mini-hysteroscopes. The author describes here a mini-hysteroscope with a diameter of less than 5 mm that can be introduced through the cervical canal without analgesia or dilatation. The majority of studies on mini-hysteroscopy focus on this category of scopes. Some mini-hysteroscopes are oval in cross-section as is the internal os.

If there is a cervical stenosis or the patient feels severe pain during passage of the cervical canal, a cervical block with or without dilation might be required.

Most mini-hysteroscopes have a working channel of 5–7 French for insertion of graspers, scissors, polyp snares or electrodes.

Valves for distention fluid have different shapes; a continuous flow system is recommended (Figs 46.1A and B). The newest development goes toward thinner and smaller resectoscopes where the mini-hysteroscopic procedures now can be accomplished with resection due to development of small loops and a variety of working electrodes. Both monopolar and bipolar electrodes are available, but the bipolar is still recommended because the use of pure saline as distention media is the safest and will minimize the risk of water intoxication. Especially endometrial sampling in postmenopausal women with bleeding can be performed with greater sensibility and specificity when the biopsy is both visually conducted as well as increased in depth and wideness (Figs. 46.1C and D).

Distention of the Cavity

Examination of and operative procedures in the uterine cavity require a distention of the cavity by a continuous flow of fluid, usually sterile saline. The continuous flow will clear the vision and flush away mucus, blood and tissue debris.

The cavity will usually distend at a fluid pressure of 50–80 mm Hg. The recommended flow is the lowest possible, which gives a sufficient distention. Too high a pressure will cause uterine contraction (pain) and loss of fluid into the abdominal cavity through the tubes. Sometimes a pressure of 125 mm Hg is necessary to obtain a clear vision.

For office hysteroscopy, a pressure bag to compress a 1L bag of saline is sufficient to carry out diagnostic hysteroscopy and biopsy. This method requires a nurse to attend to the pressure bag and maintain it at a constant pressure throughout the procedure. The pressure is normally set at around 125 mm Hg at the beginning of a procedure.

A hysteroscopic pump can maintain the pressure sufficiently to give a clear vision. In the beginning, it is set at 50–80 mm Hg, but it may be necessary to increase the pressure later.

Sterile saline is the preferred distention media, due to the low risk of water intoxication during intravasation of the fluid, and is required if bipolar electrosurgery is used. Bipolar electrodes for cutting and tissue evaporation require a conductive ion or electrolyte-rich medium to close the circuit between active and return electrode (Figs. 46.2A and B).

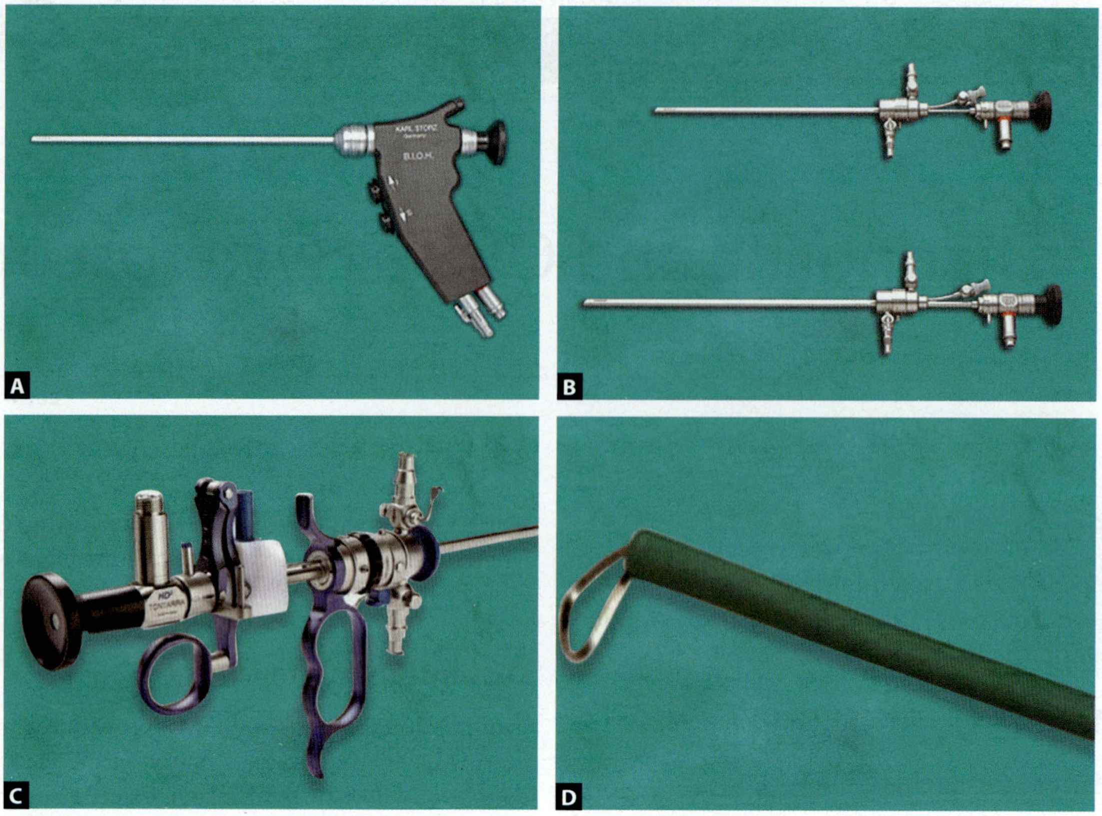

Figs. 46.1A to D: (A) Bettocchi® integrated office hysteroscope (Karl Storz); (B) Bettocchi® hysteroscopes (Karl Storz); (C) Gubini mini-resectoscope, 2,9 telescope, 5 Fr working channel—oval shape; (D) Loop for resection biopsies and minor resections.

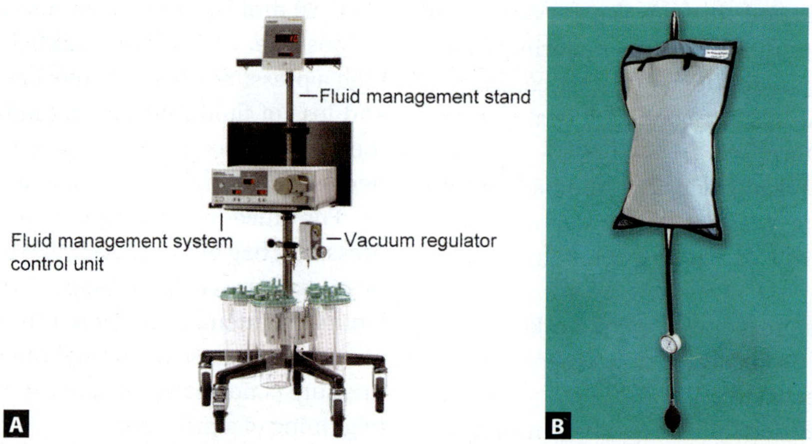

Figs. 46.2A and B: (A) Hysteroscopic pump; (B) A pressure bag.

Instruments

The following instruments are suitable for taking biopsies and removing pathologies or foreign bodies from the cavity:

- Biopsy cup grasper
- Scissors.

Bipolar electrodes (for cutting and tissue evaporation). Other devices, such as a morcellator or a polyp snare, are also available (Figs. 46.3A to D).

Electrosurgery

Bipolar mini-electrodes (5 Fr) make it possible to cut and evaporate minor pathologies in the cavity. It is a safe bipolar method performed in saline. The technique requires a 5–7 French working channel, a generator, a foot pedal and a cable. Bipolar electrodes come in both reusable and single use versions. Here, the single-use version is described because this type has special features for cutting and evaporation of the tissue (Figs. 46.3A to D).

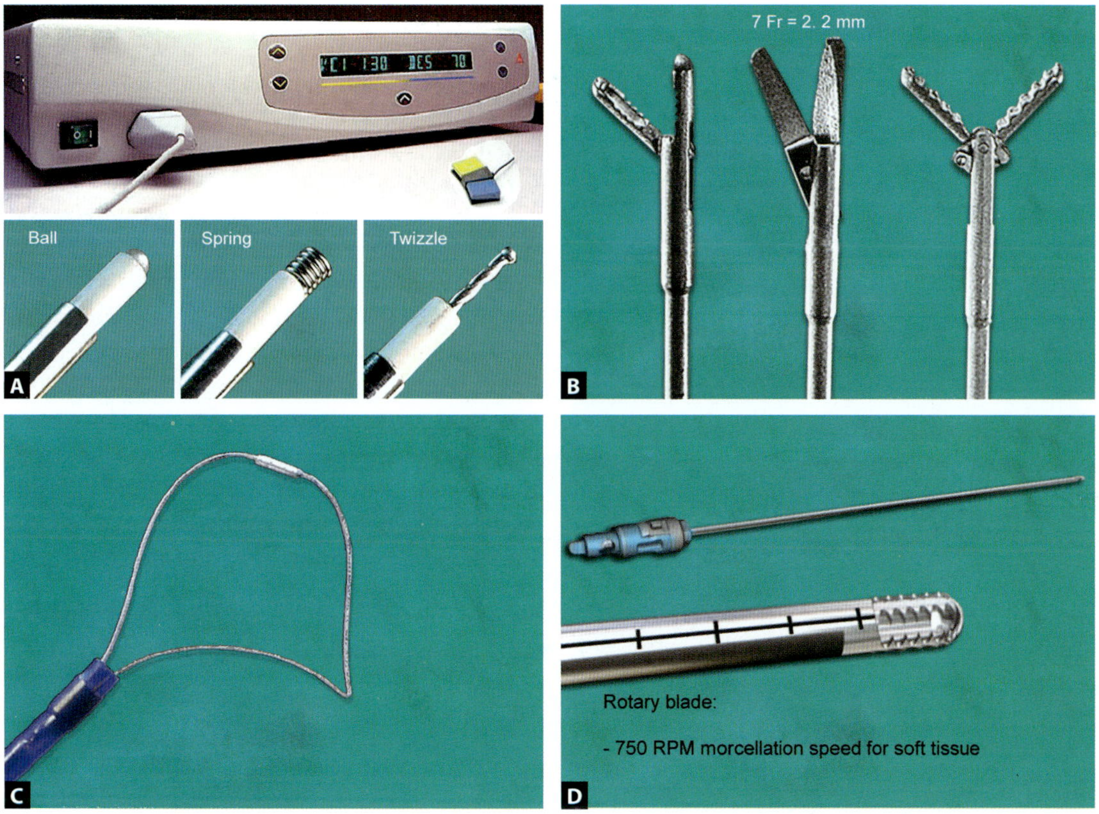

Figs. 46.3A to D: (A) Bipolar generator for the minielectrodes: Ball, spring, twizzle; (B) Biopsy cup, scissors, grasper; (C) Monopolar polyp snare; (D) Hysteroscopic morcellator.

Endoscopic Stack

As with all other endoscopic procedures, the following equipment is needed for optimal vision:

- Camera and camera box
- Light generator and light cable (white light) [some systems have narrow band imaging (NBI) light as well]
- Monitor.

Diathermy generator/cables and hysteroscopic pump (see above) (Fig. 46.4).

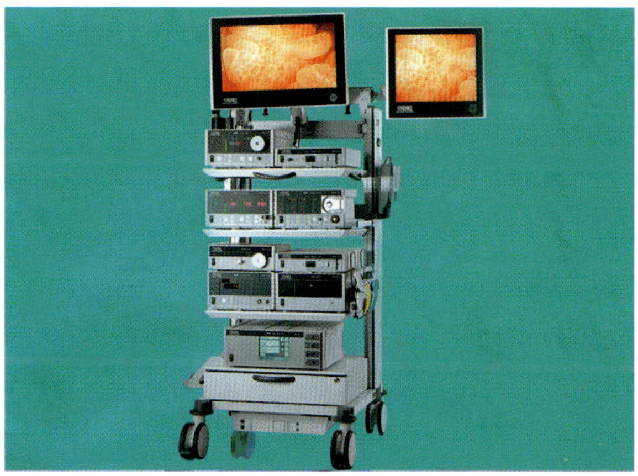

Fig. 46.4: Endoscopic stack for gynecologic endoscopic surgery (laparoscopy and hysteroscopy) with electrosurgical unit, CO_2 insufflator, light source and high-definition imaging (HDTV) monitor (Karl Storz 3D system) as well as control unit for hysteroscopic surgery (Karl Storz).

PREPARATIONS

Preoperative Diagnosis

It is important to know the kind and size of pathology you are dealing with before choosing the mini-hysteroscopic approach. Only minor pathologies can be removed with this small diameter scope, mainly because there has been no dilation of the cervical canal. The limits described for the mini-hysteroscopic technique are as follows:

- Polyps up to 20 mm
- Fibroids type 0 and 1, up to 18 mm septum (seldom limits).

Fundal pathologies are difficult to remove and require a special technique (see below). Large-size pathologies are time consuming to remove and will cause edema of the endometrium and thereby compromise vision.

Transvaginal ultrasound scan (TVS) and especially saline infusion sonography (SIS) is the golden

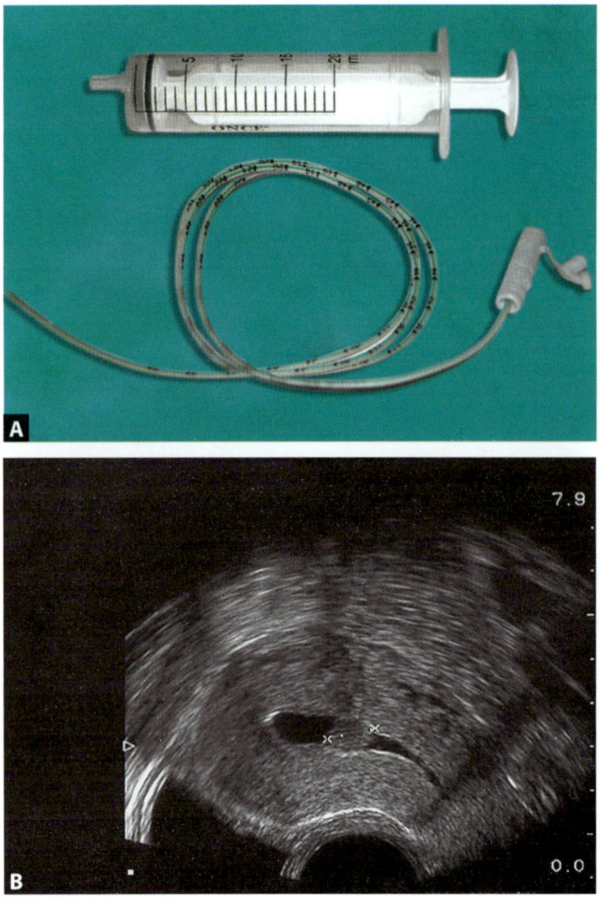

Figs. 46.5A and B: Equipment for saline infusion sonography: Sterile syringe (20 cc).

standard to assess the intracavitary conditions before hysteroscopy.

A low-cost method for SIS is a baby feeding tube 1–1½ mm in diameter inserted through the cervical os into the cavity using a tampon forceps. While performing TVS, the nurse injects sterile saline from a syringe. This way the cavity opens and pathologies can be assessed for origin, size and type. The procedure is painless if the water pressure is gradually increased (Figs. 46.5A and B).

Timing of the Procedure

In premenopausal women, the endometrium gets thick and fluffy close to the time of the menstrual period. Due to the small diameter scope, vision is easily obstructed and pathology, such as polyps, might "disappear" into the endometrium. Removal at the base of the polyp is then compromised. Bleeding will also blur vision because the small diameter flow of the channel makes flushing difficult. To avoid these difficulties, optimal timing of the procedure is right after the menstrual bleeding has finished. Medical thinning of the endometrium is also an option. Administration of continuous oral contraceptives (the pill with no pause) or a Mirena for a minimum time of respectively 2–3 months or 6 months will provide a sufficient thinning of the endometrium.

Preparation of the Patient

A well-informed patient has realistic expectations for the procedure and will comply better. The surgeon has optimal working conditions if the patient has full confidence that she is "the boss" and will be heard if she asks for a break for regaining control and breathing. If pain is observed, due to contractions of the uterus, just turn-down the pressure, wait and ask the patient to say when the pain has gone. Usually, the rest of the procedure can be performed with no discomfort.

Analgesics

"Vocal local" means the form of communication or diversion whereby the nurse is next to the patient and asks questions on anything other than the procedure or pain. When the patient is asked to talk about her job or holiday, she focuses no longer on anxiety or possible pain, but concentrates on answering the questions. This results in better working conditions for the surgeon and at the end of the day a satisfied patient.

Nevertheless, in 10% of patients a cervical block with or without dilatation is needed to pass the cervical canal and enter the uterine cavity. Apply Citanest Dental (4–6 ampoules) into the cervix with a 27 G needle, wait 5 minutes and then entry is possible. Other methods for cervical stenosis are described below (Fig. 46.6).

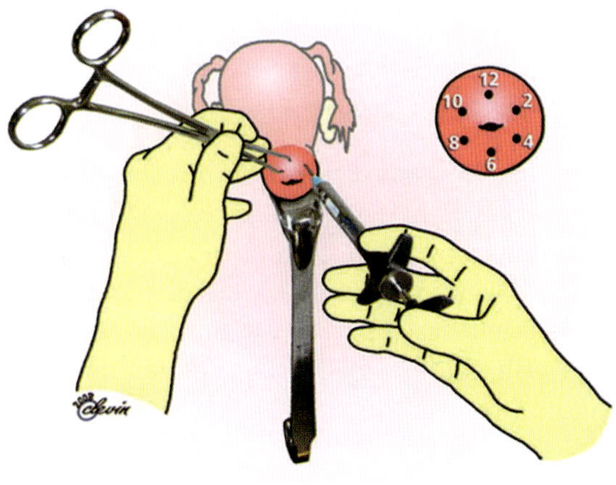

Fig. 46.6: Cervical block.

Discomfort due to contractions of the uterus after the procedure is prevented by administering 1 g of paracetamol and 400 mg of ibuprofen orally, 30 min before the procedure.

Position of the Patient and the Equipment Including the Surgeon

The patient is in a lithotomy position with a plastic bag underneath the buttocks to collect fluid (Fig. 46.7).

The endoscopic stack, the pump (fluid bag) and the table with the instruments are on the left side of the patient as a convenience for the surgeon (vice versa when the surgeon is left handed). If all cables and tubing are on one side, this makes the handling easier and the patient can get on and off the bench without struggling with cables and tubing.

To maintain a steady hand during the procedure, the surgeon can sit back to front on a wheeled chair and thereby rest the underarms on the back of the chair. By this means unintended movement of the scope can be avoided while in the cavity.

Vaginal Washing

No vaginal wash is necessary. Several scientific papers have shown that the risk of infections during mini-hysteroscopy is minimal.

No speculum or tenaculum is required because the introduction of the mini-hysteroscopy is done by the vaginoscopic approach.

Vaginoscopic Approach

By utilizing the water flow and the vision through the scope, it is possible to move along the vagina to the cervical os, through the cervical canal into the uterine cavity. Observe the movement of the scope by looking downward through the vagina to the cervical os, then looking upward through the cervical canal into the uterus (in the anteverted uterus) (Fig. 46.8).

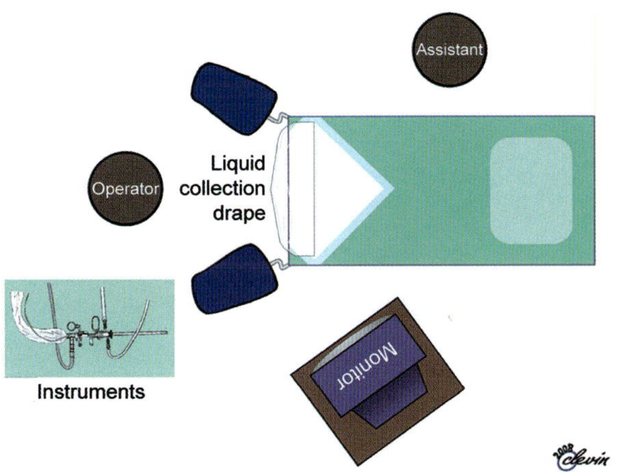

Fig. 46.7: All equipment are placed to the left of the patient.

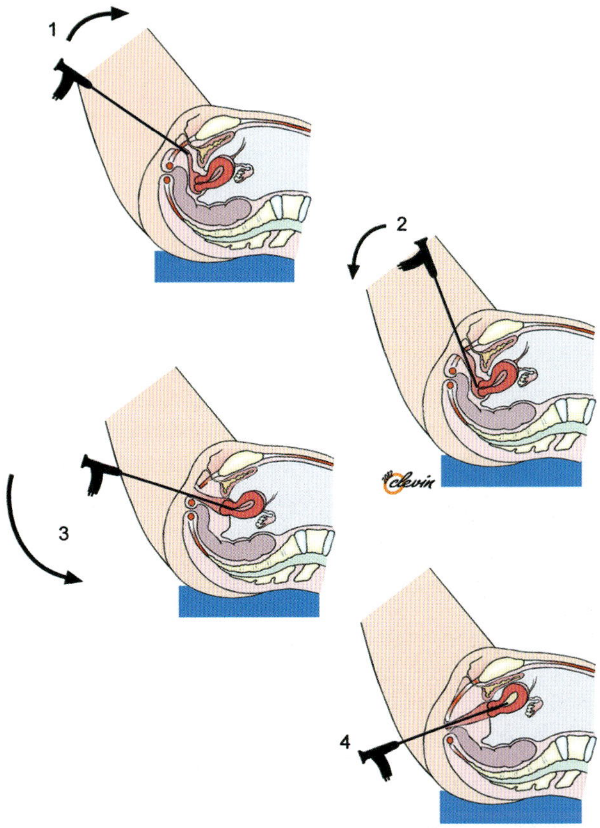

Fig. 46.8: Vaginoscopic approach.

Diagnostic Hysteroscopy

If there are difficulties in locating the cervix and the external os, go to the posterior fornix, look for the mucus and then the external os is found. In very anteverted uteri this might be difficult in the beginning (Fig. 46.9). If using an oval scope, passage of the internal os is easy by turning the scope 90° to fit the os.

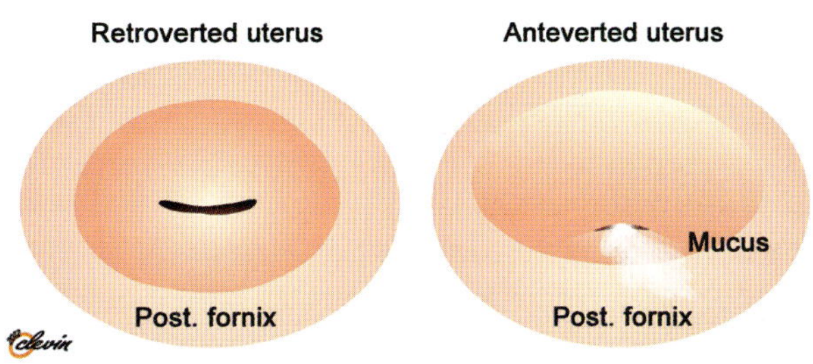

Fig. 46.9: Look for the mucus in the anteverted uterus to locate the external os.

Unlike other procedures all these structures can be examined by close-up vision:

- Vaginal mucosa
- Portio and the external os
- The cervical canal and the internal os
- The uterine cavity with the endometrium and the tubal os on both sides.

A biopsy cup can be inserted through the working channel to take visually guided endometrial biopsies. Definite diagnostic hysteroscopic criteria have not yet been developed. There is no specific description of the different pathologies. Lesions suggestive of carcinoma or complex atypical hyperplasia vary in appearance. However, irregular lesions, multiple lesions, prominent and/or bizarre blood vessels and friable/necrotic tissue are highly suggestive. Biopsies, including excision of the lesion, should be undertaken. Vaporization of any endo-metrial lesion is not recommended as the opportunity to obtain histological confirmation is lost.

Particular attention should be paid to the hormonal drug history, in particular progesterone, which induces pseudodecidualization of the endometrium, which assumes the appearance of neoplasia.

Removal of Minor Pathologies

Keeping in mind the size of the instruments, including the fact that the cervical os has not been dilated, minor pathology can be removed by either mechanical instruments, such as scissors and graspers, or in combination with bipolar electrodes.
The following lesions can be removed successfully:

- Endometrial polyps (fibroids)
- Synechiae or adhesions
- Congenital malformations, such as septa Retained tissue—typically after abortion
- Foreign bodies, such as intrauterine devices (IUDs)

  Conditions of interest affecting the cervix include:
- Cervical stenosis (cervical polyps)
- Cervical carcinoma
- Lower segment cesarean scar defects.

Operative Technique

In mini-hysteroscopy everything is small and delicate. Working with these instruments in the uterine cavity, the procedures become much easier and offer no discomfort for the patient. The instruments are inserted so that visibility is optimal. The tip of the instrument is visible. The whole scope is then moved back and forth, to the sides or turned around. This insures the best and safest procedure.

The working channel in the mini-hysteroscopes is either 5 or 7 French. Therefore, when taking out tissue with a biopsy cup or a grasper, it is not possible to retract the tissue through the working channel. Instead leave the forceps in the channel and remove the whole scope and the forceps together.

Endometrial Biopsy

For collecting an endometrial biopsy for microscopic diagnosis, the scraping technique is used. Insert the biopsy cup, open the jaws, scrape forward in the region for biopsy, then close the jaws and retract the whole scope and the biopsy cup (Fig. 46.10).

Removal of Pathology

Polyps

Polyps can be removed either by using scissors or just the biopsy cup alone to cut or grab the polyp at the base. Larger polyps have to be cut using electrodes, such as a single-use twizzle or a reusable bipolar device, which is bent at the tip (for fundal polyps).

The twizzle can be bent as well. Put it through the working channel, bend the tip, retract the twizzle to the tip of the scope and then insert the scope with the twizzle within the working channel into the uterine cavity (Fig. 46.11).

The trick is to cut the polyp at the base, i.e., at the level of the endometrium, no further and still deep enough. Larger polyps must be divided into smaller pieces otherwise they cannot be removed through the narrow non-dilated internal os (Fig. 46.12). Do not cut off the whole polyp at once, otherwise it will float around in the cavity because of the continuously running fluid and be very difficult to catch. Leave a

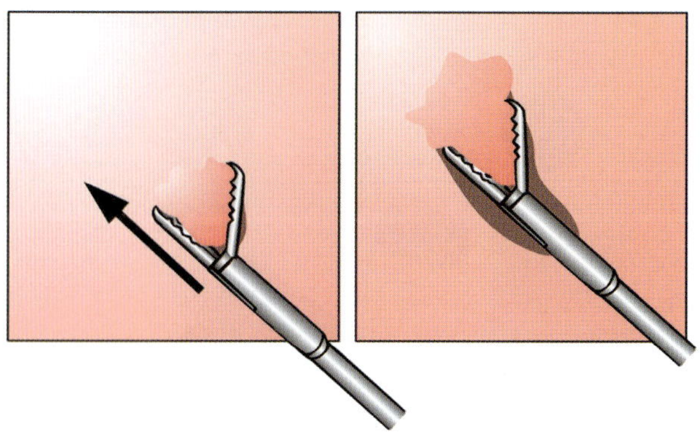

Fig. 46.10: Endometrial biopsy by the scraping technique.

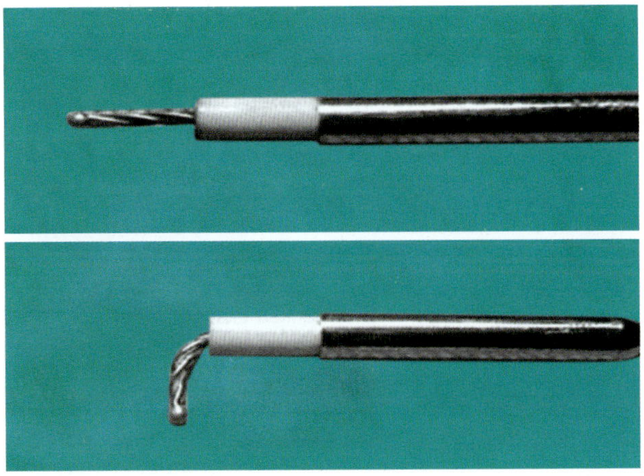

Fig. 46.11: Bending the tip of the twizzle.

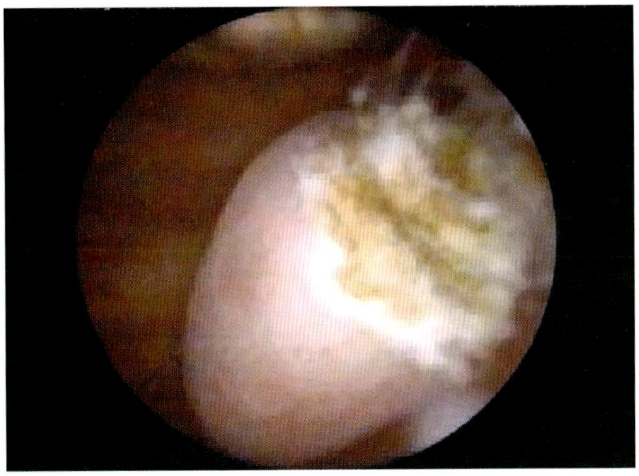

Fig. 46.13: The polyp is still attached in a small area.

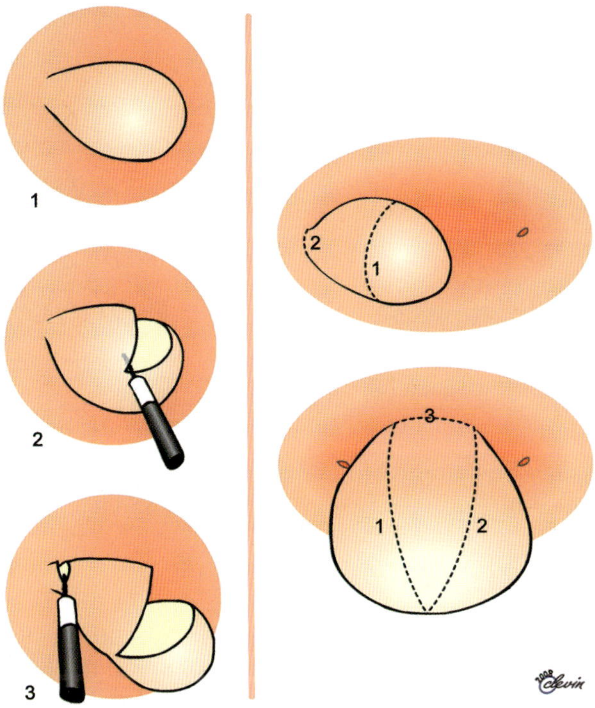

Fig. 46.12: Two slicing techniques.

small piece uncut, then grab the polyp with the biopsy cup and retract the whole scope and biopsy cup still positioned in the working channel (Fig. 46.13).

To prevent re-occurrence of the polyps, the endometrial tissue at the origin of the polyp can be evaporated with a ball or a spring electrode.

Polyps can also be removed using a polyp snare which is monopolar and then requires glycine or sorbitol as a distention fluid.

Finally, new equipment, such as the hysteroscopic morcellator, can be used but the technique requires a special hysteroscope.

Fibroids

The slicing technique can be used on fibrotic tissue as well. Slice the fibroid into pieces that can pass the internal os while retracting the scope. Due to its concave jaws the biopsy cup is optimal for removing tissue. With the grasper it is often difficult to grab the tissue and hold onto it all the way through the cervical canal.

Small bits of left over fibrotic tissue can eventually be evaporated, especially in the fundus.

A special technique is described to enucleate type 2 fibroids. By this method the endometrium over the fibroid is sliced open and, using the twizzle or another electrode to enucleate the pathology, the fibroid is then lifted out of the myometrium. This technique is rarely used as these smaller type 2 fibroids seldom cause symptoms.

Synechiae

In fertility patients where synechiae have developed after D&Cs (either due to abortion or postpartum bleeding) avoid the use of diathermy so that the endometrium can recover. If possible, use only the scissors. If not possible, then the twizzle can be used to break down the adhesions. Increasing the flow or pressure of the distention fluid will push the cavity open (but may cause short pain due to contractions of the uterus) (Fig. 46.14).

There are still no evidence-based recommendations on how to avoid re-occurrence of synechiae. It is advised to apply a copper IUD, administer oral estrogen (4 mg a day for 3–4 weeks) and/or apply prophylactic adhesion material into the cavity (hyaluronic acid).

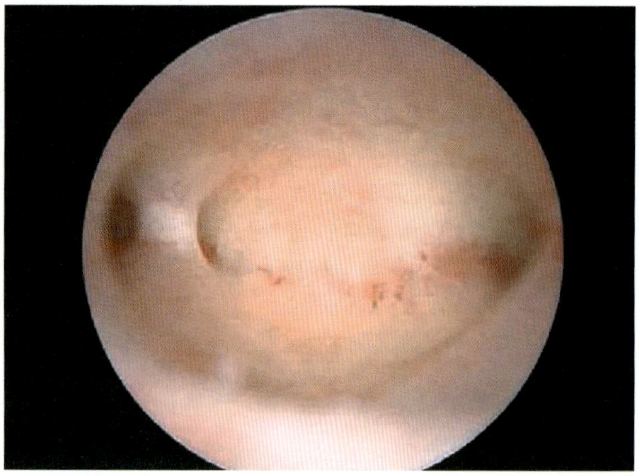

Fig. 46.14: A synechia close to the right tubal os.

Septum

Fertility patients with a uterine septum will benefit from removing the septum. This can be done in the office setting with the twizzle. A real septum [verified by magnetic resonance imaging (MRI) scan] is a fibrotic wall between the two sides of the uterine cavity. By utilizing pressure from the distention fluid and the twizzle, the septum can be cut. Stop when the vessels of the myometrium become visible. The procedure is then safe with no risk of perforation at the fundus. The septum tissue looks whiter than the myometrium (Figs. 46.15A and B).

Practical Manual for Laparoscopic and Hysteroscopic Gynecological Surgery

Hysteroscopic Sterilization

This permanent method has revolutionized anticontraceptives for women. Hysteroscopic sterilization can, as any other mini-hysteroscopic procedure, be performed without any anesthesia in the outpatient clinic or in the office. If the vaginoscopic approach during mini-hysteroscopy is mastered, this procedure is easy and with no discomfort. The endometrium

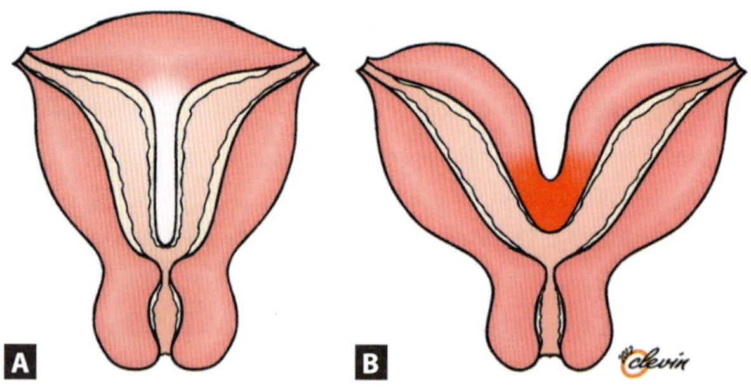

Figs. 46.15A and B: (A) Septum with fibrotic tissue (white); (B) Didelphys with well-vascularized myometrium (red).

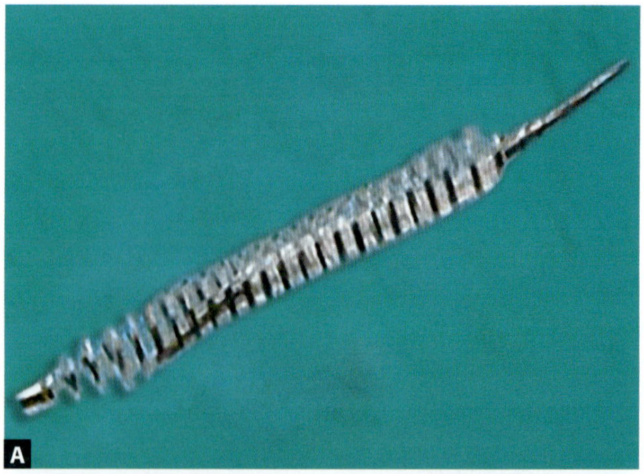

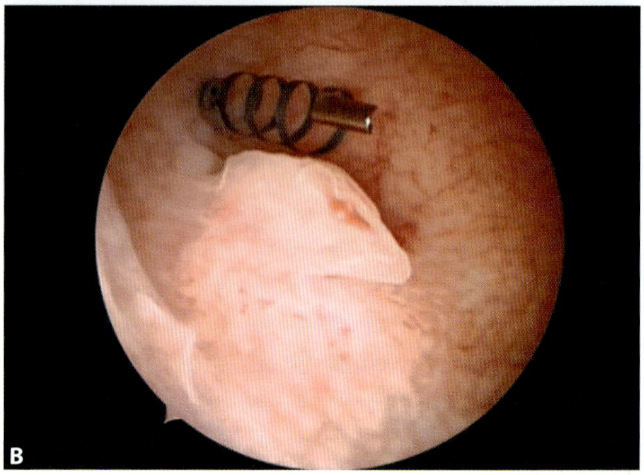

Figs. 46.16A and B: (A) The Essure device; (B) The Essure device placed in the right tube.

has to be flattened to make the tubal os visible. The procedure takes 5–10 min (Fig. 46.16A and B).

Complications

Because mini-hysteroscopy is performed in the office setting without any anesthesia (or at the most in a cervical block), there is no risk of major complications as the patient will say stop before severe complications, such as perforation or electrosurgical damage, can occur. Overload symptoms are not seen because the pressure of the distention media, in combination with the small diameter instruments, cannot open the vessels to the degree it takes to create overload.

Infections and vasovagal reactions are hardly ever seen.[1-62]

TIPS AND TRICKS

Ergonomics: Turn the chair with the back support to the front, sit opposite on it, resting the underarms on the back support (Fig. 46.17).

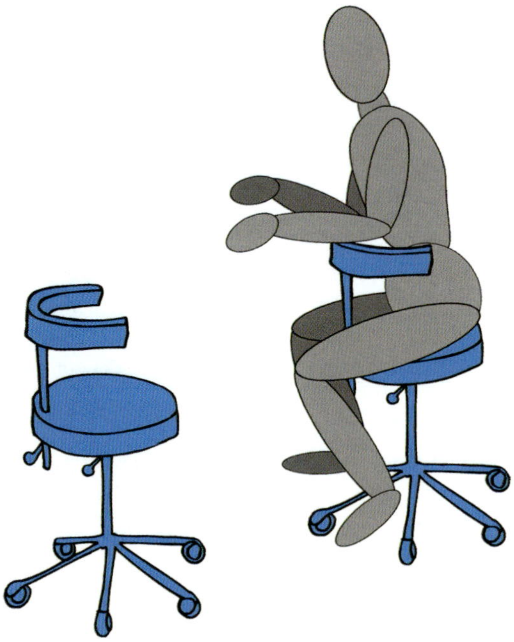

Fig. 46.17: The surgeon sitting back to front on a chair with the arms resting on the back support.

Timing: Preparation of the patient.

Cutting technique: Slice larger pathologies. Larger polyps must be divided into smaller pieces otherwise they cannot be removed through the narrow non-dilated internal os (Fig. 46.12).

Grasping technique: Do not cut off the whole polyp at once, otherwise it will float around in the cavity because of the continuously running fluid and be very difficult to catch. Leave a small piece uncut, then grab the polyp with the biopsy cup and retract the whole scope and biopsy cup, still positioned in the working channel.

Biopsy technique: Insert the biopsy cup, open the jaws, scrape forward in the region for biopsy, then close the jaws and retract the whole scope and the biopsy cup (Fig. 46.10).

Avoid pain: During entry, do not touch the myometrium, and keep down the pressure. If the uterus contracts just close the inflow and wait—the uterus will relax after a while. If necessary, place a cervical block, wait and see if dilatation is necessary.

Vocal local: Talk a lot with the staff about what Vocal Local is. At the beginning the staff is normally so interested in the procedure itself and what is seen on the screen that they forget to make the patient talk.

Stenosis of the internal os: Cut open the stenosis with the scissors or perform just a blunt dissection. It is often just some fibrotic fibers that close the os with no nerves.

Blurred vision due to blood and debris: Go to the fundus. Let the fluid rinse the cavity (have patience). If too much blood or a very thick mucosa with edema blurs the vision, make another appointment with the patient and try some kind of medical treatment for thinning the endometrium.

Fundal pathology: The twizzle can be bent. Put it through the working channel, bend the tip, retract the twizzle to the tip of the scope and then insert the scope with the twizzle within the working channel into the uterine cavity. The twizzle can be bent and straightened out around five times.

Too much light: It will diminish the possibility of differentiating the different structures in the cavity, i.e. if the light is too bright, just turn the light down on the generator.

REFERENCES

1. Bettocchi S, Ceci O, Di Venere R, et al. Advanced operative office hysteroscopy without anesthesia: analysis of 501 cases treated with 5 Fr. bipolar electrode. Hum Reprod. 2002;17(9):2435-8.
2. Di Spiezio Sardo A, Mazzon I, Bramante S, et al. Hysteroscopic myomectomy: a comprehensive review of surgical techniques. Hum Reprod Update. 2008;14(2):101-19.
3. Varma R, Soneja H, Clark TJ, et al. Hysteroscopic myomectomy for menorrhagia using Versascope bipolar system: efficacy and prognostic factors at a minimum of 1 year follow-up. Eur J Obstet Gynecol Reprod Biol. 2009;142(2):154-9.
4. Ceci O, Bettocchi S, Pellegrino A, et al. Comparison of hysteroscopic and hysterectomy findings for assessing the diagnostic accuracy of office hysteroscopy. Fertil Steril. 2002;78(3):628-31.
5. Garuti G, Mirra M, Luerti M. Hysteroscopic view in atypical endometrial hyperplasias: a correlation with pathologic findings on hysterectomy specimens. J Minim Invasive Gynecol. 2006;13(4):325-30.
6. Garuti G, Cellani F, Garzia D, et al. Accuracy of hysteroscopic diagnosis of endometrial hyperplasia: a retrospective study of 323 patients. J Minim Invasive Gynecol. 2005;12(3):247-53.
7. Arslan S, Aytan H, Gunyeli I, et al. Office hysteroscopic evaluation of endometrium: can we hit the target? Arch Gynecol Obstet. 2005;271(3):200-2.
8. Lasmar RB, Barrozo PR, de Oliveira MA, et al. Validation of hysteroscopic view in cases of endometrial hyperplasia and cancer in patients with abnormal uterine bleeding. J Minim Invasive Gynecol. 2006;13(5):409-12.
9. Tinelli R, Tinelli FG, Cicinelli E, et al. The role of hysteroscopy with eye-directed biopsy in postmenopausal women with uterine bleeding and endometrial atrophy. Menopause. 2008;15(4):737-42.

10. Bettocchi S, Di Venere R, Pansini N, et al. Endometrial biopsies using small-diameter hysteroscopes and 5F instruments: how can we obtain enough material for a correct histologic diagnosis? J Am Assoc Gynecol Laparosc. 2002;9(3):290-2.
11. Bettocchi S, Ceci O, Nappi L, et al. Operative office hysteroscopy without anesthesia: analysis of 4,863 performed with mechanical instruments. J Am Assoc Gynecol Laparosc. 2004;11(1):59-61.
12. Garuti G, Centinaio G, Luerti M. Outpatient hysteroscopic polypectomy in postmenopausal women: a comparison between mechanical and electrosurgical resection. J Minim Invasive Gynecol. 2008;15(5): 595-600.
13. Litta P, Cosmi E, Saccardi C, et al. Outpatient operative polypectomy using a 5 mm-hysteroscope without anesthesia and/or analgesia: advantages and limits. Eur J Obstet Gynecol Reprod Biol. 2008;139(2):210-4.
14. Marsh FA, Rogerson LJ, Duffy SR. A randomized controlled trial comparing outpatient versus daycase endometrial polypectomy. Br J Obstet Gynecol. 2006; 113(8):896-901.
15. Muzii L, Bellati F, Pernice M, et al. Resectoscopic versus bipolar electrode excision of endometrial polyps: a randomized study. Fertil Steril. 2007;87(4):909-17.
16. Guida M, Pellicano M, Zullo F, et al. Outpatient operative hysteroscopy with bipolar electrode: a prospective multicenter randomized to study between local anesthesia and conscious sedation. Hum Reprod. 2003;18(4):840-3.
17. Marwah V, Bhandari SK. Diagnostic and interventional microhysteroscopy with use of the coaxial bipolar electrode system. Fertil Steril. 2003;79(2):413-7.
18. Vilos GA. Intrauterine surgery using a new coaxial bipolar electrode in normal saline solution (Versapoint): a pilot study. Fertil Steril. 1999;72(4): 740-3.
19. Gulumser C, Narvekar N, Pathak M, et al. See-and-treat outpatient hysteroscopy: an analysis of 1,109 examinations. Reprod Biomed Online. 2010;20(3): 423-9.
20. Garuti G, Cellani F, Colonnelli M, et al. Outpatient hysteroscopic polypectomy in 237 patients: feasibility of a one-stop "see-and-treat" procedure. J Am Assoc Gynecol Laparosc. 2004;11(4):500-4.
21. Lindheim SR, Kavic S, Shulman SV, et al. Operative hysteroscopy in the office setting. J Am Assoc Gynecol Laparosc. 2000;7(1):65-9.
22. Hinckly MD, Milki AA. One thousand office-based hysteroscopies prior to in vitro fertilization: feasibility and findings. J Soc Laparoendosc Surg. 2004;8(2):103-7.
23. Ttocchi S, Di Spiezio Sardo A, Ceci O, et al. A new hysteroscopic technique for the preparation of partially intramural myomas in office setting (OPPIuM technique): a pilot study. J Minim Invasive Gynecol. 2009;16(6):748-54.
24. Jivraj S, Dass M, Panikkar J, et al. Outpatient hysteroscopy: an observational study of patient acceptability. Medicina (Kaunas). 2004;40(12):1207-10.
25. Moore KL, Dolley AF. Clinical Oriented Anatomy, 5th edition. London: Lippincott, Williams & Wilkins; 2006.
26. Zupi E, Luciano AA, Valli E, Marconi D, et al. The use of topical anesthesia in diagnostic hysteroscopy and endometrial biopsy. Fertil Steril. 1995;63(2):414-6.
27. Clark TJ, Voit D, Gupta JK, et al. Accuracy of hysteroscopy in the diagnosis of endometrial cancer and hyperplasia: a systematic quantitative review. J Am Med Assoc. 2002;288(13):1610-21.
28. Cooper N, Smith P, Khan K, et al. Vaginoscopic approach to outpatient hysteroscopy: a systematic review of the effect on pain. Br J Obstet Gynecol. 2010;117(5):532-9.
29. Almeida ZM, Pontes R, Costa Hde L. Evaluation of pain in diagnostic hysteroscopy by vaginoscopy using normal saline at body temperature as distention medium: a randomized controlled trial. Rev Bras Ginecol Obstet. 2008;30(1):25-30.
30. Garbin O, Kutnahorsky R, Göllner JL, et al. Vaginoscopic versus conventional approaches to outpatient diagnostic hysteroscopy: a two-center randomized prospective study. Hum Reprod. 2006; 21(11):2996-3000.
31. Guida M, Di Spiezio SA, Acunzo G, et al. Vaginoscopic versus traditional office hysteroscopy: a randomized controlled study. Hum Reprod. 2006;21(12):3253-7.
32. Paschopoulos M, Anastassopoulus P, Kaponis A, et al. Vaginoscopic versus conventional approach to outpatient hysteroscopy: a comparative randomized study. Gyneco-logical Endoscopy. 2000;51(suppl).
33. Sagiv R, Sadan O, Boaz M, et al. A new approach to office hysteroscopy compared with traditional hysteroscopy: a randomized controlled trial. Obstet Gynecol. 2006;108(2):387-92.
34. Sharma M, Taylor A, di Spiezio Sardo A, et al. Outpatient hysteroscopy: traditional versus the "no-touch" technique. BJOG. 2005;112(7):963-7.
35. Nagele F, Lockwood G, Magos AL. Randomized placebo-controlled trial of mefenamic acid for premedication at outpatient hysteroscopy: a pilot study. Br J Obstet Gynaecol. 1997;104(7):842-4.
36. Tam WH, Yuen PM. Use of diclofenac as an analgesic in outpatient hysteroscopy: a randomized, double-blind, placebo-controlled study. Fertil Steril. 2001; 76(5):1070-2.
37. Cooper NA, Khan KS, Clark TJ. Local anesthesia for pain control during outpatient hysteroscopy: systematic review and meta-analysis. BMJ. 2010; 23:340.
38. Makris N, Xygakis A, Dachlythras M, et al. Mepivacaine local cervical anesthesia for diagnostic hysteroscopy: a randomized placebo-controlled study. J Gynecol Surg. 2001;17:7-1.
39. Bellati U, Bonaventura A, Costanza L, et al. Tramadolhydrochloride versus mepivacaine hydrochloride: comparison between two analgesic procedures in hysteroscopy. Giornale Italiano di Ostetricia e Ginecologia. 1998;20:469-72.

40. Broadbent JA, Hill NC, Molnár BG, et al. Randomized placebo-controlled trial to assess the role of intracervical lignocaine in outpatient hysteroscopy. Br J Obstet Gynecol. 1992;99(9):777-9.
41. Esteve M, Schindler S, Machado SB, et al. The efficacy of intracervical lidocaine in outpatient hysteroscopy. Gynecol Endosc. 2002;11:33-6.
42. Finikiotis G, Tsocanos S. Outpatient hysteroscopy: a comparison of 2 methods of local analgesia. Aust NZJ Obstet Gynecol. 1992;32(4):373-4.
43. Al-Sunaidi M, Tulandi T. A randomized trial comparing local intracervical and combined local and paracervical anesthesia in outpatient hysteroscopy. J Minim Invasive Gynecol. 2007;14(2):153-5.
44. Lau WC, Lo WK, Tam WH, et al. Paracervical anesthesia in outpatient hysteroscopy: a randomized double-blind placebo-controlled trial. Br J Obstet Gynecol. 1999;106(4):356-9.
45. Cicinelli E, Didonna T, Schonauer LM, et al. Paracervical anesthesia for hysteroscopy and endometrial biopsy in postmenopausal women. A randomized, double-blind, placebo-controlled study. J Reprod Med. 1998;43(12):1014-8.
46. Vercellini P, Colombo A, Mauro F, et al. Paracervical anesthesia for outpatient hysteroscopy. Fertil Steril. 1994;62(5):1083-5.
47. Giorda G, Scarabelli C, Franceschi S, et al. Feasibility and pain control in outpatient hysteroscopy in postmenopausal women: a randomized trial. Acta Obstet Gynecol Scand. 2000;79(7):593-7.
48. Cicinelli E, Didonna T, Ambrosi G, et al. Topical anesthesia for diagnostic hysteroscopy and endometrial biopsy in postmenopausal women: a randomized placebo-controlled double-blind study. Br J Obstet Gynecol. 1997;104(3):316-9.
49. Costello MF, Horrowitz SD, Williamson M. A prospective randomized double-blind placebo-controlled study of local anesthetic injected through the hysteroscope for outpatient hysteroscopy and endometrial biopsy. Gynecol Endosc. 1998;7:121-6.
50. Lau WC, Tam WH, Lo WK, et al. A randomized double-blind placebo-controlled trial of transcervical intrauterine local anesthesia in outpatient hysteroscopy. Br J Obstet Gynecol. 2000;107(5):610-3.
51. Kabli N, Tulandi T. A randomized trial of outpatient hysteroscopy with and without intrauterine anesthesia. J Minim Invasive Gynecol. 2008;15(3): 308-10.
52. Shankar M, Davidson A, Taub N, et al. Randomized comparison of distention media for outpatient hysteroscopy. Br J Obstet Gynecol. 2004;111(1): 57-62.
53. De Angelis C, Santoro G, Re ME, et al. Office hysteroscopy and compliance: mini-hysteroscopy versus traditional hysteroscopy in a randomized trial. Hum Reprod. 2003;18(11):2441-5.
54. Cicinelli E, Schönauer LM, Barba B, et al. Tolerability and cardiovascular complications of outpatient diagnostic mini-hysteroscopy compared with conventional hysteroscopy. J Am Assoc Gynecol Laparosc. 2003;10(3):399-402.
55. Campo R, Molinas CR, Rombauts L, et al. Prospective multicenter randomized controlled trial to evaluate factors influencing the success rate of office diagnostic hysteroscopy. Hum Reprod. 2005;20(1):258-63.
56. Pluchino N, Ninni F, Angioni S, et al. Office vaginoscopic hysteroscopy in infertile women: effects of gynecologist experience, instrument size, and distention medium on patient discomfort. J Minim Invasive Gynecol. 2010;17(3):344-50.
57. Cicinelli E, Parisi C, Galantino P, et al. Reliability, feasibility, and safety of mini-hysteroscopy with a vaginoscopic approach: experience with 6,000 cases. Fertil Steril. 2003;80(1):199-202.
58. Garuti G, Luerti M. Hysteroscopic bipolar surgery: a valuable progress or a technique under investigation? Curr Opin Obstet Gynecol. 2009;21(4): 329-34.
59. Vilos GA, Abu-Rafea B. New developments in ambulatory hysteroscopic surgery. Best Pract Res Clin Obstet Gynecol. 2005;19(5):727-42.
60. Sutton C. Hysteroscopic surgery. Best Pract Res Clin Obstet Gynecol. 2006;20(1):105-37.
61. Bakour SH, Jones SE, O'Donovan P. Ambulatory hysteroscopy: evidence-based guide to diagnosis and therapy. Best Pract Res Clin Obstet Gynecol. 2006; 20(6):953-75.
62. Farrugia M. Modern Operative Hysteroscopy, 1st edition. Johnson & Johnson Medical S.P.A; 2008.

Laparoscopy and Hysteroscopy as Complementary Procedures

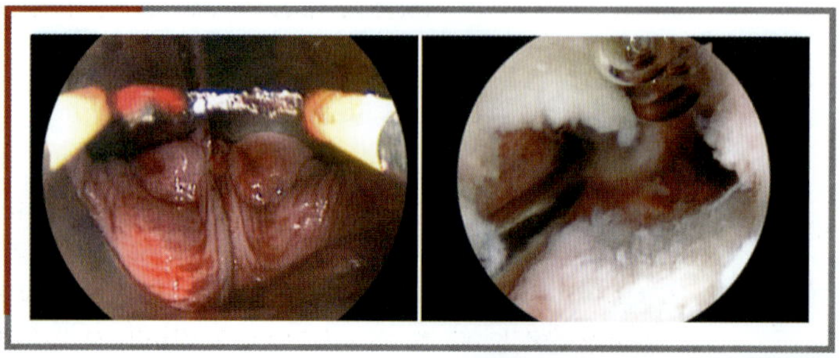

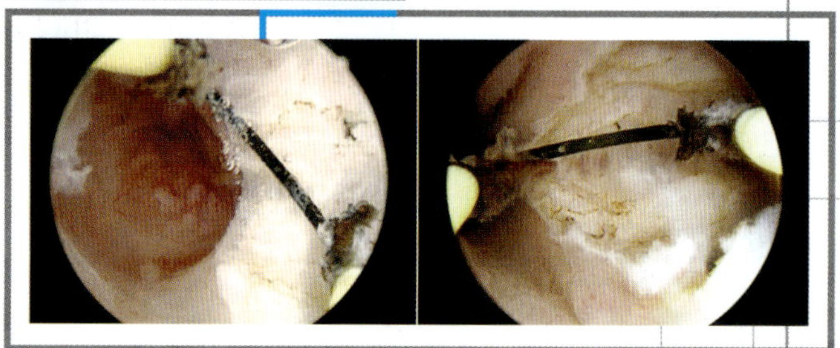

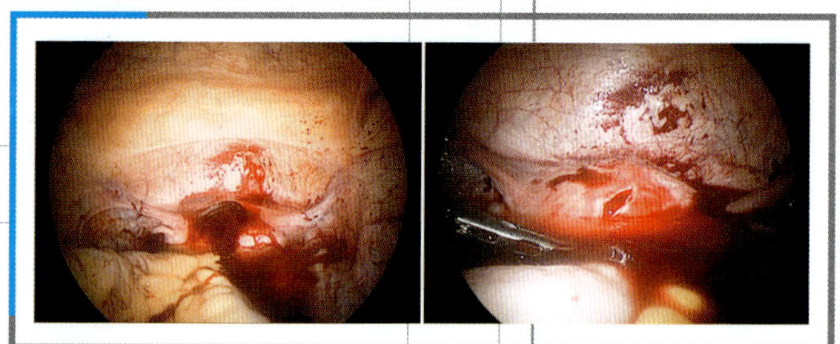

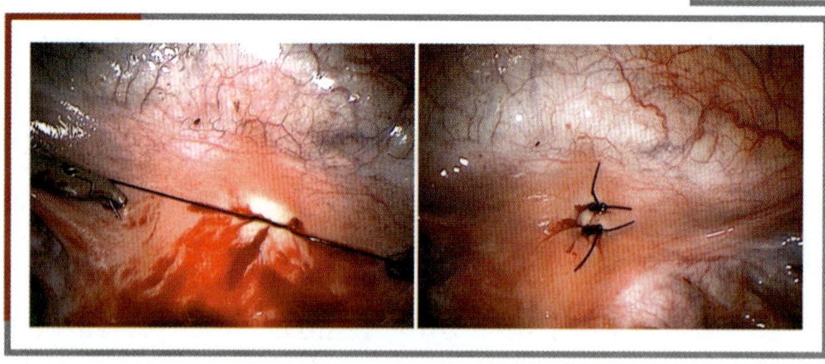

Chapter 47

Laparoscopy and Hysteroscopy as Complementary Procedures

Ibrahim Alkatout, Liselotte Mettler

BASIC CONCEPT

The basic concept of laparoscopy was developed by Kurt Semm and Liselotte Mettler in the 1980s. However, the instruments and techniques used at that time (endotherm and loop) did not keep pace with the development of the surgical techniques and the variety of surgical indications. Advancements in instruments, technical support and consistent training have considerably improved the procedure.

Laparoscopy today has become a standard operation with low complication rates and a regular learning curve. It is associated with reduced blood loss, shorter hospital stays, earlier return to normal activities and fewer infections compared to all other surgical methods. Its major advantage is the possibility to simultaneously treat comorbidities, such as endometriosis, fibroids or adhesions. Regarding family planning, complementary usage of hysteroscopy and laparoscopy might be useful to better diagnose anatomic pathologies, such as septum or adenomyosis, and allows simultaneous treatment at the highest level of safety. The final decision is made jointly by the doctor and the patient.

INTRODUCTION

Office Hysteroscopy without Anesthesia in an Ambulatory Setting

In many reproductive medical centers around the world, hysterosalpingo-contrast sonography (HyCoSy) and transvaginal hydrolaparoscopy combined with hysteroscopy have become widely accepted examinations in early infertility diagnosis without any suspicion of pathology. In cases where, primarily because of the reproductive history of the couple, a laparoscopy with chromopertubation is planned, it should be performed together with diagnostic hysteroscopy using a diagnostic hysteroscope with a small operative channel. In indications for an infertility check-up or a suspected tubal, ovarian or uterine pathology by laparoscopy, hysteroscopy complements and facilitates a complete diagnosis. If no pathology is found intrauterine, it is still possible to perform endometrial scratching as this has been shown to improve the implantation rate. An operative hysteroscopy is indicated in all infertility cases with submucosal polyps, fibroids, septum and adhesions.

Operative hysteroscopy became popular after improvements in endoscopic technology and instruments in the 1970s and after the introduction of fluid distension media in the 1980s. Since that time, the development of new hysteroscopic instruments, fiber optics and digital video equipment has continued to provide more varied, efficacious and less invasive procedures. The introduction of smaller-diameter hysteroscopes has allowed operative hysteroscopy to become a safe surgical procedure. However, besides this classic diagnostic coupling of two endoscopic procedures, hysteroscopy may also support the treatment of abnormal uterine bleeding, submucosal fibroids, uterine polyps, uterine septum, lysis of adhesions, cannulaton of fallopian tube ostia, removal of a foreign body or placental remnants and sterilization. Hysteroscopy allows the diagnosis of adenomyosis and, in its operative form, excisions and resections in patients with severe pain and who have the desire for conception. In the planning and performance of laparoscopic myomectomy and even hysterectomy, in benign cases or in genital cancer surgery,

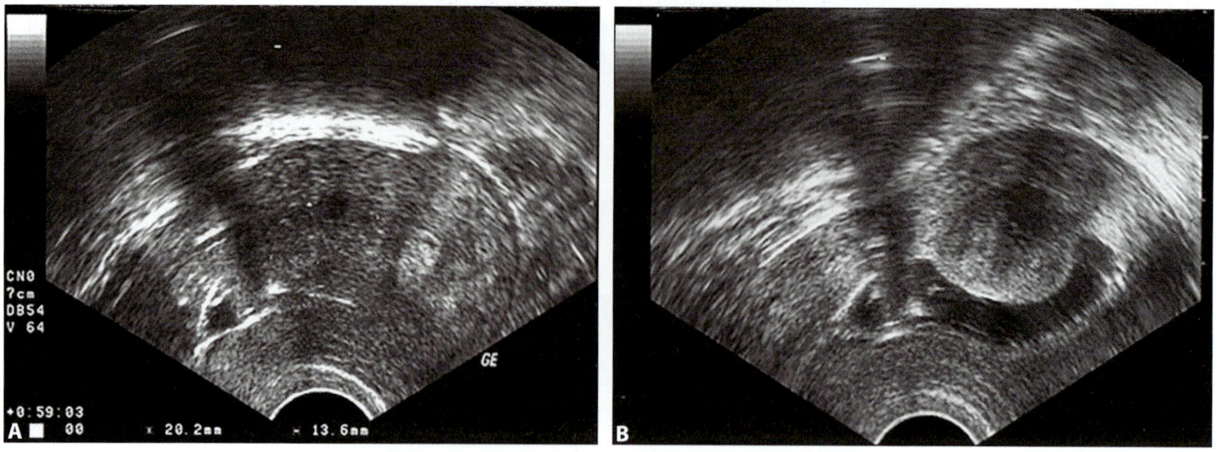

Figs. 47.1A and B: (A) Vaginal sonography showing an unclear mass in the back wall. The relation to the uterine cavity cannot be determined clearly. Therefore, it is not clear whether more or less than 50% of the myoma is in the uterine wall (Type I versus Type II myoma after Wamsteker); (B) Ultimately, hysterosalpingosonography shows a submucous myoma [European Society for Gynaecological Endoscopy (ESGE) Type I]. After application of normal saline through a 3 Charrière Nelaton catheter (balloon visible in the left lower corner) the well-demarcated tumor is visible including its infiltrating depths and the clear distance to the serosa. Furthermore, the angle between fibroid and mucosa can be measured. Below 90°, it resembles Type I and therefore can be resected by hysteroscopy.

the indications for an explorative laparoscopy are often complemented by a preliminary hysteroscopy to cover the full diagnostic spectrum.

Hysteroscopic procedures are generally considered safe, but severe complications can arise. To increase patient safety, training before performing hysteroscopic procedures should be mandatory as in all other surgical procedures.

It is the aim of this chapter to evaluate all hysteroscopic complementary situations to diagnostic and operative laparoscopy. These are the same for conventional multisite entries at laparoscopy, single port surgery, mini-laparoscopy and robotically assisted laparoscopic surgery. Furthermore, this chapter reviews the current training models available for hysteroscopy and what to consider when training.

Laparoscopy

Benign gynecological diseases that are often treated laparoscopically in combination with hysteroscopy are fibroids, endometriosis/adenomyosis uteri, sterility problems and hysteroscopic problems requiring additional laparoscopy. Nevertheless, the treatment of endometriosis is performed primarily by laparoscopy, and very seldom is hysteroscopic diagnosis (deep chip removal) or even treatment (opening of focal adenomyoma) indicated. Regarding myoma treatment, all Type 0 and Type I myomas can and should be removed by hysteroscopy. In some cases the differentiation between Type I and Type II is difficult by sonography. For this reason the use of fluid hysterosonography can be very helpful (Figs. 47.1 and 47.2) in the preoperative setup. Genital disorders are often unspecific and make a combined surgery necessary to clearly detect and treat the anomaly. In the case of intraoperative hysteroscopic problems (perforation, via falsa, unclear septum), laparoscopy clarifies the situation and offers a simultaneous treatment solution. In malignant diseases hysteroscopy plays only a role in diagnostics, e.g. in endometrial cancer, seldom in cervical cancer or unclear intrauterine masses. The main type of therapeutic surgery performed in cervical, endometrial or tubal cancer is laparoscopy or even open surgery. With regard to hysterectomies performed for benign disease, the number of abdominal hysterectomies is decreasing, the number of vaginal hysterectomies varies, but laparoscopic and robotic-assisted laparoscopic procedures are on the increase;[1] this trend is visible throughout the world.[2]

Hysteroscopy

Preoperative Considerations and Preparation

Office Hysteroscopy: Distension of the Cavity

Examination of and operative procedures in the uterine cavity require a distension of the cavity by a continuous flow of fluid, usually sterile saline. The continuous flow will clear the vision and flush away

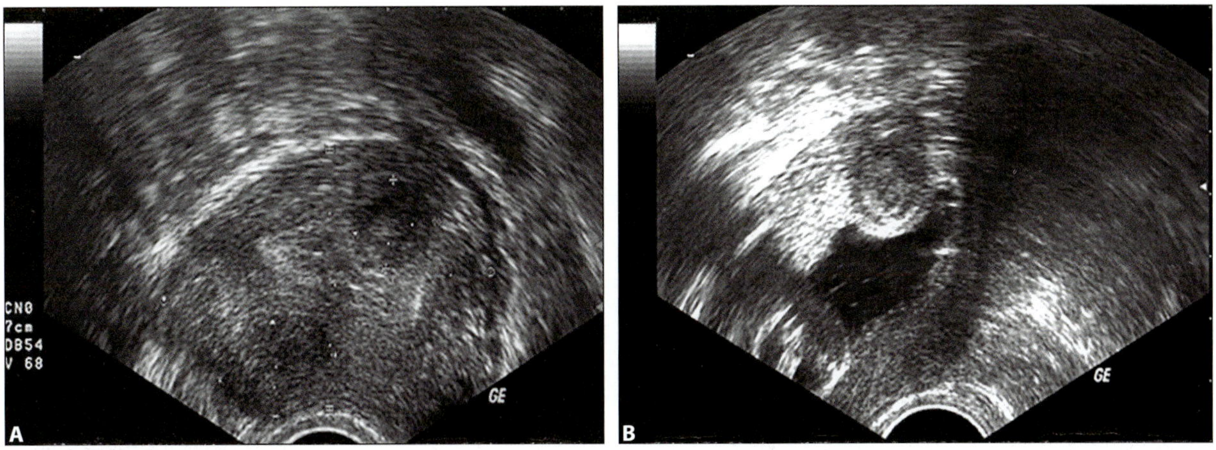

Figs. 47.2A and B: (A) Vaginal sonography showing an unclear mass in the back wall. The relation to the uterine cavity cannot be determined clearly. Therefore, it is not clear whether more or less than 50% of the myoma is in the uterine wall (Type I versus Type II myoma after Wamsteker); (B) Ultimately, hysterosalpingosonography shows an intramural myoma [European Society for Gynaecological Endoscopy (ESGE) Type II]. After application of normal saline through a 3 Charrière Nelaton catheter (balloon visible in the left lower corner) the well-demarcated tumor is visible including its infiltrating depths and the clear distance to the serosa. Furthermore, the angle between fibroid and mucosa can be measured. Over 90° resembles Type II and therefore can be resected by hysteroscopy.

Table 47.1: Advantages and disadvantages of rigid and flexible hysteroscopes in an office setup.

	Advantages	*Disadvantages*
Rigid hysteroscope	Better intrauterine visibility Shorter procedure time Better hysteroscopic view and diagnostic possibilities	More painful Discomfort at introduction
Flexible hysteroscope	Less pain	Longer procedure time More difficult to judge diagnostic findings More expensive than procedures with the rigid hysteroscope

mucus, blood and tissue debris. The cavity will usually distend at a fluid pressure of 50–80 mm Hg. The recommended flow is the lowest possible that gives a sufficient distension. Too high a pressure will cause uterine contraction (pain) and loss of fluid into the abdominal cavity through the tubes. There is low evidence that the loss of fluid in the abdominal cavity might lead to metastatic spread. Sometimes, a pressure of 125 mm Hg is necessary to obtain a clear vision.

For office hysteroscopy (Table 47.1), a pressure bag to compress a 1 L bag of saline is sufficient to carry out diagnostic hysteroscopy and biopsy. The pressure is normally set at around 125 mm Hg at the beginning of a procedure.

A hysteroscopic pump can maintain the pressure sufficiently to give a clear vision. In the beginning, it is set at 50–80 mm Hg but it may be necessary to increase the pressure later.

Sterile saline is the preferred distension media, due to the low risk of water intoxication during intravasation of the fluid, and is required if bipolar electrosurgery is used. Bipolar electrodes for cutting and tissue evaporation require a conductive ion or electrolyte-rich medium to close the circuit between active and return electrode.[3]

Diagnostic and Operative Hysteroscopy: Indications

Hysteroscopy in Infertility

The nonconception, better called sterility, and the inability to carry a child to term named infertility require investigation of the site of sperm deposition and migration to the site of fertilization in the fimbriae of the Fallopian tubes and back to the site of implantation, the uterine cavity: vagina, cervical canal, uterine cavity and Fallopian tubes. The site of oocyte or embryo implantation is inspected by the hysteroscopic view at laparoscopy. Hysteroscopy adds to the different types of laparoscopic explorations and repair and rounds up the diagnostic and therapeutic possibilities in the clinical anatomical exploration of the female genital tract.

The most common indications in patients with infertility:

- Septum dissection with uterus subseptus/septus
- Intrauterine adhesiolysis with adhesions, grades III–IV/ESGE
- Myoma resection.

Treatment of Bleeding Symptoms or Intrauterine Pathology by Hysteroscopy

Other than infertility indications, bleeding disorders in general or expected intrauterine pathologies are also treated by hysteroscopy.

With bleeding disorders:

- Myoma resection
- Polyp resection
- Endometrial ablation/endometrial resection

Special indications:

- Resection of residual placenta
- Opening or coagulation of a hamatometra in the rudimentary uterine horn.

Instrumentation and Technical Equipment

Necessary basic equipment for operative hysteroscopy should be:

- Hysteroresectoscope with matching electrode and 12° angle lenses
- Light source with cable
- Hysteromat with inflow and outflow tube
- Distending medium
- Video camera
- High-frequency unit.

Operative Hysteroscopy: Technique and Procedure of Operative Hysteroscopy

- In most indications a cervical curettage is performed as a first step.
- Dilatation of the cervical canal up to Hegar 9 (when using a smaller resectoscope for fertility surgery up to Hegar 7).
- Insertion of the outer sheath with obturator.
- Replacement of the obturator by a hysteroresectoscope with matching electrode and 12° lenses.
- Check the connections.
  - Check the correct distending medium (bipolar: Ringer's solution; monopolar: sorbitol-mannitol solution)
  - Inflow tube for the distending medium: airless and connected with the Hysteromat
  - Check the pressure and flow selection on the Hysteromat
  - Outlet tube in collect container
  - Connection with electrosurgical unit and check the power level on the high-frequency unit (preselected programs for monopolar and bipolar surgery).
  - Opening of the inflow tube and distension of the cavum uteri often an irrigation is primarily necessary because the dilatation of the cervix often causes bleedings in the cavum uteri.
  - Start of the surgery as soon as view and distension are sufficient.

Operative Hysteroscopy: Operative Steps of Concrete Hysteroscopic Procedures

Septum Dissection

Indications for septum dissection have increased in the last years. Subtle preoperative diagnostics is necessary. For a differential diagnosis between uterus bicornis and uterus septus a laparoscopy is imperative as there is a significant risk of perforation with a uterus bicornis.

Absolute Indications

Habitual abortions (2 or 3 recurrent abortions)

Relative indications

- Primary and secondary infertility
- Dysmenorrhoea (therapy-resistant).

Technique of Septum Dissection

- Dissection of the septum with the resection needle from caudal to fundal
- From time to time check the extent of the dissection using the tubal ostia as points of orientation
- With complete septa first dissect the area caudal, afterwards insert the resectoscope completely (sufficient flow), then dissection from fundal to caudal.

Diagnostics and therapeutic management of suspected uterus malformation (uterus septus/bicornis)

- Anamnesis (abortions, premature births?)
- Gynecological examination and sonography ("two-cavities-phenomenon")
- Scheduling of the surgery: ideally post menstruationem (thin endometrium)

- *Procedure of the surgery:*
  - Diagnostic hysteroscopy: cavum uteri divided into two parts
  - Diagnostic laparoscopy: fundus of the uterus smooth or small median raphe
  - Operative hysteroscopy with transcervical septum dissection.

Postoperative management after septum dissection depends on the type of septum.

With complete or wide septa or additional intrauterine adhesions

- At the end of the surgery insertion of an IUD for the prevention of intrauterine adhesions for the duration of 3 months (preferably IUD type DANA or copper-IUD with a wide surface)
  Estrogenization for 3 months to stimulate the endometrium proliferation (e.g., 2–4 mg estradiol for 21 days progestagen for 12 days)
- Follow-up hysteroscopy (possibly with IUD extraction), in most of the cases as outpatient procedure without anesthesia, possible after 3 months.

The most frequent complication of the septum dissection is perforation in the fundal area.

Management:

- Diagnostic laparoscopy
- Check for injuries of other organs (especially bowel injuries); if these cannot be definitely excluded, a laparotomy is indicated
- With bleeding: endoscopic suture for hemostasis
- Perioperative application of antibiotics
- Frequent postoperative follow-up.

Intrauterine adhesiolysis

Indications for intrauterine adhesiolysis are:

- Habitual abortions (two or more recurrent abortions)
- Primary and secondary infertility
- Hypomenorrhea/amenorrhea
- Dysmenorrhea
- Recurrent lower abdominal pain

Diagnostics and therapeutic management in the case of suspected intrauterine adhesions (Table 47.2).

- Anamnesis:
  - Bleeding characteristics
  - Preliminary intrauterine intervention
- Gynecological examination
- Vaginal sonography: endometrium structure
- Diagnostic hysteroscopy: intrauterine adhesions with description of the grade
- Operative hysteroscopy simultaneous with intrauterine adhesiolysis (if necessary, simultaneous sonography or laparoscopy)
- IUD insertion at the end of surgery (compulsory with grades III and IV according to ESGE)
- Estrogenization for 3 months for endometrium proliferation
- Follow-up hysteroscopy with IUD extraction (if necessary, further adhesiolysis).

Myoma resection: The indications for hysteroscopic myoma resection are as follows:

- Recurrent bleeding disorders resistant to therapy, in most of the cases connected with dysmenorrhoea or secondary anemia
- Bleeding disorders during oral contraception or postmenopausal hormone therapy
- Habitual abortions
- Primary and secondary infertility

The best time for surgery is without pretreatment: post-menstruationem or with pretreatment (ulipristal acetate or GnRH-analogs): 2–3 weeks after last application.

Myoma resection is similar to polyp resection. The fibroid capsule needs to be resected and often forms the relevant surgical layer. Dissecting in the capsula allows mobilization of the myoma and easier complete resection without simultaneous removal of neighboring healthy tissue. Myoma resection is performed in single pieces that are usually taken out together to keep distension and overview maximized.

Polyp resection

- Gynecological examination and vaginal sonography, if necessary progesterone test to differentiate between polyp and endometrium hyperplasia
- Diagnostic hysteroscopy and target curettage

Table 47.2: Operative therapy and prognosis of intrauterine adhesions.

	Grade I	*Grade II*	*Grades III and IV*
Operative therapy	Cutting by sheath of the hysteroscope	Cutting by microscissors	Electrosurgical adhesiolysis or by laser (operative hysteroscopy)
Successful therapy of the bleeding disorders	100%	100%	60–70%
Pregnancy rate	70–90%	70–90%	20–40%

- Operative hysteroscopy (patient should already be informed before surgery) with transcervical electrosurgical resection of the polyp.[4]

A diagnostic laparoscopy with tubal patency testing by chromopertubation, as performed with methylene blue or other dye solutions, may not detect a uterine septum, adhesions, polyps or adenomyosis and therefore hysteroscopy is a complementary procedure. Frequently, after a routine hysteroscopy at the end of a myomectomy or ovarian cyst removal in infertility patients and recurrent aborting patients, we have detected an unknown intrauterine septum. Of course, this anatomical variation has then to be simultaneously treated by a septum dissection in an infertility patient.

In many but not all cases, a laparoscopy requires antibiotic prophylaxis, such as second-generation cephalosporin. Especially long procedures, the opening of external body cavities, such as the vagina, and contact with infectious material make antibiotic prophylaxis obligatory. In cases of suspected bowel involvement, the application of metronidazole is also essential. The antibiotic should be applied about 30 min before the start of the operation.

The instruments consist of trocars, a uterine manipulator (for selected cases only), needle holders and sutures. Additionally, one needs an instrument for coagulation, graspers, scissors, window forceps and a suction irrigation unit. If a robotic set-up is available, the instruments must be adjusted accordingly. A thermofusion device with an integrated knife is optional.

Prerequisites

Obesity or comorbidities, a large uterus or a uterus with multiple myomas, ovarian cysts and adhesions are not contraindications for a laparoscopic procedure. However, in these cases, the preoperative assessment and the anesthesia procedure must be discussed with the patient in advance. The trocars may need to be placed higher in the abdominal wall and the surgeon may need more than the usual two ancillary trocars. In cases of laparoscopy combined with hysteroscopy due to genital disorder, perforation, tubal reconstruction or similar findings, trocar sizes and localization might differ. Preoperative planning includes the consideration whether laparoscopy alone, hysteroscopy alone or a combined surgery is required.

In infertility patients with severe comorbidities the operative risk has to be weighed against the expected gain through surgery. Furthermore, the necessity of weight reduction, behavioral changes, etc. needs to be discussed before surgery. Likewise, a possible origin in the male factor needs to be excluded before targeted surgery is performed.

Operative Steps of All Laparoscopic Procedures

Step 1

A vaginal examination under anesthesia is performed before using, for example, the manipulator. If no further vaginal or rectal pathologies are found, the manipulator is inserted, if required (e.g., hysterectomy, deep infiltrating endometriosis and some myoma resections). In infertility patients we usually try to avoid screwing in the cervix and keep dilation to a minimum.

Step 2

Port placement:[5] A number of entry techniques are available; direct entry under sight has become very popular in the last few years. Nevertheless, the traditional entry technique described by Kurt Semm and Liselotte Mettler at the Kiel University Department of Obstetrics and Gynaecology in the 1980s, and still used today at the Kiel School of Gynaecological Endoscopy, is shown here.

Optic Trocar

Veress Needle Technique and CO_2 Gas

To insert the Veress needle, the operating table needs to be in a horizontal position. The Trendelenburg tilt is carried out after creating a pneumoperitoneum. The most common site of entry for the Veress needle is the umbilical area. As the wall layers are thinnest at this level, a deep incision will ensure access to the peritoneal cavity. Before incising the skin it would be advisable to palpate the course of the aorta and identify the iliac bifurcation. This will permit inspection and palpation of the abdomen in order to detect any unusual masses (Figs. 47.3 to 47.6).[6]

The Veress needle must be tested to ensure that the valve springs, and that gas flow is between 6 mm Hg and 8 mm Hg. In this position the insertion of the primary instrument at a 45° angle toward the uterus involves the least risk of damaging the major vessels coursing downward retroperitoneally. The

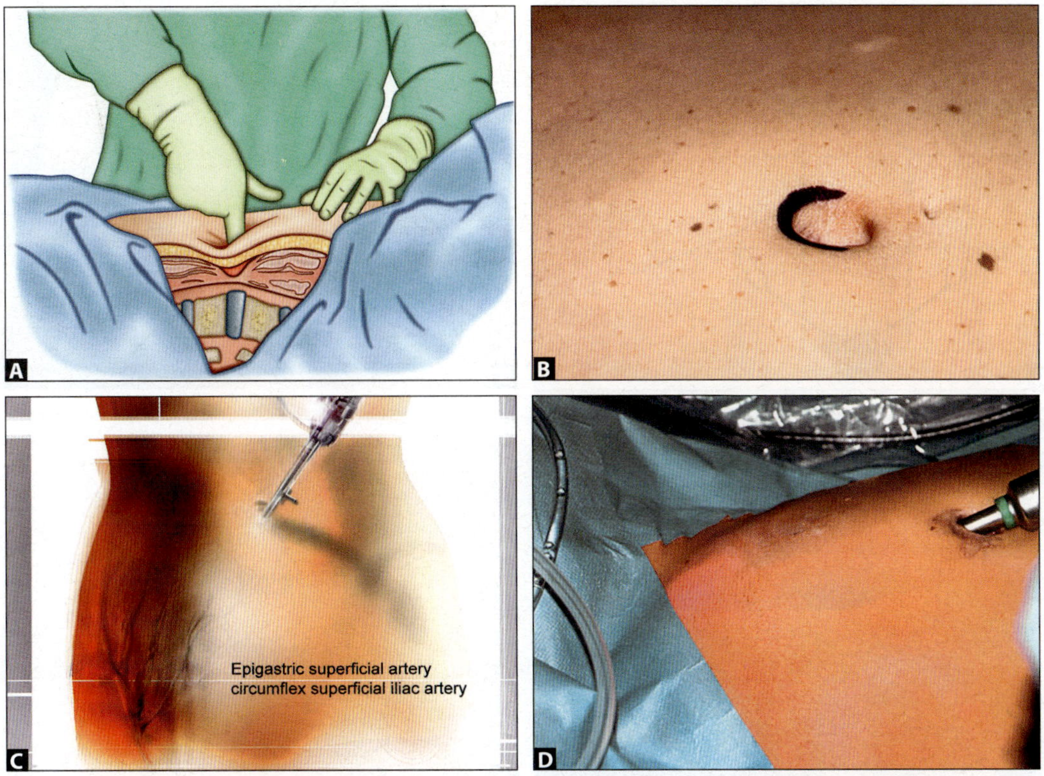

Figs. 47.3A to D: (A) Typical point of palpation in the subumbilical region. The fingertip is pointing to the promontory. Subumbilical incision and local palpation reveal the short distance from the skin to the spine; (B to D) Diaphanoscopy illuminates the region of insertion of the ancillary trocars while demarcating the superficial epigastric artery and the superficial circumflex iliac artery.

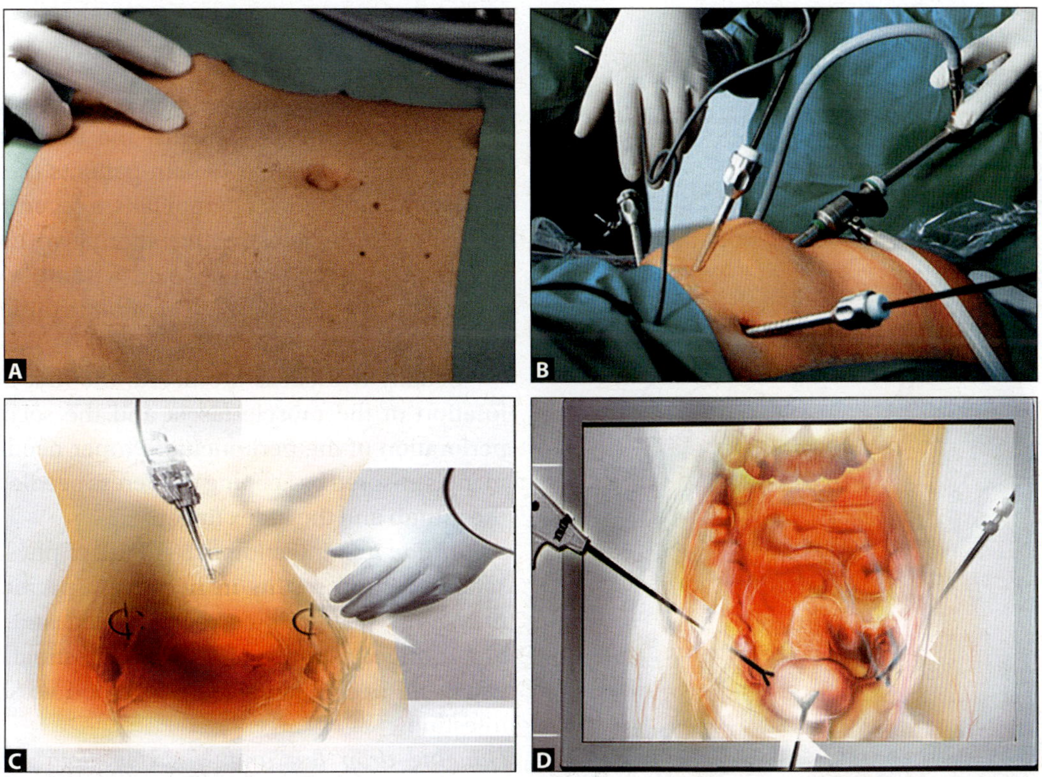

Figs. 47.4A to D: (A and C) Point of insertion from the outside (two thumbs medial to the anterior superior spine) at a 90° angle to the surface, with penetration of all layers of the abdominal wall. Trocar insertion site lateral to the lateral umbilical fold; (B and D) Overview after insertion of the laparoscope and 3 ancillary trocars.

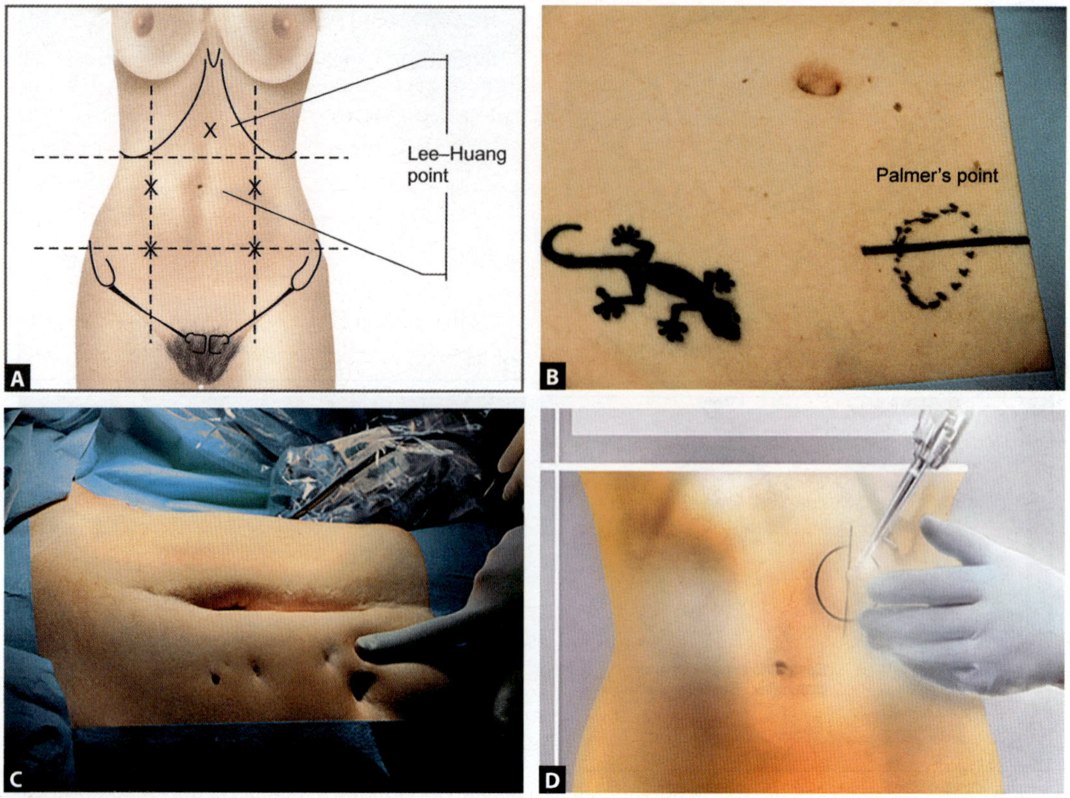

Figs. 47.5A to D: Alternative entry site showing. (A) In cases of a large uterus, especially at or above the level of the umbilicus, the Lee–Huang point. This point is recommended for video-assisted laparoscopy; or (C) In cases of anticipated adhesions in the region of Palmer's point; (B and D) Palmer's point is situated in the midclavicular line, about 3 cm below the costal margin.

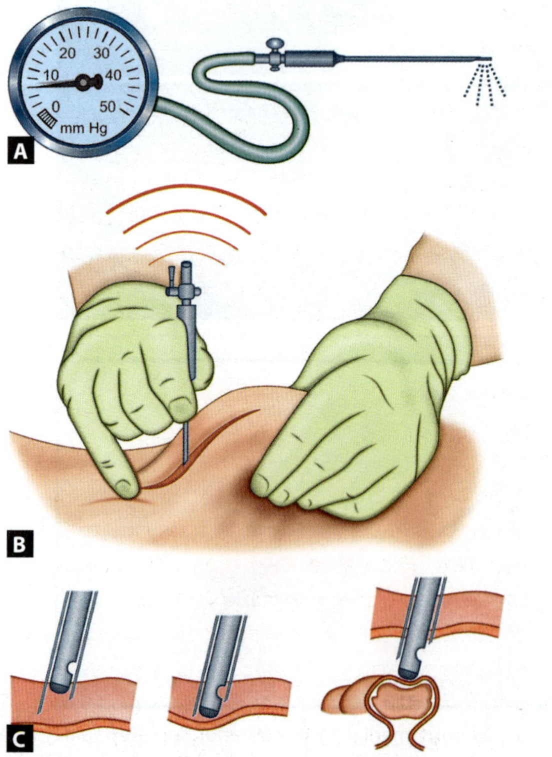

Figs. 47.6A to C: Veress needle and its insertion. The safety mechanism avoids damage or injury to the bowel or vessels.

abdominal wall should be lifted before inserting the instrument. In obese patients, the insertion angle is close to 90°, whereas in slim patients the angle is close to 45°. If the first attempt fails, a second attempt is made before selecting an alternative entry site. Before placing the Veress needle, a number of safety checks should be performed in order to minimize the risk of complications:

Usually two clicks are heard: the first after perforation of the muscle fascia and the second after perforation of the peritoneum. Proper needle placement is ensured by keeping the Veress needle between the thumb and the index finger.

Aspiration test: Injection of 5–10 mL of physiological saline solution results in negative aspiration when the Veress needle is correctly placed and yields a blood-tinged aspirate, or one with intestinal contents when the needle is placed in a blood vessel or the intestine.

Hanging drop test and "fluid in flow": With the Veress needle placed in the abdominal cavity, lifting the abdominal wall creates negative intraabdominal pressure. A drop of water is then placed on the open end of the Veress needle. If the needle is correctly positioned, the water will move down the shaft.

Any movement of the needle after placement must be avoided as this may convert a small needlepoint injury into a complex and threatening tear. After ensuring that the Veress needle has been positioned correctly, the insufflation is started. Once adequate gas flow and pressure have been achieved, the influx can be raised so that 2–3 L of CO_2 gas can be insufflated per minute until 3–6 L have been insufflated, depending on the patient's size and obesity. After an insufflation volume of about 300 mL, percussion of the liver region will confirm the *loss of liver dullness*, which is a reliable sign of proper positioning of the Veress needle and the creation of a pneumoperitoneum. Abdominal pressure should then be increased to 20–25 mm Hg before inserting the primary trocar because this maximizes the distension of the abdominal wall away from all underlying structures.[7]

The optic trocar is inserted in one or in two steps. A 10 mm optic trocar can be inserted using the Z-technique; however, in all cases with previous surgery, unknown pathology, etc. in the first step, a 5 mm optic trocar and the laparoscope are inserted to confirm the pneumoperitoneum and the absence of local adhesions. Dilation to 10 mm is achieved in the second step, either under sight or blindly, thus ensuring optimum visibility during the operation.

Step 1: Entry is performed by a Z technique in the following manner: After proceeding forward with the trocar forward to about 1.5 cm, the tip is moved to about 1.5 cm to the right at a 90° angle. The abdominal wall is lifted in the same manner as when inserting the Veress needle, and the trocar is screwed with the dominant hand straight into the abdominal wall at a 90° angle, toward the hollow of the sacrum.

Correct placement of the trocar is indicated by a hissing sound when gas escapes through the open valve of the trocar. The obturator is then removed and the trocar is held in place. Before dilating to 10 mm, a 5 mm laparoscope is introduced and rotated through 360° to check visually for any bleeding, intraabdominal abnormality or adherent bowel loops. If the surgeon suspects adherence of the bowel in the umbilical region, the primary trocar site must be visualized from a secondary port site, such as the lower abdominal wall, with a 5 mm laparoscope.

Step 2: A blunt palpation probe is placed in the 5-mm trocar; the shaft is pulled over the palpation probe and taken out. A 10 mm trocar is then screwed into the abdominal cavity.[7]

Subcostal Insufflation Technique (Palmer's Point or Lee–Huang Point)

No entry technique is entirely devoid of the risk of gas embolism or injury to vessels, intestines or the urinary tract. Palmer's point is the safest laparoscopic entry point because it is least likely to be affected by adhesions.

For all patients with a significantly higher risk of adhesions, a history of abdominal surgery including cesarean section, a large fibroid uterus, umbilical hernia, large ovarian cysts, preperitoneal gas insufflation or failed umbilical entry, Palmer described in 1974 an abdominal entry point in the midclavicular line, about 3 cm below the costal margin. Palmer's point can be used for the Veress needle as well as for small trocars. In case adhesions are suspected in the subcostal region on the left side, the Lee–Huang point in the midline is a suitable alternative (Figs. 47.5A to D).[7]

Ancillary Trocars

All ancillary trocars must be inserted with an intraabdominal pressure of 15–20 mm Hg under direct vision. The inferior epigastric vessels are visualized laparoscopically whereas the superficial vessels can be visualized by diaphanoscopy.

Once the tip of the trocar has pierced the peritoneum, it should be angulated in the direction of the uterine fundus under visual control until the port is placed correctly and the sharp tip can be removed.

Before inserting any ancillary trocars, the patient is moved into the Trendelenburg position. Premature Trendelenburg positioning may increase the risk of retroperitoneal vascular injury because the iliac vessels are located exactly in the axis of a preconceived 45° insertion angle, especially in slim patients with minimal retroperitoneal fat. The number of ancillary trocars is variable; all of them must be inserted under direct vision. If two working trocars are needed, they should be placed in the lower quadrant above the pubic hairline, lateral to the deep epigastric vessels from the interior view. From the exterior view the trocars are placed two fingers medial to the anterior superior iliac spine. Two major superficial vessels—the superficial epigastric artery and the superficial circumflex iliac artery—must be avoided. These vessels can be visualized by diaphanoscopy. When a third ancillary trocar is required, the suprapubic midline is the most common site. An alternative is the mid-abdomen on the left side. But, make sure that optic trocar and each ancillary trocar are at a sufficient

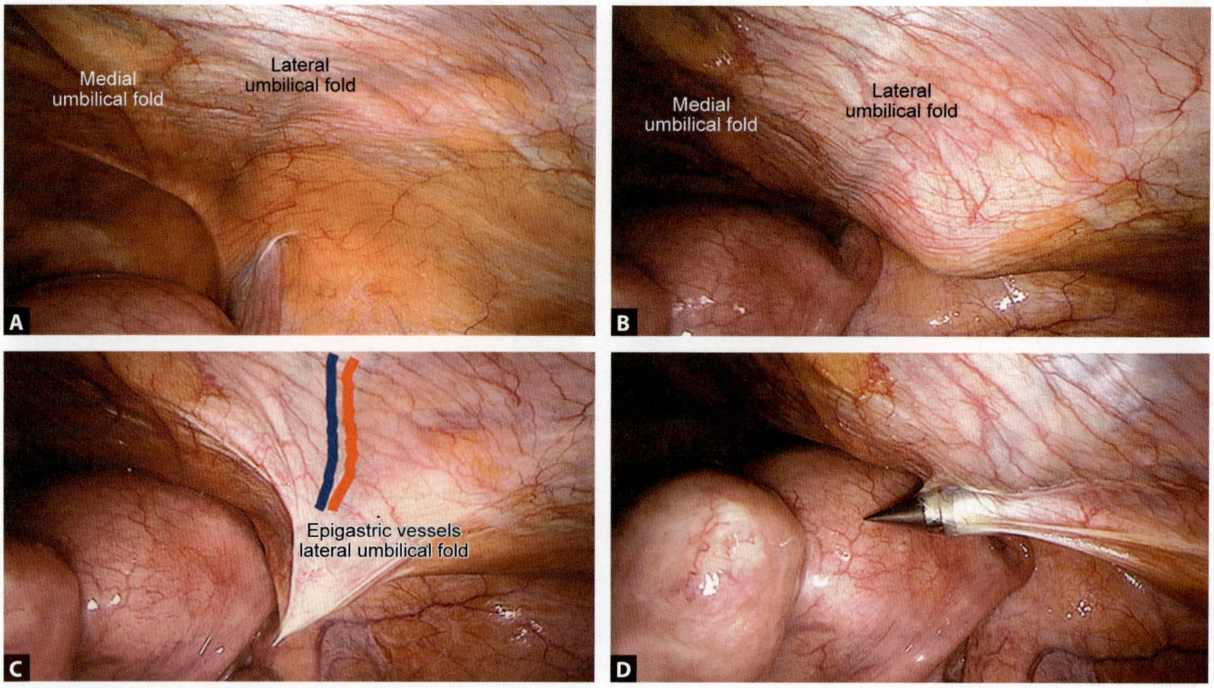

Figs. 47.7A to D: Secondary trocar placement, entry in the right lower abdomen. (A) The three different plicae are visualized; (B) The palpating finger is showing the area lateral to the lateral umbilical fold; (C) Entry of the sharp ancillary trocar lateral to the lateral umbilical fold; (D) Once the peritoneum has been penetrated, the trocar points to the fundus of the uterus to avoid injury to the major vessels and the bowel.

distance from each other. Furthermore, for precise preparation the distance of the two ancillary trocars from medial to lateral is mandatory. Diaphanoscopy cannot be relied upon to locate the deep vessels, especially in obese patients (Figs. 47.7 and 47.8).

Finger-tapping from the outside can be used to verify correct positioning of the trocar. A small skin incision should be performed before the trocar sleeve is inserted. The trocars must be inserted by the shortest route at a 90° angle to the skin surface so that the risk of injuring structures on the way to the abdominal wall is minimized. When inserting a trocar in the midline, the Foley catheter must be identified in order to avoid accidental bladder perforation.[7,8]

Step 3: Surgical Steps

Myomectomy: The etiology of fibroids shows a panorama of theories. Fibroids are composed primarily of smooth muscle cells. The uterus, stomach and bladder are all organs made of smooth muscle. Smooth muscle cells are arranged so that the organ can stretch instead of being arranged in rigid units like the cells in the skeletal muscles in arms and legs that are designed to "pull" in a particular direction.

In women with fibroids, tissue from the endometrium typically looks normal under the microscope. Sometimes, however, over submucosal fibroids there is an unusual type of uterine lining that does not have the normal glandular structure. The presence of this abnormality called aglandular funtionalis (functional endometrium with no glands) in women having menstrual symptoms is sometimes a clinical clue for their doctors to look more closely for a submucosal fibroid. A second pattern of endometrium termed chronic endometritis can also suggest that there may be a submucosal fibroid although this pattern can also be associated with other problems, such as retained products of conception and various infections of the uterus.

Based on immunohistochemical findings, it is proposed to remove fibroids in women seeking pregnancy while respecting the pseudocapsule by neurofiber sparing in the incision site. We have published that this is of utmost importance for optimal muscular healing and myometrial function in future pregnancies. In fibroids less than 5–6 cm in diameter, especially in young women wanting to achieve pregnancy, myomectomy should be performed before the myoma reaches a size causing compression of the surrounding tissues and uterine distortion, which may result in the loss of regenerative potential.

In certain cases it is good surgical and clinical practice to perform a hysteroscopy before performing

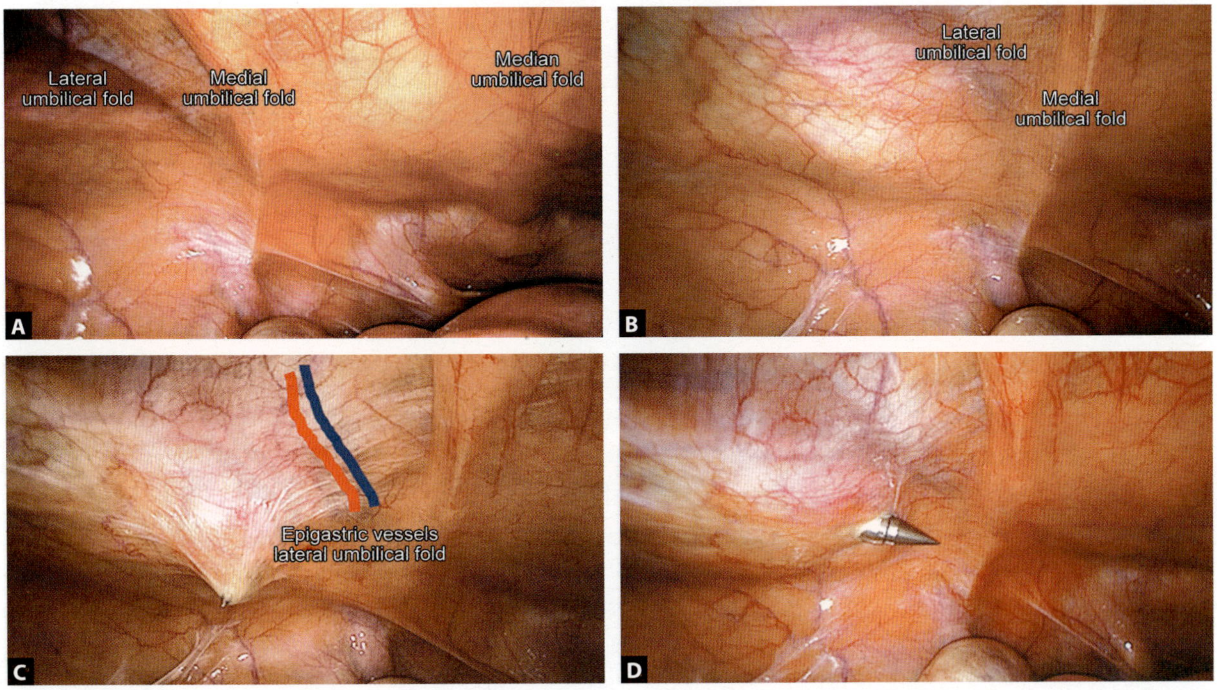

Figs. 47.8A to D: Secondary trocar placement, entry in the left lower abdomen. (A) The three plicae are visualized; (B) The palpating finger is showing the area lateral to the lateral umbilical fold; (C) Entry of the sharp ancillary trocar lateral to the lateral umbilical fold; (D) Once the peritoneum has been penetrated, the trocar points to the fundus of the uterus to avoid injury to the major vessels and the bowel.

a laparoscopic myomectomy. The advantage of the hysteroscopy for infertility patients is that the endometrial pathology can be identified and corrected and the intracavity extension of the fibroid can be noted. A chromopertubation should be performed before proceeding to myomectomy. If at laparoscopic myomectomy the blue dye solution becomes visible, this is a clear indication of the opening of the uterine cavity. Depending on the size of the myoma and the uterine scar afterward, sometimes a secondary diagnostic laparoscopy with chromopertubation is useful. A clear opening of both tubes can then be stated or excluded. Exclusion leads directly to reproductive management.

Technically, from a certain size of the myoma and especially in back wall localization, it is advisable to use a uterine manipulator to stabilize the mobile uterus during a myomectomy.

A longitudinal incision on the uterus is usually preferred for a myomectomy but, if the myoma extends laterally, a horizontal incision is also acceptable. If the uterine cavity is entered during the procedure, it has to be sutured additionally in a special layer. If the fibroid is posterior, there might be an increased risk of adhesion formation and an antiadhesive strategy needs to be adopted. The patient should always be informed that there is a low risk that the surgery may have to be converted to a laparotomy.

At laparoscopic myoma enucleation we perform an intracapsular approach with an adequate reconstruction of the uterine wall, which gives the patient a good start for further fertility results. After vasopressin-dilution injection in several wells, the capsule is incised by the cutting-side of the harmonic scalpel or any other cutting-coagulating device. Under traction the fibroid is enucleated, while the basic vessels are coagulated. The adaption of wound edges may be in one, two or three layers depending on the situation. If the uterine cavity has been opened, an extralayer of sutures has to be applied to readapt the endometrium. Conventional or barbed sutures are acceptable although we have the best experience with extracorporeal knotting of monofilament absorbable sutures.

Morcellation and extraction of the fibroid is performed with utmost care, if desired in a contained surrounding. After reconstruction of the uterine wall an antiadhesive barrier can be applied.

Post-surgery, the patient is usually advised to attempt pregnancy after 3 months to give adequate time for the uterine scar to heal. The decision on whether a pregnancy can be delivered spontaneously or by planned cesarean section is left to the surgeon and needs to be indicated in the surgical notes.

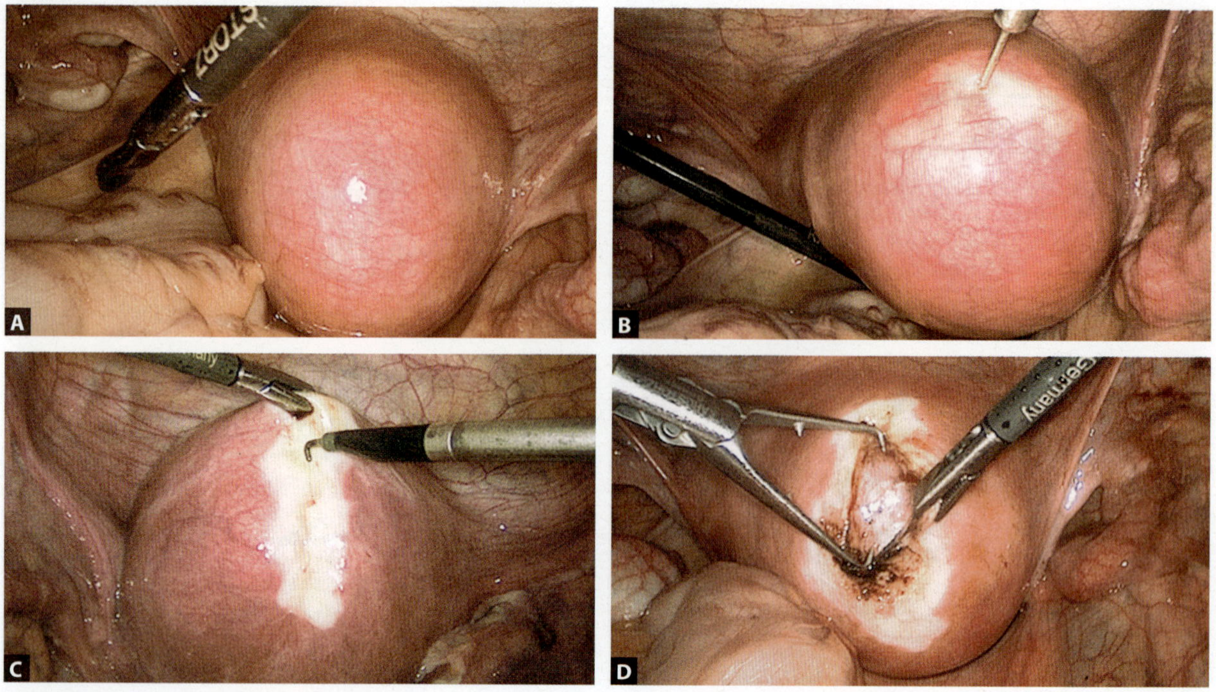

Figs. 47.9A to D: Laparoscopic myoma enucleation. (A) Situs of a fundal/anterior wall fibroid; (B) Prophylactic hemostasis with 1:100 diluted vasopressin solution (Gylcylpressin) in separate wells between the superficial and healthy tissue of the myometrium, and the capsule/fibroid surface. The purpose of the injection is to separate the pseudocapsule from the fibroid and reduce bleeding; (C) Bipolar superficial coagulation of the longitudinal incision strip and opening of the uterine wall above the myoma with a monopolar hook or needle until one reaches the myoma; (D) Grasping the fibroid and starting the enucleation. The pseudocapsule remains within the uterine wall and is pushed off bluntly.

Laparoscopic Myomectomy and Uterine Wall Reconstruction in a Stepwise Description (Figs. 47.9 to 47.14)

Endometriosis

Endometriosis is the second most common benign genital disease in women after uterine myoma. It is defined as the presence of endometrial glands and stroma outside the internal epithelial lining of the uterine cavity. The symptoms include chronic pelvic pain, dysmenorrhea, deep dyspareunia, cyclical bowel or bladder symptoms (such as dyschezia, bloating, constipation, rectal bleeding, diarrhea and hematuria), subfertility, abnormal menstrual bleeding, chronic fatigue or low back pain. The unspecific symptoms reflect the diversity of pathologies and localization as well as individual reactions to the disease. All classifications suggested so far are limited in terms of their predictive value.[9]

The interval between the first unspecific symptoms and the medical diagnosis of endometriosis is about 7 years. The condition is usually diagnosed for the first time between the ages of 20 and 40. In cases of secondary sterility, the frequency increases parallel to the time elapsed since the last pregnancy: less than 5 years 7%, 5–10 years 19%, and longer than 10 years 26%.[10]

As the pathogenesis of endometriosis is not clear, its causal treatment remains impossible. The treatment options include expectant management, analgesia, hormonal therapy, surgical intervention and a combination of medical treatment before and/or after surgery. As it has been shown that the growth of endometriosis is promoted by estrogen, various medical treatments can be used to address the condition.[11,12]

Adenomyosis of the uterus can be distinguished from endometriosis in that adenomyosis is marked by the appearance of endometrial glands and endometrial stroma within the myometrium. The spread of endometrial tissue induces hypertrophy and hyperplasia of the surrounding tissue. This leads to an enlarged, occasionally softened, and sometimes rigid uterus. Adenomyosis can be identified very clearly by imaging procedures. Nevertheless, focal adenomyosis can be easily mistaken for a leiomyoma.

Adenomyosis and Infertility

General endometriosis is associated with infertility, which can be addressed by medication and/or

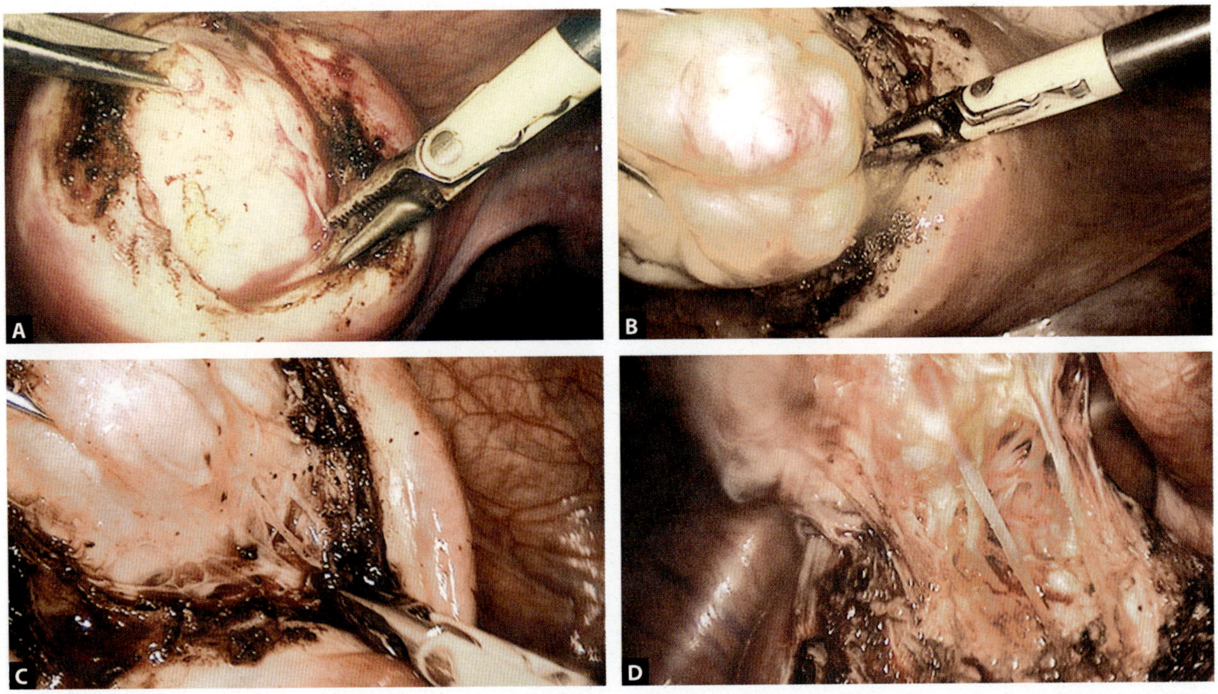

Figs. 47.10A to D: Laparoscopic myoma enucleation. (A) Traction of the fibroid with a tenaculum and blunt demarcation from the capsule; (B) Focal bipolar coagulation of basic vessels; (C) Continuous enucleation of the fibroid under traction and specific coagulation of capsule fibers containing vessels; (D) Magnification of the remaining capsule fibers to be coagulated and cut.

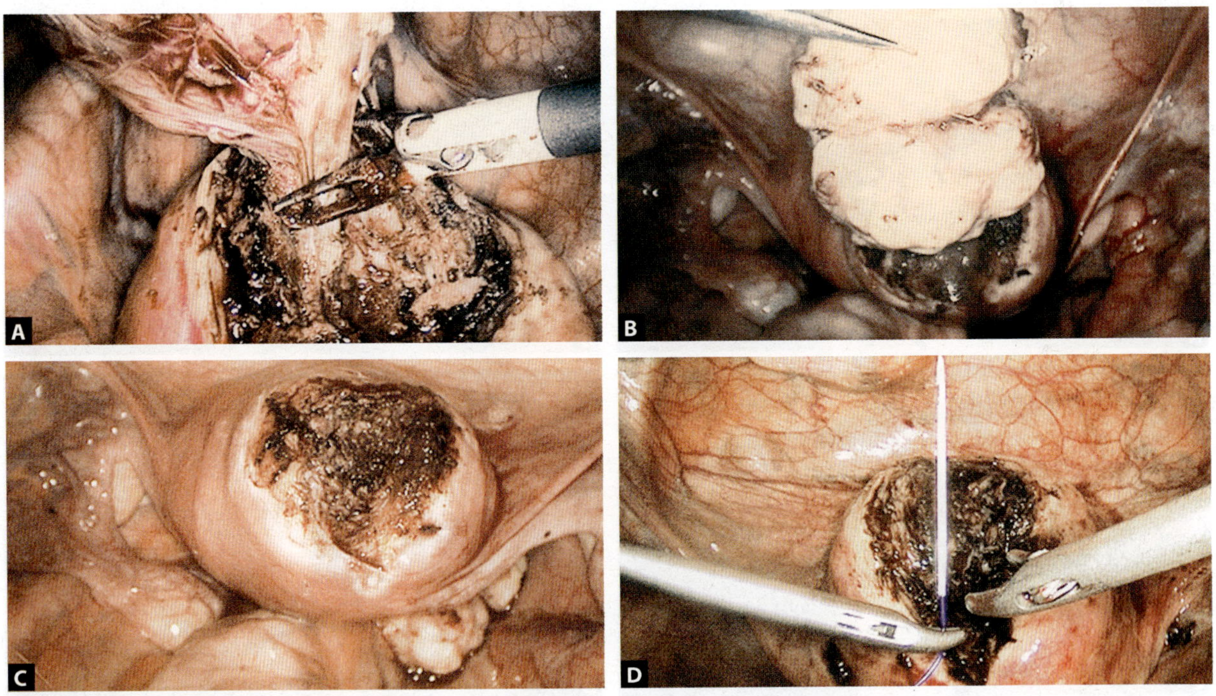

Figs. 47.11A to D: Laparoscopic myoma enucleation. (A) Final coagulation of the capsule vessels; (B) Double belly fibroid after complete enucleation; (C) Minimal coagulation of bleeding vessels under suction and irrigation; (D) Approximation of the wound edges with a straight or round sharp needle and a monofilar late-absorbable suture.

surgery. Surgery enhances the likelihood of natural conception.

The detrimental effects of adenomyosis on fertility may be due to the impairment of sperm transport, hyperperistaltic or dysperistaltic uterotubal transport. The eutopic and heterotopic endometrium of these patients might be associated with biochemical and functional alterations, leading to poor receptivity.

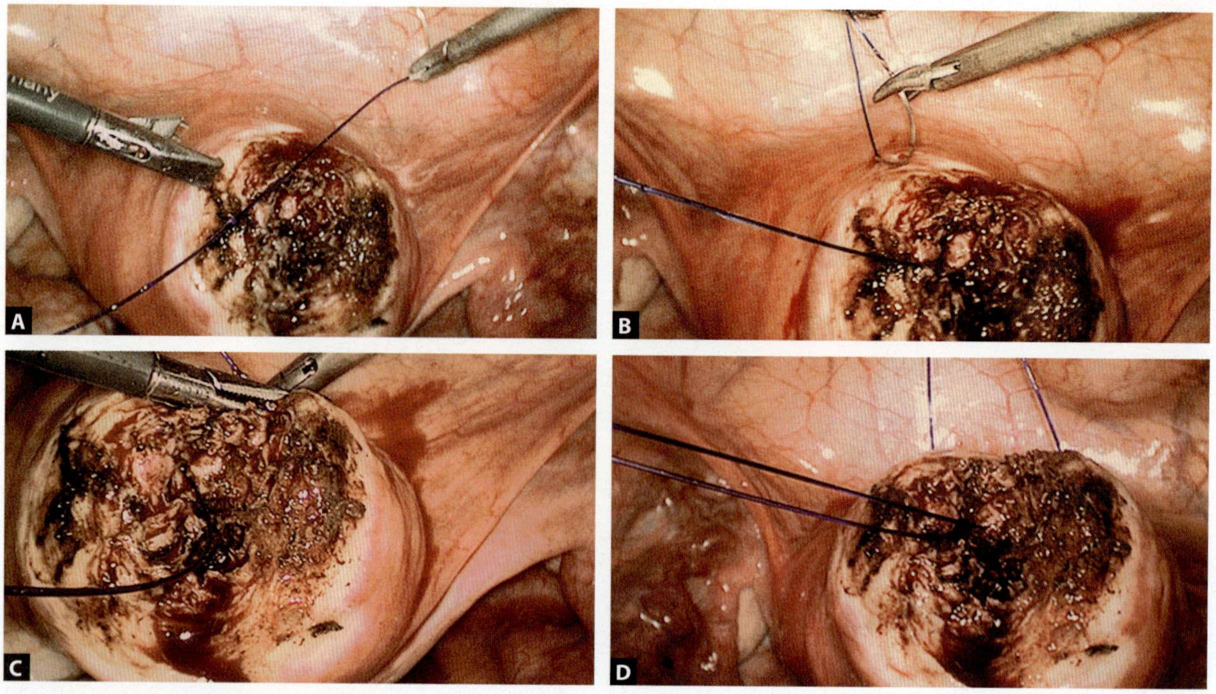

Figs. 47.12A to D: Laparoscopic myoma enucleation. (A) Advantages of a circular needle stitch: (a) The wound angle is elevated safely and completely when raised with a Manhes forceps, (b) Deeper layers of the myometrium can be grasped more easily with a circular needle; (B) Needle exit and simplified re-grasping with the right needle holder; (C) Final stitch to invert the knot; (D) Extirpation of the needle, completing the extracorporeal knot, and preparing to push down the extracorporeal knot.

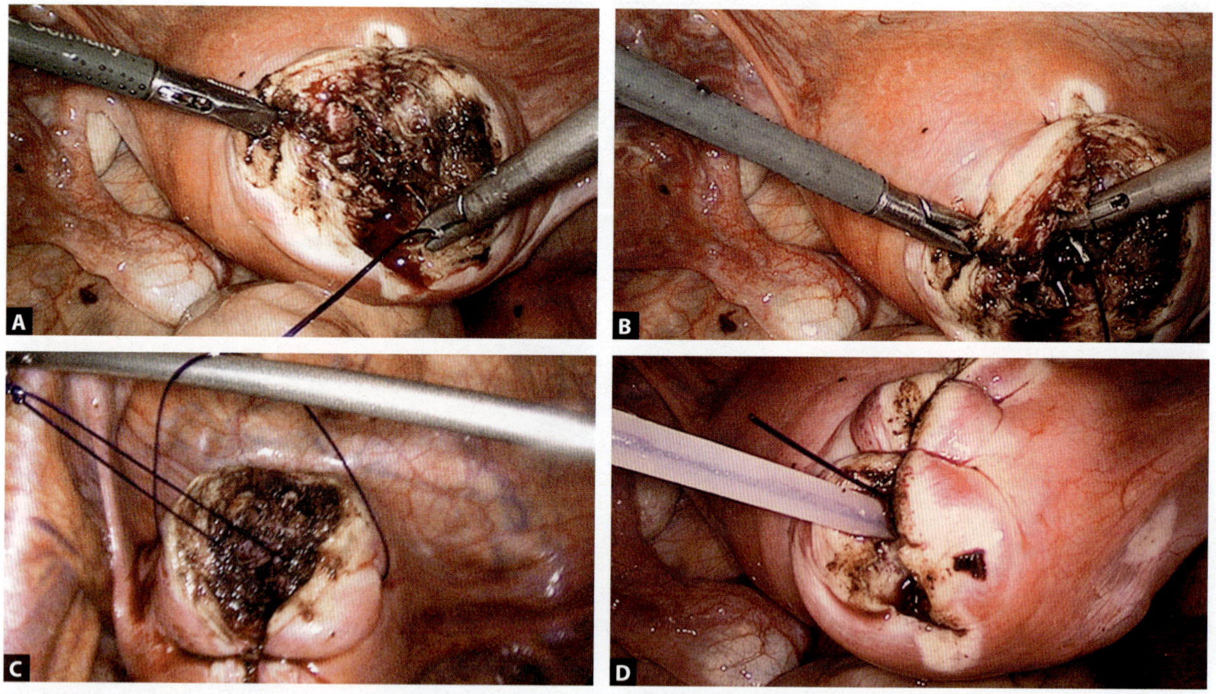

Figs. 47.13A to D: The extracorporeal "von Leffern" knot. (A) Pulling out the suture, removing the needle, half hitch; (B) Holding the knot with the left hand and reaching over with the right hand; (C) Grasping the short end from below and leading it back, exiting before the half hitch; (D) Turning back the knot. Holding the straight suture and tightening the knot.

The high spontaneous abortion rate may be due to a dysfunctional junctional zone. Adenomyosis is also known to influence the outcome of in vitro fertilization (IVF) and intracytoplasmic sperm injection (ICSI) adversely: lower rates of clinical pregnancy and implantation as well as higher rates of early pregnancy loss have been reported. The long downregulation protocol appears to exert a protective effect.[13,14]

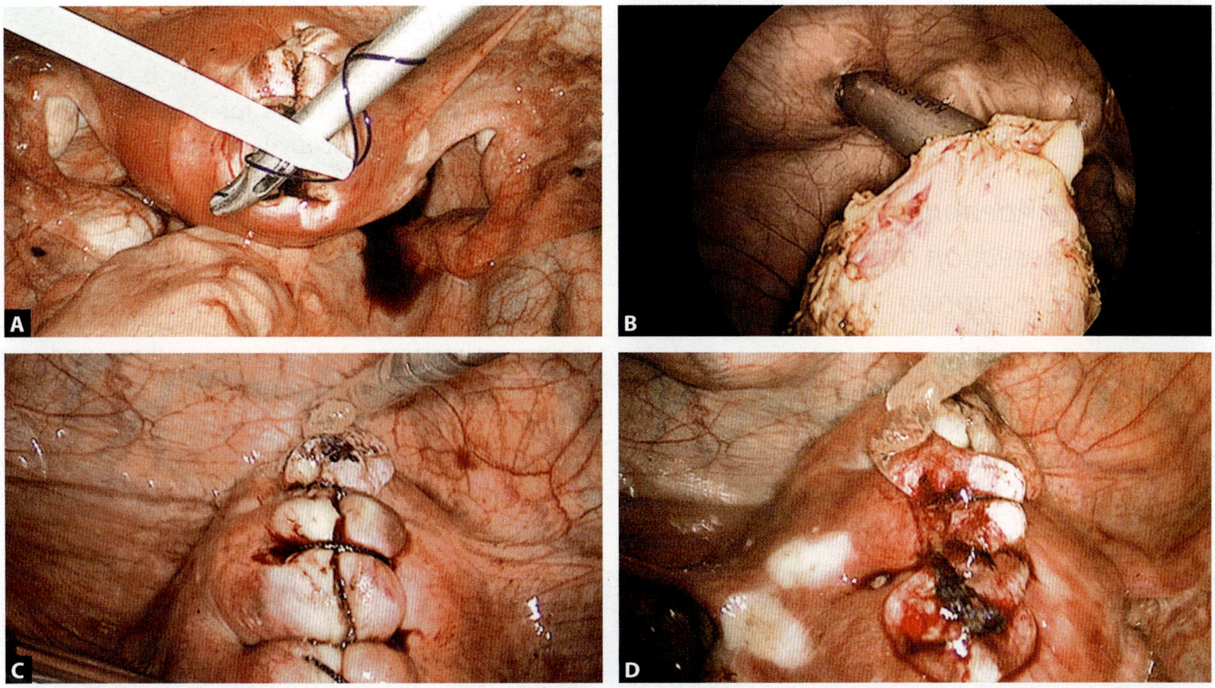

Figs. 47.14A to D: Laparoscopic myoma enucleation. (A) Second single suture starting as deep as possible in the uterine wound; (B) The needle exits on the left wound margin (immediately adjacent to the Manhes forceps); (C) Completing the stitch and preparing the extracorporeal von Leffern knot. The needle holder elevates the thread to avoid tearing the uterine wall when pulling the monofilar thread (PDS); (D) Pushing down the extracorporeal knot with a plastic pushrod into the depth of the wound to dump the knot, thus minimizing the size of the external part of the suture.

Treatment

Causal treatment of adenomyosis is difficult. Conservative medical therapy is identical to that of endometriosis. In many cases, adenomyosis of the uterus and endometriosis exist simultaneously.[15]

General Treatment of Endometriosis Combined with Adenomyosis of the Uterus

As the pathogenesis of endometriosis is not clearly understood, no causal treatment other than hysterectomy is available at the present time. The treatment options include expectant management, analgesia, hormonal medical therapy, surgical intervention and a combination of medical treatment before and/or after surgery. The therapeutic procedures may be divided into three groups: medical, surgical and combined treatment. The fact that the growth of endometriosis is assisted by estrogen has led to a variety of medical treatments.[11,12,16] The first structured therapy was introduced by Mettler and Semm. It involves diagnostic laparoscopy, removing all visible endometriosis foci as far as possible, three to six months of endocrine therapy and a subsequent second-look laparoscopy with resection of residual foci, removal of adhesions and reconstruction of organs. If the patient desires children, the gynecologist is advised to use assisted reproductive treatment.[17]

Combined treatment: Combined treatment involves diagnostic laparoscopy, removal of all visible endometriosis foci as far as possible, 3 to 6 months of endocrine therapy and a subsequent second-look laparoscopy with resection of residual foci, adhesiolysis and reconstruction of organs. When women with endometriosis and/or adenomyosis of the uterus wish to have children, the gynecologist uses endocrine down-regulation and consecutive stimulation over a prolonged period of time in combination with in-vitro fertilization.[18-23]

Surgical Treatment of Adenomyosis of the Uterus

The foremost advantage of endoscopic treatment of adenomyosis is that it permits simultaneous treatment of intraabdominal comorbidities such as endometriosis, severe adenomyosis affecting the adjacent organs (sacrouterine ligaments, cardinal ligament, bladder and/or bowel) and adhesions. Although uterine-preserving surgical strategies are still controversially discussed and their results are not consistently promising, the only conclusive treatment of adenomyosis is total hysterectomy. Since the disease is confined to the uterus, the ovaries can be preserved.

Diagnosis of Adenomyosis (Figs. 47.15 to 47.17) and Resection of Endometriosis in a Stepwise Description

The primary step in these cases is removal of all visible endometriosis spots. These may be superficial and easy to excise (Figs. 47.18 to 47.25), or adherent to more delicate structures and difficult to eliminate (Figs. 47.26 and 47.27).

Postoperative Management

The urinary catheter is removed; it remains in place only in specific cases for infectious reasons. A postoperative cystoscopy is performed in cases of severe endometriosis or adhesions in the upper part of the bladder. Early ambulation a few hours after surgery is good practice. Clear fluids can be ingested 6 hours post-surgery, followed by a light diet. Thromboprophylaxis (mechanical and medical) must be used in appropriate cases. A postoperative ultrasound scan of the renal pelvis should be performed. Ordinary light activities are permitted and the patient may return to work after 4–5 days. Sexual activity, intensive sports and heavy work should be avoided for 6–8 weeks.

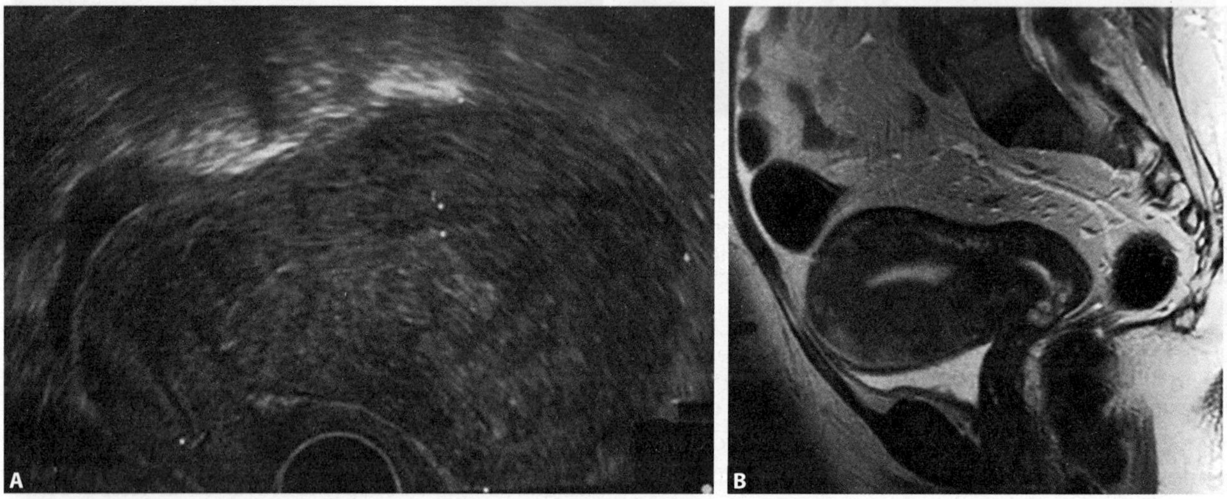

Figs. 47.15A and B: (A) Transvaginal ultrasound of the uterus. The heterogeneous anterior wall is clearly seen. Furthermore, there is a discrepancy between anterior and posterior wall thickness resembling the multiple intramural adenomyosis cysts; (B) The discrepancy is also seen in sagittal MRI. Here, a solitary myoma can be excluded as a differential diagnosis.

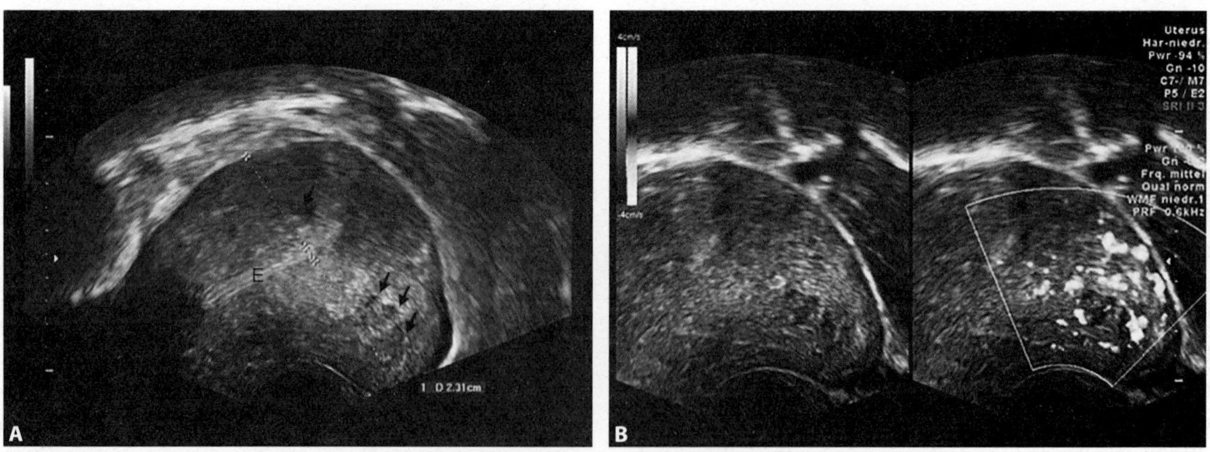

Figs. 47.16A and B: (A) Transvaginal ultrasound of the uterus. The heterogeneous anterior wall is very extended. Small intramural cysts can be demarcated. Furthermore, there is a big discrepancy between anterior and posterior wall thickness resembling the multiple intramural adenomyosis cysts. No solitary cyst or clearly demarcated myoma is described; (B) The diagnosis of adenomyosis uteri and focal adenomyosis is corroborated by Doppler signal.

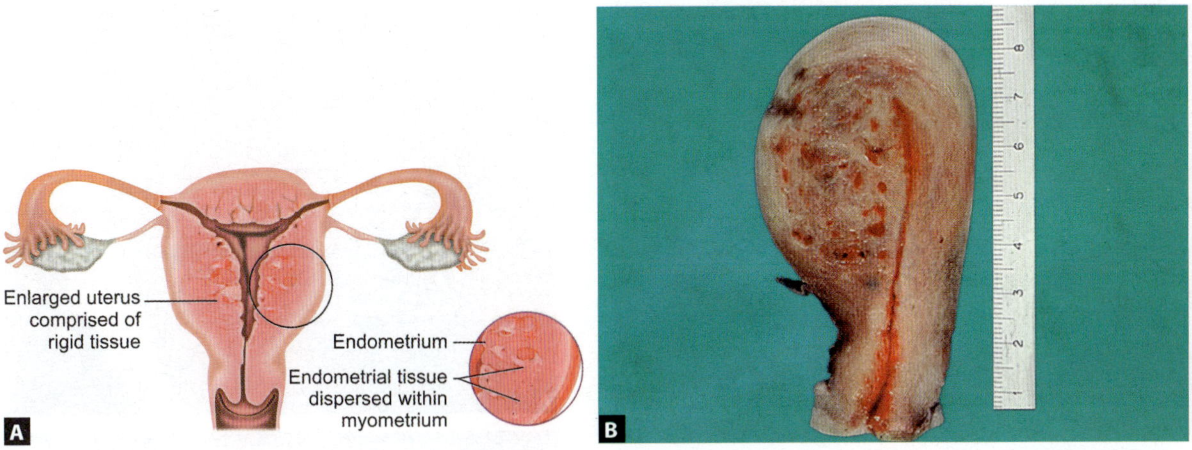

Figs. 47.17A and B: (A) Schematic illustration of an enlarged uterus with adenomyosis. Endometriosis glands are dispersed within the myometrium; (B) Anatomical specimen in a sagittal cut. The posterior wall is much thicker than the anterior wall, with endometriosis glands spread diffusely in the myometrium wall.

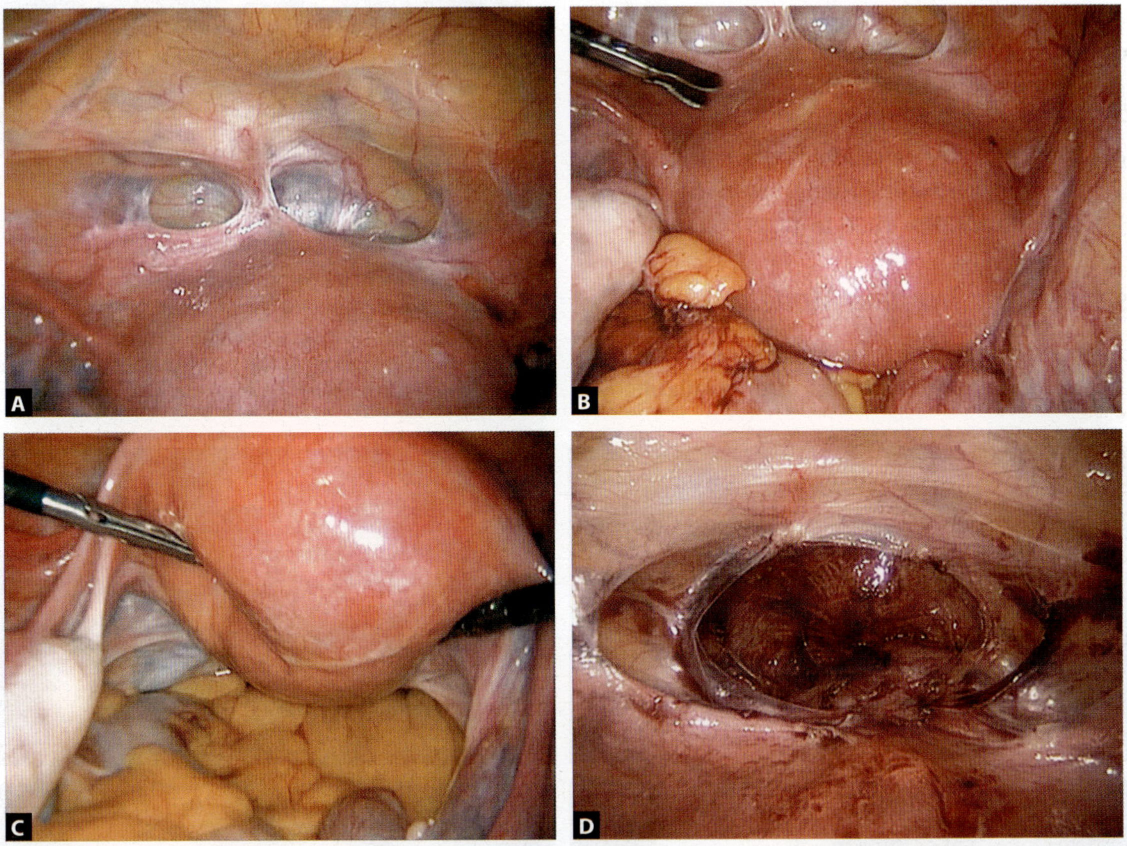

Figs. 47.18A to D: (A) Overview of the laparoscopic situs of a patient with severe dysmenorrhea; (A to C) The uterus is enlarged and soft. The anterior wall is connected to the bladder peritoneum by multiple adhesions; (D) After adhesiolysis one has the impression that the adenomyosis has grown through the uterine wall into the adjoining bladder.

Congenital Anatomical Uterine Malformations

Congenital malformations are very difficult to clearly assign. Figures 47.28 and 47.29 provide a scheme for definite description of expected or verified uterine malformations.

In the following sections the authors will introduce the importance of the knowledge of hysteroscopy and laparoscopy and their individual use with the help of three special cases.

Case 1: Uterus duplex bicornis with complete vaginal septum (Figs. 47.30 to 47.32)

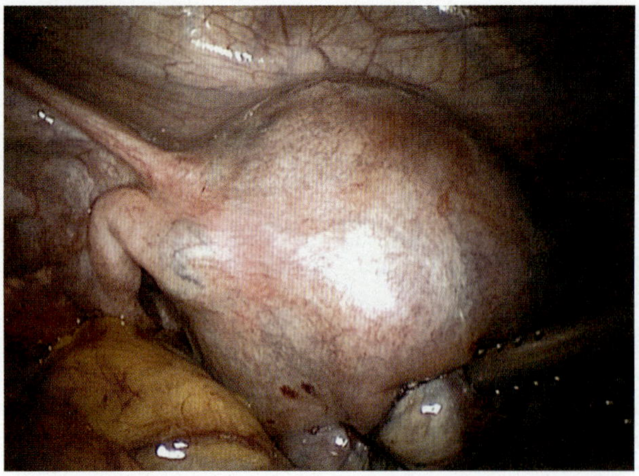

Fig. 47.19: Patient with severe dysmenorrhea and dyspareunia. The injection of blue dye exposes the intramural vessels, which seem to be massively increased. This picture is also typical of adenomyosis of the uterus.

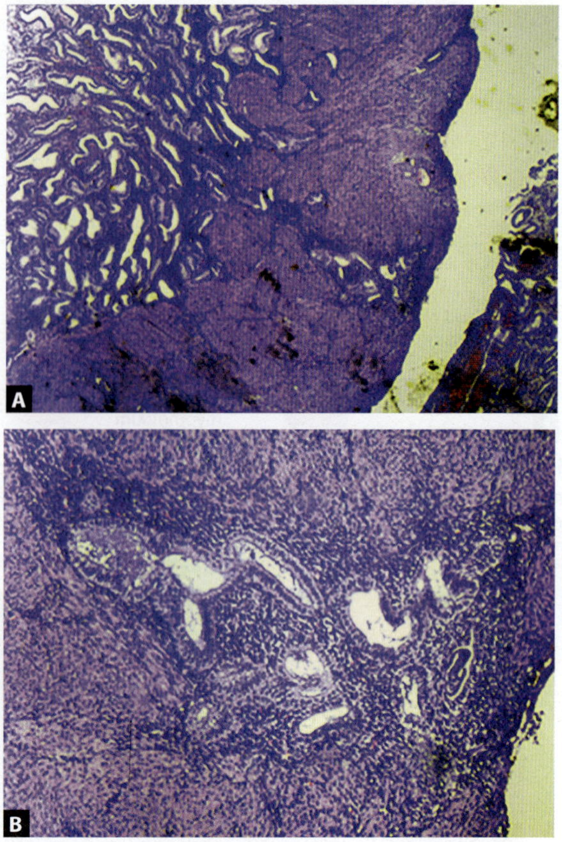

Figs. 47.20A and B: (A) Low magnification of a piece of ablated endometrium with the adjoining myometrium tissue in the early secretion phase; (B) Islets of endometrium glands in the myometrium stroma with no connection to the uterine cavity. Obviously, the endometrium is fully involved in the endocrine cycle.

Case 2: Placental remnant with curettage and hysteroscopy under laparoscopic guidance—multiple perforation (Figs. 47.33 to 47.35)

Case 3: Uterine wall defect after cesarean section—uterine wall reconstruction with the vis-à-vis maneuver (Figs. 47.36 to 47.39).

Hysteroscopic Training Models

Currently, several options for the hands-on training of hysteroscopic procedures are available. In

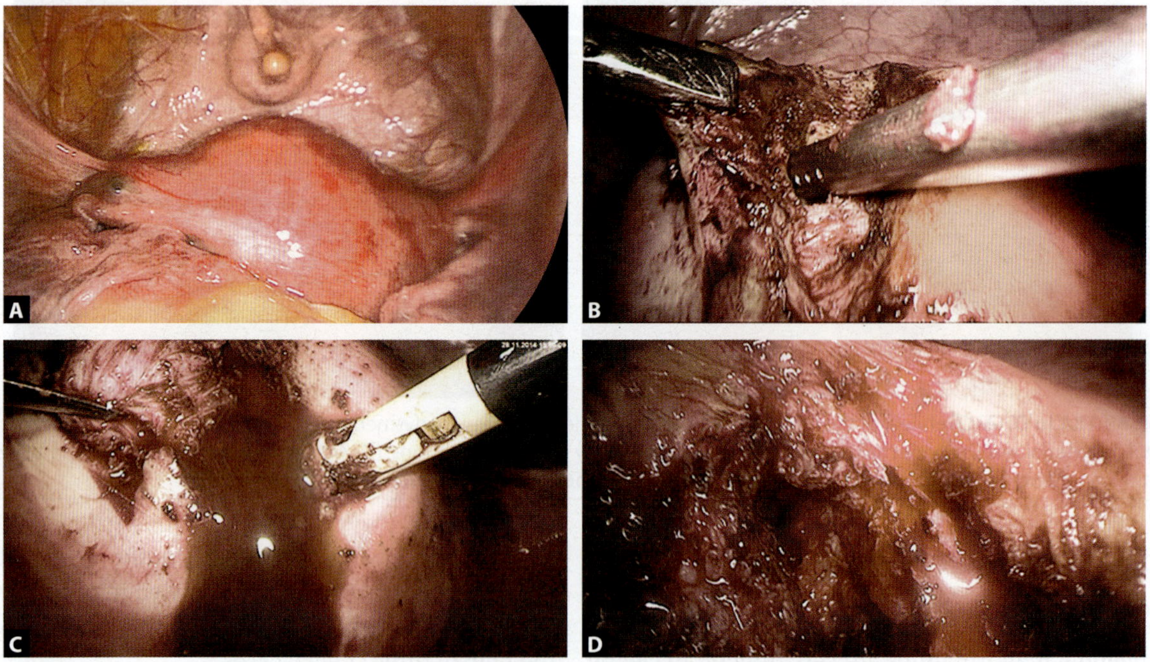

Figs. 47.21A to D: (A) Overview of an asymmetrical uterus; endometriosis is suspected at the left tube and a central space-occupying lesion is seen; (B) Opening the central intramural lesion, which was suspected to be a fibroid; (C) Chocolate-like fluid after entering the adenomyoma; (D) On the magnification even the wall layers, including the mid-endometrium tissue can be seen.

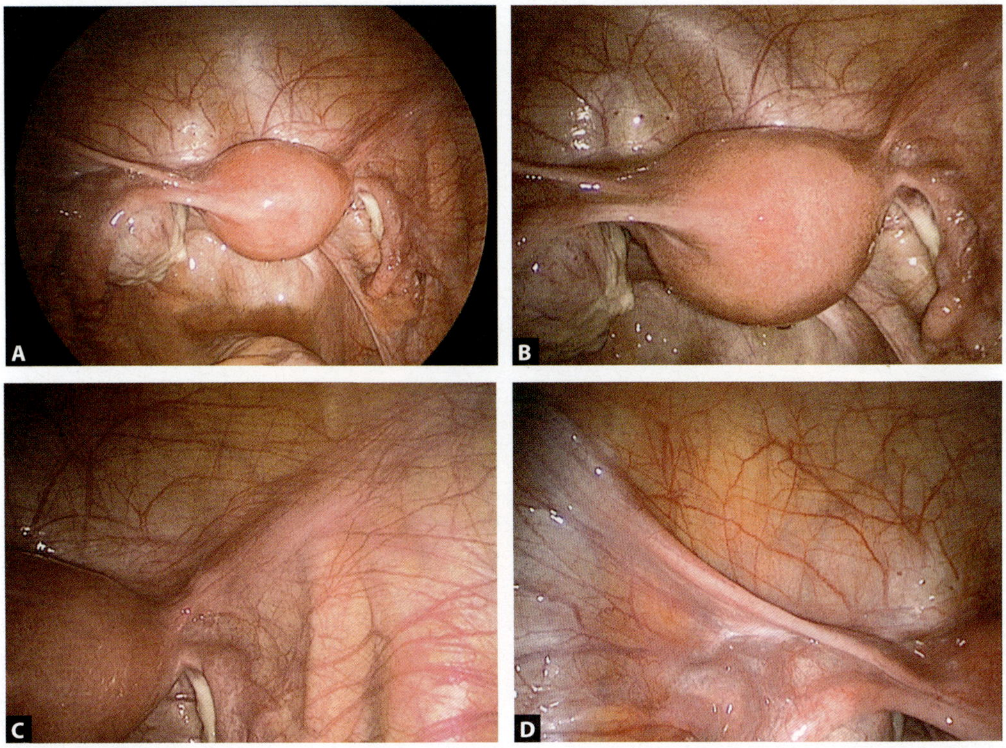

Figs. 47.22A to D: Laparoscopic overview of a patient with dysmenorrhea. (A and B) An enlarged and irregular uterus with hypervascularization of the serosa. The chronic disease has caused an asymmetry of the round ligaments; (C) The right side is much shorter than; (D) The left side.

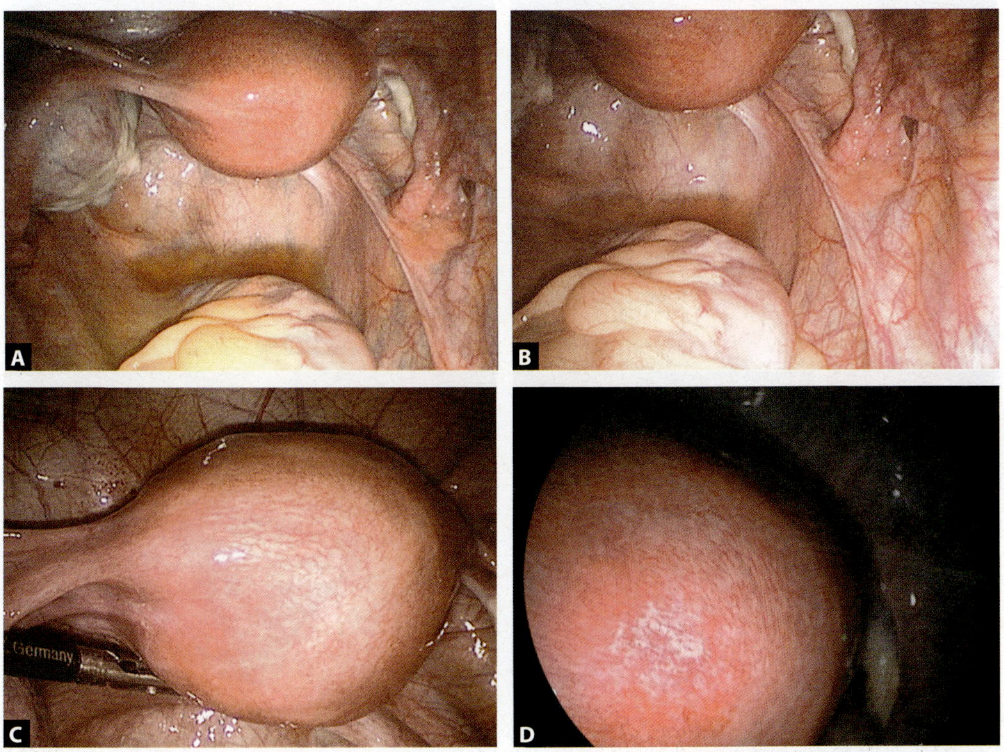

Figs. 47.23A to D: (A and C) The uterus appears to be less mobile but somehow fixed in the pelvis; (B) The peritoneum above the ureter is under tension and can be demarcated from the sacrouterine ligament; (C) The surface of the uterus is hypervascularized; (D) The outflow of the tubes seems to be steep.

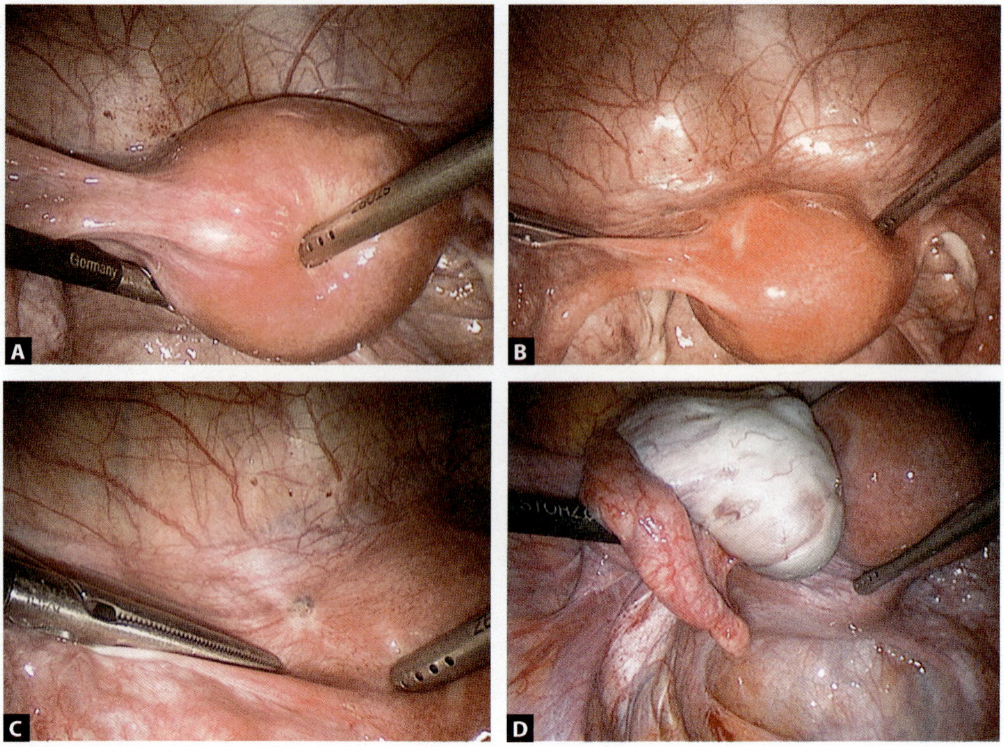

Figs. 47.24A to D: (A) Palpating the uterus with a blunt instrument shows that its consistency is less soft; (B) It is tight but hypervascular; (C) Endometriotic nodule on the lower uterine anterior wall; (D) Fixed and enlarged cystic left ovary in the ovarian fossa. The ureter can be demarcated behind the peritoneum and is lifted to the fixed area.

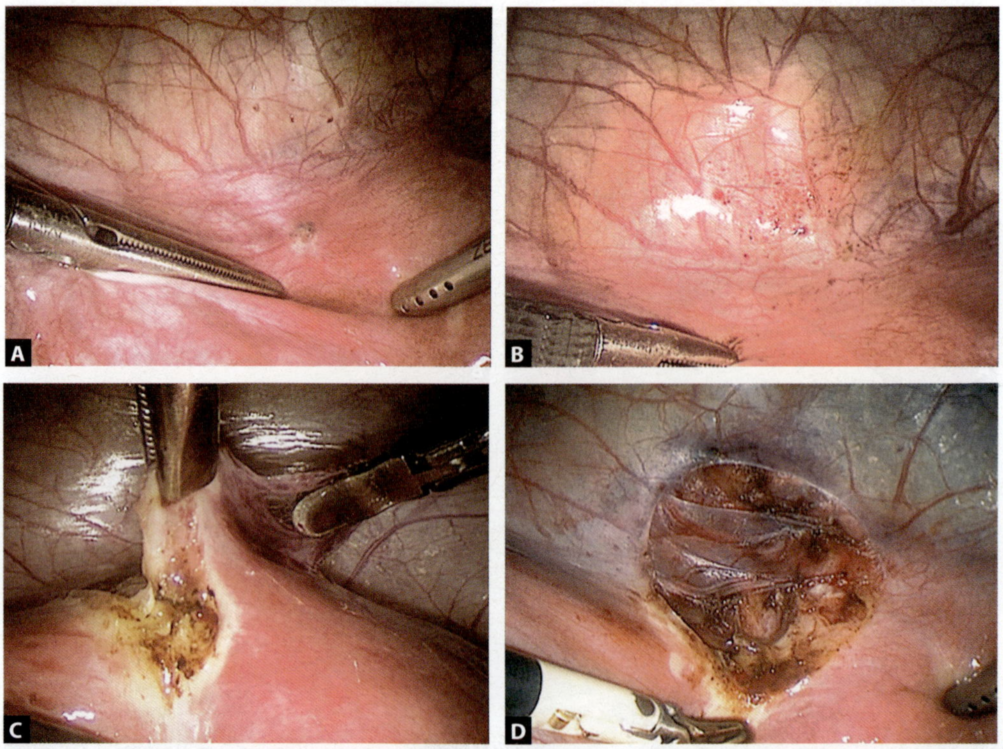

Figs. 47.25A to D: (A to D) Excision of the endometriotic nodule of the lower anterior uterine wall; (B) Even the adjacent bladder peritoneum appears to be superficially affected because it is hypervascularized and fragile.

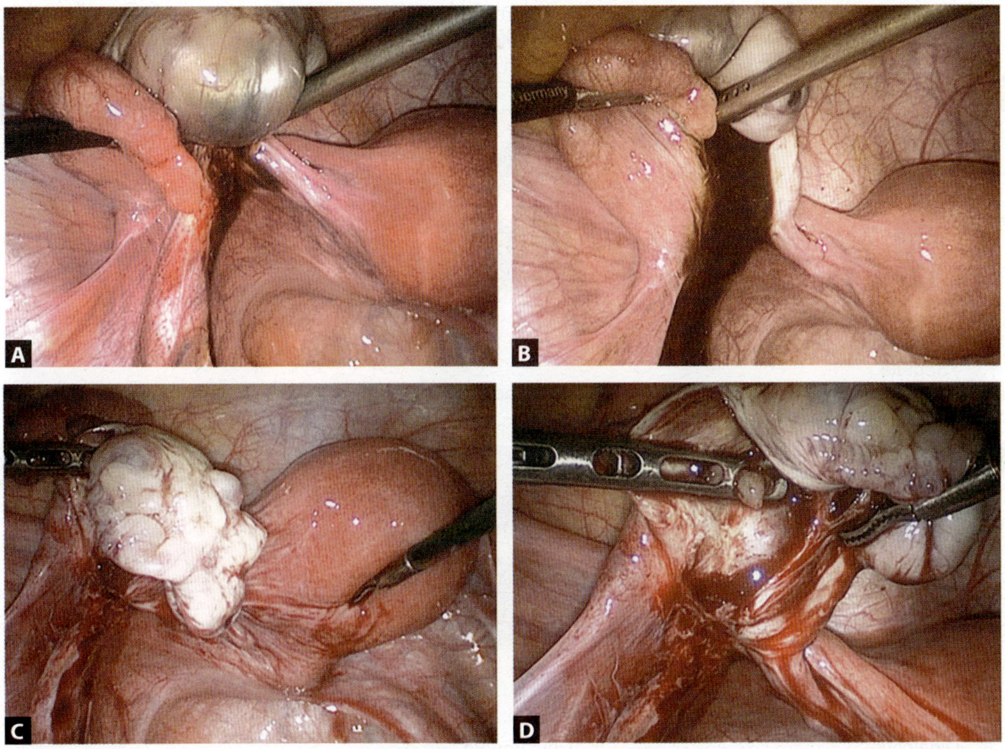

Figs. 47.26A to D: (A and B) Lifting the ovary out of the ovarian fossa and releasing it from its peritoneal adhesion leads to opening of the endometrioma; (C and D) The depths of the ovarian fossa are affected by disease, as proven by the demarcation of the peritoneal nodule. These nodules are usually connected to the cardinal ligament or the sacrouterine ligament.

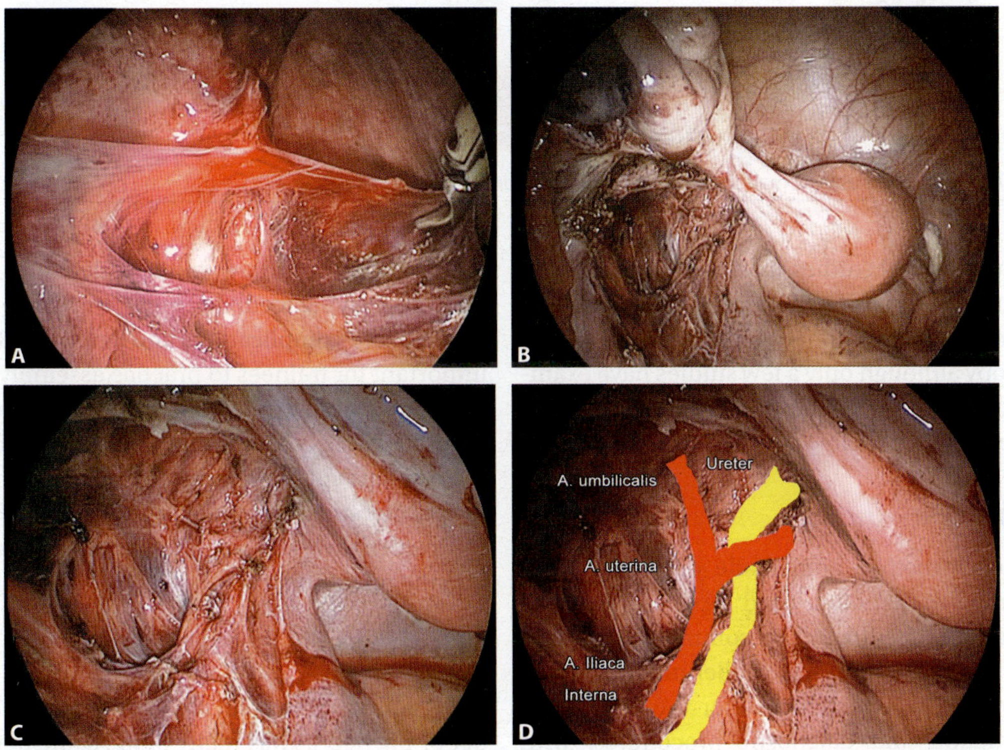

Figs. 47.27A to D: Opening the peritoneal wall for resection of the symptomatic endometriotic nodule. The ureter and vessels of the pelvic wall can be separated bluntly from the peritoneum and the endometriotic nodule. The ureter or the vessels themselves are very rarely affected. If they are, the condition calls for special surgical treatment.

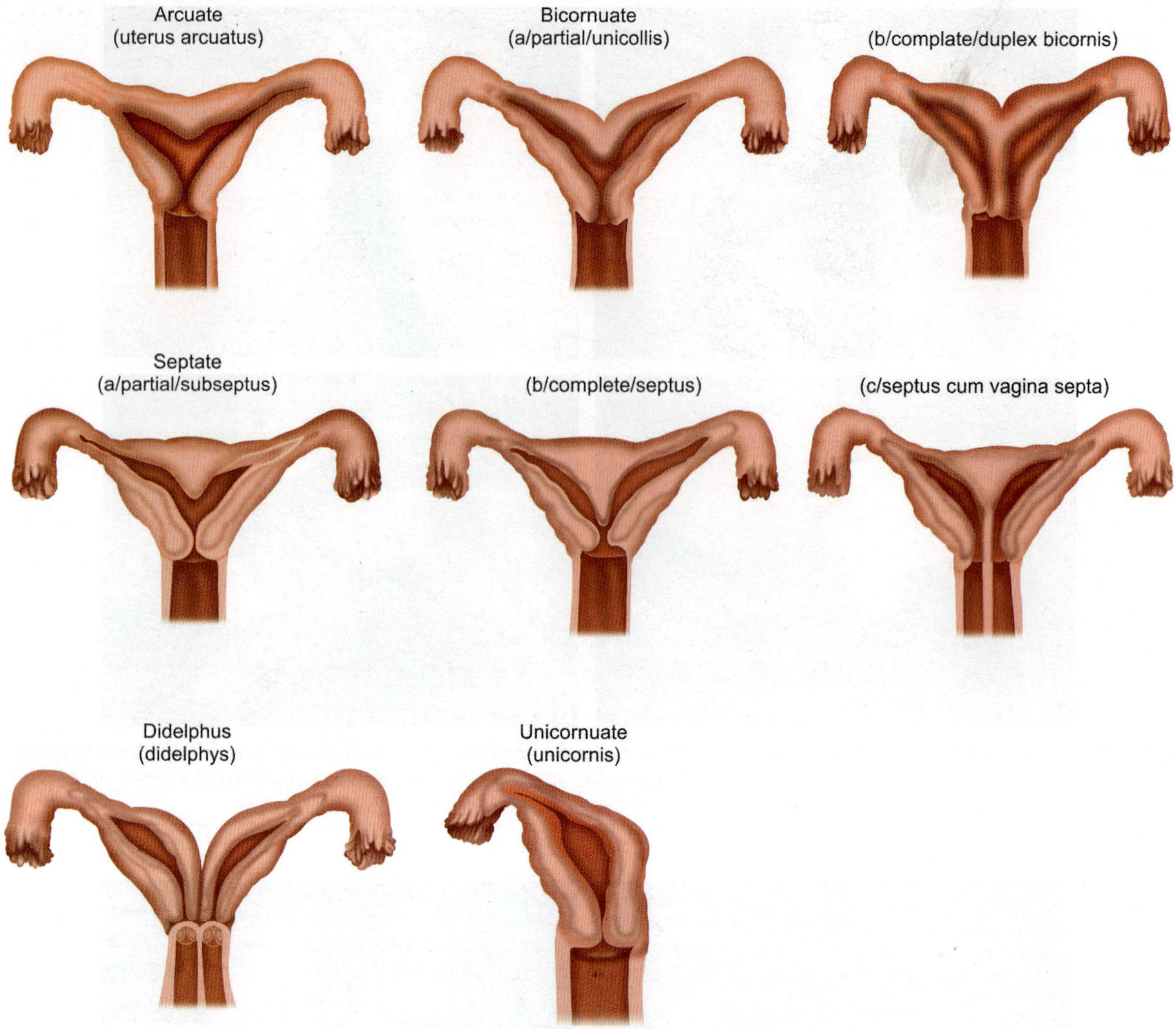

Fig. 47.28: An overview of uterine malformations by schematic drawings.

laparoscopy, several studies have shown that training on simulators leads to an improvement in operative technique. It is assumed that this is also true in hysteroscopy although only a few studies have examined this to date. The benefits and drawbacks of each option are discussed below.

Box Trainers

Box trainers, whether homemade or commercial, are a training model often used for the practice of hysteroscopic procedures. The commercial models generally consist of a uterine model made of latex, silicone or rubber, which allows for the practice of instrumentation and diagnostic procedures, with different models displaying different pathologies. Single-use models for operative procedures have also been developed. Some models also allow training the use of distension media.

Training on these models depends upon an instructor giving feedback on performance.

To avoid complications and delay in OR time, it is important for trainees to practice assembly and handling of hysteroscopic equipment, which can easily be done using a box trainer. Being able to use real instruments and train with the same equipment used in the operating room makes it easier for the trainee to transfer the skills acquired on the bench station into the operating room.

Animal Models

Using animal parts, such as cow uteri, sheep bladder or pig hearts, has many of the same benefits and drawbacks as box trainers, but most importantly they allow for highly realistic training using electrosurgical equipment. The basic principle is to use a hollow tissue organ to simulate the uterine cavity.

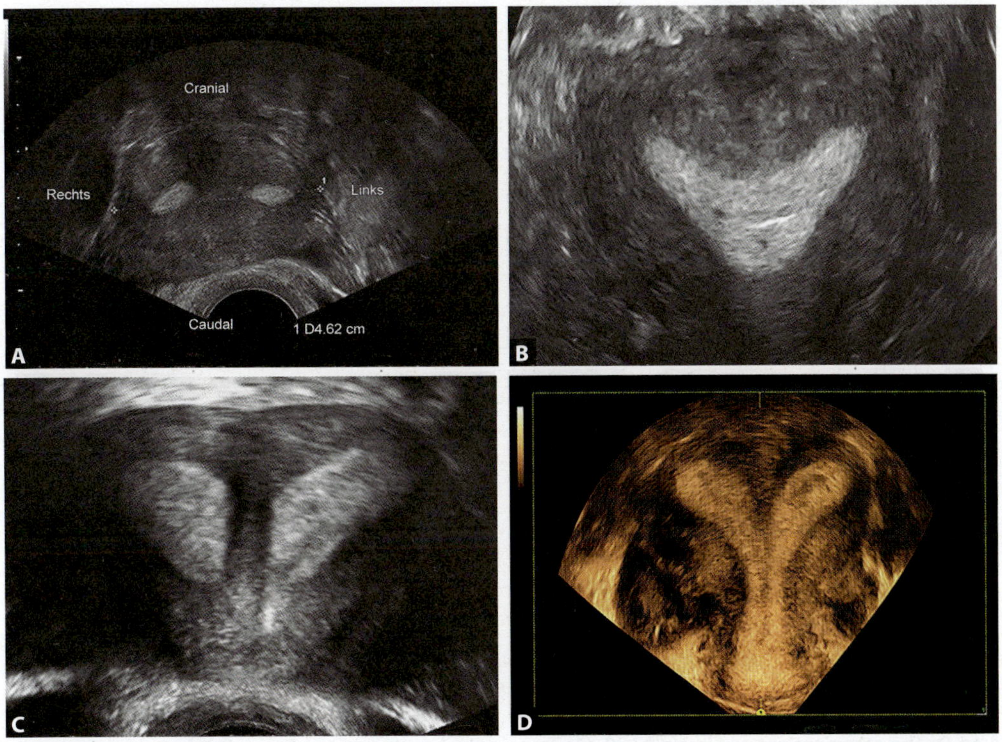

Figs. 47.29A to D: (A) The transverse scan at the fundal region of the corpus uteri clearly shows two endometrial parts separated from each other; (B) Representation of the endometrium in the fundal region by 3D sonography indicates an arcuate uterus, which explains the thicker than expected fundal uterine wall; (C) Corpus uteri, transverse scan, showing two parts of endometrium separated from each other. Suspicion of a septate uterus becomes firmer by performing continuous transverse scans from the fundal to the cervical uterine region and reverse; (D) Presentation of the whole uterus in its length by a frontal scan, using the 3D OmniView technique, impressively demonstrates the septate uterus.

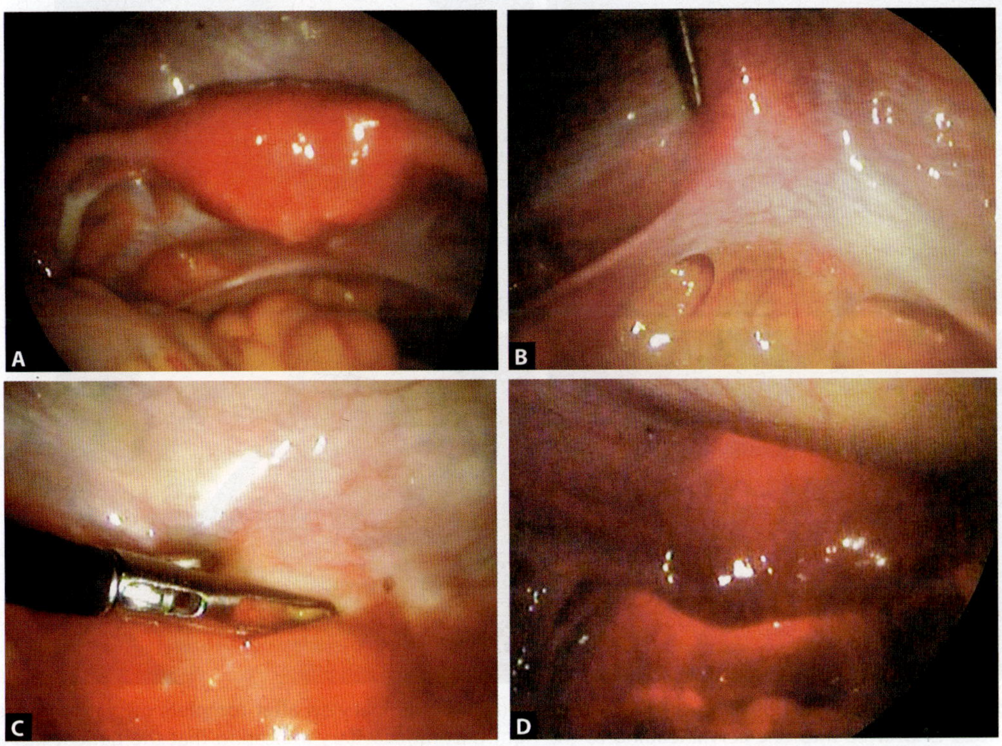

Figs. 47.30A to D: (A) Laparoscopic overview of a patient with expected septate uterus. The fundus is clear and the cervix from the intra-abdominal view seems to be single; (B) Dorsal view; (C) Ventral view; (D) Simultaneous hysteroscopy, by reducing the intra-abdominal illumination the real anatomy with at least two cornua is reflected.

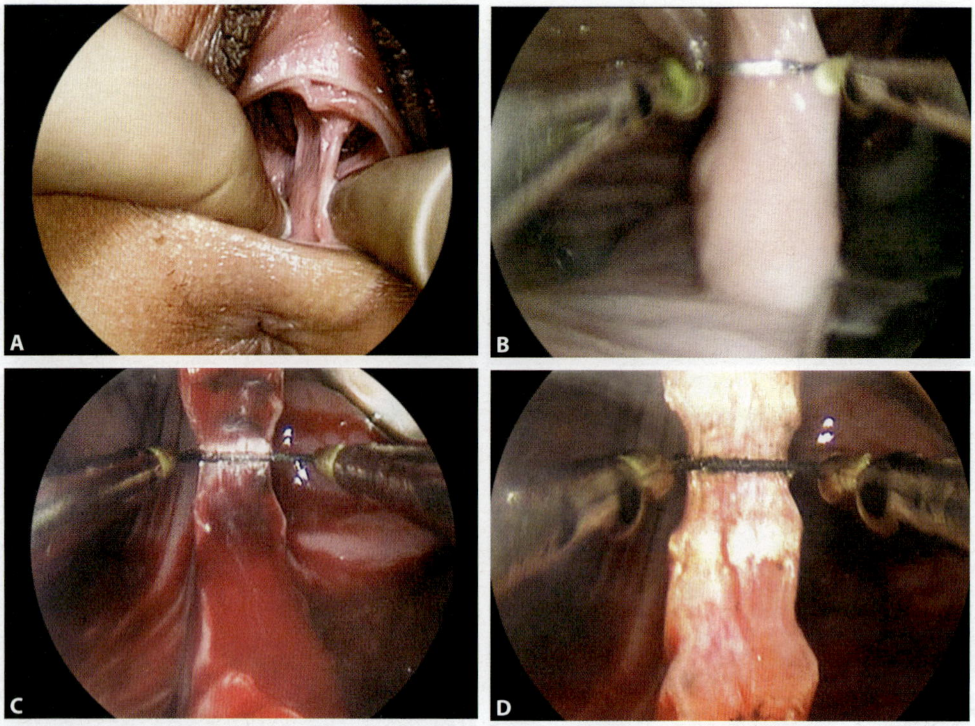

Figs. 47.31A to D: The same patient as Figure 47.30. (A) Transvaginal examination shows clearly a thick and complete vaginal septum; (B) The septum can be dissected, e.g. with a monopolar hysteroscopic loop; (C) In the depths of the vagina the septum becomes vascularized; and (D) Dissection can be continued until the two cervices are visible and reached.

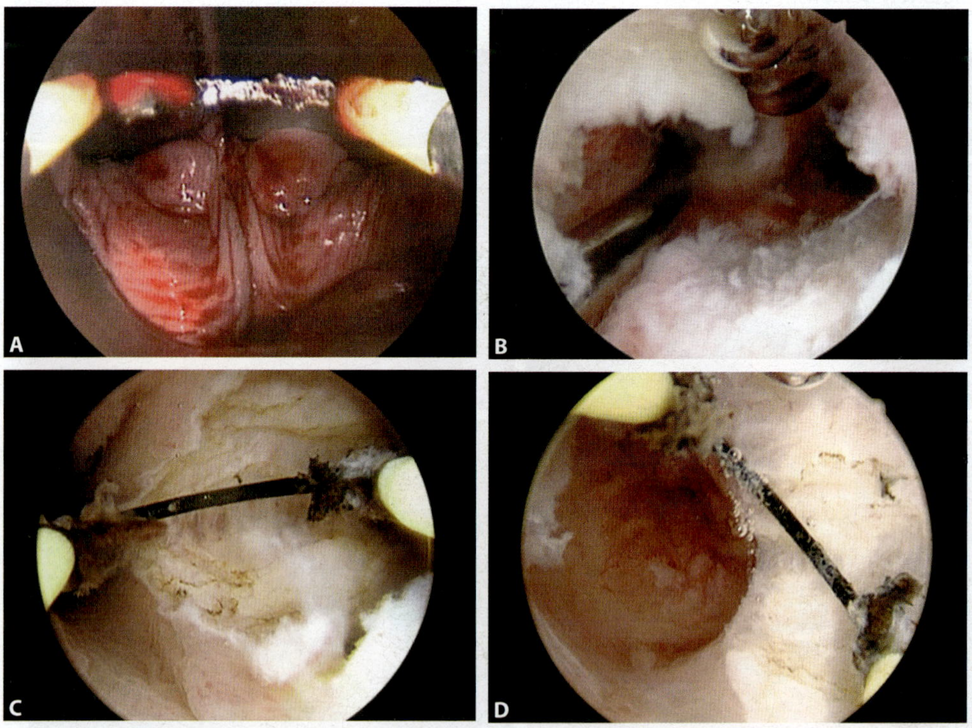

Figs. 47.32A to D: The same patient as in Figures 47.30 and 47.31. (A) Final vaginal view after complete dissection of the vaginal septum; (B) A probe is inserted into one cervix leading to the right part intracavitary indicating that the patient has a vaginal septum, two cervices and a uterine septum with a connection between the two corneal parts; (C) The broad intracavitary septum can clearly be demarcated and dissected, e.g. with a monopolar straight loop; (D) Dissection can be safely continued until reaching the fundus of the uterus as the laparoscopic view excluded the existence of a bicornuate uterus.

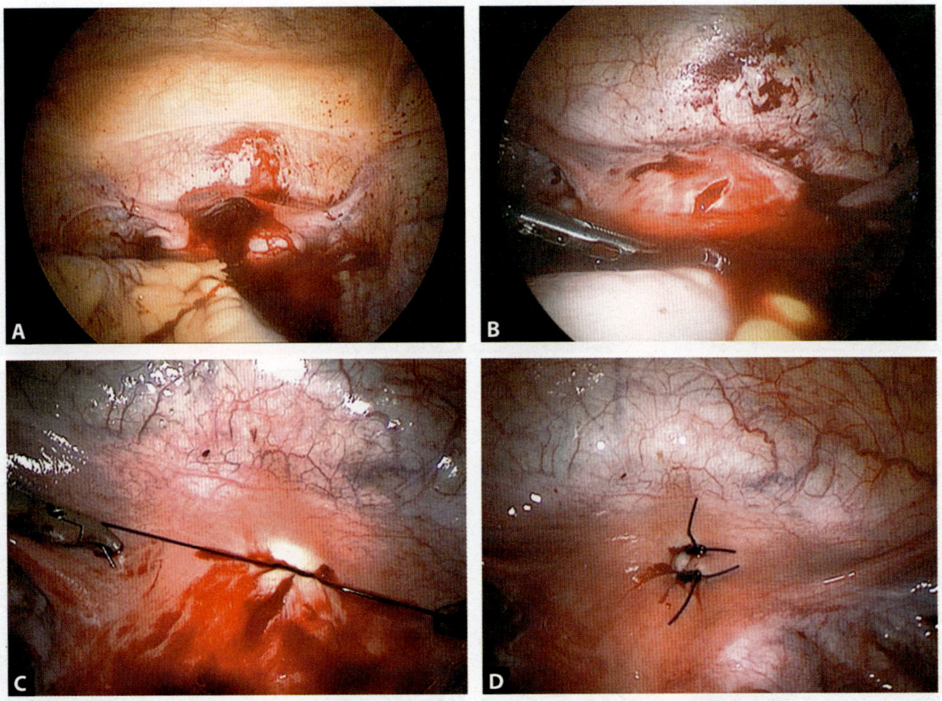

Figs. 47.33A to D: A 32-year-old patient with continuous vaginal bleeding, para I, with suspected placental remnant 5 weeks after delivery. (A and B) The soft wall of the enlarged uterus has been perforated at the anterior wall by curettage for placental remnant resection. The extent of the perforation was only recognized while doing a simultaneous laparoscopy. Active bleeding, hematoma and free fluid (hysteroscopic dilution) can be seen; (C and D) The hole can be sutured with a thick monofilament suture, performing intracorporeal knotting.

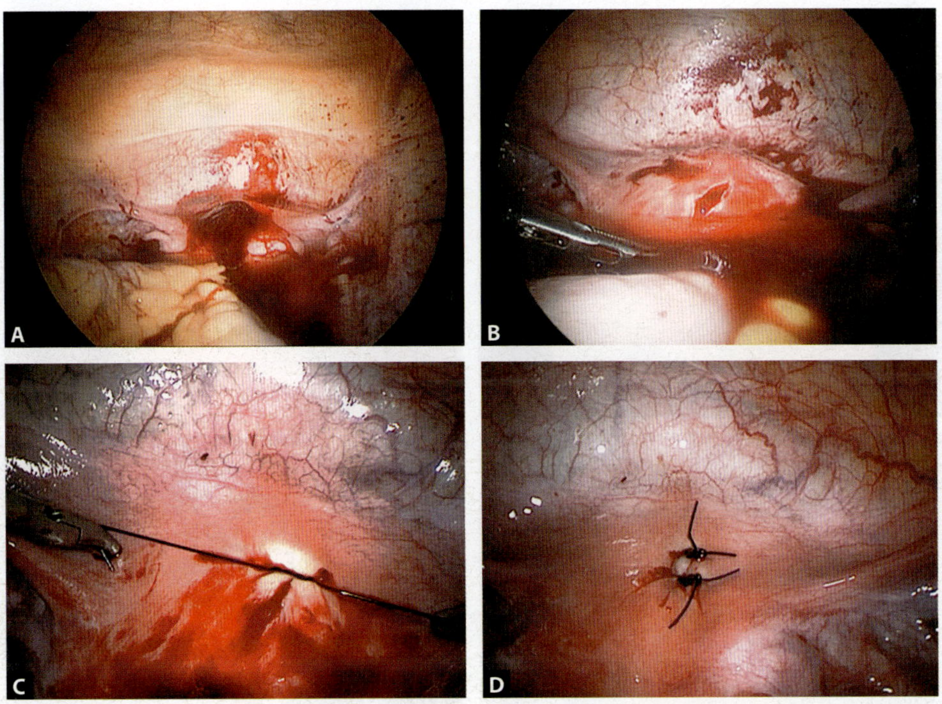

Figs. 47.34A to D: Same patient as in Figure 47.33. (A) Attempt to perform curettage under laparoscopic vision reveals a second perforation at the cervico-corporal transmission zone. Only the peritoneum of the bladder is still intact; (B) Immediate bleeding begins subperitoneally; (C) An early attempt to overcome the perforation area by performing hysteroscopy leads to a large edema in the subperitoneal space; (D) Therefore, the peritoneum needs to be opened and after complete preparation of the anterior uterine wall down to the vagina the sole hysteroscope is inserted without dilution medium and the perforation can be demarcated and overcome under laparoscopic site. The left forceps helps the distal part of the perforated tissue to be pulled on the distal part of the hysteroscope. Therewith, the distal part of the uterine corpus can be examined.

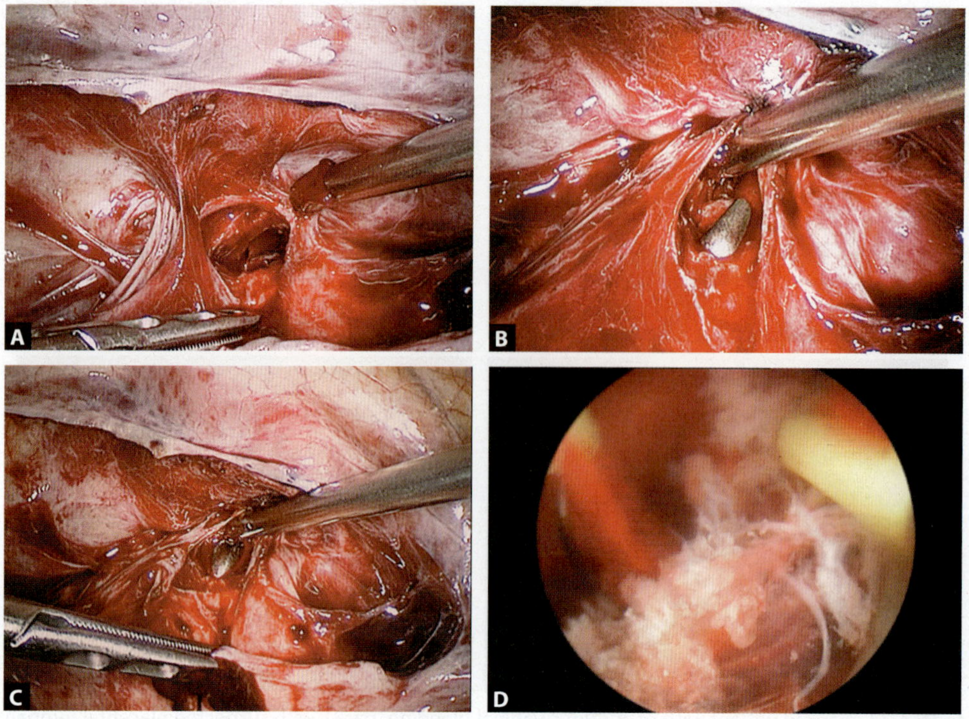

Figs. 47.35A to D: Same patient as in Figures 47.33 and 47.34. (A) After complete preparation of the uterine anterior wall only the vesicovaginal ligament is protected; (B) A probe is inserted into the cervix; and (C) Directed into the uterine cavity under laparoscopic guidance. The defect can then (after bridging of the defect by the probe) easily be closed by intracorporal full-wall thickness sutures; (D) Hysteroscopic vision of the placental remnant that can then be removed stepwise. After closure of the defect there is no more leakage and the dilution medium enables intrauterine vision.

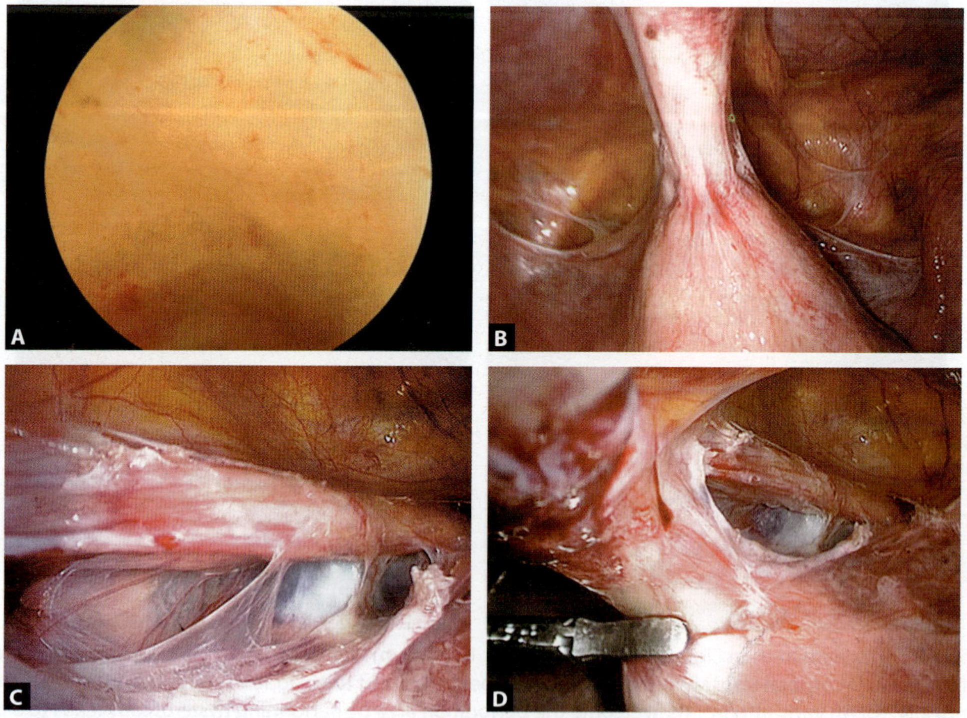

Figs. 47.36A to D: A 35-year-old patient, para I, after cesarean section in a developing country. (A) With a suspected defect of the cesarean scar. Hysteroscopy shows the margin of the intact wall and the defect that seems only to be covered by peritoneum; (B) Laparoscopic view shows a strong adhesive cord of the anterior uterine wall to the anterior abdominal wall. After opening the (C) Left; and (D) Right anterior leaf of the broad ligament the bladder can be kept at a distance and the uterine defect demarcated.

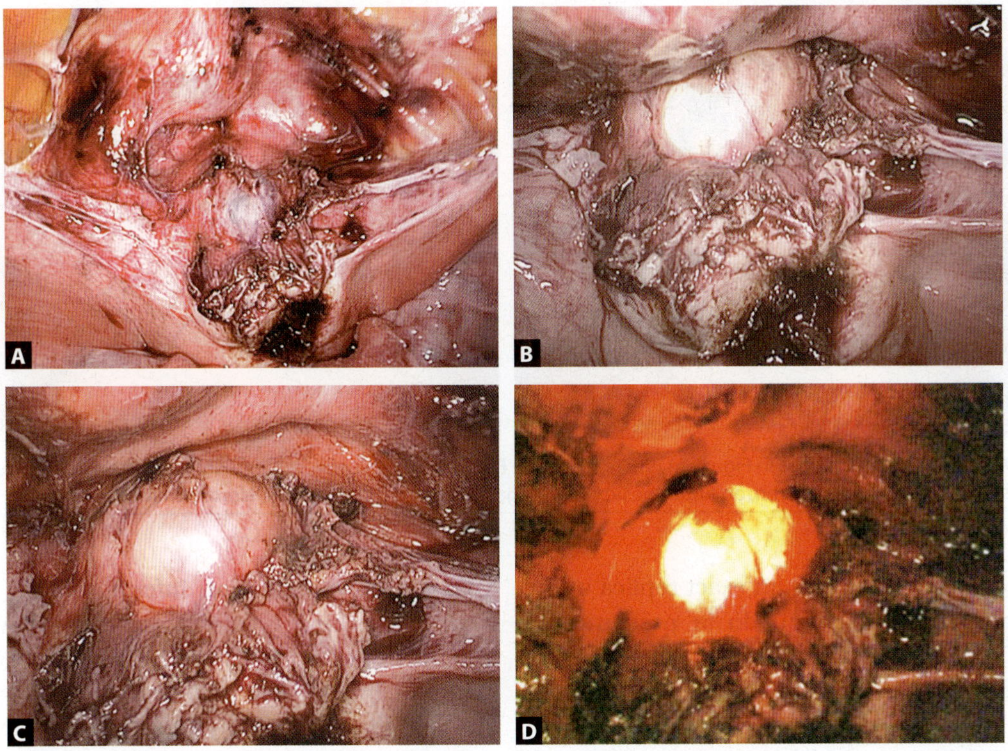

Figs. 47.37A to D: Same patient as in Figure 47.36. (A) After complete adhesiolysis the bladder is moved away from the uterus and the deep defect demarcated; (B) Simultaneous hysteroscopy is able to confirm that the whole area of the wall is defect; (C) The weak defect cover is seen after insertion of distribution fluid by hysteroscopy; (D) After dimming of the intra-abdominal light the hysteroscopic illumination becomes very expressive.

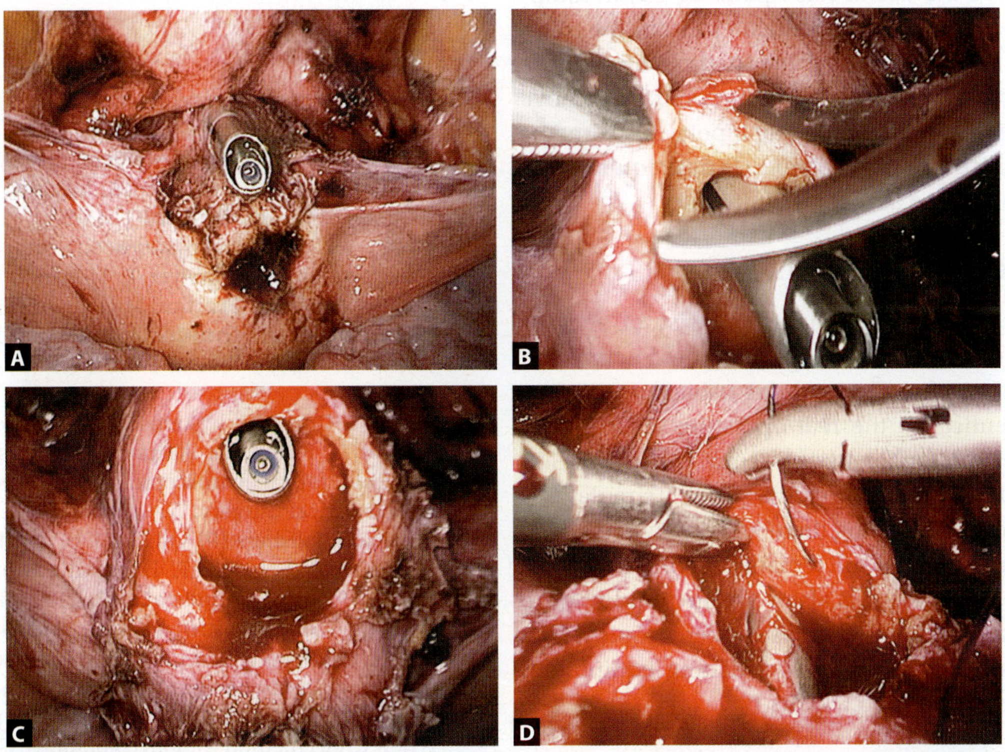

Figs. 47.38A to D: Same patient as in Figures 47.36 and 47.37. (A) Planned perforation with the hysteroscope allows; (B) Specific resection of the respective area; (C) The defect is demarcated and bridged with the hysteroscope; (D) This allows end-to-end covering.

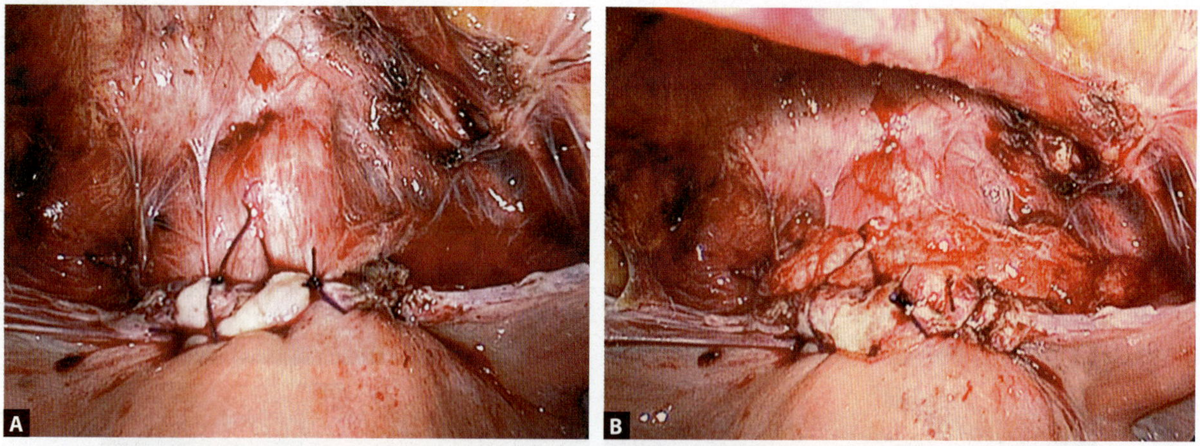

Figs. 47.39A and B: Same patient as in Figures 47.36 to 47.38. (A) Final view of the covered defect of the anterior uterine wall; (B) As the patient still wishes to have children, an antiadhesion barrier gel is applied (Hyalobarrier, Nordic Pharma, Germany).

Nevertheless, you do not get an exact replica of the anatomical structures as you do in prefabricated models. The tissue is not perfused so bleeding will not be seen as in real operations, and the poor perfusion results in higher resistance requiring a higher power setting than in real life; however, you are still able to get a realistic sense of using the equipment. It is also possible to realistically train fluid management and the use of in- and outflow valves. Animal parts for training are relatively cheap, but the setup does require the use of real operating room equipment and electrodes. It is difficult to train the treatment of specific intrauterine pathologies. These models are more useful in training general operative techniques, i.e. resection. Using bipolar instruments is easier since a return electrode is not required and saline can be used as distension media.

Virtual Reality Simulators

Virtual reality (VR) simulators consist of a computer generating a virtual operating field where you are able to perform procedures using an interface that is identical to the real operating instruments. One VR-simulator for hysteroscopy is the HystSim (VirtaMed AG, Zurich, Switzerland). This simulator is able to produce bleeding thereby increasing realism, but one problem that still remains is generating realistic force feedback. It is also possible to train more specific procedures, such as hysteroscopic sterilization and the use of new operating equipment, e.g. hysteroscopic morcellators.[24]

SUMMARY AND CONCLUSION

Hysteroscopy remains complementary to laparoscopic surgery in many explorations of the genital tract, e.g. in cases of infertility and recurrent abortions, uterine bleeding abnormalities within the reproductive and the postmenopausal age, adenomyosis, laparoscopic myomectomy and in specific cases of laparoscopic hysterectomy and explorative cancer surgery.

Furthermore, laparoscopy remains complementary to many hysteroscopic procedures and therefore, knowledge of laparoscopic surgery is mandatory for safe and professional hysteroscopic treatment.

REFERENCES

1. Kovac SR. Route of hysterectomy: an evidence-based approach. Clin Obstet Gynecol. 2014;57(1):58-71.
2. Schollmeyer T. et al. Hysterectomy trends over a 9-year period in an endoscopic teaching center. Int J Gynaecol Obstet. 2014;126(1):45-9.
3. Clevin L. Diagnostic hysteroscopy and office hysteroscopy. In: Schollmeyer T, Mettler L, Rüther D, Alkatout I, editors. Practical Manual for Laparoscopic and Hysteroscopic Gynecological Surgery. New Delhi: Jaypee Brothers Medical Publishers (P) Ltd; 2013. p. 423-33.
4. Römer T. Operative hysteroscopy. In: Schollmeyer T, Mettler L, Rüther D, Alkatout I, editors. Practical Manual for Laparoscopic and Hysteroscopic Gynecological Surgery. New Delhi: Jaypee Brothers Medical Publishers (P) Ltd; 2013. p. 437-44.
5. Schüssler B, Scheidel P, Hohl MK. Hysterektomie update. Frauenheilkunde aktuell. 2008;3:4-12.
6. Veress J. Neues Instrument zur Ausführung von Brust- und Bauchpunktionen und Pneumothoraxbehandlung. Deutsche med Wochen. 1938;64:1480-1.
7. Semm K. [Hysterectomy via laparotomy or pelviscopy. A new CASH method without colpotomy]. Geburtshilfe Frauenheilkd. 1991;51(12):996-1003.
8. Alkatout I, Mettler L, Maass N, et al. Abdominal anatomy in the context of port placement and trocars. J Turk Ger Gynecol Assoc. 2015;16(4):241-51.

9. Olive DL, Schwartz LB. Endometriosis. N Engl J Med. 1993;328(24):1759-69.
10. Engemise S, Gordon C, Konje JC. Endometriosis. Br Med J. 2010;340:c2168.
11. Hughes E, et al. Ovulation suppression for endometriosis. Cochrane Database Syst Rev. 2007;(3): CD000155.
12. Mahmood, TA, Templeton A. The impact of treatment on the natural history of endometriosis. Hum Reprod. 1990;5(8):965-70.
13. Vercellini P, Consonni D, Dridi D, et al. Uterine adenomyosis and in vitro fertilization outcome: a systematic review and meta-analysis. Hum Reprod. 2014;29(5):964-77.
14. Benagiano G, Brosens I, Habiba M. Adenomyosis: a life-cycle approach. Reprod Biomed Online. 2015; 30(3):220-32.
15. Alkatout I, Egberts JH, Mettler L, et al. [Interdisciplinary Diagnosis and Treatment of Deep Infiltrating Endometriosis.]. Zentralbl Chir. 2016;141(6):630-8.
16. Practice Committee of American Society for Reproductive Medicine. Treatment of pelvic pain associated with endometriosis. Fertil Steril. 2008;90 (5 Suppl): S260-9.
17. Schindler AE. Kombiniertes chirurgisch-hormonelles Management der Endometriose. Zentralbl Gynakol. 1999;121(7):325-9.
18. Crosignani PG, Vercellini P, Biffignandi F, et al. Laparoscopy versus laparotomy in conservative surgical treatment for severe endometriosis. Fertil Steril. 1996;66(5):706-11.
19. Jacobson TZ, Barlow DH, Garry R, et al. Laparoscopic surgery for pelvic pain associated with endometriosis. Cochrane Database Syst Rev. 2001;(4):CD001300.
20. Taylor E, Williams C. Surgical treatment of endometriosis: location and patterns of disease at reoperation. Fertil Steril. 2010;93(1):57-61.
21. Healey M, Ang WC, Cheng C. Surgical treatment of endometriosis: a prospective randomized double-blinded trial comparing excision and ablation. Fertil Steril. 2010;94(7):2536-40.
22. Yeung PP Jr, Shwayder J, Pasic RP. Laparoscopic management of endometriosis: comprehensive review of best evidence. J Minim Invasive Gynecol. 2009;16(3): 269-81.
23. Alkatout I, Mettler L, Betete C, et al. Combined surgical and hormone therapy for endometriosis is the most effective treatment: prospective, randomized, controlled trial. J Minim Invasive Gynecol. 2013; 20(4):473-81.
24. Bjerrum F. Current hysteroscopic training models. In: Schollmeyer T, Mettler L, Rüther D, Alkatout I, editors. Practical Manual for Laparoscopic and Hysteroscopic Gynecological Surgery. New Delhi: Jaypee Brothers Medical Publishers (P) Ltd; 2013. p. 41-4.

48 Operative Hysteroscopy

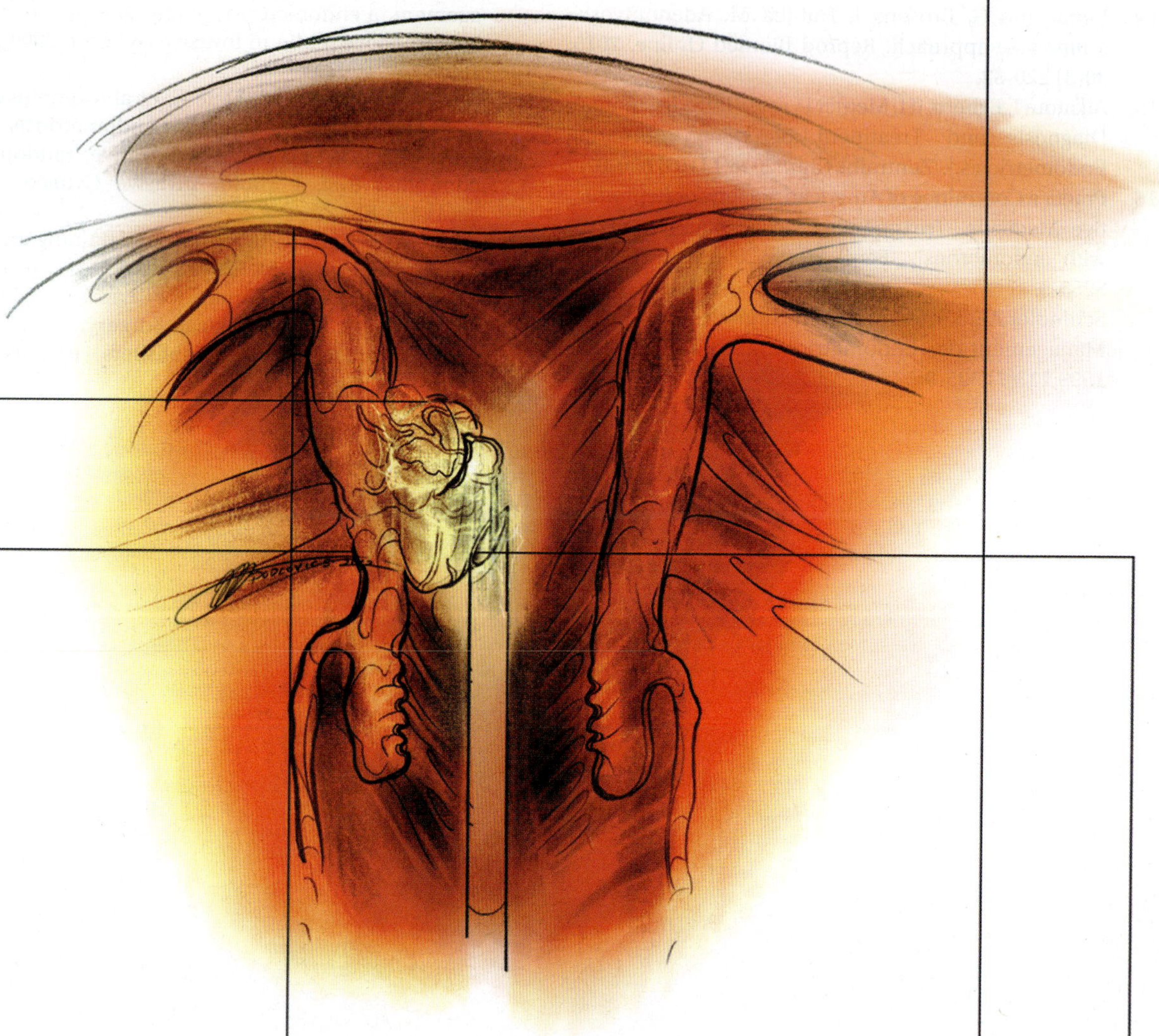

Chapter 48

Operative Hysteroscopy

Thomas Römer

INDICATIONS

In patients suffering from infertility of bleedings operative hysteroscopy is often indicated.[1]

With infertility:

- Septum dissection with uterus subseptus/septus
- Intrauterine adhesiolysis with adhesions grades III–IV/ESGE
- Myoma resection

With bleeding disorders:

- Myoma resection
- Polyp resection
- Endometrial ablation/endometrial resection

Special indications:

- Resection of residual placenta
- Opening or coagulation of a hematometra in the rudimentary uterine horn

INSTRUMENTATION AND TECHNICAL EQUIPMENT

Necessary basic equipment for operative hysteroscopy should be:

- Hysteroresectoscope with matching electrode and 12° angle lenses
- Light source with cable
- Hysteromat with inflow and outflow tube
- Distending medium
- Video camera and
- High-frequency unit.

TECHNIQUE AND PROCEDURE

- Diagnostic hysteroscopy with 5-mm-hysteroscope[2]
- Dilatation of the cervical canal up to Hegar 9 (when using a smaller resectoscope for fertility surgery up to Hegar 7)
- Insertion of the outer sheath with obturator
- Replacement of the obturator by a hysteroresectoscope with matching electrode and 12° angle lenses
- *Check the connections:*
  - Check the correct distending medium (bipolar: Ringer's solution; monopolar: sorbitol-mannitol solution).
  - Inflow tube for the distending medium—airless and connected with the Hysteromat (irrigate beforehand!).
  - Check the pressure and flow selection on the Hysteromat.
  - Outlet tube in collect container.
  - Connection with electrosurgical unit and check the power level on the high-frequency unit (preselected programs for monopolar and bipolar surgery).
- Opening of the inflow tube and distension of the cavum uteri often an irrigation is primarily necessary because the dilatation of the cervix often causes bleedings in the cavum uteri.
- Start of the surgery as soon as view and distension are sufficient.

STAFF REQUIREMENTS

A very important factor for the success of operative hysteroscopy is a well-trained surgeon.

Surgeon

- Experience in about 200 diagnostic hysteroscopies performed individually
- Knowledge of indications, contraindications and, first of all, safety aspects of operative hysteroscopy
- Knowledge of the fundamentals, safety aspects and complications of electrosurgery

- Training with animal models (handling of the equipment)
- Knowledge of potential complications and their clinical management
- Work shadowing with a surgeon experienced in operative hysteroscopy.

Surgical nurse:
- Exact knowledge of the equipment and instrumentation
- Assembly of the hysteroresectoscope
- Operation of the Hysteromat
- Distending medium (selection)
- High-frequency unit (adjustments).

Anesthesiologist:
- Knowledge of the complications of operative hysteroscopy
- Special diagnostics and therapy of the TUR-syndrome or diagnostics and management of air embolism.

SURGICAL INTERVENTIONS

Septum Dissection

Indications of septum dissection have increased in the last years. Subtle preoperative diagnostics is necessary. For a differential diagnosis between uterus bicornis and uterus septus a laparoscopy is imperative. Never perform a septum dissection without a self-performed or well-documented laparoscopy. There is risk of perforation with a uterus bicornis.

Indications

Absolute:
Habitual abortions (two or three recurrent abortions).

Relative:
- Primary and secondary infertility
- Dysmenorrhea (therapy-resistant).

Technique of Septum Dissection

- Dissection of the septum with the resection needle from caudal to fundal.
- From time to time check of the extent of the dissection using the tubal ostia as. points of orientation.
- With complete septa first dissect the area caudal, afterwards insert the resectoscope completely (sufficient flow) (Fig. 48.1).

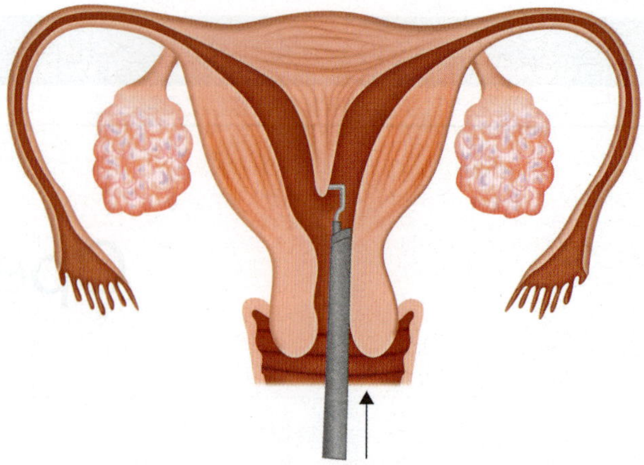

Fig. 48.1: Dissection of caudal septum.

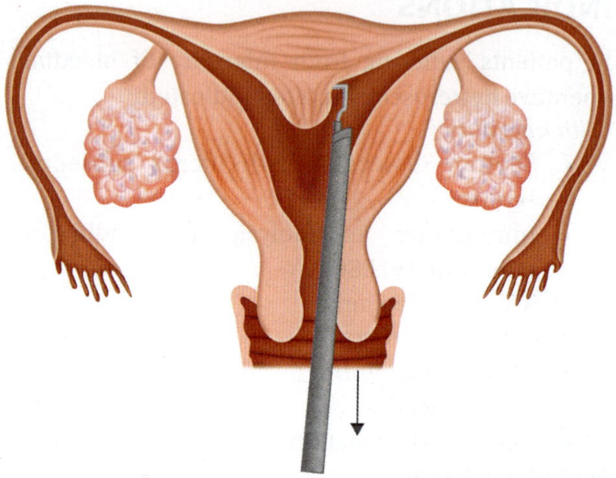

Fig. 48.2: Dissection of fundal septum.

- Then dissection from fundal to caudal (Fig. 48.2).
- Permanent orientation at the tubal ostia.

Dissection in the middle of the septum! Median dissection not up to the ostia level if median raphe is known. There is also a risk of perforation. The reconstruction of the cavum uteri as a uterus arcuatus is sufficient for the optimization of fertility. Spare the tubal ostia when dissection (about 1 cm distance with cutting current) to avoid functional disorders of the ostia.

Diagnostics and Therapeutic Management of Suspected Uterus Malformation (Uterus Septus/Bicornis)

- Anamnesis (abortions, premature births?)
- Gynecological examination and sonography ("two-cavities phenomenon")
- Scheduling of the surgery—ideally postmenstruation (thin endometrium)

- *Procedure of the surgery:*
  - *Diagnostic hysteroscopy*: cavum uteri divided into two parts
  - *Diagnostic laparoscopy*: fundus of the uterus smooth or small median raphe
  - *Diagnosis*: uterus septus
  - When indicated, simultaneous laparoscopic resection of the endometriosis
  - Operative hysteroscopy with transcervical septum dissection (with complete septa perhaps insertion of an IUD to prevent adhesions) (Fig. 48.3).[3]

Treatment with GnRH-analogs before the septum dissection does not bring any intra- or postoperative advantages and can therefore be waived if surgery is performed postmenstruationem.

Postoperative management after septum dissection depends on the type of septum.

With complete or wide septa or additional intrauterine adhesions

- At the end of the surgery insertion of an IUD for the prevention of intrauterine adhesions for the duration of 3 months (preferably IUD type DANA or copper IUD with a wide surface)
- Estrogenization for 3 months to stimulate the endometrium proliferation (e.g. 2–4 mg oestradiol for 21 days progestagen for 12 days)
- Follow-up hysteroscopy (possibly with IUD extraction); in most of the cases as outpatient procedure without anesthesia, possible after 3 months.

An IUD insertion and estrogenization is only recommended with complete septa for the prevention of possible adhesions (lack of sufficient data).

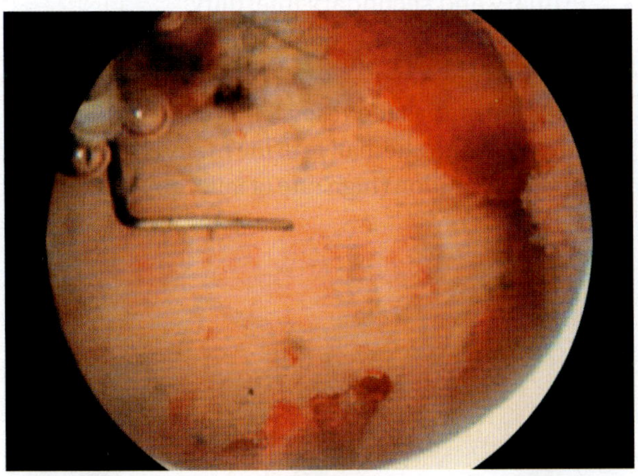

Fig. 48.3: Septum dissection. Septum has already been removed caudally. Now further orientation towards the tubal ostia and further dissection from lateral to medial and from fundal to caudal.

The most frequent complication of the septum dissection is a perforation in the fundal area.

Management

- Diagnostic laparoscopy
- Check for injuries of other organs (especially bowel injuries); if these cannot be definitely excluded, a laparotomy is indicated.
- With bleeding—endoscopic suture for hemostasis
- Perioperative application of antibiotics
- Frequent postoperative follow-up.

For the prevention of the perforation of the fundus during a hysteroscopic septum dissection we advise:

- Consideration of the median raphe (median dissection in the fundal area not as far as in the lateral area)
- With bleeding beginning from the vessels in the septum area—stop surgery because these are mainly myometrial vessels (during a teaching surgery possibly septum dissection under simultaneous sonographic or laparoscopic control)
- With indistinct orientation about the level of the dissection—simultaneous abdominal sonography
- In most of the cases laparoscopy is only useful after perforation!

In infertile patients the operative hysteroscopy should only be performed by a surgeon experienced in hysteroscopy.

Intrauterine Adhesiolysis

Indications for intrauterine adhesiolysis are:

- Habitual abortions (two or more recurrent abortions)
- Primary and secondary infertility
- Hypomenorrhea/amenorrhea
- Dysmenorrhea
- Recurrent lower abdominal pain.

It is necessary to have a strict indication for intrauterine adhesiolysis for grades III and IV because this is the most difficult operative-hysteroscopic intervention with a high rate of complications. A classification according to the grades is primarily necessary because of its therapeutic and prognostic consequences (Table 48.1).

Table 48.1: Operative therapy and prognosis of intrauterine adhesions.

	Grade I	*Grade II*	*Grades III and IV*
Operative therapy	Cutting by sheath of the microscissors	Cutting by adhesiolysis or by successful therapy of the hysteroscope (operative hysteroscopy)	Electrosurgical laser
Bleeding disorders	100%	100%	60–70%
Pregnancy rate	70–90%	70–90%	20–40%

DIAGNOSTICS AND THERAPEUTIC MANAGEMENT IN THE CASE OF SUSPECTED INTRAUTERINE ADHESIONS

- *Anamnesis:*
  - Bleeding characteristics?
  - Intrauterine intervention
- Gynecological examination
- *Vaginal sonography:*
  - Endometrium structure
- *Diagnostic hysteroscopy:*
  - Intrauterine adhesions with description of the grade
- Operative hysteroscopy simultaneous (preoperative information) with intrauterine adhesiolysis (if necessary, simultaneous sonography or laparoscopy) (Fig. 48.4)
- IUD insertion and intrauterine instillation of 5 mL hyalouronic acid at the end of surgery (compulsory with grades III and IV according to ESGE)[4]
- Estrogenization for 3 months for endometrium proliferation
- Follow-up hysteroscopy with IUD extraction (if necessary, further adhesiolysis).

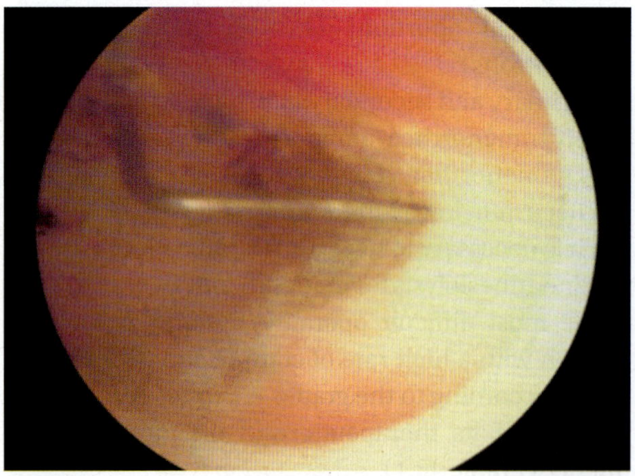

Fig. 48.4: Intrauterine adhesion grade III: Left tubal ostium exposed.

POSTOPERATIVE MANAGEMENT AFTER INTRAUTERINE ELECTROSURGICAL ADHESIOLYSIS

Compulsory

- Insertion of an IUD and intrauterine instillation of 5 mL hyalouronic acid for 3 months
- Estrogenization for 3 months[5]
- Outpatient follow-up hysteroscopy and IUD-extraction (if necessary, further adhesiolysis) 3 months after surgery.[6]

The low postoperative pregnancy and birth rate and the difficult and complicated surgery require focusing attention on the prevention of intrauterine adhesions.

Myoma Resection

Indications for hysteroscopic myoma resection:

- Recurrent bleeding disorders resistant to therapy, in most of the cases connected with dysmenorrhea or secondary anemia
- Bleeding disorders during oral contraception or postmenopausal hormone therapy
- Habitual abortions
- Primary and secondary infertility.

A hysteroscopic resection is only indicated for solitary submucous myomas. In patients with multiple intramural myomas the resection of a solitary submucous myoma is no alternative to the hysterectomy or just a temporary solution (high rate of failure) (Fig. 48.5).

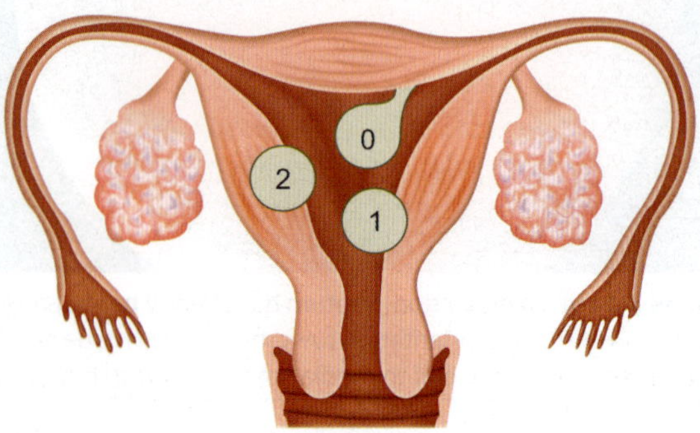

Fig. 48.5: Classification of submucous myoma 0,1,2.

Submucous Myomas and Infertility

Submucous myomas can cause implantation problems and thus reduce the pregnancy rate. Large submucous myomas cause a rise in the frequency of abortions. The closer the myoma is located to the endometrium, the higher is the probability of fertility disorders.[7,8]

Hysteroscopic Myoma Resection and Time of Surgery

The best time of surgery is without pretreatment: post menstruationem (best: first or second day without bleeding) or with pretreatment with GnRH analogs or ulipristal acetate 2–3 weeks after last injection (Fig. 48.6).[9,10]

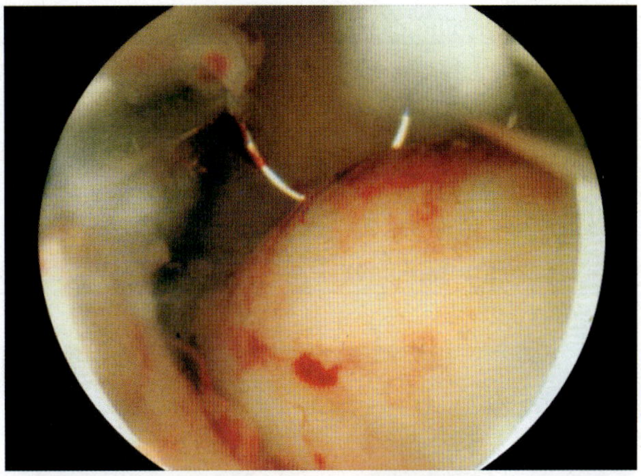

Fig. 48.6: Submucous myoma grade 1/ESGE (intramural portion <50%). Resection possible without problems. Intramural portion is pressed toward the cavity by the contraction of the uterus.

Indications for the use of GnRH-analogs or ulitpristalacetate before the hysteroscopic myoma resection are:

- In all infertile patients with submucous myomas of a diameter >3 cm
- With unfavorable position of the myoma (e.g., in the tubal corner)
- With secondary anemia caused by bleeding disorders (autoreinfusion)
- With larger intramural myomas (grade 2/ESGE)
- With myomas that cannot be completely resected during one session.

Polyp Resection

Diagnostic and Therapeutic Management of Corpus Polyps

- Gynecological examination and vaginal sonography, if necessary progesterone test to differentiate between polyp and endometrium hyperplasia)
- Diagnostic hysteroscopy and target curettage
- Follow-up hysteroscopy
- Polyp cannot be removed
- Operative hysteroscopy (patient should already be informed before surgery) with transcervical electrosurgical resection of the polyp.

Endometrialablation/Resection

The aim of the endometrial ablation is the reduction in bleeding intensity with recurrent therapy-resistant recurrent hypermenorrheas.[11,12,13]

Possibilities of endometrial ablation/-resection: (Tables 48.2 and 48.3)

- *First generation:*
  - Coagulation with the roller-ball-electrode (Fig. 48.7)
  - Resection with the cutting loop (Fig. 48.8)
  - ND: YAG-laser
- *Second generation:*
  - Hydrothermal ablation
  - Bipolar electrode (NovaSure®)
  - Microwave
  - Uterine balloon techniques for the thermal coagulation of the endometrium (e.g. Thermachoice®)

Table 48.2: Advantages and disadvantages of the endometrial ablation and resection.

	Endometrial ablation	*Endometrial resection*
Intraoperative	Roller-ball (Fig. 48.7)	Cutting loop (Fig. 48.8)
Histology	None	Yes
Risk of perforation	Lower	Higher
Intraoperative bleedings	Minimal	Considerably more
Intraoperative view	Good	Made difficult by floating resectates
Pretreatment	Necessary	Recommended

Table 48.3: Current data on long-term results of the endometrial ablation.

Author (year)	Follow-up	Patients	Rate of hysterectomy (%)	Success rate (%)
Boe–Engelsen (2006), Norway	4–10 years	386	16.6	83.4
Fürst (2007), Denmark	10 years	120	22	78
Cooper (2001), Scotland	5 years	93	19	81
Litta (2006), Italy	6–12 years	106	11.3	89.7
Römer (2010) Germany	6 years	368	11.4	89.6

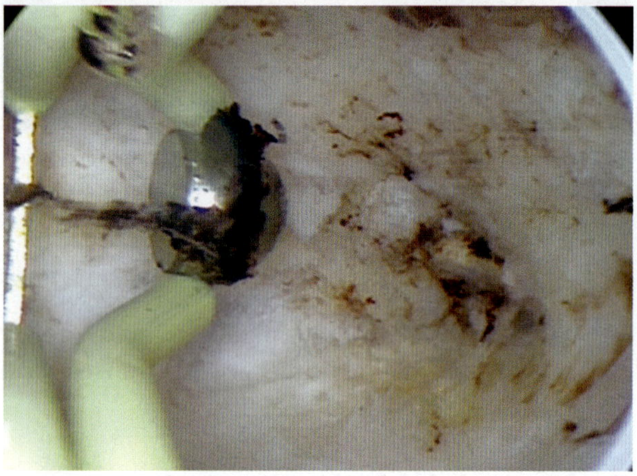

Fig. 48.7: Endometrial ablation with the bipolar coagulation electrode.

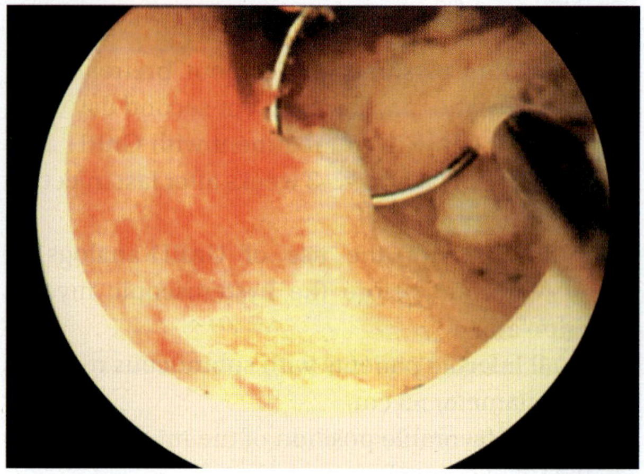

Fig. 48.8: Endometrial resection with the cutting loop: On the left: already resected endometrium (yellow-white); On the right: endometrium still to be removed (reddish).

Inclusion criteria for endometrial ablation:

- Recurrent hypermenorrhea resistant to therapy (persistent for more than 1 year, and hormonal treatment without success)
- Finished family planning
- Exclusion of complex and atypical endometrial hyperplasias and uterine cancer
- Regular genital findings or small, solitary submucous myomas (diameter <3 cm) (sonography, hysteroscopy, histology)
- Informed consent of the patient after extensive information about risks and benefits of the therapy
- Uterine probe length <10 cm

Indications for endometrial ablation

- Recurrent hypermenorrhea resistant to therapy
- Perimenopausal bleeding disorders resistant to therapy
- Bleeding disorders with coagulopathies and in patients undergoing long-term anticoagulant therapy
- Anesthesiological risk group with contraindications for a hysterectomy
- Therapy-resistant bleeding disorders during a postmenopausal hormone therapy
- Bleeding disorders and endometrium hyperplasia during a tamoxifen treatment
- Menstrual hygiene for patients seriously in need of nursing care.

Specific complications of the endometrial ablation are:

- Hematometra
- Endometritis
- Post-ablation syndrome[14]
- First symptoms of an endometrial cancer may be obscured
- Pregnancies
- Recurrences.

BIPOLAR HYSTEROSCOPY

With the development of the bipolar technique the scope of the operative hysteroscopy expands and the procedure gets even safer (Table 48.4). The decisive advantage of the bipolar hysteroscopy is that it can be performed without an electrolyte-free solution (sorbitol-mannitol solution). Instead, Ringer's or saline solution can be used. This results in lower costs of the distending medium. For risk situations (e.g., myomas of grade 2/ESGE) bipolar hysteroscopy is the current method of choice because of reduced rate of complications. Bipolar techniques

Table 48.4: Comparison of mono- and bipolar surgical techniques exemplified by the resection of a myoma grade 2/ESGE.

	Monopolar resection	*Bipolar resection*
Equipment	Standard	Additional equipment
Distending medium	Sorbitol-mannitol solution	Ringer's solution
Danger of TUR syndrome	High	No
Cost of distending medium (e.g., consumption of 3 L)	4.83 Euro	4.75 Euro
Level of training of surgeon	No difference	No difference
Second surgery	Frequent	Rare
Results with large myoma grade 2	After first surgery: about 60% success	After first surgery: about 95% success

gain increasingly in importance in the operative hysteroscopy. Bipolar techniques in hysteroscopy can contribute to solving some problems of intrauterine surgery and to increasing the safety of the patient. Preferred indications for the bipolar surgical technique are myomas grade 2/ESGE and large myomas (>4 cm). The main advantages of the bipolar myoma resection are avoidance of the TUR syndrome, e.g., electrolyte shifts, and avoidance of second or third surgeries resulting thereof. Even with the use of Ringer's solution an overload should be avoided. The fluid deficit should not exceed 3 L. Even higher caution is necessary with anesthesiological risk groups (Fig. 48.9).[15]

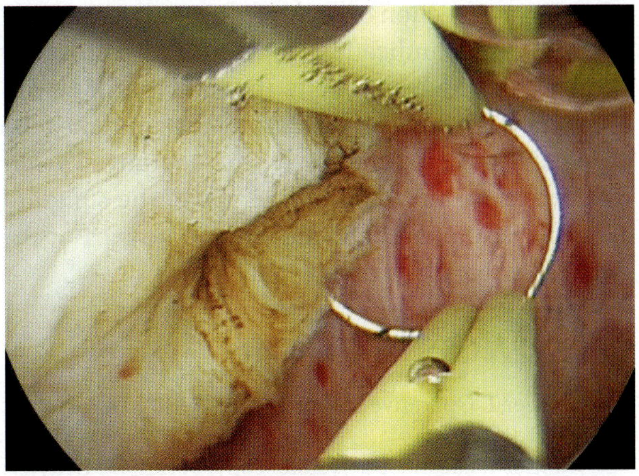

Fig. 48.9: Bipolar myoma resection.

GENERAL COMPLICATIONS OF OPERATIVE HYSTEROSCOPY: MANAGEMENT AND PREVENTION

Possible complications of the operative hysteroscopy are:[16,1]

- Perforation with injury of other pelvic organs
- Bleeding
- Infection
- TUR syndrome[17]
- Burns
- Air embolism.

The frequency of complications are listed in Table 48.5.[1]

Table 48.5: Frequency of complications with different hysteroscopic surgeries.

	Perforation	*Bleeding*	*TUR-syndrome (monopolar)*	*Infections*
Myoma resection				
Grade 2	+++	+++	+++	+
Grade 0	+	+	++	+
Polyp resection	+	+	+	+
Endometrial ablation	+	ϕ	+	+
Endometrial resection	++	+	++	+
Septum dissection	+	+	+	+
Intrauterine adhesiolysis grades III/IV	+++	+	++	+

Note: ϕ: no risk 0; +: low risk < 1%; ++: medium risk < 5%; +++: increased risk > 5%.

SUMMARY

The established indications for operative hysteroscopy are:

- Septum dissection in patients suffering from habitual abortions
- Intrauterine adhesiolysis in infertile patients
- Myoma resection of solitary submucous myomas in patients suffering from bleeding disorders and infertile patients
- Endometrial ablation and resection.

The relative indications for operative hysteroscopy are:

- Septum dissection with primary and secondary infertility and
- Myoma resection of multiple myomas.

With exact indications operative hysteroscopy is an established minimally invasive method with excellent postoperative results and thus enriches the scope of operative gynecology. The operative hysteroscopy has meanwhile become one of the standard gynecological operations and should be part of the range of surgery in every hospital.

REFERENCES

1. Römer T. Operative Hysteroscopy. Berlin: De Gruyter; 2011.
2. Römer T. Diagnostic Hysteroscopy. Berlin; De Gruyter; 2009.
3. Römer T, Lober R. Hysteroscopic correction of a complete septate uterus using a balloon technique. Hum Reprod. 1997;12(3):478-9.
4. Healy MW, Schexnayder B, Connell MT et al. Intrauterine adhesion prevention after hysteroscopy: a systematic review and meta-analysis. Am J Obstet Gynecol. 2016;215(3):267-75.
5. Bosteels J, Weyers S, Kasius J, et al. Anti-adhesion therapy following operative hysteroscopy for treatment of female subfertility. Cochrane Database Syst Rev. 2015;11:CD011110.
6. Di Spiezio Sardo A, Calagna G, et al. Prevention of intrauterine post-surgical adhesions in hysteroscopy. A systematic review. Eur J Obstet Gynecol Reprod Biol. 2016;203:182-92.
7. Bosteels J, Kasius J, Weyers S, et al. Hysteroscopy for treating subfertility associated with suspected major uterine cavity abnormalities. Cochrane Database Syst Rev. 2015;2:CD009461.
8. Shokeir TA. Hysteroscopic management in submucous fibroids to improve fertility. Arch Gynecol Obstet. 2005;273(1):50-4.
9. Ferrero S, Raca A, Tafi E, et al. Ulipristal acetate before high complexity hysteroscopic myomectomy: a retrospective comparative study. J Minim Invasive Gynecol. 2016;23(3):390-5.
10. Kamath MS, Kalampokas EE, Kalampokas TE. Use of GnRH analogues pre-operatively for hysteroscopic resection of submucous fibroids: a systematic review and meta-analysis. Eur J Obstet Gynecol Reprod Biol. 2014;177:11-8.
11. Laberge P, Leyland N, Murji A, et al. Endometrial ablation in the management of abnormal uterine bleeding. J Obstet Gynaecol Can. 2015;37(4): 362-79.
12. Lethaby A, Penninx J, Hickey M, et al. Endometrial resection and ablation techniques for heavy menstrual bleeding. Cochrane Database Syst Rev 2013;30:CD001501.
13. Sowter MC, Lethaby A, Singla A. Preoperative endometrial thinning agents before endometrial destruction for heavy menstrual bleeding. Cochrane Database Syst Rev. 2000;(3):CD 001124.
14. McClausland AM, McClausland VM. Frequency of symptomatic cornual hematometra and postablation tubal sterilization syndrome after total rollerball endometrial ablation: a 10-year follow-up. Am J Obstet Gynecol. 2002;186:1274-80.
15. Tammam AE, Ahmed HH, Abdella AH, et al. Comparative study between monopolar electrodes and bipolar electrodes in hysteroscopic surgery. J Clin Diagn Res. 2015;9(11):QC11-3.
16. Munro MG, Christianson LA, Complications of hysteroscopic and uterine resectoscopic surgery. Clin Obstet Gynecol. 2015;58(4):765-97.
17. Umranikar S, Clark TJ, Saridogan E, et al. BSGE/ESGE guideline on management of fluid distension media in operative hysteroscopy. Gynecol Surg. 2016;13(4):289-303.

Section 4

Complications in Laparoscopic and Hysteroscopic Surgery

KIEL SCH•O L

49 of Gynaecological Endoscopy

Laparoscopic
Complications and Management

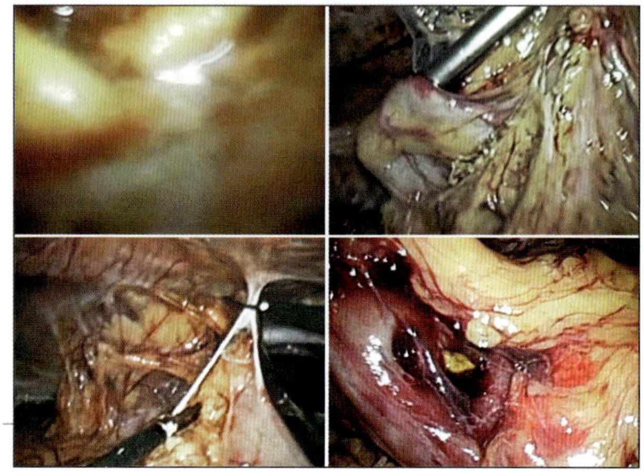

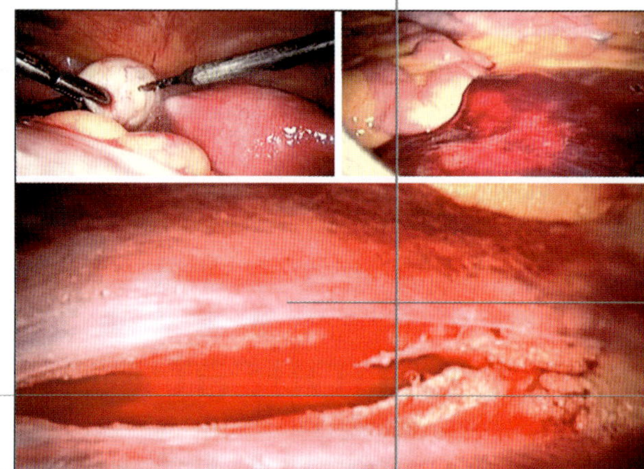

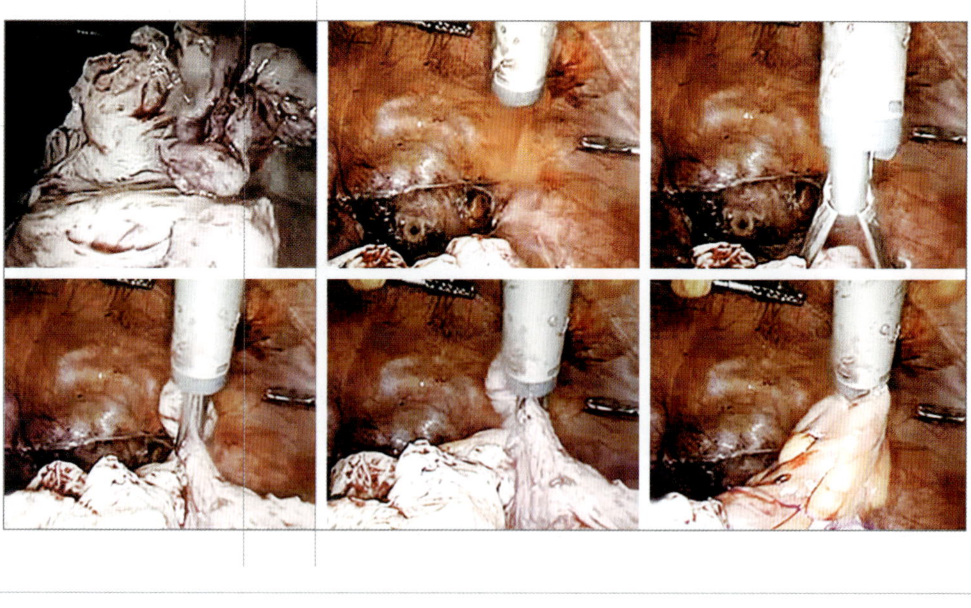

Chapter 49

Laparoscopic Complications and Management

Ibrahim Alkatout, Liselotte Mettler

INTRODUCTION

The anatomy of the human being has not changed. However, technical developments in operating materials and methods call for improvements in surgical procedures as well as the management of complications. A fundamental distinction between any operating method and laparoscopy is that, in the latter, the initial entry is usually performed in a blind fashion. Blind entry may result in vessel or organ damage, especially in patients who have undergone previous surgery. One of the difficulties associated with the entry is that the damage may not be identified immediately and then necessitate major abdominal repair. Furthermore, the improvement of surgical instruments and techniques enables the surgeon to perform even major operations by the laparoscopic approach. This is associated with renewed learning curves and a high rate of complications due to vascular, bowel, uterine or bladder damage. The improvement of surgical techniques must be accompanied by advancements in the management of complications.

The aim of this review is to address the risks of laparoscopy as well as their correct and professional management.

COUNSELING AND INFORMED CONSENT

Patients undergoing a laparoscopic procedure must be informed of the risks and potential complications as well as alternative surgical methods. Counseling before laparoscopy should include a discussion of the entry technique used and the risks associated with laparoscopic entry:[1,2] injury to the bowel, the urinary tract, blood vessels, omentum and other surrounding organs. Potential complications at a later point in time include wound infection, pain due to adhesions, and the formation of hernia.

The counseling must include the patient's individual risk depending on his or her body mass index (BMI), potential obesity or significant underweight, as well as any immunosuppression that may be present. Depending on the patient's medical history, it would be important to take anatomical malformations, midline abdominal incisions, a history of peritonitis or inflammatory bowel disease into account.[3,4]

PRECONDITIONS OF TROCAR PLACEMENT

Elevation of the abdominal wall by means of a sufficient pneumoperitoneum is a precondition for safe trocar insertion. Excepted from this rule is blind entry without a pneumoperitoneum. An insufflation pressure to 25 mm Hg can be tolerated by the patient. The optic trocar may be placed indirectly (10 mm) or in two steps: inserting a 5 mm trocar first and then dilating to 10 mm in case the surgeon anticipates any bleeding, intraabdominal abnormality or adherent bowel loops. If the surgeon suspects adherence of the bowel in the umbilical region, the primary trocar site must be visualized from a secondary port site, such as the lower abdominal wall, with a 5 mm laparoscope (Figs. 49.1A to D).[3]

All ancillary trocars must be inserted with an intra-abdominal pressure of 20–25 mm Hg under direct vision in order to achieve the maximum distance between the abdominal wall and the inner organs. The inferior epigastric vessels are visualized laparoscopically, whereas the superficial vessels can be visualized by diaphanoscopy. Thus it is ensured that the entry points are at a distance from the respective vessels (Figs. 49.2 and 49.3). The number of ancillary trocars may vary, but all of them must be

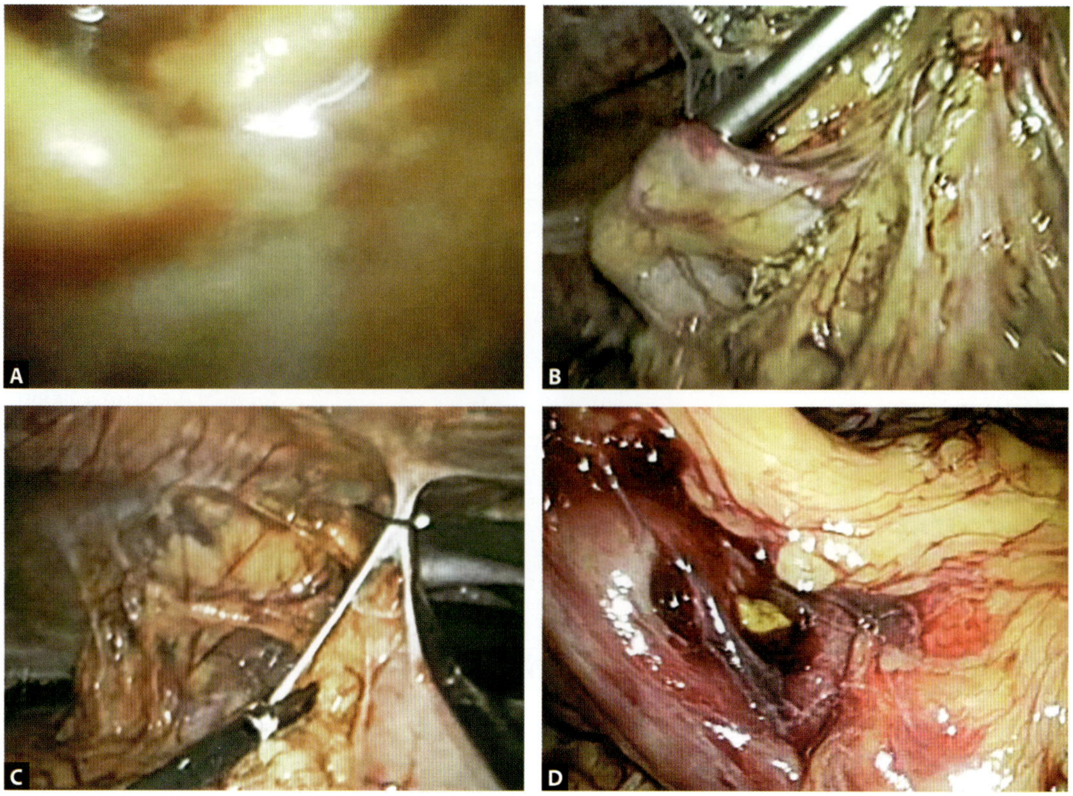

Figs. 49.1A to D: (A) Entering the primary trocar site with a 5-mm optical trocar. Stool is visible in the distant parts of the trocar; (B) The injury is clearly seen after inserting an ancillary trocar in the lower abdomen. It is important to leave the primary trocar in its respective location; (C) After mobilizing the adhesions that fixed the bowel to the abdominal wall; (D) The defect can be demarcated and sutured.

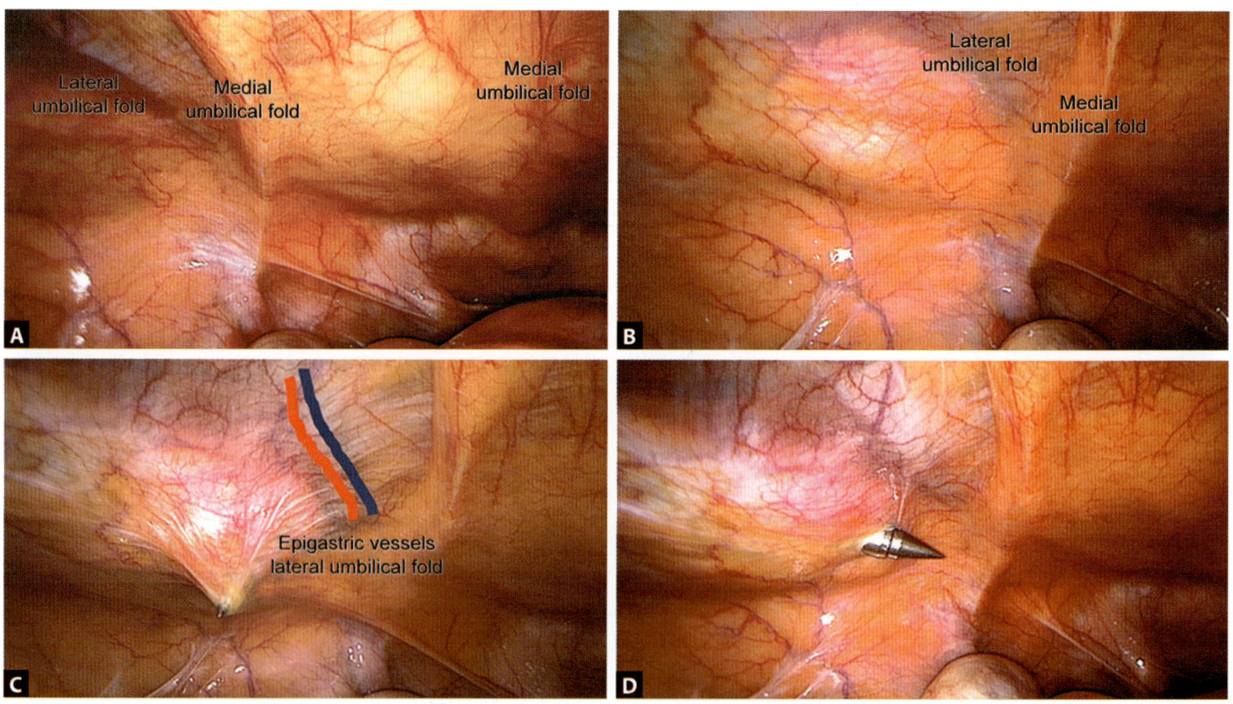

Figs. 49.2A to D: Secondary trocar placement, left lower abdominal entry. (A) The three plicae are visualized; (B) The palpating finger is showing the area lateral to the lateral umbilical fold; (C) Entry of the sharp ancillary trocar lateral to the lateral umbilical fold; (D) Once the peritoneum has been penetrated, the trocar is heading toward the fundus of the uterus and thus avoiding injury to the major vessels and the bowel.

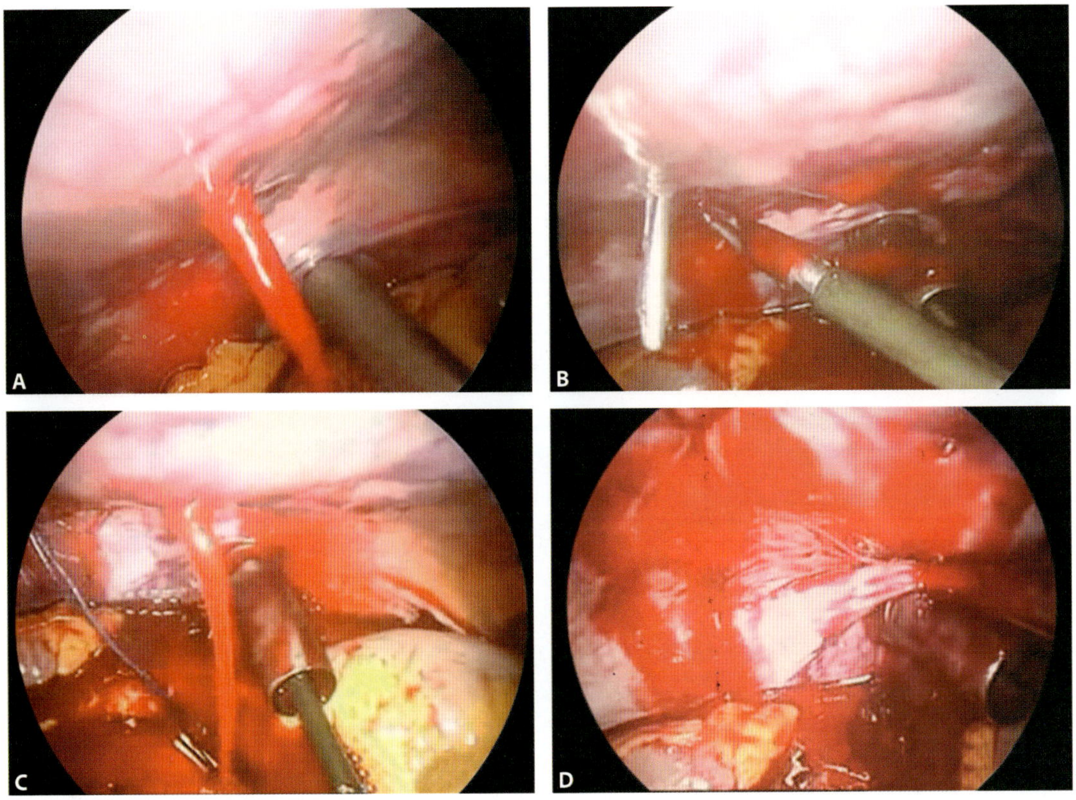

Figs. 49.3A to D: (A) Acute bleeding from the inferior epigastric artery; (B and C) The surgeon's view is obliterated within seconds. Blood is flowing at the site; the situation is obviously precarious; (B to D) The artery is closed by the inside-out suturing technique and the suture is fixed to the abdomen.

inserted under direct viewing. For safe insertion, the two major superficial vessels in this region must be avoided, i.e., the superficial epigastric artery and the superficial circumflex iliac artery.[3,5-7]

For patients with a significantly high risk of adhesions, a history of abdominal surgery, including cesarean section, a large fibroid uterus, an umbilical hernia, large ovarian cysts, preperitoneal gas insufflation or failed umbilical entry, Palmer described in 1974 an abdominal entry point in the midclavicular line, about 3 cm below the costal margin. Palmer's point can be used for the Veress needle as well as for small trocars. In patients with scars or previous operations in the upper left quadrant, the Lee–Huang point is an alternative (Figs. 49.4A to D).

Indications for the use of Palmer's point are the following:

- After two failed attempts to achieve subumbilical insufflation
- Very obese patients
- Patients who have undergone previous abdominal surgery and/or those with suspected intraabdominal adhesions.
- Patients with previous longitudinal abdominal incisions.

COMPLICATIONS IN PORT PLACEMENT

Complications of laparoscopy can be divided into *early complications*, which are recognized immediately and can be resolved instantly, and *delayed or late complications* that occur after a time interval in the postoperative period. The latter are more difficult to manage because the patients will have been discharged from the hospital or their symptoms may be unspecific.[8,9]

Classification of Laparoscopic Entry Lesions

Laparoscopic entry lesions may be classified as follows.

Type 1 Injuries

Damage to major blood vessels or the bowel in normal location, caused by entering with the Veress needle or the primary trocars (0.1–0.4 %).

Type 2 Injuries

Damage to vessels in the abdominal wall and to the bowel adherent to the abdominal wall, both caused by the Veress needle or the primary trocar. Type 2

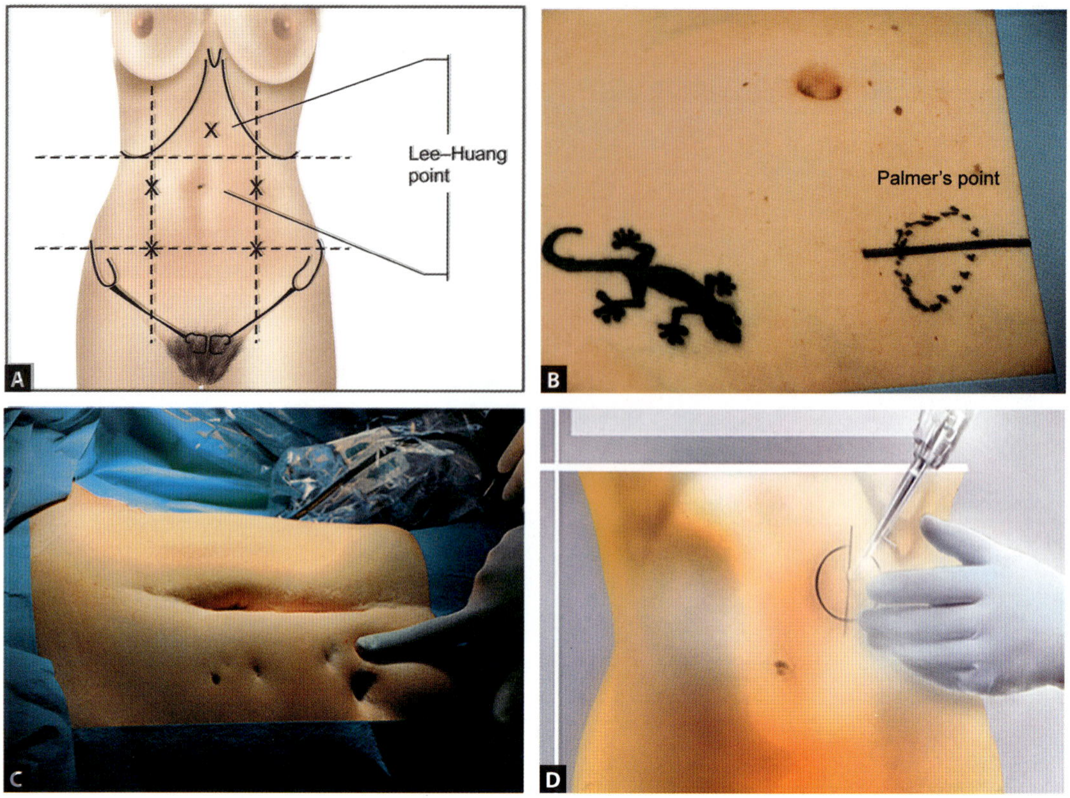

Figs. 49.4A to D: (A) The Lee–Huang point can be palpated directly beneath the xiphoid; (B to D) Alternative entry site showing Palmer's point. It is situated in the midclavicular line, about 3 cm below the costal margin, and is used in patients with known or anticipated umbilical adhesions.

lesions may occur regardless of whether the mode of access is laparotomy or laparoscopy.

Complications associated with laparoscopy vary, depending on the experience of the surgeon and the medical staff as well as the wide range of operational demands. Complication rates vary between 0.1% and 1.3%.

The establishment of laparoscopic surgery for routine procedures at university teaching hospitals as well as small county hospitals has enhanced the quality of the surgeon's work, which is now associated with a shorter learning curve. This advancement has been accompanied by a lower rate of complications. The development of laparoscopic instruments and optic transmission has also contributed to this phenomenon. More than 50% of all laparoscopic injuries are known to occur during the initial entry steps: insertion of the Veress needle or blind entry, creation of a pneumoperitoneum and insertion of the primary trocar. Accordingly, the incidence of injuries has been reduced significantly in the last three decades. Injury to the bowel occurs in 0.04%, and to major vessels in 0.02–0.04% of all laparoscopic procedures. Nevertheless, 30–50% of bowel injuries and 13–50% of all vascular injuries are not detected immediately during the operation, resulting in correspondingly high morbidity and mortality rates. Furthermore, laparoscopic surgery is frequently performed at outpatient clinics without banked human blood reserves, vascular surgical instruments and expertise. Bowel injury ranks third among the causes of death from a laparoscopic procedure, being preceded by major vessel injury and anesthesia.[10-12]

Vascular and Visceral Lesions during Port Placement

Vascular lesions may occur in the abdominal wall (superficial and epigastric vessels) or the intraabdominal aspect (vessels of the mesentery, omentum, iliac arteries and veins, or the aorta/vena cava). Vessel injury may lead to a parietal hematoma or intraperitoneal hemorrhage, depending on the injury site (Figs. 49.3 and 49.5). Even partial entrance of the Veress needle into the lumen of a vessel may cause gas embolism. Besides, CO_2 is highly soluble in plasma. Large volumes can be lethal and are

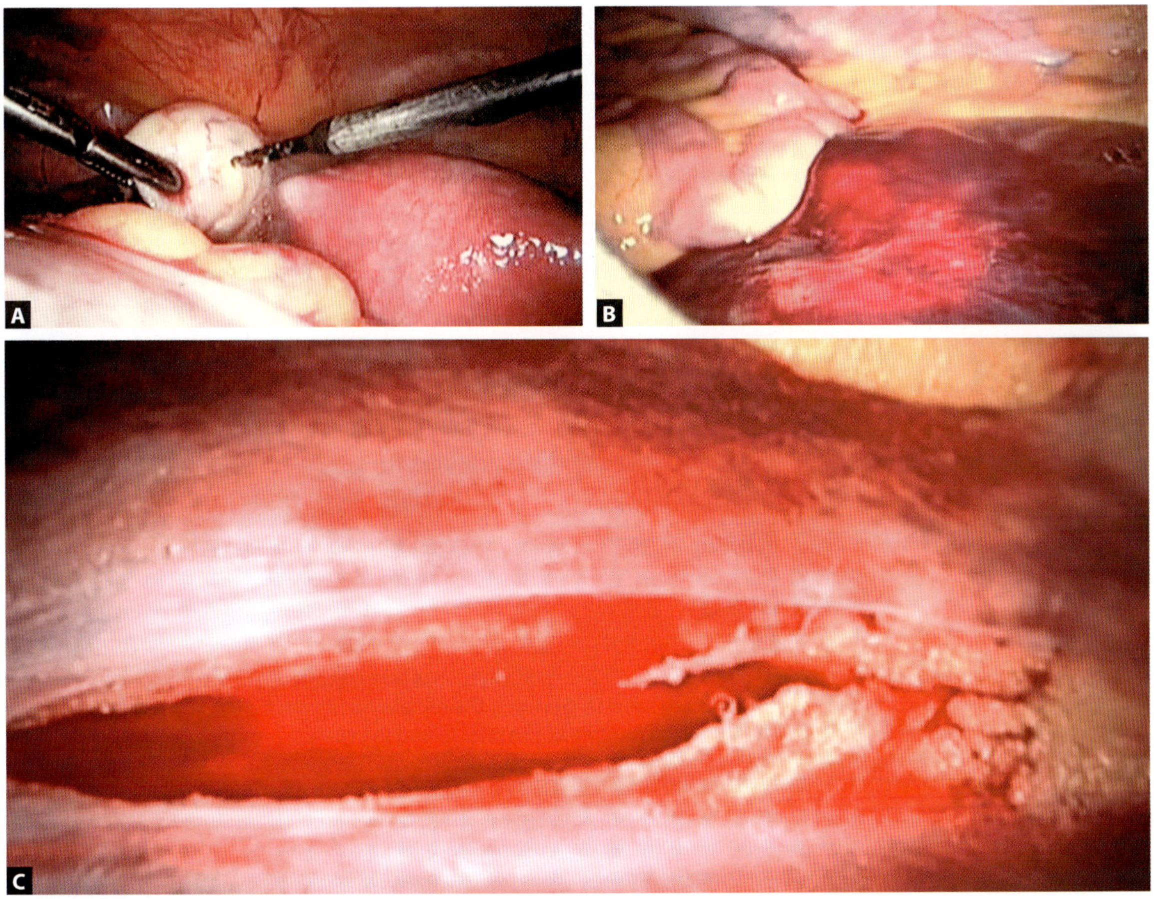

Figs. 49.5A to C: (A) Monopolar drilling of the ovary just before ending of the operation; (B) The final view reveals a massive retroperitoneal hematoma, increasing in size; (C) Detailed inspection of the retroperitoneum shows a laceration just above the vena cava.

liable to cause immediate death. Injury to the retroperitoneal space and retroperitoneal structures may occur when using excessive force to insert the Veress needle, or even when using normal force in very slim patients; such injury may also occur when the surgeon fails to follow the midline axis during insertion of the primary trocar or employs an incorrect angle relative to the abdominal wall when entering the peritoneal cavity. As the aorta and the inferior vena cava bifurcate and diverge before entering the pelvis, it is important to minimize the risk of injury.[7,13,14]

Visceral Lesions

Visceral lesions include injury to the greater omentum, the stomach, the bowel, the liver or the spleen, depending on the entry site and the level of filling of the hollow organs. Therefore, a gastric tube must be placed at the beginning of the operation, especially when using Palmer's point or the Lee-Huang point.

As the first step in ensuring a safe procedure, penetration of the bowel can be identified by the aspiration of gas or the presence of ambiguous or malodorous fluid. Injury to the liver or the spleen would lead to the aspiration of blood. Depending on the members of the interdisciplinary team, injury to visceral organs can be treated laparoscopically or, if necessary, by immediate laparotomy (Figs. 49.1 and 49.6).[6,13,15-18]

Early Complications

Early complications include bowel, vessel, bladder or ureter lesions as well as anesthesia-related or general complications, such as pulmonary embolism, massive hemorrhage after major vessel injury or intravascular insufflation, and cardiac arrest.

Early complications may also occur in hysteroscopy (Figs. 49.7 to 49.9) and cannot be entirely avoided even by the most experienced surgeon when performing a laparoscopic procedure or a laparotomy (Figs. 49.10 to 49.13). The surgeon's expertise is manifested by his speed and skill in identifying and dealing with complications.

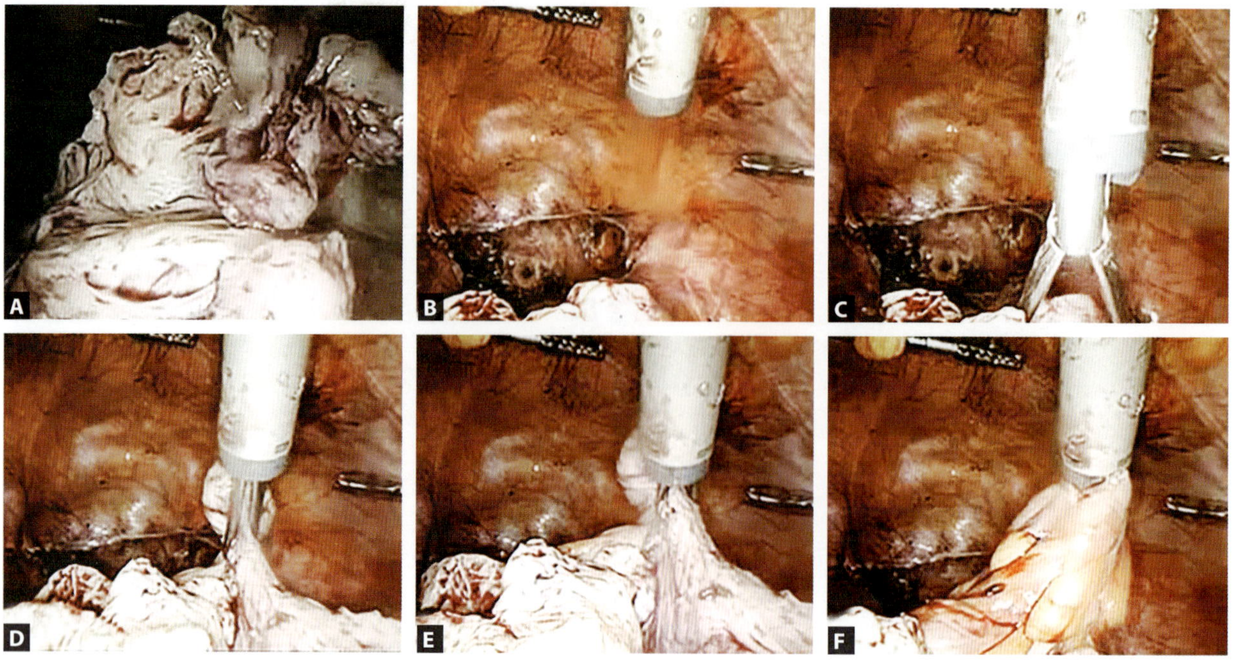

Figs. 49.6A to F: (A) Morcellation of a medium-sized uterus; (B) The morcellator has been inserted into the midline; this ensures the best overview and the greatest distance to the organs; (C and D) Grasping the remaining uterus; (E) The tenaculum has grasped a small intestinal sling, but as the area of interest is not in the middle of the picture and the camera is too far away, the problem is not identified; (F) The surgical team identifies the bowel injury only after morcellation of the intestine.

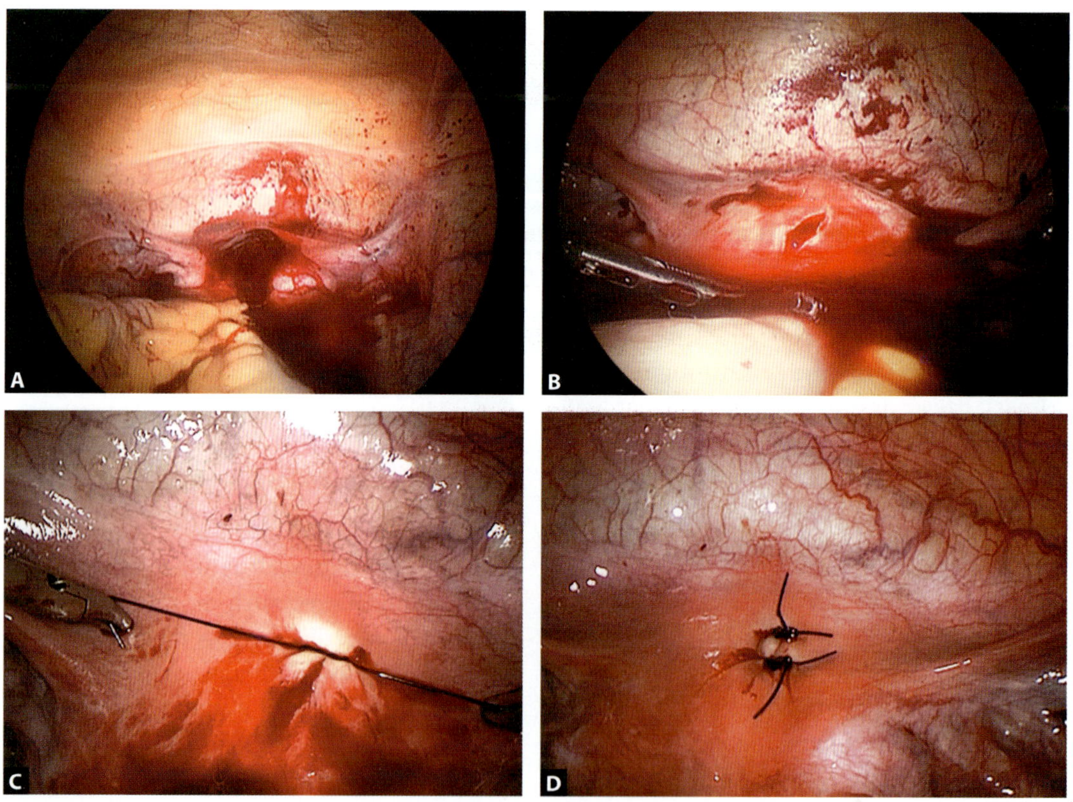

Figs. 49.7A to D: A 32-year-old patient with continuous vaginal bleeding, para 1, with suspected placental remnants 5 weeks after delivery. (A and B) The soft anterior wall of the enlarged uterus was perforated during curettage for removal of placental remnants. The extent of perforation was identified during the simultaneous laparoscopy. Active bleeding, hematoma, and free fluid (rinsing fluid used for hysteroscopy); (C and D) The hole can be closed with a thick monofilament suture and intracorporeal knotting.

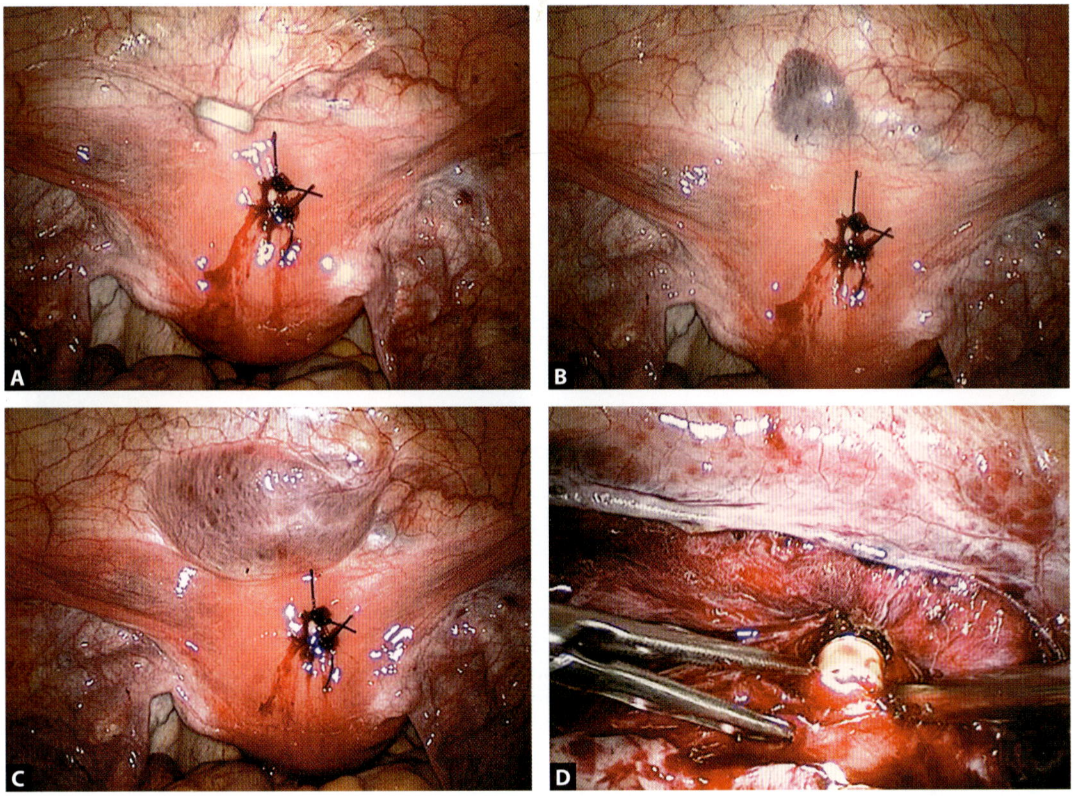

Figs. 49.8A to D: Same patient as in Figure 7. (A) Attempt to perform curettage under laparoscopic vision reveals a second perforation at the cervico-corporal transition. Only the peritoneum of the bladder has remained intact; (B) Immediate subperitoneal bleeding; (C) An early attempt to manage the area of perforation by performing a hysteroscopy leads to a large edema in the subperitoneal space; (D) The peritoneum needs to be opened. After complete exposure of the anterior uterine wall down to the vagina, the sole hysteroscope is inserted without dilution medium; the perforation is demarcated and treated under laparoscopic vision. The left forceps is used to pull the distal part of the perforated tissue onto the distal part of the hysteroscope. The distal portion of the uterine corpus can now be examined.

Vascular Lesions

Major vessel injury may occur during the operative part of the procedure, particularly during retroperitoneal dissection.[11] In the normal anatomical situation, the distal abdominal aorta and the common as well as external and internal iliac arteries lie in the retroperitoneal space. Lacerations of these vessels are fortunately rare (Fig. 49.5).

Early recognition of a major vessel injury, minimization of bleeding and conversion to laparotomy when the bleeding cannot be compressed laparoscopically, arrested or sutured, are crucial aspects of effective management. Medical hemostasis might be helpful, such as the use of TachoSil. A vascular surgeon will be needed to conclude the operation.

Bowel Lesions

Abdominal access and the creation of a pneumoperitoneum bear a significant risk of bowel injury, which is more common in laparoscopic surgery than in open surgery. Although bowel injuries are uncommon, they constitute a major cause of mortality due to laparoscopic procedures and a significant source of morbidity in connection with any laparoscopic procedure. Many intraoperative bowel lesions can be sutured; a partial excision and suturing as well as resection of lacerated areas may be necessary, including end-to-end anastomosis or a temporary ileostomy. Unlike major vessel injuries, which are seen immediately, many bowel injuries remain concealed at the time of the procedure. Patients may present postoperatively with specific or unspecific symptoms of peritonitis. Persistent pyrexia, tachycardia or an ileus in the postoperative period should raise suspicion of bowel injury. Late detection of this condition makes it a significant cause of morbidity and mortality. Bowel preparation is no longer advisable before major pelvic surgery. Injuries with healthy edges can be repaired primarily by using tension-free, single-layer, interrupted sero-submucosal 3-0 Vicryl or 4-0 PDS sutures. For more extensive injuries,

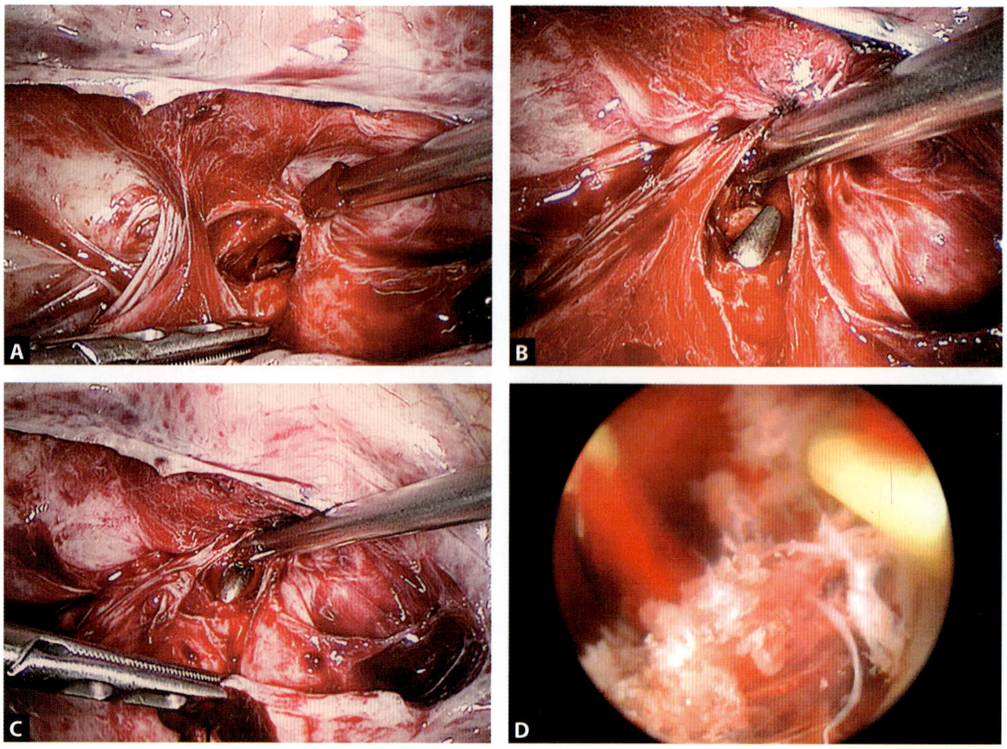

Figs. 49.9A to D: Same patient as in Figures 7 and 8. (A) After complete exposure of the anterior uterine wall, only the vesicovaginal ligament is preserved; (B) A probe is inserted into the cervix and (C) Directed into the uterine cavity under laparoscopic guidance. The defect is bridged by the probe and easily closed by performing intracorporeal full-thickness sutures to the wall; (D) Hysteroscopic view of placental remnants, which may then be removed in a stepwise manner. After closure of the defect, there is no further leakage and the dilution medium permits intrauterine vision.

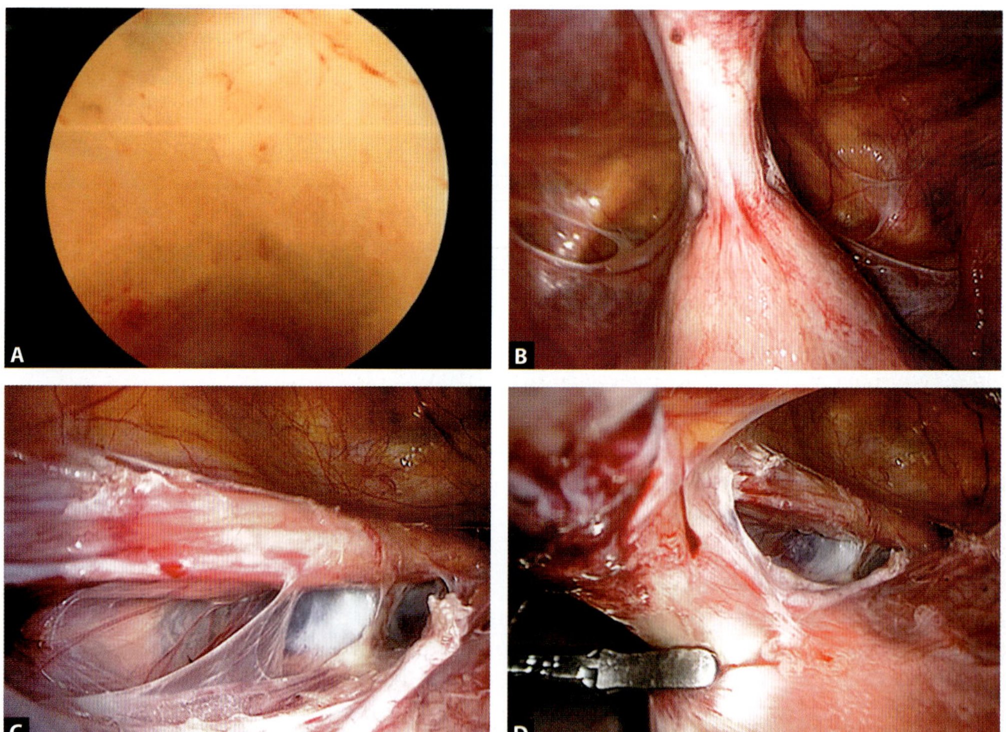

Figs. 49.10A to D: 35-year-old patient, para I: (A) After cesarean section in a developing country with a suspected defect of the cesarean scar. Hysteroscopy shows the margin of the intact wall; the defect seems to be covered by peritoneum alone; (B) The laparoscopic view shows a strong adhesive cord of the anterior uterine wall to the anterior abdominal wall; (C and D) After opening (C) the left and (D) the right anterior leaf of the broad ligament, the bladder can be kept at a distance and the uterine defect demarcated.

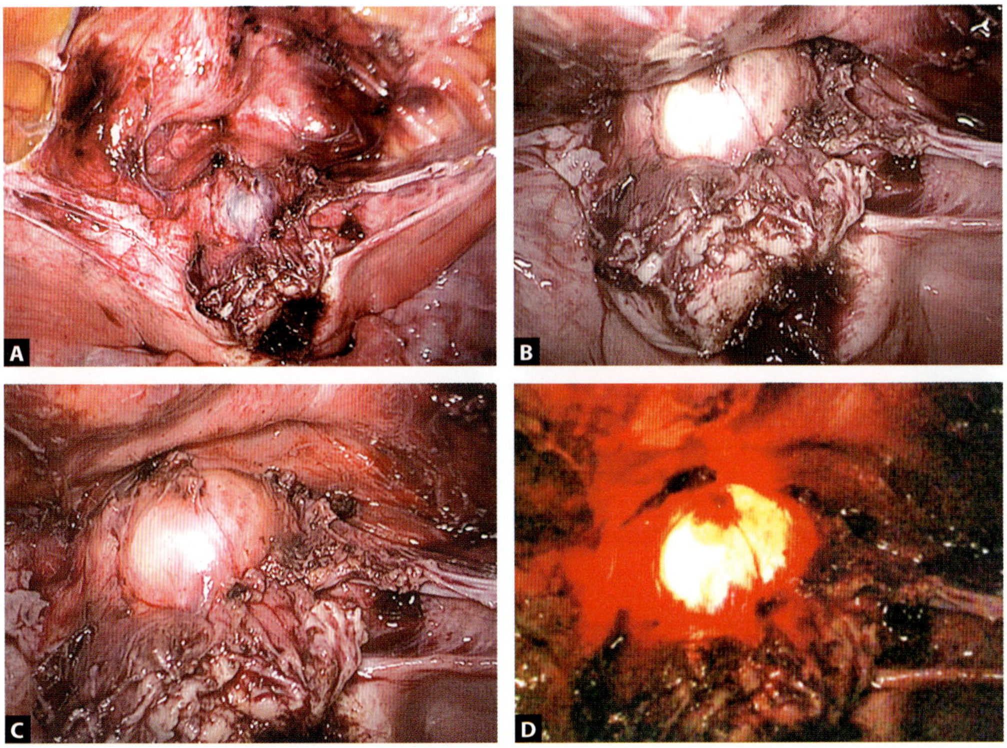

Figs. 49.11A to D: Same patient as in Figure 10. (A) After complete adhesiolysis the bladder is moved away from the uterus and the deep defect demarcated; (B) A simultaneous hysteroscopy confirms that the defect covers the entire wall; (C) The thin cover of the defect is seen after the introduction of fluid through the hysteroscope. Additionally, the defect is demarcated by the illumination fixed to the hysteroscope; (D) Once the intra-abdominal illumination has been dimmed, the hysteroscopic illumination becomes very expressive.

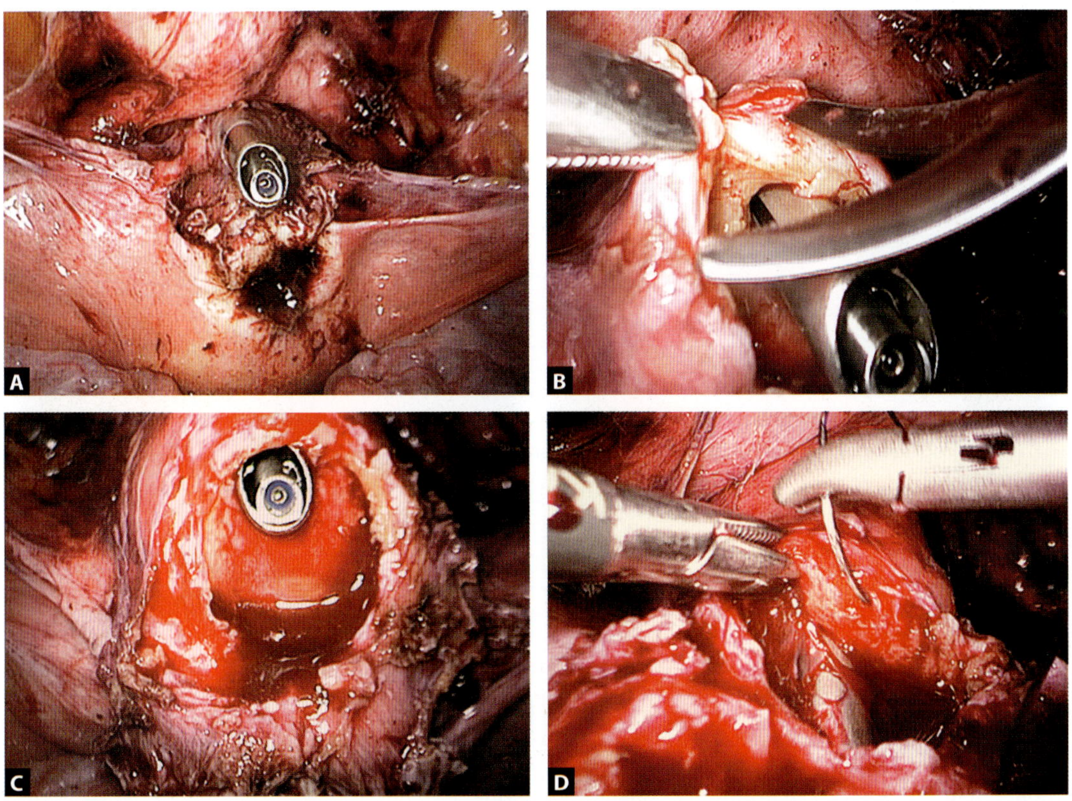

Figs. 49.12A to D: Same patient as in Figures 10 and 11. (A) Planned perforation with the hysteroscope allows; (B) Specific resection of the respective area; (C) The defect is demarcated and (D) Bridged with the hysteroscope, thus permitting end-to-end coverage.

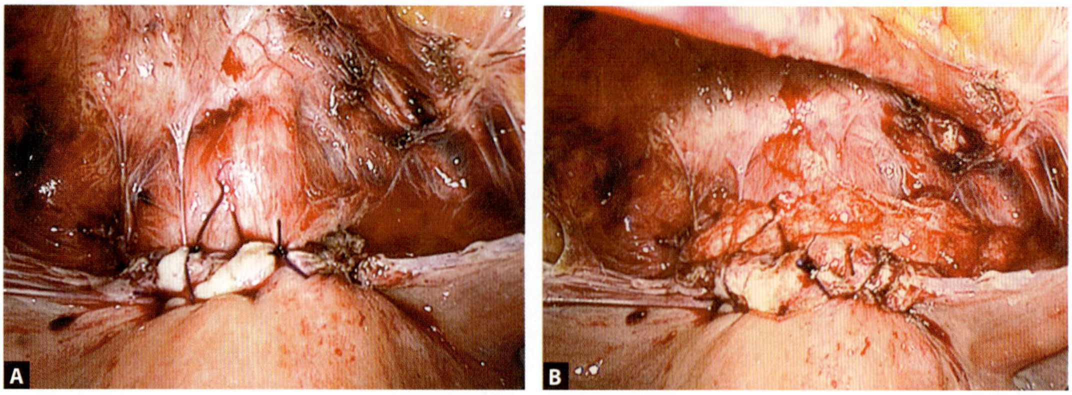

Figs. 49.13A and B: Same patient as in Figures 10 and 12. (A) Final view of the covered defect of the anterior uterine wall; (B) As the patient still wishes to have children, an antiadhesion barrier gel is applied (Hyalobarrier, Nordic Pharma, Germany).

resection and primary anastomoses may be required (Figs. 49.1 and 49.6).

Bladder and Ureter Injuries

Intraoperative viewing of the ureter is always necessary when performing surgery in the ureteric area. Dissection of the ureter becomes necessary sometimes (Figs. 49.14A to D). Routine intraoperative cystoscopies after major gynecological surgery permit early recognition and repair during the primary operation, with less morbidity for the patient. An open bladder is, of course, also detected by direct emission of urine. Sometimes the Foley catheter bag is filled with CO_2, indicating a bladder lesion.[19]

Urinary tract injuries in connection with laparoscopic surgery differ markedly from laparoscopic major vessel injury or iatrogenic intestinal injury. The former rarely results in the death of the patient, but the latter two are associated with mortality. Urinary complications are seldom the result of needle or trocar trauma (in other words, entry related). The most relevant factors related to ureteral damage are: (a) inadequate knowledge of pelvic anatomy,

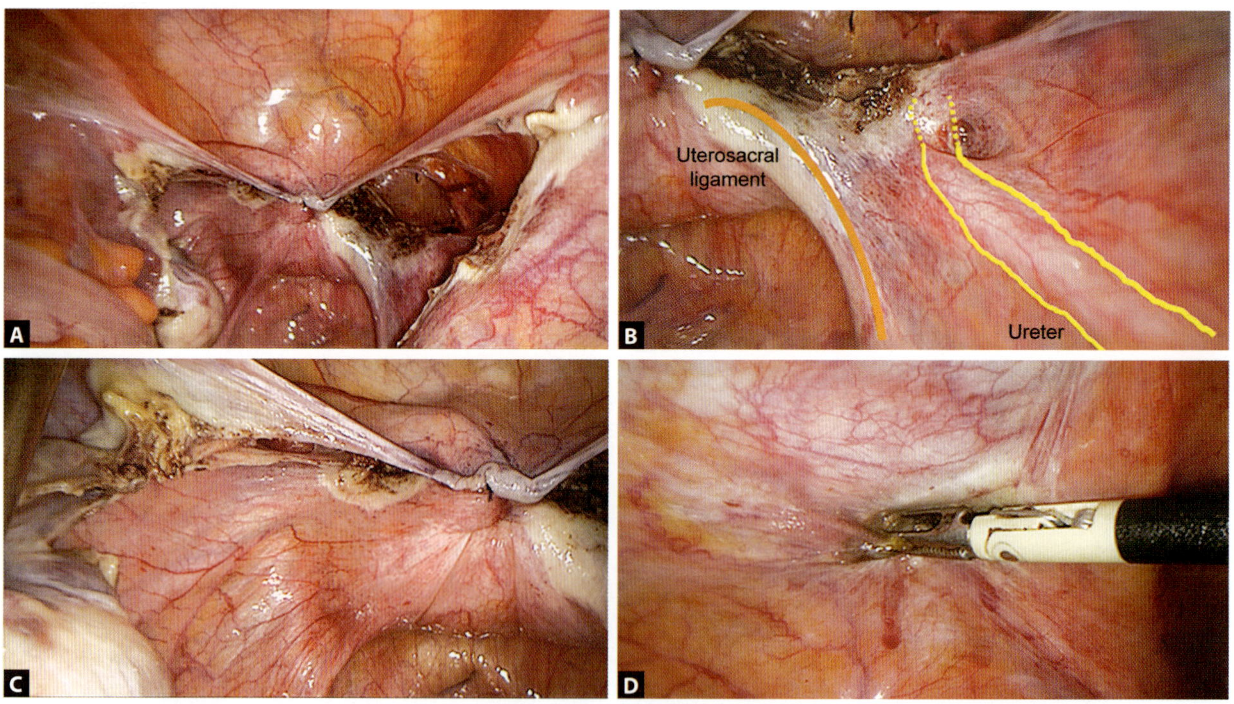

Figs. 49.14A to D: LSH: Final view after the LSH procedure. The peritoneum is closing the cervical canal and drainage is possible from both sides. Both sacrouterine ligaments are under slight tension and thus achieve suspension of the cervix. (A to C) The preserved integrity of the ureter is confirmed by observing peristalsis; (D) Coagulation of the right trocar entry point after removal.

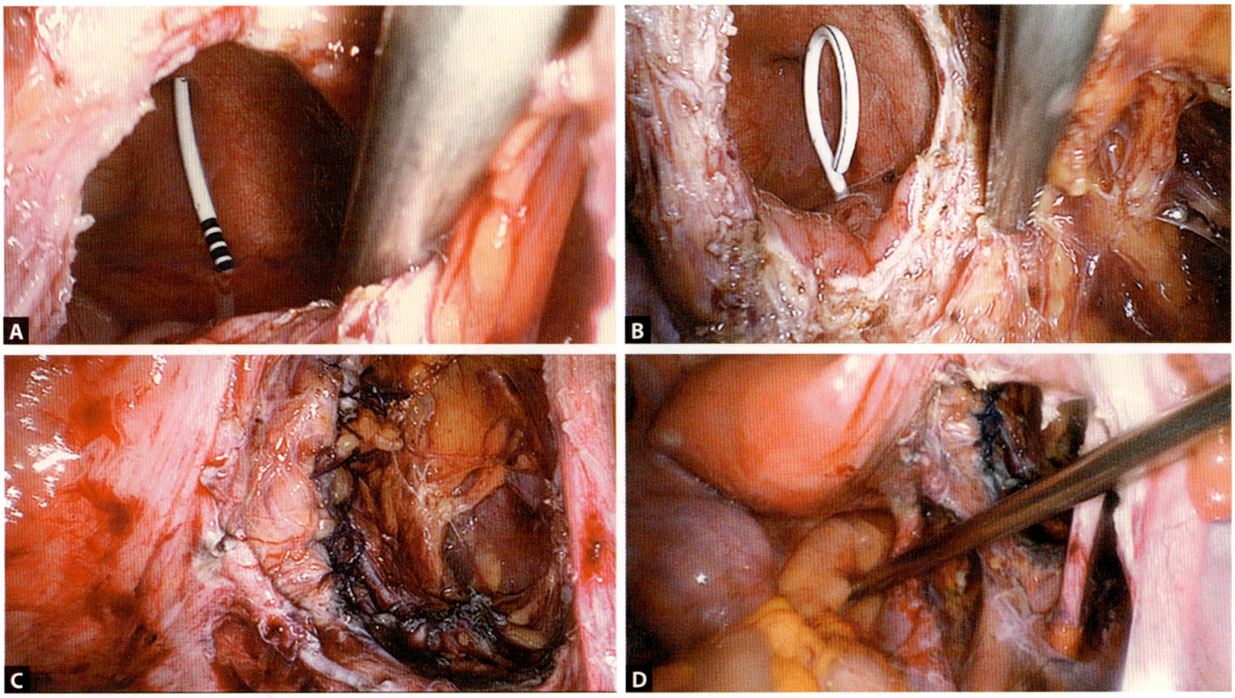

Figs. 49.15A to D: Opening the bladder usually requires the simultaneous insertion of a ureteral stent. (A and B) This is achieved via cystoscopy; (C and D) When the trigone of the bladder and the intramural pathway of the ureter are distant to the laceration, the latter can be securely closed by laparoscopy. The hole is closed by performing an interior suture line with Vicryl 3.0, using a continuous suture, and an interrupted suture line above with Vicryl 2.0 including the muscle and the peritoneum.

(b) failure to open the peritoneum and dissect retroperitoneally, (c) the use of energy devices with marginal knowledge of their physics and tissue interaction, (d) imprecise application of stapling devices and (e) pelvic adhesions, particularly dense adhesions located in and around the ovarian fossa. Injury to the ureter is greatly compounded by its late identification after the operation. Failure to perform suitable diagnostic tests (such as indigo carmine dye injection, cystoscopy, intravenous pyelogram or retrograde pyelograms) causes additional damage. Bladder injuries may be less serious than ureteral injuries, particularly when lacerations are recognized intraoperatively and repaired appropriately in a timely manner. Injury to the trigone may be avoided by performing a cystoscopy before or during closure of a bladder laceration and inserting a double-J-catheter (Figs. 49.15A to D). The risk of injury, especially to the ureter, is higher when using the laparoscopic approach and particularly in laparoscopic gynecologic operations.

Late Complications

Late complications occurring in the postoperative period are also referred to as secondary lesions and occur in 0.5% of cases; these include secondary bowel lesions associated with peritonitis and massive intra-abdominal infection (Figs. 49.16A to D). Small vascular lesions may remain unnoticed until a hematoma appears. Some ureteral lesions remain unidentified until the development of urinoma; this may occur several days after surgery. All patients must be cautioned to immediately report adverse symptoms or conditions, regardless of whether they are still in the hospital or have been discharged.

CONCLUSION AND FUTURE PROSPECTIVES

Independent of the type of entry technique used, the surgeon must be well trained in the technique of his or her preference. Furthermore, all surgeons should be familiar with alternative entry sites and techniques in order to resolve any type of obstacle or complication. The surgeon's regular attendance of standard training courses is known to shorten the learning curve.

Laparoscopic surgeons of all disciplines tend to divide laparoscopic surgery into various pillars, one of which is laparoscopic entry. During the training of young surgeons, attention should be given to laparoscopic entry alongside the more popular

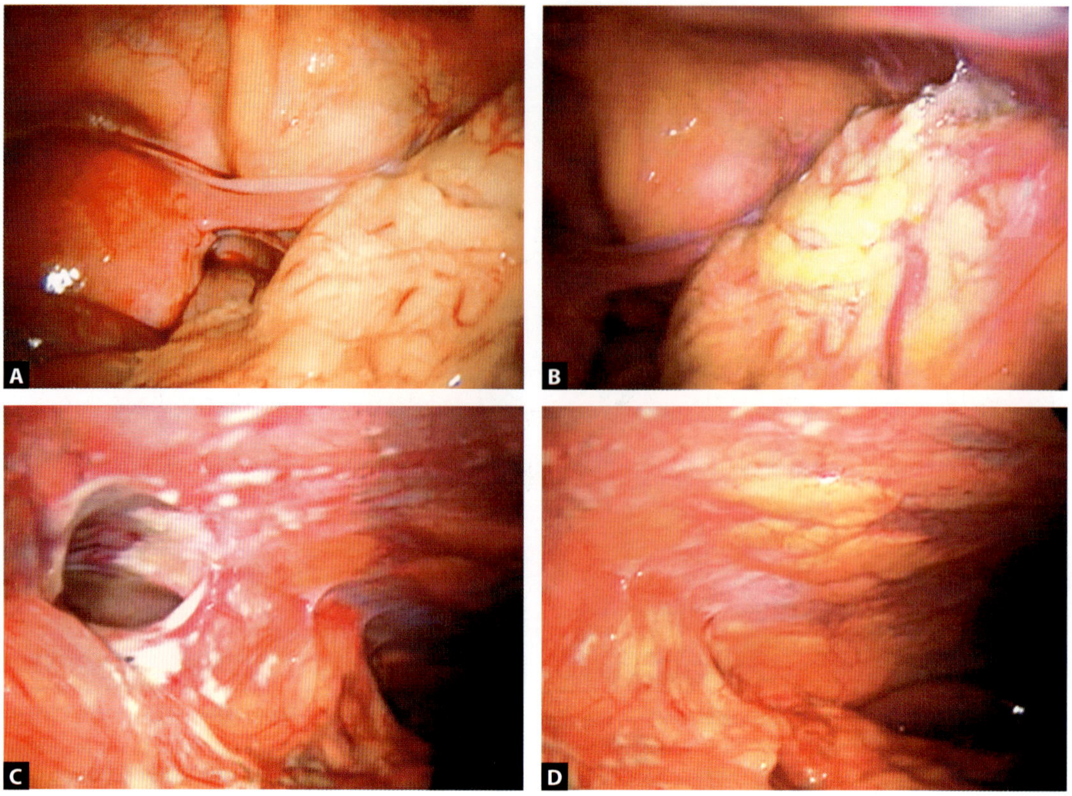

Figs. 49.16A to D: (A) Second-look laparoscopy three days after unproblematic myoma enucleation of the uterine back wall. The patient experienced bouts of high temperature and had increasing inflammation parameters. No drain was inserted. The overview shows normal pelvic anatomy and no sign of peritonitis or organ damage; (B) Atypical adhesions in the right lower abdomen (cecal region); (C) The endoscope clearly demarcates the bowel damage and signs of local peritonitis. The bowel injury probably occurred when the bowel was moved out of the operating field; (D) The upper right quadrant is also free of any signs of peritonitis.

pillars of endoscopic exposure and suturing. Awareness of potential complications, their early detection and professional treatment are essential aspects of a high-quality operating unit.[3,20,21]

All surgical procedures including port placement, even under direct vision, are associated with immanent risks.[22] Regardless of the sophisticated technological options of current times, doctors and surgeons need to work with great care and immense caution.

REFERENCES

1. Alkatout I, Bojahr B, Dittmann L, et al. Precarious preoperative diagnostics and hints for the laparoscopic excision of uterine adenomatoid tumors: two exemplary cases and literature review. Fertil Steril. 2011;95(3):1119.e1115-8.
2. Alkatout I, Stuhlmann-Laeisz C, Mettler L, et al. Organ-preserving management of ovarian pregnancies by laparoscopic approach. Fertil Steril. 2011;95(8): 2467-70.e2461-2.
3. Gynaecologists RCoOa. Preventing entry-related gynaecological laparoscopic injuries. RCOG Green-top Guideline. 2008;No.49:1-10.
4. Mettler L, Clevin L, Ternamian A, et al. The past, present and future of minimally invasive endoscopy in gynecology: a review and speculative outlook. Minim Invasive Ther Allied Technol. 2013;22(4): 210-26.
5. Pasic R. Creation of pneumoperitoneum and trocar insertion techniques. In: Pasic R, Levine R, editors. A Practical Manual of Laparoscopy: A Clinical Cookbook. Abingdon, UK: Informa Healthcare; 2007. pp. 57-74.
6. Palmer R. Safety in laparoscopy. J Reprod Med. 1974;13(1):1-5.
7. Nezhat F, Brill AI, Nezhat CH, et al. Laparoscopic appraisal of the anatomic relationship of the umbilicus to the aortic bifurcation. J Am Assoc Gynecol Laparosc. May 1998;5(2):135-40.
8. Alkatout I, Honemeyer U, Strauss A, et al. Clinical diagnosis and treatment of ectopic pregnancy. Obstet Gynecol Surv. 2013;68(8):571-81.
9. Alkatout I, Schollmeyer T, Hawaldar NA, et al. Principles and safety measures of electrosurgery in laparoscopy. JSLS. 2012;16(1):130-9.
10. Vilos GA, Vilos AG, Abu-Rafea B, et al. Three simple steps during closed laparoscopic entry may minimize major injuries. Surg Endosc. 2009;23(4):758-64.
11. Vilos GA, Ternamian A, Dempster J, et al. The Society of O, Gynaecologists of C. Laparoscopic entry: a

review of techniques, technologies, and complications. J Obstet Gynaecol Can. 2007;29(5):433-65.

12. Magrina JF. Complications of laparoscopic surgery. Clin Obstet Gynecol. 2002;45(2):469-80.
13. Hurd WW, Bude RO, DeLancey JO, et al. The relationship of the umbilicus to the aortic bifurcation: implications for laparoscopic technique. Obstet Gynecol. 1992;80(1):48-51.
14. Hurd WH, Bude RO, DeLancey JO, et al. Abdominal wall characterization with magnetic resonance imaging and computed tomography. The effect of obesity on the laparoscopic approach. J Reprod Med. 1991;36(7):473-6.
15. Semm K. New methods of pelviscopy (gynecologic laparoscopy) for myomectomy, ovariectomy, tubectomy and adnectomy. Endoscopy. 1979;11(2):85-93.
16. Semm K. [Visible control of peritoneal perforation in surgical pelviscopy]. Geburtshilfe Frauenheilkd. 1988;48(6):436-9.
17. Semm K. [Morcellement and suturing using pelviscopy—not a problem any more]. Geburtshilfe Frauenheilkd. 1991;51(10):843-6.
18. Semm K. Cutting versus conical tip designs. Endosc Surg Allied Technol. 1995;3(1):39-47.
19. Mettler L, Schollmeyer T, Tinelli A, et al. Complications of uterine fibroids and their management, surgical management of fibroids, laparoscopy and hysteroscopy versus hysterectomy, haemorrhage, adhesions, and complications. Obstet Gynecol Int. 2012;2012:791248.
20. Alkatout I, Mettler L, Beteta C, et al. Combined surgical and hormone therapy for endometriosis is the most effective treatment: prospective, randomized, controlled trial. J Minim Invasive Gynecol. Jul-Aug 2013;20(4):473-81.
21. Mettler L, Sammur W, Schollmeyer T, et al. Cross-linked sodium hyaluronate, an anti-adhesion barrier gel in gynaecological endoscopic surgery. Minim Invasive Ther Allied Technol. 2013;22(5):260-5.
22. Mettler L, Schollmeyer T, Alkatout I. Adhesions during and after surgical procedures, their prevention and impact on women's health. Womens Health (Lond Engl). 2012;8(5):495-8.

Complications of Hysteroscopy

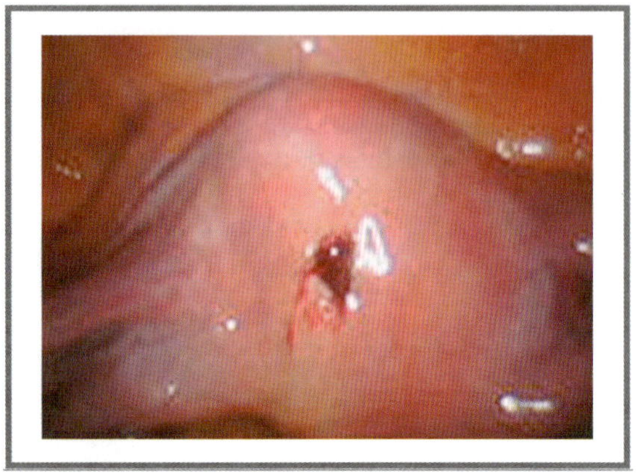

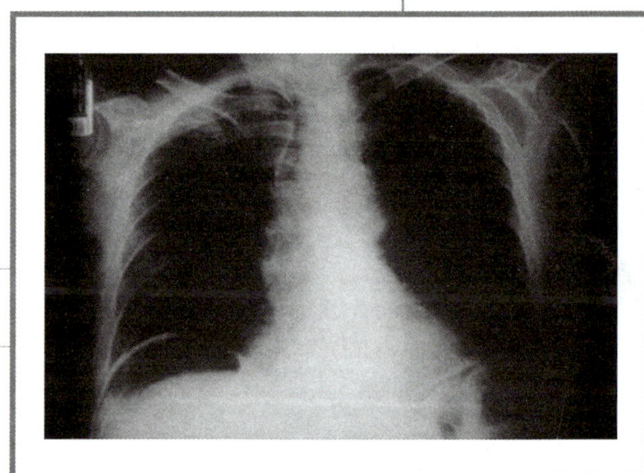

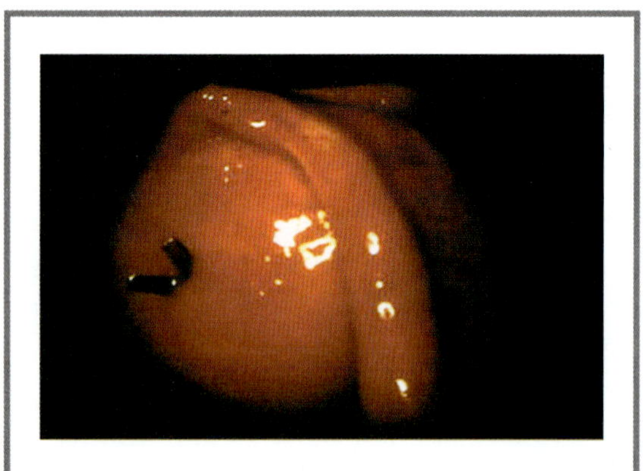

Chapter 50

Complications of Hysteroscopy

Parul Kotdawala, Nidhi Nagar

INTRODUCTION

Hysteroscopy surgery is one of the most significant additions to a gynecologist's armamentarium. After the advent of ultrasonography, hysteroscopy has perhaps made the biggest impact in gynec practice, especially gynec surgeries. A technology that can be learned easily, with a short learning curve, has given us a beautiful window to access the insides of uterus and to deal with medical problems arising from within the uterine cavity. Diagnostic and concurrent operative hysteroscopy is a tool to evaluate women with fusion defects of uterus, menstrual disorders, infertility, post-menopausal bleeding and recurrent pregnancy loss to quote just a few.

Hysteroscopy is a safe procedure, is easily learned and has excellent surgical outcomes. Adverse events associated with hysteroscopic procedures are in general rare. Complications of hysteroscopy occur more frequently in operative than in diagnostic procedure. With expanding surgical arena to undertake more complex situations we are observing the complications more often. The complications reported encompass those that occur due to the basic components of procedures like patient positioning, anesthesia and analgesia, and also those arising out of the specific surgical procedure carried out. (i.e., perforation of uterus, injuries to surrounding structures and blood vessels, circulatory overload and hyponatremia).

INCIDENCE

The complication rate in diagnostic hysteroscopy is low and was estimated by Lindemann (1989)[1] to be 0.012%. Complications from operative hysteroscopy are more common and potentially more serious. In the 1993 survey by the American Association of Gynecologic Laparoscopists (AAGL), there were 14,707 hysteroscopies reported with a complication rate of 3%. In two multicentric interviews of the American Association of Gynaecologic Laparoscopists performed by Hulka the severe complication rate decreased from 1% to 0.2 % in 3 years.[2]

Complications from operative hysteroscopy are more common and more serious (1–3%), hemorrhage (2.4%), uterine perforation (1.5%), cervical laceration (1–11%) (Taylor and Gordon, 1994),[3] uterine perforation: incidence 0.8% (Hill et al, 1992).[4] 1.29% and 2.47% when 'roller ball & loop' or 'loop alone' were used (Maresh 1996).[5] Hemorrhage: With 'loop and roller ball' or 'loop alone' 2.57% and 3.53% respectively (Maresh 1996). In a review of advanced operative procedures the overall intra-operative and post-operative rate of complication was 24% (Smith and co-workers).[6] Exact rates are difficult to determine owing to the natural tendency to report successes but not complication.

Hysteroscopic surgery, performed by a well-trained hysteroscopic surgeon, is a safe procedure with an overall complication rate of 3%. Most complications are related to cervical dilation or uterine entry techniques. Efforts therefore should be focused on identifying the patients at risk and finding novel techniques for cervical priming.[7]

There is a big difference in diagnostic hysteroscopy compared to the operative hysteroscopy, especially after the advent of office hysteroscopy. Office procedures have obviated the need for anesthesia and also the need to dilate the cervix. This has reduced two major sources of complications; the anesthesia in peri- and post-reproductive life where blood pressure and diabetes are likely to complicate the anesthesia, and the dilatation of cervix, especially in infertility patients, resulting in cervical trauma, occasional perforation and hemorrhage.

The complications of hysteroscopy surgery can be tabulated in following manner:

- *Intraoperative and early postoperative complications:*
  - Anesthesia related
  - Patient position during surgery
  - Distension media used
  - Electrosurgical accidents
  - Mechanical or traumatic complications (e.g., uterine perforation, hemorrhage)
- *Delayed complications:*
  - Infection
  - Adhesion formation
  - Failure of resolution of the presenting symptoms.

ANESTHESIA

The anesthesia risks are almost same as those from any other surgery. The specific issues encountered in hysteroscopic surgery are fluid overload, hyposmolality, hyponatremia, uterine perforation, hemorrhage and although rare gas or air embolism. Fluid overload occurs in up to 6% and can be fatal due to hyponatremia and hyposmolality. Obviously one should take all possible measures to prevent the fluid overload, to detect it early and treat it promptly. There are no controlled studies comparing different anesthetic techniques for operative hysteroscopy. The general anesthesia with intratracheal tube in place offers the advantage of immediate positive pressure ventilation and tracheal suction. However, some anesthetists prefer regional anesthesia over the general anesthesia for its advantage of conscious patient and early detection of fluid overload.

PATIENT POSITION

Lithotomy and head-low position have their own issues. Peripheral neuropathies have been associated with lithotomy position. Certain nerves are likely to be compressed in this position: the sciatic, common peroneal and saphenous nerves. The common peroneal nerve runs superficially over the fibular head and pressure from leg supports may lead to nerve injury. It is important to place padding and avoid any pressure on the nerve. The saphenous nerve may also be damaged by pressure from leg supports as it passes over the medial condyle of the tibia. Flexion and external rotation at the hip can stretch and damage the sciatic nerve. One should always consider the normal range of movement for a person and limit the positioning within that range during the surgery. In a patient under anesthesia there is tendency to go beyond normal range in a bid to obtain good exposure and access to cervix, especially in obese patient. The patient cannot complain and give a feedback that excessive movements are carried out. It is important to monitor patient positioning throughout the procedure, as the leg supports may be moved once the patient has been draped, making assessment of the movement at the hip joint more difficult. Both legs should be positioned in stirrups simultaneously to avoid inadvertent musculoskeletal injury. The lithotomy position is also associated with the uncommon complication of compartment syndrome of the lower leg. Obstruction to venous drainage also predisposes patients to development of venous thrombosis. Brachial plexus injury may result from incorrectly placed shoulder restraints or from excessive abduction of patient's arms on the hand-rest. A non-slip mattress is preferred to shoulder restraints. Injury can result from even 15 minutes in a faulty position. The anesthetist and surgeon should ensure that the patient is positioned properly.

DISTENSION MEDIA

Types of Distension Media

- Gas: CO_2
- High-viscosity fluid—Dextran 70
  - Low-viscosity fluid—Glycine-Sorbitol-Mannitol-Saline/Ringer's lactate

CO_2

Carbon dioxide has been used for diagnostic hysteroscopy, but its use is gradually decreasing, as it requires a special additional apparatus for a controlled delivery of the gas. It is rapidly absorbed by the blood circulation and released in the lungs. Related complications are metabolic changes like hypercarbia and metabolic acidosis, CO_2 or air embolism leading to respiratory collapse, cyanosis and cardiac arrest. High mechanical pressure leading to tubal rupture and diaphragmatic rupture are also reported.

To prevent these complications specific machine is required for the electronic calibration and flow rate of CO_2. Safer flow rate required is 40–50 mL/min, and should not exceed 100 mL/min. Capnography monitoring should be carried out, and a drop in $ETCO_2$ of is suggestive of embolism.

Fluid Media (Table 50.1)

High-molecular weight fluids like dextran can cause anaphylactic reactions, acute respiratory distress

Table 50.1: Comparison of various distension media for hysteroscopy surgery.

Type	*Operative use*	*Office use*	*Miscibility with blood*	*Complex procedure*	*Safety*
Gaseous					
CO_2	+	+++	+	+	++
Liquid: Nonelectrolytic					
Hyscon	+++	+++	+++	++	++
Glycine	+++	+	+	+++	+
Sorbitol	+++	+	++	+++	+
Mannitol	+++	+	++	+++	++
Liquid: Electrolytic					
NS	++	+++	+++	++	+++
RL	++	+++	+++	++	+++

syndrome, pulmonary edema, coagulopathies, oliguria and acute renal failure. Low-molecular weight fluids can be colloids (electrolyte free) and crystalloids (with electrolytes). In general the high molecular fluids are not used of late.

The colloids generally used for hysteroscopy are glycine, sorbitol and mannitol. They are used as non-conducting fluids when monopolar cautery and resectoscope are to be used. Complications related to glycine toxicity are hyperammonemia, hypervolemic, hyposmolar hyponatremia and central pontine myelinosis causing nausea, vomiting, altered mental status, muscle aches and decreased visual acuity.

The crystalloids like normal saline and Ringer's lactate are much safer and are preferred. They conduct the electricity via the electrolytes in them and are not a good option as the current dissipates when a monopolar cautery is being used. Again in presence of bleeding the blood mixes with the solution and makes the field hazy. With advent of bipolar resectoscope technology, the crystalloids are preferred media for distension. Excessive absorption of saline leading to saline overload produces a hypervolemic state.

The goals of fluid management include

- Selecting a distending medium less likely to cause complications when excessive absorption occurs.
- Minimizing systemic absorption during surgery, and
- Early recognition of excess absorption & prompt treatment.

Normal saline is associated with fewer unfavorable changes in serum sodium and osmolality than is the case when electrolyte-free media are used with monopolar systems.[8-11]

A variety of infusion pumps are available, ranging from simple devices with constant flow and pressure (at the inflow port) to instruments designed to monitor and maintain a preset intrauterine pressure. Simple pump devices continue to press fluid into the uterine cavity regardless of resistance, whereas the pressure-sensitive pumps reduce the flow rate when the preset level is reached.[12] While there is little value to using these systems for diagnostic hysteroscopy or for short procedures, maintenance of a standard intrauterine pressure is essential for longer operative interventions.

The simplest method of monitoring the amount of fluid absorption is to manually subtract the volume of fluid collected outside, from the volume infused. A good collection drape that gathers all fluid that leaks out during the procedure—both the outflow channel and all that seeps out around the scope sheath, is necessary for an accurate assessment.

The inaccuracy of manual measurement make it preferable to use an automated fluid measurement system that takes into account an exact measurement of infused volume as well as all of the potential sources of returned media. Such systems provide continuous measurement of the amount of distending media absorbed into the systemic circulation by using the weight of the infused volume.[13]

Fluid absorption is affected by the size and number of lesions removed, depth of myometrial resection, number of myometrial sinuses opened and the Intrauterine pressure. It can be minimized by keeping operating times to a minimum, avoiding entering the vascular channels and keeping fluid pressures below 80–100 mm Hg. The procedure must be abandoned if the deficit > 2 L, there is bleeding at resection or there is bleeding from intraoperative site (Fig. 50.1).

If a fluid overload with colloid distension media is suspected, the procedure is abandoned. She is transferred to urgent care and ICU facility. In consultation with the intensivist, hypertonic saline solution + loop

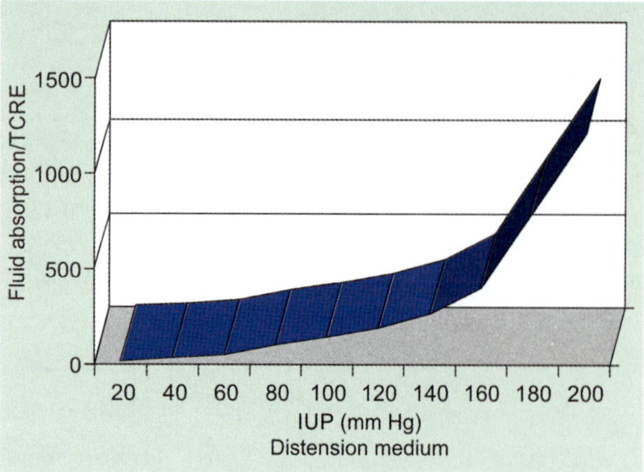

Fig. 50.1: IUP during hysteroscopic surgery and the amount of fluid overload.
Source: Royal College of Obstetricians and Gynaecologists.

diuretics are started. Serum sodium levels should be increased very slowly; 1–2 mEq/L/h and avoid 12 mEq/L in first 24 h. When pt presents with hyponatremia of >48 h postoperation rapid correction should not be attempted as it can lead to seizures and death. Central pontine myelinolysis (also described as "osmotic demyelinating syndrome") represents brain injury resulting from brain desiccation due to too rapid correction of hyponatremia.

If the overload is with saline, it will produce a simple hypervolemic state, which may be treated by insertion of a central venous line, administration of a diuretic and oxygen. Cardiac stimulants are given sparingly, only when necessary. A blood pressure cuff may be applied to each limb to occlude venous return which, in effect, performs a bloodless phlebotomy.

Significant increase in philtrum-mastoid prominence (PMP) distance when fluid absorption >1000 mL (Fig. 50.2).

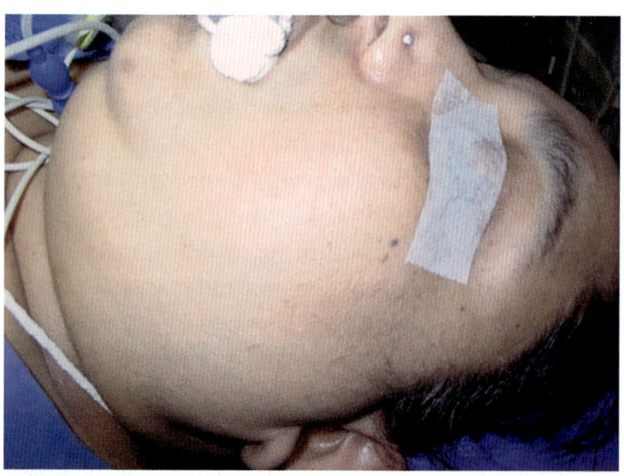

Fig. 50.2: Parotid area sign.

- Parotid area sign
- interstitial edema as a result of fluid overload
- Significant increase in philtrum- mastoid prominence (PMP) distance when fluid absorption >1000 mL
- When the fluid absorption is >1L: for every 500 mL increase in absorption, approx. 0.5 cm increase in PMP distance
- >1.5 L fluid absorption, PMP is generally 0.5 cm+ and >2 L, it is >1 cm

TIPS TO PREVENT MEDIA-RELATED COMPLICATIONS

- Intracervical injection of 8 mL of a dilute vasopressin solution (0.05 U/mL) just prior to the procedure reduces the blood flow to and from uterus, thereby containing the absorption of distension media during resectoscopic surgery. This also helps in quicker, easier and atraumatic dilatation of cervical. The anesthetist must be alerted when vasopressin is given, as systemic vasopressin may lead to cardiovascular collapse, myocardial infarction and death.[14]
- The uterine cavity distention pressure should be set as low as possible, just necessary to distend the uterine cavity for the procedure planned, and ideally should be maintained below the mean arterial pressure (MAP), ie <100 mm Hg.
- Excessive absorption of hypotonic fluids such as glycine 1.5% or sorbitol 3% can result in fluid overload and hypotonic hyponatremia, causing permanent neurologic complications or death. This risk of hypotonic encephalopathy is greater in reproductive-aged women than in postmenopausal women, perhaps due to high vascularity, or hormonal effects. An injection of GnRHa depot (3.75 mg) 2 weeks before the planned surgery helps reduce fluid absorption and overload, by suppressing the estrogens. It reduces both, systemic absorption of distension media and the impact of hyponatremic hypotonic encephalopathy. It is also associated with reduced fluid deficit among premenopausal women.[15]
- When compared with electrolyte-free media, saline appears to have a safer profile.
- The risk of systemic absorption varies with the procedure and increases when myometrial integrity is breached with procedures, such as myomectomy and transcervical resection of the endometrium (TCRE). In such instances,

patients should be counseled that more than one stage procedure may be required.

- The risks associated with distending media overload may be reduced by limiting the degree of preoperative hydration with oral or intravenous fluids.
- CO_2 is a suitable medium for the performance of diagnostic hysteroscopy but should not be used for operative hysteroscopy because of its impact on hysteroscopic visualization and the risk of CO_2 embolus.
- It is very vital that the air is purged out of the system before performing operative hysteroscopy with liquid distending medium. One should also be careful to change the liquid-containing bag before it is completely emptied during the procedure to avoid injection of air in the open blood vessels through the uterine cavity.
- A prior baseline levels of serum electrolytes including sodium, chloride and potassium in women on diuretics or with medical conditions that may predispose to electrolyte disorders shortly before the resectoscopic surgery is advisable.
- Immediate measurement of plasma electrolytes and osmolality is recommended when significant absorption of electrolyte-free distending media has occurred.
- Normal saline should be used wherever possible for operative hysteroscopic surgery to reduce the risk of hyponatremia and hyposmolarity. Normal saline should be used for distention during operative hysteroscopic procedures not requiring the use of monopolar electrosurgical instruments.
- The use of an automated fluid management system is recommended. Such systems should ideally comprise an infusion pump that allows determination and continuous monitoring of true intrauterine distention pressure and a system for accurate measurement of fluid deficit.
- An anticipated acceptable volume of the distension media should be identified considering the medical condition of the patient, and the osmolality and electrolyte content of the media prior to the surgery to alert the surgeon of possible adverse event if the surgery gets prolonged.
- In case of overload, an ultrasound check for intra-abdominal fluid collection, and laparoscopic suction of all fluid from peritoneal cavity will eliminate delayed circulatory overload.

MECHANICAL OR TRAUMATIC COMPLICATIONS

Perforation: This is a well-documented risk of operative hysteroscopy and should be discussed with the patient when obtaining informed consent. In the AAGL survey,[1] the incidence of perforation was 14 per 1,000. It was even higher during transection of lateral and fundal adhesions: 2–3 per 100.[16] Although perforation is more common with thermal energy sources, it may occur mechanically when scissors are used to transect a uterine septum, synechiae, or polyps. If it is noticed that the cautery was used after the fundal perforation, a laparoscopy or laparotomy to rule out visceral damage to abdominal organs is very important. At times, if the bleeding is significant, or if the case is of infertility, a good tight stitch is vital to attain hemostasis and also the strength to the fundus for future expansion during pregnancy. Small perforations near the cornua can occur during cornual tubal cannulation and placement of Essure device in the tubal ostia (Figs. 50.3A to C).

When to suspect uterine perforation: When the operative view suddenly disappears, when fluid deficit suddenly increases and when the hysteroscope suddenly inserts beyond fundus. The delayed symptoms of a perforation may be postoperative abdominal/pelvic excessive pain, distention, heavy vaginal bleeding, hypotension, nausea/vomiting or hematuria and thermal bowel injury. A perforation may go unrecognized.

Prevention of perforation can be achieved by performing a pelvic exam to determine uterine position before hysteroscopy, careful dilatation of cervix, use of cervical softeners like laminaria or preoperative use of misoprostol, and the use of flexible scope when available. An under vision entry in to the uterus by the office scope also reduces the chance of perforation.

When the cervix is stenotic or the uterus is acutely ante- or retroflexed, sounds and dilators can perforate the uterus. Most perforations—even those involving large dilators—usually do not require treatment, although further assessment may be necessary to rule out bowel injury. Most perforations occur in the fundal region or posterior lower segment. Infertility predisposes to cervical tears, false passages and perforation.

Laceration of the cervix: Although this is a minor complication, substantial bleeding sometimes

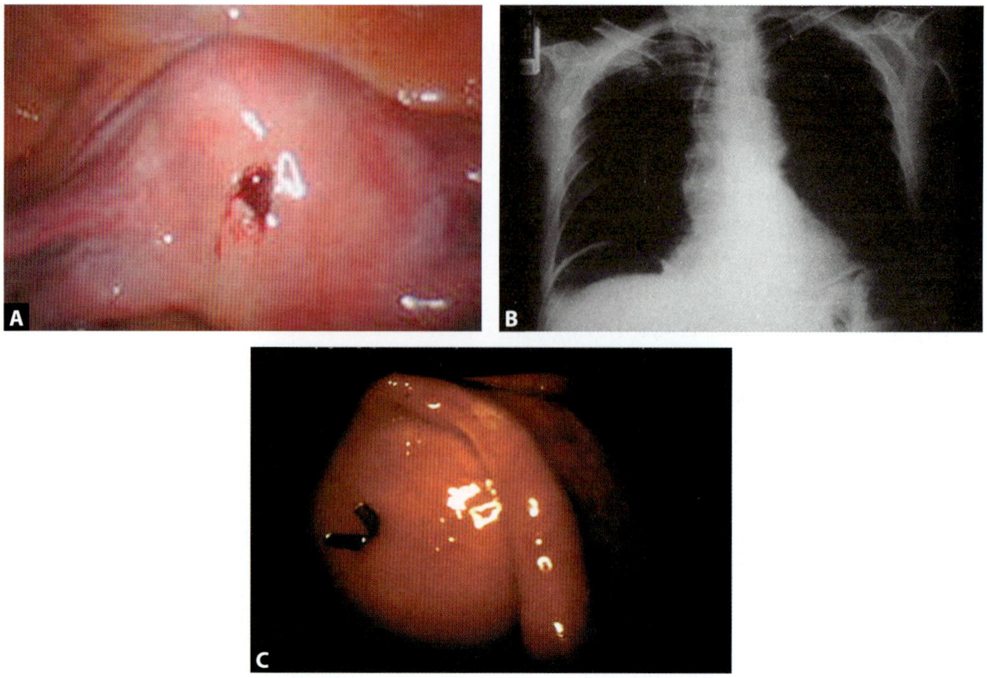

Figs. 50.3A to C: (A) Perforation at resectoscopy; (B) Gas under diaphragm; (C) Perforation by scissors.

occurs when the cervix is lacerated by the tenaculum. In these cases suturing the cervical tear may become necessary.

A false passage: This might be created while entering the uterus. Occasionally the surgeon may be fooled into thinking that the hysteroscope is in uterine cavity with adhesions, as this false passage distends. If muscle fibers are visible and the tubal ostia are not, one should assume the possibility of a false passage. The hysteroscope is withdrawn slowly to identify the location of false and the true passage. One can enter the cavity and complete the procedure. But sometimes one may need to abandon the procedure—even if no perforation is detected—to prevent distention fluid from being absorbed into the circulation through the injury. Adequate distention may not possible at this time and the repeat hysteroscopy is delayed for 2 to 3 months. Use of office hysteroscope has almost eliminated the "false passage" happening as the scope is introduced and advanced through the cervix under vision, without prior dilatation.

Bleeding: Intraoperative bleeding is rare unless vessels are lacerated or injured in cervical canal or lower uterine segment during dilatation. They may open up during myoma resection, TCRE and very occasionally during septum resection. The reported incidence is 0.5–1.9%.[17] The natural recoil and tone of the myometrium stops the bleeding soon. If it persists, a balloon tamponade using Foley's catheter with 30 cc normal saline and packing with gauze soaked in diluted vasopressin generally suffices. Of late one or two inj. of tranexamic acid is being used quite frequently to reduce the flow of bleeding.

ELECTROSURGICAL COMPLICATIONS

Most electrosurgical complications involve activation of an electrode at the time of perforation, or current diversion to the outer sheath. Thermal injuries also can be caused by overheating of the return plate. Electrode insulation failure allows current to jump to the outer sheath of the resectoscope, causing diversion of current leading to genital tract burns. To avoid this, inspect all electrodes thoroughly before surgery and use them only once. Sheath-within-a-sheath design of the resectoscope resembles a capacitor, and the high-voltage current can jump to the outer sheath without direct contact from the electrode. One way to avoid these injuries is to activate the electrode intermittently, with short bursts, rather than rolling back and forth over an area with continuous current.

POSTOPERATIVE AND LATE COMPLICATIONS

Infection is relatively rare following endometrial ablation, with a rate of 0.3–0.5% reported in most series. Cervical stenosis occurs in about 10–15% cases of TCRE, leading to collection of fluid and menstrual blood, ultimately ending in pyometra. Focal adhesions leading to formation of trapped areas due to adhesions, leading to dysmenorrhea, are also quite a significant sequel of TCRE. Endometritis, parametritis and pyometra are more common following resection of submucous myomas, with rates as high as 2% reported. This may be prevented by prophylactic antibiotics.

Intrauterine adhesions are common especially after myomectomy when two fibroids are situated on opposing uterine walls. In this case the myomectomy is better performed in stages to prevent adhesion formation. There is emerging awareness that intrauterine adhesions are quite frequent than previously thought. This happens more frequently when electric current is used on the endometrium. Many experienced surgeons are moving toward the increasing use of scissors, and limiting the use of electrocautery over the endometrium to its minimum. Some colleagues have started a policy of second look officescopy after a week, when extensive cautery was used, to check and lyse the adhesions, if enhancing the childbearing is the purpose of primary surgery. *Failure of procedure or failed resolution of symptoms*: In approximately 2% cases the procedure is either not carried out or is abandoned. A significant proportion of cases end up in "failure of resolution of the presenting symptoms." This depends upon the primary indication for the surgery and this should be discussed with the patient prior to the surgery.

Approximately 15% of the patients have an early pregnancy loss following septum resection (Taylor and Gordon, 1993) and greater risk of III stage complications. Myomectomy for menorrhagia or infertility is disappointing Because 20% have no immediate improvement and 80% fail to conceive. Endometrial ablation produces amenorrhea in 30% of the patients, satisfactory improvement in another 50%. Moreover, 10% will require further surgery within 12 months. Adhesiolysis for Asherman's syndrome is only curative in about 30–40% of cases.

IN A NUTSHELL

Hysteroscopy is a fairly safe procedure, but the technique has its share of complications. The diagnostic hysteroscopy, with the use of micro or mini-scope without dilatation of cervix, and without anesthesia and being a short procedure, is almost complications free. Operative hysteroscopy has, although uncommon, its share of serious complications. One should be alerted of major complications if the cervix is not easily dilated, if a colloid solution is to be used along with electrocautery, if the subendometrium/myometruim is going to be exposed (myoma resection, TCRE, deep septal resection), and if the surgery is taking longer time. With due precautions, and experienced team of surgeon, anesthesiologist and operating room (OR) personnel, we can minimize the incidence and severity of the complications.

REFERENCES

1. Lindemann H-J. Complications of Hysteroscopy. Antwerp: Presented to European Society of Hysteroscopy; 1986.
2. Hulka JF, Peterson HB, Phillips JM, et al. Operative hysteroscopy. AAGL 1991 membership survey. J Reprod Med. 1993;38(8):572-3.
3. Taylor PJ, Gordon AG. Practical Hysteroscopy. Oxford: Blackwell Scientific Publications; 1994. pp. 89-98.
4. Hill D, Maher P, Wood C, et al. Complications of operative hysteroscopy. Endoscopy, 1992;1:185-9.
5. Overton C, Hargreaves J, Maresh M. A national survey of the complications of endometrial destruction for menstrual disorders: the MISTLETOE study. Minimally Invasive Surgical Techniques: Laser, EndoThermal or Endoresection., Br J Obstet Gynaecol. 1997;104(12):1351-1359.
6. Smith, DC, Donohue LR, Waszak SJ. A hospital review of advanced gynecologic endoscopic procedures. Am J Obstet Gynecol. 1994;170(6):1635-42.
7. Isaacson KB. Complications of hysteroscopy. Obstet Gynecol Clin North Am. 1999;26(1):39-51.
8. Shveiky D, Rojansky N, Revel A, et al. Complications of hysteroscopic surgery: "Beyond the learning curve." J Minim Invasive Gynecol. 2007;14(2):218-22.
9. Darwish AM, Hassan ZZ, Attia AM, et al. Biological effects of distension media in bipolar versus monopolar resectoscopic myomectomy: a randomized trial. J Obstet Gynaecol Res. 2010;36(4):810-7 (Evidence I).

10. Makris N, Vomvolaki E, Mantzaris G, et al. Role of a bipolar resectoscope in subfertile women with submucousmyomas and menstrual disorders. J Obstet Gynaecol Res. 2007;33(6):849-54 (Evidence II-3).
11. Touboul C, Fernandez H, Deffieux X, et al. Uterine synechiae after bipolar hysteroscopic resection of submucosal myomas in patients with infertility. Fertil Steril. 2009;92(5):1690-3 (Evidence II-3).
12. Shirk GJ, Gimpelson RJ. Control of intrauterine fluid pressure during operative hysteroscopy. J Am Assoc Gynecol Laparosc. 1994;1(3):229-33 (Evidence II-3).
13. Hawe JA, Chien PF, Martin D, et al. The validity of continuous automated fluid monitoring during endometrial surgery: luxury or necessity? Br J Obstet Gynaecol. 1998;105(7):797-801 (Evidence II-1).
14. Istre O. Fluid balance during hysteroscopic surgery. Curr Opin Obstet Gynecol. 1997;9:219-25.
15. Role of leuprolide acetate depot in hysteroscopic surgery: a controlled study. Antonion Perino, MD et al. Fertility and Sterility; 1993; 59(3):507-510.
16. Valle RF, Sciarra JJ. Intrauterine adhesions; hysteroscopic diagnosis, classification, treatment, and reproductive outcome. Am J Obstet Gynecol. 1988; 158(6 Pt 1):1459-70.
17. Serden SP, Brooks PG. Treatment of abnormal uterine bleeding with the gynecologic resectoscope. J Reprod Med. 1991;36:697.

Index

Page numbers followed by *b* refer to box, *f* refer to figure, *fc* refer to flowchart, and *t* refer to table

A

B

C

D

I

J

K

L

N

O